The Essential Physics of Medical Imaging

FOURTH EDITION

JERROLD T. BUSHBERG, PhD

Clinical Professor of Radiology and Radiation Oncology
University of California, Davis
Sacramento, California

J. ANTHONY SEIBERT, PhD

Professor of Radiology
University of California, Davis
Sacramento, California

EDWIN M. LEIDHOLDT Jr, PhD

Clinical Associate Professor of Radiology
University of California, Davis
Sacramento, California

JOHN M. BOONE, PhD

Professor of Radiology and Biomedical Engineering
University of California, Davis
Sacramento, California

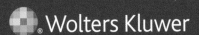

Wolters Kluwer

Philadelphia • Baltimore • New York • London
Buenos Aires • Hong Kong • Sydney • Tokyo

Not authorised for sale in United States, Canada, Australia, New Zealand, Puerto Rico, and U.S. Virgin Islands.

Executive Editor: Sharon Zinner
Development Editor: Eric McDermott
Senior Editorial Coordinator: Emily Buccieri
Marketing Manager: Kristin Ciotto
Production Project Manager: Catherine Ott
Design Coordinator: Stephen Druding
Manufacturing Coordinator: Beth Welsh
Prepress Vendor: SPi Global

Fourth Edition

Cataloging-in-Publication Data available on request from the Publisher
ISBN: 978-1975-1-0322-4

I am dedicating the fourth edition of this textbook to my brother Siri who is the very role model of an amazing teacher (albeit not in the physical sciences) and to my fellow teachers of medical physics and to the giants upon whose shoulders we all stand. Education's contribution to one's foundation, upon which they will develop their gifts, is immeasurable. As teachers, we strive to simplify the complex and make abstract concepts accessible to our students. None of this would be possible of course without the tireless efforts of those who have come before. Their contributions to our profession both grand and otherwise have all contributed in their own way to the body of knowledge upon which we rely. Let me also take this opportunity to extend my most sincere and heartfelt appreciation to all the teachers in my life, both inside and outside of academia, who have contributed so much to my education. Among the most important of these, I want to especially acknowledge my wife Lori who has contributed so much over so many years. Words are insufficient to express how grateful I am for you.

Teachers never know the true impact of their teaching or of their ability to influence the lives of others. Do our words, insights, and creative teaching methods cause a mere ripple in the pond, or do they promote such energy that the "flow of knowledge" permanently changes allowing students to forge new pathways and channels? How do we provoke and challenge students to the extent that they transform and grow? Medical physics teachers provide the power of education to today's radiology residents and biomedical engineers, thereby providing another piece of the puzzle with the hope that they will, in turn, use it to contribute to a better future for us all.

J.T.B

My parents, Nancy and Jim, have provided the values and opportunities for life, liberty, and happiness I have enjoyed throughout my existence. For each serendipitous turn of events with the ups and downs of growing up with my six brothers and one sister, they have been a steady source of support and inspiration through thick and thin, and beyond! In fact, my 96-year-old father is still showing me the ropes on how to be a thriving survivor! I truly owe them a debt of gratitude and deepest thanks—this book is dedicated to you, mom and dad!

J.A.S.

To my family, especially my parents and my grandmother Mrs. Pearl Ellett Crowgey, and my teachers, especially my high school mathematics teacher Mrs. Neola Waller, and Drs. James L. Kelly, Roger Rydin, W. Reed Johnson, and Denny D. Watson of the University of Virginia. To two superb nuclear medicine physicists, Drs. Mark W. Groch and L. Stephen Graham, who contributed to earlier editions of this book, but did not live to see this edition. And to my wife, Jacalyn Killeen, who makes it all worthwhile.

E.M.L.

This book has been a staple of my life for 3 decades, and with each edition, one marks the passage of time. With the first edition, I stepped carefully across the kitchen floor due to the scattering of Cabbage Patch Kids dolls and Hot Wheels lying about. My two children are now in their early 30s and thriving. Daughter Emily recently married her girlfriend Rachel—two beautiful young women—teachers—planning their future together. Son Julian is making plans for graduate school after living on five different continents for the past 5 years—and with this, his genuine passion and knowledge of history will be passed on to a new generation of students. After 30 years of marriage, I found myself single some years ago, adrift in a sea of introspection—while pondering my pending Medicare status. But from those uncertain waters, an angel appeared, beautiful, powerful, capable, and amazingly familiar—Lori was my high school sweetheart, and now Lori Cooper Boone and I are married and are busy making up for the 50-year gap in our love story. *De las cenizas prevalece la esperanza.*

Once again, I am honored to share front cover credits on this fourth edition with my friends Tony, Jerry, and Ed—the cuatro amigos ride again!

J.M.B.
[From the ashes, hope prevails]

There has been an
Alarming Increase
?
in the Number
of Things
I Know
Nothing About

Ashleigh Brilliant

Preface to the Fourth Edition

The first edition of this text was published in 1993, followed by subsequent editions in 2002 and 2012. With this fourth edition published in 2020, we have established a tradition of writing a new edition per decade. It is hard to even imagine the largely analog nature of medical imaging when we started this project in the early 1990s. Screen-film radiography was the most widely used modality in every section of radiology at that time, and every radiologist knew how to read a chest x-ray. The change to digital imaging and newer technologies—many of them three-dimensional—has started to supplant the once-ubiquitous two-dimensional planar radiograph. And with the increasing prevalence of these new technologies, the skill sets of radiologists have also adapted to meet the demands of image interpretation with a far more capable and complicated fleet of instruments. Instead of 1–10 images per study of the past, these higher-tech imaging systems can easily produce studies with a thousand or more images. No wonder radiologists are so busy!

Back in the early 1990s when we started this, some of the authors had darker hair, more hair, or trimmer waistlines, and we all had more time. Back then we were more involved in the operation of the imaging equipment discussed throughout the pages of this textbook. Fast-forward 30 years, our seniority and administrative responsibilities have grown and we have specialized in particular technical areas. Today, no one person is likely to be a true expert in all of the imaging modalities and subspecialty areas that comprise the science of medical imaging. Recognizing this, with this fourth edition, we have recruited about a dozen outstanding scientists who are well-known experts in their field of medical imaging science. They have helped shape the outline of specific chapters and indeed have contributed significantly to the chapters' accuracy, timeliness, and quality. The list of these authors is provided in the Contributing Authors section. Thank you all!

In the third edition, we reported that population dose data from the NCRP (NCRP 160, 2006) showed an alarming increase in radiation exposure to the U.S. population due to the increased use of computed tomography and other imaging systems with ionizing radiation. With this fourth edition, we are happy to report that according to NCRP 184, radiation dose reduction efforts over the past decade have led to a 15%–20% reduction in the annual radiation levels to the population from medical imaging procedures. It is likely that further reductions in radiation dose from medical imaging procedures will be realized with the growing use of artificial intelligence and specifically convolutional neural network techniques, which have demonstrated considerable potential for dose reduction though denoising and other methods. Requirements for radiation dose reporting (e.g., California legislation SB 1237, 2012) have also helped the imaging community better identify high-dose procedures through the reporting process, and this enhanced data-gathering effort has improved our ability to focus on dose reduction protocols.

Much of the writing of this fourth edition has occurred during the time of the global COVID-19 pandemic. This pandemic has made the entire medical imaging community realize the complexity of imaging extremely sick patients with a highly contagious and deadly disease. The reality of spending 60 minutes decontaminating a CT suite in which the scan took 15 minutes may help us all plan and prepare for the next pandemic, which the experts predict *will* happen. Should we design decontamination ports or UV lights right into the scanners, and site critical imaging systems in positive pressure rooms? The pandemic has also helped us better appreciate the power of remote viewing (and the IT professionals who help support it) in a crisis, where with the right workstation hardware at home, radiologists can perform image interpretations efficiently and quickly while practicing physical distancing measured in *miles*. The pandemic has also forced many medical professionals to communicate more efficiently using technology, and hopefully, these lessons will not be forgotten.

It is probably true that the book's title *The Essential Physics of Medical Imaging* (EPMI) was never completely accurate as both "Essentials" and "Physics" are a bit misleading. In its fourth edition, it is now well over 1,000 pages. The text also includes a thorough review of the radiation sciences related to medical imaging as well as comprehensive treatments of radiation protection and radiation biology. We also realize that the target audience has broadened from our original focus on radiologists-in-training to include biomedical engineers, medical physicists, and other imaging scientists. Hence, the breadth of discussion has grown to fully embrace this broader readership.

To address the original goal of providing a compendium of information that focuses more on the didactic needs of radiologists, other physicians, and clinical medical physicists who will be preparing for their professional board examinations, we have developed the *EPMI Study Guide* organized with three sections for each chapter. The first section contains a summary of the textbook chapter's key points and illustrations. The second section contains sample questions and explanatory answers for that chapter's material, which are keyed (hyperlinked in the e-edition) to the textbook for more in-depth information. The third section has a list of key equations, symbols, quantities, and units introduced in the chapter. We hope that the EPMI Study Guide will serve the original intent of the "Essentials" and that this textbook will complement the Study Guide for those who desire to understand the material at a deeper level.

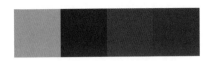

Foreword

This fourth edition of the best recognized and most widely used medical imaging physics textbook contains quite a number of welcome updates as the field has progressed dramatically since the 2012 third edition. The authors are perhaps the most qualified of any who have written a medical physics textbook with well over 130 years of combined teaching experience and 30+ years teaching an international physics review course for radiology residents. The authors include the senior vice-president of the National Council on Radiological Protection and Measurements, a Gold Medal Winner of the RSNA, an AAPM William D. Coolidge gold medal recipient, a Warren K. Sinclair medal winner for excellence in radiation science, a governor of the American Board of Radiology, and fellowships of more professional societies than I care to count. This edition also has added a number of new internationally recognized contributing authors.

There has been a significant update of all chapters but particularly involving informatics, new DICOM and HL7 standards and methods, breast imaging, tomosynthesis, radiation dosimetry, dose reduction strategies, new detectors, and innovations in MRI and ultrasound. While there has been an effort to substantially reduce the description of older technology, there has been an effort to retain and concisely present important historical concepts. There are sections on both radiation biology and radiation protection incorporating new epidemiology and recent recommendations of the NCRP and NRC.

The previous edition was just over 1,000 pages with more than 700 wonderfully clear illustrations. The new edition is approximately the same size with hundreds of new illustrations. While the title contains the word "Essential," this is a fully complete and almost an encyclopedic work, and it will be valuable for residents, fellows, graduate students, and faculty. The most welcome change is the addition of a Study Guide, which will help the reader identify crucial concepts and provide question and answer section that should be very valuable for board review. There are also hyperlinks to the main textbook in the Study Guide for further elucidation of all the subjects.

Personally, every time I see a physics book I am reminded of the saying, "Never trust atoms, they make up everything" (anonymous).

Fred A. Mettler Jr, MD, MPH
Emeritus Professor, University of New Mexico

Authors

Jerrold T. Bushberg, PhD

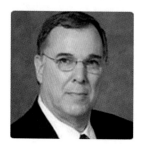

Jerrold T. Bushberg is a clinical professor of Radiology and Radiation Oncology at the University of California (UC), Davis, School of Medicine. He served as associate chair of Radiology (Radiation Biology & Medical Health Physics) until 2018 and was awarded Emeritus status by the UC Davis Chancellor as Director of Medical/Health Programs at that time. Dr. Bushberg is chair of the Board of Directors and senior vice-president of the United States National Council on Radiation Protection and Measurements. He is an expert on the biological effects, safety, and interactions of ionizing and non-ionizing radiation and holds multiple radiation detection technology patents. With over 35 years of experience, he has served as a subject matter expert and an adviser to government agencies and institutions throughout the nation and around the world including U.S. Department of Homeland Security, the U.S. EPA's Radiation Protection Division, the National Academy of Sciences, the FDA's Center for Devices and Radiological Health, the World Health Organization's Radiation Program, Geneva, and the International Atomic Energy Agency, Austria, in the areas of ionizing and non-ionizing radiation protection, risk communication, medical physics, and radiological emergency medical management. A former Commander in the U.S. Naval Reserve, among other assignments, CDR Bushberg served as Executive Officer of CBNR120 Pacific, a highly skilled multidisciplinary military emergency response and advisory team. Dr. Bushberg is an elected fellow of the American Association of Physicists in Medicine and the Health Physics Society. He has published numerous journal articles, book chapters, as well as other enduring academic material outside the domain of medical physics covering such diverse topics as emergency medical response to radiological terrorism and electromagnetic interference of wireless telecommunications systems with cardiac pacemakers. Dr. Bushberg is certified by several national professional boards with specific subspecialty certification in radiation protection and medical physics and currently serves as a director of the American Board of Medical Physics and served as its vice chair from 2015 to 2018. Dr. Bushberg has received numerous honors and awards including NCRP's Warren K. Sinclair Medal for Excellence in Radiation Science in 2014 and the Christiansen Distinguished Alumnus award from Purdue University in 2016. Before joining the faculty at UC Davis as technical director of Nuclear Medicine, Dr. Bushberg was on the faculty of Yale University School of Medicine in the Department of Radiology where his research was focused on radiopharmaceutical development. Dr. Bushberg has responsibility for medical postgraduate education in medical physics as well as ionizing and non-ionizing radiation biology and radiation protection.

J. Anthony Seibert, PhD

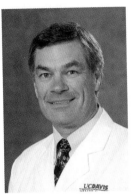

J. Anthony Seibert is a professor of diagnostic imaging physics at the University of California (UC) Davis Health in Sacramento, California. Dr. Seibert leads initiatives in x-ray fluorography, CT, digital mammography, projection imaging, interventional radiology, imaging informatics, and the tracking/assessment of radiation dose through automated registries.

Dr. Seibert received his PhD in radiological sciences from UC Irvine in 1983, with a focus on quantitative digital fluoroscopic imaging. He has served on the faculty of UC Davis since January 1983, conducting research in digital imaging, and directing education in medical physics for graduate students and radiology residents.

Dr. Seibert is a voice for medical physicists, advancing opportunities for collaboration and quality improvement among specialties. An experienced leader, Dr. Seibert has served as chair of the Society for Imaging Informatics in Medicine (SIIM) (2004–2006), third vice-president of the Radiological Society of North America (RSNA) (2009), president and chair of the American Association of Physicists in Medicine (AAPM) (2010–2012), and chair of the board of trustees of the American Board of Imaging Informatics (2012–2013). He has been active with the American Board of Radiology (ABR) since 1995, volunteering on several Diagnostic Medical Physics Committees and as chair for the Part I and Part 2 exam committees. Dr. Seibert was elected to the ABR as a Trustee for Medical Physics in 2013, and in 2017 moved to the ABR Board of Governors.

Dr. Seibert leads educational symposiums for the AAPM, the International Atomic Energy Agency, and the National Council on Radiation Protection and Measurements, where he also serves as a council member. He is a fellow of the AAPM, American College of Radiology, SIIM, and the International Organization for Medical Physics. The author of more than 120 peer-reviewed articles and 200 published abstracts, Dr. Seibert has served as a reviewer for *Medical Physics*, as well as editorial board member and reviewer for Radiology and RadioGraphics. In 2019, Dr. Seibert received the Gold Medal award from the RSNA.

Edwin M. Leidholdt Jr, PhD

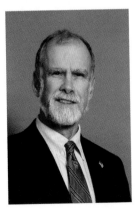

Edwin M. Leidholdt Jr, PhD, is the director of the National Health Physics Program, Veterans Health Administration (VHA), U.S. Department of Veterans Affairs (VA). His areas of expertise include technical quality assurance, error prevention, and radiation dose management in medical imaging. He is a diplomate of the American Board of Radiology in Medical Nuclear Physics and Diagnostic Radiological Physics and is a Fellow of the American College of Radiology. He received a PhD in Nuclear Engineering, a Master of Applied Mathematics, a Master of Engineering in Nuclear Engineering, and a BS in Nuclear Engineering, all from the University of Virginia. He has had a distinguished career at the VA serving in a number of professional capacities, including Radiation Safety Officer and Technical Director of Nuclear Medicine, for several VA medical centers, and as the Radiation Safety Program Manager for VHA Western Region of the VA National Health Physics Program. He is a clinical associate professor of Radiology at the University of California, Davis, and the co-author of several scientific papers, abstracts, and textbook chapters. He has been a council member of the National Council on Radiation Protection and Measurements (NCRP) since 2006 and has served on several scientific committees that led to NCRP Reports including Report No. 165, *Responding to a Radiological or Nuclear Terrorism Incident: A Guide for Decision Makers*; Statement No. 11 on *Quality Assurance Associated with Fluoroscopically-Guided Interventions Procedures*; and Report No. 185, *Evaluating and Communicating Radiation Risks for Studies Involving Human Subjects: Guidance for Researchers and Institutional Review Boards*. He is the author of highly regarded Federal Guidance Report No. 14, *Radiation Protection Guidance for Diagnostic and Interventional X-Ray Procedures*. Dr. Leidholdt served as a surface line officer in the U.S. Navy from 1971 until 1975.

John M. Boone, PhD

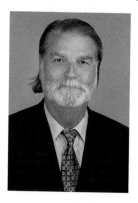

John M. Boone is a professor of Radiology and Biomedical Engineering (by courtesy) at the University of California, Davis. He has held numerous administrative positions including chief of medical physics and vice-chair for research and has directed the radiology resident physics course since 1992. Dr. Boone plays a minor role in clinical physics as a board-certified clinical medical physicist, primarily in support of Dr. Seibert's leadership in this area. In addition to his role with resident education, Dr. Boone has mentored over 20 graduate students and 10 postdoctoral fellows. Dr. Boone's primary role at UC Davis is as a researcher in medical imaging, and he has enjoyed significant external funding to support his laboratory over the past 30 years.

Dr. Boone received his undergraduate degree in Biophysics from UC Berkeley and received the MS and PhD degrees in Radiological Sciences at UC Irvine. He had faculty positions at the University of Missouri Columbia and at Thomas Jefferson University in Philadelphia before joining the faculty at UC Davis in 1992. He was elected as fellow of the American Association of Physicists in Medicine, the American College of Radiology, the Society of Breast Imaging, the Society for Photo-optical and Instrumentation Engineering (SPIE), and the American Institute for Medical and Biological Engineering. He is a commissioner of the International Commission on Radiation Units and sits on their Board of Directors. He served as president of the AAPM in 2015 and chaired the AAPM Board in 2016. He was awarded the William D. Coolidge Gold Medal from the AAPM in 2019 and also won the Butterfly Award from the Image Gently campaign that same year.

Dr. Boone has published over 225 peer-reviewed papers and has spoken nationally and internationally on a wide range of topics, in the capacity of educator and researcher. He has published extensively on radiation dosimetry for both breast imaging and whole body computed tomography. Dr. Boone chaired several AAPM committees that led to the development of the Size Specific Dose Estimate (SSDE), which will be reported on all CT systems in the near future. He has been interested in modeling x-ray spectra for breast imaging and medical/industrial radiography, and spectral models developed in his lab have been utilized worldwide by other researchers. Dr. Boone has led research on the development of cone beam breast CT systems, with nearly 600 women scanned on these prototype systems since 2004.

Contributors

Craig K. Abbey, PhD
Researcher
University of California,
  Santa Barbara
Santa Barbara, California
(*Chapter 4 Image Quality and
  Appendix G Convolution and
  Fourier Transforms*)

Stephen Balter, PhD
Professor of Clinical Radiology,
  Physics in Medicine
Columbia University
New York, New York
(*Chapter 9 Fluoroscopy*)

Wesley E. Bolch, PhD
Distinguished Professor of
  Biomedical Engineering
J. Crayton Pruitt Family
  Department of Biomedical
  Engineering
University of Florida
Gainesville, Florida
(*Chapter 16 Radionuclide
  Production,
  Radiopharmaceuticals,
  and Internal Dosimetry,
  Appendix E Effective Doses,
  Organ Doses, and Fetal
  Doses from Medical Imaging
  Procedures, and Appendix
  F Radiopharmaceutical
  Characteristics and Dosimetry*)

Lawrence T. Dauer, PhD
Associate Attending Physicist
Memorial Sloan Kettering
  Cancer Center
New York, New York
(*Chapter 21 Radiation Protection
  and Appendix I Radionuclide
  Therapy Home Care
  Guidelines*)

William D. Erwin, MS
Senior Medical Physicist
University of Texas MD
  Anderson Cancer Center
Houston, Texas
(*Chapter 18 Nuclear Imaging—
  The Gamma Camera*)

Kathryn D. Held, PhD
President
National Council on Radiation
  Protection and Measurements
Bethesda, Maryland
Associate Radiation Biologist/
  Associate Professor
Massachusetts General
  Hospital/Harvard Medical
  School
Boston, Massachusetts
(*Chapter 20 Radiation Biology*)

Youngkyoo Jung, PhD
Associate Professor of Radiology
University of California, Davis
Sacramento, California
(*Chapter 12 Magnetic
  Resonance Basics: Magnetic
  Fields, Nuclear Magnetic
  Characteristics, Tissue
  Contrast, Image Acquisition
  and Chapter 13 Magnetic
  Resonance Imaging: Advanced
  Image Acquisition Methods,
  Artifacts, Spectroscopy, Quality
  Control, Siting, Bioeffects, and
  Safety*)

Richard L. Kennedy, MSc, CIIP
Technical Director of Imaging
  Informatics
The Permanente Medical Group
Sacramento, California
(*Chapter 5 Medical Imaging
  Informatics*)

Osama Mawlawi, PhD
Professor of Imaging Physics
  and Chief of Nuclear
  medicine Physics
University of Texas MD
  Anderson Cancer Center
Houston, Texas
(*Chapter 19 Nuclear Tomographic
  Imaging—Single Photon and
  Positron Emission Tomography
  [SPECT and PET]*)

**Michael McNitt-Gray, PhD,
  DABR, FAAPM, FACR**
Professor
Department of Radiological
  Sciences
David Geffen School of
  Medicine
University of California,
  Los Angeles
Los Angeles, California
(*Chapter 10 Computed
  Tomography*)

**Charles E. Willis, PhD,
  DABR, FAAPM, FACR**
Retired Associate Professor
University of Texas MD
  Anderson Cancer Center
Houston, Texas
(*Chapter 7 Radiography*)

Acknowledgments

We are grateful to our publisher Wolters Kluwer Lippincott Williams & Wilkins and (in particular) Sharon R. Zinner who encouraged us to develop the fourth edition. We would also like to thank our editorial coordinator, Emily Buccieri, and our development editor, Eric McDermott, for their tireless efforts to bring this edition to fruition. We would also like to take this opportunity to note the passing of Jonathan Pine who served as our senior executive editor during the development of the third edition. His endless capacity to provide encouragement and assistance was truly inspirational and greatly appreciated. He is missed by many.

During the production of this work, several individuals generously gave their time and expertise. Without their help, this new edition would not have been possible. The authors would like to express their gratitude for the invaluable contributions of the following individuals:

Shadi Aminololama-Shakeri, MD
University of California, Davis

Erin Angel, PhD
Canon Medical Systems

Ramsey Badawi, PhD
University of California, Davis

John D. Boice Jr, ScD
Vanderbilt University
Vanderbilt-Ingram Cancer Center

Kevin S. Buckley, MSc
Prospect CharterCare LLC

George Burkett, MEng
University of California, Davis

Simon R. Cherry PhD
University of California, Davis

Michael Corwin, MD
University of California, Davis

Michael Cronan, RDMS
University of California, Davis

Brian Dahlin, MD
University of California, Davis

Robert Dixon, PhD
Wake Forest University

Thomas Ferbel, PhD
University of Rochester

Brian Goldner, MD
University of California, Davis

R. Edward Hendrick, PhD
University of Colorado

Andrew Hernandez, PhD
University of California, Davis

Corey J. Hiti, MD
University of California, Davis

Jiang Hsieh, PhD
General Electric Medical Systems

John Hunter, MD
University of California, Davis

Sachin Jambawalikar, PhD
Columbia University Irving Medical Center

Kalpana Kanal, PhD
University of Washington, Seattle

Frederick W. Kremkau, PhD
Wake Forest University School of Medicine

Linda Kroger, MS
University of California Davis Health System

Steven M. LaFontaine, MS
Therapy Physics, Inc.

Ramit Lamba, MD
University of California, Davis

Karen Lindfors, MD
University of California, Davis

Mahadevappa Mahesh, PhD
Johns Hopkins University

Cynthia McCollough, PhD
Mayo Clinic, Rochester

John McGahan, MD
University of California, Davis

Fred A. Mettler Jr, MD, MPH
University of New Mexico School of Medicine

Stuart Mirell, PhD
University of California at Los Angeles

Norbert Pelc, ScD
Stanford University

Nancy Pham, MD
University of California, Davis

Paul Schwoebel, PhD
University of New Mexico

D. K. Shelton, MD
University of California, Davis

Jeffrey Siewerdsen, PhD
Johns Hopkins University

Mani Tripathi, PhD
University of California, Davis

Jay Vaishnav, PhD
Canon Medical Systems

Steve Wilkendorf, RDMS
University of California, Davis

Sandra Wootton-Gorges, MD
University of California, Davis

Kai Yang, PhD
Harvard University

Contents

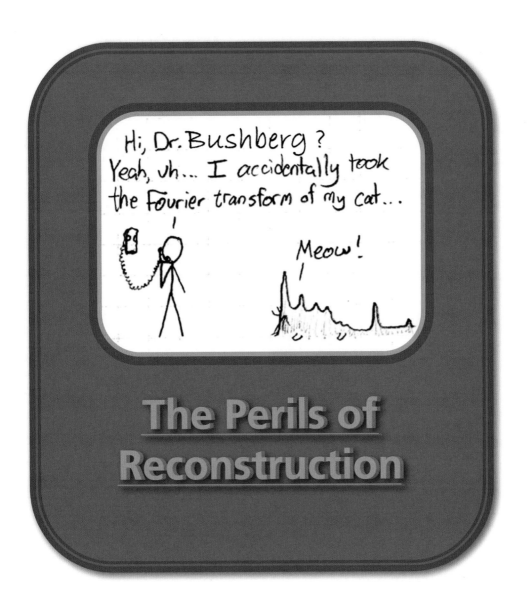

The Perils of Reconstruction

Basic Concepts

CHAPTER 1

Introduction to Medical Imaging

Radiological imaging of the intact human body requires some form of energy to enter the body, interact, and then deliver a signal to a detector, typically located outside of the body. While visible light is used in dermatology and other disciplines of medicine for observation, the primary role of radiological imaging is to produce images, which depict anatomy or physiological function well below the skin surface. In diagnostic radiology, the electromagnetic spectrum is used extensively for medical imaging, including x-rays in mammography, radiography, fluoroscopy, and computed tomography (CT); radiofrequency (RF) waves are used in magnetic resonance imaging (MRI); and γ rays in nuclear medicine. Mechanical energy from a rapidly vibrating transducer, in the form of high-frequency sound waves, is used in ultrasound imaging.

Except for nuclear medicine, all medical imaging requires that the energy used to penetrate the body's tissues also interacts with those tissues. If energy were to pass through the body and not experience some type of interaction (*e.g.*, absorption or scattering), then the detected energy would not contain any useful information regarding the internal anatomy, and thus it would not be possible to construct an image of the anatomy using that information. In nuclear medicine imaging, radioactive substances are injected or ingested, and it is the physiologically mediated biodistribution of the agent that gives rise to the information in the images.

The diagnostic utility of a medical image relates both to the technical quality of the image and to the conditions of its acquisition. In most cases, the image quality that is obtained from medical imaging devices involves compromise—better x-ray images can be made when the radiation dose to the patient is high, better magnetic resonance images can be made when the image acquisition time is long, and better ultrasound images result when the ultrasound power levels are high. However, patient safety and comfort must be considered when acquiring medical images; thus, excessive patient dose in the pursuit of a perfect image is not acceptable. This means that the power and energy levels used to make medical images require a compromise between patient safety and image quality.

1.1 THE MODALITIES

Different types of medical images are produced by varying the types of energies used to interrogate the patient, the acquisition geometry, and the scanning methods used. The different modes of making images in radiology are referred to as *modalities*. Each modality has its own niche in diagnostic and interventional radiology. One crucial aspect of medical imaging is related to how long it takes to produce the image(s). Because of patient motion, short acquisition time frames are desirable. However, the acquisition time of some imaging procedures are fundamentally limited by physics. For example, in nuclear medicine, radioactive isotopes are injected into the patient and the imaging system captures the radiation that is emitted from radioisotope decay. Because specific radioisotopes have decay constants, which are long, the scan time to produce the images is necessarily long—for example 10 minutes (min). Because the patient has involuntary motion of the lung, heart, and esophagus over this time frame, the ability to achieve high resolution will be compromised simply due to patient motion. Thus, there is a general trend that imaging modalities that require minutes for acquisition have lower resolution than modalities that can scan the patient in a few seconds.

1.1.1 Radiography

Radiography was the first medical imaging technology, made possible when the physicist Wilhelm Roentgen discovered x-rays on November 8, 1895. Roentgen also made the first radiographic images of human anatomy (Fig. 1-1). Radiography defined the field of radiology, which ultimately gave rise to radiologists, physicians who specialize in the interpretation of medical images. Radiography is performed with an x-ray source on one side of the patient and an x-ray detector on the other side. A short-duration pulse of x-rays is emitted by the x-ray tube, a large fraction of the x-ray beam interacts in the patient, and the remaining *primary* x-rays that pass through the patient reach the detector, forming a radiographic image (Fig. 1-2). The spatially homogeneous distribution of x-rays that enters the patient is modified by interactions

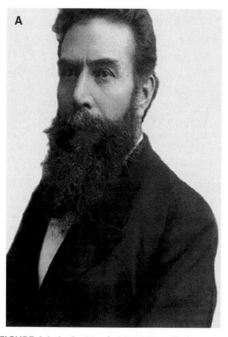
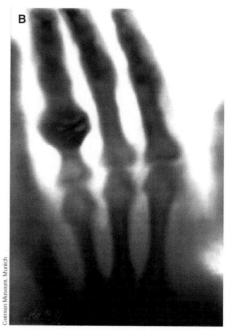

German Museum, Munich

■ **FIGURE 1-1 A.** On March 27, 2020, Wilhelm Conrad Rontgen would celebrate his 175th birthday. Roentgen discovered x-rays on a Friday evening, November 8, 1895, while experimenting with cathode rays in his laboratory in Wurzburg, Germany. He labeled the "new ray" with the letter "x" to symbolize the unknown origin and properties of the remarkable discovery for which he would receive the first Nobel Prize in Physics in 1901. Roentgen immediately noticed x-rays could have medial applications. Along with his initial paper announcing the discovery of x-rays submitted to Physical-Medical Society of Wurzburg on December 28, 1895, he sent a letter to physicians around Europe that he knew (January 1, 1896). (Imagine the Universe: Wilhelm Conrad Röentgen: https://imagine.gsfc.nasa.gov/people/Wilhelm_Roentgen.html. Accessed June 24, 2020.) **B.** He also acquired the first radiographic image of his wife's (Anna Bertha) hand with wedding ring, which was produced following a 15-min exposure on December 22, 1895. Upon seeing the bones in the radiograph of her hand Ms. Roentgen reportedly commented, "Ich habe meinen eigenen Tod gesehen": "I have seen my own death." (Used with permission from Deutsches Röntgen-Museum, Remscheid.)

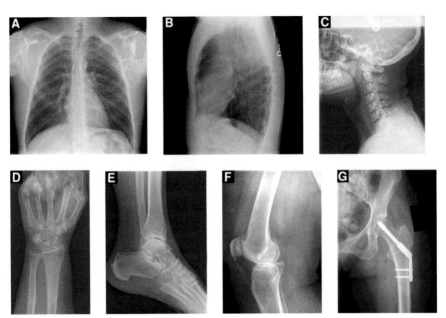

■ **FIGURE 1-2** Radiographic images remain the most prevalent type of image acquired in most radiology departments, and provide a fast, low cost view of the patient's anatomy. The anterior-posterior chest radiograph **(A)**, with the lateral chest radiograph **(B)** shown. **C.** The lateral C-spine image demonstrates the alignment of crucial bones in the neck. Images of the extremities (**D:** the distal radius and hand, **E:** the ankle, **F:** the knee) demonstrate bone fidelity and alignment. **G.** Metallic implants as seen here are readily visualized on radiographs due to the high contrast of high atomic number materials.

in the patient—both scattering and absorption events, resulting in a heterogeneous distribution of x-rays that emerges from the patient, which produces the subject contrast that is recorded by the radiographic image. Attenuation is a term that includes both absorption and scattering, and the attenuation properties of the anatomic structures inside the patient such as bone, liver, and lung are very different. These different attenuation levels provide the contrast to produce a two-dimensional image of the patient's anatomy, encoded into the radiograph. The radiographic detector of choice for a century was the screen-film cassette, but digital detector systems have now replaced screen-film radiography in most regions of the world.

1.1.2　Fluoroscopy

Fluoroscopy systems provide image sequences over time resulting in a real-time x-ray movie of the patient. Fluoroscopic systems use x-ray detector systems capable of producing images in rapid temporal sequence, typically up to 30 frames per second. The detectors are also very sensitive to low levels of radiation given that so many images are used over the course of a fluoroscopic procedure—for example, 10 min of fluoroscopy results in 18,000 images at 30 frames per second. Fluoroscopy is used for positioning intravascular catheters, visualizing contrast agents in the GI tract, and image-guided intervention including arterial stenting, placement of drainage catheters, and image-guided biopsy procedures. Fluoroscopy is used when real-time feedback is required for the medical task. While most fluoroscopy images are not recorded, recorded sequences of fluoroscopy images are used for the assessment of various motion studies, such as swallowing studies to assess peristaltic motion of the esophagus, assessment of joint movement of the knee or elbow, and several other applications.

1.1.3 Mammography

Mammography is radiography of the breast. To increase the relatively low subject contrast in breast tissues, mammography uses much lower x-ray energies than general purpose radiography, and consequently the x-ray and detector systems are designed specifically for breast imaging. A conventional screening mammogram of a compressed breast is shown in Figure 1-3A. Screening mammography is used to routinely evaluate asymptomatic women for breast cancer. Diagnostic mammography is used to facilitate the diagnosis of women with suspected breast pathology, often following a positive screening mammogram or in women with a palpable lesion.

Most digital mammography systems are capable of tomosynthesis, where the x-ray tube moves in an arc over a limited range of angles around the breast. Nine to 25 images acquired over an angular range of 15° to 50° constitute the raw data for tomosynthesis. The projection images are reconstructed in 1-mm increments through the compressed breast to yield the tomosynthesis image data set. The tomosynthesis images are parallel to the plane of the detector and reduce the superimposition of anatomy above and below the focal plane. Scrolling through the tomosynthesis images can assist the radiologist in finding patterns correlated with cancer that are otherwise hidden, as shown in Figure 1-3B. A synthetic projection mammogram can be generated by rearranging and combining the tomosynthesis data set to eliminate the need to acquire a conventional projection mammogram,

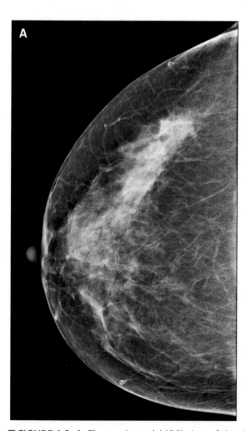
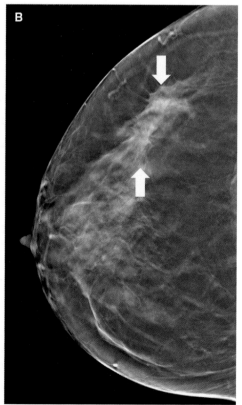

■ **FIGURE 1-3 A.** The craniocaudal (CC) view of the right breast demonstrates heterogeneously dense breast parenchyma, with no definite abnormality seen. **B.** A digital tomosynthesis acquisition (at about the same radiation dose) generates ~50 reconstructed slices in the CC view. One image clearly demonstrates two spiculated masses (solid arrows). Subsequent core biopsy of the suspicious masses reveals low grade multifocal invasive ductal carcinoma. (Courtesy of Dr. Shadi Aminololama-Shakeri MD, UC Davis Health.)

thereby reducing the overall radiation dose of the exam. This is becoming the standard of practice at many clinics.

1.1.4 Computed Tomography

CT changed the practice of medicine 50 years ago by essentially eliminating the use of exploratory surgery, which was widely used as a diagnostic procedure prior to the 1970s.

CT images are produced by acquiring numerous (~1,000) x-ray projection images over a large angular swath (typically 360°) by rotating the x-ray tube and detector around the patient. A CT detector array, opposite the x-ray source, collects the transmission projection data, and these data are synthesized by a computer into *tomographic* images of the patient using a reconstruction algorithm. CT results in high resolution thin-slice images of individual slabs of tissue along the length of the patient. CT has the ability to display three-dimensional (3D) images of the anatomy of interest, eliminating the superposition of anatomical structures, which occurs in radiography. CT images depict detailed anatomy to the physician unobstructed by normal anatomical structures, which can obscure image interpretation. While whole body CT scanners generate trans-axial images as the native image reconstruction, the thin-slice transaxial image data set can be reconfigured to produce high resolution coronal, sagittal, and multi-planar images as well.

Typical whole-body CT scanners can acquire ~0.50-mm-thick tomographic images over the desired field of view along the length of the patient. For example, a 500-mm length of the patient (1,000 × 0.5 mm images) can be imaged in less than 4 seconds (s) (40 mm wide detector array, helical acquisition with pitch = 1.0, and 0.30-s gantry rotation time). The CT image data set can reveal the presence of cancer, ruptured disks, subdural hematomas, aneurysms, and a huge assortment of other pathologies (Fig. 1-4). The CT volume data set is essentially isotropic, and coronal and sagittal CT images are routinely produced in many protocols, in addition to the traditional axial images in CT. Newly introduced high-resolution CT scanners extend the typical CT image matrix of 512 × 512 with ~0.7 mm pixel dimensions (in the axial plane) in the thorax to a 1,024 × 1,024 with 0.25 mm pixel dimensions, or even a 2,048 × 2,048 image matrix with 0.15 mm pixel dimensions (Fig. 1-4). The pixel dimensions along the length of the patient (the z dimension in coronal and sagittal images) can be adjusted from 0.5 to 5 mm in conventional CT scanners, and the high-resolution system is capable of a 0.25 mm section thickness.

Compared to standard CT image dimensions, as voxel dimensions get smaller at the same radiation dose levels, the images will become noisier—hence there is always a compromise between image noise, radiation dose, and spatial resolution. Iterative reconstruction techniques have been successful at reducing image noise using mathematical techniques, and new artificial intelligence techniques are making inroads in producing high resolution images with manageable noise levels at acceptable radiation dose levels.

There are many different acquisition modes available on modern CT scanners, including dual-energy imaging, axial and helical imaging, perfusion imaging, and prospectively gated cardiac CT. While CT is routinely used for anatomic imaging, the intravenous injection of iodinated contrast allows functional assessment of organ vascularity, perfusion, and physiological status. Because of the speed of CT acquisition and widespread availability of CT in many countries, CT has replaced radiography for many clinical indications. This trend continues. For example, intravenous pyelography (contrast radiography of the kidney) has largely been replaced by renal CT. While the radiation dose is higher, the diagnostic accuracy is improved considerably.

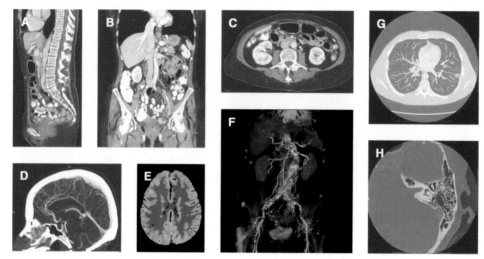

■ **FIGURE 1-4** Computed tomography images depict anatomy in cross section, including the abdomen-pelvis in **(A)** the sagittal view, **(B)** the coronal view, and **(C)** the transaxial view. **D.** A sagittal view of a contrast-enhanced head CT is shown. **E.** Perfusion CT imaging of the head allows parametric images to be calculated, as shown here. **F.** Three-dimensional rendering software allows CT volume data sets to display false-colored anatomy with impressive realism. **G.** High resolution CT can depict anatomy down to 0.15 to 0.25 mm, here showing a high-resolution contrast-enhanced chest CT displayed using maximum intensity projection (MIP), and **(H)** a high resolution CT image showing temporal bone with excellent depiction of the small boney anatomy. (Courtesy of Nancy Pham, MD and Brian W. Goldner, MD.)

1.1.5   Cone Beam Computed Tomography

The development of large field of view flat-panel x-ray detectors has led to the development of cone beam CT (CBCT) scanners, where the wider (~300 mm) flat panel detector is used in the design of the scanner instead of the relatively narrow (~40 mm) CT detector arrays of conventional CT scanners. The wide panel allows the entire CT image dataset to be acquired in one rotation of the gantry. CBCT systems are used in several specialty imaging applications, including dental imaging, orthopedic imaging (*e.g.*, knees), image-guided radiation therapy, breast imaging, and CT in angiography suites. CBCT has the advantage of being less expensive than whole body CT systems, as they are designed for niche imaging applications (Fig. 1-5). While the image quality suffers from an increase in scattered radiation to the detector and from so-called cone beam artifacts, CBCT systems often have better three-dimensional spatial resolution than most whole-body CT scanners.

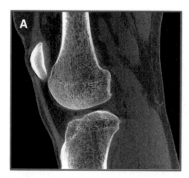
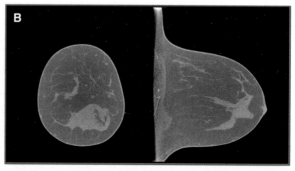

■ **FIGURE 1-5** Cone beam CT systems are inexpensive scanners typically dedicated to specific applications, with images from a commercial **(A)** orthopedic scanner and a prototype **(B)** breast CT system shown. (Image **A** is courtesy of Dr. Jeffrey H. Siewerdsen, PhD.)

1.1.6   Magnetic Resonance Imaging

MRI scanners use magnetic fields that are about 10,000 to 60,000 times stronger than the earth's magnetic field, and these fields are generated in a large cylindrical enclosure. For most imaging studies, MRI utilizes the nuclear magnetic resonance (NMR) properties of the proton—that is, the nucleus of the hydrogen atom, which is very abundant in biological tissues (each cubic millimeter of tissue contains about 10^{18} protons). The proton has an extremely small magnetic moment, and when placed in a magnetic field the magnetic moment precesses about its axis at an angular frequency proportional to the field strength. For a 3 T field, the precession frequency is about 128 million cycles per second (megahertz—MHz). Thermal energy in the tissues causes protons from unbound water to align against (antiparallel) or along (parallel) the magnetic field direction, with a slight excess of about 2–3 protons per million aligned in the parallel direction (*i.e.*, 499,999↓ to 500,002↑). Despite this small difference, a net magnetic moment is observable simply due to the enormous numbers of protons present in even a small sample of tissue.

The "resonance" in MRI refers to the coupling of the magnetic field precessional frequency of protons in tissue to the same frequency of an externally applied RF wave. In other words, the energy difference ΔE between the parallel and antiparallel spins corresponds to a specific RF frequency f, where $\Delta E = hf$. Here, h is the Planck's constant. Thus, pulsing the tissues with a precise RF frequency (using an antenna or *coil*) will pump energy into the system, which causes some protons to move from the parallel to the antiparallel state. After the RF pulse is over, the higher energy antiparallel protons will gradually flip back to the lower energy parallel state, and in the process the magnetic variations of the tissue sample occurring over a short period and at the same frequency are recorded by the coil in an unchanging magnet field. Sensitive coils surrounding the patient detect and store the MR signals for processing.

In addition to the main magnetic field coils, within the bore of the MRI system there are magnetic gradient coils that produce small linear gradients in the magnetic field across the field of view—and this slight change in magnetic field strength slightly changes the precessional frequencies of the protons in the tissues across the patient's body along the direction of the applied gradient. The MRI system uses the frequency and phase of the returning signals to determine the position. Because the signal can be attributed to specific locations (x, y, z) in the body due to the application of magnetic field gradients, an image can be produced based upon the variations in amplitude of the generated signals from each location.

MRI produces a set of tomographic images depicting slices through the patient, in which each voxel in the image depends on the both the number of protons (proton density) and magnetic properties of the tissue in that voxel. Because different types of tissue such as fat, white and gray matter in the brain, cerebral spinal fluid, and cancer all have different local magnetic properties, images made using MRI demonstrate high sensitivity to biochemical variations in soft tissue and therefore can produce high contrast images. Due to the solid structure and lack of free, unbound protons, bone structures do not generate MR signals, but the bone marrow does.

MRI has demonstrated exceptional utility in neurological imaging of the head and spine, and in musculoskeletal applications such as imaging the knee or shoulder after athletic injury (Fig. 1-6). MR is also used for breast and abdominal imaging. MR elastography has recently been introduced by combining MR imaging with mechanical waves produced by a wave generator to create a visual map (elastogram) showing the stiffness of body tissues that can be correlated with normal or disease properties. Fast image acquisition techniques have made it possible to produce images in much

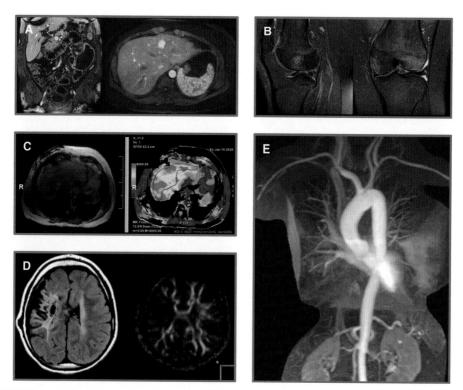

■ **FIGURE 1-6** Magnetic resonance images provide excellent anatomic contrast, tissue stiffness, diffusion, and blood flow information. **A.** MR images of the abdominal cavity in the coronal and axial planes. **B.** Multiplanar MRI of the left knee: sagittal (left) and coronal (right) fat saturation images for anterior cruciate ligament evaluation. **C.** MRI elastography measures stiffness and is a good predictor of liver fibrosis. Left: axial abdominal image. Right: corresponding elastogram, with color scale illustrating a measure of stiffness. **D.** MR evaluation of the brain. Left: Axial fluid-attenuated inversion recovery (FLAIR) sequence; Right: Diffusion Tensor Imaging reconstruction demonstrating neural tract diffusion directions, color encoded as red, left-right; green, anterior-posterior; blue, superior-inferior. **E.** MR angiography sequence with gadolinium contrast depicting the coronal view of the vasculature in the chest and abdomen. (Courtesy of Michael T. Corwin, MD and Nancy Pham, MD.)

shorter time, allowing imaging of the motion-prone thorax and abdomen. MRI scanners can also monitor blood flow through arteries (MR *angiography*), as well as blood flow in the brain (*functional* MR), which leads to the ability to measure brain function correlated to a task (*e.g.*, finger tapping, response to audible or visual stimuli, etc.). In MRI neuroradiology applications, diffusion weighted imaging of the brain can create sophisticated three-dimensional cerebral *diffusion tensor images*, making it possible to estimate the location, orientation, and anisotropy of the brain's white matter tracts.

A specific MR acquisition sequence allows for analyses of metabolic products in the tissue, known as MR spectroscopy. Indeed, spectroscopy using NMR is a method that has been used for 70 years in analytical chemistry laboratories and is the basic physics underlaying to MRI spectroscopy. In MR spectroscopy, a single voxel or multiple voxels may be analyzed using specialized MRI sequences to evaluate the biochemical composition of tissues in a precisely defined volume. The spectroscopic signal can be diagnostic for tumors or other pathology.

1.1.7 Ultrasound Imaging

Mechanical energy in the form of high frequency "ultra" sound can be used to generate images of the anatomy of a patient. A short-duration pulse of sound is generated by an ultrasound *transducer* that is in direct physical contact with the patient being imaged. The short pulse travels into the tissue and is reflected by internal structures in the body such as boundaries between tissues. A fraction of the pulse returns to the transducer as an echo, while the pulse continues to interact with tissue boundaries at greater depth. Over a short time period on the order of a millisecond, the transducer, acting as a receiver, records the amplitude and time delay of the echoes for a given direction of the pulse. The process is repeated at a slightly different location and direction of the ultrasound pulse. Repetition allows interrogation of a portion of the patient in the intended anatomical area, creating an ultrasound image. This mode of operation of an ultrasound device is called *pulse echo* imaging. Modern ultrasound transducers have multiple elements, which can individually (or in groups) transmit and receive ultrasound energy. Using these arrays, the ultrasound beam is electronically swept over a portion of the patient's anatomy, line by line. The direction of the ultrasound beam from the surface of the transducer is steered using phase delays from individual transducer elements, allowing scanning with no physical rotation of the transducer head. Each line is initiated with a short mechanical pulse; reflected sound energy returns as echoes from each pulse of ultrasound, and these are recorded as a function of time. These data are synthesized to produce a brightness mode (B-mode) ultrasound image of a planar section of tissues.

Ultrasound is weakly reflected by interfaces, such as the surfaces and internal structures of abdominal organs allowing for good penetration of the pulse, and strongly reflected by pockets of air and high-density bone. Because ultrasound does not use ionizing radiation, it is preferred for imaging obstetrical patients (Fig. 1-7). An interface between tissue and air is highly reflective, and thus very little sound

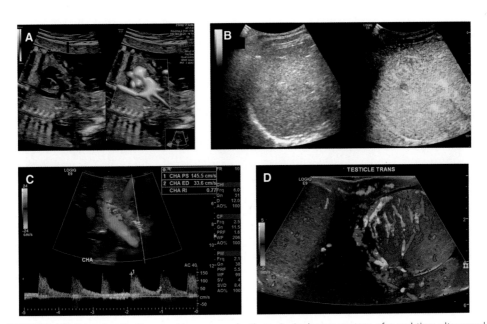

■ **FIGURE 1-7** Examples of ultrasound image examinations. **A.** An image capture of a real-time ultrasound video clip of a normal fetal aortic arch is shown. Left: a grayscale image; Right: a color-flow image demonstrates the direction of blood flow. **B.** Real-time ultrasound sequence of the liver. Left: without contrast; Right: with ultrasound contrast, demonstrating a hypoechoic lesion corresponding to a focal metastasis only seen after contrast injection. **C.** Color flow image and pulsed Doppler of the porta hepatis region of the liver. The larger color-filled structure is the portal vein. The Doppler cursor is placed on the smaller structure identified as the common hepatic artery, generating the Doppler spectral display on the bottom of the figure demonstrating pulsatile flow. **D.** Transverse ultrasound image demonstrating the normal testis on the left side and increased color flow noted on the right side within the testis secondary to inflammation (orchitis). (Courtesy of John P. McGahan, MD)

energy can penetrate into an air-filled cavity. Therefore, ultrasound imaging has less utility in the thorax where the air in the lungs presents a barrier that the ultrasound beam cannot penetrate. The interface between tissue and bone is also highly reflective, making brain imaging impractical in most cases.

Doppler Ultrasound

Doppler ultrasound makes use of the well-known Doppler effect. The Doppler effect results in a train whistle being higher in pitch as the train approaches the listener, and lower in pitch as the train whistle sounds off into the distance. The same phenomenon occurs at ultrasound frequencies, and the change in frequency (the Doppler shift) is used to measure the velocity of blood flow. Both the speed and direction of blood flow can be measured spatially, and a color flow image is produced, which typically shows blood flow in one direction as red, and in the other direction as blue Figure 1-7.

1.1.8   Nuclear Medicine Imaging

Nuclear medicine is the branch of radiology in which a radioactive atom is either injected without binding it into a radiopharmaceutical (*e.g.*, Iodine-131), or more commonly a radioactive atom is bound to some radiopharmaceutical agent and is given to the patient orally, by injection, or by inhalation. Once this agent has been distributed in the body by physiological processes, a radiation detector (gamma camera) is used to acquire images from the x- and/or γ-rays emitted during radioactive decay of the agent. Note that γ rays, by definition, are emitted from the nucleus and x-rays are emitted from a shuffling of atomic electrons, and radioactive decay can involve either or both of these types of emissions.

Nuclear medicine imaging is a form of functional imaging. Rather than providing solely anatomical information of the patient, nuclear medicine images provide information regarding the physiological conditions in the patient. For example, a radioactive thallium tracer tends to concentrate in normal heart muscle, while accumulation in infarcted or ischemic areas of the heart is reduced. Such abnormalities appear as "cold spots" on a nuclear medicine image and can be indicative of damaged heart tissue. Thyroid tissue has great affinity for iodine, and administering radioactive iodine produces a quantitative image of the thyroid. If thyroid cancer has metastasized in the patient outside of the organ, then "hot spots" indicating their location may be seen on the nuclear medicine images. Much of nuclear medicine imaging uses metastable technetium, Technetium-99m (^{99m}Tc), as this agent has excellent physical properties (energy, decay mode, half-life) for nuclear imaging.

Nuclear Medicine Planar Imaging

The energy of γ rays used in nuclear imaging is typically higher than x-ray energies used in radiography, and hence the gamma camera detector is thicker (*i.e.*, 10 mm thick NaI) to better absorb these higher energy photons. In nuclear medicine imaging, photons are measured individually, photon by photon, and this is known as *photon-counting*, which contrasts to most x-ray detection systems, which are *energy-integrating*. The photon-counting mode of nuclear cameras also allows the energy of each detection event to be quantified, which is necessary for scattered radiation rejection. In nuclear imaging, the gamma camera is placed quite near the patient (who was previously injected with a radiotracer) and a planar projection image is acquired over a time frame of about 30 s, or sometimes the patient is imaged until some number of photons (*e.g.*, 200,000, or 1,000,000, *etc.*) have been acquired. Planar nuclear images are essentially two-dimensional maps of the three-dimensional radioisotope distribution in the patient taken at a specific angle or orientation, and so they are *projection* images. These images are used directly for diagnosis, but a series of projection images acquired around a patient constitute the basic data set needed for producing single photon emission computed tomography (SPECT) images.

Gamma cameras require a collimator, which is positioned over the surface of the detector, in order to focus the γ-ray image incident upon it. If there were no collimator, the image would simply be a bright blur. The most common collimator is a sheet of thick lead with lots of parallel holes in it, and there are other types of collimators as well. While a collimator is necessary, it does reduce the sensitivity of nuclear imaging by about a factor of 10,000 (Fig. 1-8).

Single Photon Emission Computed Tomography (SPECT)

SPECT is the tomographic counterpart of nuclear medicine planar imaging, just like CT is the tomographic counterpart of radiography. In SPECT, a nuclear camera records x- or γ-ray emissions from the patient from a series of different angles

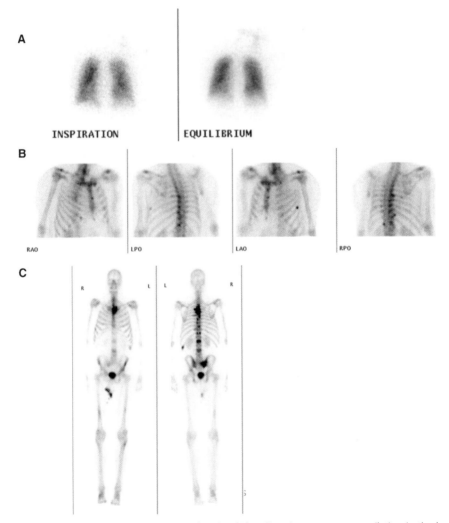

■ **FIGURE 1-8** Planar gamma camera images showing **(A)** radioactive xenon gas ventilation in the lungs, **(B)** thoracic bone scan, and **(C)** widespread metastatic disease in a patient with prostate cancer.

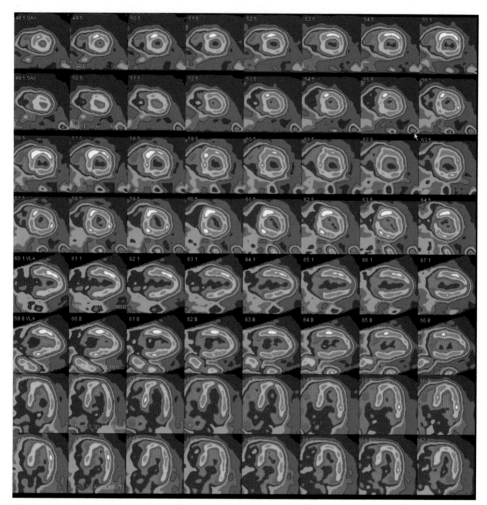

■ **FIGURE 1-9** Single photon emission computed tomography (SPECT) images of the heart are shown, at different section locations and different projections.

around the patient. These projection data are used to reconstruct a series of tomographic emission images. SPECT images provide diagnostic functional information similar to nuclear planar examinations; however, their tomographic nature allows physicians to better visualize the precise distribution of the radioactive agent, and to make a better assessment of the function of specific organs or tissues within the body (Fig. 1-9). Similar radiopharmaceutical agents are used in both planar nuclear imaging and SPECT.

Positron Emission Tomography (PET)

Positrons are positively charged electrons, e^+, and are emitted by many neutron-deficient isotopes such as Fluorine 18 (written as either ^{18}F or F-18), ^{15}O, and ^{13}N. When an e^+ is emitted, it interacts quickly with an available negatron, e^-, and both are converted into pure energy resulting in two 511 keV photons with trajectories almost exactly 180° apart. These emissions are called *annihilation radiation* but are often referred to as γ rays. Their notation as γ rays is somewhat controversial as some sources define γ rays as being emitted exclusively from atomic nuclei. To capture both of these photons, paired detectors with coincidence circuitry are positioned around the patient. When a detector pair record events within a very narrow time window

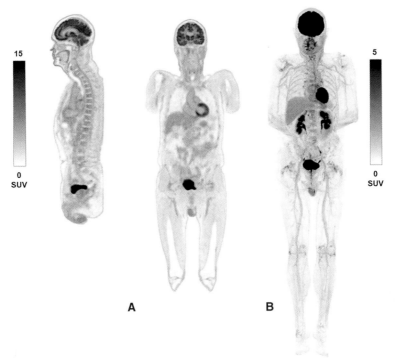

A   **B**

■ **FIGURE 1-10** EXPLORER total-body positron emission tomography (PET) images using the radiotracer [18]FDG in a normal subject. Single sagittal slice **(A)** and a maximum intensity projection image **(B)**. (Courtesy Drs. Ramsey Badawi, Simon Cherry, and Yasser G Abdelhafez.)

(*e.g.*, 4–6 ns)—which can be thought of as "exactly the same time," it is assumed that the pair of recorded events resulted from the same annihilation event. Since the positions of the detection events on each detector are both recorded, and the geometry between the two detectors is known, a line of response can be drawn between those two detection locations and after millions of such events are recorded, these data can be used to reconstruct the three-dimensional activity distribution. This mode of detection leverages the two-photon emission and detection such that a collimator is not needed—and this increases the sensitivity of PET imaging by several orders of magnitude compared to conventional nuclear medicine imaging, which requires a collimator. Most modern PET detectors have sufficient temporal resolution to measure the difference in arrival time of the two annihilation photons, thus providing a rough estimate of the position along the line of response where the annihilation event occurred—this is known as "time-of-flight" capability and when this added information is incorporated into the reconstruction process, image noise is reduced.

A recent advance in PET imaging technology is the development of a PET imaging system (EXPLORER) capable of imaging the entire body simultaneously (Fig. 1-10). Developed by UC Davis scientists and a multi-institutional consortium, EXPLORER can acquire 40 times more signal in the same time, scan up to 40 times faster, or use up to 40 times less injected activity than conventional PET imaging systems. This makes it possible to reconstruct images with unprecedented image quality, to conduct repeated studies in an individual, or to dramatically reduce dose in pediatric studies. This high-sensitivity scanner can also create video and acquire whole body dose distribution data just after injection to evaluate the early behavior of radiolabeled drugs. These data provide never-before seen kinetic information about the uptake and redistribution of radiopharmaceuticals that may provide new clinically relevant insights into disease development progression and treatment.

PET has many advantages in certain clinical and research settings, starting with the sensitivity gain arising from elimination of the collimator. In addition, many of the elements that emit positrons (carbon, oxygen, nitrogen, fluorine) are more physiologically relevant than isotopes used in conventional nuclear imaging such as ^{99m}Tc. The most widely used tracer in PET is ^{18}F-labeled fluorodeoxyglucose—^{18}FDG—which is accumulated in tissues of high glucose metabolism such as primary tumors and metastatic lesions. Therefore, PET scans of cancer patients can in many cases assess the extent of cancer metabolism, and indeed can monitor this metabolism before and after therapeutic interventions such as drug or radiation therapy to further assess response to therapy.

1.1.9 Combined Imaging Modalities

PET studies are often combined with CT images acquired immediately before or after the PET scan. Indeed, all PET scanners are now sold as PET/CT systems. The CT images provide data for the PET reconstruction algorithm to correct for attenuation making the PET image more quantitative, and the CT information also provides anatomical context onto which the PET image information is positioned as a color overlay. PET/CT combined imaging has applications in oncology, cardiology, neurology, and infection and has become a routine diagnostic tool for cancer staging (Fig. 1-11). Other combinations include SPECT/CT for reasons indicated

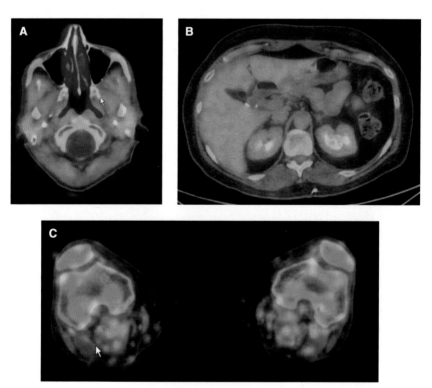

■ **FIGURE 1-11** It is common to overlay colorized PET image data that show functional activity onto the fiducially aligned CT image, which provides an anatomical backdrop. Here, PET/CT images of the **(A)** head, **(B)** abdomen, and lower extremities **(C)** are shown. The yellow areas indicate regions of high uptake of fluorodeoxyglucose.

for PET/CT modalities, and PET/MR, which combines the excellent soft-tissue contrast capabilities of MR with the functional and metabolic capabilities of PET in the fused images.

1.2 DIGITAL IMAGING BASICS

Computers were developed before digital images, and while there are exceptions, modern computers package data into bits, bytes, and words. A bit is a single binary concept (a single switch that is on [1] or off [0]), and a byte is comprised of 8 bits. Because each bit can have 2 states (on or off), a byte can hold 2^8 (*i.e.*, 256) numbers, which run from 0 to 255. A standard *word* is comprised of 2 bytes, or 16 bits. A *word* therefore can hold 2^{16} numbers, ranging from 0 to 65,535. Unlike typical scientific prefixes (where for example "kilo" means 1,000), prefixes in computer terms such as kilo, mega, and giga are power-of-two multipliers, so kilo = 1,024 (2^{10}), mega = 1,048,576 (2^{20}), and so on.

Digital images are ubiquitous in modern living, due to the ever-present cell phone camera. The photographic images acquired on a cell phone are acquired using complementary metal-oxide semiconductor (CMOS) technology, where a small computer chip with a digital matrix of perhaps 4,000 × 3,000 detector elements (dexels) can produce an image with 12 million picture elements (pixels). Photographic images are color and so each pixel is encoded using three (or more) channels, typically red, green, and blue (RGB), using typical photographic file formats such as JPEG or TIFF. Over 16 million colors can be produced using three 8-bit color channels per pixel ($2^{(8+8+8)} = 2^{24} = 16.8$ million).

Some digital radiography systems also use CMOS technology with a scintillator (such as cesium iodide or gadolinium oxysulfide), which converts x-rays to light. During the radiographic image acquisition, the light emitted from the scintillator strikes the dexels of the CMOS system, which leads to the production of unbound electrons in proportion to the light intensity and integration time, and these electrons form a charge, which is digitized by an *analog to digital converter* (ADC), resulting in a grayscale value for the corresponding pixel. Medical images are "black and white" or monochrome at the acquisition phase, but in some cases (*e.g.*, color flow in ultrasound or PET/CT) can be colorized at display. Grayscale refers to the number of different levels of gray that can be depicted by each pixel, and most digital image formats corresponding to the different image modalities use two bytes per pixel. This means that grayscale for each pixel can run from 0 to 65,535; however rarely does a medical imaging device have the fidelity that would require this "bit-depth." For example, radiographic images are typically digitized to have 10, 12, or 14 usable bits per pixel—depending on the technology. Some ultrasound images use 8 bits. CT and MRI images are 12 bits, allowing 4,096 shades of gray. SPECT and PET images typically use 12 bits as well.

The digital images that are acquired from the imaging systems are stored on a computer as a digital image file. As an example, a CT image is typically 512 × 512 pixels, but there are two bytes per pixel, so one image requires 512 × 512 × 2 bytes = 524,288 bytes or 512 kilobytes of disk storage. Most digital images in medicine are stored in a DICOM (digital imaging communication) file format, and to use the CT image example, it will contain the 524,288 bytes for the image data but there will be perhaps 1,000–2,000 other bytes added to this to encode the so-called DICOM header. Of course, a given CT scan will produce hundreds of CT images (or more), and so the typical disk space (for 800 CT images, for example) would be 400 megabytes.

1.3 IMAGE PROPERTIES

1.3.1 Image Formation

Transmission imaging refers to imaging in which the energy source (*e.g.*, x-ray tube) is on one side of the body, the energy passes through the body, and a detector measures the energy distribution on the other side of the body. X-ray imaging modalities (*i.e.*, radiography, mammography, fluoroscopy, CT) are transmission imaging modalities. In nuclear medicine, the source of radiation is injected into the patient and therefore the detected image data are produced by the emission of radiation from inside the patient. Hence, nuclear imaging (both PET and SPECT) is an example of *emission imaging*. In MR imaging, a pulse of RF radiation is tuned to have resonance absorption in protons in the patient; a fraction of this RF energy is absorbed, which disturbs the spin lattice equilibrium, and tissue magnetization induces signals within the patient. Thus, MRI is also a form of *emission* imaging. The vast majority of clinical ultrasonography involves sending mechanical energy into the patient with returning echoes generating *emissions* from reflective surfaces in the patient. Some ultrasound system geometries use a source transducer with a receiver transducer on the other side of the body part being imaged, and this geometry would be considered *transmission* imaging.

Projection imaging refers to the case where each point on the image corresponds to information along a straight-line trajectory through the patient, and this could be a parallel trajectory, or converging or diverging geometries. Radiography is a diverging projection imaging modality, and nuclear images using a parallel hole collimator are parallel projections of image data. In SPECT, PET, and x-ray CT, the raw data is acquired as projection images around some angular range about the patient, and the 3D images are computed from the many projection images acquired at those different angles.

1.3.2 Contrast

Contrast manifests as differences in the grayscale values in an image and is dependent on detected subject contrast (inherent in the characteristics of the object), digital processing of the signals (to enhance the contrast for human viewing), and display contrast (the way the processed signals are mapped into brightness and contrast on the monitor). A uniformly gray image has no contrast, whereas an image with large differences between dark gray and light gray demonstrates high contrast.

The subject contrast in x-ray imaging (radiography, fluoroscopy, mammography, and CT) is produced by differences in tissue composition and corresponding differences in local x-ray attenuation coefficient. The attenuation coefficient is dependent upon the density (g/cm^3) and the effective atomic number (Z_{eff}) of the individual tissues in the patient. The energies of the x-ray photons in the beam (adjusted by the operator) also affect subject contrast. Because bone has a markedly different effective atomic number ($Z_{eff} \approx 13$) than soft tissue ($Z_{eff} \approx 7$), due to its high concentration of calcium ($Z = 20$) and phosphorus ($Z = 15$), bones attenuate x-rays more readily than soft tissue and produce high subject contrast on x-ray based modalities—especially at low x-ray energies where atomic number-dependent attenuation is higher. Subject contrast describes the contrast inherent to the examination, but detector properties can change this. After an image is acquired, digital manipulation and processing enhances the contrast with subsequent digital window and level adjustments to fine-tune the contrast in the displayed image.

The chest radiograph is the most common radiographic procedure performed. High x-ray energies are used to lower the subject contrast of bone relative to soft tissue so that rib shadows are reduced, while the lung parenchyma still maintain good subject contrast due to the large difference in density between the air sacs in the lung and the surrounding soft tissue (Fig. 1-2).

The subject contrast in CT is higher than projection x-ray imaging modalities due to its tomographic reconstruction and the elimination of out-of-plane structures in the CT image. This is complemented by the higher signal to noise ratio in CT achieved with higher radiation dose levels compared to radiography. During the reconstruction process, the attenuation values are normalized to water attenuation to create Hounsfield units that manifest the contrast differences in the tomographic image. Adjustment of display contrast provides excellent flexibility of overall contrast of CT images that can be tuned for specific visualization of soft tissue, bone, and lung structures.

Nuclear medicine images (planar images, SPECT, and PET) are maps of the spatial distribution of radioisotopes in the patient. Thus, contrast in nuclear images depends upon the tissue's ability to concentrate the radioactive material, the background isotope accumulation in the surrounding tissues, and the imaging system's ability to record and display that information. PET and SPECT have much better contrast than planar nuclear imaging because, like CT, the images are not obscured by out-of-plane structures.

Contrast in MR imaging is related primarily to the proton density and to relaxation phenomena (*i.e.*, how fast a group of protons changes its tissue magnetization properties). Proton density is influenced by the mass density (g/cm^3), so MRI can produce images that look somewhat like CT images. Proton density differs among tissue types, and in particular adipose tissues have a higher proportion of protons than other tissues, due to the high concentration of hydrogen in fat ($CH_3(CH_2)_nCOOH$). Two different relaxation mechanisms (spin/lattice and spin/spin), characterized by time constants T_1 and T_2, respectively, are present in tissue. The relative weighting of T_1, T_2, and proton density images is achieved by manipulating the timing of the RF pulse sequence and magnetic field gradients in the MRI system. Through the clever application of different pulse sequences, blood flow can be detected using MRI techniques, giving rise to an MR angiogram. Contrast mechanisms in MRI are complex, and provide dramatic contrast levels in many cases, which is the signature utility of MR as a diagnostic tool.

Contrast in ultrasound imaging is largely determined by the acoustic properties of the tissues being imaged. The difference between the *acoustic impedances* (tissue density × speed of sound in tissue) of two adjacent tissues or other substances affects the relative amplitude of the returning ultrasound signals. Hence, contrast is quite apparent at tissue interfaces where the differences in acoustic impedance are large. Thus, ultrasound images display unique information about patient anatomy not provided by other imaging modalities. Doppler ultrasound imaging can reveal the amplitude and direction of blood flow by analyzing the frequency shift in the reflected signal, and thus with Doppler imaging, motion is the source of contrast.

1.3.3 Spatial Resolution

Just as each modality has different mechanisms for providing contrast, each modality also has different abilities to resolve fine detail in the patient. *Spatial resolution* refers to the ability to see small detail, and an imaging system has *higher* spatial resolution if it can demonstrate the presence of *smaller* objects in the image. The *limiting spatial resolution* is the size of the smallest object that an imaging system can resolve.

Table 1-1 lists the limiting spatial resolution of each of the imaging modalities used in medical imaging. The wavelength of the energy used to probe the object is a fundamental limitation of the spatial resolution of an imaging modality. For example, optical microscopes cannot resolve objects smaller than the wavelengths of visible

TABLE 1-1 RESOLUTION OF MEDICAL IMAGING SYSTEMS BY MODALITY

MODALITY	LIMITING SPATIAL RESOLUTION (line pairs/mm)	APPROXIMATE RESOLVABLE SIZE (mm)
Mammography	7.3	0.07
Digital radiography	3.5	0.14
Ultrasound (10 MHz)	3.2	0.16
Fluoroscopy (flat panel)	2.5	0.20
High resolution computed tomography	2.4	0.21
Computed tomography	1.2	0.42
Magnetic resonance imaging	1.0	0.50
Ultrasound (3.5 MHz)	1.0	0.50
EXPLORER total body PET	0.33	1.52
Conventional PET	0.17	2.94
Planar gamma camera and SPECT	0.01	5.00

Note: The human eye resolves high contrast objects of approximately 0.1 mm (5 lp/mm) at a viewing distance of ~25 cm and as small as 0.02 mm (30 lp/mm) on close inspection at ~5 cm.

light, about 400 to 700 nm. The wavelength of x-rays depends on the x-ray energy, but even the longest x-ray wavelengths are tiny—about 1 nm. This is far from the actual resolution in x-ray imaging, but it does represent the theoretical limit on the spatial resolution using x-rays. In ultrasound imaging, the wavelength of sound is the fundamental limit of spatial resolution. At 3.5 MHz, the wavelength of sound in soft tissue is about 500 μm. At 10 MHz, the wavelength is 150 μm.

MRI poses a paradox to the wavelength-imposed resolution rule—the wavelength of the RF waves used (at 1.5 T, 64 MHz) is 470 cm, but the spatial resolution of MRI is typically better than a millimeter. This is because the spatial distribution of the paths of RF energy is not used to form the actual image (contrary to ultrasound, light microscopy, and x-ray images). Localization of the protons is achieved by application of a gradient magnetic field that spatially encodes position by variations in precessional frequency. A multi-frequency output signal is detected and decoded by a mathematical process known as Fourier transformation to determine the spatial position along the applied gradient direction.

The mechanisms for generating contrast and the spatial resolution properties differ amongst the modalities, providing a wide range of diagnostic tools for radiologists. The proper choice of image modality for a given patient's needs requires an understanding of the specific clinical condition being evaluated, including anatomical location, tissue characteristics, and patient history, as well as understanding the physical principles of each image modality. The following chapters of this book are aimed at giving the medical practitioner and students of medical imaging technology just that knowledge.

SUGGESTED READING AND REFERENCES

NCRP Report 160. *Ionizing Radiation Exposure of the Population of the United States* (NCRP Report No. 160). Bethesda, MD: National Council on Radiation Protection and Measurements; 2009.

NCRP Report 184. *Medical Radiation Exposure of Patients in the United States* (NCRP Report No. 184). Bethesda, MD: National Council on Radiation Protection and Measurements; 2019.

CHAPTER 2

Radiation and the Atom

Radiation simply refers to energy that propagates through space or matter. Two categories of radiation of importance in medical imaging are electromagnetic radiation (EMR) and sub-atomic particulate radiation. Several forms of EMR are used in diagnostic imaging.

Diagnostic imaging began with the discovery of x-rays. X-rays are used in the most common medical imaging examinations, including radiography, fluoroscopy, and computed tomography. When electrons are accelerated across a high electrical potential difference in an x-ray tube and strike a target electrode, a small fraction of the electrons (but still a very large number) interact with atomic nuclei in the target, producing a vast quantity of x-rays.

In diagnostic nuclear medicine, radiopharmaceuticals (chemicals or other substances labeled with radioactive materials) are administered to patients. Gamma rays, characteristic x-rays, or pairs of annihilation photons (depending upon the radioactive material) are emitted as a result of unstable nuclei of the radioactive atoms transforming to more stable energy states during the process of radioactive decay (nuclear transformation). The radiation from the patients is detected and the resultant information is used to create images showing the distribution of the radiopharmaceuticals in the patients.

Visible light, another form of EMR, is produced when x-rays, γ-rays, or charged particles interact with scintillators in radiation detectors in x-ray and nuclear medicine imaging devices. Radiofrequency EMR, near the FM frequency band, is used to excite protons and receive signals in magnetic resonance imaging (MRI).

2.1 CLASSICAL ELECTROMAGNETISM

Classical electrostatics is a branch of physics that studies the interactions between stationary electric charges using an extension of the classical Newtonian model. The sources of magnetic fields were identified and studied later as a separate topic. Undoubtedly one of the most profound contributions to science that is on par with those of Newton, Planck, and Einstein were the contributions of James Maxwell. Maxwell took the experimental laws of Coulomb, Gauss, Faraday, and Ampere and unified electricity, magnetism, and optics into a symmetric coherent set of equations. The more than 20 equations developed by Maxwell were reduced to the four more commonly used mathematical expressions of the Laws of Maxwell by British physicist Oliver Heaviside. These four equations, known collectively as Maxwell's Equations, describe how electric and magnetic fields propagate and interact, and how they are influenced by objects they encounter. Many if not all of the aspects of electromagnetic fields are covered in introductory physics classes and include such topics as Gauss' law that relates the distribution of electric charge to the resulting electric field; Coulomb's law that describes the force between two stationary, electrically charged particles; Faraday's law of electromagnetic induction that describes how an electric current produces a magnetic field and vice versa; and Ampere's law that relates magnetic field strength to the electric current that produces it. Many of these and other fundamental principles of physics are reviewed in Appendix A. Maxwell's equations set the stage for the era of modern physics, laying the foundation even for such fields as special relativity and quantum mechanics. One of the revelations to come out of quantum mechanics was the concept that a particle that is bound (confined spatially) can only take on certain discrete values of energy, called *energy levels*. This contrasts with classical particle physics, in which a particle or system can have any amount of energy. These energy levels are commonly used to describe how much energy is required to eject electrons from different orbitals in atoms, ions, or molecules, which are bound by the electric field of the nucleus, but can also refer to energy levels of nuclei or vibrational or rotational energy levels in molecules. Einstein introduced the idea that light itself is made of such discrete units of energy, a theory that was later validated empirically. The term *photon* was given to describe these discrete quantities or "packets" of electromagnetic energy. The energies of photons are commonly expressed in units of electron volts (eV). The evolution of this discovery and its implications continues in Section 2.3. One electron volt is defined as the energy acquired by an electron as it traverses an electrical potential difference (voltage) of one volt in a vacuum. Multiples of eV common to medical imaging are keV (1,000 eV) and MeV (1,000,000 eV).

2.2   ELECTROMAGNETIC RADIATION

Radio waves, visible light, x-rays, and γ-rays correspond to different frequencies of EMR. Such radiation carries no mass, is largely unaffected at low energies by either electric or magnetic fields, and has a constant speed in each medium. Although EMR propagates through matter, it does not require matter for its propagation. Its maximal speed (2.998×10^8 m/s) occurs in a vacuum. In matter such as air, water, or glass, its speed is reduced by the refractive index of the material. EMR travels in straight lines unless it is altered in direction through interactions with matter, a process referred to as *attenuation*. Attenuation (the removal of EMR from its straight-line trajectory) can occur (1) by multiple *scattering* events within atoms or even atomic nuclei, (2) through the *absorption* (removal of the radiation) by atoms or nuclei, or (3) at energies beyond a million eV, through a *transformation* of a photon, into particulate matter (*e.g.*, energy to mass conversion of a photon to electron and positron pairs near the field of a nucleus).

Unlike a Newtonian universe, in the context of special relativity, the time-lapse between two events is not invariant from one observer to another but rather is dependent on the relative speeds of the observers. Also, rather than seeing time and the three dimensions of space as separate entities, they are interwoven into a single continuum known as "spacetime." We can use some of Newton's ideas to describe many of the physical interactions that occur with radiation in medical imaging. However, it is important to understand that Newton did not realize that we live in a spacetime continuum, nor that $E = mc^2$, and it is these ideas that describe such things as the transformation of mass into energy. The most common example of this in medical imaging occurs shortly after a positive electron (positron) is emitted during each decay of the radioisotope F-18. The rest mass of the positron and that of another electron are converted into the two oppositely directed 511 keV annihilation radiation photons used in positron emission tomography (PET).

More than 100 years have passed since English scientists used a total solar eclipse to prove a revolutionary new theory of gravity—the brainchild of Albert Einstein that would turn this exceptional scientist into a superstar whose name is synonymous with genius. Nobel laureate J.J. Thompson (credited with the discovery of the electron) called general relativity "one of the greatest achievements in human thought." In Einstein's general theory of relativity, gravity is treated as a phenomenon resulting from the curvature of the fabric of spacetime. This curvature is caused by and is proportional to the presence of mass. Einstein's general theory predicted, among other things, that gravitational fields warp the fabric of spacetime causing light to bend as it simply follows the shortest path in the spacetime domain. However, the degree of bending predicted was so small per unit mass that it would require a truly massive object (like our sun) to be observable. The total solar eclipse in 1919 provided the opportunity for British astronomer Arthur Eddington to ascertain that the light rays from distant stars had been diverted off their paths by the gravitational field of the sun by the amount predicted in Einstein's theory.

2.2.1 Electromagnetic Radiation Spectrum

EMR is commonly characterized by its wavelength (λ) and frequency (ν), or energy (E) that equals $h\nu$, where h is Planck's constant ($6.62607004 \times 10^{-34}$ m² kg/s). Naturally occurring and technologically generated EMR can be produced over a continuous spectrum of a wide range of wavelengths, frequencies, and energies that are collectively referred to as the EM spectrum. For convenient reference, the EM spectrum is divided into categories that include the radio spectrum (involving transmissions from technologies such as AM, FM, and TV broadcasting; cellular and cordless telecommunication systems; as well as other wireless data and power transfer and communications technologies); infrared radiation (i.e., radiant heat); visible light, ultraviolet (UV) radiation; and x- and Gamma (γ) rays (Fig. 2-1).

2.2.2 Wave Characteristics of Electromagnetic Radiation

Any wave (EM or mechanical, such as sound) can be characterized by its *amplitude* (maximal height), *wavelength* (λ), *frequency* (ν), and *period* (τ). The intensity of the wave is proportional to the square of the amplitude. The wavelength is the distance between any two identical points on adjacent cycles. The time required to complete one cycle of a wave is the period. The number of periods that occur per second is the frequency ($1/\tau$). Phase is the temporal shift of one wave relative to another. Some of these quantities are depicted in Figure 2-2. The speed (c), wavelength, and frequency of all EM waves in a vacuum are related by

$$c = \lambda v. \qquad [2\text{-}1]$$

Because the speed of EMR is constant in a given medium, its frequency and wavelength are inversely proportional to each other. Wavelengths of x-rays and γ-rays are typically measured in fractions of *nanometers* (nm), where 1 nm $= 10^{-9}$ m. Frequency is expressed in *hertz* (Hz), where 1 Hz $= 1$ cycle/s.

The speed (v) of any wave in a medium with refractive index (n) is described by

$$v = c/n. \qquad [2\text{-}2]$$

EMR propagates as a pair of oscillating and mutually reinforcing electric and magnetic fields that are orthogonal (perpendicular) to one another and to the direction of propagation, as shown in Figure 2-3.

Problem: Find the frequency of blue light with a wavelength of 400 nm in a vacuum.
Solution: From Equation 2-1

$$v = \frac{c}{\lambda} = \frac{(3 \times 10^8 \text{ m/s})(10^9 \text{ nm/m})}{400 \text{ nm}} = 7.5 \times 10^{14} / \text{s} = 7.5 \times 10^{14} \text{ Hz}.$$

2.2.3 Penetration of Electromagnetic Radiation in Tissue

To interrogate the physical or chemical structure of organs and tissues within the body through imaging with EMR, the energy of the EMR must be able to penetrate and interact with the organ and tissue of interest. The interactions must produce signals that

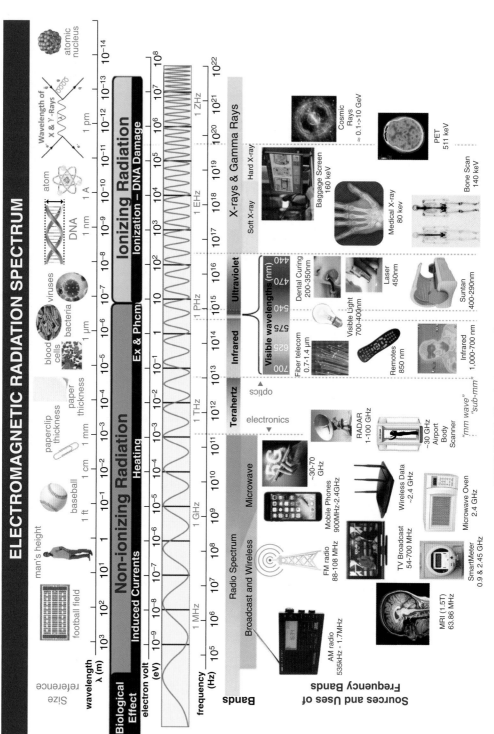

■ **FIGURE 2-1** The electromagnetic spectrum.

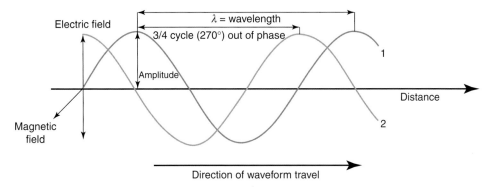

■ **FIGURE 2-2** Characterization of EM waves, of equal wavelength and amplitude, but with wave #2 having a 3/4 cycle phase difference. The magnetic field component is not shown for clarity (see Fig. 2-3).

can be captured on an image receptor or other device to reveal the nature of the interactions in a way that can help differentiate between normal tissue and the presence of disease. As seen in Figure 2-4, after traversing 25 cm of soft tissue, a beam of EMR (the interrogating signal) in the low frequency or low energy portion of the spectrum is rapidly attenuated, transmitting only 1% of the incident beam at 300 MHz (1 m). However, at lower frequencies in the TV and FM broadcast portion of the spectrum (including the ~64 MHz signals received from hydrogen nuclei in a 1.5 Tesla [T] MRI), much less attenuation takes place. At the higher frequency or photon energy portions of the EMR spectrum, where x- and γ-rays are used in medical imaging, the opposite relationship holds between frequency, photon energy, and attenuation, because as the frequencies and photon energies increase, the fraction of the incident radiation transmitted increases. Nevertheless, as will be discussed in several upcoming chapters, as the photon energy of the EMR increases, there is a trade-off between the ability of the radiation to penetrate the anatomy of interest, the detection efficiency of the image receptor, and the amount of "noise," or decrease in available contrast observed in the final image.

2.3 BEHAVIOR OF ENERGY AT THE ATOMIC SCALE: ONE OF THE MOST IMPORTANT DISCOVERIES IN THE HISTORY OF SCIENCE

At the turn of the 19th century, physicists were trying to define the mathematical relationship between the color of light emitted by some objects as they were heated (*i.e.*, color spectrum) and the object's temperature. Using classical mechanics and

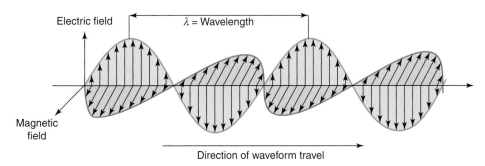

■ **FIGURE 2-3** Electric and magnetic field components of EM radiation.

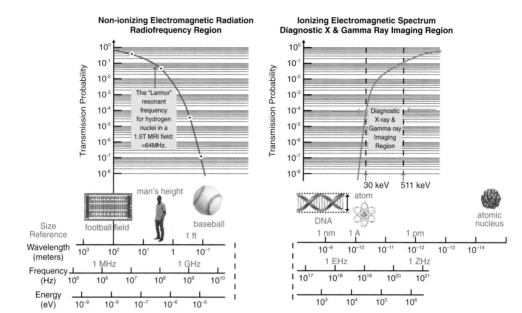

■ FIGURE 2-4 Attenuation of electromagnetic energy in the radiofrequency and diagnostic x- and γ-ray regions of the electromagnetic spectrum as it is transmitted through 25 cm of soft tissue. The Larmor (or precessional) frequency of the hydrogen nuclei in a 1.5 tesla (T) magnetic resonance imaging (MRI) system is ~64 MHz that provides a measurable signal to generate images of soft tissue as discussed in Chapter 12. Diagnostic x-ray and γ-ray energies between ~30 keV and 511 keV have sufficient transmission probability to generate images as discussed in Chapters 7–10, 18 and 19.

electromagnetism, they envisioned that, at equilibrium, energy is shared evenly amongst all the accessible modes of motion (e.g., translation, rotation, vibration). This led to them to conclude that a continuous relationship existed between the energy of the modes of motion (degrees of freedom), such as the frequencies of vibrations, and the colors of the emitted light. At low temperatures, the vibrations were slower and therefore emitted more red light, but at higher temperatures, the vibrations were faster and emitted more blue light. Lord Rayleigh and Sir James Jeans developed an equation (Rayleigh-Jeans law) that implied that the radiated power per unit frequency should be proportional to the square of the frequency. While this law accurately predicted experimental results at low frequency, the intensity of EMR predicted at higher frequencies of the EM spectrum was far greater than observed. Worse yet, the intensity of EMR appeared to approach infinity as frequency increased! The failure of Rayleigh-Jeans law to accommodate this discrepancy showed that there was something wrong with the law, with classical electromagnetic theory, or with both. The problem was that in classical physics everything (mass, energy, speed, time, etc.) was observed to be continuous and could be added or divided into infinitesimally smaller quantities.

2.3.1 Energy Quanta and the Photon

During that same time, German physicist Max Planck was also examining the nature of light and thermodynamics, and struggled with the possibility of having an infinite number of vibrational states at low energy. Planck observed that matter absorbed or emitted energy only in restricted amounts. In 1900, out of frustration, desperation, and no doubt partly ingenuity, he proposed a radical concept, that particles could only vibrate, be emitted or absorbed at energies that corresponded to multiples of some minimal finite discrete packets of energy he called *quanta*. This minimum energy was defined by the product of the frequency of vibration and a constant, h, as $E_{min} = h\nu$. Today, these discrete finite (*i.e.*, particle-like) packets of EM energy are called *photons*. The energy of a photon is given by

$$E = h\nu = \frac{hc}{\lambda},$$ [2-3]

where Planck's constant $(h) = 6.626 \times 10^{-34}$ J-s $= 4.136 \times 10^{-18}$ keV-s. When E is expressed in keV and λ in nanometers (nm),

$$E\,(\text{keV}) = \frac{1.24}{\lambda\,(\text{nm})}.$$ [2-4]

This incredibly small constant h of 6.62618×10^{-34} J-s was not only consistent with the experimental data at all frequencies of EMR but it also had the effect of limiting the amount of energy the high-frequency vibrations could hold. This was an astonishing discovery because it challenged the idea that all forms of energy were continuous and could be transferred in any amounts. While the inventor of what would be known as the quantum hypothesis did not realize it at the time, Planck's discovery would open up a completely new field of research in physics called quantum mechanics, responsible for a great diversity of new technologies (*e.g.*, cell phone, personal computer, DVD, and MRI) that make modern life and healthcare possible—and even reduces to classical physics in the appropriate regime.

2.3.2 Particle Characteristics of Electromagnetic Radiation

Prior to the advent of quantum mechanics, the classical wave description of EMR could not accommodate the observation that, upon absorbing EMR, the kinetic energies of electrons ejected from an atom (referred to as *photoelectrons*) depended on the energy (or wavelength) of the incident radiation, rather than the intensity or number of incident photons per unit area (*i.e.*, fluence). In 1905, Albert Einstein resolved this issue by postulating that Planck's quanta were acting like physical particles—namely photons. For this bold elucidation, of what is now known as the *photoelectric effect*, Albert Einstein received the Nobel Prize in Physics in 1921.

2.3.3 Wave-Particle Duality

As previously discussed, there are two equally correct ways of describing EM radiation—as waves and as photons—the discrete particle-like packets or quanta of energy. A central tenet of quantum mechanics is that all particles exhibit wave-like properties and all waves exhibit particle-like properties. This "*wave-particle duality*," initially proposed in 1924 by future Nobel Laureate Louis de Broglie, addresses the inadequacy of classical Newtonian mechanics in fully describing the behavior of atomic and sub-atomic objects. Wave characteristics are more apparent when EMR interacts with objects having dimensions similar to the photon's wavelength. For example, light photons with wavelengths of ~4–7×10^{-7} m are separated into colors by a diffraction grating of tracks on a compact disc (CD) where the track separation $(1.6 \times 10^{-6}$ m) is of the same order of magnitude as the wavelength of light, as shown in Figure 2-5A. Particle characteristics of EMR, on the other hand, are more evident when an object's dimensions (*e.g.*, an electron of 10^{-18} m) are much smaller than the photon's wavelength. For example, light photons, produced through the interaction of γ-rays with the NaI crystal in a nuclear medicine gamma camera, interact with the

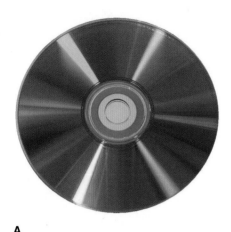
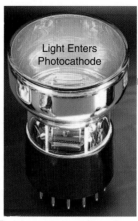

Light Enters
Photocathode

Relative Size

A **B**

■ **FIGURE 2-5** Wave- and particle-like properties of light. **A.** A CD is pressed with tracks (either with bit pits, or just a groove for photosensitive dye), followed by a aluminized covering layer. Colors on the CD are produced as light waves interact with the periodic structure of the tracks on a CD. The effect seen on the CD is similar to a diffraction grating effect, but in this case the reflected light diffracts into several beams of different frequencies (color) traveling in different directions. **B.** The imaging chain in nuclear medicine begins when γ-rays interact with the NaI crystal of a gamma camera (not shown) producing light. The NaI crystal is optically coupled to the surface of a number of PMTs like the one shown above. Just below the glass surface of the PMT, light photons strike the photocathode, ejecting electrons in a classical billiard ball (particle-like) fashion. This process is the photoelectric effect described by Einstein for which he was awarded the Nobel Prize in Physics in 1921. Additional details regarding the photoelectric effect as it applies to higher energy EMR (x-ray and γ-rays) is provided in Chapter 3. The ejected electrons are subsequently accelerated and amplified in the PMT, thereby increasing the gain of the signals used to localize the γ-ray interactions. Nuclear medicine imaging systems are discussed in Chapters 18 and 19.

photomultiplier tubes (PMTs, Fig. 2-5B) and can eject electrons from atoms in the photocathode material. The PMTs, which are optically coupled to the crystal, direct the ejected electrons via a focusing electrode toward a series of dynodes where electrons are multiplied thus providing an amplified electrical signal for the formation of an image (discussed in Chapter 18).

The particle-like behavior of x-rays is also exemplified by the classical "billiard-ball" type of collision between an x-ray photon and an orbital electron in *Compton scattering.* Similarly, the x-ray photon's energy is completely absorbed and results in the ejection of a tightly bound inner shell electron (a *photoelectron*) in the *photoelectric effect.* Each of these interactions is important in medical imaging and will be discussed further in Chapter 3.

2.4 IONIZING AND NON-IONIZING RADIATION

An atom or molecule that has lost or gained one or more electrons and has a net electrical charge and is called an ion (*e.g.*, sodium ion or Na$^+$). Some but not all electromagnetic and particulate radiations can cause ionization. In general, photons of higher frequency than the far UV region of the spectrum (*i.e.*, wavelengths shorter than 200 nm) have sufficient energy per photon to remove bound electrons from atomic shells, thereby producing ionized atoms and molecules. Radiation in this portion of the spectrum (*e.g.*, x-rays and γ-rays) is called *ionizing radiation.* EMR with photon energies in and below the UV region (*e.g.*, visible, infrared, terahertz, microwave, and radio waves) is called *non-ionizing radiation.*

The threshold energy for ionization depends on the type and state of matter. The minimum energies required to remove the outermost electron of an atom in

TABLE 2-1 **PROPERTIES OF PARTICULATE RADIATION**

PARTICLE	SYMBOL	ELEMENTARY CHARGE	REST MASS (amu)	ENERGY EQUIVALENT (MeV)
Alpha	α, $^4\text{He}^{2+}$	+2	4.00154	3,727
Proton	p, $^1\text{H}^+$	+1	1.007276	938
Electron	e^-	−1	0.000549	0.511
Negatron (beta minus)	β^-	−1	0.000549	0.511
Positron (beta plus)	β^+	+1	0.000549	0.511
Neutron	n^0	0	1.008665	940

An elementary charge is a unit of electric charge where 1 is equal in magnitude to the charge of an electron. The amu, atomic mass unit, is defined as 1/12th the mass of a carbon-12 atom.

its ground state is referred to as the *ionization energy*. For calcium (Ca), glucose ($C_6H_{12}O_6$), and liquid water (H_2O), these thresholds are 6.1, 8.8, and 11.2 eV, respectively. As water is the most abundant (thus most likely) molecular target for radiation to interact within the body, a practical radiobiological demarcation between ionizing and nonionizing EMR is approximately 11 eV. While 11 eV is the lowest photon energy able to ionize water, in a random set of ionization events in a medium, the average energy expended per ion pair (W) is larger than the minimum ionization energy due to non-ionizing energy losses from excitation and small kinetic energy transfers. For water and tissue-equivalent gas, W is about 30 eV. Particles such as high-speed electrons, protons, and α particles (discussed below) can also produce ionization. Energetic charged particles and EM radiation interactions are discussed further in Chapter 3.

2.5 PARTICULATE RADIATION

The physical properties of the most important particulate radiations associated with medical imaging and radionuclide therapy are listed in Table 2-1. Protons are found in the nuclei of all atoms. A proton has a positive electrical charge that is identical to that of the nucleus of a hydrogen atom. An electron in atomic orbit has a negative electrical charge, equal in magnitude to that of a proton, and has approximately 1/1,800 the mass of a proton. Electrons emitted by the nuclei of radioactive atoms are referred to as *beta particles*. Except for their nuclear origin, these negatively charged beta-minus particles (β^-) are indistinguishable from ordinary orbital electrons. However, there are also positively charged electrons, referred to as beta-plus particles (β^+) or *positrons*. Positrons are a form of "leptonic[1]" antimatter that ultimately combines with electrons in a unique transformation in which their "Lorenz-invariant[2]" rest mass (m)

---

[1] In the standard model of elementary particle physics matter is composed of two kinds of particles: hadrons and leptons. Whereas hadrons are composed of other elementary particles (quarks, anti-quarks, etc.), leptons are elementary point-like particles without internal structure that exist on their own. According to the standard model, there are six types of leptons: electron, electron neutrino, muon, muon neutrino, tau, and tau neutrino. For each of these, the neutrino carries a neutral charge and is nearly massless, while their counterparts all have a negative charge and a distinct mass.

[2] A quantity that does not change due to a Lorentz transformation; a quantity that is independent of the inertial frame (a reference frame in which an object stays either at rest or at a constant velocity). In all cases m can be thought of as having the center of momentum energy $\vec{p}$ (collection of relative momenta/velocities) of zero.

is converted through annihilation to an equivalent amount of energy in the form of two high-energy photons. This mass-energy conversion and its relevance to medical imaging are discussed briefly below and in greater detail in Chapters 3 and 15. Unless otherwise specified, common usage of the term beta particle refers to β^-, whereas β^+ particles are usually referred to as positrons. A neutron is an uncharged nuclear particle that has a mass slightly greater than that of a proton. Neutrons are released in nuclear fission and are used to produce radionuclides (Chapter 16). An alpha particle (α) consists of two protons and two neutrons; giving it a +2 charge and is thus identical to the nucleus of a helium atom ($^4He^{2+}$). Many radioactive elements with large atomic numbers, such as uranium, thorium, and radium, emit α particles. Following emission, the α particle eventually acquires two electrons from the surrounding medium and becomes an uncharged helium atom (^4He). When α particles are external to the body they typically do not have sufficient energy to pass through the stratum corneum (outermost layer of the epidermis) and are harmless. However, α particles can cause extensive localized cellular damage within our bodies due to the dense ionization they produce and because of the increased difficulty in restoring biological fidelity to damaged molecules compared to sparsely ionizing radiation (e.g., x- and γ-rays). The emission of α particles during radioactive decay is discussed in Chapter 15, and the radiobiological aspects of internally deposited α particles are discussed in Chapter 20.

2.6 MASS-ENERGY EQUIVALENCE

Within months of Einstein's ground-breaking work uniting the concepts of space and time in his special theory of relativity, he theorized that mass and energy were just two aspects of the same entity and are, in fact, interchangeable. In all rest frames, the quantity $E^2 = (pc)^2 + (mc)^2$ for a system of particles, where E, p, and c are the total energy, momentum, and speed of light, respectively and for which mass m can be shown to be the system's Lorentz-invariant rest mass, (i.e., a fixed value that is conserved, or independent of the systems' rest frame). In classical physics, there are two separate conservation laws, one for mass and one for energy. While these separate conservation laws provided satisfactory accommodations for the behavior of objects moving at relatively low speeds, they fail in processes in which particle speed approaches that of light. For example, the production of pairs of 511 keV photons created as a result of the rest mass annihilation of e^+e^- that are used in position emission tomography (PET), could not be understood if not for Einstein's insight that neither mass nor energy is necessarily conserved separately but can be transformed, one into the other, and it is only the total invariant mass of the system, (i.e., system's total energy and momentum) that is conserved. The relationship between the mass and the energy in any system is expressed in one of the most famous equations in science:

$$E = mc^2, \tag{2-5}$$

when energy E in joules (J) (where 1 kg m²/s² = 1 J) represents the energy equivalent to mass m at rest and c is the speed of light in a vacuum (2.998×10^8 m/s), the energy equivalent of an electron with a rest mass (m) of 9.109×10^{-31} kg is

$$E = mc^2,$$
$$E = (9.109 \times 10^{-31} \, kg)(2.998 \times 10^8 \, m/s)^2,$$
$$E = 8.187 \times 10^{-14} \, J = (8.187 \times 10^{-14} \, J)(1 \, MeV/1.602 \times 10^{-13} \, J),$$
$$= 0.511 \, MeV = 511 \, keV.$$

Due to mass–energy equivalence, the rest energy of the system is simply the invariant mass times the speed of light squared. Similarly, the total energy of the system is its total (relativistic) mass times the speed of light squared.

A common unit of mass used in atomic and nuclear physics is the atomic mass unit (amu), defined as $\frac{1}{12}$ of the mass of an atom of ^{12}C. One amu is equivalent to 931.5 MeV of energy. The conversion between mass and energy occurs in other phenomena discussed later in this book including e^+e^- pair production, radioactive decay, and annihilation radiation in positron emission tomography discussed in Chapters 3, 15, and 19, respectively.

2.7 STRUCTURE OF THE ATOM

2.7.1 The Nature of Atomic Constituents

The atom is the smallest unit of an element in which its chemical identity is maintained. The atom is composed of an extremely dense positively charged nucleus, containing protons and neutrons, and an extranuclear cloud of light, negatively charged electrons. In its normal state, an atom is electrically neutral because the number of protons equals the number of electrons. The radius of an atom is approximately 10^{-10} m, whereas that of the nucleus is only about 10^{-14} m. The atom corresponds therefore to a largely unoccupied space in which the volume of the nucleus is only 10^{-12} (a millionth of a millionth) the volume of the atom. If the empty space in an atom could be removed, a cubic centimeter of protons would have a mass of approximately 4 million metric tons! The number of electrons in the valence shell of the atom determines its reactivity, or the tendency to form chemical bonds with other atoms. A single electron separates fluorine (a highly toxic pale yellow and extremely reactive diatomic gas) from neon (a colorless, odorless, inert monatomic gas).

2.7.2 Electron Orbits

The Bohr Model

In the Bohr model of the atom (Niels Bohr 1913), electrons orbit around a dense positively charged nucleus at fixed distances (Bohr radii). Bohr combined the classical Newtonian laws of motion and Coulomb's law of electrostatic attraction with notions of quantum theory. In this model of the atom, each electron occupies a discrete energy state in a given electron shell. These electron shells are assigned the letters K, L, M, N, ..., with K denoting the innermost shell, in which the electrons have the lowest (*i.e.*, most negative) energy states or, said another way, the highest binding energy. The shells are also assigned the quantum numbers 1, 2, 3, 4, ..., with the quantum number 1 designating the K shell. Each shell can contain a maximum number of electrons given by $2(n^2)$, where n is the quantum number of the shell. Thus, the K shell ($n = 1$) can only hold 2 electrons, the L shell ($n = 2$) can hold $2(2^2)$ or 8 electrons, and so on, as shown in Figure 2-6. The outer electron shell of an atom, the valence shell, determines the chemical properties of the element. Despite its great success in atomic physics, the development of quantum mechanics led to major changes and refinements in the Bohr model.

Quantum Mechanical Model

One of the most basic consequences of quantum mechanics is that there is a wave associated with all matter, including electrons in an atom. In 1925, Schrödinger developed the wave equation that offered the most intuitive mathematical descriptions of

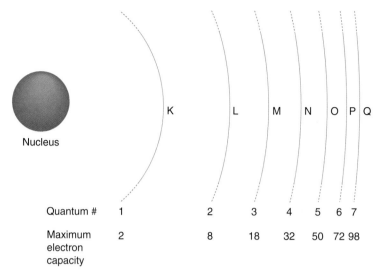

Quantum #	1		2	3	4	5	6	7

Maximum electron capacity	2		8	18	32	50	72	98

■ **FIGURE 2-6** Electron shell designations and orbital filling rules.

how subatomic particles behave and their wave-like motion. Quantum theory is based on an operator formalism for interactions in which the energy operator (the Hamiltonian[3]) operating on a wave function[4] provides the eigenvalues[5] for the allowed energies of the system. The Schrödinger wave equation provides the atomic structure where the location of an orbital valence electron is accurately described in terms of the probability it will occupy a given location within the atom with both wave and particle properties. At any given moment, there is even a probability, albeit extremely low, that an electron can be within the atom's nucleus. However, the highest probabilities are associated with Bohr's original atomic radii.

An electron can have only certain discrete energies inside an atom that agree with the experimental observation of the line spectra in which atoms exhibit and account for the characteristic red and yellow light that neon and sodium bulbs produce. Heisenberg received the Nobel Prize for the discovery of quantum mechanics in 1932, while Schrödinger shared the 1933 Nobel Prize for Physics with British physicist Paul Dirac, who predicted the existence of antiparticles such as the positron from the energy spectrum he obtained when he included the requirements of Einstein's relationship among energy, mass, and momentum.

2.7.3   Electron Binding Energy

The energy required to remove an orbital electron completely from the atom is called its *orbital binding energy*. Thus, for radiation to be ionizing, the energy transferred to

---

[3]In, quantum mechanics, a Hamiltonian is an operator corresponding to the sum of the kinetic energies plus the potential energies for all the particles in the system.

[4]A mathematical function used in quantum mechanics to describe the propagation of the wave associated with a particle or group of particles. The wave function (Ψ) is a solution to Schrödinger's equation, given the boundary conditions that describe the physical system in which the particle is found. The square of the value of the wave function (Ψ^2) is the probability of finding the particle described by a specific wave function at a specific point in space at a specific time.

[5]In a matrix, an eigenvector is a vector whose direction remains unchanged when a linear transformation (*i.e.*, scaling or stretching the matrix) is applied to it. Each eigenvector (which points in a direction of the stretch) is paired with a corresponding so-called eigenvalue, which represents the factor by which it is stretched.

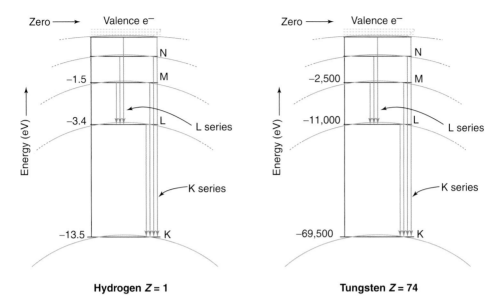

■ **FIGURE 2-7** Energy-level diagrams for hydrogen and tungsten. The energy necessary to separate electrons (ionize) in particular orbits from the atom (not drawn to scale) increases with Z and decreases with distance from the nucleus. Note that zero energy represents the point at which the electron is experiencing essentially no Coulombic attractive force from the protons in the nucleus (often referred to as a "free" electron). For a bound electron to reach that state, energy has to be absorbed. The energy states of the electrons within the atom must be below zero and as represented therefore by negative numbers. The vertical lines represent various transitions (*e.g.*, K and L series) of the electrons from one energy level to another.

the electron must equal or exceed its binding energy. Due to the closer proximity of the electrons to the positively charged nucleus, the binding energy of the K shell is greater than that of outer shells. For a particular electron shell, binding energy also increases with the number of protons in the nucleus (*i.e.*, atomic number). In Figure 2-7, electron binding energies are compared for hydrogen ($Z = 1$) and tungsten ($Z = 74$). A K shell electron of tungsten with 74 protons in the nucleus is much more tightly bound (~69,500 eV) than the K shell electron of hydrogen orbiting a nucleus with a single proton (~13.6 eV). The energy required to move an electron from the innermost electron orbit (K shell) to the next orbit (L shell) is the difference between the binding energies of the two orbits (*i.e.*, $E_{bK} - E_{bL}$ equals the transition energy).

Hydrogen:

$$13.6 \text{ eV} - 3.4 \text{ eV} = 10.2 \text{ eV}.$$

Tungsten:

$$69,500 \text{ eV} - 11,000 \text{ eV} = 58,500 \text{ eV} (58.5 \text{ keV}).$$

2.8 RADIATION FROM ELECTRON TRANSITIONS

When an electron is removed from its shell by an x-ray or γ-ray photon or via interaction with a charged particle, a vacancy is created in that shell. This vacancy is usually filled by an electron from an outer shell, leaving a vacancy in the outer shell that in turn can be filled by an electron transition from a more distant shell. This series of transitions is called an *electron cascade*. The energy released in each transition is equal to the difference in binding energy between the original and final shells of the electron. This energy can be released by the atom as characteristic x-rays or Auger electrons.

2.8.1   Characteristic X-rays

Electron transitions between atomic shells can result in the emission of radiation in the visible, UV, and x-ray portions of the EM spectrum. The energy of this radiation is a unique "characteristic" of each atom since the electron binding energies depend on the atom's atomic number (Z). Emissions from transitions exceeding 100 eV are called *characteristic* or *fluorescent* x-rays. Characteristic x-rays are named according to the orbital in which the vacancy occurred. For example, the radiation resulting from a vacancy in the K shell is called a K-characteristic x-ray, and the radiation resulting from a vacancy in the L shell is called an L characteristic x-ray. If the vacancy in one shell is filled by the adjacent shell, it is identified by a subscript α (*e.g.*, $L \rightarrow K$ transition = K_α, $M \rightarrow L$ transition = L_α). If the electron vacancy is filled from a nonadjacent shell, the subscript beta is used (*e.g.*, $M \rightarrow K$ transition = K_β). The energy of the characteristic x-ray ($E_{x\text{-ray}}$) is the difference between the electron binding energies (E_b) of the respective shells:

$$E_{x\text{-ray}} = E_{b \text{ vacant shell}} - E_{b \text{ transition shell}}. \qquad [2\text{-}6]$$

Thus, as illustrated in Figure 2-8A, an M to K shell transition in tungsten would produce a K_β characteristic x-ray of

$$E(K_\beta) = E_{bK} - E_{bM},$$
$$E(K_\beta) = 69.5 \text{ keV} - 2.5 \text{ keV} = 67 \text{ keV}.$$

2.8.2   Auger Electrons and Fluorescent Yield

An electron cascade does not always result in the production of a characteristic x-ray. A competing process that predominates in low Z elements is *Auger electron emission*, in which the energy released is transferred to an orbital electron, typically in the same shell as the cascading electron (Fig. 2-8B). The ejected Auger electron possesses kinetic energy equal to the difference between the transition energy and the binding energy of the ejected electron.

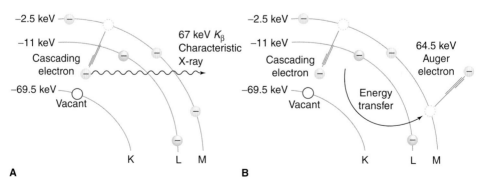

■ **FIGURE 2-8** De-excitation of a tungsten atom. An electron transition filling a vacancy in an orbit closer to the nucleus will be accompanied by either the emission of characteristic radiation **(A)** or the emission of an Auger electron **(B)**.

The probability that the electron transition will result in the emission of a characteristic x-ray is called the *fluorescent yield* (ω). Thus, $1 - \omega$ is the probability that the transition will result in the ejection of an Auger electron. Auger emission dominates in low Z elements and with electron transitions in outer shells of heavy elements. The K-shell fluorescent yield is essentially zero (less than 1%) for elements with $Z < 10$ (*i.e.*, the elements comprising the majority of soft tissue), being about 15% for calcium ($Z = 20$), about 65% for iodine ($Z = 53$), and approaching 80% for $Z > 60$.

2.9 THE ATOMIC NUCLEUS

2.9.1 Composition of the Nucleus

The nucleus is composed of protons and neutrons, known collectively as *nucleons*. The number of protons in the nucleus is the *atomic number* (Z), and the total number of protons and neutrons within the nucleus is the *mass number* (A). It is important not to confuse the mass number with the atomic mass, which is the actual mass of the atom. For example, the mass number of oxygen-16 is 16 (8 protons and 8 neutrons), whereas its atomic mass is 15.9994 amu. The notation specifying an atom with the chemical symbol is X is $^{A}_{Z}X_{N}$ where N is the number of neutrons in the nucleus. In this notation, Z and X are redundant because the chemical symbol identifies the element and thus the number of protons. For example, the symbols H, He, and Li refer to atoms with $Z = 1, 2,$ and 3, respectively. The number of neutrons is calculated as $N = A - Z$. For example, iodine $^{131}_{53}I_{78}$ is usually written as ^{131}I or as I-131. The charge on an atom is indicated by a superscript to the right of the chemical symbol. For example, Ca^{2+} indicates that the calcium atom has lost two electrons and therefore has a net charge of $+2$.

2.9.2 Classification of Nuclides

Species of atoms characterized by the number of protons and neutrons are called *nuclides*. Isotopes, isobars, isotones, and isomers are families of nuclides that share specific properties (as indicated in Table 2-2). An easy way to remember these relationships is to associate the **p** in iso*p*es with the same number of protons, the **a** in iso*a*rs with the same atomic mass number (A), the **n** in iso*n*es with the same number of neutrons, and the **e** in isom*e*r with the different nuclear energy states.

TABLE 2-2 NUCLEAR FAMILIES: ISOTOPES, ISOBARS, ISOTONES, AND ISOMERS

FAMILY	NUCLIDES WITH SAME	EXAMPLE
Isotopes	Atomic number (Z) (# of protons)	I-131 and I-125: $Z = 53$
Isobars	Mass number (A)	Mo-99 and Tc-99: $A = 99$
Isotones	Number of neutrons (A − Z)	$_{53}$I-131: $131 - 53 = 78$ $_{54}$Xe-132: $132 - 54 = 78$
Isomers	Atomic and mass numbers but different energy states in the nucleus	Tc-99m and Tc-99: $Z = 43$ $A = 99$ Energy of Tc-99m > Tc-99: $\Delta E = 142$ keV

Note: See text for description of the bold red and italicized letters in the nuclear family terms.

2.9 The Atomic Nucleus

Four Classical Forces of Nature

Forces acting within the Atom	Relative Strength	Representations	Range	Particle Mediator (mass)	Examples
• **Strong Force:** The repulsive Coulomb force of protons within a nucleus is overcome by the *strong* but short-range nuclear force that provides transformations among nucleons through meson exchange.	1	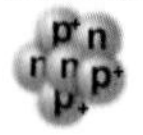	Diameter of the nucleus ≈10^{-14}–10^{-15} m	Mesons (≈0.135–9.5 GeV/C²)	Holds the atom's nucleus together
• ***Electromagnetic Force:*** Electrons are bound to nuclei through the *coulombic* (electrostatic) attractive forces.	10^{-2}	$F_g = \dfrac{k\,q_1\,q_2}{r^2}$	Infinite	Photons (0)	Holds atoms together and provides for formation of chemical bonds
• ***Weak Force:*** Neutrons can decay into protons nuclei through *weak* nuclear force, emitting an electron or beta minus (β-) particle and an anti-neutrino (v̄).	10^{-4}	$n \longrightarrow p^+ + \beta^- + \bar{v}$	0.1% diameter of a proton ≈10^{-18} m	W & Z bosons (≈86 & ≈97 amu)	Exchange force in radioactive decay and triggers nuclear fusion in stars
• ***Gravity:*** Strong planetary force, but very weak at the subatomic atomic level.	10^{-38}	$F_G = \dfrac{G\,m_1\,m_2}{r^2}$	Infinite	Graviton (< ≈10–22 eV/C²)	Holds your feet on the ground and the universe together

■ **FIGURE 2-9** We are most familiar with the attractive force of **gravity**, where F is the force due to gravity between two masses (m_1 and m_2), which are a distance r apart; G is the universal gravitational constant 6.673 × 10^{-11} Nm²/kg². Somewhat less familiar but easily observed (*e.g.*, static electricity) is the **electromagnetic force** where the relationships between the force and the variables are similar to gravity except that the electromagnetic force is between two charges (q_1 and q_2), which are a distance r apart, can be either attractive (if they are oppositely charged) or repulsive (if they have the same charge) and where the constant of proportionality k_e is Coulomb's electrostatic constant 8.99 × 10^9 Nm²/C². The remaining two forces work at the level of the atomic nucleus and, despite their central role in the structure of all matter, are far beyond the reach of human senses. The **weak force** is responsible for radioactive decay, specifically beta decay, where a neutron within the nucleus changes into a proton and an electron (beta-minus particle) and an anti-neutrino ($\bar{v}$) are ejected from the nucleus. Last, but not least, is the **strong force** that acts between nucleons (n-p, n-n, and p-p) through the exchange of mesons and is the strongest known force in the universe. However, it only operates over extremely short (subatomic) distances. The strong force binds elementary particles together in clusters to make more-familiar subatomic particles, such as protons and neutrons. The strong force is also responsible for holding the nucleus together by overcoming the substantial electrostatic repulsive forces between protons held together in an unimaginably small volume. While the description is adequate for our understanding of the discussion of radioactivity, a particle physicist would describe the strong force in a bit more detail noting that the strong force is responsible for making up nucleons (protons [p] and neutrons [n], the components of atomic nuclei) from quarks (a type of elementary particle and a fundamental constituent of matter), whose interaction is enabled by the exchange of gluons (an elementary particle that acts as the exchange particle for the strong force between quarks mediating the electric charge).

2.9.3 Nuclear Forces and Energy Levels

Two main forces (electromagnetic and the strong force) act in opposite directions on particles in the nucleus. The electromagnetic repulsive force between two protons next to each other is substantial (on the order of about 20 lbs). While that may not sound like much in our world, in the subatomic world it is massive. If we could suddenly remove the force holding the two protons together in our theoretical example, they would fly away from each other at a speed of 8,000 miles per second! The electromagnetic repulsive force between the protons is overcome by a factor of about 130 by the attractive nuclear strong force that operates over an extremely short range via the exchange of mesons. Mesons are composed of a quark and antiquark pair[6]) and are the carriers of the nuclear strong force among all nucleons. Compared to electrostatic forces that extend (albeit weakly) over vast distances, the exchange or *strong force,* that holds the nucleus together is a contact force that operates only over very short (nuclear) distances (less than 10^{-15} m), beyond which it drops to zero. These forces, along with the weak force associated with radioactive decay (discussed below) and gravity represent the four fundamental forces of nature, Figure 2-9.

The nucleus has energy levels that are analogous to orbital electron shells, although often much higher in energy. The lowest energy state is called the *ground*

---

[6]The quarks are held together by particles, called gluons, that act as forces carriers between the quarks.

state of an atomic nucleus. Nuclei with energy in excess of the ground state are said to be in an *excited state*. The average half-life of excited states for most radionuclides is on the order of 10^{-16} seconds. Nuclei whose excited states have longer half-lives 100 to 1,000 times longer than the half-lives of typical excited nuclear states, ordinarily greater than 10^{-9} seconds are referred to as *metastable*. Metastable states are denoted by the letter m after the mass number of the atom (*e.g.*, Tc-99m).

2.10 NUCLEAR STABILITY AND RADIOACTIVITY

Only certain combinations of neutrons and protons in the nucleus are stable. On a plot of Z versus N, stable nuclides fall along a "line of stability" for which the N/Z ratio is approximately 1 for low Z nuclides and approximately 1.5 for high Z nuclides, as shown in Figure 2-10. A higher neutron-to-proton ratio is required in heavy elements to offset the Coulomb repulsive forces between protons. Only four nuclides with odd numbers of neutrons and odd numbers of protons are stable, whereas many more nuclides with even numbers of neutrons and even numbers of protons are stable. The number of stable nuclides identified for different combinations of neutrons and protons is shown in Table 2-3. Magnetic properties of the nucleus are influenced by spin and charge distributions intrinsic to the proton and neutron. Nuclides with an odd number of nucleons are capable of producing a nuclear magnetic resonance signal, an essential characteristic of MRI, that is discussed in Chapter 12.

While atoms with unstable combinations of neutrons and protons do exist, over time they will undergo transformations in their atomic nuclei rendering them less unstable or stable. Two kinds of instability are referred to as neutron excess and neutron deficiency (*i.e.*, proton excess). Such nuclei have excess internal energy compared with a stable arrangement of neutrons and protons. They achieve stability by the conversion of a neutron to a proton or vice versa, and these events are accompanied by the emission of energy. The emissions include either or both particulate and EM radiations. Nuclides that decay (*i.e.*, transform) to more stable nuclei are said to be *radioactive*, and the transformation process is called *radioactive decay* (or radioactive disintegration). There are several types of radioactive decay, and these are discussed in Chapter 15.

A nucleus can undergo several decays before a stable configuration is achieved. These "decay chains" are often found in nature. For example, the decay of uranium 238 (U-238) is followed by 13 successive decays before the stable nuclide, lead 206 (Pb-206), is formed. The radionuclide at the beginning of a particular decay sequence is referred to as the *parent*, and the nuclide produced by the decay of the parent is referred to as the decay product or progeny, which may be either stable or radioactive. Historically the term *daughter* has also been used to refer to the decay products of radionuclides.

2.10.1 Gamma (γ) rays

Radioactive decay often leaves the nucleus of the atom in an excited state. The EMR emitted from the nucleus as the excited state transitions to a lower (more stable) energy state is referred to as *gamma-rays*. This energy transition is analogous to the emission of characteristic x-rays following electron transitions. However, γ-rays (by definition) emanate from the nucleus. Because the spacing of energy states within the nucleus is usually considerably larger than those of atomic orbital electron energy states, γ-rays are often much more energetic than characteristic x-rays. When this nuclear de-excitation takes place in an isomer (*e.g.*, Technetium Tc-99m), it is an *isomeric transition* (discussed in Chapter 15). In isomeric transitions, the nuclear energy state is reduced without affecting the A or Z.

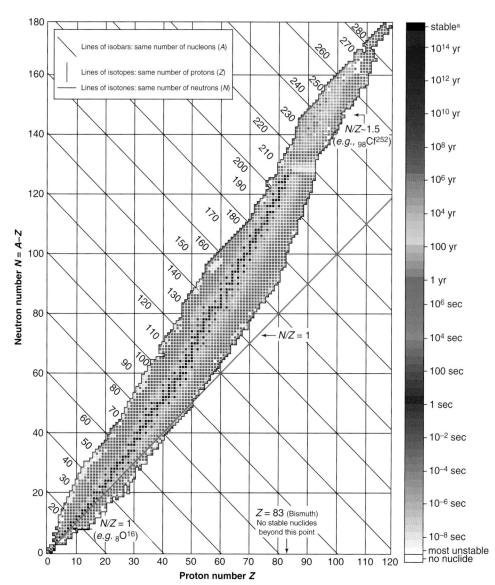

■ **FIGURE 2-10** A plot of the nuclides where the number of protons (*i.e.*, atomic number or *Z*) and neutrons of each nuclide are shown on the *x*- and *y*-axes, respectively. The outlined area containing all the black and colored squares represents the range of known nuclides. The stable nuclides are indicated by small black squares, whereas the colored squares represent radioactive (*i.e.*, unstable) nuclides or *radionuclides*. The stable nuclides form the so-called *line of stability* in which the neutron-to-proton ratio is approximately 1 for low *Z* nuclides and increases to approximately 1.5 for high *Z* nuclides. The color code indicates the physical half-life (The physical half-life is a characteristic constant of a radionuclide indicating the time required for a quantity of radioactive atoms to decay to the point where the number of radioactive atoms remaining are equal to one half of their initial value [see Chapter 3].) of each of the radionuclides. Note that all nuclides with *Z* > 83 (bismuth) are radioactive and that, in general, the further the radionuclide is from the line of stability, the more unstable it is, and the shorter the half-life it has. Radionuclides to the left of the line of stability are neutron rich and are likely to undergo beta-minus decay, while radionuclides to the right of the line of stability are neutron poor and thus often decay by positron emission or electron capture. Extremely unstable radionuclides and those with high *Z* often decay by α-particle emission. These concepts are discussed in further detail in Chapter 15. (ªThe colored bar on the right side of this figure is a color key for the half-life of the nuclides displayed on the chart. They should not be confused as representing a right "Y" axis of the figure.)

TABLE 2-3 DISTRIBUTION OF STABLE NUCLIDES AS A FUNCTION OF NEUTRON AND PROTON NUMBER

NUMBER OF PROTONS (Z)	NUMBER OF NEUTRONS (N)	NUMBER OF STABLE NUCLIDES
Even	Even	165
Even	Odd	57 (NMR signal)
Odd	Even	53 (NMR signal)
Odd	Odd	4 (NMR signal)
	Total	279

NMR, nuclear magnetic resonance.

2.10.2 Internal Conversion Electrons

Nuclear de-excitation does not always result in the emission of a γ-ray. An alternative form of de-excitation is *internal conversion*, in which the de-excitation energy is completely transferred to an orbital (typically K, L, or M shell) electron. The conversion electron is ejected from the atom, with a kinetic energy equal to the difference between the γ-ray and the electron binding energy. The vacancy produced by the ejection of the conversion electron will be filled by an electron cascade and associated characteristic x-rays or via emission of Auger electrons as described previously. The internal conversion energy transfer is analogous to the emission of an Auger electron in lieu of a characteristic x-ray energy emission. However, the kinetic energy of the internal conversion electron is often much greater than that of Auger electrons due to the greater energy associated with most γ-ray emissions compared to characteristic x-ray energies.

2.11 NUCLEAR BINDING ENERGY AND MASS DEFECT

The energy required to separate an atom into its constituent parts is the *atomic binding energy*. It is the sum of the orbital electron-binding energies. The *nuclear binding energy* is the energy needed to dissociate a nucleus into its constituent parts and is the result of the strong forces acting between nucleons. Compared with the nuclear binding energy, the orbital electron binding energy is negligible. When two subatomic particles approach each other under the influence of this strong nuclear force, their total energy decreases, and the lost energy is emitted in the form of radiation. The total energy of the bound particles is, therefore, less than that of the separated free particles.

The binding energy can be calculated by subtracting the mass of the atom from the total mass of its constituent protons, neutrons, and electrons; this mass difference is called the *mass defect*. For example, the mass of an N-14 atom, which is composed of 7 electrons, 7 protons, and 7 neutrons, is 14.00307 amu. The total mass of its constituent particles in the unbound state is

$$
\begin{aligned}
\text{mass of 7 protons} &= 7 \times 1.007276 \text{ amu} = 7.050932 \text{ amu} \\
\text{mass of 7 neutrons} &= 7 \times 1.008665 \text{ amu} = 7.060655 \text{ amu} \\
\text{mass of 7 electrons} &= 7 \times 0.000549 \text{ amu} = \underline{0.003843 \text{ amu}} \\
\text{mass of component particles of } ^{14}\text{N} &= 14.115430 \text{ amu.}
\end{aligned}
$$

Hence, the mass defect of the ^{14}N atom or the difference between the mass of its constituent particles and its atomic mass is 14.11543 amu − 14.003074 amu = 0.112356 amu. According to the formula for mass-energy equivalence (Eq. 2-5), this mass defect is equal to 0.112356 amu × (931.5 MeV/amu) = 104.7 MeV.

An extremely important observation is made by carrying the binding energy calculation a bit further. The total binding energy of the nucleus can be divided by the mass number *A* to obtain the average binding energy per nucleon. Figure 2-11 shows the average binding energy per nucleon for stable nuclides as a function of mass number. The fact that this curve reaches its maximum near the middle elements and decreases at either end predicts that large quantities of energy can be released from a small amount of matter. The two processes by which this can occur are called *nuclear fission* and *nuclear fusion*.

2.11.1 Nuclear Fission and Fusion

Nuclear fission is a process by which a nucleus with a large atomic mass captures a thermal (low kinetic energy) neutron and splits into two usually unequal parts called *fission fragments*, each with an average binding energy per nucleon greater than that of the original nucleus. In this reaction, the total nuclear binding energy increases. The change in the nuclear binding energy is released as EM and particulate radiation and as kinetic energy of the fission fragments. Fission is typically accompanied by the release of several energetic neutrons. These neutrons deposit their kinetic energy (slow down) by scattering from atomic nuclei as they as they traverse the surrounding medium until they are captured by atomic nuclei. If a neutron is captured by a fissionable nucleus, it may cause another fission, continuing the process. A nuclear reactor is a device that can maintain a self-sustaining nuclear fission chain reaction. Nuclear reactors are said to have achieved criticality when a controlled and balanced self-sustaining chain reaction proceeds with each fission event, releasing a sufficient mean number of neutrons to maintain an ongoing series of reactions. For example, the absorption of a single thermal neutron by the nucleus of a U-235 atom can result in the instantaneous fission of U-236 into two fission fragments (*e.g.*, Kr-82 and Ba-141 or Sn-131 and Mo-102) and two or three neutrons with large kinetic energies as shown in Figure 2-11. This reaction results in a mass defect equivalent to approximately 200 MeV, which is released as the kinetic energy of the fis-

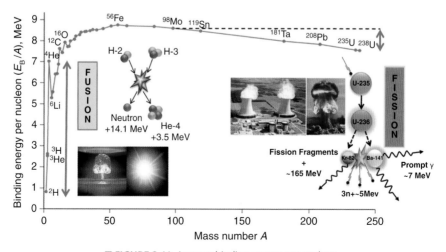

■ FIGURE 2-11 Average binding energy per nucleon.

sion fragments (~165 MeV); neutrons (~5 MeV); *prompt* (instantaneous) γ-radiation (~7 MeV); and radiation from the decay of the fission products (~23 MeV). The probability of fission increases with neutron flux, which is the number of neutrons per cm^2/s. Fission is used in nuclear-powered electrical generating plants and is the physical principle that permitted the development of the "atom" bombs. The use of nuclear fission for the production of radionuclides used in Nuclear Medicine is discussed in Chapter 16.

Energy is also released from the fusion (combining) of light atomic nuclei. For example, the fusion of deuterium (^2H) and tritium (^3He) nuclei results in the production of ^4He and a neutron. As can be seen in Figure 2-11, the ^4He atom has a much higher average binding energy per nucleon than either tritium (^3H) or deuterium (^2H). The energy associated with the mass defect of this reaction is ~17.6 MeV. Exceptionally high kinetic energies are required to overcome the substantial Coulombic repulsive forces during fusion. The fusion of hydrogen nuclei in stars, under the influence of extreme gravitational forces resulting in extraordinarily high temperatures, is the first step in subsequent self-sustaining fusion reactions that produce ^4He. The *H-bomb* is a fusion device that uses the detonation of an atom bomb (a fission device) to generate the temperature and pressure needed for fusion. Such bombs are also referred to as "thermonuclear" weapons. While the use of fission as a heat source to create steam to drive turbines creating electricity in Nuclear Power plants has been commercially successful for over 60 years, the promise of economical, clean energy from fusion-based commercial power plants remains to be demonstrated.

CHAPTER **3**

Interaction of Radiation with Matter

This chapter introduces the concepts and principles that govern x- and γ-ray photon interactions with matter and the energetic electrons those interactions set into motion. It considers the fate of these electrons as they subsequently transfer and distribute their kinetic energy in the material they traverse. These electrons transfer their kinetic energy to the surrounding medium by interacting with surrounding atoms via excitation, ionization, and radiative emissions. The photon interactions to be discussed include Rayleigh and Compton scattering and photoelectric absorption. The metrics commonly used to describe the change in intensity and quality of x- and γ-rays by attenuation as they traverse matter are presented. Energy deposited from radiation per unit mass is the definition of the quantity *Absorbed Dose*. There are many "dose" terms used in medical imaging, radiation biology, and radiation protection, each with its own specific meaning and application. Unfortunately, absorbed dose and many other dose-related terms (including KERMA, Equivalent Dose, Imparted Energy, Effective Dose, and others) are often used incorrectly. The definitions of these terms, their intended applications, and related concepts are discussed below and throughout the book.

3.1 PARTICLE INTERACTIONS

Particles of ionizing radiation include charged particles, such as alpha particles (α^{+2}), protons (p^+), beta particles (β^-), positrons (β^+), and energetic extranuclear electrons (e^-), and uncharged particles, such as neutrons. The behavior of heavy charged particles (*e.g.*, alpha particles and protons) is different from that of lighter charged particles such as electrons and positrons.

3.1.1 Excitation, Ionization, and Radiative Losses

Energetic charged particles interact with matter by electrical (*i.e.*, coulombic) forces and lose kinetic energy via *excitation*, *ionization*, and *radiative losses*. Excitation and ionization occur when charged particles lose energy by interacting with orbital electrons in the medium. These interactional, or *collisional*, losses occur due to the coulombic forces exerted on charged particles when they pass in proximity to the electric field generated by the atom's electrons and protons. Excitation is the transfer of some of the incident particles' energy to electrons in the absorbing material, promoting them to a different orbital with a higher energy level. The main difference between orbitals and energy levels is that orbitals show the most probable pathway of an electron that is in motion around the nucleus whereas energy levels show the relative locations of orbitals according to the amount of energy they possess. In excitation, the energy transferred to an electron does not exceed its binding energy. Following excitation, the electron will return to a lower energy level, with the emission of the excitation energy in the form of electromagnetic radiation or Auger electrons. This process is referred to as *de-excitation* (Fig. 3-1A). If the transferred energy exceeds

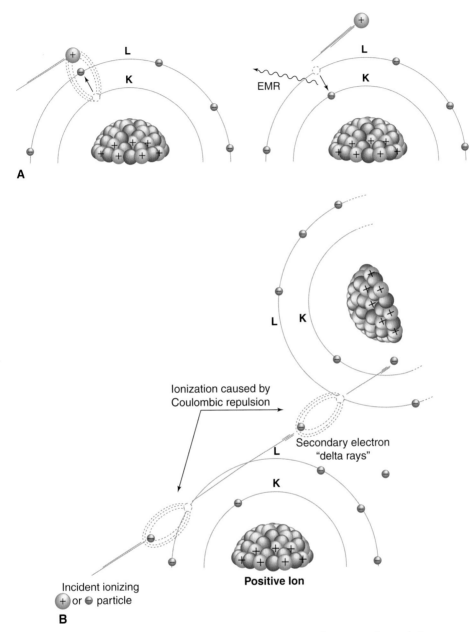

A

Ionization caused by
Coulombic repulsion

Secondary electron
"delta rays"

Positive Ion

Incident ionizing
⊕ or ⊖ particle

B

■ **FIGURE 3-1 A.** Excitation (left) and de-excitation (right) with the subsequent release of electromagnetic radiation. **B.** Ionization and the production of delta rays.

the binding energy of the electron, ionization occurs, whereby the electron is ejected from the atom (Fig. 3-1B). The result of ionization is an *ion pair* consisting of the ejected electron and the positively charged atom. Sometimes, the ejected electrons possess sufficient energy to produce further ionizations called *secondary ionization*. These electrons are called *delta rays*.

Approximately 70% of the energy deposition of energetic electrons in soft tissue occurs via ionization. However, as electron energy decreases the probability of energy loss via excitation increases. For a very low energy electron (~40 eV) the probabilities of excitation and ionization are equal and with further reductions in electron energy, the probability of ionization rapidly diminishes becoming zero (in tissue) below the first ionization state of liquid water at approximately 11.2 eV. So, while the smallest binding energies for electrons in carbon, nitrogen, and oxygen are less than 10 eV, the average energy deposited per ion pair produced in air (mostly nitrogen and oxygen) and soft tissue (mostly hydrogen, carbon, and oxygen) is approximately 34 and 22 eV, respectively. The energy difference is the result of the excitation process. Medical imaging with x-rays and γ-rays results in the production of energetic electrons by mechanisms discussed later in this chapter. It should be appreciated that, owing to the relatively modest amount of energy necessary to produce a secondary electron, each of these energetic electrons will result in an abundance of secondary electrons as it deposit its energy in tissue. For example, a 10 keV electron will result in the production of over 450 secondary electrons, most with energies between 10 and 70 eV.

Specific Ionization

The average number of primary and secondary ion pairs produced per unit length of a charged particle's path is called the *specific ionization*, expressed in ion pairs (IP)/mm. Specific ionization increases with the square of the electrical charge (Q) of the particle and decreases with the square of the incident particle velocity (v); thus,

specific ionization $\propto \dfrac{Q^2}{v^2}$. A larger charge produces a greater coulombic field; as the

particle loses kinetic energy, it slows down, allowing the coulombic field to interact at a given location for a longer period of time. The kinetic energies of alpha particles emitted by naturally occurring radionuclides extend from a minimum of about 4.05 MeV (Th-232) to a maximum of about 10.53 MeV (Po-212). The ranges of alpha particles in matter are quite limited and, for the alpha particle energies mentioned above, their ranges in air are 2.49 and 11.6 cm, respectively. In tissue, the alpha particle range is reduced to less than the diameters of a dozen or so cells (~30 to 130 μm). The specific ionization of an alpha particle can be as high as approximately 7,000 IP/mm in air and about 10 million IP/mm in soft tissue. The specific ionization as a function of the particle's path is shown for a 7.69-MeV alpha particle from ^{214}Po in air (Fig. 3-2). As the alpha particle slows, the specific ionization increases to a maximum (called the *Bragg peak*), beyond which it decreases rapidly as the alpha particle acquires electrons and becomes electrically neutral, thus losing its capacity for further ionization. The large Bragg peak associated with heavy charged particles produced by specialized accelerators is used at some medical facilities to provide this treatment in lieu of surgical excision or conventional radiation therapy. For example, there are about 30 proton centers currently in the United States, many more in the around the world as well as at least 8 carbon ion therapy centers. By adjusting the kinetic energy of heavy charged particles, a large radiation dose can be delivered at a

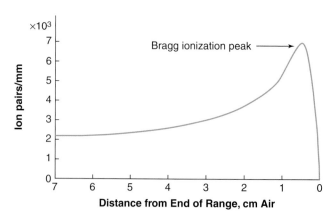

■ **FIGURE 3-2** Specific ionization (ion pairs/mm) in air of a 7.69-MeV alpha particle from ^{214}Po as a function of distance from the end of its range. The rapid increase in specific ionization reaches a maximum (Bragg peak) and then drops off sharply as the particle kinetic energy is exhausted and the charged particle is neutralized.

particular depth and over a fairly narrow range of tissue containing a lesion. On either side of the Bragg peak, the dose to tissue is substantially lower. Compared to heavy charged particles, the specific ionization of electrons is much lower (in the range of 5 to 10 IP/mm of air).

Charged Particle Tracks

Another important distinction between heavy charged particles and electrons is their paths in matter. Electrons follow tortuous paths in matter as the result of multiple scattering events caused by coulombic deflections (repulsion and/or attraction). The sparse tortuous ionization track of an electron is illustrated in Figure 3-3A. On the other hand, the larger mass of a heavy charged particle results in a dense and usually linear ionization track (Fig. 3-3B). The *path length* of a particle is defined as the distance the particle travels. The *range* of a particle is defined as the depth of penetration of the particle in matter. As illustrated in Figure 3-3, the path length of the electron almost always exceeds its range, whereas the typically straight ionization track of a heavy charged particle results in the path length and range being nearly equal. Additional information on the pattern of energy deposition of charged particles at the cellular level and their radiobiological significance is presented in Chapter 20.

Linear Energy Transfer

While specific ionization reflects all energy losses that occur before an ion pair is produced, the linear energy transfer (LET) is a measure of the average amount of energy deposited locally (near the incident particle track) in the absorber per unit path length. LET is often expressed in units of keV or eV per μm. The LET of a charged particle is proportional to the square of the charge and inversely proportional to the particle's kinetic energy (*i.e.*, LET $\propto Q^2/E_k$). The LET of a particular type of radiation describes the local energy deposition density, which can have a substantial impact on the biologic consequences of radiation exposure. In general, for a given absorbed dose, the dense ionization tracks of "high LET" radiations (alpha particles, protons, etc.) deposit their energy over a much shorter range and are much more damaging to cells than the sparse ionization pattern associated with "low LET" radiations. Low LET radiation includes energetic electrons (*e.g.*, β^- and β^+) and ionizing electromagnetic radiation (γ- and x-rays, whose interactions set electrons into motion). By way of perspective, the exposure of patients to diagnostic x-rays results in the production of energetic electrons with an average LET of approximately 3 keV/μm in soft tissue, whereas the average LET of 5-MeV alpha particles in soft tissue is approximately

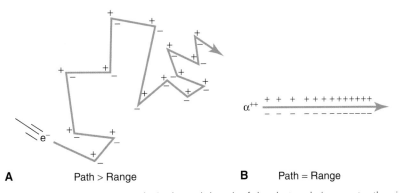

A   Path > Range   **B**   Path = Range

■ **FIGURE 3-3 A.** Electron scattering results in the path length of the electron being greater than its range. **B.** Heavily charged particles, like alpha particles, produce a dense, nearly linear ionization track, resulting in the path and range being essentially equal.

100 keV/μm. Despite their typically much higher initial kinetic energies, the range of high LET radiation is much less than that of low LET radiation. For example at the point where an alpha particle and electron traversing tissue have the same kinetic energy, say 100 keV, their ranges from that point will be 1.4 and 200 μm, respectively.

Scattering

Scattering refers to an interaction that deflects a particle or photon from its original trajectory. A scattering event in which the total kinetic energy of the colliding particles is unchanged is called *elastic*. Billiard ball collisions, for example, are elastic (disregarding frictional losses). When scattering occurs with a loss of kinetic energy (*i.e.*, the total kinetic energy of the scattered particles is less than that of the particles before the interaction), the interaction is said to be *inelastic*. For example, the process of ionization can be considered an elastic interaction if the binding energy of the electron is negligible compared to the kinetic energy of the incident electron (*i.e.*, the kinetic energy of the ejected electron is equal to the kinetic energy lost by the incident electron). If the binding energy that must be overcome to ionize the atom is not insignificant compared to the kinetic energy of the incident electron (*i.e.*, the kinetic energy of the ejected electron is less than the kinetic energy lost by the incident electron), the process is said to be inelastic.

Radiative Interactions—Bremsstrahlung

While most electron interactions with the atomic nuclei are elastic, electrons can undergo inelastic interactions in which the path of the electron is deflected by the positively charged nucleus, with a loss of kinetic energy. This energy is instantaneously emitted as electromagnetic radiation (*i.e.*, x-rays). Energy is conserved, as the energy of the radiation is equal to the kinetic energy lost by the electron.

The radiation emission accompanying electron deceleration is called *bremsstrahlung*, a German word meaning "braking radiation" (Fig. 3-4). The deceleration of the high-speed electrons in an x-ray tube produces the bremsstrahlung x-rays used in diagnostic imaging.

Total bremsstrahlung emission per atom is proportional to Z^2, where Z is the atomic number of the absorber, and inversely proportional to the square of the mass of the incident particle, that is, Z^2/m^2. Due to the strong influence of the particle's mass, bremsstrahlung production by heavier charged particles such as protons and alpha particles will be less than one-millionth of that produced by electrons.

The energy of a bremsstrahlung x-ray photon can be any value up to and including the entire kinetic energy of the deflected electron. Thus, when many

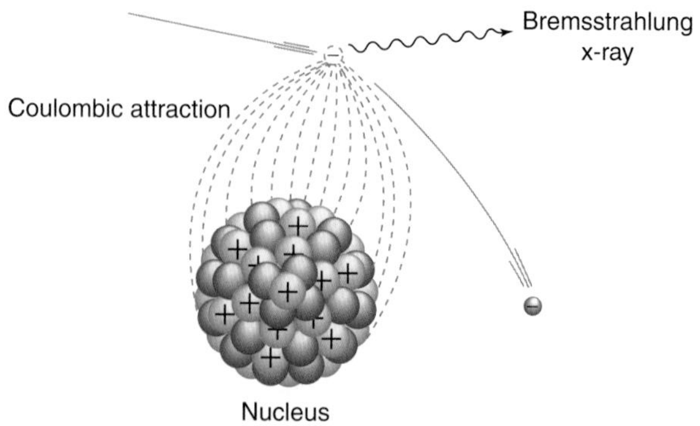

■ **FIGURE 3-4** Radiative energy loss via bremsstrahlung (braking radiation).

Coulombic attraction

Bremsstrahlung x-ray

Nucleus

electrons undergo bremsstrahlung interactions, the result is a continuous spectrum of x-ray energies. This radiative energy loss is responsible for the majority of the x-rays produced by x-ray tubes and is discussed in greater detail in Chapter 6.

Positron Annihilation

The fate of positrons (β^+) is unlike that of negatively charged electrons (e^- and β^-) that ultimately become bound to atoms. As mentioned above, all energetic electrons (positively and negatively charged) lose their kinetic energy by excitation, ionization, and radiative interactions. When a positron (a form of antimatter) reaches the end of its range, it interacts with a negatively charged electron, resulting in the annihilation of the electron-positron pair and the complete conversion of their rest mass to energy in the form of two oppositely directed 0.511-MeV *annihilation photons*. This process occurs following radionuclide decay by positron emission (see Chapter 15). Imaging of the distribution of positron-emitting radiopharmaceuticals in patients is accomplished by the detection of the annihilation photon pairs during positron emission tomography (PET) (see Chapter 19). The annihilation photons are not often emitted at exactly 180° apart because there is often a small amount of residual momentum in the positron when it interacts with the oppositely charged electron. This *noncolinearity* is not severe (~0.5°), and its blurring effect in the typical PET imaging system is not clinically significant.

3.1.2 Neutron Interactions

Unlike protons and electrons, neutrons, being uncharged particles, cannot cause excitation and ionization via coulombic interactions with orbital electrons. They can, however, interact with atomic nuclei, sometimes liberating charged particles or nuclear fragments that can directly cause excitation and ionization (Fig. 3-5). Neutrons often interact with atomic nuclei of light elements (*e.g.*, H, C, O) by scattering in "billiard ball"–like collisions, producing recoil nuclei that lose their energy via excitation and ionization. In tissue, energetic neutrons interact primarily with the hydrogen in water, producing recoil protons (hydrogen nuclei). Neutrons may also be captured by atomic nuclei. Neutron capture results in a large energy release (typically 2 to 7 MeV) due to the large binding energy of the neutron. In some cases, one or more neutrons are reemitted; in other cases, the neutron is retained, converting the atom into a different isotope. For example, the capture of a neutron by a hydrogen atom (^{1}H) results in deuterium (^{2}H) and the emission of a 2.22-MeV γ-ray, reflecting the increase in the binding energy of the nucleus:

$$^1H + {}^1n \rightarrow {}^2H + \gamma \quad \gamma\text{-ray energy } (E_\gamma) = 2.22 \text{ MeV}.$$

Some nuclides produced by neutron absorption are stable, and others are radioactive (*i.e.*, unstable). As discussed in Chapter 2, neutron absorption in some very

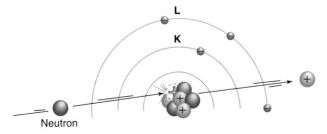

■ **FIGURE 3-5** Schematic example of collisional energy loss. An uncharged particle (neutron) interacts with the atomic nucleus of an atom resulting in the ejection of a proton. This interaction results in the transformation of the atom into a new element with an atomic number (*Z*) reduced by 1.

heavy nuclides such as ^{235}U can cause nuclear fission, producing very energetic fission fragments, neutrons, and γ-rays. Neutron interactions important to the production of radiopharmaceuticals are described in greater detail in Chapter 16.

3.2 X-RAY AND GAMMA (γ)-RAY INTERACTIONS

When traversing matter, photons will penetrate without interaction, scatter, or be absorbed. There are four major types of interactions of x-ray and γ-ray photons with matter, the first three of which play a role in diagnostic radiology and nuclear medicine: (1) Rayleigh scattering, (2) Compton scattering, (3) photoelectric absorption, and (4) pair production.

3.2.1 Rayleigh Scattering

In Rayleigh scattering, the incident photon interacts with and excites the *total atom*, as opposed to individual electrons as in Compton scattering or the photoelectric effect (discussed later). This interaction occurs mainly with very low energy x-rays, such as those used in mammography (15 to 30 keV). During the Rayleigh scattering event, the electric field of the incident photon's electromagnetic wave expends energy, causing all of the electrons in the scattering atom to oscillate in phase. The atom's electron cloud immediately radiates this energy, emitting a photon of the same energy but in a slightly different direction (Fig. 3-6). In this interaction, electrons are not ejected, and thus, ionization does not occur. In general, the average scattering angle decreases as the x-ray energy increases. In medical imaging, detection of the scattered x-ray will have a deleterious effect on image quality. However, this type of interaction has a low probability of occurrence in the diagnostic energy range. In soft tissue, Rayleigh scattering accounts for less than 5% of x-ray interactions above 70 keV and at most only accounts for about 10% of interactions at 30 keV. Rayleigh interactions are also referred to as "coherent" or "classical" scattering.

3.2.2 Compton Scattering

Compton scattering (also called inelastic or nonclassical scattering) is the predominant interaction of x-ray and γ-ray photons in the diagnostic energy range with soft

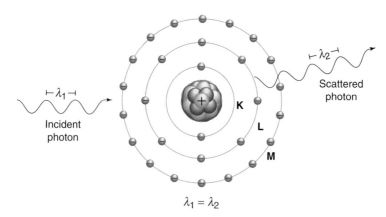

■ **FIGURE 3-6** Rayleigh scattering. The diagram shows that the incident photon λ_1, interacts with an atom and the scattered photon λ_2 is being emitted with the same wavelength and energy. Rayleigh scattered photons are typically emitted in the forward direction fairly close to the trajectory of the incident photon. *K, L,* and *M* are electron shells.

tissue. In fact, Compton scattering not only predominates in the diagnostic energy range above 26 keV in soft tissue but also continues to predominate well beyond diagnostic energies to approximately 30 MeV. This interaction is most likely to occur between photons and outer ("valence")-shell electrons (Fig. 3-7). The electron is ejected from the atom, and the scattered photon is emitted with some reduction in energy relative to the incident photon. As with all types of interactions, both energy and momentum must be conserved. Thus, the energy of the incident photon (E_o) is equal to the sum of the energy of the scattered photon (E_{sc}) and the kinetic energy of the ejected electron (E_{e-}), as shown in Equation 3-1. The binding energy of the electron that was ejected is comparatively small and can be ignored.

$$E_o = E_{sc} + E_{e-} \qquad [3\text{-}1]$$

Compton scattering results in the ionization of the atom and a division of the incident photon's energy between the scattered photon and the ejected electron. The ejected electron will lose its kinetic energy via excitation and ionization of atoms in the surrounding material. The Compton scattered photon may traverse the medium without interaction or may undergo subsequent interactions such as Compton scattering, photoelectric absorption (to be discussed shortly), or Rayleigh scattering.

The energy of the scattered photon can be calculated from the energy of the incident photon and the angle (with respect to the incident trajectory) of the scattered photon:

$$E_{sc} = \frac{E_o}{1 + \dfrac{E_o}{511 \text{ keV}}\left(1 - \cos\theta\right)}, \qquad [3\text{-}2]$$

where E_{sc} = the energy of the scattered photon, E_o = the incident photon energy, and θ = the angle of the scattered photon.

As the incident photon energy increases, both scattered photons and electrons are scattered more toward the forward direction (Fig. 3-8). In x-ray transmission imaging, these photons are much more likely to be detected by the image receptor.

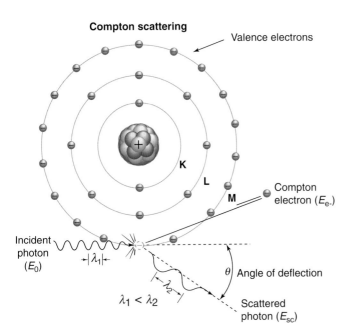

Compton scattering

Valence electrons

K

L

M

Compton electron (E_{e-})

Incident photon (E_0)

λ_1

$\lambda_1 < \lambda_2$

θ Angle of deflection

Scattered photon (E_{sc})

■ **FIGURE 3-7** Compton scattering. The diagram shows the incident photon with energy E_o, interacting with a valence-shell electron that results in the ejection of the Compton electron (E_e) and the simultaneous emission of a Compton scattered photon E_{sc} emerging at an angle θ relative to the trajectory of the incident photon. K, L, and M are electron shells.

■ FIGURE 3-8 Graph illustrates relative Compton scatter probability as a function of scattering angle for 20-, 80-, and 140-keV photons in tissue. Each curve is normalized to 100%. (Courtesy of John M. Boone, PhD, Department of Radiology, School of Medicine, University of California, Davis.)

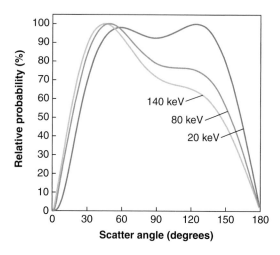

In addition, for a given scattering angle, the fraction of energy transferred to the scattered photon decreases with increasing incident photon energy. Thus, for higher energy incident photons, the majority of the energy is transferred to the scattered electron. For example, for a 60° scattering angle, the scattered photon energy (E_{sc}) is 90% of the incident photon energy (E_o) at 100 keV but only 17% at 5 MeV. When Compton scattering occurs at the lower x-ray energies used in diagnostic imaging (15 to 150 keV), the majority of the incident photon energy is transferred to the scattered photon. For example, following the Compton interaction of an 80-keV photon, the minimum energy of the scattered photon is 61 keV. Thus, even with maximal energy loss, the scattered photons have relatively high energies and tissue penetrability. In x-ray transmission imaging and nuclear emission imaging, the detection of scattered photons by the image receptors results in a degradation of image contrast and an increase in random noise. These concepts, and many others related to image quality, will be discussed in Chapter 4.

The laws of conservation of energy and momentum place limits on both scattering angle and energy transfer. For example, the maximal energy transfer to the Compton electron (and thus, the maximum reduction in photon energy) occurs with a 180° photon scatter (backscatter). In fact, the maximal energy of the scattered photon is limited to 511 keV at 90° scattering and 255 keV for a 180° scattering event. These limits on scattered photon energy hold even for extremely high-energy photons (e.g., therapeutic energy range). The scattering angle of the ejected electron cannot exceed 90°, whereas that of the scattered photon can be any value including a 180° backscatter. In contrast to the scattered photon, the energy of the ejected electron is usually absorbed near the scattering site.

The incident photon energy must be substantially greater than the electron's binding energy before a Compton interaction is likely to take place. Thus, the relative probability of a Compton interaction increases, compared to Rayleigh scattering or photoelectric absorption, as the incident photon energy increases. The probability of Compton interaction also depends on the electron density (number of electrons/g × density). Except for hydrogen, the total number of electrons/g is fairly constant in tissue; thus, the probability of Compton scattering per unit mass is nearly independent of Z, and the probability of Compton scattering per unit volume is approximately proportional to the density of the material. Compared to other elements, the absence of neutrons in the hydrogen atom results in an approximate doubling of electron density. Thus, hydrogenous materials have a higher probability of Compton scattering than anhydrogenous material of equal mass.

3.2.3 The Photoelectric Effect

In the photoelectric effect, all of the incident photon energy is transferred to an electron, which is ejected from the atom. The kinetic energy of the ejected *photoelectron* (E_{pe}) is equal to the incident photon energy (E_o) minus the binding energy of the orbital electron (E_b) (Fig. 3-9, left).

$$E_{pe} = E_o - E_b \qquad\qquad [3\text{-}3]$$

In order for photoelectric absorption to occur, the incident photon energy must be greater than or equal to the binding energy of the electron that is ejected. A table of electron binding energies and other data important to medical imaging for elements $1-100$ is listed in Appendix C. The ejected electron is most likely one whose binding energy is closest to, but less than, the incident photon energy. For example, for photons whose energies exceed the *K*-shell binding energy, photoelectric interactions with *K*-shell electrons are most probable. Following a photoelectric interaction, the atom is ionized, with an inner-shell electron vacancy. This vacancy will be filled by an electron from a shell with lower binding energy. This creates another vacancy, which, in turn, is filled by an electron from an even lower binding energy shell. Thus, an electron cascade from outer to inner shells occurs. The difference in binding energy is released as either characteristic x-rays or Auger electrons (see Chapter 2). The probability of characteristic x-ray emission decreases as the atomic number of the absorber decreases, and thus, characteristic x-ray emission does not occur frequently for diagnostic energy photon interactions in soft tissue. The photoelectric effect can and does occur with valence shell electrons such as when light photons strike the high *Z* materials that comprise the photocathode (*e.g.*, cesium, rubidium, and antimony) of a photomultiplier tube. These materials are specially selected to provide weakly bound electrons (*i.e.*, electrons with a low work function), so when illuminated the photocathode readily releases electrons (see Chapter 17). In this case, no inner shell electron cascade occurs and thus no characteristic x-rays are produced.

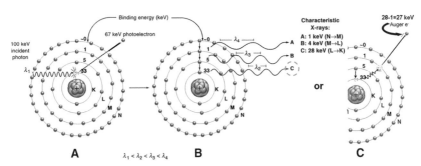

■ FIGURE 3-9 Photoelectric absorption. Left: The diagram shows that a 100-keV photon is undergoing photoelectric absorption with an iodine atom. **A.** In this case, the *K*-shell electron is ejected with a kinetic energy equal to the difference between the incident photon energy and the *K*-shell binding energy (100 keV − 33 keV = 67 keV). **B.** The vacancy created in the *K* shell results in the transition of an electron from the *L* shell to the *K* shell. The difference in their binding energies (*i.e.*, 33 keV − 5 keV) results in a 28-keV K_α characteristic x-ray. This electron cascade will continue, resulting in the production of other characteristic x-rays of lower energies. Note that the sum of the characteristic x-ray energies equals the binding energy of the ejected photoelectron (33 keV). **C.** An alternative (competing) process that can occur is the transfer of the difference in binding energy (transition energy), that would otherwise have been emitted as a characteristic x-ray (in this case the 28 keV) to an electron in the same atom whose binding energy is less than the transition energy. The figure shows the 28-keV K_α transition energy being transferred to an "M" shell electron that is ejected from the atom as an *Auger* electron with a kinetic energy equal to the transition energy minus its binding energy (28 keV − 1 keV = 27 keV). The probability of Auger electron emission increases relative to characteristic x-ray emission as the transition energy decreases.

EXAMPLE: The K- and L-shell electron binding energies of iodine are 33 and 5 keV, respectively. If a 100-keV photon is absorbed by a K-shell electron in a photoelectric interaction, the photoelectron is ejected with a kinetic energy equal to $E_o - E_b = 100 - 33 = 67$ keV. A characteristic x-ray or Auger electron is emitted as an outer-shell electron fills the K-shell vacancy (*e.g.*, L to K transition is $33 - 5 = 28$ keV). The remaining energy is released by subsequent cascading events in the outer shells of the atom (*i.e.*, M to L and N to M transitions). Note that the total of all the characteristic x-ray emissions in this example equals the binding energy of the K-shell photoelectron (Fig. 3-9, right).

Thus, photoelectric absorption results in the production of

1. A photoelectron
2. A positive ion (ionized atom)
3. Characteristic x-rays or Auger electrons

The probability of photoelectric absorption per unit mass is approximately proportional to Z^3/E^3, where Z is the atomic number, and E is the energy of the incident photon. For example, the photoelectric interaction probability in iodine ($Z = 53$) is $(53/20)^3$ or 18.6 times greater than in calcium ($Z = 20$) for a photon of a particular energy.

The benefit of photoelectric absorption in x-ray transmission imaging is that there are no scattered photons to degrade the image. The fact that the probability of photoelectric interaction is proportional to $1/E^3$ explains, in part, why image contrast decreases when higher x-ray energies are used in the imaging process (see Chapters 4 and 7). If the photon energies are doubled, the probability of photoelectric interaction is decreased eightfold: $(\frac{1}{2})^3 = 1/8$.

Although the probability of the photoelectric effect decreases, in general, with increasing photon energy, there are exceptions. For every element, the probability of the photoelectric effect, as a function of photon energy, exhibits sharp discontinuities called *absorption edges* (see Fig. 3-10). The probability of interaction for photons of energy just above an absorption edge is much greater than that of photons of energy slightly below the edge. For example, a 33.2-keV x-ray photon is about six times as likely to have a photoelectric interaction with an iodine atom as a 33.1-keV photon.

As mentioned above, a photon cannot undergo a photoelectric interaction with an electron in a particular atomic shell or subshell if the photon's energy is less than the binding energy of that shell or subshell. This causes a dramatic decrease in the probability of photoelectric absorption for photons whose energies are just below the

■ **FIGURE 3-10** Photoelectric mass attenuation coefficients for tissue ($Z_{effective} = 7$), and iodine ($Z = 53$) as a function of energy. The abrupt increase in the attenuation coefficients called "absorption edges" occur due to increased probability of photoelectric absorption when the photon energy just exceeds the binding energy of inner-shell electrons (*e.g.*, K, L, M, ...), thus increasing the number of electrons available for interaction. This process is very significant in high-Z elements, such as iodine and barium, for x-rays in the diagnostic energy range.

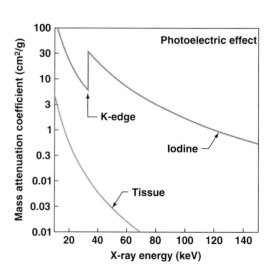

binding energy of a shell. Thus, the photon energy corresponding to an absorption edge is the binding energy of the electrons in that particular shell or subshell. An absorption edge is designated by a letter, representing the atomic shell of the electrons, followed by a roman numeral subscript denoting the subshell (e.g., K, L_I, L_{II}, L_{III}). The photon energy corresponding to a particular absorption edge increases with the atomic number (Z) of the element. For example, the primary elements comprising soft tissue (H, C, N, and O) have absorption edges below 1 keV. The element iodine ($Z = 53$), commonly used in radiographic contrast agents to provide enhanced x-ray attenuation, has a K-absorption edge of 33.2 keV (Fig. 3-10). The K-edge energy of the target material in most x-ray tubes (tungsten, $Z = 74$) is 69.5 keV. The K- and L-shell binding energies for elements with atomic numbers 1 to 100 are provided in Appendix C, Table C-3.

The photoelectric process predominates when lower energy photons interact with high Z materials (Fig. 3-11). In fact, photoelectric absorption is the primary mode of interaction of diagnostic x-rays with image receptors, radiographic contrast materials, and radiation shielding, all of which have much higher atomic numbers than soft tissue. Conversely, Compton scattering predominates at most diagnostic and therapeutic photon energies in materials of lower atomic number such as tissue and air. At photon energies below 50 keV, photoelectric interactions in soft tissue play an important role in medical imaging. The photoelectric absorption process can be used to amplify differences in attenuation between tissues with slightly different atomic numbers, thereby improving image contrast. This differential absorption is exploited to improve image contrast through the selection of x-ray tube target material and filters in mammography (see Chapter 8).

3.2.4 Pair Production

Pair production can only occur when the energies of x-rays and γ-rays exceed 1.02 MeV. In pair production, an x-ray or γ-rays interacts with the electric field of the nucleus of an atom. The photon's energy is transformed into an electron-positron pair (Fig. 3-12A). The rest mass energy equivalent of each electron is 0.511 MeV, and this is why the energy threshold for this reaction is 1.02 MeV. Photon energy in excess of this threshold is imparted to the electron (also referred to as a negatron or beta minus particle) and positron as kinetic energy. The electron and positron lose their kinetic energy via excitation and ionization. As discussed previously, when the

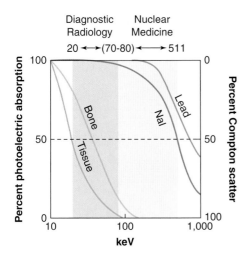

■ **FIGURE 3-11** Graph of the percentage of contribution of photoelectric (left scale) and Compton (right scale) attenuation processes for various materials as a function of photon energy. When diagnostic energy photons (i.e., diagnostic x-ray effective energy of 20 to 80 keV; nuclear medicine imaging photons of 70 to 511 keV) interact with materials of low atomic number (e.g., soft tissue), the Compton process dominates.

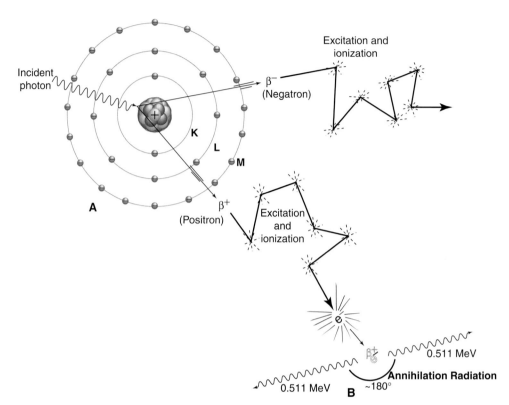

■ **FIGURE 3-12** Pair production. **A.** The diagram illustrates the pair production process in which a high-energy incident photon, under the influence of the atomic nucleus, is converted to an electron-positron pair. Both electrons (positron and negatron) expend their kinetic energy by excitation and ionization in the matter they traverse. **B.** However, when the positron comes to rest, it combines with an electron producing the two 511-keV annihilation radiation photons. *K*, *L*, and *M* are electron shells.

positron comes to rest, it interacts with a negatively charged electron, resulting in the formation of two oppositely directed 0.511-MeV annihilation photons (Fig. 3-12B).

Pair production does not occur in diagnostic x-ray imaging because the threshold photon energy is well beyond even the highest energies used in medical imaging. In fact, pair production does not become significant until the photon energies greatly exceed the 1.02-MeV energy threshold.

3.3 ATTENUATION OF X-RAYS AND γ-RAYS

Attenuation is the removal of photons from a beam of x-rays or γ-rays as it passes through matter. Attenuation is caused by both absorption and scattering of the primary photons. The interaction mechanisms discussed in the previous section, in varying degrees, cause the attenuation. At low photon energies (less than 26 keV), the photoelectric effect dominates the attenuation processes in soft tissue. However, as previously discussed, the probability of photoelectric absorption is highly dependent on photon energy and the atomic number of the absorber. When higher energy photons interact with low *Z* materials (*e.g.*, soft tissue), Compton scattering dominates (Fig. 3-13). Rayleigh scattering occurs in medical imaging with low probability, comprising about 10% of the interactions in mammography and 5% in chest radiography. Only at very high photon energies (greater than 1.02 MeV), well beyond the range of diagnostic and nuclear radiology, does pair production contribute to attenuation.

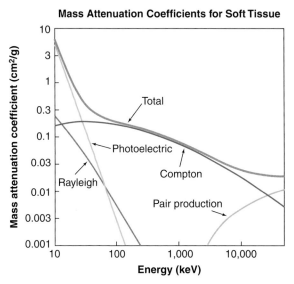

Mass Attenuation Coefficients for Soft Tissue

■ **FIGURE 3-13** Graph of the Rayleigh, photoelectric, Compton, pair production, and total mass attenuation coefficients for soft tissue ($Z \approx 7$) as a function of photon energy.

3.3.1 Linear Attenuation Coefficient

The fraction of photons removed from a monoenergetic beam of x-rays or γ-rays per unit thickness of material is called the *linear attenuation coefficient* (μ), typically expressed in units of inverse centimeters (cm⁻¹). The number of photons removed from the beam traversing a very small thickness Δx can be expressed as

$$n = \mu N \Delta x, \qquad [3\text{-}4]$$

where n is the number of photons removed from the beam, and N is the number of photons incident on the material.

For example, for 100-keV photons traversing soft tissue, the linear attenuation coefficient is 0.16 cm⁻¹. This signifies that, for every 1,000 monoenergetic photons incident upon a 1-mm (0.1 cm) thickness of tissue, approximately 16 will be removed from the beam, by either absorption or scattering.

As the thickness increases, however, the relationship is not linear. For example, it would not be correct to conclude from Equation 3-4 that 6 cm of tissue would attenuate 960 (96%) of the incident photons. To accurately calculate the number of photons removed from the beam using Equation 3-4, multiple calculations utilizing very small thicknesses of material (Δx) would be required. Alternatively, calculus can be employed to simplify this otherwise tedious process. For a monoenergetic beam of photons incident upon either thick or thin slabs of material, an exponential relationship exists between the number of incident photons (N_0) and those that are transmitted (N) through a thickness x without interaction:

$$N = N_0 e^{-\mu x}. \qquad [3\text{-}5]$$

Thus, using the example above, the fraction of 100-keV photons transmitted through 6 cm of tissue is

$$N/N_0 = e^{-(0.16 \text{ cm}^{-1})(6 \text{ cm})} = 0.38.$$

This result indicates that, on average, 380 of the 1,000 incident photons (*i.e.*, 38%) would be transmitted through the 6-cm slab of tissue without interacting. Thus, the actual attenuation ($1 - 0.38$ or 62%) is much lower than would have been predicted from Equation 3-4.

The linear attenuation coefficient is the sum of the individual linear attenuation coefficients for each type of interaction:

$$\mu = \mu_{\text{Rayleigh}} + \mu_{\text{photoelectric effect}} + \mu_{\text{Compton scatter}} + \mu_{\text{pair production}}. \qquad [3\text{-}6]$$

In the diagnostic energy range, the linear attenuation coefficient decreases with increasing energy except at absorption edges (*e.g.*, K-edge). The linear attenuation coefficient for soft tissue ranges from approximately 0.35 to 0.16 cm^{-1} for photon energies ranging from 30 to 100 keV.

For a given thickness of material, the probability of interaction depends on the number of atoms the x-rays or γ-rays encounter per unit distance. The density (ρ, in g/cm^3) of the material affects this number. For example, if the density is doubled, the photons will encounter twice as many atoms per unit distance through the material. Thus, the linear attenuation coefficient is proportional to the density of the material, for instance:

$$\mu_{\text{water}} > \mu_{\text{ice}} > \mu_{\text{water vapor}}.$$

The relationship among material density, electron density, electrons per mass, and the linear attenuation coefficient (at 50 keV) for several materials is shown in Table 3-1.

3.3.2 Mass Attenuation Coefficient

For a given material and thickness, the probability of interaction is proportional to the number of atoms per volume. This dependency can be overcome by normalizing the linear attenuation coefficient for the density of the material. The linear attenuation coefficient, normalized to unit density, is called the *mass attenuation coefficient*.

$$\text{Mass Attenuation Coefficient } (\mu/\rho) \left[\text{cm}^2/\text{g}\right]$$
$$= \frac{\text{Linear Attenuation Coefficient } (\mu) \left[\text{cm}^{-1}\right]}{\text{Density of Material } (\rho) \left[\text{g/cm}^3\right]} \qquad [3\text{-}7]$$

The linear attenuation coefficient is usually expressed in units of cm^{-1}, whereas the units of the mass attenuation coefficient are usually cm^2/g.

TABLE 3-1 MATERIAL DENSITY, ELECTRONS PER MASS, ELECTRON DENSITY, AND THE LINEAR ATTENUATION COEFFICIENT (AT 50 keV) FOR SEVERAL MATERIALS

MATERIAL	DENSITY (g/cm³)	ELECTRONS PER MASS (e/g) × 10²³	ELECTRON DENSITY (e/cm³) × 10²³	μ AT 50 keV (cm⁻¹)
Hydrogen gas	0.000084	5.97	0.0005	0.000028
Water vapor	0.000598	3.34	0.002	0.000128
Air	0.00129	3.006	0.0038	0.000290
Fat	0.91	3.34	3.04	0.193
Ice	0.917	3.34	3.06	0.196
Water	1	3.34	3.34	0.214
Compact bone	1.85	3.192	5.91	0.573

The mass attenuation coefficient is *independent* of density. Therefore, for a given photon energy,

$$\mu_{water}/\rho_{water} = \mu_{ice}/\rho_{ice} = \mu_{water\ vapor}/\rho_{water\ vapor}.$$

However, in radiology, we do not usually compare equal masses. Instead, we usually compare regions of an image that correspond to irradiation of adjacent volumes of tissue. Therefore, density, the mass contained within a given volume, plays an important role. Thus, one can radiographically visualize ice in a cup of water due to the density difference between the ice and the surrounding water (Fig. 3-14).

To calculate the linear attenuation coefficient, the density ρ of the material is multiplied by the mass attenuation coefficient to yield the linear attenuation coefficient. For example, the mass attenuation coefficient of air, for 60-keV photons, is 0.186 cm^2/g. Under typical room conditions (1 atmosphere of pressure 21°C, 30% humidity), the density of air is 0.001196 g/cm^3. Therefore, the linear attenuation coefficient of air under these conditions is

$$\mu = (\mu/\rho)\,\rho = (0.186\ cm^2/g)(0.001196\ g/cm^3) = 0.000222\ cm^{-1}.$$

To use the mass attenuation coefficient to compute attenuation, Equation 3-5 can be rewritten as

$$N = N_o e^{-\left(\frac{\mu}{\rho}\right)\rho x}. \tag{3-8}$$

Because the use of the mass attenuation coefficient is so common, scientists in this field tend to think of thickness, not as a linear distance x (in cm), but rather in terms of mass per unit area ρx (in g/cm^2). The product ρx is called the *mass thickness* or *areal thickness*.

3.3.3   Half-Value Layer

The half-value layer (HVL) is defined as the thickness of material required to reduce the intensity (*e.g.*, air kerma rate) of an x-ray or γ-ray beam to one half of

■ **FIGURE 3-14** Radiograph (acquired at 125 kV with an anti-scatter grid) of two ice cubes in a plastic container of water. The ice cubes can be visualized because of their lower electron density relative to that of liquid water. The small radiolucent objects seen at several locations are the result of air bubbles in the water. (Reprinted with permission from Bushberg JT. The AAPM/RSNA physics tutorial for residents. X-ray interactions. *RadioGraphics*. 1998;18:457-468. Copyright © Radiological Society of North America. doi: 10.1148/radiographics.18.2.9536489.)

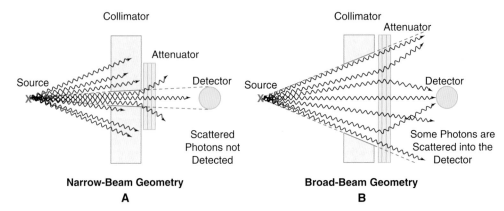

Narrow-Beam Geometry
A

Broad-Beam Geometry
B

■ **FIGURE 3-15 A.** Narrow-beam geometry means that the relationship between the source shield and the detector is such that almost no scattered photons interact with the detector. **B.** In broad-beam geometry, scattered photons may reach the detector; thus, the measured attenuation is less compared with narrow-beam conditions.

its initial value. The HVL of a beam is an indirect measure of the photon energies (also referred to as the *quality*) of a beam when measured under conditions of *narrow-beam geometry*. Narrow-beam geometry refers to an experimental configuration that is designed to exclude scattered photons from being measured by the detector (Fig. 3-15A). In *broad-beam geometry*, the beam is sufficiently wide that a substantial fraction of scattered photons remain in the beam. These scattered photons reaching the detector (Fig. 3-15B) result in an underestimation of the attenuation coefficient. Most practical applications of attenuation (*e.g.*, patient imaging) occur under broad-beam conditions. The tenth-value layer (TVL) is analogous to the HVL, except that it is the thickness of material that is necessary to reduce the intensity of the beam to a tenth of its initial value. The TVL is often used in x-ray room shielding design calculations (see Chapter 21).

For monoenergetic photons under narrow-beam geometry conditions, the probability of attenuation remains the same for each additional HVL thickness placed in the beam. Reduction in beam intensity can be expressed as $(\frac{1}{2})^n$, where n equals the number of HVLs. For example, the fraction of monoenergetic photons transmitted through 5 HVLs of material is

$$\frac{1}{2} \times \frac{1}{2} \times \frac{1}{2} \times \frac{1}{2} \times \frac{1}{2} = (1/2)^5 = 1/32 = 0.031 \text{ or } 3.1\%.$$

Therefore, 97% of the photons are attenuated (removed from the beam). The HVL of a diagnostic x-ray beam, measured in millimeters of aluminum under narrow-beam conditions, is a surrogate measure of the penetrability of an x-ray spectrum.

It is important to understand the relationship between μ and HVL. In Equation 3-5, N is equal to $N_o/2$ when the thickness of the absorber is 1 HVL. Thus, for a monoenergetic beam,

$$N_o/2 = N_o e^{-\mu(\text{HVL})},$$
$$1/2 = e^{-\mu(\text{HVL})},$$
$$\ln(1/2) = \ln e^{-\mu(\text{HVL})},$$
$$-0.693 = -\mu(\text{HVL}),$$
$$\text{HVL} = 0.693/\mu. \qquad [3\text{-}9]$$

For a monoenergetic incident photon beam, the HVL can be easily calculated from the linear attenuation coefficient, and vice versa. For example, given

1. $\mu = 0.35 \text{ cm}^{-1}$

$$\text{HVL} = 0.693/0.35 \text{ cm}^{-1} = 1.98 \text{ cm},$$

2. HVL = 2.5 mm = 0.25 cm

$$\mu = 0.693/0.25 \text{ cm} = 2.8 \text{ cm}^{-1}.$$

The HVL and μ can also be calculated if the percent transmission is measured under narrow-beam geometry.

EXAMPLE: If a 0.2-cm thickness of material transmits 25% of a monoenergetic beam of photons, calculate the HVL of the beam for that material.

STEP 1. $0.25 = e^{-\mu(0.2 \text{ cm})}$

STEP 2. $\ln 0.25 = -\mu(0.2 \text{ cm})$

STEP 3. $\mu = (-\ln 0.25)/(0.2 \text{ cm}) = 6.93 \text{ cm}^{-1}$

STEP 4. $\text{HVL} = 0.693/\mu = 0.693/6.93 \text{ cm}^{-1} = 0.1 \text{ cm}$

HVLs for photons from three commonly used diagnostic radionuclides (^{201}Tl, ^{99m}Tc, and ^{18}F) are listed for tissue and lead in Table 3-2. Thus, the HVL is a function of (1) photon energy, (2) geometry, and (3) attenuating material.

Effective Energy

X-ray beams in radiology are *polyenergetic,* meaning that they are composed of a spectrum of x-ray energies. The determination of the HVL in diagnostic radiology is a way of characterizing the penetrability of the x-ray beam. The HVL, usually measured in millimeters of aluminum (mm Al) in diagnostic radiology, can be converted to a quantity called the *effective energy.* The effective energy of a polyenergetic x-ray beam is an estimate of the penetration power of the x-ray beam, expressed as the energy of a monoenergetic beam that would exhibit the same "effective" penetrability. The relationship between HVL (in mm Al) and effective energy is given in Table 3-3. The effective energy of an x-ray beam from a typical diagnostic x-ray tube is one third to one half the maximal value.

Mean Free Path

One cannot predict the range of a single photon in matter. In fact, the range can vary from zero to infinity. However, the average distance traveled before interaction can

TABLE 3-2 HVLs OF TISSUE, ALUMINUM, AND LEAD FOR X-RAYS AND γ-RAYS COMMONLY USED IN NUCLEAR MEDICINE

	HALF VALUE LAYER (mm)	
PHOTON SOURCE	*Tissue*	*Lead*
70 keV x-rays (^{201}Tl)	37	0.2
140 keV γ-rays (^{99m}Tc)	44	0.3
511 keV γ-rays (^{18}F)	75	4.1

Note: These values are based on the narrow-beam geometry attenuation and neglecting the effect of scatter. Shielding calculations (discussed in Chapter 21) are typically for broad-beam conditions. Tc, technetium; Tl, thallium; F, fluorine.

TABLE 3-3 HVL AS A FUNCTION OF THE EFFECTIVE ENERGY OF AN X-RAY BEAM

HVL (mm Al)	EFFECTIVE ENERGY (keV)
0.26	14
0.75	20
1.25	24
1.90	28
3.34	35
4.52	40
5.76	45
6.97	50
9.24	60
11.15	70
12.73	80
14.01	90
15.06	100

Al, aluminum.

be calculated from the linear attenuation coefficient or the HVL of the beam. This length, called the *mean free path* (MFP) of the photon beam, is

$$\text{MFP} = \frac{1}{\mu} = \frac{1}{0.693/\text{HVL}} = 1.44 \text{ HVL}. \qquad [3\text{-}10]$$

Beam Hardening

The lower energy photons of the polyenergetic x-ray beam will preferentially be removed from the beam while passing through matter. The shift of the x-ray spectrum to higher effective energies as the beam transverses matter is called *beam hardening* (Fig. 3-16). Low-energy (soft) x-rays will not penetrate the entire thickness of the body; thus, their removal reduces patient dose without affecting the diagnostic quality of the exam. X-ray machines remove most of this soft radiation with filters, thin plates of aluminum, copper, or other materials placed in the beam. This added filtration will result in an x-ray beam with higher effective energy and thus a greater HVL.

The homogeneity coefficient is the ratio of the first to the second HVL and describes the polyenergetic character of the beam. The first HVL is the thickness

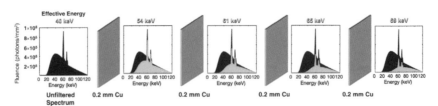

■ **FIGURE 3-16** Tungsten anode x-ray spectra generated using the TASMICS spectral model for 120 kV (3 mm inherent Al filtration) and four successive copper filters with a thickness of 0.2 mm each. Beam hardening results from preferential absorption of lower energy photons (gold spectra) as the x-rays traverse the copper filters. The effective energy of each of the beams is indicated above. (Courtesy of Andrew M. Hernandez Ph.D., UC Davis Health.)

that reduces the incident intensity to 50%, and the second HVL reduces it to 25% of its original intensity (*i.e.*, 0.5 × 0.5 = 0.25). For most diagnostic x-ray imaging, the homogeneity coefficient of the x-ray spectrum is between 0.5−0.7. However for special applications such as conventional projection mammography with factors optimized to enhance the spectral uniformity of the x-ray beam the homogeneity coefficient can be as high as 0.97. A monoenergetic source of γ-rays has a homogeneity coefficient equal to 1.

The maximal x-ray energy of a polyenergetic spectrum can be estimated by monitoring the homogeneity coefficient of two heavily filtered beams (*e.g.*, 15th and 16th HVLs). As the coefficient approaches 1, the beam is essentially monoenergetic. Measuring μ for the material in question under heavy filtration conditions and matching it to known values of μ for monoenergetic photons permits an estimation of the beam's maximal energy.

3.4   ABSORPTION OF ENERGY FROM X-RAYS AND γ-RAYS

3.4.1   Radiation Units and Measurements

The International System of Units (SI) provides a common system of units for science and technology. The system consists of seven base units: meter (m) for length, kilogram (kg) for mass, second (s) for time, ampere (A) for electric current, kelvin (K) for temperature, candela (cd) for luminous intensity, and mole (mol) for the amount of substance. In addition to the seven base units, there are *derived units* defined as combinations of the base units. Examples of derived units are m/s for speed and kg/m^3 for density. Details regarding derived units used in the measurement and calculation of radiation dose for specific applications can be found in the publications of the International Commission on Radiation Units and Measurements (ICRU) and the International Commission on Radiological Protection (ICRP). Several of these units are described below, whereas others related to specific imaging modalities or those having specific regulatory significance are described in the relevant chapters.

3.4.2   Fluence, Flux, and Energy Fluence

The number of photons or particles passing through a unit cross-sectional area is referred to as the *fluence* and is typically expressed in units of cm^{-2}. The fluence is given the symbol Φ.

$$\Phi = \frac{\text{Photons}}{\text{Area}} \qquad [3\text{-}11]$$

The fluence rate (*e.g.*, the rate at which photons or particles pass through a unit area per unit time) is called the *flux*. The flux, given the symbol $\dot{\Phi}$, is simply the fluence per unit time.

$$\dot{\Phi} = \frac{\text{Photons}}{\text{Area} \cdot \text{Time}} \qquad [3\text{-}12]$$

The flux is useful in situations in which a photon beam is on for extended periods of time, such as in fluoroscopy. Flux has the units of (photons/[cm^2 s])

The amount of energy passing through a unit cross-sectional area is referred to as the *energy fluence*. For a monoenergetic beam of photons, the energy fluence (ψ) is simply the product of the fluence (Φ) and the energy per photon (E).

$$\Psi = \Phi \left(\frac{\text{Photons}}{\text{Area}} \right) \times E \left(\frac{\text{Energy}}{\text{Photon}} \right) \qquad [3\text{-}13]$$

The units of Ψ are energy per unit area, J/m^2, or joules per m^2. For a polyenergetic spectrum, the total energy in the beam is tabulated by multiplying the number of photons at each energy by that energy and adding these products. The energy fluence rate or energy flux is the energy fluence per unit time.

3.4.3 Kerma

As a beam of indirectly ionizing (i.e., uncharged) radiation (*e.g.*, x-rays or γ-rays or neutrons) passes through a medium, it deposits energy in the medium in a two-step process:

Step 1. Energy carried by the photons (or other indirectly ionizing radiation) is transformed into kinetic energy of charged particles (such as electrons). In the case of x-rays and γ-rays, the energy is transferred by photoelectric absorption, Compton scattering, and, for very high energy photons, pair production.

Step 2. The directly ionizing (charged) particles deposit their energy in the medium by excitation and ionization. In some cases, the range of the charged particles is sufficiently large that energy deposition is some distance away from the initial interactions.

"Kerma" is an acronym for *Kinetic Energy Released in MAtter*. Kerma is defined as the kinetic energy transferred to charged particles by indirectly ionizing radiation per unit mass E_{tr}/m, as described in Step 1 above. The SI unit of kerma is the joule per kilogram with the special name of *gray* (Gy), where 1 Gy = 1 J/kg. For x-rays and γ-rays, kerma can be calculated from the mass-energy transfer coefficient of the material and the energy fluence.

Mass Energy Transfer Coefficient

The mass-energy transfer coefficient is given the symbol:

$$\left(\frac{\mu_{tr}}{\rho} \right).$$

The mass-energy transfer coefficient is the mass attenuation coefficient multiplied by the fraction of the energy of the interacting photons that is transferred to charged particles as kinetic energy. As was mentioned above, energy deposition in matter by photons is largely delivered by the energetic charged particles produced by photon interactions. The energy in scattered photons that escape the interaction site is not transferred to charged particles in the volume of interest. Furthermore, when pair production occurs, 1.02 MeV of the incident photon's energy is required to produce the electron-positron pair and only the remaining energy ($E_{photon} - 1.02$ MeV) is given to the electron and positron as kinetic energy. Therefore, the mass-energy transfer coefficient will always be less than the mass attenuation coefficient.

For 20-keV photons in tissue, for example, the ratio of the energy transfer coefficient to the attenuation coefficient (μ_{tr}/μ) is 0.68, but this reduces to 0.18 for 50-keV photons, as the amount of Compton scattering increases relative to photoelectric absorption.

Calculation of Kerma

For a monoenergetic photon beam with an energy fluence Ψ and energy E, the kerma K is given by

$$K = \Psi E \left(\frac{\mu_{tr}}{\rho} \right)_E, \qquad [3\text{-}14]$$

where $\left(\dfrac{\mu_{tr}}{\rho} \right)_E$ is the mass-energy transfer coefficient of the absorber at energy E.
The SI units of energy fluence are J/m^2, and the SI units of the mass-energy transfer coefficient are m^2/kg, and thus their product, kerma, has units of J/kg (1 J/kg = 1 Gy).

3.4.4 Absorbed Dose

The quantity *absorbed dose* (D) is defined as the energy (E) imparted by ionizing radiation per unit mass of irradiated material (m):

$$D = \frac{E}{m}. \qquad [3\text{-}15]$$

Unlike kerma, absorbed dose is defined for all types of ionizing radiation (*i.e.*, directly and indirectly ionizing). However, the SI unit of absorbed dose and kerma is the same (gray), where 1 Gy = 1 J/kg. The traditional unit of absorbed dose is the *rad* (an acronym for radiation absorbed dose). One rad is equal to 0.01 J/kg. Thus, there are 100 rads in a gray, and 1 rad = 10 mGy.

If the energy imparted to charged particles is deposited locally and the bremsstrahlung produced by the energetic electrons is negligible, the absorbed dose will be equal to the kerma. For x-rays and γ-rays, the absorbed dose can be calculated from the mass-energy absorption coefficient and the energy fluence of the beam.

Mass-Energy Absorption Coefficient

The mass-energy transfer coefficient discussed above describes the fraction of the mass attenuation coefficient that gives rise to the initial kinetic energy of electrons in a small volume of the absorber. The mass-energy absorption coefficient will be the same as the mass-energy transfer coefficient when all transferred energy is locally absorbed. However, energetic electrons may subsequently produce bremsstrahlung radiation (x-rays), which can escape the small volume of interest. Thus, the mass-energy absorption coefficient may be slightly smaller than the mass-energy transfer coefficient. For the energies used in diagnostic radiology and for low-Z absorbers (air, water, tissue), the amount of radiative losses (bremsstrahlung) is very small. Thus, for diagnostic radiology,

$$\left(\frac{\mu_{en}}{\rho} \right) \cong \left(\frac{\mu_{tr}}{\rho} \right).$$

The mass-energy absorption coefficient is useful when energy deposition calculations are to be made.

Calculation of Dose

The distinction between kerma and dose is slight for the relatively low x-ray energies used in diagnostic radiology. The dose in any material is given by

$$D = \Psi E \left(\frac{\mu_{en}}{\rho} \right)_E. \qquad [3\text{-}16]$$

The difference between the calculation of kerma and dose for air is that kerma is defined using the mass-energy transfer coefficient, whereas dose is defined using the mass-energy absorption coefficient. The mass-energy transfer coefficient defines the energy transferred to charged particles, but these energetic charged particles (mostly electrons) in the absorber may experience radiative losses, which can exit the small volume of interest. The coefficient

$$\left(\frac{\mu_{en}}{\rho}\right)_E,$$

takes into account the radiative losses, and thus

$$\left(\frac{\mu_{tr}}{\rho}\right)_E \geq \left(\frac{\mu_{en}}{\rho}\right)_E.$$

3.4.5 Exposure

The amount of electrical charge (Q) produced by ionizing electromagnetic radiation per mass (m) of air is called *exposure* (X):

$$X = \frac{Q}{m}.$$ [3-17]

Exposure is expressed in the units of charge per mass, that is, coulombs per kg (C/kg). The historical unit of exposure is the roentgen (abbreviated R), which is defined as

$$1\,R = 2.58 \times 10^{-4}\,C/kg\ (exactly).$$

Radiation beams are often expressed as an exposure rate (R/h or mR/min). The output energy fluence of an x-ray machine can be measured and expressed as an exposure (R) per unit of current times exposure duration (milliampere second or mAs) under specified operating conditions (*e.g.*, 5 mR/mAs at 70 kV for a source-image distance of 100 cm, and with an x-ray beam filtration equivalent to 2 mm Al).

Exposure is a useful quantity because ionization can be directly measured with air-filled radiation detectors, and the effective atomic numbers of air and soft tissue are approximately the same. Thus, exposure is nearly proportional to dose in soft tissue over the range of photon energies commonly used in radiology. However, the quantity of exposure is limited in that it applies only to the interaction of ionizing photons (not charged particle radiation) in air (not any other substance).

The exposure can be calculated from the dose to air. Let the ratio of the dose to air (D_{air}) to the exposure (X) in air be W, and substituting in the above expressions for D_{air} and X yields

$$W = \frac{D_{air}}{X} = \frac{E}{Q}.$$ [3-18]

W, the average energy deposited per ion pair in air, is approximately constant as a function of photon energy. In the absence of a minor correction for photon energy (less than 1%) the value W is 33.97 eV/ion pair or 33.97 J/C (Moretti, 1992).

In terms of the traditional unit of exposure, the roentgen, air kerma is

$$K_{air} \approx D_{air} \approx W \times X\left(\frac{2.58 \times 10^{-4}\,C}{kg \cdot R}\right).$$

or

$$K_{air}(Gy) \approx 0.00876 \left(\frac{Gy}{R} \right) \times X. \qquad [3\text{-}19]$$

Thus, one R of exposure results in approximately 8.76 mGy of air kerma at 20 keV (see Table 3-6). The quantity exposure is still in common use in the United States, but the equivalent SI quantity of air kerma is used exclusively in most other countries. These conversions can be simplified to

$$K_{air}(mGy) \cong \frac{X(mR)}{114.2 \ (mR/mGy)}. \qquad [3\text{-}20]$$

$$K_{a,r}(\mu Gy) \cong \frac{X(\mu R)}{114.2 \ (\mu R/\mu Gy)} \qquad [3\text{-}21]$$

3.5 IMPARTED ENERGY, EQUIVALENT DOSE, AND EFFECTIVE DOSE

3.5.1 Imparted Energy

The total amount of energy deposited in matter, called the *imparted energy* (ε), is the product of the dose and the mass over which the energy is imparted. The unit of imparted energy is the joule.

$$\varepsilon = (J/kg) \times kg = J \qquad [3\text{-}22]$$

For example, assume a head computed tomography (CT) scan delivers a 30-mGy dose to the tissue in each 5-mm slice. If the scan covers 15 cm, the dose to the irradiated volume is 30 mGy; however, the imparted (absorbed) energy is approximately 15 times that in a single scan slice.

Other modality-specific dosimetric quantities such as the CT dose index (CTDI), the dose-length product (DLP), the size-specific dose estimate (SSDE) used in computed tomography, dose per entrance skin air kerma (ESAK) for radiographic examinations, and kerma-area-product (KAP or P_{KA}) and reference point air kerma ($K_{a,r}$) used in fluoroscopy will be introduced in context with their imaging modalities and discussed again in greater detail in Chapter 11. Mammography-specific dosimetric quantities such as the mean glandular dose (MGD) are discussed in Chapter 8. The method for calculating doses from radiopharmaceuticals used in nuclear imaging utilizing the Medical Internal Radionuclide Dosimetry (MIRD) scheme is discussed in Chapter 16. Dose quantities such as the total effective dose equivalent (TEDE) used by the Nuclear Regulatory Commission (NRC) and other dose metrics defined by regulatory agencies are presented in the Radiation Protection chapter (Chapter 21).

3.5.2 Equivalent Dose

Not all types of ionizing radiation cause the same biological damage per unit absorbed dose. To modify the dose to reflect the relative effectiveness of the type of radiation in producing biologic damage, a *radiation weighting factor* (w_R) was established by the ICRP as part of an overall system for radiation protection (see Chapter 21). High LET radiations that produce dense ionization tracks cause more biologic damage per unit

TABLE 3-4 RADIATION WEIGHTING FACTORS (w_R) FOR VARIOUS TYPES OF RADIATION

TYPE OF RADIATION	RADIATION WEIGHTING FACTOR (W_R)
X-rays, γ-rays, beta particles, and electrons	1
Protons	2
Neutrons (energy-dependent)[a]	2.5–20
Alpha particles and other multiple-charged particles	20

Note: For radiations principally used in medical imaging (x-rays and γ-rays) and beta particles, w_R = 1; thus, the absorbed dose and equivalent dose are equal (*i.e.*, 1 Gy = 1 Sv).
[a]w_R values are a continuous function of energy with a maximum of 20 at approximately 1 MeV, a minimum of 2.5 at 1 keV, and 5 at 1 BeV. (Adapted from ICRP Publication 103. The 2007 Recommendations of the International Commission on Radiological Protection. *Ann ICRP.* 37(2–4):49-79, Copyright © 2007 ICRP, published by Elsevier Ltd. doi: 10.1016/j.icrp.2007.10.005.).

dose than low LET radiations. This type of biological damage (discussed in greater detail in Chapter 20) can increase the probability of stochastic effects like cancer and thus are assigned higher radiation weighting factors. The product of the absorbed dose (D) and the radiation weighting factor is the *equivalent dose* (H).

$$H = Dw_R \qquad [3\text{-}23]$$

The SI unit for equivalent dose is joule per kilogram with the special name of the *sievert* (Sv), where 1 Sv = 1 J/kg. Radiations used in diagnostic imaging (x-rays and γ-rays) as well as the energetic electrons set into motion when these photons interact with tissue or when electrons are emitted during radioactive decay have a w_R of 1: thus, 1 mGy × 1 (w_R) = 1 mSv. For heavy charged particles such as alpha particles, the LET is much higher, and thus, the biologic damage and the associated w_R are much greater (Table 3-4). For example, 10 mGy from alpha radiation may have the same biologic effectiveness as 200 mGy of x-rays.

The w_R used to calculate equivalent dose is not intended to reflect the relative effectiveness of different types of radiation to induced tissue reactions (sometimes referred to as non-stochastic or deterministic effects) following high (greater than 1 Gy) acute radiation doses. The increase in the severity of tissue reactions from high LET radiations relative to low LET radiations should be reflected in tissues and radiation specific, relative biological effectiveness factors (RBEs). The specific value of an RBE for a particular radiation type, tissue, and biological endpoint may be significantly different from the radiation weighting factors (or older quality factors) used in routine radiation protection that are based on stochastic endpoints. Generally, RBE values for tissue reactions are lower than those for stochastic effects (ICRP Publication 103, 2007). The concept of RBE applied to stochastic effects is discussed in Chapter 20.

The quantity H replaces an earlier but similar quantity, the *dose equivalent*, which is the product of the absorbed dose and the *quality factor* (Q) (Eq. 3-24). The quality factor is similar to w_R.

$$H = DQ \qquad [3\text{-}24]$$

The need to present these out-of-date dose quantities arises because regulatory agencies in the United States have not kept pace with current recommendations of national and international organizations for radiation protection and measurement. The traditional unit for both the dose equivalent and the equivalent dose is the rem. A sievert is equal to 100 rem, and 1 rem is equal to 10 mSv.

TABLE 3-5 TISSUE WEIGHTING FACTORS ASSIGNED BY THE INTERNATIONAL COMMISSION ON RADIOLOGICAL PROTECTION (ICRP REPORT 103)

ORGAN/TISSUE	w_T	% OF TOTAL DETRIMENT
Breast	0.12	
Bone marrow	0.12	
Colon[a]	0.12	72
Lung	0.12	
Stomach	0.12	
Remainder[b]	0.12	
Gonads[c]	0.08	8
Bladder	0.04	
Esophagus	0.04	16
Liver	0.04	
Thyroid	0.04	
Bone surface	0.01	
Brain	0.01	4
Salivary gland	0.01	
Skin	0.01	
Total	**1.0**	**100**

[a]The dose to the colon is taken to be the mass-weighted mean of upper and lower large intestine doses.
[b]Shared by remainder tissues (14 in total, 13 in each sex) are adrenals, extrathoracic tissue, gallbladder, heart, kidneys, lymphatic nodes, muscle, oral mucosa, pancreas, prostate (male), small intestine, spleen, thymus, uterus/cervix (female).
[c]The w_T for gonads is applied to the mean of the doses to testes and ovaries. (Adapted from ICRP Publication 103. The 2007 Recommendations of the International Commission on Radiological Protection. *Ann ICRP.* 37(2–4):49-79, Copyright © 2007 ICRP, published by Elsevier Ltd. doi: 10.1016/j.icrp.2007.10.005.)

3.5.3 Effective Dose

Biological tissues vary in their sensitivity to the effects of ionizing radiation. Tissue weighting factors (w_T) were also established by the ICRP as part of their radiation protection system to assign a particular organ or tissue (T) the proportion of the detriment[1] from stochastic effects (*e.g.*, cancer and hereditary effects, discussed further in Chapter 20) resulting from irradiation of that tissue compared to uniform whole-body irradiation (ICRP Publication 103, 2007). These tissue weighting factors are shown in Table 3-5. The sum of the products of the equivalent dose to each organ or tissue irradiated (H_T) and the corresponding weighting factor (w_T) for that organ or tissue is called the *effective dose* (E).

$$E\,(\mathrm{Sv}) = \sum_T \left[w_T \times H_T(\mathrm{Sv}) \right] \qquad [3\text{-}25]$$

The effective dose is expressed in the same units as the equivalent dose (Sv).

The w_T values were developed for a reference population of equal numbers of both genders and a wide range of ages. Thus effective dose applies to a population,

---

[1]The total harm to health experienced by an exposed group and its descendants as a result of the group's exposure to a radiation source. Detriment is a multidimensional concept. Its principal components are the stochastic quantities: probability of attributable fatal cancer, weighted probability of attributable non-fatal cancer, weighted probability of severe heritable effects, and length of life lost if the harm occurs.

TABLE 3-6 RADIOLOGICAL QUANTITIES, SYSTEM INTERNATIONAL (SI) UNITS, AND TRADITIONAL UNITS

QUANTITY	DESCRIPTION OF QUANTITY	SI UNITS (ABBREVIATIONS) AND DEFINITIONS	TRADITIONAL UNITS (ABBREVIATIONS) AND DEFINITIONS	SYMBOL	DEFINITIONS AND CONVERSION FACTORS
Exposure	Amount of ionization per mass of air due to x-rays and γ-rays	C/kg	Roentgen (R)	X	$1\ R = 2.58 \times 10^{-4}\ C\ kg^{-1}$ $1\ R = 8.7566\ mGy$ air kerma at 20 keV[b] $1\ R = 8.7654\ mGy$ air kerma at 60 keV[b] $1\ R = 8.7708\ mGy$ air kerma at 100 keV[b]
Absorbed dose	Amount of energy imparted by radiation per mass	Gray (Gy) $1\ Gy = J/kg$	rad $1\ rad = 0.01\ J/kg$	D	$1\ rad = 10\ mGy$ $100\ rad = 1\ Gy$
Kerma	Kinetic energy transferred to charged particles per unit mass	Gray (Gy) $1\ Gy = J/kg$	—	K	—
Air kerma	Kinetic energy transferred to charged particles per unit mass of air	Gray (Gy) $1\ Gy = J/kg$	—	K_{air}	$1\ mGy = 0.1142\ R$ at 20 keV[b] $1\ mGy = 0.1141\ R$ at 60 keV[b] $1\ mGy = 0.1140\ R$ at 100 keV[b] $1\ mGy \cong 0.140\ rad$ (dose to skin)[a] $1\ mGy \cong 1.4\ mGy$ (dose to skin)[a]
Imparted energy	Total radiation energy imparted to matter	Joule (J)	—	ε	Dose (J/kg) × mass (kg) = J
Dose equivalent (defined by ICRP in 1977)	Absorbed dose weighted for the biological effectiveness of the type(s) of radiation (relative to low LET **photons and electrons) to produce stochastic health effects** in humans	Sievert (Sv)	rem	H	$H = QD$ $1\ rem = 10\ mSv$ $100\ rem = 1\ Sv$
Equivalent dose (defined by ICRP in 1990 to replace dose equivalent)	Absorbed dose weighted for the biological effectiveness of the type(s) of radiation (relative to low LET photons and electrons) to produce stochastic health effects in humans	Sievert (Sv)	rem	H	$H = w_R D$ $1\ rem = 10\ mSv$ $100\ rem = 1\ Sv$

Effective dose equivalent (defined by ICRP in 1977)	Dose equivalent, weighted for the biological sensitivity of the exposed tissues and organs (relative to whole body exposure) to stochastic health effects in humans	Sievert (Sv)	rem	H_E	$H = \sum_T w_T H_T$
Effective dose (defined by ICRP in 1990 to replace effective dose equivalent and modified in 2007 with different w_T values)	Equivalent dose, weighted for the biological sensitivity of the exposed tissues and organs (relative to whole body exposure) to stochastic health effects in humans	Sievert (Sv)	rem	E	$E = \sum_T w_T H_T$

[a]Includes backscatter (discussed in Chapters 9 and 11).
[b]These reflect the adjustment to the average amount of energy (J) deposited in dry air at standard temperature and pressure per coulomb (C) of charge released as a function of incident photon energy (W_{eff}/e) from 33.97 (defined for Co-60 γ-rays 1.17 and 1.33 MeV) to 33.8579, 33.8919, and 33.9123 at photon energies of 20, 60, and 100 keV, respectively. (Data from Moretti CJ. Changes to the National Physical Laboratory primary standards for x-ray exposure and air kerma. *Phys Med Biol.* 1992;37(5):1181-1183 and Buhr H, et al. Measurement of the mass energy-absorption coefficient of air for x-rays in the range from 3 to 60 keV. *Phys Med Biol.* 2012;57(24):8231-8247.)
ICRP, International Commission on Radiological Protection.

not to a specific individual, and should not be used as the patient's dose for the purpose of assigning risk. This all too common misuse of effective dose, for a purpose for which it was never intended and does not apply, is discussed in further detail in Chapter 11. ICRP's initial recommendations for w_T values (ICRP Publication 26, 1977) were applied as shown in Equation 3-25, the product of which was referred to as the *effective dose equivalent* (H_E). Many regulatory agencies in the United States, including the NRC, have not as yet adopted the current ICRP Publication 103 w_T values. While there is a current effort to update these regulations, they are, at present, still using the old (1977) ICRP Publication 26 dosimetric quantities (sadly, this is exactly what we said 10 years ago in the 3rd edition).

3.6 SUMMARY

The interaction of x- and γ-rays with matter results in a cascade of energetic electrons. These electrons transfer their kinetic energy to the surrounding medium via excitation, ionization, and radiative emissions. X-ray attenuation by various tissues and objects in the body, as well as primary x-rays whose photons traverse the body without interacting and are recorded on the image receptor, constitute the fundamental basis of x-ray transmission imaging. The photoelectric effect (PE), Compton scattering (CS), and even (to a minor degree) Rayleigh scattering contribute to image formation. The differences in attenuation by CS reflect differences in electron density (closely related to mass density), while differences in attenuation by PE reflect differences chiefly in atomic number. Adjusting the average photon energy of the x-ray beam by kV selection and beam filtration determines the relative amounts of PE and CS interactions, with higher photon energies decreasing the relative impact of PE. The usefulness of CS for generating attenuation differences is largely due to the use of anti-scatter grids or other methods to prevent most scattered photons from contributing to the image. However, to the degree the grid fails to eliminate CS photons that reach the image receptor, image noise is increased, and image contrast is degraded. In addition, CS becomes the source of radiation responsible for unnecessary doses to patients and medical staff. When a primary photon interacts via the PE, image degradation caused by scatter is not an issue, since the photon is completely absorbed. On the other hand, following absorption and photoelectron ejection in tissue, low energy characteristic x-rays, or worse (from a radiobiological perspective), Auger electrons, will be produced. Both produce more densely ionizing tracks over a very short range in tissue than their higher energy counterparts and (with the exception of mammography in particular) neither contribute to image formation.

In nuclear medicine emission imaging, the effects of attenuation are mostly deleterious, causing the deposition of radiation dose, attenuating photons that would otherwise contribute to the images. Non-uniform attenuation in nuclear medicine is one cause of sub-optimal image quality.

Altering the trajectory of radiation by attenuation results in a harder beam by selectively removing lower energy x-rays in the bremsstrahlung spectrum, with higher effective energy and greater ability to penetrate dense objects. Quantitative assessment of the penetrating capability of an x-ray beam by measurement and calculation of the results expressed as the half-value layer in mm of Al is one of the most frequently used metrics of x-ray beam quality control used worldwide.

SUGGESTED READING AND REFERENCES

Bushberg JT. The AAPM/RSNA physics tutorial for residents. X-ray interactions. *RadioGraphics*. 1998;18:457-468.

International Commission on Radiation Units and Measurements. Fundamental quantities and units for ionizing radiation. *J ICRU*. 2011;11(1); Report 85.

International Commission on Radiological Protection. Recommendations of the ICRP. *Ann ICRP*. 2007;37(2-4):Publication 103.

Moretti CJ. Changes to the National Physical Laboratory primary standards for x-ray exposures and air kerma. *Phys Med Biol*. 1992;37(5):1181-1183.

Image Quality

The quality of medical images is related to how well they convey specific anatomical or functional information to the interpreting physician such that an accurate diagnosis can be made. Radiological images acquired with ionizing radiation can be made less grainy (*i.e.*, lower noise) by simply turning up the radiation levels used. However, the important diagnostic features of the image may already be clear enough, and the additional radiation dose to the patient is an important concern. Diagnostic medical images, therefore, require thoughtful consideration in which image quality is not necessarily *maximized* but rather is *optimized* to perform the specific diagnostic task for which the exam was ordered.

While diagnostic accuracy is the most rigorous measure of image quality, measuring it can be quite difficult, time-consuming, and expensive. In principle, measurement of diagnostic accuracy requires a clinical trial with patient cohorts, well-defined scanning protocols, an adequate sample of trained readers, and procedures for obtaining the ground truth status of the patients. Such studies most certainly have their place in the evaluation of medical imaging methodology, but they also can be a substantial overkill if one is simply deciding between a detector with a pixel pitch of 80 μm and another with 100 μm.

As a result, the vast majority of image quality assessments are not determined from direct measurement of diagnostic accuracy. Instead, they are based on surrogate measures that are linked by assumption to diagnostic accuracy. For example, if we can improve the resolution of a scanner without affecting anything else, then we might assume that diagnostic accuracy improves, or at least does not get any worse. In cases where noise and resolution trade off against each other, image quality measures based on a ratio may be used. This forms the basis for the contrast-to-noise ratio (CNR) and signal-to-noise ratio (SNR) measures. In other situations, a simplified reading procedure is used. These can be used to produce a contrast-detail diagram or a receiver operating characteristic (ROC) curve.

This chapter is intended to elucidate these topics. It is also meant to familiarize the reader with the specific terms used to describe the quality of medical images, and thus the vernacular introduced here is important as well. This chapter, more than most in this book, appeals to mathematics and mathematical concepts, such as convolution and Fourier transforms. Some background on these topics can be found in Appendix G, but to physicians in training, the details of the mathematics should not be considered an impediment to understanding but rather as a general illustration of the concepts. To engineers or image scientists in training, the mathematics in this chapter are a necessary basic look at imaging system analysis.

4.1 SPATIAL RESOLUTION

Spatial resolution describes the level of detail that can be seen on an image. In simplistic terms, the spatial resolution relates to how small of an object can be visualized on a particular imaging system, assuming that other potential limitations of the system (*e.g.,* object contrast or noise) are not an issue. However, more rigorous mathematical methods based on the spatial frequency spectrum provide a measure of how well the imaging system performs over a continuous range of object dimensions.

Low-resolution images are typically seen as blurry. Objects that should have sharp edges appear to taper off from bright to dark and small objects located near one another appear as one larger object. All of this will generally make identifying subtle signs of disease more difficult. In this section, we will describe some of the reasons why medical images have limited resolution, how blur is modeled as a point spread function (PSF), and how this leads in turn to the concept of a modulation transfer function (MTF).

4.1.1 Physical Mechanisms of Blurring

There are many different mechanisms in medical imaging that cause blurring, and some of these mechanisms will be discussed in length in subsequent chapters. It is important to understand that every step of image generation, acquisition, processing, and display can impact the resolution of an image. This makes resolution a relevant topic of consideration throughout the imaging process.

Most x-ray images are generated by electrons impacting an anode at high velocity. The area in which this happens is called the focal spot of the x-ray tube. The width of the focal spot causes points in the field of view to have a width when they are projected onto a detector. This is called focal-spot blur. Similar phenomena occur in other imaging modalities. In PET imaging, positrons diffuse away from the point of radioactive decay before they annihilate, leading to positron range blurring. In ultrasound imaging, the finite width of a transmission aperture limits the focal width of the resulting pulse leading to aperture blur. These examples show how imaging systems have resolution limitations even before they have imaged anything.

Detectors are also a source of blur in imaging systems. When an x-ray or γ-ray strikes an intensifying screen or other phosphors, it produces a burst of light photons that propagate by optical diffusion though the screen matrix. For thicker screens, the diffusion path toward the screen's surface is longer, and more lateral diffusion occurs, which results in a broader pattern of light reaching the surface of the screen and consequently more blurring. Furthermore, the digital sampling that occurs in detectors results in the integration of the 2D signal over the surface of the detector element, which can be thought of as detector sampling blur.

It is often the case that image data are processed and displayed in ways that suppress noise. This can be accomplished by any of a number of smoothing operations that employ averaging over multiple detector elements or image pixels. These operations usually involve a trade-off between how much noise is suppressed, and how much blur is added to the imaging system.

Blurring means that image intensity, which should be confined to a specific location, is spread over a region. Various spread functions are used to characterize the impact of physical blurring phenomena in medical imaging systems. A common mathematical approach to modeling spread relies on the idea of convolution.

4.1.2 Convolution

Convolution is an integral calculus procedure that accurately describes mathematically what the blurring process does physically under the assumption that the spread function is not changing with position, a property known as shift-invariance. The convolution process is also an important mathematical component of image reconstruction, and understanding the basics of convolution is essential to a complete understanding of imaging systems. Below, a basic description of the convolution process is provided, with more details provided in Appendix G.

Convolution in 1D is given by

$$G(x) = \int_{-\infty}^{\infty} H(x')k(x-x')dx' = H(x) \otimes k(x),$$ [4-1]

where $\otimes$ is the mathematical symbol for convolution. This equation describes the convolution of an input function, $H(x)$, with a convolution kernel, $k(x)$. Convolution can occur in two or three dimensions as well, and the extension to multidimensional convolution is straightforward: x becomes a two- or three-dimensional vector representing spatial position, and the integral becomes two- or three-dimensional as well.

As a way to better understand the meaning of convolution, let us sidestep the integral calculus of Equation 4-1 and consider a discrete implementation of convolution. In this setting, the input function, H, can be thought of as an array of numbers, or more specifically, a row of pixel values in a digital image. The convolution kernel can be thought of as an array of weights. In this case, we will assume there are a total of five weights each with a value of 0.20 (this is sometimes referred to as a five-element "boxcar" average).

Figure 4-1 shows how these discrete values are combined, resulting in the output column of averaged values, G. In pane A, the first five numbers of H are multiplied by the corresponding elements in the kernel, and these five products are summed, resulting in the first entry in column G. In pane B, the convolution algorithm proceeds by shifting down one element in column H, and the same operation is computed, resulting in the second entry in column G. In pane C, the kernel shifts down another element in the array of numbers, and the same process is followed. This shift, multiply, and add procedure is the discrete implementation of convolution—it is one of the ways this operation can be executed in a computer program. The integral in Equation 4-1 can be thought of as the limit as there are more and more (ever smaller) pixels and weights.

A plot of the values in columns H and G is shown in Figure 4-2, and H, in this case, is the value 50 with randomly generated noise added to each element. The values of G are smoothed relative to H, and that is because the elements of the convolution kernel, in this case, are designed to perform data smoothing—essentially by averaging five adjacent values in column H. Notice that the values of G are generally

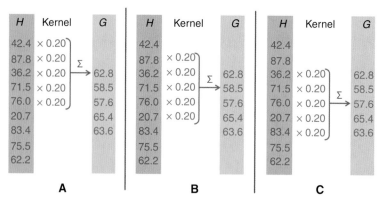

■ **FIGURE 4-1** The basic operation of discrete convolution is illustrated. In the three panes **(A–C)**, the input array H is convolved with a five-element boxcar kernel, k, resulting in the output array, G. The different panes show the convolution kernel, and the output value, advancing by one index element at a time. The entire convolution is performed over the complete length of H.

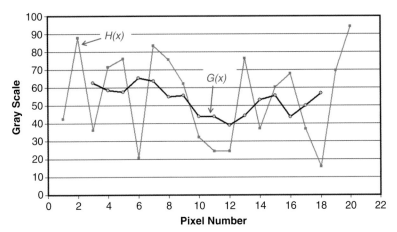

■ **FIGURE 4-2** A plot of the noisy input data in $H(x)$, and of the smoothed function $G(x)$, where x is the pixel number (x = 1, 2, 3, …). The first few elements in the data shown on this plot correspond to the data illustrated in Figure 4-1. The input function $H(x)$ is random noise distributed around a mean value of 50. The convolution process with the boxcar average results in substantial smoothing, and this is evident by the much smoother $G(x)$ function that is closer to this mean value.

closer to the mean value than the original values of H, indicating some suppression of the noise.

However, there is generally a price to be paid for smoothing away noise. To illustrate this, consider Figure 4-3. In this case, we will assume that the deviation from the value of 50 is not due to noise. Instead, these points represent some sort of fine structure in the image. Here, the effect of the boxcar average is to blur these points. On the left side of the plot, the single-pixel structure gets turned into a 5-pixel "blob" after this convolution. And the 3-pixel structure on the right side gets turned into a 7-pixel blob that has completely lost the appearance of a valley between two high points. Thus, the boxcar filter spreads the intensity of these fine features over many more pixels and can erase potentially important features. It is also worth noting that the peak intensity of the features has been lowered considerably.

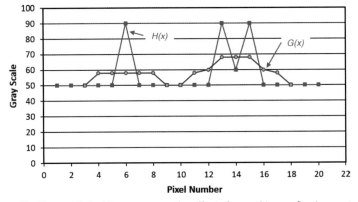

■ **FIGURE 4-3** Unlike Figure 4-2, in this case, we see the effect of smoothing on fine image structure (signal). Here the departures from the mean value of 50 are because of fine structure in the image. The boxcar average lowers peak image intensity and spreads it out over a wider region. It completely removes the valley between the two peaks on the left.

Point Spread Function (PSF)

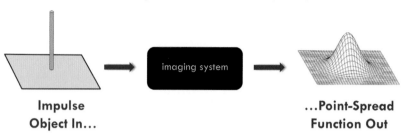

**Impulse
Object In...**

**...Point-Spread
Function Out**

■ **FIGURE 4-4** An impulse stimulus to an imaging system is illustrated (left), and the response of the imaging system, the point spread function (PSF), is shown (right). The spread of intensity in the PSF is used to model sources of blur in the image. This PSF is rotationally symmetric.

4.1.3 The Spatial Domain: Spread Functions

In radiology, images vary in size from small spot images acquired in mammography (~50 mm × 50 mm) to the chest radiograph, which is 350 mm × 430 mm. These images are viewed in the spatial domain, which means that every point (or pixel) in the image represents a position in 2D or 3D space. The spatial domain refers to the two dimensions of a single image or the three dimensions of a volumetric image such as computed tomography (CT) or magnetic resonance images (MRI). Several metrics that are measured in the spatial domain and characterize the spatial resolution of an imaging system are discussed below.

The Point Spread Function

The PSF is the most basic measure of the resolution properties of an imaging system, and it is perhaps the most intuitive as well. A point source (or impulse) is input to the imaging system, and the PSF is (by definition) the response of the imaging system to that point input (Fig. 4-4). The PSF is also called the impulse response function. The PSF is most commonly used for 2D imaging modalities, where it is described in terms of the x and y dimensions of a 2D image, PSF(x, y). The diameter of the "point" input should theoretically be infinitely small, but practically speaking, the diameter of the point input should be smaller than the width of a detector element in the imaging system being evaluated.

To produce a point input on a planar imaging system such as in digital radiography or fluoroscopy, a sheet of attenuating metal such as lead, with a very small hole in it,[1] is placed covering the detector, and x-rays are produced. High exposure levels need to be used to deliver a measurable signal, given the tiny hole. For a tomographic system, a small-diameter wire or fiber can be imaged with the wire placed normal to the tomographic plane to be acquired.

An imaging system with the same PSF at all locations in the field of view is called *shift-invariant*, while a system that has PSFs that vary depending on the position in the field of view is called *shift variant* (Fig. 4-5). In general, medical imaging systems are considered shift-invariant to a first approximation—even if some small shift variant effects are present. Pixelated digital imaging systems have finite detector elements (dexels), commonly in the shape of a square, and in some cases, the detector element is uniformly sensitive to the signal energy across its surface.

---

[1]In reality, PSF and other resolution test objects are precision-machined tools and can cost thousands of dollars.

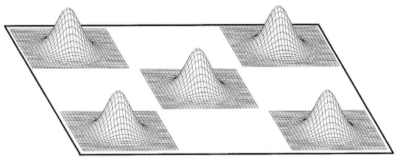

Shift-Invariant Imaging System

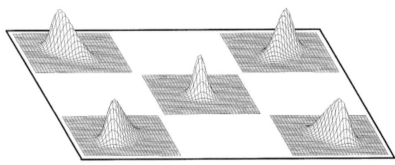

Shift-Variant Imaging System

■ **FIGURE 4-5** A shift-invariant imaging system is one in which the PSF remains constant over the field of view of the imaging system, as shown in the upper panel. A shift-variant system has a different PSF, depending on the location in the field of view, as shown in the lower panel.

This implies that if there are no other factors that degrade spatial resolution, the digital sampling matrix will impose a PSF, which is in the shape of a square (Fig. 4-6) and where the dimensions of the square are the dimensions of the dexels. The PSF describes the extent of blurring that is introduced by an imaging system, and this blurring is the manifestation of physical events during the image acquisition and subsequent processing of the acquired data.

The Line Spread Function

When an imaging system is stimulated with a signal in the form of a line, the line spread function (LSF) can be evaluated. For a planar imaging system, a slit in some attenuating material can be imaged and would result in a line on the image (Fig. 4-7). Once the line is produced on the image (*e.g.*, parallel to the y-axis), a profile through that line is then measured perpendicular to the line (*i.e.*, along the x-axis). The profile is a measure of grayscale as a function of position. Once this profile is normalized such that the area is unity, it becomes the $LSF(x)$.

From the perspective of making measurements, the LSF has advantages over the PSF. First of all, a slit will generally pass more x-ray photons than a small hole, so the measurement does not require turning up the x-ray intensity as high. There are also some tricks that can be played with the orientation of the slit that allows for very fine sampling of the LSF. We will discuss this topic shortly. However, there are some disadvantages too. The LSF is a somewhat indirect measurement of spread, and it requires some analysis to relate it to the PSF. Additionally, the LSF only makes measurements at the orientation of the slit. If the underlying PSF is asymmetric, the LSF will need to

■ **FIGURE 4-6** A 2D "RECT" function is shown (see Appendix G), illustrating the PSF of a digital imaging system with square detector elements of width *a*, in the absence of any other blurring phenomenon. This PSF is the best possible for a digital imaging system.

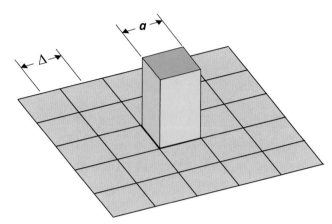

be acquired at multiple orientations to capture the asymmetry. For digital x-ray imaging systems that have a linear response to x-rays such as digital radiography, the profile can be easily determined from the digital image using appropriate software. Profiles from ultrasound and MR images can also be used to obtain an LSF in those modalities, as long as the signal is converted linearly into grayscale on the images.

For a system with good spatial resolution, the LSF will be quite thin, and thus on the measured profile, the LSF may only be a few pixels wide. Consequently, the LSF measurement may suffer from coarse pixel sampling in the image. One way to avoid this is to place the slit at a small angle (*e.g.*, 2° to 8°) to the detector element columns during the physical measurement procedure. Then, instead of taking one profile through the slit image, several profiles are taken at different locations vertically (Fig. 4-8) and the data are synthesized into a *presampled LSF*. Due to the angulation of the slit, the profiles taken at different vertical positions intersect the slit image at different horizontal displacements through the pixel width—this allows the LSF to be synthesized with sub-pixel spacing intervals, and a better sampled LSF measurement results.

The Edge Spread Function

In some situations, PSF and LSF measurements are not ideally suited for a specific imaging application, where the edge spread function (ESF) can be measured. Instead of stimulating the imaging system with a slit image as with the LSF, a sharp edge is presented. The *edge gradient* that results in the image can then be used to measure the ESF(*x*). The ESF is particularly useful when the spatial distribution characteristics of glare or scatter phenomenon are the subject of interest—since a large fraction of the field of view is stimulated, low-amplitude effects such as glare or scatter (or both) become appreciable enough in amplitude to be measurable. By comparison, exposure to the tiny area of the detector receiving signal in PSF or LSF measurements would not be sufficient to cause enough optical glare or x-ray scatter to be measurable. A sharp edge is also less expensive to manufacture than a point or slit phantom,

■ **FIGURE 4-7** The line impulse function that is input to the imaging system (by imaging a slit for example) leads to an image that has the line-spread function when a profile along the *x*-axis is taken.

Line Spread Function (LSF)

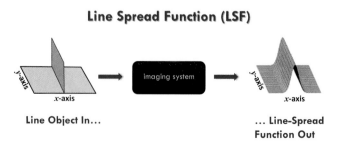

Line Object In...   **... Line-Spread Function Out**

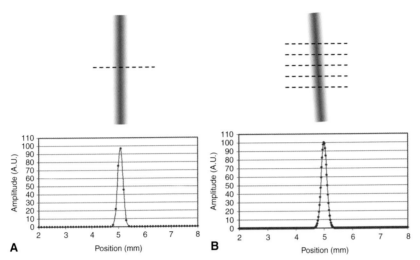

FIGURE 4-8 A. The conventional approach to measuring the LSF involves the acquisition of a slit image along the y-axis, and a profile (grayscale versus position) across it (in the x-axis) is evaluated. This approach is legitimate but is limited by the sampling pitch of the detector. **B.** An alternative approach to computing the LSF was proposed by Fujita. Here, the slit image is acquired at a slight angle (~5°) relative to the y-axis. At any row along the vertical slit, a single LSF can be measured. However, because of the angle, a composite LSF can be synthesized by combining the LSFs from a number of rows in the image. The angle of the slit creates a small differential shift of the LSF from row to row—this can be exploited to synthesize an LSF with much better sampling than the pixel pitch. This oversampled LSF is called the presampled LSF.

and even spherical test objects can be used to measure the ESF, which is useful when characterization of the spatial resolution in three dimensions is desired.

Examples of all three spatial domain spread functions are shown in Figure 4-9.

Relationships Between Spread Functions

There are mathematical relationships between the spatial domain spread functions PSF, LSF, and ESF. The specific mathematical relationships are described

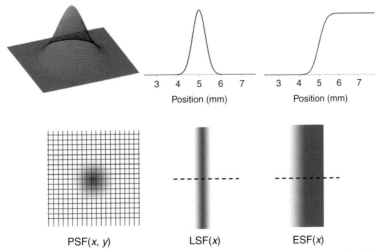

FIGURE 4-9 The three basic spread functions in the spatial domain are shown—the PSF(x, y) is a 2D spread function. The LSF and ESF are both 1D spread functions. There is a mathematical relationship between the three spread functions, as discussed in the text.

here, but the take-home message is that under most circumstances, given a measurement of one of the spread functions, the others can be computed. This feature adds to the flexibility of using the most appropriate measurement method for characterizing an imaging system. These statements presume a rotationally symmetric PSF, but in general, that is the case in many (but not all) medical imaging systems.

The LSF and ESF are related to the PSF by the convolution equation. The LSF can be computed by convolving the PSF with an impulse function that is spread over a line[2]:

$$LSF(x) = PSF(x,y) \otimes LINE(y).$$ [4-2]

Because a line is purely a 1D function, the convolution shown in Equation 4-2 reduces to a simple integral

$$LSF(x) = \int_{y=-\infty}^{\infty} PSF(x,y)dy.$$ [4-3]

Convolution of the PSF with an edge[3] results in the ESF

$$ESF(x) = PSF(x,y) \otimes EDGE(y).$$ [4-4]

In addition to the above relationships, the LSF and ESF are related as well. The ESF is the integral of the LSF, and this implies that the LSF is the derivative of the ESF,

$$ESF(x) = \int_{x'=-\infty}^{x} LSF(x')dx',$$ [4-5]

where x' is a variable of integration.

One can also compute the LSF from the ESF, and the PSF can be computed from the LSF; however, the assumption of rotational symmetry with the PSF is necessary unless multiple orientations of the LSF are used.

4.1.4   The Frequency Domain: Modulation Transfer Function

The PSF, LSF, and ESF are apt descriptions of the resolution properties of an imaging system in the spatial domain. Another useful way to express the resolution of an imaging system is to make use of the spatial *frequency domain*. If a sine wave has a period of P (the length it takes to complete a full cycle of the wave), then the spatial frequency of the wave is $f = 1/P$. As this relationship would suggest, a sine wave with a larger period has a smaller spatial frequency and vice versa.

The frequency domain is accessed through the Fourier Transform, which decomposes a signal into sine waves that, when summed, replicate that signal. Once a spatial domain signal is Fourier transformed, the results are considered to be in the frequency domain. The Fourier Transform is a powerful theoretical tool for mathematical analysis of imaging systems, but here we will mostly focus on interpreting the results of this analysis. A more detailed mathematical description of the Fourier Transform can be found in Appendix G.

In Figure 4-10, let the solid black line be a trace of grayscale as a function of position across an image. Nineteenth-century French mathematician Joseph Fourier developed a method for decomposing a function such as this grayscale profile into the

---

[2]The Line function is like an impulse in the x direction and constant in the y direction. So, Line(y) approaches ∞ near $y = 0$, and is 0 elsewhere.
[3]Edge(y) = 1, where $y > 0$, = 0, elsewhere.

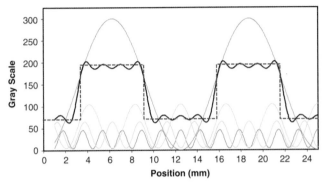

■ **FIGURE 4-10** The basic concept of Fourier analysis is illustrated. The solid black lines are the sum of the four sets of sine waves (shown towards the bottom of the plot) and approximate the two RECT functions (dashed lines). Only four sine waves are summed here, but with a more complete set, the RECT functions could be almost perfectly matched. The Fourier transform breaks any arbitrary signal down into the sum of a set of sine waves of different phase, frequency, and amplitude.

sum of a number of sine waves. Each sine wave has three parameters that characterize its shape: amplitude (a), frequency (f), and phase (ψ), where

$$g(x) = a\sin(2\pi\,fx + \psi).$$
[4-6]

Figure 4-10 illustrates the sum of four different sine waves (*solid black line*), which approximates the shape of two rectangular functions (*dashed lines*). Only four sine waves were used in this figure for clarity; however, if more sine waves (i.e., a more complete Fourier *spectrum*) were used, the shape of the two rectangular functions could in principle be matched.

The Fourier transform, FT[], converts a spatial signal into the frequency domain, while the inverse Fourier transform, FT^{-1}[], converts the frequency domain signal back to the spatial domain. An important result of linear systems theory is that convolution is equivalent to multiplication in the spatial frequency domain. Referring back to Equation 4-1, the function G(x) can be alternatively computed as

$$G(x) = FT^{-1}\left\{FT\big[H(x)\big] \times FT\big[k(x)\big]\right\}.$$
[4-7]

Equation 4-7 computes the same function G(x) as in Equation 4-1, but compared to the convolution procedure, in most cases, the Fourier transform computation runs faster on a computer. Therefore, image processing methods that employ convolution filtration procedures such as in CT are often performed in the frequency domain for computational speed. Indeed, the kernel used in CT is often described in the frequency domain (descriptors such as *ramp, Shepp-Logan, bone kernel, B41*), so it is more common to discuss the shape of the kernel in the frequency domain (i.e., FT[k(x)]) rather than in the spatial domain (i.e., k(x)), in the parlance of clinical CT. Inverse Fourier transforms are used in MRI to convert the received time-domain signal into a spatial signal. Fourier transforms are also used in ultrasound imaging and Doppler systems. All in all, Fourier computations are a routine part of the signal and image processing components of medical imaging systems.

The Modulation Transfer Function

Conceptual Description

Imagine that it is possible to stimulate an imaging system spatially with a pure sinusoidal waveform, as illustrated in Figure 4-11A. The system will detect the incoming sinusoidal signal at frequency f, and as long as the frequency is not too high (relative

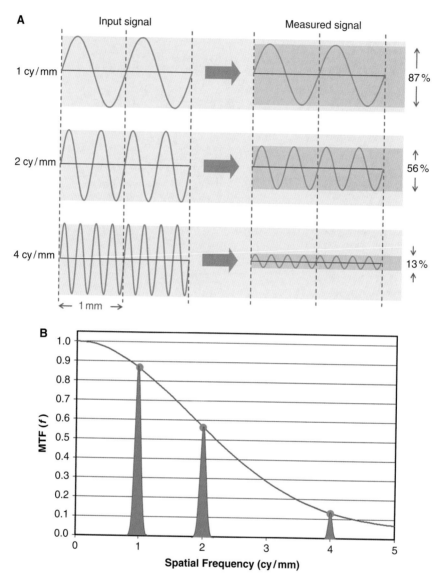

■ **FIGURE 4-11 A.** Sinusoidal input signals incident on a detector (intensity as a function of position) at three different frequencies are shown as input functions (left). The signals measured by the imaging system are shown on the right. The frequency is the same as the inputs in all cases, but the amplitude of the measured signal is reduced compared to that of the input signal. This reduction in amplitude is a result of resolution losses in the imaging system, which are greater with signals of higher frequencies. For the input at 1 cycle/mm, the original 100% amplitude was attenuated to 87%, and with the 2- and 4-cycle/mm input functions, the resulting signal amplitudes were reduced to 56% and 13%, respectively. **B.** This figure shows the amplitude reduction as a function of spatial frequency shown in **A.** At 1 cycle/mm, the system reduced the contrast to 87% of the input. For 2 and 4 mm⁻¹, the signal was modulated as shown. This plot shows the MTF, which illustrates the spatial resolution of an imaging system as a function of the spatial frequency of the input signal.

to the Nyquist frequency, discussed below), it will produce an image at that same frequency but in most cases with reduced contrast (Fig. 4-11A, right side). The loss of contrast is the result of resolution losses (*i.e.*, blurring) in the imaging system, and can also be thought of as a modulation of the amplitude of the input sinusoid. For input signals with frequencies of 1, 2, and 4 cycles/mm (shown in Fig. 4-11A), the measured signals after passing through the imaging system were 87%, 56%, and 13% of the inputs, respectively. For any one of these three frequencies measured individually, if the Fourier transform was computed on the recorded signal, the result would be a peak at the corresponding frequency. Three such peaks are shown in Figure 4-11B, representing three individually acquired (and then Fourier transformed) signals. The amplitude of the peak at each frequency reflects the contrast transfer (retained) at that frequency, with contrast losses due to resolution limitations in the system.

Interestingly, due to the characteristics of the Fourier transform, the three sinusoidal input waves shown in Figure 4-11A could be acquired simultaneously by the detector system, and the Fourier Transform could separate the individual frequencies and produce the three peaks at $F = 1, 2,$ and 4 cycles/mm shown in Figure 4-11B. Indeed, if an input signal contained more numerous sinusoidal waves (10, 50, 100, …) than the three shown in the figure, the Fourier transform would still be able to separate these frequencies and convey their respective amplitudes from the recorded signal, ultimately resulting in the full, smooth MTF curve shown in Figure 4-11B. Thus the MTF shows how much signal passes through an imaging system as a function of the spatial frequency of the signal.

Limiting Resolution

The MTF gives a rich description of spatial resolution as a function of frequency, and it is the accepted standard for the mathematical characterization of spatial resolution. However, it is sometimes useful to have a single numerical value that characterizes the resolution limit of an imaging system. The *limiting spatial resolution* is often considered to be the frequency at which the MTF crosses the 10% level (see Fig. 4-12), or some other agreed-upon and specified level.

Nyquist Frequency

Let's look at an example of an imaging system where the center-to-center spacing (pitch) between each detector element (dexel) is Δ (in mm). In the corresponding image, it would take two adjacent pixels to display a full cycle of a sine wave (Fig. 4-13)—one pixel for the upward lobe of the sine wave, and the other for the downward lobe. This wave is the highest frequency that can be accurately measured on the imaging system. The period of this sine wave is 2Δ, and the corresponding spatial frequency is $F_N = 1/2\Delta$. This frequency is called the Nyquist frequency (F_N), and it sets an upper bound on the spatial frequency that can be detected for a digital

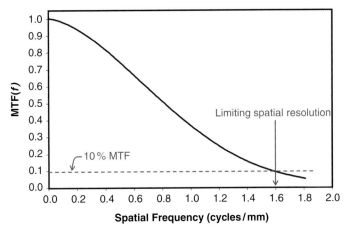

■ **FIGURE 4-12** The limiting spatial resolution is the spatial frequency at which the amplitude of the MTF decreases to some agreed-upon level. Here the limiting spatial resolution is shown at 10% modulation, and the limiting spatial resolution is 1.6 cycles/mm.

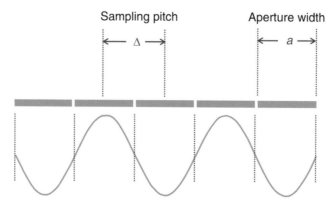

■ **FIGURE 4-13** This figure illustrates a side view of detector elements in a hypothetical detector panel. Detectors whose center-to-center spacing (pitch) is about equal to the detector width are very common, and these represent contiguous detector elements. The sampling pitch affects aliasing in the image, while the aperture width of the detector element influences the spatial resolution (the LSF and MTF). A sine wave (shown) where each period just matches the width of two detector elements is the highest frequency sine wave that can be resolved with these detectors due to their sampling pitch.

detector system with detector pitch Δ. For example, for $\Delta = 0.05$ mm, $F_N = 10$ cycles/mm, and for $\Delta = 0.25$ mm, $F_N = 2.0$ cycles/mm.

If a sinusoidal signal greater than the Nyquist frequency were to be incident upon the detector system, its true frequency would not be recorded, but rather it would be *aliased*. Aliasing occurs when frequencies higher than the Nyquist frequency are imaged (Fig. 4-14). The frequency that is recorded is lower than the incident frequency, and indeed the recorded frequency appears to *wrap around* the Nyquist frequency. For example, for a system with $\Delta = 0.100$ mm, and thus $F_N = 5.0$ cycles/mm, sinusoidal inputs of 2, 3, and 4 cycles/mm are recorded accurately (along the frequency axis) because they obey the Nyquist Criterion. Since the input functions are single frequencies, the Fourier transform appears as a spike at that frequency, as shown in Figure 4-15. For sinusoidal inputs with frequencies greater than the Nyquist frequency, the signal wraps around the Nyquist frequency—a frequency of 6 cycles/mm ($F_N + 1$) is recorded as 4 cycles/mm ($F_N - 1$), and a frequency of 7 cycles/mm ($F_N + 2$) is recorded as 3 cycles/mm ($F_N - 2$), and so on. This is seen in Figure 4-15 as well. Aliasing is visible when there is a periodic pattern that is imaged, such as an x-ray antiscatter grid, and aliasing appears visually in many cases as a Moiré pattern.

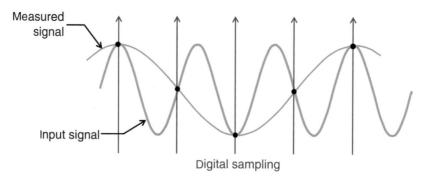

■ **FIGURE 4-14** The concept of aliasing is illustrated. The input sine wave (green) is sampled at each of the arrows, but the Nyquist criterion is violated here because the input sine wave frequency is higher than the Nyquist frequency. Thus, the sampled image data will be aliased and have the appearance of a lower frequency sine wave in the measured signal.

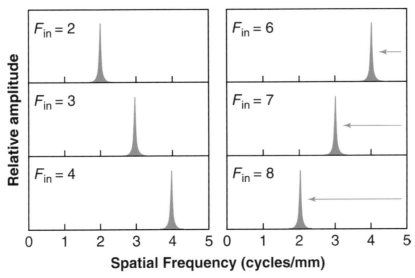

■ **FIGURE 4-15** For a single-frequency sinusoidal input function to an imaging system (sinusoidally varying intensity versus position), the Fourier transform of the image results in an impulse at the measured frequency. The Nyquist frequency in this example is 5 cycles/mm. For the three input frequencies in the left panel, all are below the Nyquist frequency and obey the Nyquist criterion, and the measured (recorded) frequencies are exactly what was input into the imaging system. On the right panel, the input frequencies were higher than the Nyquist frequency, and the recorded frequencies in all cases were aliased—they wrapped around the Nyquist frequency—that is, the measured frequencies were lower than the Nyquist frequency by the same amount by which the input frequencies exceeded the Nyquist frequency.

The Presampled MTF

Aliasing can pose limitations on the measurement of the MTF, and the finite size of the pixels in an image can cause sampling problems with the measured LSF that is used to compute the MTF (Eq. 4-3). Figure 4-8 shows the angled slit method for determining the presampled LSF, and this provides a methodology for computing the so-called presampled MTF, which represents blurring processes up to the point at which the signal is sampled. Using a single line perpendicular to the slit image (Fig. 4-8A), the sampling pitch of the LSF measurements is Δ, and the maximum frequency that can be computed for the MTF is then $1/2\Delta$. However, for many medical imaging systems, it is quite possible that the MTF has non-zero amplitude beyond the Nyquist limit of $F_N = 1/2\Delta$.

In order to measure the presampled MTF, the angled-slit method is used to synthesize the presampled LSF. By using a slight angle between the long axis of the slit and the columns of detector elements in the physical measurement of the LSF, different (nearly) normal lines can be sampled (Fig. 4-8B). The LSF computed from each individual line is limited by the Δ sampling pitch, but multiple lines of data can be used to synthesize an LSF, which has much better sampling than Δ. Indeed, oversampling can be performed by a factor of 5 or 10 (*etc.*), depending on the measurement procedure, the slit-angle relative to the (x, y) matrix, and how long the slit is. The details of how the presampled LSF is computed are beyond the scope of the current discussion; however, by decreasing the sampling pitch from Δ to, for example, $\Delta/5$, the Nyquist limit goes from F_N to $5F_N$, which is often sufficient to accurately measure the presampled MTF.

Field Measurements of Resolution Using Resolution Templates

Spatial resolution should be monitored on a routine basis for many imaging modalities. However, measuring the LSF or the MTF is more detailed than necessary for routine quality assurance purposes. For most clinical imaging systems, the evaluation of spatial resolution using resolution test phantoms is adequate for routine quality

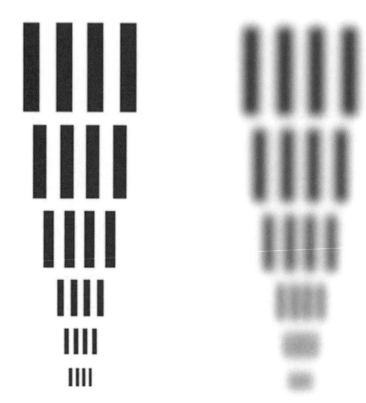

■ **FIGURE 4-16** Line pair phantoms are used for practical estimates of the spatial resolution in field tests of clinical imaging equipment. An ideal test phantom (left) is imaged, and the system blurs the image of the object as shown here (right). The observer reads the spatial frequency (not indicated here) corresponding to the smallest set of bars that were visible individually, and this measurement is considered the *limiting spatial resolution*.

assurance purposes. The test phantoms are usually line-pair phantoms (Fig. 4-16) or star patterns. The test phantoms are imaged, and the images are viewed to estimate the limiting spatial resolution of the imaging system. This is typically reported as line-pairs per mm, which is synonymous with spatial frequency. There is a degree of subjectivity in such an evaluation, but in general, viewers will agree within acceptable limits. These measurements are routinely performed on fluoroscopic equipment, radiographic systems, nuclear cameras, and in CT.

4.2 CONTRAST RESOLUTION

Contrast resolution refers to the ability to render subtle differences in grayscale. Contrast resolution is not a concept that is focused on physically large or small objects per se (that is the concept of spatial resolution); rather, contrast resolution relates more to anatomical structures (such as tumors) that produce changes in signal intensity (as reflected in the image pixel values). Small differences in signal intensity can make it difficult for a radiologist or other image reader to confidently detect and characterize that structure, especially when it is presented in a noisy background.

Contrast is defined in terms of a background intensity, S_0, and some sort of target intensity, S_1, as

$$C_s = \frac{(S_0 - S_1)}{S_0}.$$

[4-8]

The measure of intensity, S, is being left somewhat vague at this point since contrast can be defined at various points in the imaging process. The meaning of S will change depending on what stage of the process is being evaluated.

4.2.1 Subject Contrast

Subject contrast is the fundamental contrast that arises in the signal after it has interacted with the patient, but before it has been detected. The example of projection radiography is illustrated in Figure 4-17. In this case, an approximately spatially uniform x-ray beam is incident upon the patient. The x-rays interact with the tissues of the body through various mechanisms, resulting in many of the x-rays being attenuated. The differential attenuation, depending on what structures the x-ray beam passes through, forms the basis of subject contrast. Although this beam cannot be measured in reality until it reaches a detector, the concept of subject contrast is useful for assessing the feasibility of imaging different structures in the body, and for understanding how much contrast may be expected in subsequent stages in the formation of an image.

In terms of Equation 4-8, in projection radiography, S is photon fluence. Typically, S_0 would represent the fluence of a beam path that does not include some structure of interest (A in Fig. 4-17), and S_1 does include the structure (B in Fig. 4-17). Assuming that the structure is more attenuating than the surrounding tissue, $S_0 > S_1$, which means that contrast runs from 0 to 1 (*i.e.*, 0% to 100%). But negative contrast is possible for less attenuating structures. It is worth noting that the choice of S is not set in stone. For example, if we were considering CT rather than projection radiology, S could be the linear attenuation coefficient at a given point instead of photon fluence.

Subject contrast has intrinsic factors and extrinsic factors—the intrinsic component of subject contrast relates to the actual anatomical or functional changes in the

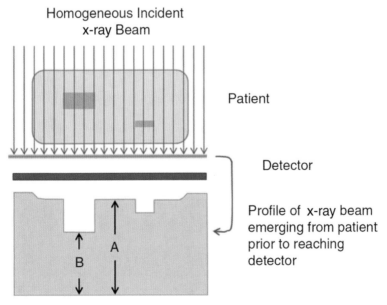

■ FIGURE 4-17 A uniform field of x-rays are transmitted through a simple "patient," resulting in a heterogeneous pattern of x-rays, which then are incident upon the x-ray detector. Subject contrast is defined as the differences in the x-ray beam fluence at the detector.

patient's tissues, which give rise to contrast. That is, the patient walks into the imaging center with intrinsic, physical, or physiological properties that give rise to subject contrast. For a single pulmonary nodule in the lung, for example, the lesion is of greater density than the surrounding lung tissue, and this allows it to be seen on chest radiography or thoracic CT or thoracic MRI. The lesion may also exhibit higher metabolism, and thus, when a sugar molecule labeled with a radioisotope is injected into the patient, more of that biomarker will accumulate in the lesion than in the surrounding lung due to its greater metabolism, and the radioisotope emission resulting from this concentration difference results in subject contrast.

Extrinsic factors in subject contrast relate to how the image-acquisition protocol can be optimized to enhance subject contrast. Possible protocol enhancements include changing the x-ray energy spectrum, using a different radiopharmaceutical, injecting an iodine (CT) or gadolinium (MR) contrast agent, changing the delay between contrast injection and imaging, changing the pulse sequence in MR, or changing the angle of an ultrasound probe with respect to a vessel in Doppler imaging. These are just a few examples of ways in which subject contrast can be optimized; many more parameters are available for optimization.

4.2.2   Detector Contrast

When the incident beam of energy from the imaging system reaches the detector(s), it is transduced into a signal through many possible physical processes, which can have an impact on the contrast of structures of interest. Figure 4-18 illustrates this process by showing two different detector responses that relate to how the incident signal is recorded (y-axis) as a function of the incident signal striking the detector (x-axis). A linear response is seen for Detector 1, and a non-linear response to x-rays is seen for Detector 2. The signal levels that define subject contrast in Figure 4-18 (S_0 and S_1) are shown, and where these signal levels meet each curve is projected (dashed lines) to the vertical axis. The contrast recorded at the detector is a consequence of the characteristic curve of the detector.

4.2.3   Image Contrast

The detector contrast acts to modulate the subject contrast, but for modern medical imaging equipment, it is nearly always the case that the acquisition procedure ultimately results in the capture of digital image data. Most medical images have bit depths ranging from 10, 12, and even 14 bits, which run from 1,024, 4,096, to 16,384 shades of gray, respectively. Modern displays, however, are only capable of

■ **FIGURE 4-18** This figure illustrates the characteristic curves for two detector systems. These plots show the effect of different detector response functions. For an input signal (x-axis) with a given subject contrast (S_0 and S_1), the linear signal levels on Detector 1 are dramatically different than the non-linear response on Detector 2.

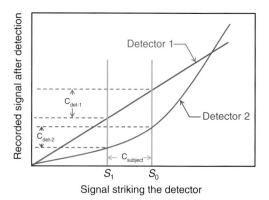

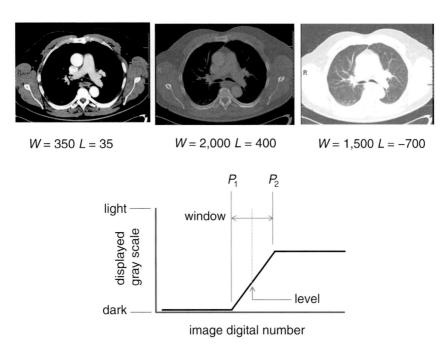

$W = 350\ L = 35$ $W = 2{,}000\ L = 400$ $W = 1{,}500\ L = -700$

■ **FIGURE 4-19** A digital image is represented as a matrix of grayscale values in the memory of a computer, but the look-up table (LUT) describes how that grayscale is converted to actual intensity on a display. Three different "window/level" settings are shown in the lung CT images at the top (Left: soft tissue window; middle: bone window; right: lung window), with display LUTs defined by the Window and Level values. The diagram shows how these parameters determine the LUT. The image data is saturated to black at $P_1 = L - W/2$ and is saturated white at $P_2 = L + W/2$.

displaying 8-bit (256 shades of gray) to 10-bit (1,024 shades of gray) information. The display computer converts the high bit depth image to a range of grayscales visible on the monitor, and there is a *look-up table* (LUT) that is used to make this conversion. The LUT transforms the intensity of each pixel of the image stored in memory on the computer, ultimately to be displayed as grayscale on the monitor.

The most commonly used LUT in radiological imaging is the so-called window/level approach, shown in Figure 4-19 for a thoracic CT image. The variable W represents the number of display units shown in the image, and the variable L represents the display units that the window is centered on. This causes saturation to black below $L - W/2$ (labeled point P_1) and saturation to white above $L + W/2$ (point P_2). Because display monitors cannot generally depict the depth of grayscale from an entire image, it is routine for the interpreting physician to change the window/level settings for a given image, so that the entire range of grayscale on the acquired image can be evaluated during multiple viewings. While freely changing the window and level setting is possible on most image workstations, several preset window and level settings are generally used to expedite viewing (*e.g.*, soft-tissue window, bone window, and lung window in Fig. 4-19).

4.3 NOISE AND NOISE TEXTURE

While spatial resolution and contrast resolution are predominantly descriptors for the accuracy of imaging, noise relates directly to precision. In the case of x-ray and γ-ray imaging, which are typically *quantum-limited,* precision can almost always be improved by collecting more photons (quanta) to produce the image by increasing the time of image acquisition, increasing the intensity of the source, or both. In MRI and ultrasound, a number of redundant signal measurements are made and are averaged together to improve precision and reduce noise.

Sources of Image Noise

In much the same way that there are multiple potential sources of blur and contrast in an imaging system, there are also multiple potential sources of noise that originate from different random components of the imaging process.

Quantum Noise

Quantum noise in imaging describes randomness in a signal that arises from randomness in the number of photons used in the imaging process. The term, *quanta*, refers to any number of particles or objects that can be counted, such as electrons, x-ray photons, optical photons, or even brush strokes on impressionist paintings. Human vision is subject to quantum noise, although typical visual experience is so quantum rich that we cannot usually perceive the relatively small fluctuations in the number of photons reaching our photoreceptors. Radioactive decay—which leads to γ-ray production—is a random process, as is x-ray production. The number of photons generated in a short time window will fluctuate from moment to moment. These fluctuations represent quantum noise.

For reasons described below, these fluctuations will be relatively larger when fewer photons are being generated, and thus quantum noise is typically made worse at low levels of photon production. In the radiology department, to reduce radiation dose to the patient, x-ray and γ-ray imaging systems attempt to use as few quanta as reasonably possible to form an image. Indeed, the numbers of quanta are so low that for most medical images involving x-rays or γ-rays, appreciable quantum noise is evident in the images; fluoroscopy or planar nuclear images are the best examples of this.

Anatomical Noise

Anatomical noise refers to the contrast in the image that is generated by patient anatomy that may be present in an image but is not important for the diagnosis. Here we are considering patient-to-patient differences in the arrangement of tissues as a random effect. For example, in abdominal angiography, the vascular system is the anatomy of interest, and other sources of image contrast such as bowel gas, the bones of the spine, and organ parenchyma may act to obscure the vascular anatomy of interest. Using digital subtraction angiography (DSA), images are acquired before and after the injection of a vascular contrast agent, and these images are subtracted, revealing only the vascular anatomy (DSA). Chest radiographs are acquired for the evaluation of the pulmonary anatomy and the mediastinum, but the ribs and spine are a source of anatomical noise. Using dual-energy subtraction techniques (Fig. 4-20), the ribs (and other bones) can be subtracted revealing only the pulmonary contrast in the image. Both temporal (*e.g.*, DSA) and dual-energy subtraction methods are performed primarily to reduce anatomical noise.

One of the underappreciated aspects of modern tomographic imaging, such as CT, MRI, and ultrasound, is that these images eliminate overlapping anatomical structures, and this can substantially lessen the impact of anatomical noise by reducing or eliminating the superposition of normal tissue structures. Much of the *power of tomography*, then, is in its ability to reduce anatomical noise. Several approaches capitalize on the temporal, energy, or spatial characteristics of the image formation process to manage the effects of anatomical noise.

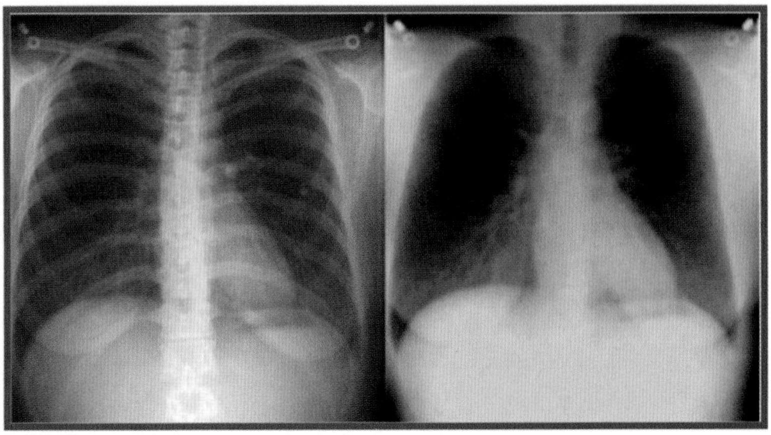

Digital Subtraction Angiography to Remove Ribs

■ **FIGURE 4-20** Anatomical noise refers to anatomy in the patient that is not pertinent to the specific imaging examination. For example, ribs are a source of anatomical noise in a chest radiograph, where the lung parenchyma is the anatomy of interest. Ribs can be digitally removed using dual-energy x-ray imaging techniques.

Electronic Noise

Electronic detector systems can be analog or digital or a combination of the two, but the flow of electrons (current) is a common detector phenomenon that transports the signal from one point in the imaging chain to other points. Some of these electrons result from actual signal detection events, but there are also electrons that contaminate the signal that can be from thermal sources, shot noise, and other electronic noise sources. If the electrons associated with noise are added into the signal prior to amplification circuits, then their noise contribution will be amplified as well. In some imaging situations, especially when signal levels are low, the added noise can be substantial and can contribute appreciably to the overall noise levels in the image. Many times, the noise contribution will differ spatially, and this represents non-stationary noise. There are many ways to reduce electronic noise, including cooling the detector system to reduce thermal noise, adding noise reduction circuitry (*e.g.*, double correlated sampling), or electronic shielding to reduce stray signal induction.

Electronic noise is a real problem in some clinical applications, such as the use of thin-film transistor (TFT) panels for fluoroscopy or cone-beam CT, or in very low dose CT situations.

Structured Noise

Most pixelated detectors have parallel channels for reading out the array of detector elements, and this reduces readout time. Each channel uses its own amplifier circuits and these circuits cannot be perfectly tuned with respect to each other. As a result, groups of detector elements that are read out may have different offset noise and gain characteristics, and these phenomena cause structured or fixed pattern noise in digital detector systems (Fig. 4-21). This form of structured noise is due to random effects in the manufacture of detectors and is typically corrected in the early stages of processing detector signals. The key to correcting for structured noise is that it is spatially constant over time. This allows the offset and gain factors for individual detector elements to be characterized by exposing the detector to radiation in the absence of an object (the so-called *gain* image). The *offset* image is measured with no radiation incident on the detector. These two calibration images can then be used to

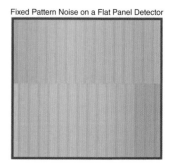

■ **FIGURE 4-21** Structured noise represents a reproducible pattern that reflects differences in the gain of individual detector elements or groups of detector elements. Because of its reproducibility, structured noise can be corrected by calibrating the detector.

Fixed Pattern Noise on a Flat Panel Detector

correct for structured noise using a flat field correction algorithm.[4] Because the structured noise pattern can change over time, for many imaging systems it is routine to acquire the offset and gain images necessary for calibration frequently—hourly, daily, or monthly, depending on the system.

4.3.2 Mathematical Characterizations of Noise

We will assume that readers are familiar with the basic ideas of probability theory. Here, a short discussion of statistical concepts is presented as a preliminary to a more focused discussion on noise in medical imaging. In particular, we will assume that readers are familiar with the concept of an *expected* value, often referred to as a mean value or the long-run average. In the case of a continuously defined random variable, like the "bell-shaped" normal distribution, the expected value of a random variable, y, is given by

$$\mu_y = \langle y \rangle = \int yp(y)\,dy, \tag{4-9}$$

where the angle brackets are used to indicate a mathematical expectation defined by the integral and $p(y)$ is the probability density function that describes the uncertainty in y.

In the case of discrete random variables, like a photon-counting detector, y can only take values that are non-negative whole numbers, and in this case, the expectation is given by a sum instead of an integral,

$$\mu_y = \langle y \rangle = \sum_{y=0}^{\infty} y\Pr(y), \tag{4-10}$$

where $\Pr(y)$ is the probability of observing y counts (with a probability of zero for any value of y that is not a whole number). For example, if y represents a Poisson number of photons, then

$$\Pr(y) = \frac{e^{-Q}Q^y}{y!}, \tag{4-11}$$

where the Poisson parameter, Q, represents the expected value (i.e., $\mu_y = Q$) of the distribution. For the more mathematically inclined, it is a good exercise to derive this using Equations 4-10 and 4-11. It is also worth noting that even though the observed value, y, must be a discrete number, the mean value does not have to be. It is perfectly

---

[4] $I_{corrected} = g\dfrac{I_{raw} - I_{offset}(r)}{I_{gain} - I_{offset}(g)}$ where g is the mean gray scale of the denominator, and the offsets are for the raw (r) and gain (g) images, respectively.

reasonable to have a Poisson random variable with a mean value of $Q = 3.5$, even though this value cannot actually be observed in y.

Equations 4-9 and 4-10 give the expected value of y, but expectations can also be applied to more complex functions of a random variable. For example, the variance of y is defined as

$$\sigma_y^2 = \left\langle (y - \mu_y)^2 \right\rangle = \int (y - \mu_y)^2 p(y)\,dy, \qquad [4\text{-}12]$$

for a continuously defined random variable, with a similar expression involving sums used when y is discrete. By definition, the standard deviation, σ_y, is the square root of the variance. Whereas the mean value can be thought of as describing the "location" of a random variable (i.e., what values it is centered on), the standard deviation and variance are both used as measures of the "spread."

An important property of the Poisson distribution in Equation 4-11 is that the variance of a Poisson random variable is equal to the mean ($\sigma_y^2 = \mu_y = Q$). This relationship is important for understanding why quantum noise is considered a greater factor when photons are less abundant. On an absolute scale, a larger variance means more noise, and so it would seem that quantum noise should be a problem when the mean number of photons (i.e., Q) is large. However, it is common to characterize noise magnitude on a relative scale as the ratio of the standard deviation to the mean (this is also called the *coefficient of variation*). In this case, we have $\sigma_y / \mu_y = 1/\sqrt{Q}$, which gets smaller as Q gets larger. Alternatively, the ratio, $\mu_y/\sigma_y = \sqrt{Q}$ can be thought of as a signal-to-noise ratio, in which the mean number of photons μ_y is regarded as the measure of signal, and σ_y is regarded as the measure of noise. Because of the mean-variance equivalence of the Poisson distribution, this grows as the square root of the mean number of photons. Thus, in low-count regimes (smaller Q) the SNR is lower and the coefficient of variation is larger.

Pixel Variance

Now, let y represent the value of a given image pixel located at a particular point in an image. We will assume that there is quantum and electronic noise in the imaging process and so this value may be considered a random variable. If the scanner were run again on exactly the same object, the value of this pixel would very likely be different. The pixel noise in the image value is the difference between the measured value, y, and the conceptual value of the *noiseless* data. Typically, noiseless data are defined as the mean value, and so the observed pixel value is defined as

$$y = \mu_y + \varepsilon, \qquad [4\text{-}13]$$

where ε represents the contribution of noise. This equation is useful, even though it is not really practical. It is not practical, because, for any real system, we will never really know μ_y, so we cannot explicitly calculate the noise as $y - \mu_y$. In fact, if we knew what μ_y was, we would not really need to obtain the noisy measurement, y, in the first place. But the equation is useful because it shows us how to think about noise. If a repeat measurement were made, we would likely get a different value of y, even though μ_y is unchanging, because ε changes with each acquisition. Understanding image noise consists of characterizing the statistical properties of ε.

The most basic statistical property related to image noise is its variance, or equivalently its standard deviation. Like the mean value, this quantity is not directly observable. However, it can be estimated. One way to do this is to repeatedly scan a test object. Let y_n be the pixel value in the nth repetition ($n = 1, \ldots, N$). We can estimate the mean value from the sample average

$$\hat{\mu}_y = \frac{1}{N}\sum_{n=1}^{N} y_n.$$ [4-14]

Note that the caret (^) indicates that this number is an estimate of μ_y. The sample average can be used in turn to estimate the variance of y as

$$\hat{\sigma}_y^2 = \frac{1}{N-1}\sum_{n=1}^{N}(y_n - \hat{\mu}_y)^2.$$ [4-15]

Both $\hat{\mu}_y$ and $\hat{\sigma}_y^2$ are based on noisy measurements (the y_n values), so these estimates are noisy themselves. But as N gets larger, these sample estimates are known to get closer and closer to the actual values of μ_y and σ_y^2. So even though we cannot directly observe noise in an image pixel, we can estimate its variance or standard deviation using this sort of repeated measurement procedure.

But it can take a lot of repeat scans to get a good estimate. For example, it can take hundreds of repeat scans to get an estimate, that is within 10% of the true σ_y^2. As a result, variance estimates from several pixels in a region are often averaged together to get a single more precise estimate of noise magnitude that is representative of the region. It is important to realize that this approach makes an assumption that the variance is at least approximately the same over the region being averaged. This idea, that the local statistical properties in a region are the same, is called *stationarity*, and here we are assuming a stationary variance. If stationarity does not hold, then the variance at a given pixel may be quite different than the representative value.

It is also possible to estimate noise magnitude from a single image, using data from multiple pixels instead of multiple replications. This replaces the y_n values in Equations 4-14 and 4-15 with values from different pixels. However, this approach makes the assumption of a stationary mean value (i.e., μ_y is unchanging) over the pixels being used in addition to the assumption of a stationary variance. This assumption is therefore only appropriate in regions where we would expect uniform image intensity, although there are more advanced methods that can attempt to correct for non-uniform backgrounds.

Noise Texture and the Autocovariance Function

Pixel variance or standard deviation are useful ways to characterize the magnitude of noise in an image. But noise texture is also important because it can have a strong effect on how well structures can be visualized in an image. As an example, consider Figure 4-22, which shows 3 different noise fields (highpass noise, white noise, and lowpass noise) that all have the same mean pixel value and pixel variance. These look considerably different, and as we shall see below, they relate to different kinds of noise found in imaging systems. More importantly, a small target placed in the center of the image gets harder to see going from left to right. We will return to this point below.

The differences in the noise textures in Figure 4-22 are due to dependencies between nearby pixels. Figure 4-23 shows scatterplots of the intensity of a pixel and the intensity of its diagonal neighbor. The highpass-noise plot on the left shows a fairly subtle negative relationship between the two pixels; when the first pixel has a higher value (pushed up by a positive noise value), then the second pixel tends to have a lower value. This can be quantified by the correlation coefficient, which is -0.22 in this case, indicating this negative association. The white-noise scatterplot in the middle of the figure is round, with a correlation coefficient of 0, indicating no linear relationship between the two. In this case, if the noise pushes the value of a pixel up, it has no effect on the value of its diagonal neighbor. The lowpass noise on

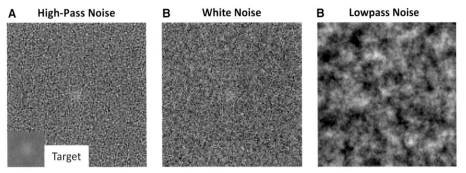

| A   High-Pass Noise | B   White Noise | B   Lowpass Noise |

Target

■ **FIGURE 4-22** The panel shows noise fields with different noise textures. All three fields have the same mean value and the same pixel variance. The difference between the textures is due to different patterns of covariance between the local pixels. Note that the small target placed in the center of the images appears to get more difficult to detect as the textures go from highpass noise **(A)** to white noise **(B)**, to lowpass noise **(C)**.

the right side of the figure shows a stronger positive relationship between the pixels, with a correlation coefficient of 0.85. In this case, when the noise pushes the value of one pixel up, it also tends to increase the value of its diagonal neighbor.

Most characterization of noise texture is based on these sorts of pairwise comparisons. Instead of the correlation coefficient used above, noise texture is often described using the *covariance* between pairs of pixel values. Since we are thinking of the pixels as being elements of one image, this is referred to as *auto-covariance*, a term that would not apply to the covariance between a pixel from a CT image and another pixel from a PET image (this would be called the *cross-covariance*). Let y represent the value of one pixel and z represent the value of another pixel. The covariance between these two pixels is given by the expected value,

$$\Sigma_{yz} = \langle (y - \mu_y)(z - \mu_z) \rangle, \qquad [4\text{-}16]$$

where μ_y and μ_z are the mean values of y and z respectively. Note that the order of the variables is meaningless, so $\Sigma_{zy} = \Sigma_{yz}$. If y and z happen to be the same pixel, then Equation 4-16 turns into Equation 4-12, and the covariance is just the pixel variance. So covariance is a generalization of the idea of variance to situations where there are multiple measured values (pixel values here). For this reason, a matrix of covariance values between all possible pairs of pixels is sometimes referred to as the variance-covariance matrix.

Covariance between pixel values can also be estimated from repeated scans, as it was for the pixel variance in Equation 4-15. Let y_n and z_n be the two pixel values of interest in the nth repeated image ($n = 1, ..., N$). The covariance estimate is given by

$$\hat{\Sigma}_{yz} = \frac{1}{N-1} \sum_{n=1}^{N} (y_n - \hat{\mu}_y)(z_n - \hat{\mu}_z), \qquad [4\text{-}17]$$

where $\hat{\mu}_y$ and $\hat{\mu}_z$ are the estimates of the sample means shown in Equation 4-14. Here we also see that if y and z happen to be the same pixel, then $z_n = y_n$ (and $\hat{\mu}_z = \hat{\mu}_y$), and Equation 4-17 simplifies to become Equation 4-15, showing that $\hat{\Sigma}_{yy} = \hat{\sigma}_y^2$. Note that the correlation coefficient referred to above in describing the scatterplots in Figure 4-23 can be computed by normalizing $\hat{\Sigma}_{yz}$ in Equation 4-17 by the product of $\hat{\sigma}_y$ and $\hat{\sigma}_z$ computed according to Equation 4-15.

Spatial averaging can be used here as well to improve the estimate when only limited numbers of repeat images are available. So now let us imagine that y represents a pixel in a 2D image, say $y = I[27, 45]$ (*i.e.*, the 27th-pixel position horizontally and the 45th position vertically), and z represents its diagonal neighbor, $z = I[28, 46]$, with

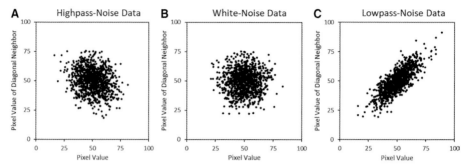

■ **FIGURE 4-23** Scatterplots showing the value of a pixel on the x-axis, and then the value of its diagonal neighbor (incremented by one in both horizontally and vertically) on the y-axis. For the highpass-noise texture **(A)**, these values have a mildly negative orientation. For the white-noise texture **(B)**, the scatterplot looks round with no particular trend. For the lowpass-noise texture **(C)**, there is a clear positive trend in the pixel values. These pixel correlations are the basis for the different appearances of the textures in Figure 4-22.

the y_n and z_n being extracted from replicate images, I_n. We can estimate the covariance between these two points, using Equation 4-17, and then average it together with the covariance between I[28, 45] and I[29, 46], and other nearby pairs of diagonal neighbors. This approach assumes that the covariance between diagonal neighbors is not changing over the set of pairs being used in the average, an assumption of *stationary covariance*. This approach, like variance estimation, can also be extended to a single image if we can make the additional assumption of a stationary mean value.

So far, we have been looking at the covariance as a relationship between two pixels. However, to really describe noise texture, we need to consider all possible pairs of pixels. That is a lot of pixel pairs. In the relatively small images used in Figure 4-22, there are a total of 16,384 ($=128^2$) pixels. The number of unique pixel pairs (including self-pairs) is 134,225,920. But many of these pixels are relatively far apart, and so the covariance will likely be negligible, and furthermore, we can often restrict our interest to a region of the image that is stationary to a good approximation. When this can be done, the covariance of one pixel and all its neighbors represents the regional texture of the noise, which is a much more compact representation of the pixel relationships than a list of millions of covariances. This covariance map is the autocovariance function of the noise.

Figure 4-24 shows the three autocovariance functions that describe the noise textures in Figure 4-22. The middle point in each of these is the pixel variance, which is the largest value. In the lowpass-noise texture, the nearby points are also quite bright, indicating the positive covariance we see in the scatterplot in Figure 4-23. For the

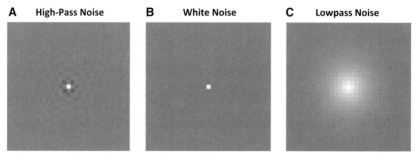

■ **FIGURE 4-24** The panel shows autocovariance functions for the different noise textures in Figure 4-22. The central point in each autocovariance function is the pixel variance, which is identical for all three textures. However, moving away from the center, covariance in the highpass-noise textures **(A)** is seen to oscillate and decay to zero (uniform grey). In the white-noise textures **(B)**, covariance immediately drops to zero. In the lowpass-noise textures **(C)**, covariance slowly and uniformly decays to zero.

white-noise texture, the covariance for all other pixel pairs is zero. This means that each pixel is uncorrelated with all the others. For the highpass-noise texture, the covariance values oscillate and decay moving away from the central pixel.

The autocovariance function characterizes statistical dependencies between pixels spatially (*i.e.*, as a function of the relative position between pixel pairs) in much the same way that a PSF characterizes blur spatially, relative to a point source. And, like the PSF, this leads to a meaningful interpretation in the spatial frequency domain that will be described below.

Noise Power Spectrum

Quite simply put, the noise power spectrum (NPS) is the Fourier transform of the autocovariance function. This terse statement belies quite a bit of more advanced mathematics. For example, the NPS is always real-valued (*i.e.*, not a complex number), and always non-negative. But why should the Fourier transform of the auto-covariance function necessarily have these properties? (The answer has to do with concepts related to the symmetry of autocovariance.) These topics are beyond the scope of this chapter, but the NPS is such a useful and ubiquitous characterization of noise texture that it is worth understanding its interpretation separate from the theoretical foundations needed to derive it.

The intuitive understanding of NPS is that it describes the contribution of different spatial frequencies to the image noise. With this in mind, Figure 4-25 plots the noise power spectra for the noise textures in Figure 4-22. Note that these are 2-dimensional textures, and so noise power spectra are also 2D. However, these noise textures were approximately *isotropic*, and so the NPS is rotationally symmetric and can be represented by a single frequency axis. Plots like these are a common way to present the NPS. Plots using linear axes and log-log axes are shown since both forms of plots are used.

The highpass noise texture has an NPS plot that is increasing linearly across the frequency range. So, it has more noise power at high spatial frequencies, and hence the name—highpass noise (it tends to pass more high-frequency noise on to the image). This particular form of highpass noise is also sometimes referred to as *ramp-spectrum* noise, because of the linear rise in noise power. Ramp-spectrum noise

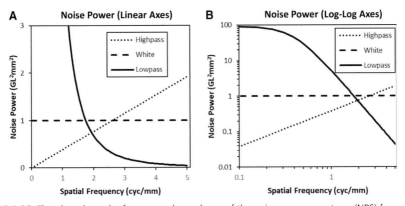

■ FIGURE 4-25 The plots show the frequency dependence of the noise-power spectrum (NPS) for each of the three textures in Figure 4-22. The power spectra are isotropic (rotationally invariant) and hence they can be represented by a single radial frequency. In the linear-axis plot **(A)**, we see that the highpass-noise NPS rises linearly with frequency, the white-noise NPS is flat, and the lowpass-noise NPS decays rapidly. On log-log axes **(B)**, the power-law nature of the NPS for all three textures is evident from the linear profiles (above 0.5 cycle/mm for the lowpass-noise NPS).

is closely related to noise in tomographic images, where white noise in the detector becomes ramp-spectrum noise in the reconstruction.

The white-noise texture has a flat NPS plot, showing equal power at all spatial frequencies. This is the definition of white noise. White noise is closely related to quantum and electronic noise at the level of the detector. To a first approximation, these lead to independent effects in each detector pixel (*i.e.*, an autocovariance function as in the middle of Fig. 4-24), which gives the flat NPS.

The lowpass-noise texture has very high power at low spatial frequencies, falling off drastically with increasing frequency. In this case, the power spectrum falls off as frequency cubed ($1/f^3$), which makes it similar to the power spectrum of breast tissue in a projection mammogram. This kind of power-law NPS is commonly used to describe anatomical noise in medical imaging, and "natural scenes" more generally.

The enormous range of this plot makes it difficult to show on linear axes, and for this reason, NPS plots involving anatomical noise are often plotted on log-log axes (meaning the log of the *x*-axis and the log of the *y*-axis), as on the right side of Figure 4-25. On log-log axes, a straight line indicates a power-law relationship, and we can see that all three of the noise textures are power laws, although the lowpass NPS levels off at the lowest spatial frequencies (a true $1/f^3$ power-law goes to infinity as the frequency goes to zero). At the higher frequencies, the lowpass noise has a slope of -3 on the plot (*i.e.*, it drops by 3 orders of magnitude in power for every order of magnitude gained in spatial frequency). The white noise NPS is a flat line with a slope of zero, indicating that noise power is proportional to f^0, a constant. The ramp-spectrum noise has a positive slope of 1 (noise power is proportional to f^1).

4.4 RATIO MEASURES OF IMAGE QUALITY

In the three preceding sections, spatial resolution and contrast resolution were used to characterize accuracy, and noise properties were used to characterize precision. When we consider the quality of images in these terms, we need to balance effects on accuracy against the effects on precision. This has led to various ratio measures in which the numerator is related to some property of the signal, and the denominator is related to the noise.

4.4.1 Contrast-to-Noise Ratio

The CNR is an object *size–independent* measure of the signal level in the presence of noise. Take the example of a disk as the object (Fig. 4-26). The contrast in this example is the difference between the average grayscale of a region of interest (ROI) in the disk $(\hat{\mu}_s)$ and that in an ROI in the background $(\hat{\mu}_{bg})$, and the noise can be calculated from the (typically larger) background ROI as well. Thus, the CNR is given by

$$\text{CNR} = \frac{\left(\hat{\mu}_s - \hat{\mu}_{bg}\right)}{\hat{\sigma}_{bg}}. \tag{4-18}$$

The CNR metric describes the signal amplitude relative to the magnitude of noise in an image, and this is particularly useful for simple objects in white noise. Because the CNR is computed using the difference in mean values between the signal region and the background, this metric is most applicable when test objects that generate a homogeneous signal level are used—that is, where the mean grayscale in the signal ROI is representative of the entire object. And since it accounts for noise effects as

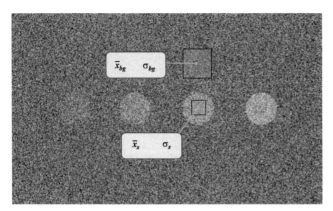

■ **FIGURE 4-26** The CNR concept is illustrated. The CNR is an area-independent measure of the contrast, relative to the noise, in an image, typically measured from a phantom with multiple contrasts as is shown here. The CNR is useful for optimizing image acquisition parameters for generic objects of variable sizes and shapes. The CNRs in this figure (in the disks running from left to right) are 0.39, 1.03, 1.32, and 1.70.

Mean BG = 127.5332
Noise = 10.2949
Steps are 5, 10, 15, 20

a pixel standard deviation, it is most appropriate when noise texture is relatively unchanged by whatever parameter of the imaging process is being evaluated. Example uses of the CNR metric include optimizing the x-ray tube potential of an imaging study to maximize bone contrast at a fixed dose level, computing the dose necessary to achieve a given CNR for a given object, or computing the minimum concentration of contrast agent that could be seen on given test phantom with a fixed radiation dose.

4.4.2   Signal-to-Noise Ratio

A signal-to-noise ratio can be defined in a variety of ways depending on how signal and noise are quantified. In fact, the CNR described above can be thought of as a SNR with contrast as the measure of signal and pixel standard deviation as the measure of noise. Another SNR metric is like the CNR, except that the size and shape of an object are explicitly included in the computation. This SNR does not require the test object that generates the signal to be homogeneous; however, the background does need to be homogeneous in principle—a series of Gaussian "blobs" are used as signals to illustrate this point (Fig. 4-27). The numerator in the SNR is the signal integrated over the entire dimensions of the object of interest. The signal amplitude of each pixel is the amount in which this patch of the image is elevated relative to the mean background signal—thus, for a mean background of μ_{bg}, the net signal at each pixel $[i, j]$ in the image is $I[i, j] - \mu_{bg}$. The denominator is the pixel standard

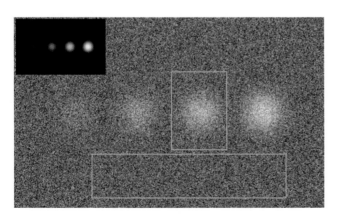

■ **FIGURE 4-27** Signal regions with Gaussian-based intensities are shown. The SNR has a fundamental relationship with detectability, and the Rose Criterion states that if SNR > 5, the signal region will be detectable in most situations.

deviation in the homogeneous background region of the image (σ_{bg}), and thus the SNR represents the integrated signal over an ROI, which encapsulates the object of interest, divided by the noise

$$\text{SNR} = \frac{\sqrt{\Sigma_{i,j}(I[i,j] - \mu_{bg})^2}}{\sigma_{bg}}. \qquad [4\text{-}19]$$

The SNR is estimated using the sample mean, $\hat{\mu}_{bg}$ and standard deviation, $\hat{\sigma}_{bg}$ defined in Equations 4-14 and 4-15. It does require that the estimate of $\hat{\mu}_{bg}$ be accurate, and thus it should be computed over as large a region as possible.

This SNR can be a meaningful metric that describes the conspicuity of an object—how well it will be seen by the typical observer. Indeed, Albert Rose recognized this and was able to demonstrate that if SNR $\geq$ 5, then an object will almost always be recognized (detected), but that detection performance continuously degrades as SNR approaches zero. This is called the *Rose Criterion*. But it should also be recognized that it does not account for noise texture, and so it is not appropriate in situations where the NPS is changing substantially. As an example, consider the three noise textures in Figure 4-22, with the small Gaussian target in the middle. The signal and pixel standard deviation are the same in all three textures, which leads to a common value of SNR = 7.1. This suggests that the target should be readily visible for all three textures, even though the target gets considerably harder to see in the rightmost (lowpass noise) image.

4.4.3   SNR in the Frequency Domain: Noise Equivalent Quanta

We have seen how the spatial frequency concepts of MTF and NPS are used to characterize blur and noise texture in the spatial frequency domain. Given the important role of these phenomena on image quality, it should not be surprising to find them in measures of image quality. They play an explicit role in the definition of a frequency SNR.

In this case, we can hypothesize a signal that is confined to a single spatial frequency. The degree to which the signal is passed into the image is determined by the signal strength, the MTF of the signal frequency, and then whatever gain is implemented by the signal detector. The noise that masks this signal will be determined by the NPS of the particular frequency. The result is an SNR defined for a particular frequency, f, as

$$\text{SNR}(f) = g\frac{\text{MTF}(f)}{\sqrt{\text{NPS}(f)}}, \qquad [4\text{-}20]$$

where g is the gain factor defined as the mean pixel value in the ROI. The frequency SNR is also used to describe the efficiency of imaging systems as described below.

In the analysis of x-ray imaging systems, the square of the frequency SNR is also known as the *Noise Equivalent Quanta* (NEQ(f) = SNR$^2(f)$), a name derived from the idea that it represents the number of quanta needed to achieve the observed SNR. For the Poisson distribution described in Section 4.3.2, it was seen that SNR^2 was equivalent to the mean number of observed photons, with small numbers leading to low SNR. The NEQ makes this concept applicable to images in a frequency-specific way. The frequency SNR and NEQ are theoretically satisfying because they balance the MTF, which represents the amount of signal passed by an imaging system, against the NPS, which represents the amount of noise that is generated during the imaging process.

4.4.4 Detective Quantum Efficiency

Both the SNR and NEQ measures defined above measure the quality of the imaging process. However, it may be of interest to focus on the detection step in particular, independent of other factors. For example, in an x-ray imaging system, NEQ can be increased by simply turning up the mAs of the x-ray tube. This may not be helpful if we are interested in characterizing the detector or comparing two different detectors. The detective quantum efficiency (DQE) is a way to isolate the detector's impact on image quality in a frequency-dependent manner for quantum-limited imaging systems.

The idea behind DQE is that the SNR described in Equation 4-20 (and by extension the NEQ as well) can be regarded as describing the "output" SNR from the detector ($\mathrm{SNR_{OUT}}(f)$). To quantify the role of the detector, we need to normalize this by the "input" SNR of the x-ray field that is incident to the detector ($\mathrm{SNR_{IN}}(f)$). For a field with Poisson statistics, $\mathrm{SNR_{IN}^2}$ is simply the photon fluence, q, which is the expected number of quanta falling on the detector divided by the area, at all frequencies. DQE is defined as the ratio of the squared SNRs,

$$\mathrm{DQE}(f) = \frac{\mathrm{SNR_{OUT}^2}(f)}{\mathrm{SNR_{IN}^2}}. \qquad [4\text{-}21]$$

In terms of the MTF and NPS of the imaging system, the DQE(f) is given by

$$\mathrm{DQE}(f) = \frac{g^2 \mathrm{MTF}^2(f)}{q\mathrm{NPS}(f)} = \frac{\mathrm{NEQ}(f)}{q}. \qquad [4\text{-}22]$$

The DQE(f) has become the standard by which the performance of planar x-ray imaging systems is measured in the research environment. It is an excellent description of the dose efficiency of an x-ray detector system—that is how effectively the imaging system captures the incoming quanta to form the image at each frequency.

At zero frequency ($f = 0$), and in the absence of appreciable electronic noise, the DQE(0) converges to the detector's *quantum detection efficiency*, the QDE. The QDE reflects the global efficiency of x-ray detection, neglecting other elements in the imaging chain that inject or amplify noise. It is typically derived from purely physical considerations. Assume an x-ray spectrum, $\phi(E)$, that quantifies the density of imaging photons (photons/unit energy), a detector material with an energy-dependent linear attenuation coefficient, $\mu(E)$, and thickness, T, the QDE of the detector is then given by

$$QDE = \frac{\int_E \phi(E)\left[1 - e^{-\mu(E)T}\right]dE}{\int_E \phi(E)dE}. \qquad [4\text{-}23]$$

The numerator gives the fraction of photons stopped by the detector, integrated over all energies, and the denominator is the total photon fluence. The correspondence of Equation 4-23 with DQE(0) links the mathematical evaluation of image quality to the material properties of the detector.

4.5 IMAGE QUALITY MEASURES BASED ON VISUAL PERFORMANCE

The methods above provide quantitative measures of image quality on the basis of properties of the imaging system and the kinds of objects that are being imaged. While these measures are appropriate for answering many questions about imaging systems, as the focus of interest gets more task-specific, there often comes a point at which a demonstration of improved accuracy by actual image readers is needed. Even at this stage, it is often still desirable to avoid a full clinical trial. The methods described below show how reader-based evaluations of performance can be used for image quality assessment in a setting that can be considerably less costly than a clinical trial.

4.5.1 Contrast-Detail Diagrams

The contrast-detail diagram, or *CD diagram*, is a conceptual, visual method for combining the concepts of spatial resolution and contrast resolution. A standard CD phantom is illustrated in Figure 4-28A. Here, the disk diameter decreases toward the left, so the greatest detail (smallest disks) is along the left column of the CD diagram. The contrast of each disk decreases from top to bottom, and thus the bottom row of the CD diagram has the lowest contrast—and the disks in the bottom row will, therefore, be most difficult to see, especially in a noisy image. Figure 4-28B shows the same disks, but with some resolution loss and with increased noise and with the CD diagram superimposed on the image. It is important to remember that the most difficult disk to see is at the lower left (smallest with lowest contrast), and the easiest disk to see is at the upper right (largest with highest contrast) on this CD diagram. The line (see Fig. 4-28B) on a CD diagram is the line of demarcation, separating the disks that you can see from the ones that you cannot see. To the left and below the line are disks that cannot be seen, and above and to the right of the line are disks that can be seen. Figure 4-28C shows the CD diagram with even more noise, and in this image, the line of demarcation (the CD curve) has changed because the increased noise level has reduced our ability to see the disks with subtle contrast levels.

Figure 4-28 illustrates CD diagrams superimposed over the actual test images. Figure 4-29 illustrates pairs of CD diagrams on the same plot to facilitate comparison. The curves in these plots correspond to two imaging systems (System 1 and System 2), but how can the differences in these two imaging systems be interpreted? Let us assume

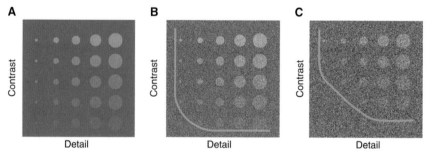

■ **FIGURE 4-28** Contrast-detail diagrams are illustrated. **A.** The (noiseless) CD phantom is illustrated, where disks are smaller to the left and have less contrast toward the bottom. **B.** Some resolution loss and added noise are present, and the smallest and lowest contrast disk can no longer be seen with confidence. The yellow line is the line of demarcation between disks that can be seen (upper right) and those that cannot be seen (lower left). **C.** More noise is added, and more of the subtle disks (including the entire, low-contrast bottom row) cannot be reliably seen.

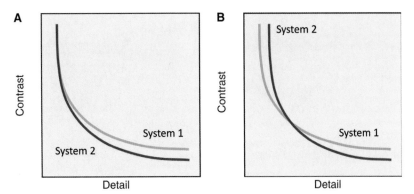

■ **FIGURE 4-29** **A.** CD curves are shown. Both curves demonstrate the same detail (in the limit of high-contrast objects), but System 2 extends to lower contrast. One explanation is that System 2 corresponds to a higher dose version of System 1. **B.** System 2 has less detail but more contrast resolution than System 1 and one explanation would be that System 2 corresponds to an image that was smoothed, relative to the image corresponding to System 1.

that System 2 in Figure 4-29A represents a standard radiographic procedure and System 1 represents a low-dose radiograph. The dose does not change the detail in the image, and thus the two curves come together in the upper left (where the contrast is the highest) to describe the same level of detail. However, because System 2 produces an image that is acquired with higher radiation dose—the noise in the image is less, and the CD diagram shows that this system has better contrast resolution—because disks lower down on the CD diagram (*i.e.*, with lower contrast) can be seen relative to System 1.

Figure 4-29B shows another example of a CD diagram. In this case, let us assume that the two systems being compared use two different image processing procedures for the same image. Let the System 1 curve represent the original acquired data of the CD phantom and let the System 2 curve represent an image that has been smoothed using image processing techniques. The smoothing process blurs edges (reduces detail) but reduces image noise as well (increases contrast resolution). Thus, relative to System 1, the System 2 curve has less detail (does not go as far left as the System 1 curve) due to the blurring procedure but has better contrast resolution (The System 2 curve goes lower on the CD diagram) because blurring reduces noise.

The use of CD diagrams unites the concepts of spatial resolution, contrast resolution, and noise on the same graph. It is a subjective visual test, and so it is excellent in conveying the relationships visually, but it is not an objective measure of performance.

4.5.2 Receiver Operating Characteristic Curves

The ROC curve is considered an objective evaluation of detection performance for a *binary task* in which cases are divided into one of two possible classes (*e.g.*, normal and abnormal). It includes not only the quality of an imaging system for a specific task but the skill of the interpreting physician (or computer algorithm) in assessing this data.

The starting point of ROC analysis is the 2 × 2 *decision matrix* (sometimes called the truth table), shown in Figure 4-30. The patient either has the suspected disease (actually abnormal) or not (actually normal), and this gold standard is considered the "truth." The diagnostician makes a binary decision—whether the patient is normal or abnormal. The 2 × 2 decision matrix defines the terms *true positive (TP)*, *true negative (TN)*, *false positive (FP)*, and *false-negative (FN)*. Most of the work in performing patient-based ROC studies is the independent confirmation of the "truth," which may require biopsy confirmation, long-term patient follow-up, or other methods to determine the actual condition of the patient.

■ **FIGURE 4-30** The 2 × 2 truth table is illustrated. This combines the decisions rendered with the underlying truth state of the patient.

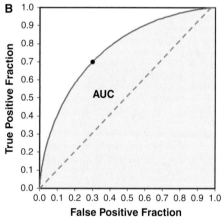

In most radiology applications, the criteria that inform a decision to label a patient as abnormal is not just one feature, but is rather an overall impression derived from a number of factors, including gestalt, diagnostic reasoning, contextual information such as family history or symptoms, and even consultation. We can think of a decision variable as distilling all of these processes into a single number that represents the suspicion of disease. Figure 4-31A illustrates the concept that the decision

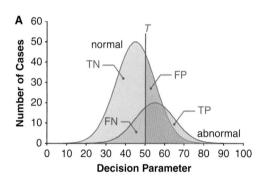

■ **FIGURE 4-31** The underlying data that explain ROC analysis are shown **(A)**. Histograms of normal and abnormal populations of patients are illustrated as a function of an underlying level of suspicion, but the observer needs to set a decision threshold (vertical line, *T*) such that cases to the right are "called" abnormal, and cases to the left of the threshold are diagnosed as normal. These data are not always observable for real-world human observer ROC measurements. Nonetheless, this concept informs the analysis of decision making. The two populations and the single threshold value define the TP, FN, TN, and FP. These values are used to compute *sensitivity* and *specificity*, as defined in the text, which are used to define one point on the ROC curve **(B)**. An ROC curve is defined as the TPF (sensitivity) as a function of FPF (1 − specificity), and the ROC curve corresponding to the distributions shown in Figure 4-31A is shown. The black dot is the point on the curve defined by the current position of the threshold (*T*). To compute the entire ROC curve, the threshold needs to be swept across the x-axis, which will lead to the computation of many pairs of points needed to draw the entire ROC curve. The dashed line shows an ROC curve for an observer who merely guesses at the diagnosis uninformed by the image or any other source of patient-specific information; it represents the minimum performance. The area under the curve (AUC) is often used as a shorthand metric for the overall performance shown on an ROC curve. AUC values run from 0.5 (dotted line, pure guessing) to 1.0—a perfect ROC curve runs along the left and top axes, bounding the entire area of the unit square.

variable will be distributed somewhat differently for patients that are normal (left curve) and those that are abnormal (right curve). The generic descriptors *normal* and *abnormal* are used here, but these can be more specific for a given diagnostic task. For example, for mammography, the abnormal patients may have breast cancer and the normal patients do not. In many cancer imaging applications, the decision variable is referred to as a *probability of malignancy* score.

In difficult imaging tasks, overlap occurs between normal and abnormal findings, representing the ambiguity in the image information. Even though there may be some ambiguity due to the overlap of the two curves, the radiologist is usually responsible for diagnosing each case one way or another (*e.g.*, to decide to biopsy or not). Hence, the patient is either determined to be *normal* or *abnormal*—a binary decision. In this case, the diagnostician sets his or her own *decision threshold* T (Fig. 4-31A). Cases to the right of the decision threshold are considered abnormal, and cases to the left of the threshold are considered normal.

The two distributions shown in Figure 4-31A are not generally observable; they are often a model of the diagnostic thinking of the image reader. But what can be observed are the values of TP, TN, FP, and FN in the truth table. From these values, properties of the reader can be inferred. Using the values of TP, TN, FP, and FN, the true-positive fraction (TPF), also known as the *sensitivity*, can be calculated as

$$TPF = sensitivity = \frac{TP}{TP + FN}. \qquad [4-24]$$

The TPF is the probability that a positive case will be greater than T, and hence correctly labeled "Abnormal" by the reader. The true-negative fraction (TNF), also known as the *specificity,* can be determined as follows:

$$TNF = specificity = \frac{TN}{TN + FP}. \qquad [4-25]$$

The TNF is the probability that a negative case will be correctly labeled by the reader as normal. The false-positive fraction (FPF) can be determined as well,

$$FPF = \frac{FP}{TN + FP}, \qquad [4-26]$$

which is the probability that a negative case will be labeled "abnormal." It can be seen that the FPF $= 1 - $ TNF, just as the false-negative fraction (FNF) is FNF $= 1 - $ TPF.

An ROC curve (see Fig. 4-31B) is a plot of the TPF as a function of the FPF, which is also the sensitivity as a function of $1 - $ specificity. It can be seen in Figure 4-31A that the selection of one threshold value results in defining specific values of TP and FP, such that one value of sensitivity (Eq. 4-24) and one value of specificity (Eq. 4-25) can be calculated. This contributes to one point on the ROC curve, the *black dot* in Figure 4-31B. The same logic could also be used to define TNF and FNF, although these are redundant with TPF and FPF and so are not shown on the ROC curve. In order to compute the entire ROC curve, which is defined by all possible pairs of (FPF, TPF) values, the threshold value (T) in Figure 4-31A has to be swept over the entire width of the two distributions. As the threshold is moved higher, the dot on the ROC curve will move downward and to the left along the curve.

For some ROC computations where (often, computer-generated) data similar to that shown in Figure 4-31A are available, the threshold T can be stepped across the data sets allowing direct computation of the ROC curve (as was done to make these plots). For ROC studies involving human observers, the data similar to that shown in Figure 4-31A are not typically available. Instead, the human observer is asked to use five or more different confidence levels as decision thresholds. Often these are given descriptive labels such as *definitely normal*, *probably normal*, *uncertain*, *probably abnormal*, and *definitely abnormal*. Using the data derived from this test, four different 2 × 2 truth tables can be established, depending on which of the five categories are considered as normal and which are considered abnormal. For example, we could specify that only the "definitely normal" responses are counted as a normal response, and all others are counted as abnormal. Or, we could count the "definitely normal" and "probably normal" categories and normal responses, etc. The four 2 × 2 truth tables produced in this manner result in four different pairs of sensitivity-specificity values. These four points can be used to estimate the full ROC using a mathematical ROC model to fit the data.

The ROC curve is plotted on a unit square (area = 1.0). Pure guessing results in a TPF = FPF, which is a diagonal line (Fig. 4-31B, *dashed line*). The area under the ROC curve is often referred to simply as AUC, and this value is a number that ranges from 0.5 (the diagonal line of pure guessing) to 1.0 (perfect detection performance) and is often referred to as a metric of observer performance. The AUC of the ROC curve shown in Figure 4-31B is 0.77.

The ROC curve is typically estimated on a reader-by-reader basis (and then analyzed statistically), and as such it is a description of the performance of a given observer at a given task (*e.g.*, Dr. Smith in mammography, Dr. Jones in head MRI). Although the ROC *curve* describes their theoretical performance as if they were able to dramatically vary their threshold value, in reality, Dr. Smith has a typical *operating point* at a diagnostic task such as mammography, and this operating point resides somewhere along the ROC curve. Take the ROC curve shown

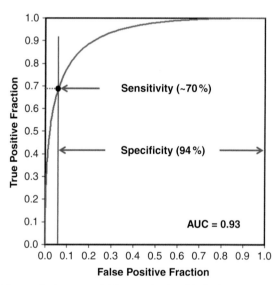

■ **FIGURE 4-32** An ROC curve is shown, and this curve is plausible for breast cancer screening using mammography. The ROC curve describes the theoretical performance of a skilled observer, but this observer will generally operate at a given point on the curve, called the operating point (black dot). This figure demonstrates the trade-offs of decision performance. Compared to the operating point shown, the radiologist could increase sensitivity but generally, this will come at a reduction in specificity—the operating point will move upward and to the right along the curve. More cancers will be detected (sensitivity will be increased), but far more women will be called back and asked to undergo additional imaging procedures and potentially biopsies (reduced specificity). Conversely, reducing the false-positive fraction (increasing specificity) comes at a price of reduced sensitivity for detecting cancers.

in Figure 4-32, which has an AUC of about 0.93, a realistic value for screening mammography. It is known that the call back rate in screening mammography is approximately 6% (depends on the radiologist), and this corresponds very nearly to a specificity of 94% (100% − 6%). The operating point at this specificity is shown in Figure 4-32, and it can be seen that the corresponding sensitivity is about 70%. The radiologists can move their operating point along the ROC curve, but for an experienced radiologist, the curve is pretty much fixed for a given modality and patient population. To increase their sensitivity, the specificity would have to decrease (increasing the FPF), increasing the call back rate, and probably increasing the negative biopsy rate as well. These observations demonstrate the fundamental trade-off that diagnosticians make in setting the operating point on their ROC curve for difficult tasks.

The widespread use of specificity and sensitivity as performance measures in the medical literature is partly because these parameters are independent of disease *incidence*. Notice in Figure 4-31A, the abnormal population is smaller than the normal population (the area of the abnormal curve is smaller). The ROC curve computation (using sensitivity and specificity metrics) remains the same, regardless of the relative numbers in the normal and abnormal populations. There are several other parameters related to observer performance that are not independent of incidence.

Accuracy is defined as the probability of making a correct decision,

$$\text{Accuracy} = \frac{\text{TP} + \text{TN}}{\text{TP} + \text{TN} + \text{FP} + \text{FN}}, \qquad [4\text{-}27]$$

which sounds like a simple and reasonable way to evaluate performance. However, care must be used in interpreting accuracy, because it combines normal and abnormal responses and it is dependent on disease *incidence*. For example, due to the low incidence of breast cancer cases in a screening population, a breast imager could invariably improve accuracy by just calling all cases negative, and not even looking at the mammograms. Because the incidence of breast cancer in the screening population is low (~5/1,000), with all cases called negative (normal), TN would be very large (~995 per 1,000), FP and TP would be zero (since all cases are called negative, there would be no positives), and accuracy would be approximately 99.5%. Although the specificity would be 100%, the sensitivity would be 0%—obviously a useless test in such a case. For these reasons, accuracy, as defined in Equation 4-27, is rarely used as a metric for the performance of a diagnostic test.

The *positive predictive value* (PPV) refers to the probability that the patient is actually abnormal (TP) when the diagnostician *says* the patient is abnormal (TP + FP),

$$\text{Positive predictive value} = \frac{\text{TP}}{\text{TP} + \text{FP}}. \qquad [4\text{-}28]$$

Conversely, the negative predictive value (NPV) refers to the probability that the patient is actually normal (TN) when the diagnostician *says* the patient is normal (TN + FN),

$$\text{Negative predictive value} = \frac{\text{TN}}{\text{TN} + \text{FN}}. \qquad [4\text{-}29]$$

The PPV and NPV of a diagnostic test (such as an imaging examination with radiologist interpretation) are useful metrics for referring physicians as they weigh the information from a number of diagnostic tests (some of which may be contradictory) for a given patient, in the process of determining their diagnosis.

SUGGESTED READING AND REFERENCES

Barrett HH, Swindell W. *Radiological Imaging: The Theory of Image Formation, Detection, and Processing.* vols. 1 and 2. New York, NY: Academic Press; 1981.

Bracewell RN. *The Fourier Transform and Its Applications.* New York, NY: McGraw-Hill; 1978.

Boone JM. Determination of the presampled MTF in computed tomography. *Med Phys.* 2001;28:356-360.

Dainty JC, Shaw R. *Image Science.* New York, NY: Academic Press; 1974.

Fugita H, Tsai D-Y, Itoh T, et al. A simple method for determining the modulation transfer function in digital radiography. *IEEE Trans Med Imaging.* 1992;MI-11:34-39.

Hasegawa BH. *The Physics of Medical X-Ray Imaging.* 2nd ed. Madison, WI: Medical Physics; 1991.

International Commission on Radiation Units and Measurements. ICRU Report No. 87: Radiation dose and image-quality assessment in computed tomography. *J ICRU.* 2012;12(1):1-149.

Metz CE. Basic principles of ROC analysis. *Semin Nucl Med.* 1978;8:283-298.

Rose A. *Vision: Human and Electronic.* New York, NY: Plenum Press; 1973.

5

Medical Imaging Informatics

In healthcare, medical informatics represents the process of collecting, analyzing, storing, and communicating information (data) that is crucial to the provision and delivery of appropriate patient care critical for health and well-being, as well as for education and research. These data are comprised of many sources such as doctors' notes in free-form text, quantitative and qualitative measurements of various basic tests including blood evaluations, electrocardiograms, projection radiographs, more complex tests such as genetic surveys, CT, MRI, PET, and other advanced evaluations. Informatics has grown substantially over the past decade to address the issues of uncertainty in handling data by converting analog input sources to digital format and ensuring an authoritative source for patient demographics and records through the implementation of digital databases and the electronic health record (EHR). Advances in computer networks and access to the Internet provide rapid mechanisms for acquisition, archiving, retrieval, concurrent sharing, and data mining of relevant medical information.

Medical *imaging* informatics is a sub-field of medical informatics that addresses aspects of image generation, processing, management, transfer, storage, distribution, display, perception, privacy, and security. It overlaps many other disciplines such as electrical engineering, computer and information sciences, medical physics, and perceptual physiology and psychology, and has evolved chiefly in radiology, although other specialties including pathology, cardiology, dermatology, surgery—in fact, the majority of clinical disciplines—generate digital medical images as well. Certainly, imaging informatics is an important and growing part of health and medicine.

An important part of imaging informatics includes ontologies (the basic communications lexicons), standards (critical pathway to ensure interoperability of different informatics systems), computers and networking (the information highway and communication medium), and the picture archiving and communications system (PACS) infrastructure (image distribution, analysis, diagnosis, and archive). PACS implementation details, including operational considerations, image display technology/calibration, and quality control issues, constitute the largest section of this chapter. The lifecycle of a radiology exam from the initial order to report distribution and action by the referring physician demonstrates the imaging informatics infrastructure and use cases necessary to achieve the goals of patient-centric care. Privacy and Security, Big Data and Data Plumbing, image and non-image analytics, business aspects of informatics, and the wider description of clinical informatics complete the topics covered in this chapter.

5.1 ONTOLOGIES, STANDARDS, PROFILES

5.1.1 Ontologies

An ontology is a collection of content terms and their relationships to represent concepts in a specific branch of knowledge; relevant to this book are those for medical imaging. Different levels of usage include the definition of a common vocabulary, the standardization of terms and concepts, schemas for transfer and sharing of information, representation of knowledge, and the structures for constructing queries and their responses. Benefits of ontologies include enhancing interoperability between information systems; facilitating the transmission, reuse, and sharing of structured content; as well as integrating knowledge and data. There are many ontologies found in the field of medicine and medical imaging for the electronic exchange of clinical health information. SNOMED-CT (Systematized Nomenclature of Medicine—Clinical Terms) is a standardized, multilingual vocabulary of clinical terminology that is used by physicians and other health care providers supported by the National Library of Medicine within the United States Department of Health and Human Services. In the United States, it is designated as the national standard for additional categories of information in the EHR and health information exchange transactions. It allows healthcare providers to use different terms that mean equivalent things when implementing software applications. For instance, myocardial infarction (MI), heart attack, and MI are interpreted as the same issue by a cardiologist, but to software, these are all different. SNOMED-CT enables semantic interoperability and supports the exchange of normalized clinically validated health data between different providers, researchers, and others in the healthcare environment. Resources include subsets to identify the most commonly used medical codes and terms. This can assist in identifying diseases, signs, and symptoms for subsequent classification, as explained in the next paragraph.

The International Statistical Classification of Diseases and Related Health Problems (ICD), is sponsored by the World Health Organization and is in its tenth revision (ICD-10). This is a manual that contains codes for diseases, signs and symptoms, abnormal findings, and external causes of injury or disease. Individual countries use the ICD-10 coding for reimbursement and resource allocation in their health systems and to develop their own schemas and strategies. In the United States, variant manuals developed by the Centers for Medicare and Medicaid Services (CMS) are called ICD-10 Clinical Modification, (ICD-10-CM) with over 69,000 diagnosis codes and Procedure Coding System (ICD-10-PCS) with over 70,000 procedure codes for inpatient procedures. The ICD-10 content is used to (1) assign codes for procedures, services, conditions, and diagnoses for categorizing conditions and diseases; (2) form the foundation for health care decision making and statistical analysis of populations; and (3) bill for services performed in the hospital inpatient setting.

The Current Procedural Terminology (CPT) is a medical code manual published by the American Medical Association, used to describe the procedures performed on the patient during the interaction including diagnostic, laboratory, radiology, and surgical procedures. Physicians bill and are paid for services performed in a hospital, office setting, or other places of service based on these codes. Often, human coding teams or automated software tools assist in the verification and validation of codes for specific procedures for reimbursement. These codes are more complex than the ICD codes and are typically updated yearly.

In radiology, specific medical terminology and vocabularies are used to describe the anatomy, procedures, and protocols used in day-to-day diagnosis of medical images; however, there are many procedure names and descriptions that are practice-specific. For instance, one group may call a procedure a thorax CT angiogram, while another may call the same procedure a chest CTA. To faithfully exchange health information requires a common terminology to ensure accurate recording and to enhance consistency of data to facilitate medical decision support, outcomes analysis, and quality improvement initiatives. Since 2005 the Radiological Society of North America (RSNA) has gathered radiology professionals and standards organizations to generate a radiology-specific lexicon of terms called RadLex (Radiology Lexicon), and a RadLex Playbook that assigns RPID (RadLex Playbook IDentifier) tags to those terms (RSNA, 2020a). RadLex has been widely adopted in radiology and for use in registries, such as the American College of Radiology (ACR) Dose Index Registry (DIR). By providing standard names and codes for radiologic studies, the playbook facilitates a variety of operational and quality improvement efforts such as workflow optimization, radiation dose tracking, and image exchange. A more widely adopted and broader standard that covers tests and measurements in many medical domains is called LOINC (Logical Observation Identifiers Names and Codes), initiated in 1994 by the Regenstrief Institute, a distinguished medical research organization part of Indiana University. A harmonized effort to unify these ontologies has been established by both sponsors to use LOINC codes as the primary identifiers for radiology procedures (LOINC, 2019). A more comprehensive and widely adopted vocabulary standard will assist in making radiology procedure data more accessible to clinicians when and where they need it.

5.1.2 Standards Organizations

The acquisition, transfer, processing, diagnosis, and storage of medical imaging information is a complex process—no single system in an Information Technology (IT) environment can provide all the functionality necessary for safe, high quality, accurate, and efficient operations. Information systems must, therefore, share data and status with each other. This requires either proprietary interfaces (expensive to implement, difficult to maintain, and tightly controlled by the vendor) or IT standards, which are consensus documents that openly define information system behavior. The American National Standards Institute (ANSI) is the United States organization that coordinates standards development and accredits Standards Development Organizations (SDOs) as well as designates technical advisory groups to the International Organization for Standardization (ISO). In healthcare, two of the most important SDOs are Health Level 7 (HL7) and the National Electrical Manufacturers Association (NEMA). Standards, as applied to medical imaging informatics, have evolved over the years through consultation and consensus of key stakeholders, including manufacturers of medical imaging equipment, manufacturers of medical data software and systems such as the Radiology Information System (RIS), EHR (also known as the electronic medical record—EMR), PACS, professional societies, and end-users who participate, contribute, and update the standards content to ensure interoperability and communication amongst healthcare information systems and devices. Standards define communications protocols, structures, and formats for textual messages, images, instructions, payload deliveries, transactions, and a host of other information for technical, semantic, and process interoperability. IT standards relevant for imaging include Internet standards, the HL7 standard, and the Digital Imaging and Communications in Medicine (DICOM) standard.

5.1.3 Internet Standards

Computer networking and the Internet are successful because of hardware, protocol, and software standards that have been developed by the Internet Engineering Task Force (IETF) of the Internet Society (https://www.internetsociety.org). The Internet is the global system of interconnected computer networks that use the Internet protocol suite *transmission control protocol/Internet protocol* (TCP/IP) to link devices worldwide. There are many Internet standards relevant to imaging. HyperText Transfer Protocol (HTTP) is an application protocol for distributed, collaborative hypermedia information systems, and is the foundation of data communication for the World Wide Web, one of many application structures and network services foundational to the Internet. HyperText Markup Language (HTML) is the standard markup language for documents designed to be displayed in a web browser. Uniform Resource Locator (URL), also known as a web address, specifies the syntax and semantics for location and access of resources via the Internet. Network Time Protocol (NTP) is used to synchronize clocks in computer systems so that messages are interpreted in the appropriate time frame. Simple Mail Transfer Protocol (SMTP) and Internet Message Access Protocol (IMAP) are the basis for email transactions on the Internet. Multipurpose Internet Message Extensions (MIME) protocol allows extension of email messages to include non-textual content including medical images. Transport Layer Security (TLS) and its predecessor Secure Sockets Layer (SSL) define cryptographic mechanisms for securing the content of Internet transactions. The Syslog Protocol is used to convey event notification messages for audit trail and logging purposes. Extensible Markup Language (XML) is a free, open standard for encoding structured data and serializing it for communication between systems and is the method of choice for most new standards development for distributed systems.

5.1.4 DICOM

DICOM is a set of standards-based protocols for exchanging and storing medical imaging data, as actual images and text associated with images. Managed by the Medical and Imaging Technical Alliance (MITA), a division of NEMA, it is structured as a multi-part document and its Parts are numbered as listed in Table 5-1

TABLE 5-1 PARTS OF THE DICOM STANDARD[a]

The structure of the DICOM standard is divided into parts 1–21.
Part 1: Introduction and Overview
Part 2: Conformance
Part 3: Information Object Definitions
Part 4: Service Class Specifications
Part 5: Data Structures and Encoding
Part 6: Data Dictionary
Part 7: Message Exchange
Part 8: Network Communication Support for Message Exchange
Part 10: Media Storage and File Format for Media Interchange
Part 11: Media Storage Application Profiles
Part 12: Media Formats and Physical Media for Media Interchange
Part 14: Grayscale Standard Display Function
Part 15: Security and System Management Profiles
Part 16: Content Mapping Resource
Part 17: Explanatory Information
Part 18: Web Services
Part 19: Application Hosting
Part 20: Imaging Reports using HL7 Clinical Document Architecture
Part 21: Transformations between DICOM and other Representations

[a]Note: DICOM Parts 9 and 13 are now formally rescinded and no longer available.

(DICOM, 2020). Understanding how these Parts relate to one another is key to navigating the DICOM Standard, as it now constitutes many thousands of pages. (For example, one may refer to a "Part 10 file" as Part 10 defines DICOM file formats.) DICOM is recognized by the International Organization for Standardization as the ISO 10252 standard. DICOM is an open, public standard, and information for developing DICOM-based software applications is defined and regulated by public committees and is now, practically speaking, universal for image exchange for medical imaging modalities. Ever evolving, the standard is maintained in accordance with the procedures of the DICOM Standards Committee through working groups (WGs), standard development processes, public comment, and WG approvals. Proposals for enhancements or corrections (CPs) may be submitted to the Secretariat. Supplements and corrections to the Standard are balloted and approved several times a year. When approved as final text, the change is official and goes into effect immediately. Vendors creating devices or software claiming to support the DICOM standard are required to conform to strict and detailed protocol definitions and must provide documentation of the specific DICOM services and data types supported in a DICOM Conformance Statement as defined by Part 2 of the Standard. DICOM is critical to interoperability and communication of medical imaging and associated data between medical imaging systems and imaging databases. Essentials of DICOM use are covered in Section 5.4.

With the widespread and growing use of the Internet, one area of increasing attention is to the development of web-based tools and Application Programming Interface (API) designs for DICOM, called DICOMWeb—the DICOM standard for web-based medical imaging, consisting of services defined for sending, retrieving, and querying for images and related information. The intent is the provision of a web-browser friendly mechanism for storing, querying, and accessing images using REST (representational state transfer) architectural styles for hypermedia systems and RESTful interfaces so that the applications can be simple, lightweight, and fast.

5.1.5 HL7

HL7 refers to a set of international standards for the exchange, integration, sharing, and retrieval of electronic health information that supports clinical practice and management, delivery, and evaluation of health services. HL7 International is the ANSI-accredited organization for developing HL7 standards. Its high-level goals are to develop coherent, extendible standards that permit structured, encoded healthcare information to be exchanged between computer applications and to meet real-world requirements. The domains that the standard covers are extensive, and the interoperability is achieved through messages and documents. There are two versions of HL7 in current use. Most health systems use HL7 Version 2 (now up to V2.8.2) for their data, which is a version developed in the 1980s before the Internet became mainstream. HL7 is cryptic to the uninitiated, although it is required training in informatics as it is the ubiquitous standard for automated textual information exchange in healthcare IT. Although an exhaustive discussion of HL7 is beyond the scope of this text, one should be familiar at least with the three most common *message types* as they pertain to the imaging chain, respective to PACS: (1) *ORU*—Results; (2) *ORM* — Orders; (3) *ADT*—Admission, Discharge, and Transfer. Two of the common *segment types* are also important: (1) *OBR*—Observation Request; and (2) *OBX*—Observation/Result.

A comprehensive list of message types and segments (HL7, 2007) and general information regarding HL7 can be found at the HL7 website (HL7, 2020). Sample HL7 messages and segments are shown in Section 5.4, Lifecycle of a Radiology Exam.

HL7, compared to DICOM, is much less formally structured (thus allowing tremendous flexibility, but also creating the need to redefine almost every implementation explicitly). As a result, a major amount of effort in healthcare is devoted to the development, documentation, and maintenance of HL7 interfaces. HL7 integration engineering represents a significant fraction of the technical work in healthcare informatics overall, and work is under way to attain a more general model of interoperability.

HL7 Version 3, initiated in 1995 with a formal standard available in 2005, is based on object-oriented principles and XML encoding syntax for messaging, including processes, tools, and rules for the unambiguous understanding of code sources and domains that are being used. Clinical Document Architecture (CDA) is an XML-based markup standard to specify encoding, structure, and semantics of clinical documents for exchange that are human-readable. In the United States, a further restraint on the CDA standard is termed the Continuity of Care Document (CCD), which requires a mandatory textual part for easy interpretation, and a structured part to provide a framework for using coding systems such as SNOMED and LOINC.

Like DICOMWeb, a development in the HL7 community is a new standard called Fast Health Interoperability Resources (FHIR—pronounced "fire") and based on modern web services and RESTful interfaces approach that uses APIs and open-standard file formats such as XML or JSON (JavaScript Object Notation) to store and exchange data. FHIR can fill the needs of the previous HL7 standards (V2, V3, CDA) and provides additional benefits in the ease of interoperability, interfaces, and access to data.

5.1.6 IHE

Integrating the Healthcare Enterprise (IHE) was founded by the RSNA in 1999 and joined by the Healthcare Information Management and Systems Society (HIMSS) soon thereafter. Now, IHE International consists of over 150 member organizations including professional societies, SDOs, government agencies, industry, and academic centers. IHE does not generate IT standards but promotes their use to solve specific complex problems of healthcare information system interoperability and develops "integration profiles" that describe the details of the proposed standards-based solutions. There are many "domains" in which the IHE is organized, similar to a clinical enterprise, such as Radiology, Cardiology, Patient Care Coordination, Patient Care Devices, Pathology and Laboratory Medicine, etc. New domains are added as fields of healthcare adopt the IHE process. Two committees responsible for the work product within a domain are the Planning Committee to strategize the direction and coordination of activities from proposals received, and the Technical Committee to develop an integration profile that describes the specific problem, the standards used to solve the problem (*e.g.*, HL7 and DICOM), and the specifics of the solution. After review within IHE, the integration profile is released for public comment, comments are received/reviewed, and then the profile is tested in a "connectathon," which is a vendor-neutral, monitored testing event. After appearing in the connectathon, the profile is then incorporated into the technical framework of that domain.

For Radiology, there are many integration profiles such as scheduled workflow (SWF), patient information reconciliation (PIR), production and display of mammography images (MAMMO), radiation exposure monitoring (REM), and cross-enterprise document sharing of images (XDS-I). For instance, the latter profile is important in ensuring the proper transfer of medical data and images across enterprises and businesses. Vendors claiming conformance to IHE technical frameworks must provide an integration statement that specifies which IHE actors (the units of functionality) are provided and in which integration profiles they participate. Purchasers of medical imaging equipment can use conformance to the IHE technical framework as a contractual obligation and as an effective shorthand in a request for purchase document that avoids the complexities of specifying standards and methods to achieve a given interoperability. A major benefit of the IHE integration profiles is that a single integration profile can require conformance with DICOM, HL7, and other standards. A commitment by a vendor to support that integration profile will commit the vendor to conforming to the various standards included in that single integration profile. Verification of successful interoperability requires quality control testing, as described in Section 5.3.9—PACS Quality Control.

5.2 COMPUTERS AND NETWORKING

5.2.1 Hardware

Computer hardware includes the physical parts or components of a computer, such as the power supply, cooling fans, case, and motherboard. The motherboard is the main component, with integrated circuitry and backplane connectors that connect all other parts of the computer, including the central processing unit (CPU), graphics processing unit (GPU), random access memory (RAM), graphics, network, and sound cards, expansion cards, and storage devices (both fixed and removable) for temporary or permanent storage. Input and output peripherals are housed externally to the main computer and include a mouse and a keyboard, touchpad (for laptop computers), webcams, microphones, speakers, display monitors, and printers.

The configuration and capability of a computer are important considerations to ensure performance and throughput requirements for a radiologist workstation with the need to view large images and large datasets quickly and efficiently. The CPU processing performance is increased by using multi-core processors (from 2 to 16 and more) on one CPU chip by handling asynchronous events, interrupts and using simultaneous multi-threading to share actual CPU resources. Clock speed governs how fast the CPU can execute instructions and is measured in gigahertz (GHz)—typical values are between 1 to 5 GHz. The GPU is a specialized electronic circuit designed to rapidly manipulate and accelerate the manipulation/processing of images by processing large blocks of data in parallel, making them much more efficient than CPUs in doing such tasks. RAM stores the code and data that are being actively accessed by the CPU and GPU modules. With medical images and ever-expanding sizes and amount of image data, a configuration of a minimum of 16 GB RAM and perhaps 32–64 GB and greater is recommended, depending on the applications of a particular system to ensure that an entire study with relevant prior studies and multiple applications (PACS, RIS, Reporting, EHR, etc.) can be available without having to send information back and forth from slower data access on solid-state or spinning disk storage media. Size and type of computer storage media must be configured with enough capacity, typically in the multi-terabyte range, and network card bandwidth (*e.g.*, 1 Gb/s or higher) must be matched to avoid bottlenecks in data transfer. Portable storage devices such as universal serial bus (USB) drives and Secure Digital (SD) cards use flash memory—a non-volatile computer memory storage medium that can be electronically erased and re-programmed, offering fast read and write access times (although slower than RAM). These storage devices offer capacities in the 100s of gigabyte range, with many exceeding terabytes.

5.2.2 Software and Application Programming Interface

Software refers to the programs, consisting of sequences of instructions, which are executed by a computer. Software is commonly categorized as application programs or systems software.

An *applications program*, commonly referred to as an *application*, is a program that performs a specific function or functions for a user. Examples of applications are e-mail programs, word processing/presentation programs, web browsers, image display, and speech recognition programs.

System software is designed to run on computer hardware and as a platform for other software. It refers to the files and programs that make up the computer's *operating system* (OS), such as Microsoft Windows, Mac OS, and Linux Ubuntu. System files contain libraries of system services, functions, device drivers, system preferences, and many other configuration files. The system software is the interface between the hardware and specific user applications to manage memory, input/output devices, internal and peripheral devices, system performance, and error messages. Driver software makes it possible for connected components to perform their intended tasks as directed by the OS. Such components include a keyboard, mouse, display card, network card, and soundcard. Firmware is operational software embedded within a memory chip for the OS to identify and run commands to manage and control activities of any single hardware component. The most important firmware is the BIOS (Basic Input/Output System) or UEFI (Unified Extended Firmware Interface) on a motherboard. This loads first as a computer is powered up to wake up all hardware (processor, memory, disk drives) and to run the bootloader to install the OS.

Programming language translators are intermediate programs called compilers, assemblers, and interpreters. They allow software programmers to translate high-level language source code that humans can understand, such as Java, C++, and Python, into machine-language code that computer processors can understand. Machine code is written in a number system of base 2, with either a 0 or a 1 representing an "on-off" switch called a "bit" at a computer memory location, and typically sequenced in 8-bit chunks called a byte. A word is the largest unit of data that can be addressed on memory (i.e., register size). Expressed in bits, the size of word with which a processor can handle data in average consumer laptop computers today is 32 to 64 bits.

Utility software is a type of system software that sits between the OS and application software and is intended for computer diagnostic and maintenance tasks. Examples include anti-virus, disk partition, file compression/defragmentation, and firewall algorithms to ensure optimal function and security of the computer.

System services and libraries are a specific API to provide access to tools and resources in an OS that enables developers to create software applications by specifying how software components can access and leverage aspects of the OS. An API defines the correct way to request services from an OS or other application and expose data within different contexts and across different channels. Private APIs have specifications for a specific company's products and services that are not shared, public or open APIs can be used by any third party without restrictions, and partner APIs are used by specific parties that have a sharing agreement. They are also classified as local, web, or program APIs. Local APIs offer OS services to application programs to provide database access, memory management, security, and network services. An example is the Microsoft.NET framework. Web APIs are designed to represent resources like HTML pages and addressed using the HTTP protocol; thus, any web URL activates a web API. Web APIs are often called REST or RESTful because the publisher of the REST interface does not save data internally between requests. This allows many users to request information independently and intermingled, similar as they are on the Internet. Simple programming tools or even no programming at all can be used for data access using the REST model. When APIs need to communicate between different nodes on a network, a mechanism called a Remote Procedure Call (RPC) can be employed, as well. Modern Operating Systems provide a rich set of remotely accessible system services. An extension to provide security and fully distributed software components is part of a broader Service Oriented Architecture (SOA). SOA refers to architectures designed with a focus on services. Begun in the 1990s, the classic approach of SOA architectures was based upon complex services to build complex systems. SOA has evolved to encompass microservices, which represent a more recent subset by implementing applications as a set of simple independently deployable services using modern JavaScript. Web services and RESTful interfaces are also under the umbrella of SOA.

5.2.3 Networks and Gateways

Computer networks permit the transfer of information between computers, allowing computers to enable services such as the electronic transmission of messages (e-mail), transfer of computer files, and use of distant computers. Networks, based upon the distances they span and degree of interconnectivity, may be described as local area networks (LANs) or wide area networks (WANs). A *LAN* connects computers within a department, a building such as a medical center, and perhaps neighboring buildings, whereas a *WAN* connects computers at large distances from each other. Most WANs today consist of multiple LANs connected by medium or long-distance communication links. The largest WAN in aggregate is the Internet itself.

Networks have both hardware and software components. A connection must exist between computers so that they can exchange information. Common connections include coaxial cable, copper wiring, optical fiber cables, and electronic connections such as radio wave and microwave communication systems used by Bluetooth and Wi-Fi communication links. Optical fiber cables have several advantages over cables or wiring carrying electrical signals, particularly with long-distance connections, including no electrical interference, lower error rates, greater transmission distances without the need for repeaters to read and retransmit the signals, and highest transmission rates. The benefit of wireless communication systems such as Wi-Fi is the freedom from hard-wired connections, although transmission rates are typically lower than a direct connection. Software components are also required between the user application program and the hardware of the communications link, necessitating network protocols for communication and provision of services. Both hardware and software must comply with established protocols to achieve successful transfer of information.

In most networks, multiple computers share communication pathways. Network protocols facilitate this sharing by dividing the information to be transmitted into *packets.* Some protocols permit packets of variable size, whereas others permit only packets of a fixed size. Each packet has a header containing information identifying its destination. Large networks usually employ switching devices to forward packets between network segments or even between entire networks. Each device on a network, whether a computer or switching device, is called a *node,* and the communications pathways between them are called *links.* Each computer is connected to a network by a network adapter, also called a network interface, installed on the I/O bus of the computer, or incorporated on the motherboard. Each interface between a node and a network is identified by a unique number called a *network address.* A desktop computer usually has only a single interface, but a server generally has multiple interfaces to facilitate redundancy and throughput management. A switching device connecting two or more networks may have an address on each network.

The maximal data transfer rate of a link or a connection is called the *bandwidth,* a term originally used to describe the data transfer capacities of analog communications channels. An actual network may not achieve its full nominal bandwidth because of overhead or inefficiencies in its implementation. The term *throughput* is commonly used to describe the maximal data transfer rate that is achieved. Bandwidth and throughput are usually described in units of megabits per second (10^6 bps = 1 Mbps) or gigabits per second (10^9 bps = 1 Gbps). These units should not be confused with megabytes per second (MBps) and gigabytes per second (GBps)—recall that a *byte* consists of eight *bits.* Note that the raw network bandwidth must also accommodate overhead from various protocols (packet framing, addressing, etc.) so the actual delivered data bandwidth will be lower than network bandwidth. The former is sometimes referred to as "payload capacity" and involves many other factors beyond basic network architecture.

The *latency* is the time delay of a transmission between two nodes. In a packet-switching network (a network that groups data into packets that contain a header to define the destination and a payload that carries the information), it is the time required for a small packet to be transferred. It is determined by factors such as the total lengths of the links between the two nodes, the speeds of the signals, and the delays caused by any intermediate repeaters and packet switching devices.

Networks are commonly designed in layers, each layer following a specific protocol. Figure 5-1 shows the International Standards Organization (ISO) Open Systems Interconnection (OSI) model of a network consisting of seven layers. Each layer in the OSI stack provides a service to the layer above. The top layer in the stack is the Application Layer (Layer 7 in Fig. 5-1). Application programs, commonly called *applications,* function at this layer. Applications are programs that perform useful tasks and are distinguished from systems software, such as an OS. On a workstation, applications include the programs, such as an e-mail program, word processing program, web browser, or a program for displaying medical images, with which the user directly interacts. On a server, an application is a program providing a service to other computers on the network. The purpose of a computer network is to allow applications on different computers to exchange information.

Network communications begin at the Application Layer. The application passes the information to be transmitted to the next lower layer in the stack. The information is passed from layer to layer, with each layer adding information, such as addresses and error-detection information, until it reaches the Physical Layer (Layer 1 in Fig. 5-1). The Physical Layer sends the information to the destination computer, where it is passed up the layer stack to the application layer of the destination computer or

■ **FIGURE 5-1** International Standards Organization (ISO) Open Systems Interconnect (OSI) 7-layer network model is a conceptual framework used to describe the functions of a networking system. It characterizes computing functions to support interoperability between different products and software and defines 7 layers of network architecture. This is foundational to understanding concepts such as Layer 3 switching (discussed below).

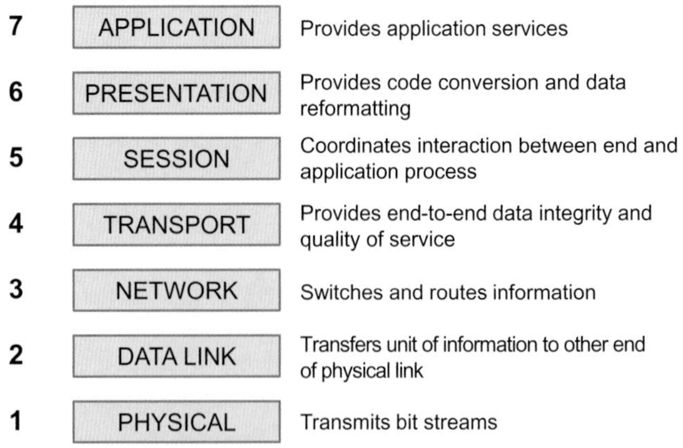

7	APPLICATION	Provides application services
6	PRESENTATION	Provides code conversion and data reformatting
5	SESSION	Coordinates interaction between end and application process
4	TRANSPORT	Provides end-to-end data integrity and quality of service
3	NETWORK	Switches and routes information
2	DATA LINK	Transfers unit of information to other end of physical link
1	PHYSICAL	Transmits bit streams

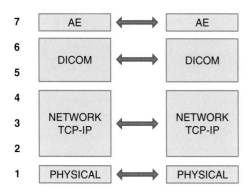

7	AE	⟷	AE
6			
5	DICOM	⟷	DICOM
4			
3	NETWORK TCP-IP	⟷	NETWORK TCP-IP
2			
1	PHYSICAL	⟷	PHYSICAL

■ **FIGURE 5-2** The OSI 7-layer framework is used to model the interconnection of medical imaging equipment. DICOM uses the OSI upper layer service to separate the exchange of DICOM messages at the Application Layer from the communication support provided by the lower layers. The DICOM upper layer augments TCP/IP and combines the upper layer protocols into a simple to implement single protocol on general networks. This is an essential property of the modern Standard—avoiding proprietary network architectures (which were once common).

device. As the information is passed up the layer stack, each layer removes the information appended by the corresponding layer on the sending computer until the information sent by the application on the sending device is delivered to the intended application on the receiving device.

The lower network layers (Layers 1 and 2 in Fig. 5-1) are responsible for the transmission of packets from one node to another over a LAN or point-to-point link and enable computers or devices with dissimilar hardware and OSs to be physically connected. As shown in Figure 5-2, the Physical Layer transmits physical signals over a communication channel (*e.g.*, the copper wiring, optical fiber cable, or radio link connecting nodes) using a protocol that describes the signals (*e.g.*, voltages, near-infrared signals, or radio waves) sent between the nodes. Layer 2, the Data Link Layer, encapsulates the information received from the layer above into packets for transmission across the LAN or point-to-point link. The packets are transferred to Layer 1 for transmission using a protocol that describes the packet formats, functions such as media access control (determining when a node may transmit a packet on a LAN), and error checking of packets received over a LAN or point-to-point link. These tasks are usually implemented in hardware.

Between the lower layers in the protocol stack and the Application Layer are intermediate layers that mediate between applications and the network interface. These layers are usually implemented in software and incorporated in a computer's OS. Many intermediate level protocols are available, their complexity depending upon the scope and complexity of the networks they are designed to serve.

LAN protocols are typically designed to permit the connection of computers over limited distances. On some small LANs, the computers are all directly connected and so only one computer can transmit at a time and usually only a single computer accepts the information. This places a practical limit on the number of computers and other devices that can be placed on a LAN without excessive network congestion. The congestion can be relieved by dividing the LAN into *segments* connected by packet switching devices, such as bridges, switches, and routers, that only transmit information intended for other segments.

The most used LAN protocols are the various forms of Ethernet. Before transmission over Ethernet, information to be transmitted is divided into packets, each with a header specifying the addresses of the transmitting and destination nodes. Ethernet is "contention-based", meaning that a node ready to transmit a packet first "listens" to determine if another node is transmitting. If none is, it attempts to transmit. If two nodes inadvertently attempt to transmit at nearly the same moment, a collision occurs. Each node then ceases transmission, waits a randomly determined but traffic-dependent time interval, and again attempts to transmit. Media access defining collision control is important, particularly for heavily used networks.

Modern forms of Ethernet are configured in a star topology (Fig. 5-3) with a switch as the central node. The switch does not broadcast the packets to all nodes. Instead, it stores each packet in memory, reads the address on the packet, and then forwards the packet only to the destination node. Thus, the switch permits several pairs of nodes to simultaneously communicate at the full bandwidth of the network. Fast Ethernet (100 Base-TX) permits data transfer rates up to 100 Mbps. More common are Gigabit Ethernet and Ten Gigabit Ethernet, which provide bandwidths of one and ten Gbps, respectively.

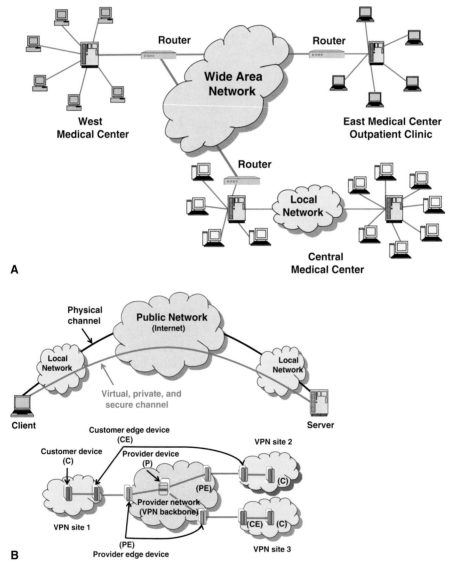

■ **FIGURE 5-3 A.** Wide area networks are commonly formed by linking together two or more local area networks (LANs) using routers and links. Routers connect and relay packets to intended destinations. Most often, the public Internet with a virtual private network is used, in lieu of older leased T1 and T3 links between LANs. **B.** The public internet is leveraged to allow clients to interact with servers through a node to node private and secure channel connection. This is achieved as part of carrier-provided VPNs as shown on the lower half of the figure, using "edge devices" to provide secure connections to each local area network and ensuring quality of service using multiprotocol label switching.

An extended LAN connects facilities, such as the various buildings of a medical center, over a larger area than can be served by a single LAN segment by connecting individual LAN segments. Links, sometimes called "backbones," of high bandwidth media such as Gigabit or Ten Gigabit Ethernet, may be used to carry heavy information traffic between individual LAN segments.

For Wi-Fi, there are several standards that dictate theoretical and actual speeds of most current Wi-Fi networks, certified by the Institute for Electronics and Electrical Engineers (IEEE), with the 802.11 standard. Depending on network cards and connections, the lowest speed will dictate the overall throughput of connected systems. The 802.11ac standard, often referred to as Gigabit Wi-Fi, operates in the 5-GHz band. Future Wi-Fi standard implementation of 802.11ax (Wi-Fi 6) portends even greater speeds, with multiple streams of channels and a throughput of over 10 Gbps depending on the transmitter and receiver configurations. With the ubiquitous availability of cell phones and cellular networks and advances in the use of spectrum bands (those frequencies that are licensed by the cellular companies), a move to a fifth-generation (5G) mobile network is being introduced, to drastically increase the maximum speed of connections and decrease the latency over that of the common 4G mobile network. It is worth noting that 5 GHz Wi-Fi has nothing to do with 5G mobile networks.

WANs are formed by linking multiple LANs by devices called *routers* as shown in Figure 5-3A. Routers are specialized computers or switches designed to route packets among networks by performing packet switching, reading the packet information, determining the intended destinations, and, by following directions in routing tables, forwarding the packets toward their destinations. Each packet may be sent through several routers before reaching its destination. Routers communicate with each other to determine optimal routes for packets.

Routers follow a protocol that assigns each interface in the connected networks a unique network address distinct from its LAN address. Routers operate at the Network Layer (Fig. 5-2) of the network protocol stack. The dominant routable protocol today is the IP, described below.

The Internet Protocol Suite, commonly called TCP/IP, is a packet-based suite of protocols used by many large networks and the Internet. TCP/IP permits information to be transmitted from one computer to another across a series of networks connected by routers. TCP/IP is specifically designed for internetworking, that is, linking separate networks that may use dissimilar lower-level protocols. TCP/IP operates at protocol layers above those of lower-layer protocols such as Ethernet. The two main protocols of TCP/IP are the *Transmission Control Protocol (TCP)*, operating at the Transport Layer and the *Internet Protocol (IP)*, operating at the Network Layer (Layers 4 and 3, respectively, in Fig. 5-1). An enhancement to this basic model involves what is termed Layer 3 Switching, generally in the context of VLANs (Virtual LANs). Increasingly, VLANs are becoming the preferred model for PACS network architectures but are beyond the scope of this text (Meraki, 2020).

Communication begins when an application passes information to the Transport Layer, along with information designating the destination computer and the application on the destination computer, which is to receive the information. The Transport Layer, following TCP, divides the information into packets, attaches to each packet a header containing information such as a packet sequence number and error-detection information, and passes the packets to the Network Layer. The Network Layer, following IP, may further subdivide the packets. The Network Layer adds a header to each packet containing information such as the source address and the destination address. The Network Layer then passes these packets to the Data Link Layer (Layer 2 in Fig. 5-1) for transmission across the LAN or point-to-point link to which the computer is connected.

The Data Link Layer, following the protocol of the specific LAN or point-to-point link, encapsulates the IP packets into packets for transmission. Each packet is given another header containing information such as the LAN address of the destination computer. For example, if the lower level protocol is Ethernet, the Data Link Layer encapsulates each packet it receives from the Network Layer into an Ethernet packet. The Data Link Layer then passes the packets to the Physical Layer, where they are converted into electrical, infrared, or radio signals and transmitted.

Each computer and router is assigned an *IP address.* Under IP Version 4 (IPv4), an IP address consists of a 32-bit number in dot-decimal notation consisting of four groups of 3 whole numbers, each separated by a period. Each group can have a value ranging from 0 to 255, making a theoretical maximum value of 255.255.255.255. In reality the actual maximum is 239.255.255.255 because certain groups of addresses are reserved for specific operational Internet functions. Each part represents a group of 8 bits of the address, thus permitting 2^{32} or over 4 billion distinct addresses. The high order bits (two bytes) of the address represent the network prefix and the low-order bits (two bytes) identify the subnet and the individual computer or device on the network as illustrated in Figure 5-4 (top). With the proliferation of Internet devices, IP version 6 (IPv6) uses a 128-bit number providing up to 2^{128} or approximately 3.4×10^{38} addresses, likely to be enough for the foreseeable future (Fig. 5-4, bottom). Currently, these two versions of the IP are in simultaneous use; however, each version defines the format of the address differently. IP addresses typically refer to the addresses defined by IPv4, per current historical prevalence. IP addresses do not have meaning to the lower network layers. IP defines methods by which a sending computer determines, for the destination IP address, the next lower layer address, such as a LAN address, to which the packets are to be sent by the lower network layers.

IP is referred to as a "connectionless protocol" or a "best-effort protocol." This means that the packets are routed across the networks to the destination computer following IP, but some may be lost on the way. IP does not guarantee delivery or even require verification of delivery. On the other hand, TCP is a connection-oriented protocol providing reliable delivery. Following TCP, Network Layer 4 of the sending computer initiates a dialog with Layer 4 of the destination computer, negotiating matters such as packet size as shown in Figure 5-2. Layer 4 on the destination computer requests the retransmission of any missing or corrupted packets, places the packets in the correct order, recovers the information from the packets, and passes it up to the proper application.

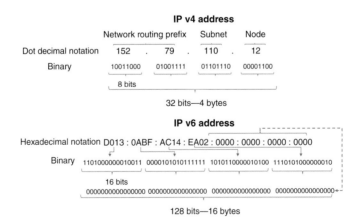

■ **FIGURE 5-4** Internet Protocol addresses. Top: IP version 4, shown in "Dot-decimal notation" as four components—the first two represent the network routing prefix, the third the subnet, and the fourth the specific node connection. Each is shown as the binary equivalent requiring 8 bits, for a total of 32 bits or 4 bytes to represent the specific address. IPv4 can address 2^{32} unique locations. Bottom: IP version 6, shown in colon hexadecimal notation as 8 hexadecimal components—the leading 4 components are currently used, each representing 16 bits of unique address locations. The latter 4 components are currently nulled for future use. In all, IP v6 can address 2^{128} unique locations.

The advantages of designing networks in layers should now be apparent. LANs conforming to a variety of protocols can be linked into a single internet by installing a router in each LAN and connecting the routers with point-to-point links. The point-to-point links between the LANs can also conform to multiple protocols. All that is necessary is that all computers and routers implement the same WAN protocols at the middle network layers. A LAN can be replaced by one conforming to another protocol without replacing the software in the OS that implements TCP/IP and without modifying application programs. A programmer developing an application need not be concerned with details of the lower network layers. TCP/IP can evolve without requiring changes to applications programs or LANs. Each network layer must conform to a standard in communicating with the layer above and the layer below.

A router performs packet switching that differs from switches that merely forward identical copies of received packets. On a LAN, the packets addressed to the router are those intended for transmission outside the LAN. The LAN destination address on a packet received by the router is that of the router itself.

The *Internet* (with a capital letter "I") is an international network of networks using the TCP/IP protocol. A network using TCP/IP within a single company or organization is sometimes called an *intranet*. The Internet is not owned by any single company or nation. The main part of the Internet consists of national and international backbone networks, consisting mainly of fiber optic links connected by routers, provided by major telecommunications companies. These backbone networks are interconnected by routers. Large organizations can contract for connections from their networks directly to the backbone networks. Individual people and small organizations connect to the Internet by contracting with companies called Internet service providers (ISPs), which operate regional networks that are connected to the Internet backbone networks.

IP addresses, customarily written in dot-decimal format (*e.g.*, 152.79.110.12), are inconvenient. Instead, host names, such as http://www.ucdmc.ucdavis.edu, are used to designate a specific computer attached to the network. The domain name system (DNS) is an Internet service consisting of servers that translate host names into IP addresses.

The Internet itself may be used to link geographically separated LANs into a WAN. Encryption and authentication can be used to create a virtual private network (VPN) within the Internet. However, a disadvantage to using the Internet to link LANs into a WAN was the historical inability of the Internet to guarantee a high quality of service. Disadvantages to the general public Internet today include lack of reliability, inability to guarantee required bandwidth, and inability to give critical traffic priority over less important traffic. For critical applications, such as PACS and teleradiology, quality of service is the major reason why "hard" leased lines were the prevailing mechanism used to link distant sites. Now it is possible to contract specifically for connectivity from major carriers defining specific Service Level Agreements (SLAs) and Quality of Service (QoS) as part of carrier-provided VPNs (Fig. 5-3B). Older technologies such as hardware X.25, Frame Relay, or T1 have generally now been superseded (or encapsulated) by protocols such as MPLS (Multiprotocol Label Switching). MPLS defines the path between nodes rather than between explicit point-to-point endpoints.

5.2.4 Servers

A *server* is a computer on a network that provides a service to other computers on the network. A computer with a large array of magnetic disks that provides data storage for other computers is called a file server. There are also print servers, application servers, database servers, e-mail servers, web servers, and cloud servers. Most servers are now established in a "virtual machine" environment, where the virtual machine (VM) is based on a computer architecture to provide the functionality and emulation of a physical computer in a centralized location. The implementation may involve specialized hardware, software, or a combination. VM instances can allow multiple OSs such as Windows and Linux; provide multiple CPUs to a specific software instance; allocate storage space; and meet unique needs as necessary in an enterprise environment. This provides flexibility, efficiency, and ability to reallocate and expand/shrink resources as necessary to meet the needs of the informatics computing infrastructure. A cloud server is a virtual server running in a cloud computing environment that is hosted and delivered on a cloud computing platform via the Internet and can be accessed remotely. Configuration of such a server for a PACS server-side rendering environment requires several component servers to handle tasks within the image database such as: data extraction, DICOM conversion, image rendering, storage, and load balancing. A computer on a network that makes use of a server is called a *client* and is typically a workstation.

Two common terms used to describe client-server relationships are *thick client* and *thin client.* "Thick client" describes the situation in which the client computer provides most information processing and the function of the server is mainly to store information, whereas "thin client" describes the situation in which most information processing is provided by the server and the client mainly serves to display the information. An example would be the production of volume rendered images from a set of CT images. In the thin client relationship, the volume rendered images would be produced by the server and sent to a workstation for display, whereas in a thick client relationship, the images would be produced by software and/or a graphics processor installed on the workstation. The thin client relationship can allow the use of less capable and less expensive workstations and enable specialized software and hardware, such as a graphics processor and multiple Graphics Processor Units (GPUs), on a single server comprised of several CPUs for specific tasks and large amounts of RAM to be used by several or many workstations.

5.2.5   Cloud Computing

The cloud computing paradigm represents the practice of using a network of remote servers and software hosted on the Internet to deliver a service. An example of a Cloud computing provider is the email service Gmail provided by Google, while an example of a Cloud storage provider is Dropbox. Medical imaging software vendors are also using the Cloud to provide client services and databases over the Internet for storage and archiving of imaging and associated data to a server that is maintained by a cloud provider. Clients send files to the cloud server instead of or in addition to local storage. Cloud storage can be used as a backup in the event of local failures.

When describing cloud-provisioned services, terms such as "SaaS" (Software as a Service), IaaS (Infrastructure as a Service) and PaaS (Platform as a Service) are often used. These are often used together to extend local PACS and vendor-neutral archive (VNA) storage (see Section 5.3.4) capacity into the Cloud as external resources.

Benefits of cloud computing and storage include (1) the ability to cut back on operating costs for in-house hosting solutions and storage; (2) accessibility to files, images, and documents from anywhere there is a usable Internet connection with necessary sign-on credentials and access; (3) recovery to retrieve any files or data from the cloud that have been damaged or lost on a local computer; (4) automated syncing of changes made to one or more files across all affiliated devices; (5) increased layers of security and redundancy usually implemented by third-party cloud providers to prevent files from ending up in the wrong hands or from being lost; and (6) dramatic economies of scale pricing (low-tier/higher latency, such as Amazon Web

Services (AWS) Glacier can cost as little as $5/TB/yr at scale for large volumes). Some disadvantages of cloud computing and services include the following: (1) a dependence on an Internet connection with upload and download speed and latency issues; (2) hard drives and physical storage devices are often still needed for many applications requiring very high-performance access; (3) end-user customer support is often lacking; (5) after migrating data, concern about privacy and who owns the information could be a major issue for medically sensitive data.

The concept of the "cloud" allows faster information deployment with little management and little supervision oversight and promises much greater expansion and use in the future. The advantages and disadvantages of cloud services should be considered prior to opting for implementation for specific applications. Additionally, cloud storage architectures such as Amazon's AWS, or Microsoft Azure are increasingly being leveraged for lower-access VNA or PACS storage tiers as well as part of DR (Disaster Recovery) models. Historically external cloud storage services were avoided by most healthcare organizations where long-term record retention was required, but services such as AWS and Azure have largely dispelled these concerns. These services are now both persistent and secure.

5.2.6 Active Directory

Lightweight Directory Access Protocol (LDAP) is an open, vendor-neutral, industry-standard application protocol for accessing and maintaining directory information services over an IP network. Active Directory is a directory service developed by Microsoft for the Windows domain networks and is included in most Windows Server OSs as a set of processes and services that instantiate LDAP as well as Kerberos for security. A server running Active Directory Domain Service (AD DS) authenticates and authorizes all users and computers in a Windows domain network and assigns and enforces security policies for all computers on the network. It is also used to install or update software.

5.2.7 Internet of Things

The Internet of Things (IoT) encompasses everything connected to the Internet with a unique identifier (UID), and the ability to collect and share data about their environment and the way they are used over a network without requiring human interaction. IoT includes an extraordinary number of objects, from self-driving cars, to home light switches, to fitness devices, and more. In the healthcare environment, IoT has numerous applications, from remote monitoring to smart sensors, to medical device integration for dialysis machines and all imaging modalities in a Radiology Department. While there are many benefits, there are also challenges, chiefly about data security and device management. Interoperability is a key attribute for IoT to deliver better patient care, but also a huge potential liability with remote access and cybersecurity concerns about control of devices, breaches of privacy and loss or corruption of data. The health and safety of patients are at risk when IoT devices are not regularly patched and updated, particularly for devices outside a hospital network.

5.3 PICTURE ARCHIVING AND COMMUNICATIONS SYSTEM

5.3.1 PACS Infrastructure

A PACS is a collection of software, interfaces, display workstations, and databases for the storage, transfer, and display of medical images. A PACS consists of a digital archive to store images, display workstations to permit physicians to view the images, and a computer network to transfer images and related information between the imaging devices and the archive and between the archive and the display workstations. A database program tracks the locations of images and related information in the archive and software permits the selection and manipulation of images for interpretation by radiologists and consultation by referring physicians. PACS can replicate images at multiple display workstations simultaneously and be a repository for several years' images. For efficiency of workflow and avoidance of errors, the PACS exchanges information with other information systems, such as the EHR, RIS, and other information systems on the hospital, clinic, or teleradiology network. A web server is typically part of the PACS to provide images to referring clinicians within the enterprise network. A schematic of a PACS with sub-components and simple connectivity is illustrated in Figure 5-5.

PACSs vary widely in size and scope. For example, a PACS may be limited to a nuclear medicine department, the ultrasound section, mammography, or a cardiac catheterization laboratory. Such a small single-modality PACS is sometimes called a *mini-PACS*. Mini-PACSs may exist in a large medical enterprise that has adopted an enterprise-wide PACS if the enterprise PACS lacks functionality needed by specialists such as mammographers, nuclear medicine physicians, or ultrasound specialists (Fig. 5-6). On the other hand, a PACS may incorporate all imaging modalities in a system of several medical centers and affiliated clinics (see Fig. 5-3A). Another model is a federated PACS model, allowing independent PACS functionality at different sites and sharing of DICOM images and information through a software federation manager. Furthermore, a PACS must make images available to the ER, ICUs, and referring

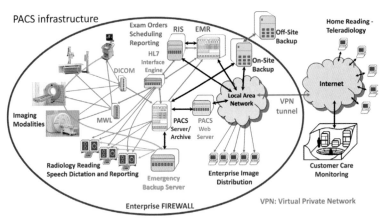

■ **FIGURE 5-5** Modern PACS infrastructure. The PACS is interconnected to the imaging modalities and information systems including the RIS and the EHR. The RIS provides the patient database for scheduling and reporting of image examinations through HL7 transactions and provides modality worklists (MWLs) with patient demographic information to the modalities, allowing technologists to select patient-specific scheduled studies to ensure accuracy. After a study is performed, image information is sent to the PACS in DICOM format and reconciled with the exam-specific information (accession number). Radiologist reporting is performed at the primary diagnostic workstations and transmitted to the RIS via HL7 transactions. An emergency backup server ensures business continuity (orange line directly connecting the modalities) in the event of unscheduled PACS downtime. For referring physicians and remote reading radiologists (teleradiology applications) a webserver is connected to the Internet—access is protected by a Virtual Private Network (VPN) to obtain images and reports. Users within the medical enterprise have protected access through a LAN. Also depicted are an "off-site" backup archive for disaster recovery and real-time customer care monitoring to provide around the clock support. A mirror archive provides on-site backup within the enterprise firewall with immediate availability in case of failure of the primary archive.

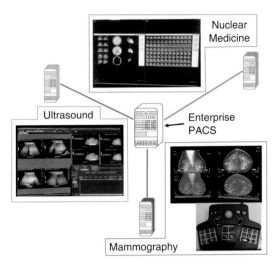

■ FIGURE 5-6 Mini PACS provide modality-specific capabilities for handling images in ways that are not available in a generalized enterprise PACS. Established mini PACS include *Mammography* with navigation enhancements through a proprietary electronic panel and robust hanging protocols; *Ultrasound* for handling video sequences more efficiently and facilitating structured reports; *Nuclear Medicine* for improving display of smaller images with unique contrast/brightness adjustments, and support of quantitative evaluations of uptake and physiological rate constants.

physicians. The goal is to store all images in a medical center or healthcare system on PACS, with images available to interpreting and referring clinicians through the EHR or thin-client workstations within the enterprise, with the PACS receiving requests for studies from the RIS, and with the PACS providing information to the RIS on the status of studies, and images available on the EHR. Another goal, far from being achieved, is to make medical images and related reports available regionally and nationwide, regardless of where they were acquired.

Image display is a key component in the imaging chain and a significant component of the PACS. An interpretation workstation for large matrix images (digital radiographs, including mammograms) is commonly equipped with two high-luminance 54-cm diagonal 3 or 5 megapixels (MP) displays, in the portrait orientation, to permit the simultaneous comparison of two images in near full spatial resolution (Fig. 5-7). A "navigation" consumer-grade display (or displays) provides access to the RIS database, patient information, reading worklist, digital speech recognition/voice dictation system, EHR, and the Internet. Images are distributed throughout the enterprise and viewed on many different types of displays. Characteristics of the different display types used for viewing are discussed in terms of technical specifications, human visual performance, gray level calibration, and quality control in Section 5.3.7.

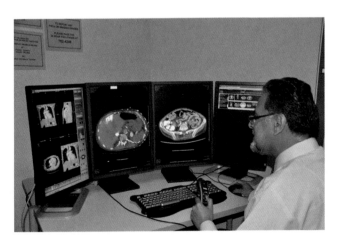

■ FIGURE 5-7 Interpretation workstation containing two 1.5k by 2k pixel (3 megapixel) portrait-format color displays for high resolution and high luminance image interpretation, flanked by two 1.9k by 1k (2 MP) color "navigation" displays (left and right) for PACS access, patient worklist, timeline, and thumbnail image displays;, digital voice dictation reporting, and EMR and RIS information access. The keyboard, mouse, and image navigation and voice dictation device assist Ramit Lamba, M.D., in his interpretation duties.

5.3.2   Image Distribution

Computer networks permit exchanges of images and related information between the imaging devices and the PACS, between the PACS and display workstations, and between the PACS and other information systems such as the RIS and EHR. A PACS may have its own LAN or LAN segment, or it may share another LAN, such as a medical center LAN. The bandwidth requirements depend upon the imaging modalities and their composite workloads. For example, a LAN adequate for a nuclear medicine or ultrasound miniPACS may not be adequate to support an entire imaging department. (The former might be adequate at 100 Mbps, where the latter may require 10 Gbps.) Network traffic typically varies cyclically throughout the day. Network traffic also tends to be "bursty"; there may be short periods of very high traffic, separated by periods of low traffic. Network design must consider both peak and average bandwidth requirements and the delays that are tolerable. Network segmentation, whereby groups of imaging, archival, and display devices that communicate frequently with each other are placed on separate segments, is commonly used to reduce network congestion. Network media providing different bandwidths may be used for various network segments. For example, a network segment serving nuclear medicine will likely have a lower bandwidth requirement than a network segment serving CT scanners or Mammography. With the larger size and number of images and video streams being produced, a larger network bandwidth such as 1 to 10 Gbps is essential to reduce the number of transient slowdowns of network speed throughout a workday.

5.3.3   Image Compression

The massive amount of data in radiological studies (Table 5-2) poses considerable challenges regarding storage and transmission. Image compression reduces the number of bytes in an image or set of images, thereby decreasing the time required to transfer images and increasing the number of images that can be stored. There are two categories of compression: *reversible*, also called bit-preserving, lossless, or recoverable compression; and *irreversible*, also called lossy or non-recoverable, compression. In reversible compression, once the data is uncompressed, the image is identical to the original. Typically, reversible compression of medical images provides compression ratios from about two to three up to five to one, depending on the complexity of the image information. Reversible compression takes advantage of redundancies in data. It is not possible to store random and equally likely bit patterns in less space without the loss of information. However, medical images incorporate considerable redundancies, permitting them to be converted into a more compact representation without loss of information. For example, although an image may have a dynamic range (the difference between maximal and minimal pixel values) requiring 12 bits per pixel, pixel values usually change only slightly from pixel to adjacent pixel and so changes from one pixel to the next can be represented by just a few bits. In this case, the image could be compressed without a loss of information by storing the differences between adjacent pixel values instead of the pixel values themselves. Dynamic image sequences, because of similarities from one image to the next, permit high compression ratios.

   In irreversible compression, some information is lost and so the uncompressed image will not exactly match the original image. However, irreversible compression permits much higher compression; ratios of 15-to-1 or higher are possissble with very little loss of image quality. With some standard compression schemes such as the Joint Photographic Experts Group (JPEG), an image can be compressed to a 30:1 ratio with a remarkable reduction in size. To the casual observer, the images appear similar.

TABLE 5-2 TYPICAL RADIOLOGIC IMAGE FORMATS AND STORAGE REQUIREMENTS PER STUDY

MODALITY IOD—DESCRIPTION	PIXEL FORMAT (APPROXIMATE)	BITS PER PIXEL	EXAM STUDY SIZE (MB)
CR—Computed Radiography	$2,000 \times 2,500$	10 to 12	28.5
DX—Digital Radiography	$3,000 \times 3,000$	12 to 16	40.5
MG—Mammography	$3,000 \times 4,000$	12 to 16	65.3
BTO—Digital Breast Tomosynthesis	$2,000 \times 3,000$	12 to 16	450.0
RF—Fluoroscopy	512^2 or $1,024^2$	8 to 12	37.0
XA—Fluoroscopy Guided Intervention	512^2 or $1,024^2$	8 to 12	34.9
CT—Computed Tomography	512^2	12	235.6
MR—Magnetic Resonance Imaging	64^2 to 512^2	12	151.0
US—Ultrasound	512^2 to 900×1450	8	137.8
NM—Nuclear Medicine/SPECT	64^2 or 128^2	8 or 16	116.0
PT/CT—Positron Emission Tomography/CT	128^2 to 512^2	16	416.1

Pixel format is an estimate of the typical image matrix size for an image. Average study size is based on one calendar quarter of imaging studies at a major health group in Northern California. Mammography data represent projection radiographs of the breast. Breast tomosynthesis study sizes are from a different source where the data represent the average size of a breast tomosynthesis screening study (4 sequences) using lossless compression to store projection (BPO) and tomographic (BTO) images. Ultrasound studies (video clips) are compressed with conventional JPEG algorithms in a lossy format from the modality. PT represents PET/CT combination studies. Not shown are future systems such as Total Body PET/CT where a typical exam will have 1.9 GB of data, and high resolution CT, where matrix sizes are 4 times and 16 times larger than the conventional CT acquisition, increasing the data size by the same factor. Overall storage requirements over a given time period can be estimated by the product of the exam study size and the number of expected exams for each modality.

However, with close inspection, a significant amount of image information can be lost (Fig. 5-8). Currently, there is controversy on how much compression can be tolerated. Research shows that the amount of compression is strongly dependent upon the type of examination, the compression algorithm used, and the way that the image is displayed. In some cases, images that are irreversibly compressed and subsequently decompressed are preferred by radiologists over the original images, due to some reduction of image noise with the compression algorithms. Legal considerations also affect decisions on the use of irreversible compression in medical imaging. Diagnostically acceptable irreversible compression refers to compression that does not affect a particular diagnostic task and may be used under the direction of a qualified physician. Practically speaking, this means that any artifacts generated by the compression scheme should not be perceptible by the viewer or are at such a low level that they do not interfere with interpretation. The US Food and Drug Administration (FDA) requires that an irreversible compressed image, when displayed, must be labeled with a message stating the approximate compression ratio and/or quality factor. In addition, the type of compression scheme (JPEG, JPEG-2000) should also be indicated.

The FDA, under the authority of the federal Mammography Quality Standards Act, does not allow irreversible compression of digital mammography for retention, transmission, or final interpretation, though irreversibly compressed images from prior studies may be used for comparison purposes if deemed of acceptable image quality by the interpreting physician. In particular, the FDA does not permit mammograms compressed by lossy methods to be used for final interpretation, nor does it accept the storage of mammograms compressed by lossy methods to meet the requirements for retention of original mammograms. The FDA does permit interpretation of digital mammograms compressed by lossless methods and considers the storage of such

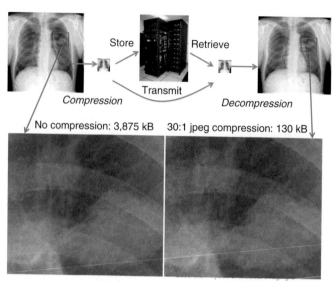

■ **FIGURE 5-8** Image compression reduces the number of bytes in an image to reduce image storage space and image transmission times. At a display workstation, an image retrieved from the archive over the network requires image decompression, which restores the images to full physical size (number of pixels) and number of bytes. Shown above is a chest image with lossless compression (left), and 30:1 jpeg lossy compression (right). Although the minified images (above) look similar, the magnified views (below) illustrate loss of image fidelity and non-diagnostic image quality with too much lossy compression.

mammograms to meet the requirement for retention of original mammograms. The reader should refer to current guidance from the FDA on this topic (FDA, 2020).

5.3.4 Archive and Storage

An archive is a location containing records, documents, and other objects of historical importance. In the context of a PACS, the archive is a long-term storage of medical images on disks and tapes in DICOM format. In the context of enterprise storage, the archive is generally on a Vendor-Neutral Archive (VNA) that is a repository for all kinds of data, including DICOM and non-DICOM images, non-image data (e.g., EKG traces), and other content. Archiving of data and images is typically performed in a compressed format for efficient use of storage and network resources. Many lossless image compression implementations are vendor proprietary, making the archive inaccessible to non-vendor access except through a translator program that outputs standard DICOM formats. Archived data is protected from disk failures through the use of RAID (Redundant Array of Independent Disks) and from natural disasters or other catastrophes by creating a backup mirror copy in a separate location to ensure business continuity and access to data. The storage size required for a PACS or enterprise archive depends on patient workload, types of modalities, and the length of time images are to be stored and can range from terabytes (2^{12}) to petabytes (2^{15}) to exabytes (2^{18}) and beyond. The amounts of storage required for individual images and typical studies from the various imaging modalities are listed in Table 5-2. Certainly, the size and complexity of the archive are dependent on the infrastructure and characteristics of the healthcare enterprise it supports.

The PACS archive may be centralized, or it may be distributed, that is, stored at several locations on a network. In either case, there must be archive management software on a server. The archive management software includes a database program that contains information about the stored studies and their locations in the archive and indexes these based on the most common metadata for rapid retrieval. The archive management software communicates over the network with imaging devices sending studies in for storage and sends copies of the studies received from imaging devices to the storage devices, including backup storage. The transfers between imaging devices and the PACS must conform to the DICOM standard. The archive management software must also obtain studies from the storage devices and send either the studies or selected images from them to workstations requesting studies or images for display. In PACS with hierarchical storage, the archive management software transfers studies between the various levels of archival storage, based upon factors such as the recentness of the study and, when a new study is ordered, prefetches relevant older studies from near-line storage to online storage to reduce the time required for display.

In some PACS, studies or images from studies awaiting interpretation and relevant older studies are requested by viewing workstations from the PACS archive as needed ("on-demand") during viewing sessions, but this can slow the workflow process of the interpreting physician. Alternatively, studies may be obtained ("prefetched") from the archive and stored on a display workstation or local file server, prior to the interpretation session, ready for the interpreting physician's use. The prefetch method requires the interpretation workstations or server to have more local storage capacity, whereas the on-demand method requires a faster archive and faster network connections between the archive and the interpretation workstations. An advantage to the on-demand method is that a physician may use any available workstation to view a particular study, whereas to view a particular study with the prefetch method, the physician must go to a workstation that has access to the locally stored study. When images are fetched on-demand, the first image should be available for viewing within about two seconds. Once images reside on the workstation's disk or local server, they are nearly instantaneously available.

On-demand systems may send all the images in entire studies to the workstation, or they may just send individual images when requested by the viewing workstation. The method of sending entire studies at once requires greater network bandwidth and more storage capacity on the viewing workstation and causes greater delay before the first images are displayed. On the other hand, providing only individual images upon request by the viewing workstation reduces the delay before the first image or images are displayed, but places more demand on the archive server to respond to frequent requests for individual images.

Server-side rendering in a cloud-based computing model is a growing option with current PACS, whereby thin client viewers (often zero-footprint, generally implemented in HTML-5) access an on-line server or server farm and archive. All of the processing and display is performed at the server location and only the results are pushed to the thin client. This type of arrangement generally reduces the overall network bandwidth of a hospital network because the images need only be sent to the PACS archive once, and the users can access the content with a thin client and have the server provide the image-only display results, in lieu of sending the full complement of image data to each thick-client workstation. The benefits of such centralization are hardware resource optimization, reduced software maintenance, no requirement for client management on the desktop, fast image viewing since only compressed images and not the full dataset are sent over the network, ability to scale to enterprise imaging (all of the image-based "-ologies"), and improved security, as hardware and software assets are easily firewalled, maintained, and protected. Appropriate sizing of servers, having enough concurrent software licenses, and server redundancy must be ensured to provide reliable host availability.

Two common storage schemes include hierarchical and on-line. In hierarchical storage, recent images are stored on arrays of high-performance magnetic hard disk drives or solid-state drives, and older images are stored on slower but more capacious archival storage media, such as lower-performance drives or automated magnetic tape libraries. *On-line storage* describes the fraction of studies with immediate and rapid access for viewing. *Near-line storage* refers to storage at remote disk farms or automated libraries of magnetic tape, from which studies may be retrieved *albeit* less rapidly. *Off-line storage* refers to storage not directly accessible (requiring some human intervention to be made available). With the lowered cost of storage media, *off-line* mechanisms are generally no longer used as primary storage tiers, but often still employed as disaster recovery mechanisms. With magnetic tape capacities already at 30 terabytes (TB) (LTO-8 compressed, at around a $100 per cartridge) and planned to exceed 100 TB (LTO-10 compressed), many sites utilize off-site magnetic tape storage for cost-effective disaster recovery. When hierarchical storage is used, the system must automatically copy ("prefetch") relevant older studies from near-line to on-line storage to be available without delay for comparison when new studies are viewed. An alternative to hierarchical storage is to store all images on arrays of magnetic or solid-state disk drives. As these become full, more disk arrays are added to the system, which has become feasible because of the increasing capacities of disk drives and the decreasing cost per unit storage capacity. This method is referred to as "everything online" storage.

A VNA is typically constructed to provide access to all enterprise images and data of clinical relevance, whether the content is DICOM compliant or formatted in another way, such as optical images from a dermatology clinic that may be encoded in a JPEG format or documents in a PDF (Portable Document Format) file structure. These objects are stored in a standard format with a standard interface and cataloged on a database so that they can be accessed in a vendor-neutral manner by other systems. A VNA decouples the PACS and workstations at the archival level and provides a means to coalesce access to mini-PACS and image databases. Availability to all encounter-based image workflows (situations without an order for imaging) is also achieved, associating content with the correct patient in the medical record on an Enterprise-wide basis. This provides a unified archive and access to such data, while still allowing proprietary front-end appliances and software to send information if they are compliant with rules/profiles set up by entities such as the IHE effort.

5.3.5 DICOM, HL7, and IHE

Connecting imaging devices to a PACS with a network, by itself, does not achieve the transfer of images and related information. This would permit the transfer of files, but medical imaging equipment manufacturers and PACS vendors could (and in the past did) use proprietary formats for digital images and related information. In the past, some facilities solved this problem by purchasing all equipment from a single vendor; others had custom software developed to translate one vendor's format into another's format. To help overcome problems such as these, the ACR and the NEMA jointly sponsor a set of standards called *Digital Imaging and Communications in Medicine* (DICOM) to facilitate the transfer of medical images and related information. Other professional societies work to develop medical specialty–specific DICOM standards. Many other national and international standards organizations recognize the DICOM standards.

DICOM includes standards for the transfer, using computer networks, of images and related information from individual patient studies between devices such as imaging devices and storage devices. DICOM specifies standard formats for the images and other information being transferred, services that one device can request from another, and messages between the devices. DICOM does not specify formats for the storage of information by a device itself, although a manufacturer may choose to use DICOM formats for this purpose. DICOM also includes standards for exchanging information regarding workflow; standards for the storage of images and related information on removable storage media, such as optical disks; and standards for the consistency and presentation of displayed images. A description and complete listing of the DICOM standard is available (DICOM, 2020).

DICOM specifies hierarchical formats for information objects, such as "patients," "studies," and "images" (sometimes referred to as "PSSI" Patient/Study/Series/Image or Instance). These are combined into composite Information Object Definition (IOD) entities, such as the CT (computed tomography), CR (computed radiography), DX (digital x-ray), MG (digital mammography x-ray), US (ultrasound), MR (magnetic resonance imaging), and NM (nuclear medicine) IODs. DICOM specifies standard services that may be performed on information objects, such as storage, query and retrieve, storage commitment, print management, and media storage. The concept of a Service-Object-Pair (SOP) is defined by the union of an IOD and a DICOM message service element (DIMSE), for example, an SOP might be "Store a CT study." A Service Class is a collection of related SOPs with a specific definition of a service supported by cooperating devices to perform an action on a specific IOD class (Fig. 5-9). Two

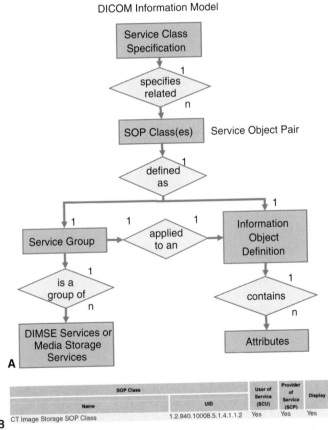

■ FIGURE 5-9 A. DICOM information model—Service/Object relationship. The Service Class specification (top rectangle) defines the services—operations such as moving, storing, finding, or printing that can be performed on data objects that DICOM can manage. The service group is comprised of DICOM Message Service Element (DIMSE) services such as "C-move," "C-store," "C-find," etc., as described in Part 4 of the DICOM standard. Data objects have Information Object Definitions (IODs) with attributes defining the object (e.g., a CT series containing images). A specific combination of a Service and an Object is termed a Service-Object-Pair (SOP), middle rectangle, which constitutes the basic unit of DICOM operability. Model shown above is adapted from the DICOM standard in Part 3.3. (DICOM PS3.3-2003, by permission). **B.** An example might be a SOP that combines "C-Move" service with "CT" IOD. In a Conformance Statement, this might be represented as shown, attesting that the implementation can both send and receive CT images. The "UID" is a Unique Identifier associated with this particular SOP class, describing a DICOM transfer syntax.

TABLE 5-3 COMMON DICOM VOCABULARY TERMS AND ACRONYMS

IOD: Information Object Definition	Modality-specific attributes (*e.g.*, the structure of a DICOM image)
AE: Application Entity AET: Application Entity Title	Applications (programs and devices) that communicate via DICOM; title = "name" of device
Service	Action to perform on an object, such as: *store, get, find, echo*
SOP: Service-Object-Pair	Union of an IOD and a DICOM message service element (DIMSE): *e.g.*, "Store a CT study"
Service Class: Collection of related SOPs	Specific definition of a supported service to perform an action on a specific class of information object; *e.g.*, SCU—Service Class User—invokes operations SCP—Service Class Provider—performs operations
Conformance Statement	Associated with a specific DICOM implementation—specifies what can and can't be performed; a public document provided by the vendor
Association	First phase of communication between AE and SOP classes, requiring IP address, port number, and AET
DICOM Metadata	Data that contains information about other data, e.g., patient, study, series, image data and attributes
UID: Unique Identifier	Provides the capability to uniquely identify a wide variety of items. For instance DICOM transfer syntax, which has a registered root of "1.2.840.10008" followed by a suffix unique to the item.

service operations are defined: Service Class User (SCU)—invokes operations, and Service Class Provider (SCP)—performs operations. Table 5-3 lists a subset of common DICOM vocabulary terms and acronyms that are widely used by PACS administrators.

DICOM provides standards for workflow management, such as modality worklist (MWL) by listing patients and validated demographic information to be merged with images from specific imaging devices, and Performed Procedure Step (PPS), for communicating information about the status of a procedure. The DICOM Grayscale Standard Presentation State (GSPS) is provided for capturing and storing a technologist's or a radiologist's adjustments of image presentation and annotations on key images for a *specific patient's study*. Adjustments such as roaming and zooming, cropping, flipping, window width and window level settings, and input annotations such as arrows and clinical notes are recorded (Fig. 5-10). Presentation states are

Original   Manipulated

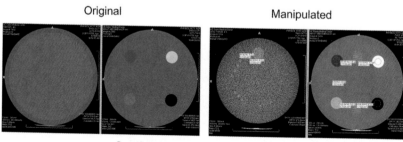

Specific to images in the study and series

■ **FIGURE 5-10** The Grayscale Softcopy Presentation State (GSPS) is a DICOM Information Object Descriptor that specifies how a radiologist or other viewer manipulates images for diagnosis and reporting, independent of the original display. This is a patient-study specific IOD that stores information on lookup table (LUT) transformations, electronic shuttering of radiographic images, rotation, flipping, magnification, annotation, and overlay displays.

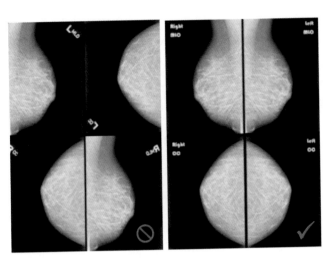

■ **FIGURE 5-11** "Hanging Protocols" such named for the historical hanging of film on an alternator in a specific arrangement that the radiologist is familiar with, in order to allow efficient reading and analysis of multiple images on a workstation display from the PACS. It is designed to radiologist preference according to the modality, order and orientation of images, window width and window level optimized settings, and other aspects of the study. It is not specific to a particular patient's images, however. That is the role of the Grayscale Softcopy Presentation State (GSPS) standard discussed in Figure 5-10.

stored with the image set on the PACS. When the images are viewed, key images appear with the adjustments and annotations made by the technologist or radiologist during the evaluation of the images. *Hanging protocols* are another implementation within the DICOM standard that are not specific to a patient, but to the way a radiologist prefers images from *specific modalities* to be presented and sequenced in a given format and order, respectively (Fig. 5-11). Parameters such as anatomical laterality, anatomical projection, current versus previous studies, acquisition protocol (*e.g.*, multiple protocols in an MRI study), location on the display, and many others assist the radiologist in efficiently navigating the study in a logical and known way to make a diagnosis.

DICOM is compatible with common computer network protocols. DICOM is an upper layer (Application Layer) standard and so is completely independent of lower-layer network protocols, such as LAN protocols. DICOM adopts the Internet Protocol Suite (TCP/IP). DICOM will function on any LAN or WAN, provided that the intermediate network layer protocol is TCP/IP.

All vendors of medical imaging and PACS equipment permit exchanges of information that conform to parts of the DICOM standard. *A DICOM conformance statement* is a formal statement, provided by a vendor, describing a specific implementation of the DICOM standard. It specifies the services, information objects, and communications protocols supported by the implementation. The structure of this statement is formally defined in Part 2 of the Standard, and the ability to review Conformance Statements is an important skill in Imaging Informatics. Generally, all Conformance Statements should be reviewed before equipment purchase.

There are practical issues regarding DICOM that are worthy of emphasis. First, DICOM applies not just to a PACS but also to each imaging device that exchanges information with the PACS. Hence, issues of DICOM conformance and functionality must be considered when purchasing individual imaging devices, as well as when purchasing or upgrading a PACS. Another issue is that DICOM is a set of standards, not a single standard. When purchasing an imaging device or a PACS, the contract should specify the specific DICOM standards with which conformance is desired. For example, support for DICOM MWLs, PPS, and Storage Commitment should be provided in most cases, in addition to image store. Furthermore, there may be more than one DICOM standard that will permit information transfer, but all may not be equally useful. For example, digital radiographs may be transferred as the older

DICOM CR image object or the newer DX image object. However, the old CR image object contains much less mandatory information regarding procedure, projection, laterality, etc. Also, the CR image object does not clearly define the meaning of pixel values. Even though use of the CR image object will permit image transfer, the lack of information about the image will hinder the use of automatic hanging protocols and optimal display of image contrast. This is one of many examples demonstrating the need for understanding the standard and conformance statements.

It is necessary to have communication among the PACS, the RIS, the EHR, and other information systems and services. The RIS supports functions within a radiology department such as ordering and scheduling procedures, maintaining a patient database, transcription, reporting, and bill preparation. The RIS is not always a separate system—it is now likely to be part of the EHR. The RIS provides worklists of scheduled studies to the operator's consoles of the imaging devices, thereby reducing the amount of manual data entry and the likelihood of improperly identified studies.

Communication among the RIS, LIS (Laboratory Information System), EHR, and PACS is implemented using the HL7 standard for the electronic exchange of alphanumeric medical information, such as administrative information, clinical laboratory data, and radiology diagnostic reporting. HL7 to DICOM translation, for instance, is a step in the RIS to PACS communication providing study MWLs to the imaging devices, through a device known as a PACS "broker." HL7, like DICOM, applies to the Application Layer in the network protocol stack. An HL7 interface engine is used to connect and synchronize messages to and from the databases making up the informatics infrastructure, as discussed in "Lifecycle of a Radiology Exam," Section 5.4.

Finally, IHE is the organization that provides interoperability profiles using DICOM and HL7 standards to achieve specific PACS functionality with other information systems. This allows users to specify a certain IHE profile without having to understand the nuances of the DICOM or HL7 requirements that are necessary for interoperability. Examples are given in the PACS quality control section.

5.3.6 Downtime Procedures, Data Integrity, Other Policies

Medical management of a patient can be delayed or be put on hold when a PACS is down or unavailable, particularly in specialties such as emergency medicine and surgery that rely heavily on the availability of images. Maintaining business continuity requires a well-defined set of policies and procedures as well as a reliable primary system and backup architecture for redundancy to ensure patient safety and minimize operational inefficiencies or system unavailability.

Downtime procedures are a crucial part of overall procedures for a PACS and must account for unscheduled or scheduled events. In a catastrophic event such as flood, fire, or earthquake, disaster recovery procedures may be enacted to re-establish image availability. Typical downtime lasts from minutes to several hours or more. Even 1 hour of unplanned downtime is unacceptable when patients are affected.

There are "planned" and "unplanned" downtime events that will impact the delivery of images, reports, and other information. Planned downtime is scheduled ahead of time when software upgrades, bug fixes, or patches are needed for maintenance operations. In this situation, the obvious times for scheduling are at the least disruptive time of the day (usually in the early morning hours and/or on weekends). Considerations are to allocate more time than anticipated (have a buffer for problems that may arise), have a roll-back plan in the event the upgrade fails or introduces other unintended issues that are unacceptable, and increase staffing prior to the start of the downtime to reduce the number of unread studies, and after downtime to reduce radiologist workload.

Unplanned downtime caused by an unexpected failure can be mitigated by configuring a system with redundancy where feasible and assessing system architecture by identifying every unique point of failure, with the understanding that a critical function should have a high priority in achieving redundancy—the more critical the function, the higher the priority to create redundancy. Potential sources of unplanned downtime include hardware failures (servers, disk drives, power supplies, interface cards); software failures (virus, malware attacks, new patches, new drivers, corrupted file systems); electrical disruptions (uninterruptible power supply/backup generator failures); heating, ventilation, air conditioning failures; information system failures (PACS, EHR, RIS, HL7 integration engine); and network failures (switches, cables, Internet).

Maintaining business continuity and patient care requires contingency plans in these situations that allow for re-routing of data to emergency backup servers and associated viewing workstations that have direct access. For both planned and unplanned downtime, a single point of communication such as a service or radiology front desk should be in place to ensure the appropriate individuals are handling communication with end-users. In addition, a departmental website should contain links to all downtime policies and procedures.

Technical considerations include (1) having a comprehensive and verified data backup before any upgrades; (2) maintaining multiple workstations and spares; (3) managing a web-based viewer to run on a thick-client PACS workstation rather than changing the configuration on each workstation; (4) utilizing a backup (sometimes referred to as a Business Continuity System or BCS) PACS to ensure availability of current and future exam workflow; (5) maintaining a DICOM router to send images to multiple destinations; (6) implementing a fault-tolerant PACS, that has no single point of failure.

Operationally, procedures should be in place to reduce the potential for data integrity issues that will inevitably occur when the MWL is unavailable, such as how to manually enter patient demographics into the modality. Also, if images fail to be sent from the modality, procedures on how to locate exams and manually send them to the PACS upon resumption of service is crucial.

5.3.7 PACS Quality Control

There are many challenges to implementing, using, maintaining, upgrading, and replacing a PACS. An important goal is achieving efficient workflow. There are far too many issues regarding the efficiency of workflow to be listed here; this paragraph merely lists several important objectives. Prior to image acquisition by an imaging device, little manual entry of information should be required by imaging technologists. This can be facilitated by utilizing "modality worklists" generated by the RIS and sent to the modality. Worklists of studies to be interpreted, arranged by factors such as modality and priority, should be provided to interpreting physicians. Images should be displayed promptly, ideally within two seconds, to referring and interpreting physicians. Little or no manipulation of images should be routinely necessary; automated hanging protocols should display the images in the expected order, orientation, magnification, and position. Software tools should be available to technologists to help identify studies that are not assigned to the proper patient, are mislabeled, or require image manipulation. Image interpretation is made more efficient by a digital speech recognition system that promptly displays the dictated report for review and approval by the interpreting physician before he or she interprets the next study. These systems greatly decrease the turn-around time of diagnostic reports and are a major benefit to the referring physician and ultimately to the patient.

PACS Maintenance and Quality Control Challenges

Major challenges include the following:

1. Initial and recurring equipment purchase or lease costs.
2. Expensive technical personnel to support the PACS.
3. Training new users in system operation.
4. Achieving communication among equipment from several vendors.
5. Achieving information transfer among digital information systems (PACS, RIS, EHR).
6. Maintaining the security of images and related information and compliance with the Health Insurance Portability and Accountability Act (HIPAA) Regulations (Sections 5.6.2 and 5.9.2)
7. Equipment failures can impede the interpretation and distribution of images and reports.
8. Digital storage media longevity and obsolescence.
9. Maintaining access to images and data during PACS upgrades.
10. Maintaining access to archived images and related data if: converting to a new archival technology, the PACS vendor goes out of business, the PACS vendor ceases to support a particular PACS, or the PACS system is replaced with one from a different vendor.
11. Locating misidentified studies.
12. Multiple PACS in a single healthcare enterprise.
13. Obtaining and importing images from outside the healthcare enterprise.
14. Providing images and reports to healthcare providers outside the healthcare enterprise.
15. Providing adequate software tools for specialists such as orthopedic surgeons and cardiologists.
16. Ensuring adequate display capabilities including resolution and luminance.
17. Ensuring appropriate image viewing conditions, reading room environment, and ergonomics.

This list is far from complete. Of course, the desirable strategy is to enhance the advantages and minimize the disadvantages. Benefits will expand as experience with these systems increases. Furthermore, the rapidly increasing capabilities and falling costs of the technology used in PACS will continue to increase performance while reducing overall cost.

Of note are the last two items on the list, implicating the requirements and overcoming the challenges of the viewing environment and *display* technical specifications for specific use cases (diagnostic, modality, clinical specialist, EHR workstations). Human image perception must be considered to optimize the grayscale display performance. Calibration of displays to match the visual response is necessary to achieve similar perception of contrast differences across all different display types. Periodic evaluation of display calibration is key to maintaining optimal performance over the lifetime of the equipment. The next four sub-sections expand upon these issues.

Image Display Technical Considerations

In medical imaging, the purpose of the display may be to permit technologists to visually assess the adequacy of acquired images, for physicians to interpret images, or to guide physicians performing interventional procedures. The designs of display systems should consider the human visual system and optimization of information transfer to the viewer.

The display system consists of a display interface also known as the computer "video interface" or "graphics adapter." One or more displays are connected to the display interface by a cable or cables that carry electrical signals, and software to control the display system. The display interface and display(s) may be consumer-grade commercial products, or they may be more expensive medical grade devices designed for the high-fidelity display of medical images.

A display system may be designed to display color images or only monochrome (grayscale) images. A system that can display color images can also display grayscale images. Nearly all general-purpose commercial, professional, and medical-grade liquid crystal display (LCD) systems are designed to display images in color. In grayscale radiological images, each pixel value is typically represented by a single integer, commonly stored in 8 bits (one byte) or 16 bits (two bytes), representing $2^8 = 256$ or $2^{16} = 65,536$ shades of gray from black to white, although fewer than 16 of the bits may be used in the latter situation. For example, the range of CT numbers requires only 12 bits $= 4,096$, but 2 bytes are still required to represent the pixel values because of computer addressing schemes requiring a byte address. In color images, each pixel is commonly represented by 8 bits for each color representing three bytes, which designate the intensities of the red, green, and blue light to be generated for that pixel.

A computer's display interface converts a digital image into a signal on the display. The computer's CPU sends the digital contents of the image under the control of an application program to the display memory. These digital values are sequentially addressed and converted into a corresponding analog voltage to generate the specific pixel brightness. For color LCD flat-panel displays, the pixels are physical structures that typically consist of three subpixels, whose light intensities for red, green, and blue colors are independently controlled. The liquid crystal (LC) material of an LCD does not produce light. Instead, it modulates the intensity of light from a uniform light source, containing fluorescent tubes or light-emitting diode (LED) sources in the back of the display. Between the light source and the display surface is a layer of LC material and a thin-film-transistor (TFT) array placed between two glass plates with a light polarizing filter on each side of the glass/LC/TFT array assembly (Fig. 5-12).

Light emitted from the backlight source is unpolarized, where the oscillations of the electromagnetic radiation comprising the light waves are randomly oriented. A polarizing filter permits components of light waves oscillating in one direction to pass through its layer, but absorbs components oscillating in the perpendicular direction. When a second polarizing filter is placed in the beam of polarized light, the intensity of the beam transmitted through the second filter depends on the orientation of the second filter with respect to the first. If both filters have the same orientation, the intensity of the beam transmitted through both filters is almost the same as that transmitted through the first. However, if the second filter is rotated with respect to the first, the intensity of the transmitted light is reduced. When the second filter is oriented so that its polarization is perpendicular to that of the first filter, almost no light is transmitted. In an LCD, the polarizing filters are typically oriented perpendicular to each other; thus there is no transmission of light unless there is a mechanism to change the orientation of the polarized light through the LC assembly. The TFT array electronically controls the orientation of the LC layer pixel by pixel in the display device.

An LC material consists of long organic molecules and has properties of both a liquid and a crystalline material. For example, it flows like a liquid. On the other hand, the molecules tend to align parallel to one another. The material has additional properties that are used in LCDs. If a layer of LC material is in contact with a surface with fine grooves, the molecules align with the grooves. If an electric field is present, the molecules will align with the field. If polarized light passes through a layer of LC material, the LC material can change the polarization of the light by modulating the electric field. Each pixel or subpixel of an LCD has a pair of electrodes attached to a TFT array

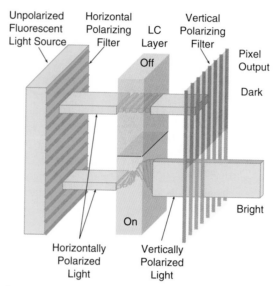

■ **FIGURE 5-12** Electronic components of an LCD display. Two pixels of a grayscale backlit LCD display are shown to illustrate brightness modulation. On each side of the LC layer in each pixel is a transparent electrode—a thin-film-transistor (TFT) array that is used for applying voltage to each pixel across the full display area. In the top pixel, no voltage is applied across the LC layer. The polarization of the light is unchanged as it passes through the LC layer, causing most of the light to be absorbed by the second polarizing filter and thereby producing a dark pixel. In the bottom pixel, a voltage is applied across the LC layer. The applied voltage causes the molecules in the LC layer to twist. The twisted molecules change the polarization of the light, enabling it to pass through the second filter with an intensity that increases with the applied voltage. With full voltage on the LC layer, the output light is vertically polarized, causing the pixel to transmit the brightest luminance. (The bars shown in the polarizing filters are merely an artist's rendition to indicate the direction of the polarization, as is depicting the polarized light as a ribbon.) Variations in grayscale are achieved by varying the voltage provided to each LCD pixel.

substrate. Applying a voltage to the electrodes produces an electric field that changes the orientation of the LC molecules and the polarization of the light, the amount of which depends on the voltage magnitude. The second polarizing filter oriented in a perpendicular direction does not pass light if no voltage is applied, or maximum light when the light is re-oriented by the LC in the perpendicular direction, as shown in Figure 5-12. As the voltage applied to the pixel is incrementally increased, the LC molecules incrementally twist, changing the polarization of the light and decreasing the fraction absorbed by the second filter, thereby making the pixel incrementally brighter.

A color LCD has an additional layer containing color filters. Each pixel consists of three subpixels, one containing a filter transmitting only red light, the second transmitting only green light, and the third transmitting only blue light. Mixtures of red, green, and blue light can create the perception of most colors. Because these color filters absorb light, they reduce the luminance of the display, in comparison to an equivalent monochrome LCD, by about a factor of three.

Flat-panel displays are matrix controlled, with one conductor serving each row of pixels and one serving each column. For a three-megapixel (MP—a common way to indicate the approximate number of addressable pixels) grayscale display (matrix of 2,048 by 1,536 pixels) only 2,048-row pathways and 1,536 column pathways (if there are not subpixels) are required. A signal is sent to a specific pixel by simultaneously providing voltages to the row conductor and the column conductor for that pixel.

The intensity of each pixel must be maintained while signals are sent to other pixels. In active-matrix LCDs, each pixel or subpixel has a transistor and capacitor.

The electrical charge stored on the capacitor maintains the voltage signal for the pixel or subpixel while signals are sent to other pixels. The transistors and capacitors are constructed on a sheet of glass or quartz coated with silicon. This sheet is incorporated as a layer within the LCD. Active matrix LCDs are also called TFT displays. TFT technology, without the polarizing filters and LC material, is used in flat-panel x-ray image receptors and is discussed in Chapter 7.

Organic light-emitting diode (OLED) panels are an alternative display technology. Unlike LCD backlit displays that use attenuation of a bright uniform source through a variable attenuating LC panel, OLEDs are made from organic materials that emit light when electricity is applied through them. They are more efficient, simpler to make, thinner, and can even be made flexible. The basic structure of an OLED is an emissive layer sandwiched between a negative electrode (cathode) and a positive electrode (anode). An OLED panel is made from a substrate, a backplane containing electronics, a front plane (organic materials and electrodes), and an encapsulation layer. The latter is needed to keep the organic materials free of moisture and oxygen from the environment. Currently, OLED displays are made by evaporating gases in a vacuum chamber to deposit the organic materials in a specific pattern. For electronics with an active matrix TFT and storage capacitors similar to that of an LC display, the panel is referred to as an active matrix (AMOLED) display.

With current technology, AMOLED panels have better contrast, higher brightness, fuller viewing angle, and a wider color range than do LCD panels, with lower power consumption. However, they cost more to make and the material lifetime and efficiency (particularly of the blue organic material) are significant issues inhibiting adoption. Nevertheless, as manufacturing processes and material sciences evolve, there will certainly be increasing numbers of AMOLED displays for medical imaging applications in the future.

Displays are partitioned into four categories: Diagnostic, Modality, Clinical Specialist, and EHR (AAPM, 2019a). *Diagnostic displays* are characterized by having higher luminance, better uniformity, smaller pixels, wider viewing angles, self-calibrating backlight intensity, larger numbers of bits to render grayscale levels for improved precision and accuracy, self-calibration to the DICOM Grayscale Standard Display Function (GSDF; as explained later), FDA approval as a "medical grade" display, and a typical 5-year warranty. *Modality displays* use mainstream technologies that are suited to provide adequate screen sizes, often touch-screen capabilities, high-end specifications, and higher luminance output, but typically a warranty that is part of the modality maintenance agreement. These displays are often neglected in terms of their calibration and performance, which often puts the technologist at a disadvantage when attempting to adjust an image dataset prior to sending it to the PACS for diagnostic interpretation. *Clinical specialist displays* are used by physicians (*e.g.*, in an Emergency Department) to review patient images for the purpose of making healthcare decisions prior to receiving a radiologist finalized report, and therefore should perform similarly to diagnostic displays. Generally, however, these displays are of lower quality and therefore must be evaluated to ensure reasonable consistency with calibration and quality control. *EHR displays* are used in conjunction with patient images following the primary interpretation by a radiologist, and are typically standard consumer model displays without calibration, luminance performance requirements, or ambient lighting considerations. These displays are of variable quality, lower luminance, and can have poor off-axis viewing capability due to the type of LCD panels used in the manufacturing process.

With higher quality and capability comes a corresponding higher cost, with prices varying a factor of 5 to 10 times between these display types. Backlight longevity at a specific luminance level is the typical limiting factor for LCDs. Medical-grade displays for interpretation can typically provide maximal luminances of about 600 to 1,000 cd/m^2 when new and are usually calibrated to provide luminances of about 400 to 600 cd/m^2 that can be sustained for tens of thousands of operating hours by measuring and adjusting the backlight intensity over time. The "headroom" allotted between the maximal and calibrated luminances, and continuous calibration adjustment is a distinguishing factor of a medical-grade display compared to a consumer or "prosumer" grade display, allowing for a typical performance warranty of 5 years, compared to 3 years or 1 year for the latter types, and is a major reason for cost differences.

The formats of digital radiological images are selected to preserve the clinical information acquired by the imaging devices. The numbers of rows and columns of pixels in an image are determined by the spatial resolution and the field-of-view of the imaging device, whereas the number of bits used for each pixel is determined by the contrast resolution of the imaging device. Thus, imaging modalities providing high spatial resolution (*e.g.,* mammography) and with large fields of view (*e.g.,* radiography) require large numbers of pixels per image, whereas modalities providing lower spatial resolution (*e.g.,* CT) or small fields of view (*e.g.,* ultrasound) can use fewer pixels. Modalities providing high contrast resolution (*e.g.,* x-ray CT) require many bits per pixel (*e.g.,* 12 bits), whereas modalities with low contrast resolution such as ultrasound require fewer bits per pixel (*e.g.,* 8 bits). Typical formats of digital images are listed in Table 5-2.

The necessary dimensions of the active face of a display and its pixel format (number of rows and columns of pixels or, equivalently, the pixel pitch, defined as the distance from the center of a pixel to the center of an adjacent pixel in the same row or column) depend upon the pixel matrix sizes of the images produced by the modalities whose images will be displayed, the distance from the viewer's eyes to the display surface, and the spatial resolution of the human visual system.

A radiologist should view an entire image at or near maximal spatial resolution. To avoid a reduction in spatial resolution when an image is viewed, a display should have at least as many pixels in the horizontal and vertical directions as the image. On the other hand, it serves no purpose to provide spatial resolution that is beyond the ability of the viewer to discern. The distance from a person's eyes to the face of a workstation display commonly ranges from about 50 to 60 cm. The viewer may lean closer to the display for short periods to see more detail, but viewing at a distance much closer than about 55 cm for long periods is uncomfortable.

Imaging modalities impose specific requirements on workstation displays. Most displays provide color capability (with some exceptions for high-resolution 5 MP displays for mammography). Another format is the ~76-cm (30–32 inches) diagonal display, available with 4, 6, 8, 10 or 12 MPs, designed to replace a pair of 54-cm diagonal displays. Such a monitor provides a seamless addressable viewing area to view radiographs side by side in portrait mode. Workstations for viewing CT and MRI images, fluorographs, angiographic images, nuclear medicine and ultrasound can permit smaller pixel format displays (*e.g.,* 2 MP) for full image viewing without pixel interpolation.

Most non-interpreting physicians typically use standard commercial personal computers with consumer-grade color displays, although some, such as orthopedic surgeons and emergency department physicians, may require specialized diagnostic workstation capabilities.

Human Perception and Image Viewing Conditions

The PACS is the interface between the physician and the image. Efficient and accurate transfer of image content requires optimization of display characteristics, such as resolution, contrast, and brightness to prevent human perception from becoming the

A   Frequency variations at fixed contrast

B   Contrast variations at fixed spatial frequency

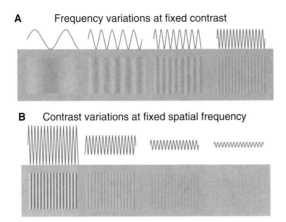

■ **FIGURE 5-13** Sinusoidal luminance test patterns are used by researchers to assess the perception of contrast as a function of spatial frequency and average luminance. **A.** Four different spatial frequencies with the background luminance equal to the average luminance of the pattern are shown. **B.** Four different contrast levels at a fixed frequency. Sinusoidal lines (in blue) above the patterns show the change in luminance as amplitude and frequency variations.

weak link in the imaging chain. To assess perceived contrast and spatial resolution, scientists studying human vision commonly use test images containing a sinusoidal luminance pattern centered in an image of constant luminance equal to the average luminance of the sinusoidal pattern (Fig. 5-13). The photometric quantity[1] describing the brightness of a display (or other light source) is *luminance*. Luminance is the rate of light energy emitted or reflected from a surface per unit area, per unit solid angle, corrected for the photopic[2] spectral sensitivity of the human eye. The SI unit of luminance is the candela per square meter (cd/m^2). Perceived brightness is not proportional to luminance; for example, the human visual system will perceive a doubling of luminance as only a small increase in brightness. Brightness and contrast of grayscale medical images result from the luminance in relation to the image gray level values.

Contrast may be defined as

$$C = (L_{max} - L_{min}) / L_{avg},$$

where L_{max} is the maximal luminance in the pattern, L_{min} is the least luminance, and L_{avg} is the average luminance. The smallest luminance difference ($L_{max} - L_{min}$) that is detectable by half of a group of human observers is known as a *just noticeable difference* (JND). The threshold contrast is the JND divided by L_{avg}. Contrast sensitivity is defined as the inverse of the threshold contrast. Figure 5-14 is a graph of contrast sensitivity as a function of spatial frequency (cycles per mm at a 60-cm viewing distance) from a typical experiment. Studies have shown that people with good vision perceive image contrast best at about five cycles per visual degree. The threshold contrast is reduced to about a tenth of the maximum at about 20 cycles per visual degree and reduced to less than one hundredth of the maximum at about 40 to 50 cycles per visual degree (Barten, 1999). At a 60-cm viewing distance, a visual degree is equivalent to a distance of 10.5 mm (10.5 mm = 60 cm × tan 1°) on the face of the display. Thus, at a 60-cm viewing distance, a person with good vision perceives contrast best at about half a cycle per mm, perceives contrast reduced to less than a tenth of this at about two cycles per mm, and perceives very little contrast beyond about four cycles per mm. Two cycles per mm is approximately equivalent to 4 pixels per mm, or a

---

[1]Photometric quantities and units describe the energy per unit time carried by light, modified to account for the spectral sensitivity of the human eye. A person with normal vision perceives a given radiance of green light as being brighter than, for example, an equal radiance of red or blue light.

[2]The word "photopic" refers to the normal daylight color vision of the human visual system. The photopic spectral sensitivity differs from the scotopic spectral sensitivity of dark-adapted night vision. This change in spectral sensitivity between photopic vision, where the cones are relatively more sensitive to the longer wavelengths, and scotopic vision where rods are relatively more sensitive to the shorter wavelengths (with peaks at 555 nm and 505 nm, respectively) is called the Purkinje shift.

■ **FIGURE 5-14** Contrast sensitivity of the human visual system as a function of spatial frequency. Visual requirements for high-fidelity display. (Adapted from Flynn MG. Visual requirements for high-fidelity display. In: *Advances in Digital Radiography: Categorical Course in Diagnostic Radiology Physics*. Oak Brook, IL: Radiological Society of North America; 2003:103-107.)

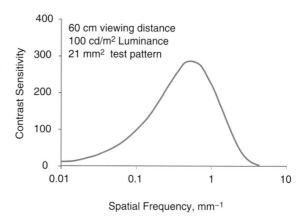

pixel pitch of 1 mm per 4 pixels = 0.25 mm and four cycles per mm is approximately equivalent to 8 pixels per mm, or a pixel pitch of 1 mm per 8 pixels = 0.125 mm.

Proper ambient viewing conditions, where interpretation workstations are used, are needed to permit the interpreting physicians' eyes to adapt to the low luminances of the displays, to avoid a loss in contrast from diffuse reflections from the faces of the displays, and to avoid specular reflections on the display's faces from bright objects. The photometric quantity *illuminance* describes the rate of light energy, adjusted for the photopic spectral sensitivity of the human visual system, impinging on a surface, per unit area. In areas used for viewing clinical images from displays, the illuminance should be low (20–50 lux), but not so low as to interfere with other necessary tasks, such as reading printed documents, or to require a major adjustment in adaption when looking at a display after looking at another object, or vice versa (Krupinski, 2006). A reading room should have adjustable indirect lighting and should not have windows unless they can be blocked with opaque curtains or shutters. When more than one workstation is in a room, provisions should be made, either by placement or by using partitions, to prevent displays from casting reflections on each other.

Displays are characterized by parameters including spatial resolution, contrast resolution, aspect ratio, dynamic range, luminance response, uniformity of luminance, noise, lag, and refresh rate. Luminance response of a medical display is the most important factor, defined by three luminance measures (ACR, 2017): (1) ambient luminance, L_{amb}, is the brightness of a display that is turned off in the presence of diffusely reflected room lighting, and should be less than one fourth of the luminance of the darkest gray level; (2) minimum luminance, L_{min}, is the luminance of the darkest gray level, should not be extremely low because the contrast response of the adapted human visual system is poor in the very dark regions of the image, and in a reading environment is modified as $L'_{min} = L_{min} + L_{amb}$; (3) maximum luminance, L_{max}, is the luminance of the maximum gray level and is modified as $L'_{max} = L_{max} + L_{amb}$.

The perceived contrast characteristics of a displayed image depend on the Luminance Ratio (LR) equal to the ratio of L'_{max} to L'_{min}. Note that the LR is not the same as the contrast ratio reported by display manufacturers, which are often touted to be greater than 1,000 to 1. A good display must support a large LR, but if greater than 350 will exceed the adapted human visual system response across the grayscale range as shown in Figure 5-15. Most effective is an LR equal to 350 and no lower than 250; ideally all displays are adjusted to give the same ratio.

The maximum brightness of a display, depends on the types of images to be displayed, the room lighting conditions, and the intended use (interpretation versus viewing). L'_{max} for interpretation workstation displays should be at least 350 cd/m²,

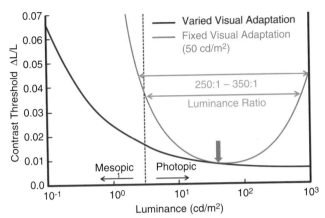

FIGURE 5-15 Human contrast sensitivity threshold is illustrated as a function of luminance. The blue line represents the visually adapted eye across a range of luminances. The red line represents the human visual response to differences in contrast as a function of luminance at a fixed nominal level, in this case 50 cd/m². The luminance values plus the ambient light values from the minimum to the maximum (the luminance ratio) should be contained within a range of 250–350 to encompass human visual response, as shown by the range limits (green horizontal lines). The vertical dashed line represents a zone of luminance at which the photopic (cone vision) and mesopic (combination of cone and rod vision) are used in visualizing a scene. Scotopic (rod vision) is used in dark scenes.

for mammography displays at least 420 cd/m², and displays used for other purposes at least 250 cd/m² (ACR, 2017). The corresponding L'_{min} for these display classes should be at least 1.0 cd/m², 1.2 cd/m², and 0.8 cd/m², respectively, to achieve a LR of 350:1. For brighter displays, the L'_{min} should be adjusted upward. Displays used in mammography have L_{max} typically ranging from 600 to 1,000 cd/m².

The luminance values of intermediate gray levels should follow the same response function for all displays in a facility. The *display function* describes the luminance produced as a function of the magnitude of the digital signal (sometimes called a "digital driving level") or analog signal sent to the display, and can greatly affect the perceived contrast of the displayed image. The inherent display function of a display is non-linear, varies from display to display, and changes with time. Furthermore, individual displays differ in L'_{max} and L'_{min}. There are controls for "brightness" and "contrast" to adjust the shape of the display function, but on most medical image interpretation displays, these are unavailable to the user. If the displays have different display functions, an image may have a different appearance, even when more than one display is attached to a single workstation. As image appearance is often modified by a technologist using a review workstation prior to transfer to the PACS, if the modality display has a display function significantly different from that of the interpretation workstation, the interpreting physician may see contrast displayed quite differently than the technologist intended.

DICOM GSDF

The DICOM GSDF was created to standardize the display of image contrast. The GSDF pertains to grayscale (monochrome) images and not color images, although it does pertain to grayscale images with color displays. The goals of the GSDF are to:

1. Provide applications with a predictable transformation of digital pixel values (called "presentation values," abbreviated as "P-values") to luminance
2. Provide a similar display of contrast on displays and printed media
3. Provide *perceptual linearization*, that is, equal differences in the pixel values received by the display system should be perceived as equal by the human visual system

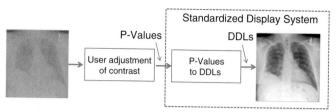

■ **FIGURE 5-16** This diagram shows an original image that is adjusted to create presentation (P) values submitted to a lookup table (LUT), labeled "P-values to DDLs," so that the net display function provided by the LUT conforms to the DICOM Grayscale Standard Display Function (GSDF). The DICOM GSDF does not replace adjustment of contrast by the user.

The display function can be modified to any desired shape using a lookup table (LUT) transformation in the workstation video card. The LUT contains an output pixel value for each possible pixel value in an image. In the DICOM GSDF, the input pixel values provided to the LUT are called "presentation values," as shown in Figure 5-16, and the output values of the LUT that are provided to the display system are called "digital driving levels." Thus, by using an LUT for each video card segment driving the display, the net display function (display and LUT) will conform to the GSDF.

Figure 5-17 shows the response model, which specifies luminance as a function of a parameter called "JND index"; "JND" is an acronym for "just-noticeable difference," discussed earlier in this section. DICOM Part 14 defines the JND index as "The input value to the GSDF, such that one step in JND Index results in a Luminance difference that is a Just-Noticeable Difference." The shape of the GSDF is based on a model of the human visual system. A detailed explanation of this model is beyond the scope of this book; refer to references (DICOM, 2011; Flynn, 2003).

Only a portion of the GSDF curve that lies between the minimal and maximal calibrated luminance of a display is used as the display function. For example, as shown in Figure 5-17, if the L'_{min} and L'_{max} of a display are 1.0 and 250 cd/m², the portion of the DICOM GSDF contained in the segment encompassing 1.0 and 250 cd/m² is used as the display function. The presentation values p, from 0 to the maximal possible presentation value (typically $2^N - 1$, where N is the number of bits used for a presentation value), are linearly related to the values of JND index j for that segment:

$$j = j_{min} + p(j_{max} - j_{min})/p_{max},$$

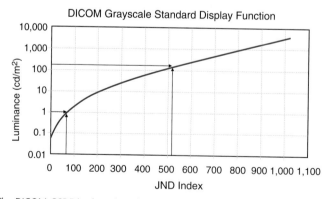

■ **FIGURE 5-17** The DICOM GSDF is plotted as the log of the luminance versus the Just Noticeable Difference (JND) Index. A segment of the curve from the minimum to the maximum luminance values of a specific display device is used as the calibrated display function; for instance, the arrows point to the operating range of the LCD display whose response is shown in Figure 5-19. The calibrated response falls along a subset of the full GSDF curve.

where j_{min} is the smallest JND index in the rectangle, j_{max} is the largest JND index in the rectangle, and p_{max} is the maximum possible presentation value. Thus, a presentation value of 0 is assigned the lowest luminance of the display, which is the lowest luminance in the part of the GSDF within the segment. The maximum possible presentation value p_{max} is assigned the maximal calibrated luminance of the display, which is the maximal luminance in the segment. Each intermediate presentation value p is assigned the luminance on the GSDF corresponding to the JND index j determined from the equation above.

Display Calibration

The calibration of a display to the GSDF is usually performed automatically by the workstation itself, using specialized software and a calibrated photometer that sends a digital luminance signal to the workstation display. The photometer is aimed at a single point on the face of the display (Fig. 5-18). The software, starting with a digital driving level of zero, increases the digital driving levels provided to the display system in a stepwise fashion and the photometer sends to the software the measured luminance for each step, thereby measuring the display function of the display system. The software then calculates the values to be placed in the LUT that will cause the LUT and display system, acting together, to conform to the GSDF. Some displays are equipped with photometers and can automatically assess luminance and GSDF calibration (Fig. 5-18, bottom).

Shown in Figure 5-19 is the characteristic response of an uncalibrated display, depicting lower luminance values that diverge substantially from the GSDF and a low contrast test pattern that shows poor contrast rendition in the darker areas of the displayed image. After calibration to the DICOM GSDF, the contrast is greatly improved, especially important in the darker, low brightness areas of an image for an object of minimal contrast. Subtle differences potentially important for a differential diagnosis can otherwise be lost.

Workstation displays must be evaluated periodically to ensure all have calibrated luminances and the same display characteristics to ensure conformance to the DICOM GSDF. The maximal luminance of a display degrades with the amount of "on" time and with the brightness of displayed images. Turning LCD displays off when not being used for an extended period of time can significantly prolong longevity; however, displays may take some time to stabilize from a cold start, so a common strategy is to place them into a "standby" mode. Displays should be replaced when their maximal luminances fall below the recommended value. Many medical-grade LCD

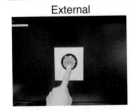

Monitor Calibration Sensors
External

Internal

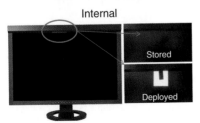

Stored

Deployed

■ **FIGURE 5-18** A display can be calibrated by using a photometer that measures the luminance of a range of digital driving levels (DDLs) from minimum to maximum under software control. The photometer sends the digitized luminance values to the computer, the DDLs are analyzed, and an LUT that conforms to the GSDF log-luminance curve is downloaded to the video display driver. The upper picture shows a display with a photometer manually placed at the center of the viewing area. The lower picture shows a medical-grade display with a built-in internal photometer that calibrates automatically.

■ **FIGURE 5-19** The characteristic response as a function of digital driving number on an uncalibrated display is shown by the white curve, and the DICOM GSDF is shown as the red curve. After calculating the adjustment lookup table and downloading to the video display driver, the subsequent conformance measurement indicates performance matching the GSDF. On the right are the corresponding images of a low contrast "Briggs" test pattern, demonstrating the improvement in contrast for the patterns in the darker areas of the image for the calibrated display.

Characteristic response

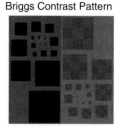

Briggs Contrast Pattern

GSDF calibration results

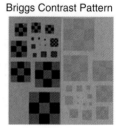

Briggs Contrast Pattern

displays have built-in sensors to measure luminances under software control and send information of GSDF conformance across a network to a web-based database server, greatly simplifying the task of monitoring display performance on a periodic basis (typically semi-annually or annually).

Test patterns, such as the Society of Motion Picture and Television Engineers (SMPTE) Test Pattern and the American Association of Physicists in Medicine (AAPM) TG18-OIQ (Fig. 5-20) are useful for semi-quantitative assessments of display

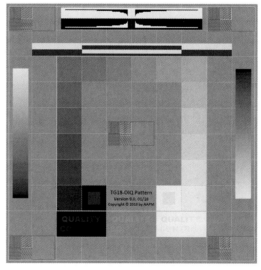

■ **FIGURE 5-20** Qualitative verification of display calibration. The AAPM TG18 OIQ (overall image quality) video test pattern has 18 luminance regions from 0 to 100%. At the ends are 0%/5% and 95%/100% contrast patches representing a difference of 13 digital numbers for an 8-bit display (256 gray levels). On the row below in the dark, midrange, and bright luminance areas are the letters "Quality Control" with a background contrast difference of 14 to 1 gray levels (1 level per letter). Spatial resolution modules of high and low contrast in the corners and the center, linear ramps on the sides for evaluating contouring and bit-depth artifacts, and dark-bright transition zones at the top are included in the test pattern. An alternate, simpler video test pattern is the Society of Motion Picture Television Engineers (SMPTE) pattern (not shown). (The AAPM TG18 OIQ pattern is used with permission from Ehsan Samei, PhD, Duke University Medical Center, and the American Association of Physicists in Medicine Samei E, Badano A, Chakraborty D, et. al. AAPM On-Line Report No. 03, April 2005.)

performance. The AAPM also has available a set of test images for display quality control and evaluation (AAPM, 2019a) that can be used as open-source material.

The refresh rate of an LCD display does matter when displaying dynamic images such as ultrasound videoclips. The frame refresh rate needed to provide the appearance of continuous motion is a minimum of 25 frames per second. The presence of lag in LCD displays, caused by the time required to change the electrical charges stored by the small capacitors in individual pixels, can reduce perceived temporal resolution, particularly for low-cost consumer grade displays. Displays add both spatial and temporal noise to viewed images.

Validating Patient Demographics with Acquired Images

Another important quality assurance task is ensuring that acquired studies are properly associated with the correct patients in the PACS, RIS, and EHR. Problems can occur if an error is made in manually entering patient identifying information, if a technologist selects the wrong patient identifier from a MWL, if an imaging study is performed on an unidentified patient, or if a patient's name is changed, such as after marriage. These can result in imaging studies stored in a PACS that are not associated with the proper patients. Procedures should be established to identify such incorrectly associated studies and to associate them with the proper patients. Collectively, these processes—Order entry at the EHR, Order processing and accessioning at the RIS, Modality Worklist to the Modality, Image acquisition, and RIS reconciliation, and Interpretation—should result in a seamless end-to-end "lifecycle" of the imaging study, which will be described more completely in the next section to eliminate repetitive human entry of data, which introduces error. These processes (Fig. 5-21) are described in the IHE profile called SWF, as was mentioned previously in Section 5.1.6, one of the earliest and fundamental of the Radiology IHE profiles (IHE, 2006).

In most modern EHR/RIS/PACS integrations, there are quality checks in place to assure demographic integrity at multiple points of the imaging chain, such as comparing the receipt of a valid Order to the DICOM images acquired, both in terms of Patient as well as Study context. If errors do occur, typically because of non-standard workflow, processes detect these errors and queue them for manual resolution by imaging staff. This is often termed Exception processing, such as where a Patient (incorrect MRN) or Study (incorrect Accession) mismatch occurs. These will generally require human review

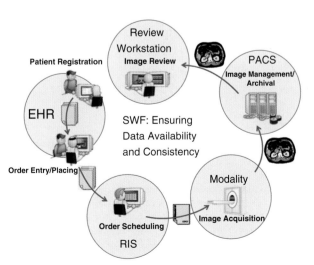

■ FIGURE 5-21 The Scheduled Workflow (SWF) IHE profile integrates the ordering, scheduling, imaging acquisition, storage, and viewing activities associated with radiology exams. This involves several steps through the information systems databases and a combination of HL7 messaging and DICOM services to achieve efficient workflow. (Adapted with permission from IHE, 2006. *Scheduled Workflow, SWF.* Integrating the Healthcare Enterprise. https://wiki.ihe.net/index.php/Scheduled_Workflow. Accessed May 31, 2020.)

and decision actions. Increasingly, however, artificial intelligence (AI) (such as anatomy/feature recognition) is becoming a part of this process to assist in error recovery.

An additional workflow path needs to be considered, where non-standard workflow is required to support emergent imaging, such as trauma or for unidentified patients as shown in Figure 5-22. IHE defines a profile for this called PIR (IHE, 2008) also previously mentioned. This is an essential addition to SWF, since compliance with standardized workflow cannot supersede critical patient care delivery. Additionally, PIR instantiates the process for correcting human workflow errors outside of trauma use cases as well.

Together, these two IHE profiles are essential to maintaining demographic data quality in the imaging lifecycle. [Note: SWF and PIR are now merged into SWF.b in recognition of their interdependence.]

Interoperability Assessment of Medical Imaging Acquisition Systems

Other considerations for Quality Control occur during the commissioning of medical imaging modalities. The functionality of a diagnostic medical imaging system extends beyond the acceptance testing of the unit itself and depends on the interoperability with the PACS, RIS, post-processing software, and clinical viewers. This requires end-to-end evaluation of image quality and associated image information from the ordering system to the archive and relevant systems where the images are viewed, processed, or modified (AAPM, 2019a). Tests that should be considered are listed in Table 5-4.

Compared to the time of analog imaging and paper-based documentation, the complex digital environment of today stretches beyond the medical imaging acquisition system for post-processing, storage, and display of images and image information, which in turn creates challenges for ensuring image fidelity and information accuracy. Interoperability assessment depends on specific equipment, infrastructure, and

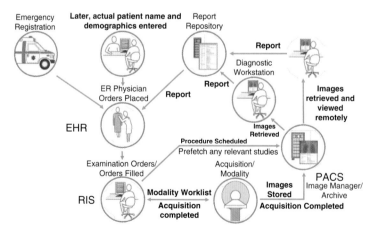

■ **FIGURE 5-22** Patient Information Reconciliation (PIR) is an IHE profile that supports non-standard workflow resulting from emergent imaging of a trauma case of an unidentified patient as the example above shows. In this situation, the patient has orders for an imaging exam scheduled as a "Doe" with typical routing for acquisition and reporting as an urgent case. After the report is released, the reconciliation of the fictitious name to the actual name and demographics of the patient occurs later, by orchestration of the PACS and RIS/EHR using HL7 and DICOM standards through the PIR profile. (Adapted with permission from IHE, 2008. *Patient Information Reconciliation, PIR*. Integrating the Healthcare Enterprise. https://wiki.ihe.net/index.php/Patient_Information_Reconciliation. Accessed May 31, 2020.)

TABLE 5-4 INTEROPERABILITY ASSESSMENT TESTS

1.	DICOM Modality Worklist configuration and Information Display is accurate
2.	Procedure or RIS Code Mapping is properly loaded into the imaging modality
3.	Images appear in a timely fashion and are associated with the correct worklist
4.	Exams and image labeling have appropriate appearance
5.	Quantitative measurement consistency is validated between systems and viewers
6.	Patient demographics are correct and editing (if allowed) is validated downstream
7.	Image orientation and laterality are properly encoded in the DICOM metadata
8.	Fidelity of information in the DICOM header is maintained with information exchange
9.	DICOM structured reports (SR) are accurate and mapped correctly
10.	Post-processing functionality is consistent across systems and reproducible
11.	Downtime procedures and alternative connectivity channels are validated

From AAPM. *Interoperability Assessment for the Commissioning of Medical Imaging Acquisition Systems, Report of AAPM Task Group 248.* American Association of Physicists in Medicine; 2019b. https://www.aapm.org/pubs/reports/detail.asp?docid=180. Accessed August 10, 2020.

utilization. Validation of interoperability is critical for ensuring optimal and safe patient care.

5.4 LIFECYCLE OF A RADIOLOGY EXAM

An encounter with an ailing patient is described in the following section, illustrating the various messaging and interactions that are necessary with the informatics infrastructure to ensure registration, evaluation, scheduling, image acquisition, diagnosis, and care of the patient. Figure 5-23 illustrates a simple informatics infrastructure and messaging pipeline that exists for supporting the communications through an HL7 *Interface Engine* to orchestrate HL7 messages between the relevant databases involved in delivering the information necessary to image a patient and follow up with reading, diagnosing, and reporting the findings. Communication amongst the various enterprise information systems such as the EHR, LIS, RIS, PACS,

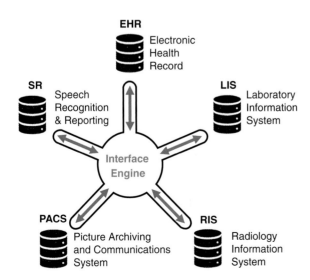

EHR
Electronic Health Record

SR
Speech Recognition & Reporting

LIS
Laboratory Information System

Interface Engine

PACS
Picture Archiving and Communications System

RIS
Radiology Information System

■ **FIGURE 5-23** Several information system databases are necessary to deliver timely assistance and care for a patient undergoing an imaging examination. These systems communicate on the Local Area Network bi-directionally with HL7 messaging through an Interface Engine, which routes HL7 messages based upon internal content to specific target databases. Each database system plays a role in the lifecycle of a radiology encounter with a patient for an imaging examination by creating, sending, using, and storing information useful for the care of the patient.

```
HL7 Admit, Discharge, Transfer (ADT) A04 Message
MSH|^~\&|ADT1|MCM|LABADT|MCM|198808181126|SECURITY|ADT^A04|MSG00001|P|2.4
EVN|A04-|198808181123
PID|||PATID1234^5^M11||DOE^JOHN^A^III||19610615|M-||2106-3|3200 N ELM
     STREET^^ANYWHERE^NC^27401-1020|GL|(999)123-1212|(999)123-3434~(999)277-
     3114||S||PATID12345678^2^M10|123456789|9-87654^NC
NK1|1|DOE^BARBARA^K|SPO|||||20011105
NK1|1|DOE^MICHAEL^A|FTH
PV1|1|I|2000^2012^01||||004777^SMITH^SIDNEY^J.|||SUR||-||1|A0-
AL1|1||^PENICILLIN||PRODUCES HIVES~RASH
AL1|2||^CAT DANDER
DG1|001|I9|1550|MAL NEO LIVER, PRIMARY|19880501103005|F||
PR1|2234|M11|111^CODE151|COMMON PROCEDURES|198809081123
ROL|45^RECORDER^ROLE MASTER LIST|AD|CP|KATE^SMITH^ELLEN|192705011201
GT1|1122|1519|BILL^GATES^A
IN1|001|A357|1234|BCMD|||||132987
IN2|ID1551001|SSN12345678
ROL|45^RECORDER^ROLE MASTER LIST|AD|CP|KATE^ELLEN|199505011201
```

■ **FIGURE 5-24** An HL7 Admit, Discharge, Transfer (ADT) message contains a standardized method of encoding ASCII information with pipes (|), delimiters (^) and content that is common for all databases to allow decoding the information into their proprietary databases. This is an A04 message for registering a patient at the EHR. The information contains many tags such as MSH-message header segment, PID (Patient Identification and Medical Record Number) segment, AL1—Allergies (e.g., in this case to penicillin and cat dander) segment, DG1—diagnosis segment—in this case, malignant neoplasm of the liver from another (primary) anatomic site. This content is sent to the Interface Engine and passed on to the relevant databases for notification and awareness of the patient's presence.

and Speech Recognition (SR) systems is accomplished with the HL7 standard for contextual interactions and services. The DICOM standard is used for communication and services between the imaging modalities and the PACS.

5.4.1 Registration and Order Entry

When a patient arrives as an *Inpatient*, the first encounter is with the registration desk to enter patient demographic information into the EHR. This initiates an HL7 "ADT" (Admit, Discharge, Transfer) message specific to registration (an A04 message) that is delivered to the network Interface Engine and sent to pertinent databases that will be part of the patient care encounter. The A04 content includes the patient name, home address, medical record number, insurance information, and other pertinent information such as allergies, and current diagnoses encoded in the message (Fig. 5-24). The patient's physician logs onto the EHR, receives information regarding patient status, and then orders appropriate laboratory and diagnostic imaging tests. An order for a complete blood count triggers an HL7 "ORM" (Order Message) that is specifically sent from the EHR to the LIS to perform the lab work. At the same time, an order for a diagnostic ultrasound exam is initiated, which sends another ORM message to the RIS to schedule the patient for the requested procedure. This order message contains content specifying an HL7 "OBR" (Observation Request) for a limited ultrasound abdominal right upper quadrant exam and typically includes the reason for the exam, such as abdominal pain (Fig. 5-25). Each of the HL7 messages contains standardized trigger

```
HL7 Order (ORM) O01 Message
MSH|^~\&|EPIC|EPIC|||20140418173314|1148|ORM^O01|497|D|2.3||
PID|1||20891312^^^^EPI||PATIENT DOE ER^^A^^MR.^||19661201|M||Cauc|505 S.
    HAMILTON AVE^^ANYTOWN^WI^53505^US^^^DN |DN|(999)123-4567|(999)123-
    5678||S|| 11480003|123-45-7890||||^^^WI^^
PD1|||FACILITY(EAST)^^12345|1173^WELBY^JOHN^A^^^ PV1|||^^^CARE HEALTH
    SYSTEMS^^^^^|||
    |1173^WELBY^JOHN^A^^^||||||||||||610613||||||||||||||||||||||||||V
ORC|NW|987654^EPIC|76543^EPC||Final||^^^20140418170014^^^^||20140418173314|1
    148^PATIENT^ER^^A^^MR.^||1173^WELBY^JOHN^A^^^|1133^^^222^^^^^|(999)123-
    4567||
OBR|1|363463^EPC|1858^EPC|73610^US ABD LIM RUQ^^^US ABD
    ||||||||||1173^WELBY^JOHN^A^^^|(999)1234567||||||||Final||^^^2014041817
    0014^^^^|||||6064^DOCTOR^J^^^^||11480010^1A^EAST^X-RAY^^^|^|
DG1||I10|S82^ABD PAIN^I10|ABD PAIN||
```

■ **FIGURE 5-25** The patient is evaluated by a physician who uses the EHR to order tests such as a blood analysis and an ultrasound exam. In this example, an HL7 order (ORM) O01 message is generated to request a limited ultrasound abdomen exam as shown in the Observation Request (OBR) segment and the reason why the exam is ordered in the DG1 segment.

events, segments, data types, and tables. The interface engine routes messages based on the content and can split messages into multiple subtypes to specific databases.

5.4.2 RIS and Scheduling

The RIS is used to manage orders, protocols, exam scheduling, and technologist workflow. Specific workflows vary depending on the modality (*e.g.*, US, CT, MRI), patient status (inpatient, outpatient, emergency), and type of exam requested. For outpatients, the scheduling template contains specific time slots, the lengths of which depend on the modality and exam type, which allows some rigidity for pre-scheduling. For inpatients and emergency room patients there are often no set schedules, but priorities based upon patient condition and urgency to get the diagnosis for patient treatment. The type of acquisition protocol, the reason for the exam, and priority are the mechanisms that allow for the appropriate scheduling to occur.

The RIS sends an HL7 ORM message to the EHR, Speech Recognition/Reporting System, and PACS interfaces as appropriate to schedule the imaging examination. An "accession number" unique to the exam is assigned at this time. Once the patient is scheduled, a second message is sent from the RIS to the PACS to indicate the location and time of the exam.

5.4.3 Modalities and Modality Worklist

All imaging modalities (CT, US, MR, PET/CT, radiography, fluoroscopy, interventional) are connected to the enterprise network and provide communication links; however, these devices are built around the DICOM standard, and do not directly respond to HL7 messages. Each modality communicates directly with the PACS or RIS/EHR through an HL7 to DICOM "broker" to receive a MWL, which contains patient names

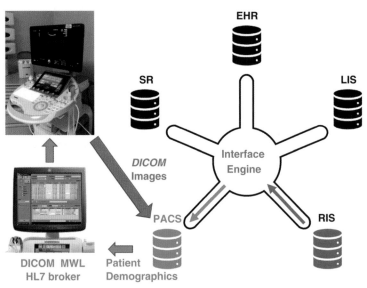

■ **FIGURE 5-26** To schedule the patient, the RIS generates an HL7 message routed to the PACS indicating the availability of the patient to be imaged. The imaging modality, however, does not use HL7 messaging for handling image acquisition and archiving events. A PACS "HL7-DICOM broker" interface generates a DICOM Modality Worklist on the modality. The technologist identifies the patient and selects the name from the list, ensuring reproducible demographic information appended to the DICOM metadata associated with the patient images at the modality (green arrows). The study is performed, and the DICOM images are sent to the PACS for review and storage (red arrow).

made available at the technologist console to allow the selection of a specific patient and corresponding unique demographics for the examination—in this example, ultrasound (Fig. 5-26). This eliminates errors of manual data entry that could otherwise result in a mismatch of patient identifiers on the informatics databases between the PACS, RIS, and EHR, and provides easy access to order information. The MWL can be configured for an inpatient/outpatient setting, hospital location, exam type, patient demographics, and other parameters by using filters that limit the list to a small number of pertinent selections. In the PACS each patient study is identified by a unique number called the accession number, generated and assigned by the RIS. The accession number is one of three identifiers used to reconcile content that is cross-referenced; the others are the patient identifier (medical record number) and the patient name. If there is a mismatch, an "exception" is generated that requires action by a PACS administrator, technologist, or clerk to reconcile the issue so that the patient's data and images are available through the database worklist and search tools. A "lost study" can still occur if the technologist mistakenly associates an imaging study with the wrong patient in a worklist.

5.4.4 Exam Acquisition and Storage

The imaging procedure is initiated at the modality—this is where the DICOM standard comes fully into play. Modality-specific attributes of acquired images are contained in the DICOM IOD that defines the metadata associated with individual images and image attributes, series and series information, study and accession number and the patient demographics. UID labels within the metadata are present to uniquely identify a wide variety of items across countries, sites, vendors, and equipment—information on UIDs can be found in the DICOM standard documentation. An ultrasound IOD will have attributes in the metadata specific to ultrasound and ultrasound exam attributes.

For each device on the network, an *Application Entity* (AE) title is configured to allow applications (programs and devices) to communicate via DICOM using a "Service" to perform on an "Object" (*e.g.*, the IOD). DICOM services include *store, get, find,* and *echo.* A SOP—*Service-Object-Pair*—is a combination of a DICOM service and DICOM object, defined by the union of an IOD and a DIMSE; for instance, in this case, the SOP might be "Store an Ultrasound Study." A *Service Class* is a specific definition of a service supported by cooperating devices to perform an action on a specific class of Information Object, including a *Service Class User* (SCU) that invokes operations, and a *Service Class Provider* (SCP) that performs operations. In the current example, the ultrasound device is the SCU and the PACS is the SCP. The DICOM services that can be performed and cannot be performed are detailed in the vendor's DICOM *Conformance Statement*, a required public document provided by the vendor of the implementation. A DICOM *Association* is the first phase of communication between AEs and SOP classes requiring the IP address, port number, and AE title of each entity. If specific SOP classes are not available in either DICOM implementation, the requested association will fail. Just because a vendor indicates "DICOM compliance" there is no guarantee of specific functionality. Details of functionality are described in the vendor's Conformance Statement—even then, some capabilities may be considered optional, so it is often up to negotiation to ensure data transfer. New data classes (*e.g.*, digital tomosynthesis of breast images—see Chapter 8) can also be a cause of failure that takes vendors time to comply with successful implementation of specific SOP classes.

During the exam technologist acquires images and can send on-the-fly image updates to the PACS and to a radiologist in-waiting at a diagnostic workstation for study verification. Modality Performed Procedure Step (MPPS) DICOM messages can be sent to the PACS or RIS to indicate when the exam is started, first images acquired, and last images acquired, and to indicate that the exam is completed. Images at this

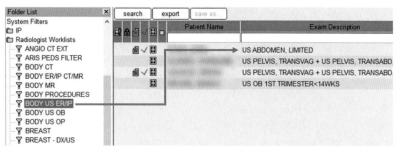

■ FIGURE 5-27 Radiologist worklist provides the radiologist a list of available completed examinations generated through the PACS or RIS. This worklist is continuously updated throughout the day. Filters are used to identify a subset of studies to be read by a specific radiologist or group of radiologists by section, anatomical site, clinic, patient status, etc. For this selected list, the exams available to be interpreted for Body Ultrasound from the Emergency Room or Inpatient scans are shown, and the limited ultrasound of the abdomen is selected.

time are stored on the PACS—however, getting access to the images for viewing and diagnosis through the various electronic databases requires further communication and interoperability.

5.4.5 Radiologist Worklist, Speech Recognition, and Report Generation

The radiologist at the PACS workstation identifies studies assigned for diagnosis based upon information in the Radiologist Worklist, from either a PACS or RIS generated list of patients and images for diagnosis. Worklist filters allow selectivity in types of sub-specialty sections, modalities, anatomical site, patient age (*e.g.*, pediatric versus adult), patient status, clinic location and many other specific attributes (Fig. 5-27). The worklist is continuously updated throughout the day—as studies are read, the entries drop off the list and other newly acquired studies appear. Radiologist worklists also permit the prefetching of relevant previous studies for comparison.

Once a study is selected, the images from the PACS are displayed in a specific arrangement using defined hanging protocols for the exam type (see Section 5.3), using the information in the DICOM metadata associated with each image, series, and patient study (Fig. 5-28). Contemporaneously, the radiologist gains access to the EHR for pertinent patient history, results from pathology workup, blood tests, and other details that assist in developing a differential diagnosis based upon display of the images. As information is ingested and synthesized by the radiologist, the speech recognition system is activated as a separate interconnected software program. Voice commands and free text are entered to generate a report through speech to text recognition; alternatively, structured radiology templates are often used as a guide for specific modality and exam types to provide a checklist for the evaluation parameters, findings, impression and conclusions in a standardized format. The information assembled by the voice recognition system is packaged into an HL7 Observation (ORU) R01 message for the patient diagnosis contained in the Observation result (OBX) segment and forwarded to the target databases for appending to the patient record in the PACS, RIS, and EHR, as shown in Figures 5-28 and 5-29.

5.4.6 Structured Reporting

The term "structured reporting" relates to concepts that might mean different things to different individuals. For example, a radiologist may think of a document with a hierarchy of headings containing text, codes, and keywords to summarize the findings of a diagnostic report. In terms of making a series of measurements, as in an

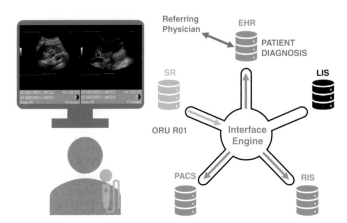

■ **FIGURE 5-28** From the radiologist worklist, a study is selected and displayed on the diagnostic workstation. Assembled information for the radiologist is the patient history, current images, pertinent prior images, and access to the speech recognition system. After review, the radiologist dictates the report; the content is converted to text by the speech recognition system and is packaged into an HL7 observation message (ORU). This message is forwarded to the Interface Engine and distributed to the pertinent target databases for appending to the patient record. In this case the message is accepted and updated by the PACS, RIS, and EHR.

obstetric ultrasound example, a software programmer might visualize a nested hierarchy of numeric measurements (*e.g.*, head diameter, femur length—each identified with individual codes, then aggregated to provide an estimate of gestational age). These and other examples describe unifying concepts of the DICOM SR including (1) the presence of lists and hierarchical relationships; (2) use of coded/numerical content and plain text; (3) use of relationships between concepts; (4) presence of embedded references to images and other objects (Clunie, 2000). A DICOM SR is defined more by its construction and less by what it contains. It does not need to be complex, nor always intended for direct rendering into a form that humans can read. The SR encodes only what is meant and is required to be unambiguous. So, it is not just a report, but more generally a structured document. Besides being stored and transferred with the images that were used to generate it, the DICOM SR is a structured document that contains text with links to other data such as images, waveforms, and spatial or temporal coordinates.

```
HL7 Unsolicited Transmission of an Observation (ORU) R01 Message
MSH|^~\&|System1||||200707090801||ORU^R01|3542196||2.3
PID|1|000-0000|||"DOE"|1922974|151-76-5760||||||||||||N
PV1|1|2|||||||| ||||||N|| ||
IN1|1|P||||
ORC|RE||2060059||||^^^200707061707^^ ||202007051013|DIONA |||""||||1007
OBR|||2060059|999991^US ABDOMEN, LIMITED|
    |200707061707|200707061621|200707061707|||""|""|||
ZOR|1|1831236|X|1|01|66696|2| |""|""|""|
ZEX|1|2060059|5|G|CC11043257 |R/O MMT|1004959042 CASE # VERIFIED ONLINE
DGC|APRV^APPROVED|202007090801|||||||||||0|0|0|0|N|N|N|N|N|""|""|""|""|""||EO
    K
OBX|1|TX|||PROCEDURE: US ABDOMEN, LIMITED~ ~HISTORY: Acute abdominal pain of
    unknown origin.~ ~TECHNIQUE: Real-time ultrasound scanning of the abdomen
    was performed by the sonographer. Representative static images and video
    clips were submitted for review.~ ~FINDINGS: Liver: Multiple echogenic
    well-circumscribed structures throughout the liver, largest in the right
    lobe measuring 2.1 x 1.6 x 2.1 cm, the largest in the left lobe measuring
    1.2 x 0.9 x 1.2 cm. The liver is overall not significantly enlarged. ~
    ~IMPRESSION:~ ~1. Multiple echogenic well-circumscribed structures
    throughout the liver, consistent with hepatic hemangiomas. 2. Liver size is
    within normal limits. …||||||F
```

■ **FIGURE 5-29** The HL7 Observation ORU—R01 message contains the pertinent information for the patient diagnosis in the Observation result (OBX) segment. When the study has been completed and the diagnosis rendered, the results are received by the EHR and accessed by the referring physician for continuance of patient care and treatment. The lifecycle for this instance is complete.

The encoding of a DICOM SR object is defined by the DICOM Standard, with SR IODs consisting of a document header and document body. The header metadata attribute values are grouped into modules such as Patient, General Study, Clinical Study, etc. and contain details about the patient, study, series, equipment, and the document content. The document body is the information that is stored in the DICOM SR Content Tree and encoded in the SR Document Content Module. Details are beyond the scope of this chapter. For further reading, an in-depth review is available in the DICOM Standard documentation, PS 3.16. An example of a structured report with ultrasound measurements encountered in an obstetric exam is shown in Chapter 14, Ultrasound, Figure 14-42.

The informatics community and radiology stakeholders are now just beginning to fully leverage further capabilities of DICOM SR for increasing accuracy and efficiency. Principal uses are currently in radiation dose (RDSR) and ultrasound (where biometric measurements are an essential quantitative component), but use cases are expanding. Measurement and tracking of lesions, volume analytics, protocol descriptions, and key image/feature identification are all potential applications of DICOM Structured Reporting as well as the construction of richer report content. (See Report Distribution, Section 5.4.8.)

5.4.7 Billing

Once an examination is completed with the signing of the interpretive report, payment for the procedure is initiated via an HL7 message to the EHR and RIS from the reporting system. Information related to each bill is reviewed by either human coders or billers or automated processes (see Section 5.9.1) to identify the procedures performed, the appropriate CPT and/or ICD-10 codes, and any modifiers that are needed to successfully match through network messaging and active monitoring.

Most radiology services or procedures are typically comprised of a professional component and a technical component, even though the procedure is described by a single CPT code. The professional component is billed on behalf of the physician (radiologist) and may include supervision, the diagnosis and interpretation, and a written report. The technical component of the service includes the use of equipment, personnel, supplies, and costs related to the performance of the examination.

5.4.8 Report Distribution—Completion of the Exam Lifecycle

A web server, interfaced to the PACS, RIS, and EHR, generally maintains information about patient demographics, reports, and images. The server permits queries and retrievals of information from the PACS database. Physicians obtain images and reports from the webserver using workstations with commercial web browsers. A major advantage of using web-based technology is that the workstations need not be equipped with specialized software for image display and manipulation; instead, these programs can be sent from the webserver with the images or the server itself can provide this function. It is particularly desirable, for healthcare systems that have implemented EHRs, that relevant images can be accessed *via* the EHR. Healthcare professionals at remote sites such as doctors' offices or small clinics or at home can connect to the EHR via the Internet, typically through secure VPNs.

In summary, the workflow of a patient encounter with radiology is a several step process and involves many events that require orchestration through multiple interactions amongst many separate databases and use of HL7 and DICOM standards to complete the transactions. Many of these steps are diagrammed in Figure 5-30.

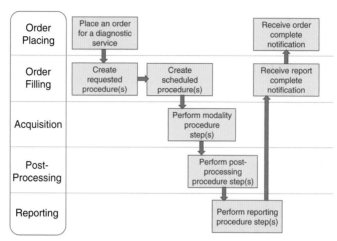

■ FIGURE 5-30 Workflow steps in radiology for an examination are a several step process that requires multiple interactions between database systems and synchronization of events for order placing, order filling, acquisition, post-processing, and reporting.

5.5 RADIOLOGY FROM OUTSIDE THE DEPARTMENT

5.5.1 Clinical Decision Support and Computerized Provider Order Entry

In an era of healthcare reform and a push to meet appropriate use guidelines for tests, implementation of clinical decision support (CDS) software has been mandated by the Protecting Access to Medicare Act (PAMA) of 2014. As part of PAMA, the CMS requires that physicians ordering advanced diagnostic imaging services consult Appropriate Use Criteria (AUC) through a Clinical Decision Support Mechanism (CDSM), an interactive, electronic tool that communicates AUC information to the users and assists them in making the most appropriate treatment decision for a patient's specific clinical condition by scoring the choice of exam against the AUC. AUC is evidence-based criteria developed or endorsed by professional medical societies or other Provider-Led Entities (PLEs) that go through a qualification process to become a qualified PLE (QPLE). There are specific requirements for developing and modifying AUC, requiring a peer-review process, literature review, and assessment of the evidence. QPLEs must publicly post their process for AUC development or modification to their website. Ultimately, CDS is supposed to help clinicians by eliminating inappropriate procedures, and help physicians adhere to practice guidelines, with a goal to deliver healthcare of the highest quality, safety, efficiency, and effectiveness for patients. Initially, eight clinical priority areas (listed as of November 2016) are coronary artery disease, suspected pulmonary embolism, headache (traumatic and non-traumatic), hip pain, low back pain, shoulder pain (to include suspected rotator cuff injury), cancer of the lung, and cervical or neck pain. An AUC consultation must occur through a qualified CDSM and report AUC consultation information (scores for the specific procedures ordered) on the professional and facility claims for the service. There are many more details that are found at the CMS.gov website (CMS, 2020a).

5.5.2 Reporting

The current standard radiology report, as Dr. Curtis Langlotz observed, has not fundamentally changed since the first radiographs were created to diagnose disease, despite tremendous advancement in acquisition modality technology (Langlotz, 2015). Still principally narrative in structure and transmitted as text, radiology reporting has not tracked technology development in other areas such as the Web. Although we would be surprised now to experience an online advertisement for a product without hyperlinks to other information, enable ordering, display additional views—this is the current state of radiology reporting. Rich multimedia content is expected with advertising media and increasingly in many other communication use cases.

By contrast, radiology reports typically still contain only narrative text based on specialized vocabulary and often including many conditional statements. The anticipated evolution of this state is towards the Multimedia Enhanced Radiology Report (MERR), more aligned with current experience in other communication areas (Fig. 5-31) (Folio et al., 2018). Reference links to key images or annotations (via IHE Key Image Notes, KIN profile), structured exchange and storage (Simple Image and Numeric Report, SINR profile), and other tools facilitate a much richer and more informative report than is now the norm. These profiles are specified in great detail in the IHE Radiology Technical Framework (IHE, 2020).

5.5.3 Reading Room

The reading room is a rapidly evolving topic. For many years the idea of the "Reading Room" was both familiar and relatively unchanged from the era of film Radiology (film alternators were replaced with workstations and analog voice recorders with speech recognition, but basically all else in the reading environment remained unchanged). But now, more reading is done in individual offices and increasingly remotely, including Radiologist homes. The construct of the dedicated "reading room" is rapidly giving way to a distributed model of interpretation. Several principal technologies or practice changes are enabling or driving this change:

1. The availability of high-performance computing hardware at a much lower cost (CPU, GPU, memory, and graphics following Moore's Law)
2. The decreased costs of diagnostic displays (with "prosumer" grade displays rapidly approaching the performance of current bespoke diagnostic displays)

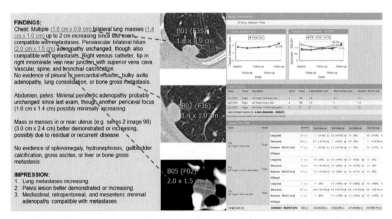

■ **FIGURE 5-31** The Multimedia Enhanced Radiology Report provides a narrative of findings and associated images that visually show the details as well as quantitative content to demonstrate longitudinal outcomes through measurements and graphs—in this case a continuing evaluation of lung metastases and patterns of evolving size. (Reproduced with permission from Folio LR, Machado LB, Dwyer AJ. Multimedia-enhanced radiology reports: concept, components, and challenges. *Radiographics*. 2018;38(2):462-482. Copyright © Radiological Society of North America. doi: 10.1148/rg.2017170047.)

3. Availability of vastly higher commercial bandwidth through a standard home or remote office ISP
4. High-performance VPNs, through either hardware (VPN appliances) or software, enabling fully secure remote reading
5. The development of wide-scale virtual Radiology practices disassociated and independent from specific hospital enterprises or healthcare organizations ("Nighthawk" and "Virtual Radiology" as independent services)

While in the past, much discussion and technology were devoted to what was considered "Teleradiology," the meaning of this term is rapidly changing. In a fully network-based distributed and virtualized Radiology practice, what exactly does the "Tele" now imply? Informatics and PACS operations need to adapt to these changes—mastering much more effective remote support and management technology than those of previous generations.

5.5.4 Social Media

While applications like Facebook or Instagram are very familiar as social media, the concept in the context of Informatics needs to be considered more widely. All widely shared electronic information in the imaging community can be considered part of the more general use case of a virtual community for Informatics. Shared Wikis, virtual conferences and presentations, online messages, and messaging forums (Aunt Minnie, Linked In, Slack, etc.), video teleconferencing, can all be considered part of the larger sense of social media. While there will always be strong value in physical meetings and conferences, the community is rapidly moving to a model de-emphasizing physical presence in favor of virtual presence. Factors such as environmental (carbon footprint) and medical (emerging pandemics) are additional drivers to the virtualization of collaboration in Informatics.

5.6 SECURITY AND PRIVACY

Critical requirements regarding medical imaging and PACS are ensuring information security and patient privacy through data integrity, authentication, non-repudiation, and availability. Privacy, also called confidentiality, refers to denying persons, other than intended recipients, access to confidential information. Integrity means that information has not been altered, either accidentally or deliberately. Authentication permits the recipient of information to verify the identity of the sender and the sender to verify the identity of the intended recipient. Non-repudiation prevents a person from later denying an action, such as approval of payment or approval of a report. Availability means that information and services are available when needed. This section describes the requirements for security and privacy with these goals in mind.

5.6.1 Layers of Security

Achieving security requires a triad of safeguards, namely physical, technical, and administrative (Fig. 5-32). *Physical safeguards* are those that prevent or limit access to protected information by unauthorized individuals. Examples include isolating devices from public access; allowing access by authorization; backing up, restoring, and disposing of information where appropriate; and complete decommissioning/destroying old computers, disk drives, and devices. *Technical safeguards* include implementation of firewalls with limited access through VPN tunnels; encryption

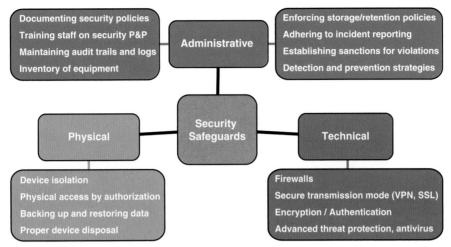

Documenting security policies
Training staff on security P&P
Maintaining audit trails and logs
Inventory of equipment

Administrative

Enforcing storage/retention policies
Adhering to incident reporting
Establishing sanctions for violations
Detection and prevention strategies

Physical

Security Safeguards

Technical

Device isolation
Physical access by authorization
Backing up and restoring data
Proper device disposal

Firewalls
Secure transmission mode (VPN, SSL)
Encryption / Authentication
Advanced threat protection, antivirus

■ **FIGURE 5-32** Security safeguards entail a three-pronged approach, including administrative, physical, and technical components with a summary of key points.

of data at rest on media and in-flight; authentication mechanisms including passwords, biometric and dual-factor methods; protection against malware such as Trojan Horses, Viruses, Worms, Spyware, Malicious codes; and monitoring/tracking software (malware crawlers, anti-virus software). *Administrative safeguards* are the policies, procedures and staffing processes that represent active operating measures to protect the privacy and security of health information. These include documenting security policies, cybersecurity training, maintaining audit trails and logs, enforcing storage and retention policies, having an up to date inventory of medical imaging devices, regular patching of software and OSs, monitoring policies to detect anomalies/intrusions; establishing sanctions for violations, and developing strategies for detection and prevention.

5.6.2 Security Threats

A major and common vulnerability inherent to the use of computers is that, in some cases, the OS, application programs, and other important information are often stored on a single disk; an accident could cause all of them to be lost. The primary threats to information and software on digital storage devices or media are mechanical or electrical malfunction, such as a disk head crash; human error, such as the accidental deletion of a file or the accidental formatting of a disk (potentially causing the loss of all information on the disk); and malicious damage or "ransomware" whereby a hacker who has access can encrypt critical information and demand a financial ransom to provide a decryption key. To reduce the risk of information loss, important files should be copied ("backed up") onto magnetic disks, optical disks, or magnetic tape at regularly scheduled times, with the backup copies stored in a distant secure location.

Programs written with malicious intent are a threat to computers. The most prevalent of these are computer viruses. A virus is a string of instructions hidden in a program. If a program containing a virus is loaded into a computer and executed, the virus copies itself into other programs stored on mass storage devices. If a copy of an infected program is sent to another computer and executed, that computer becomes infected. Although a virus may not cause harm, many do, such as the deletion of all files on the disk on Friday the 13th. Viruses that are not intended to cause damage may interfere with the operation of the computer or cause damage because they are poorly written. A computer cannot be infected with a virus by the importation of data alone or by the user reading an e-mail message. However, a computer can become infected if an infected file is attached to an e-mail message and if that file is executed.

Malicious programs also include Trojan horses, programs that are presented as being of interest so people will load them onto computers, but have hidden purposes; worms, programs that automatically spread over computer networks; time bombs, programs or program segments that do something harmful, such as change or delete information, on a future date; key loggers, programs that record everything typed by a user, which can later be viewed for information of use, such as login names, passwords, and financial and personal information; and password grabbers, programs that ask people to log in and store the passwords and other login information for unauthorized use. A virus, worm, or Trojan horse may incorporate a time bomb or key logger. The primary way to reduce the chance of a virus infection or other problems from malicious software is to establish a policy forbidding the loading of storage media and software from untrustworthy sources. Commercial virus-protection software, which searches files on storage devices and files received over a network for known viruses and removes them, should be used. The final line of defense, however, is the saving of backup copies. Once a computer is infected, it may be necessary to reformat all disks and reload all software and information from the backup copies. A related threat is a denial of service attack, the bombardment of a computer or network with so many messages that it cannot function. Denial of service attacks are commonly launched from multiple computers that are being controlled by malicious software.

Computer networks pose significant security challenges. Unauthorized persons can access a computer over the network and, on some LANs, any computer on the network can be programmed to read the traffic. If a network is connected to the Internet, it is vulnerable to attack by every "hacker" on the planet.

5.6.3   Security Considerations

Sophisticated computer OSs provide security features including password protection and the ability to grant individual users different levels of access to stored files for availability. Measures should be taken to deny unauthorized users' access to all enterprise systems. Passwords should be used to deny access, directly and over a network. Each user should be granted only the privileges required to accomplish needed tasks. For example, technologists who acquire and process studies and interpreting physicians should not be granted the ability to delete or modify system software files or patient studies, whereas the system manager must be granted full privileges to all files on the system.

The goal of availability is to ensure that acquired studies can be interpreted and stored images can always be viewed. Availability is achieved using reliable components and media, fault-tolerant and risk-informed design and installation, provisions for prompt repair, and an emergency operation and disaster recovery plan. A design that continues to function despite equipment failure is said to be fault-tolerant. The design of a PACS must consider the fact that equipment will fail. Fault tolerance usually implies redundancy of critical components. Not all components are critical. For example, in a PACS with a central archive connected by a network to multiple workstations, the failure of a single workstation would have little adverse effect, but failure of the archive or network could prevent the interpretation of studies.

An essential element of fault tolerance is for the PACS and associated systems to create and maintain copies of all information on separate and remote storage devices for backup and disaster recovery. Offsite storage for disaster recovery, perhaps leased from a commercial vendor, is an option. The value of a study declines with time after its acquisition and so, therefore, does the degree of protection required against its loss. A very high degree of protection is necessary until it has been interpreted.

An important distinction should be made between Disaster Recovery (DR) and Business Continuity (BC). The former is essential to prepare for catastrophic events, but the latter critically needs to be part of standard PACS or RIS operations. As one IT pundit stated: "Business Continuity is what you do while you are working on Disaster Recovery." Business Continuity (or Business Continuity Systems, BCS) are generally implemented as parallel workflows or systems that can sustain essential business functions either during an unplanned event (disaster, unscheduled downtime) or planned event (scheduled downtimes for upgrades or patching). These can be either smaller alternate systems (servers and storage sufficient for reduced immediate clinical requirements) or as sophisticated (and expensive) as fully parallel redundant systems. But for 24/7/365 imaging operations, both are essential components of an overall availability plan.

The design of the PACS and the policies and procedures for its use should take into account the probability and possible consequences of risks, such as human error; deliberate attempts at sabotage, including computer viruses, worms, and denial of service attacks; fire; water leaks; and natural disasters such as floods, storms, and earthquakes. Examples are installing a redundant PACS archive far from the primary archive, preferably in another building, and, in an area vulnerable to flooding, not installing a PACS archive in a basement or ground floor of a building. Provisions for repair of a PACS are also important. A failure of a critical component is less serious if it is quickly repaired. Arrangements for emergency service should be made in advance of equipment failure.

Unintentional alteration of information can be detected by use of an error detecting code, called a hash algorithm. A sending computer calculates the error detecting code from the information to be transmitted over a network and sends the code along with the transmitted information. The receiving computer calculates the error detecting code from the information it receives and compares the code it calculated to the code sent with the information. If the two codes match, there is a high degree of assurance that the information was transmitted without error. Protection against intentional modification can be achieved by encrypting both the transmitted information and the hash algorithm.

Not only must the confidentiality and integrity of information be protected during transmission across a network, but the computers on the network must be protected from unauthorized access via the network. A simple way to protect a network is to not connect it to other networks. However, this may greatly limit its usefulness. For example, at a medical center, it is useful to connect the network supporting a PACS to the main hospital network. The main hospital network typically provides a link to the Internet as well.

A *firewall* can enhance the security of a network or network segment. A firewall is a program, router, computer, or even a small network that is used to connect two networks to provide security. Many services can be provided by a firewall. One of the simplest is packet filtering, in which the firewall examines packets reaching it. It reads their source and destination addresses and the applications for which they are intended and, based upon rules established by the network administrator, forwards, or discards them. For example, packet filtering can limit which computers a person

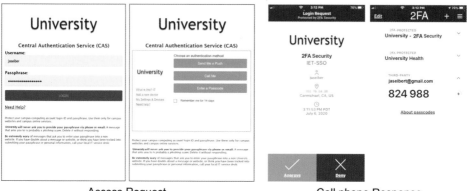

Access Request   Cell phone Response

■ **FIGURE 5-33** Two-factor authentication increases security by requiring a password for the initial access request (first factor) that sends a request to a device such as a cell phone in possession of the requestor. The cell phone, with its own security access, has a software app to respond (second factor). This response may be a simple acknowledgment, or a third-party request for authentication with a revolving 6-digit random number (as shown on the right) available for a given time span, for example, within one minute. Otherwise, a new number is generated, inactivating the old access number.

outside the firewall can access and can forbid certain kinds of access. Different rules may be applied to incoming and outgoing packets. Thus, the privileges of users outside the firewall can be restricted without limiting the ability of users on the protected network to access computers past the firewall. Firewalls also can maintain records of the traffic across the firewall, to help detect and diagnose attacks on the network. A firewall, by itself, does not provide complete protection and thus should merely be part of a comprehensive computer security program.

Authentication is usually performed based upon factors specific to an authorized user. Three major factors include something you know (*e.g.*, passwords), something you possess (*e.g.*, a cell phone with a security app), and something inherent to your person (*e.g.*, a biometric fingerprint or retina scan). Single-factor authentication allows access with one factor. To provide a higher level of security, particularly for remote access, two-factor authentication (2FA) requires a minimum of two independent factors. For instance, when requesting VPN access to a PACS from one's home, not only is a login password required, but after acceptance of the correct password, a push of information to the user's cell phone (which itself has an access authentication factor) activates the 2FA app to acknowledge the login request (Fig. 5-33). The user responds, which sends back to the VPN server an acknowledgment allowing access to the LAN through the firewall. Where 2FA was once the stuff of spy films, it is now relatively ubiquitous (such as common smartphone fingerprint or facial recognition).

Strategies for a PACS and Enterprise Imaging Security Plan

1. Perform a risk analysis.
2. Establish written policies and procedures for information security.
3. Train staff in the policies and procedures.
4. Backups—Maintain copies of important programs and information in case the data on a single device are lost. Backup copies should be stored in a secure location remote from the primary storage.
5. Install commercial anti-virus software on all computers to identify and remove common viruses and periodically update the software to recognize the signatures of recent viruses.
6. Forbid the loading of removable media (*e.g.*, USB flash drives, and optical disks from the homes of staff) and programs from non-trustworthy sources and forbid activating attachments to unexpected e-mail messages.

7. Authenticate users, directly and over a network or a modem, by passwords. Use secure passwords and consider 2FA (additional factors such as a possession such as a cell phone with a security app, or a biometric such as a fingerprint).
8. Terminate promptly the access privileges of former employees.
9. "Log off" workstations, particularly those in non-secure areas, when not in use.
10. Grant each user only sufficient privileges required to accomplish needed tasks and only access to information to which the user requires access.
11. Secure transfer—Encrypt information transferred over non-secure networks.
12. Secure storage—Physically secure media (*e.g.*, store it in a room to which access is controlled) or encrypt the information on it.
13. Erase information on or destroy removable media and storage devices before disposal or transfer for reuse. On most OSs, deleting a file merely removes the listing of the file from the device directory. The information remains stored on the device or media.
14. Install "patches" to the OS to fix security vulnerabilities.
15. Install "firewalls" at nodes where your LAN is connected to other networks.
16. Audit trails—Each access to protected healthcare information must be recorded.
17. Establish emergency operations and disaster recovery plans.

It is important to recognize that the imaging modalities, RIS, PACS MWL broker, speech recognition software, and peripheral equipment also require similar considerations over the total product lifecycle of the devices. This is an extraordinary undertaking that requires careful planning and a well-documented approach to security concerns. Fortunately, a framework of such a security protection plan is available from the National Institute of Standards and Technology (NIST) to ensure safe clinical practice and business continuity. The NIST Cybersecurity Framework (NIST, 2018) describes five pillars of security (Identify, Protect, Detect, Respond, Recover) in detail, with definitive references to national and international standards to combat outside attacks and limit vulnerabilities to a changing cybersecurity landscape. The Food and Drug Administration (FDA) has responsibility for oversight of medical imaging equipment and is working in cooperation with a consortium of imaging system manufacturers through the Medical Imaging Technology Alliance (MITA) to enhance the security requirements of such systems (MITA, 2016). Ultimately, it is the responsibility of the users (the healthcare enterprise) to adopt the recommendations of NIST, FDA and MITA to ensure a safe and secure medical imaging environment.

5.6.4   Privacy: HIPAA and HITECH

The federal Health Insurance Portability and Accountability Act of 1996 (HIPAA) and associated federal regulations (45 CFR 164) create standards to impose security requirements for "electronic protected healthcare information." The HIPAA Privacy Rule standards address the use and disclosure of individuals' health information (known as "protected health information"—PHI) by entities subject to the Privacy Rules. These individuals and organizations are called "covered entities" and include healthcare providers, health plans, healthcare clearinghouses, and business associates. The business associate must sign a legal document called a Business Associate Agreement (BAA) with the healthcare entity that specifies each party's responsibilities when it comes to PHI. A major goal of the Privacy Rule is to strike a balance that permits important uses of information while protecting the privacy of people seeking care. A covered entity is permitted, but not required to use and disclose PHI without an individual's authorization under certain circumstances, including disclosure to the individual, treatment-payment-healthcare operations, and public interest and benefit activities for national priority purposes, among several situations.

The HIPAA Security Rule protects a subset of information covered by the Privacy Rule, specifically with respect to "electronic protected health information—ePHI," which is all individually identifiable health information a covered entity creates, receives, maintains, or transmits in electronic form. It does not apply to PHI transmitted orally or in writing. Compliance with the Security Rule requires all covered entities to do the following:

1. Ensure the confidentiality, integrity, and availability of all ePHI
2. Detect and safeguard against anticipated threats to the security of the information
3. Protect against reasonably anticipated impermissible uses or disclosures
4. Certify compliance by the workforce.

The security measures described above largely conform to HIPAA security regulations, but do not include all such requirements. Furthermore, the regulations are subject to change. Hence, a covered entity responsible for a security program should refer to the current regulations (HIPAA, 2020a).

The Health Information Technology for Economic and Clinical Health (HITECH) Act was created in 2009 to motivate the implementation of EHRs and supporting technology in the United States (HIPAA, 2009). The HITECH Act anticipated the expansion in the exchange of ePHI between doctors, hospitals, and other entities that store ePHI for the sole reason of cutting down on the cost of healthcare by sharing. The HITECH Act expanded the scope of privacy and security protections available under HIPAA compliance by increasing the potential legal liability for non-compliance and for more stringent enforcement. With expanded electronic access, breaches of patient privacy by healthcare entities entrusted to maintain and protect such data can lead to substantial fines and action by the United States government.

5.6.5   De-identification of Protected Health Information

The HIPAA Privacy Rule provides the standard for de-identification of PHI, where health information is not individually identifiable if it does not identify an individual and if the covered entity has no reasonable basis to believe that the information can be used to identify an individual. Removing patient ePHI is required for performing research on clinical information and images. De-identification is defined under HIPAA (section 164.514(b)) as being one of two methods (Fig. 5-34): (1) the Statistical Method requires an "expert" statistician to document that there is a small

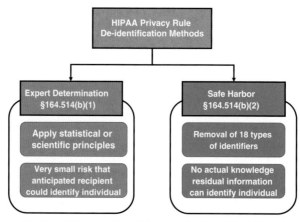

■ **FIGURE 5-34** De-identification of Protected Health Information in a patient's imaging exam and records can be achieved by Expert Determination or the Safe Harbor method, per the HIPAA privacy rule statutes.

TABLE 5-5 IDENTIFIERS TO BE REMOVED FROM ePHI TO BE DESIGNATED AS DE-IDENTIFIED BY THE SAFE HARBOR METHOD

1. Names (this includes names of the individual and his or her relatives, employers, or household members)

2. Geographic subdivisions smaller than a state, with exceptions for the use of part of the zipcode

3. All dates, except year, and all ages over 89

4. Telephone numbers

5. Fax numbers

6. Email addresses

7. Social security numbers

8. Medical record numbers

9. Health plan beneficiary numbers

10. Account numbers

11. Certificate or license numbers

12. Vehicle identifiers and license plate numbers

13. Device identifiers and serial numbers

14. URLs

15. IP addresses

16. Biometric identifiers

17. Full-face photographs and any comparable images

18. Any other unique, identifying characteristic or code

likelihood that a given record could be traced back to the patient; (2) the Safe Harbor method details 18 features that must be removed from the electronic information (Table 5-5). Researchers must request and receive permission from the local Institutional Review Board (IRB) to gain access to properly de-identified data prior to initiation of investigations. In some clinical trials and other defined research projects, not all of the 18 elements or more than the 18 elements need to be removed to be considered compliant with de-identification, as defined by specialized use of PHI by the IRB prior to any use.

5.7 "BIG DATA" AND DATA PLUMBING

5.7.1 Data: Data Types and Locations—"Big Data"

As imaging becomes an increasingly important part of machine learning (ML) as well as content for various new advanced analytics tools, we are also increasingly seeing PACS brought into the arena of what we are now calling "Big Data," encompassing multiple domains in the enterprise. The definitions of this term vary somewhat, but in general, converge on the requirements to access very large datasets (in the case of PACS) beyond traditional processes and methods that cannot scale effectively to the requirements of the new use cases. An example is where enormous datasets of images (tens or many hundreds of thousands of images, represented by many terabytes) might be required to build ML algorithms. This sort of task is generally beyond the scope of traditional PACS, which are built to support a linear processing pipeline (acquire, view, store, followed by some limited retrospective viewing access). To scale up to the new use cases and requirements, significantly more massive parallel processing capabilities will be required than are generally now in place for PACS.

Another challenge is that the DICOM standard for image transfer and, generally, storage of images in PACS does not necessarily align well with the protocols now employed in "Big Data" analytics. The representation of metadata in DICOM files (Part 10 objects) generally requires intermediate processing to facilitate efficient access by enterprise analytics tools. One mechanism to resolve this is to extract and create a separate representation of metadata in formats such as JSON more amenable to enterprise analytics. However, this creates two "silos" of metadata representation and ideally will ultimately be replaced by solutions that can represent imaging data equally effectively for both clinical imaging as well as enterprise analytics.

Yet another challenge is that many, if not most, traditional PACS are based on standard commercial relational databases (RDMS, Relational Database Management Systems) and typically only accessible by SQL (Structured Query Language). These function well for the clinical interpretation use case, but do not necessarily scale effectively into big data, where other, and newer, data models are often employed. Access by NoSQL or NewSQL is increasingly being requested to support enterprise analytics as well as support for cloud-specific protocols such as Amazon (DocumentDB) and Microsoft (Azure Storage Services).

5.7.2   Data Plumbing

There is a challenge that the nature of classic (DIMSE based) DICOM, while well suited for the current medical interpretation use case, is much less suited for massive parallel access and extraction required for machine learning/deep learning (ML/DL) development. For example, the development of a new lung nodule detection algorithm might require thousands of chest images, including indexed curation and annotation of findings. This is a task not well suited to existing PACS and will require new architecture to support effectively.

Additionally, to support the operational application of ML/DL, existing DICOM pipelines are also not effectively scalable. For example, an institution might, and generally will in the future, opt to support a portfolio of such applications, each suited for a specific use case. The problem presents as "getting the right image to the right algorithm and presented in the right context." An interpreting physician might well need a collection of such algorithms as tools or aids depending on suspected or prior diagnosis, clinical history, and anatomy of concern. Some institutions are already supporting myriad such algorithms and are facing a significant scaling challenge to support appropriate routing.

One opportunity is moving beyond DIMSE-based DICOM to web-based access, represented by the DICOMWeb suite of services. This can facilitate "as needed or appropriate" query and access, lighter than DIMSE-based DICOM, and can now be supported by RESTful (Representational State Transfer, as covered in Sections 5.1.4 and 5.2.2) web services, specifically suited to this task by some of the characteristics of REST (statelessness, cacheability, and the ability to dynamically code on-demand on the client-side, among others.)

Another opportunity is in applying more sophisticated rules engine capability and intelligence to PACS image management than traditional PACS have required. This can, and likely will, even extend to AI itself being applied to the routing and distribution of images ("right image to the right algorithm") as well as an intelligent selection of presentation context ("right algorithm presented in the right context"). For example, only certain series in an MR might be needed for a specific algorithm (thus need for series-level routing based on feature recognition) or that based on prior history available in the EHR or RIS, a specific set of oncology-based algorithms, might need to be applied predictively in PET/CT.

However, if these algorithms are to provide clinical value, they must be presented to the interpreting physician both effectively and rapidly if they are to be accepted and adopted widely. If these tools significantly reduce the efficacy of radiological interpretation, they will be unlikely to be adopted. These are the challenges for PACS to adapt to new and emerging functional requirements for "data plumbing."

5.8 ALGORITHMS FOR IMAGE AND NON-IMAGE ANALYTICS

5.8.1 Basic Image Processing

A display system must be able to display a range of pixel values from the minimum pixel value to the maximum value in the image. For displaying the image, a range of light intensities is available, from the darkest to the brightest luminance values. Many choices exist regarding how the mapping from pixel value to luminance is performed. A mapping can be selected that optimizes the contrast of important features in the image, thereby increasing their conspicuity. Alternatively, if this mapping is poorly chosen, the conspicuity of these features can be reduced.

LUTs are commonly used by medical image processing and display computers to affect the display of image contrast. Such use of an LUT may be a method of image processing. However, it is intimately connected with displaying images and so is discussed here. An LUT is simply a table containing a value for each possible pixel value in an image. For example, if each pixel in an image could have one of 4,096 values, a LUT would have 4,096 elements. In practice, each pixel value in the transformed image is determined by selecting the value in the LUT corresponding to the pixel value in the unmodified image. For example, if the value of a pixel in the unmodified image is 1,342, the value of the corresponding pixel in the transformed image is the 1,342nd value in the LUT. Figure 5-35 illustrates the use of an LUT.

An LUT may be applied to transform image contrast at more than one point in the chain from image acquisition to image display. For example, a digital radiography system may use an LUT to modify the acquired pixel values, which are proportional to the detected x-ray signals (the "original" or DICOM "For Processing" image), to cause the display of contrast to optimize human visualization of the content through

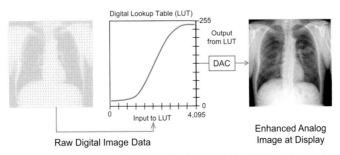

■ **FIGURE 5-35** Display interface showing function of a lookup table (LUT). An image is transferred to the memory of the display interface. The display interface selects pixel values in a raster pattern, and sends the pixel values, one at a time, to the LUT. The LUT produces a digital value indicating display intensity to the Digital to Analog Converter (DAC). The DAC converts the display intensity from a digital value to an analog form (*e.g.*, a voltage).

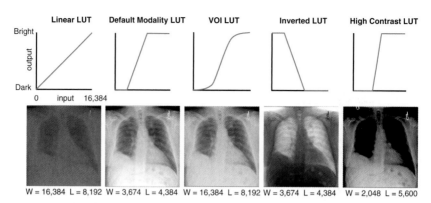

■ **FIGURE 5-36** Graphs of five digital lookup tables (LUT), for the same 14 bit digital image and corresponding "window" and "level" settings. From left to right, the first is a linear LUT that preserves the way the image was originally acquired. Typically, the useful image data occupies only a small range of values for this 14-bit image, and thus contrast is low. The second is the "default modality LUT" that is assigned by the modality, based upon an optimized grayscale range. Note that a large fraction of the range of the image is set to zero (dark) or largest output (maximal brightness), and that a small range of values is mapped from the dark to the bright values on the display. The third is the "Value of Interest" LUT (VOILUT), which encompasses the full range of input values and maps the output according to the capabilities of the display. Typically, this LUT is a sigmoidally shaped curve, which softens the appearance of the image in the dark and bright regions. The fourth LUT inverts image contrast. Shown here is the inverted second image. The fifth image demonstrates windowing to enhance contrast in underpenetrated parts of the image by increasing the slope of the LUT. Note that this causes the loss of all contrast in the highly penetrated regions of the lung.

a Value of Interest (VOI) LUT. Similarly, a medical-grade image display system may employ an LUT to modify each pixel value to compensate for the different display functions of individual displays as described by the DICOM GSDF (Section 5.3.7). Figure 5-36 shows five LUTs in graphical form.

5.8.2 Advanced 3D Visualization and Printing

Multiplanar Reconstruction

Multiplanar reconstruction (MPR) is the reformatting of a volumetric dataset (*e.g.*, a stack of axial images) into tomographic images by selecting pixel values from the dataset that correspond to the desired tomographic image planes. MPR is commonly used to produce images that are parallel to one or more of the three orthogonal planes: axial, coronal, and sagittal. In many cases (especially CT), the data are acquired in the axial plane. A coronal image can be formed from such a dataset by selecting a specific row of pixel values from each axial image. Similarly, a sagittal image can be created by selecting a specific column of pixel values from each axial image. Oblique reconstructions (arbitrary planes that are not orthogonal to the axial plane), "slab" (thicker plane) presentations, and curved MPR images are also commonly produced. The latter are obtained along user-determined curved surfaces through the volumetric dataset that follows anatomic structures such as the spine, aorta, or a coronary artery. In MPR, particularly in creating oblique and curved images, some pixels of the MPR images may not exactly correspond to the locations of values in the volumetric dataset. In this case, the pixel values in the MPR images are created by interpolation of the values in the nearest pixels in the volumetric dataset. Figure 5-37 (top row) shows axial, sagittal, and coronal MPR images.

Maximum intensity projection (MIP) is a method of forming projection images by casting "rays" through a volume dataset and selecting the maximal pixel value along each ray. The rays may be parallel, or they may diverge from a point in space;

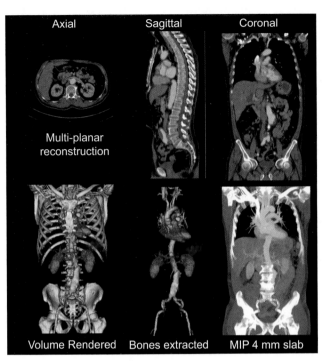

■ **FIGURE 5-37** CT angiography and data reformatting. Top row—Left: The native axial slices from the top of the shoulder to the bottom of the pelvis. Middle: Sagittal reformat from the axial data. Right: Coronal reformat. Bottom row—Left: volume rendered dataset, showing bone and contrast-filled vessel anatomy. Middle: Bones selectively removed to show contrast filled vessels. Right: 4-mm slab coronal Maximum Intensity Projection image. Compare with thin (1 mm) thick coronal plane image in the top row.

in either case, each ray intersects the center of one pixel in the projection image. This method is extremely useful for depicting high signals in a volume (*e.g.*, contrast CT or MRI studies) for vascular angiography or demonstrating calcified plaque in the vasculature, for instance. A variation is thin or thick slab MIP, using MPR projections and a selectable number of image slices (a slab), displaying the maximum values obtained along rays projected through the slab. An example MIP image is shown in Figure 5-37 (bottom right image).

Viewing in Three Dimensions

Volume rendering (VR) uses a stack of 2D images to be viewed as a 3D object. Two approaches are shaded surface displays (SSDs), called surface rendering and VR. In both approaches, the first step is to segment the volume set into different structures (*e.g.*, bones and soft tissue). Segmentation may be done entirely by the computer or with guidance by a person. Segmentation is simplest when there are large differences in the pixel values among the tissues or other objects to be segmented.

SSD provides a simulated 3D view of surfaces of an object or objects in the volume dataset. Surfaces are identified by marking individual voxels as belonging or not belonging to the surface, creating a binary dataset by using simple thresholding to exclude unwanted tissues or by using gradient edge detection methods. The computer calculates the observed light intensity in the SSD image by calculating the reflections from simulated direct and diffuse light sources. The surface may be displayed in shades of gray or in color, such as flesh-tone for "fly-through" colonoscopy image sequences. SSD algorithms are computationally efficient; however, a major disadvantage of SSDs is that only a very small fraction of the information in the original image dataset is displayed. Furthermore, errors may occur in the identification of the surface to be displayed.

Volume Rendering

VR, in contrast to SSD and MIP, uses a more complete set of the voxels within the stacked axial images. In VR, each voxel in the image volume of a stacked tomographic image set is assigned an opacity ranging from 0% to 100% and a color. A voxel assigned an opacity of 0% will be invisible in the final image, and assigning a voxel an opacity of 100% will prevent the viewing of voxels behind it. A voxel with an opacity between 0% and 100% will be visible and will permit the viewing of voxels behind it. The voxels in the volume image set are segmented into those corresponding to various organs, tissues, and objects (e.g., bone, soft tissue, contrast-enhanced blood vessels, air, fat) based upon specific ranges of pixel values (e.g., CT numbers or MRI digital values), perhaps also using assumptions about anatomy and/or guidance by a person. Then, opacity values and colors are assigned to voxels containing specific tissues. The assignments of these artificial characteristics to the voxels containing specific tissues are selected from predefined templates for specific imaging protocols and organ systems (e.g., CT angiogram, pulmonary embolism, or fracture). Next, as in MIP image formation, a set of rays, parallel or diverging from a point, are cast through the volume dataset, with each ray passing through the center of a pixel in the volume rendered image. Each pixel value in the volume rendered image is calculated from the opacities and colors of the voxels along the ray corresponding to that pixel. VR provides a robust view of the anatomy and depth relationships. Simulated lighting effects may be added, and specific anatomy such as bone may be selectively removed to visualize underlying anatomy. Figure 5-37 shows volume rendered images on the bottom row, with the full anatomy depicted in the anterior view, and bones removed on the adjacent image.

VR, on the other hand, displays only a small fraction of the information in the initial image dataset, although much more than SSD or MIP. Furthermore, segmentation errors can occur, causing errors in the displayed anatomy. Additionally, the color assignments, while appearing realistic, are arbitrary and can be misleading because of erroneous tissue classification. Nevertheless, VR is useful for surgical planning and provides images that are easy for referring physicians to understand.

Three-Dimensional Printing

A further step in the use of volumetric imaging is to create 3D physical models from acquired CT or MRI datasets using 3D printing technology. Commercially available 3D printed medical devices are used as instrumentation as an aid to surgeons to assist with surgical planning and proper surgical placement of devices; for implants such as cranial plates or hip joints; for external prostheses such as hands; for medical training/simulation; and education and teaching. These devices are manufactured with complex geometry or features that match a patient's unique anatomy. Future research includes a 3D printing process to use biomaterials and bioprinting to manufacture living organs such as the heart or liver.

3D printing is the process of making an object by depositing materials one very small layer at a time. It starts with creating a 3D blueprint from medical imaging tomographic datasets to obtain object-specific source data for the generation of 3D models. From the volume-rendered data, a software program renders the surface geometry into triangular tiles in a process called tessellation to describe the surface in a "STL" file format (Note—there are other file formats as well). The STL file is then opened in a dedicated "slicer," a piece of 3D printing software that converts digital 3D models into printing instructions to create the object. The slicer chops up the STL file into a large number (100s to 1,000s) of flat horizontal layers and calculates how much material the printer will need to extrude and the length of time to completion. User-configured settings can control the quality and time of the output, which can take from minutes to several hours and more. All information is bundled into a code file containing the native language of the 3D printer. The separate 2D layers are reassembled as a 3D object by depositing a succession of thin layers of material (plastic, composites, metals) thus building the model one layer at a time.

5.8.3 Radiomics

Radiomics is a relatively new field that describes the process of the conversion of digital medical images into mineable high-dimensional data that can potentially reveal information (biomarkers) reflecting underlying pathophysiology through quantitative image analysis. Steps to invoke the practice of radiomics includes acquiring the images under known conditions; identifying areas or volumes in the images that may contain prognostic value; segmenting the volumes by delineating borders through manual or computer-assisted or AI algorithms; extracting and qualifying descriptive features from the volume; creating a relational database from such information, and mining these data to develop classifier models to predict outcomes either alone or in combination with additional information. Such information includes demographic, clinical, comorbidity, or genomic data (Gillies, 2015).

There are many challenges to implementing radiomics processes. One is reproducibility achieved through using common standards to ensure adequate image quality during the acquisition, similar tools for analysis, and transparency in the methods and benchmarks used. Access to Big Data (Section 5.7) is a concern and whether this will be a key to understanding fundamental questions or confounding the analysis, and whether computational bottlenecks could inhibit the use of such data. Data sharing amongst groups could be impacted by ensuring compliance with HIPAA and having to potentially deal with restricted PHI that could hinder the investigations. Gaps in standards and guidelines for analyses and reporting can result in difficulties in extracting useful information. Informatics tools and the development of methods to capture radiomic data in a structured radiology report is a key goal. The Quantitative Imaging Biomarkers Alliance (QIBA) group sponsored by the RSNA seeks to improve the value and practicality of quantitative image biomarkers by reducing the variability across devices, sites, patients and time (QIBA, 2020).

Radiomics has great promise to identify key biomarkers in tomographic images from CT, MR, ultrasound, and PET studies, applicable to a wide range of diseases and pathophysiology. In conjunction with AI and data mining (discussed next) radiomic analysis is likely to advance the precision in diagnosis, assessment of prognosis, and prediction of therapy response.

5.8.4 Artificial Intelligence

AI is a wide-ranging branch of computer science concerned with building smart algorithms capable of performing tasks that typically require human intelligence. AI has been around for decades, but recent advances in computer power and algorithms have resulted in significant progress in matching human intelligence, albeit in narrow, non-generalizable applications. Natural language processing (NLP) and ML methods have demonstrated remarkable progress in image recognition tasks by allowing us to train an AI algorithm to predict outputs, given a set of inputs, without hard-coded rules.

Natural Language Processing

NLP is a branch of AI that deals with the interaction between computers and humans using the natural language. The ultimate objective of NLP is to read, decipher, understand, and make sense of the human languages in a valuable manner. Most NLP techniques rely on ML to derive meaning from human languages.

We should distinguish NLP from basic text search (although these are sometimes conflated in marketing materials). NLP in the modern sense is not based on explicitly programmed rule sets but now employs tools such as deep neural networks.

Interestingly, specialized lexicons such as generally found in Radiology reporting can often produce more consistent results than general language models, due to the specialization of vocabulary and semantics.

Machine Learning and Deep Learning

Computer-aided detection (CAD), also known as computer-aided diagnosis, uses a computer program and heuristic algorithms to detect features likely to be of clinical significance in images. Its purpose is not to replace the interpreting physician, but to assist by calling attention to structures that might have been overlooked. For example, software is available to automatically locate structures suggestive of masses, clusters of microcalcifications, and architectural distortions in mammographic images (Chapter 8). CAD can improve the sensitivity of the interpretation, but also may reduce the specificity. (Sensitivity and specificity are defined in Chapter 4.) CAD techniques and algorithms are now largely in the realm of AI applications that in general provide a more robust sensitivity, specificity, and accuracy.

ML allows computers to learn by themselves in a supervised or unsupervised learning environment. Supervised learning involves using large numbers of inputs such as curated image datasets containing image annotations, markups with known outputs based upon outcome data. Unsupervised learning uses datasets without any specified structure. The "brain" for one type of AI algorithm is based upon a neural network with an example structure shown in Figure 5-38. The network is composed of three different types of layers: The Input Layer, the Hidden Layer(s), and the Output Layer. The Input Layer receives input data and passes the inputs to the first Hidden Layer. All neurons in adjacent layers are interconnected in a feed-forward direction. The Hidden Layers perform mathematical computations on the inputs. A challenge for the designer of the neural network is to determine the number of Hidden Layers and the number of neurons for each layer. The output layer returns the output data.

How does the AI algorithm learn? Each connection between neurons is associated with a weight that dictates the importance of the input value to the neuron in the next layer. The initial weights are set randomly. Each neuron has an activation function, to standardize the output from the neuron. Once a set of data has passed through all layers, the output data are returned through the output layer. Training the neural network is an iterative process of giving inputs from the datasets and comparing the outputs with the outputs from the datasets. Since the AI is untrained, its

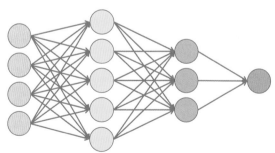

Input Layer   Hidden Layer 1   Hidden Layer 2   Output Layer

■ **FIGURE 5-38** Structure of a convolutional neural network, consisting of an "input layer," "hidden layer(s)," and an output layer. Each layer can consist of one or many nodes, depending on the task and number of input and output interfaces, and are interconnected to adjacent layer nodes. Each connection is assigned a positive or negative weight, initially randomized but with a "training set" of known input and output layers. Iterations based upon evaluation of the data give feedback to adjust the weights until a desired accuracy is obtained. Once "trained" the neural net is applied to never seen cases for testing and evaluation of success.

outputs will be incorrect. Comparing how different the AI's outputs were from the real outputs allows the creation of a cost function, which would ideally be zero, so the effort is to reduce the cost function by changing the weights of the connections between neurons. One way would be to randomly change the weights until the cost function is low, a very inefficient process. A better way is to use a technique called gradient descent that allows an efficient way to find the minimum of the cost function. It works by changing the weights in small increments after each dataset iteration. By computing the derivative (gradient) of the cost function with a certain set of weight values, the direction of the minimum can be determined. After every iteration through the dataset, the weights between neurons are adjusted. To minimize the cost function, multiple iterations through the dataset are needed, thus requiring a lot of curated data and large amounts of computational power. When in place, updating the weights gradient descent is performed automatically. Once the AI algorithm is trained on the training set, it is then tested on the unknowns from a similar set of data to evaluate its performance by using methods such as ROC analysis (Chapter 4).

There is a lot of promise with ML and AI that can perform better than humans on specific tasks with a narrow focus, for instance, a specific single organ segmentation from a cross-sectional dataset. The limitations are (1) lack of generalizability, requiring a large number of AI algorithms tuned for specific applications; (2) extensive effort to mark up and curate datasets that are used for training AI algorithms; and (3) access to large enough datasets that can be used in the training set that can function in a sensitive, specific, and accurate way on unknown cases.

The impact and challenges of AI are explained as an opinion piece in a review article (Hosny, 2018). Significant work and effort on expanding AI in radiology is manifested in the large number of publications and radiology-based medical journals specifically focused on AI and ML (*e.g.*, the RSNA has started a journal, Radiology: Artificial Intelligence with cutting edge content and commentary on state-of-the-art and future directions). Embracing AI as an adjunct as opposed to a replacement for radiologists is the current thought in which AI will provide a value-add to current practice.

5.9 THE BUSINESS OF INFORMATICS

5.9.1 Revenue Cycle

Healthcare, as with any industry or service, requires funding to sustain operations. For Imaging, there are various business models to sustain required revenue for operations, but in general all are related in some manner to a relatively granular and structured accounting of images and reports (as well as interventional procedures). In the United States, this is primarily aligned with an established collection of procedures defined by the AMA called the Current Procedural Terminology, or CPT. This is now further formalized by the CMS as the Healthcare Common Procedure Coding System or HCPCS, as the basis for all Medicare and Medicaid reimbursement. Further, each procedure in these coding systems is assigned a relative workload weight (for both technical and professional services) termed a Relative Value Unit or RVU. Thus, the workload weighting (and ultimately reimbursement) for a Chest CT is higher than that for a Chest Radiograph, reflecting both the relative infrastructure cost (CT scanner cost versus a general radiography system cost) as well as the relative level of Radiologist effort to interpret hundreds of volumetric images for a Chest CT versus one or two projection radiographs for a Chest Radiograph.

The importance of these coding systems extends well beyond just direct CMS reimbursement, however, as they are widely adopted by other payors (as well as internal reimbursement models such as integrated delivery networks). CMS currently (in 2019) coordinated with providers for the care of over 100 million patients, thus defining the majority foundation for medical reimbursement overall in the United States (UCLA, 2020).

To appropriately align the procedures to be performed and interpreted in imaging to the metrics used to assign value to them (and thus drive reimbursement) is termed the Revenue Cycle (Orders, Procedures, Billing, Reimbursement, etc.), and the technology applied is termed Revenue Cycle Management (RCM). An exhaustive review of this is well beyond the scope of this text, but informatics teams must recognize the role of the systems supported in this context. Increasingly, factors such as decision support (discussed in the following section) also need to be considered in the imaging lifecycle, as well as alignment or reconciliation of the various exam code dictionaries that are foundational to RIS, PACS, and EHR/EMRs.

Structured reporting by templates also increasingly serves an important role in RCM, as reimbursement is tied to the completeness and appropriateness of the report, respective to the order and coding applied. Report templates can, and do, greatly assist the Radiologist to report on all aspects of the procedure and not just where lesions or malignancies may be found.

Another aspect of RCM that intersects Informatics is the increasing use of automation for procedural coding. While historically much medical coding was entirely performed manually by specialized staff, more and more is being automated either by alignment to structured report templates or by NLP as part of Computer Assisted Coding (CAC) automation.

While it might seem that Imaging Informatics would be separate from the specialized environment of medical billing and Revenue Cycle, these are increasingly becoming aligned and interdependent to support the financial health of imaging in healthcare.

5.9.2   Impact of Regulations on Informatics

In previous sections, we have mentioned various government and professional agencies and organizations that impact Imaging. Several legislative acts and regulations currently and increasingly relate to Imaging and need to be considered within the scope of Imaging Informatics.

The Office of the National Coordinator for Health Information Technology (ONC) as part of Health and Human Services (HHS) is a key resource as a forum and communications organ for various federal initiatives and regulations as they relate to technology. While the formal regulations are generally found in the specific legal and administrative documents that define them, the ONC is a particularly valuable resource for beginning the navigation of the often quite complex processes defined by these agencies, regulations, acts, and initiatives (ONC, 2020a).

An essential early Federal Act relating to healthcare IT was the Health Insurance Portability and Accountability Act, or HIPAA. This was put into effect in 1996 and defined, among many things, the formal definition of Personally Identifiable Information (PII). PII is defined specifically within HIPAA and should be considered a superset of what we now term Protected Health Information (PHI), the latter term is now more common within the context of Health Information Technology. HIPAA also protects the rights of patients to access their own healthcare data, as well as formally defining those data elements that need to be redacted when de-identifying or anonymizing medical data. Understanding HIPAA and PHI constraints are now essential for Informatics workers. Significant financial penalties apply to violations and large breaches and can be as high as several million dollars to the organization in the case of large breaches. Thus, HIPAA is now essential technical knowledge for all Informatics professionals.

An important distinction was made in the Act between Anonymization and De-identification. Anonymization is the removal or replacement of protected data elements in such a manner that effectively eliminates the possibility to link a record back to the originating source. However, for use cases such as clinical trials, it is generally necessary to be able to reference the original data, albeit securely. This is generally accomplished by indexing the dataset with relation to what HIPAA defines as an Honest Broker. So, the use case, for example, of CTs supporting a clinical trial, it would still possible to reference the actual patient even though the CT images themselves contained no PHI.

One technique defined by HIPAA that needs to be understood by all Informatics professionals is that of the Safe Harbor Method, which defines 18 data elements that must be removed to meet HIPAA security (Table 5-5). Some of these are probably obvious, such as Patient Name, Medical Record Number, or Date of Birth, but others are covered and less obvious, such as Device identifiers and serial numbers, or IP addresses for devices. Particularly for compliantly de-identifying DICOM data, it is critical to understand these constraints.

The Health Information Technology for Economic and Clinical Health Act (HITECH Act) of 2009 was an investment initiative to promote technology in healthcare, first and foremost the adoption of electronic health records or EHRs (which will be discussed in more detail in the next section). Further, it delineated more specific aspects of patient data security and information exchange (also discussed further in the following section). Specific financial incentives were provided for by the Act, as well as criteria for certification of the technologies to be employed. The initial funding for the various aspects of HITECH Act was $36.5 billion over 6 years, initially as an incentive, but converted to a penalty for Medicare should providers or systems ultimately fail to adopt the defined technology.

A key concept of the HITECH Act was termed Meaningful Use (MU). This defined not just the adoption of the applicable technology (as with EHRs) but the actual quantification of the benefits of said technology.

A quite recent CMS regulation that will impact Imaging workflow and Imaging Informatics is the PAMA of 2014, discussed in Section 5.5.1. This is intended to define the appropriate use for advanced imaging prior to it being performed (CT, MR, NM, PET with some exceptions) by defining Appropriate Use Criteria (AUC) and validating the technology for implementing this, referred to as Clinical Decision Support System (CDS or CDSM). Further, it defines the process by which a CDSM can be formally qualified (termed a qCDSM). Currently, PAMA is scheduled to go into full effect in 2022 and is now in the testing phase at most organizations. Most often, this is being implemented as part of an EMR/EHR ordering process, Computerized Provider Data Entry (CPOE). There is still significant debate about the efficacy of CDS/CDSM in driving ordering appropriateness, but as they are further deployed more data will certainly be available (ACR, 2020).

The above Acts and Regulations are listed roughly in chronological order, and hopefully, it is demonstrating a continuum and chronology of these, each building on the prior for technology and structure. All of these are important to Imaging and Imaging Informatics and while few of us are likely to become experts in all these areas, it is critical to have basic awareness and knowledge of them.

5.10 BEYOND IMAGING INFORMATICS

Imaging Informatics resides as a discipline within of Medical Informatics. In turn, Medical Informatics exists—using the American Medical Informatics Association (AMIA) definition—as "The science of how to use data, information and knowledge to improve human health and the delivery of health care services" (AMIA, 2020).

By extension, imaging informatics involves the specific applications of Medical Informatics within medical imaging. However, while in the past this field was often somewhat segregated from Medical Informatics in dealing with the unique challenges of managing digital imaging (DICOM, PACS, etc.) it has increasingly become integrated with the larger scope. It would be rare now to find any EMR or EHR that lacked integration with PACS, and in fact, many think of the "Image enabled EHR" as the desired standard of practice. The distinction of PACS and the EHR in terms of user experience begins to blur in much the same manner as the historical distinction between RIS and the EHR has largely disappeared. (And in fact, some EHRs now wholly subsume the workflow functions of the RIS.) PACS generally remains separated from the EHR infrastructure by the special demands of managing very large volumes of pixel data efficiently and rapidly. While an EHR might involve many terabytes of textual data, a PACS may well involve many petabytes of image data. Different data structures and schema are generally required to efficiently support these distinct use cases, although some EHRs now support limited internal image management such as patient photos or smaller volume imaging use cases such as visible light photography (dermatology, etc.) While there is ongoing debate regarding the role of PACS versus the EHR, in general, the integration of these two systems is still accomplished by PACS web services supporting visualization from within the patient chart rather than actual image storage within the EHR. (*i.e.*, PACS still manages image modality image ingestion and storage and in turn, provides visualization services to the EHR.) This may change in the future but currently remains the general model for integration of imaging and the EHR.

5.10.1 EMR and EHR

The terms EMR and EHR are sometimes used interchangeably but are distinct. An EMR is defined (by the ONC—Office of the National Coordinator for Health Information Technology) as: "The digital version of the paper chart in the clinician's office. An EMR contains the medical and treatments in one practice."

In contrast, the ONC's definition of an EHR is: "EHRs focus is on the total health of the patient—going beyond standard clinical data collected in the provider's office and inclusive of a broader view on a patient's care. EHRs are designed to reach out beyond the health organization that originally collects and compiles the information. They are built to share information with other health care providers, such as laboratories and specialists, so they contain information from all the clinicians involved in the patient's care." The ONC (and thus other government agencies in the US) prefer the term EHR as the more comprehensive of the two terms (ONC, 2019).

5.10.2 HIEs

Thus, if the difference between an EMR and an EHR is comprehensive coverage of an entire patient health record, the latter implies interoperability of EMRs where the patient treatment history may span different healthcare organizations. This brings us to the concept of an HIE—Health Information Exchange. This goal was explicitly included in Part 1 of the CMS within MU and associated financial incentives (CMS, 2020a).

While many EHRs, to attain certification status by the CMS, have implemented interoperability by internal mechanisms, the goal for interoperability clearly demands open standards that can be implemented or adopted by all vendors, across all organizations. This remains, however, an elusive goal due to the parallel requirements of rigorous patient information security.

As a means of attaining interoperability while still retaining patient information security, many intermediate exchanges (HIEs) have been developed. These are often implemented as "brokers" to attain information exchange, and thus interoperability. The ONC and CMS define three distinct models for health information exchange:

1. Directed Exchange: From provider/organization to another provider/organization. This is often thought of as a "push" model of exchange. This is also generally the simplest model to implement since it does not require a provider/organization to provide external access to data.
2. Query-Based Exchange: Facilitates a provider/organization to find and retrieve patient information from other providers/organizations. This is often thought of as a "pull" model of information exchange. This is a more sophisticated model and requires a more complex construction of trust relationships between disparate IT systems.
3. Consumer-mediated Exchange: This facilitates the patient themselves to access, retrieve and transmit their own health records. These are, interestingly, currently more common for medical imaging than for the general use case for text-based health information due to the general adoption of DICOM as both an image structure as well as an exchange protocol.

Since agreements and shared technology are required for HIEs, these have often been implemented within specific States or as regional exchanges. Many such RHIOs (Regional Health Information Organizations) now exist providing limited geographic interoperability (ONC, 2020b).

5.10.3 Image Sharing

As mentioned above, medical image exchange (and digital medical imaging in general) enjoys the advantage of a universally accepted set of standards for data structure and messaging—DICOM. While parallel ontological standards exist for textural medical data—LOINC, SNOMED, etc.—DICOM enjoys the benefit of being the lexicon for effectively all medical imaging now both internally and externally. That said, it would seem that universal interoperability for medical image exchange would be straightforward, but unfortunately, this is still not the case. Many solutions for image exchange between organizations are offered in the current commercial market space, but they lack interoperability between these solutions. (*i.e.*, interoperability is achieved within a single vendor solution shared by a group of organizations but not between different vendor solutions.) This has led to what Dr. David Mendelson has termed the "Tribalization of image exchange" dilemma.

Significant work has been and is being done to overcome this obstacle. The RSNA has sponsored an initiative to demonstrate intra-vendor operability called the RSNA Image Share and to validate interoperability (RSNA, 2020b).

This, in turn, has evolved to what is now called the Sequoia Project to further the goals of image exchange interoperability based on open standards. The metaphor of this organization's name is based on the fact that a giant sequoia tree must rely on others to attain and sustain its height—via the root structure and shared canopy—and cannot survive in isolation (Sequoia, 2020). (Indeed, an apt metaphor for the goal of universal healthcare information exchange.)

This organization is now recognized by the ONC as the principal Recognized Coordinating Entity (RCE) for image exchange. This structure is now termed by the ONC as a TEFCA—Trusted Exchange Framework and Common Agreement—and will be the likely foundation for future reimbursement initiatives through CMS as a national infrastructure (ONC, 2020c).

As work towards open standards, frameworks, and infrastructure progresses, we will ultimately be able to overcome the "Tribalism" of image exchange technologies and solutions currently existing.

5.10.4 Clinical Informatics

As discussed at the beginning of this section, Imaging Informatics exists as a specialty of Medical or Clinical Informatics, and increasingly as an integrated part of the larger discipline. PACS and RIS can no longer operate independently but have become an essential part of the overall quest for the community-wide interoperative and image-enabled EHR.

SUGGESTED READING AND REFERENCES

AAPM. *Display Quality Assurance, Report of AAPM Task Group 270*. American Association of Physicists in Medicine; 2019a. https://www.aapm.org/pubs/reports/detail.asp?docid=183. Accessed October 28, 2019.

AAPM. *Interoperability Assessment for the Commissioning of Medical Imaging Acquisition Systems, Report of AAPM Task Group 248*. American Association of Physicists in Medicine; 2019b. https://www.aapm.org/pubs/reports/detail.asp?docid=180. Accessed August 17, 2020.

ACR. *ACR-AAPM-SIIM Technical Standard for Electronic Practice of Medical Imaging*. American College of Radiology. Practice Parameters and Technical Standards; 2017. https://www.acr.org/ACR/Files/elec-practice-medimag

ACR. *ACR-AAPM-SIIM Practice Parameter for Electronic Medical Information Privacy and Security*. American College of Radiology. Practice Parameters and Technical Standards; 2019. https://www.acr.org/Clinical-Resources/Practice-Parameters-and-Technical-Standards/Practice-Parameters-by-Modality. Accessed June 1, 2020.

ACR. *Clinical Decision Support*. American College of Radiology; 2020. https://www.acr.org/Clinical-Resources/Clinical-Decision-Support. Accessed June 16, 2020.

AMIA. *What is Informatics?* American Medical Informatics Association; 2020. https://www.amia.org/fact-sheets/what-informatics?gclid=EAIaIQobChMI6MfLwPXt6QIV1BatBh3_WA0PEAAYBCAAEgIx-_D_BwE. Accessed June 15, 2020.

Barten PGJ. *Contrast Sensitivity of the Human Eye and Its Effects on Image Quality*. Bellingham, WA: SPIE Optical Engineering Press; 1999.

Code of Federal Regulations. 45 CFR Part 164, HIPAA Privacy and Security Regulations.

Clunie DA. *DICOM Structured Reporting*. Bangor, PA: PixelMed Publishing; 2000.

CMS. *Appropriate Use Criteria Program*. Centers for Medicare and Medicaid Services; 2020a. https://www.cms.gov/Medicare/Quality-Initiatives-Patient-Assessment-Instruments/Appropriate-Use-Criteria-Program. Accessed June 12, 2020.

CMS. *Promoting Interoperability Programs*. Centers for Medicare and Medicaid Services; 2020b. https://www.cms.gov/Regulations-and-Guidance/Legislation/EHRIncentivePrograms/index?redirect=/EHRIncentivePrograms/30_Meaningful_Use.asp. Accessed June 15, 2020.

DICOM. *Digital Imaging and Communications in Medicine (DICOM) Part 1: Introduction and Overview, PS 3.1-2020*. National Electrical Manufacturers Association; 2020. https://www.dicomstandard.org/current. Accessed June 1, 2020.

DICOM. *Digital Imaging and Communications in Medicine (DICOM) Part 14: Grayscale Standard Display Function*. PS 3.14-2011. National Electrical Manufacturers Association; 2011.

FDA. *Mammography Record Retention: What should I keep and for How Long?* 2020. https://www.fda.gov/radiation-emitting-products/mqsa-insights/mammography-record-retention-what-should-i-keep-and-how-long. Accessed June 12, 2020.

Flynn MG. *Advances in Digital Radiography: Categorical Course in Diagnostic Radiology Physics*. Oak Brook, IL: Radiological Society of North America; 2003:103-107.

Folio LR, Machado LB, Dwyer AJ. Multimedia-enhanced radiology reports: concept, components, and challenges. *RadioGraphics*. 2018;38(2):462-482.

Gillies RJ, Kinahan PE, Hricak H. Radiomics: images are more than pictures, they are data. *Radiology*. 2016;278(2):563-577.

Goo JM, Choi JY, et al. Effect of monitor luminance and ambient light on observer performance in soft-copy reading of digital chest radiographs. *Radiology*. 2004;232(3):762-766.

HIPAA. *HITECH Act Enforcement Interim Final Rule*. 2009. https://www.hhs.gov/hipaa/for-professionals/special-topics/hitech-act-enforcement-interim-final-rule/index.html. Accessed June 16, 2020.

HIPAA. *Health Insurance Privacy and Accountability Act. Code of Federal Regulations, 45 CFR Part 164*. Department of Health and Human Services; 2020a. https://www.hhs.gov/hipaa/index.html

HIPAA. The De-identification Standard—Section 164.514 of the HIPAA Privacy Rule; 2020b.

HL7. Health Level 7 International: Data Definition Tables. Appendix A, Version 2.6; 2007. https://www.hl7.org/special/committees/vocab/V26_Appendix_A.pdf. Accessed May 31, 2020.

HL7. Health Level 7 International: General Information and website; 2020. https://www.hl7.org/. Accessed May 31, 2020.

Hosny A, Parmar C, Quakenbush J, Schwartz LH, Aerts HJWL. Artificial intelligence in radiology. *Nat Rev Cancer*. 2018;18(8):500-510.

IHE. *Scheduled Workflow, SWF. Integrating the Healthcare Enterprise*. 2006.https://wiki.ihe.net/index.php/Scheduled_Workflow. Accessed May 31, 2020.

IHE. *Patient Information Reconciliation, PIR*. Integrating the Healthcare Enterprise; 2008. https://wiki.ihe.net/index.php/Patient_Information_Reconciliation. Accessed May 31, 2020.

IHE. Radiology Technical Framework Profiles. 2020. https://www.ihe.net/ihe_domains/radiology/. Accessed June 16, 2020.

Krupinski EA. Technology and perception in the 21st-century reading room. *J Am Coll Radiol*. 2006;3:433-440.

Langlotz C. *The Radiology Report: A Guide to Thoughtful Communication for Radiologists and Other Medical Professionals*. Scotts Valley, CA: CreateSpace; 2015. ISBN-10: 1515174085.

LOINC. LOINC/RSNA Radiology Playbook File, Version 2.67, released 12 December 2019. https://loinc.org/downloads/accessory-files/#rsna. Accessed June 10, 2020.

Meraki. Layer 3 vs Layer 2 Switching. Cisco, Incorporated; 2020. https://documentation.meraki.com/MS/Layer_3_Switching/Layer_3_vs_Layer_2_Switching. Accessed June 14, 2020.

MITA. *Cybersecurity for Medical Imaging*. Medical Imaging Technology Alliance, a division of NEMA; 2016. https://www.nema.org/Standards/Pages/Cybersecurity-for-Medical-Imaging.aspx. Accessed May 31, 2019.

NIST. *Framework for Improving Critical Infrastructure Cybersecurity*. National Institute of Standards and Technology; 2018. https://www.nist.gov/publications/framework-improving-critical-infrastructure-cybersecurity-version-11. Accessed May 31, 2020.

ONC. *EMR vs EHR—What's the Difference?*. Office of the National Coordinator for Health Information Technology; 2019. https://www.healthit.gov/buzz-blog/electronic-health-and-medical-records/emr-vs-ehr-difference. Accessed June 15, 2020.

ONC. Office of the National Coordinator for Health Information Technology: About ONC and What We Do. 2020a. https://www.healthit.gov/topic/about-onc. Accessed June 16, 2020.

ONC. Office of the National Coordinator for Health Information Technology—Electronic Health Information Exchange (HIE). 2020b. https://www.healthit.gov/topic/health-it-and-health-information-exchange-basics/what-hie. Accessed June 15, 2020.

ONC. Office of the National Coordinator for Health Information Technology—Recognized Coordinating Entity. 2020c. https://rce.sequoiaproject.org/. Accessed June 15, 2020.

QIBA. *Radiological Society of North America*. The Quantitative Imaging Biomarkers Alliance; 2020. https://www.rsna.org/en/research/quantitative-imaging-biomarkers-alliance. Accessed June 16, 2020.

RSNA. *Informatics RadLex, Current version 4.0*. Radiological Society of North America; 2020a. http://radlex.org. Accessed June 10, 2020.

RSNA. *Image Share*. Radiological Society of North America; 2020b. https://www.rsna.org/en/practice-tools/data-tools-and-standards/image-share-validation-program. Accessed June 15, 2020.

Samei E, Badano A, Chakraborty D, et al. *Assessment of Display Performance for Medical Imaging Systems, Report of the American Association of Physicists in Medicine (AAPM) Task Group 18*. Madison, WI: Medical Physics Publishing. AAPM On-Line Report No. 03, April 2005.

Sequoia. The Sequoia Project. 2020. https://sequoiaproject.org/about-us/. Accessed June 15, 2020.

UCLA. Office of Compliance Services: Revenue Cycle and Billing Terminology and Definitions. 2020. https://www.uclahealth.org/compliance/workfiles/Training/RevenueCycleandBillingBasics.pdf. Accessed June 16, 2020.

Diagnostic Radiology

6

X-ray Production, Tubes, and Generators

X-rays are produced when highly energetic electrons interact with matter, converting some or all of their kinetic energy into electromagnetic radiation. The *x-ray tube insert* contains an electron source, a vacuum environment, and a target electrode; an external power source provides high voltage (potential difference) to accelerate the electrons. The x-ray tube insert is mounted within a *tube housing*, which includes a metal enclosure; protective radiation shielding; *x-ray beam filters* for shaping the x-ray spectrum; and *collimators*, which define the size and shape of the x-ray field. The *x-ray generator* supplies the tube potential to accelerate the electrons, a filament circuit to control tube current, and an exposure timer. These components work in concert to produce a beam of x-ray photons with controlled *fluence* (number of incident photons per unit area), *energy fluence* (energy weighted number of photons per unit area), and a well-collimated trajectory. In terms of nomenclature used in this chapter, the fluence and energy fluence are scalar radiometric quantities. The term *exposure* is a dosimetric quantity describing the amount of charge in coulombs (C) released in a known mass of air (unit of C/kg) and is expressed in terms of the energy fluence and energy absorption integrated over energy. The *exposure rate* is the increment of exposure in a time interval (unit of C/kg/s).

This chapter describes the x-ray production process, characteristics of the x-ray beam, x-ray tube design, x-ray generator components, and factors that affect exposure and exposure rate.

6.1 PRODUCTION OF X-RAYS

6.1.1 Bremsstrahlung Spectrum

X-rays are produced from the conversion of kinetic energy of electrons into electromagnetic radiation when they are decelerated by interaction within a target material. A simplified diagram of an x-ray tube (Fig. 6-1) illustrates these components. An electrical potential difference (the SI unit of potential difference is the volt, V) of 20,000 to 150,000 V (20 to 150 kV) is applied between the electrodes. The negative pole of the voltage source is applied to the *cathode*, which is also the *source* of electrons, and the positive pole is applied to the *anode*, the *target* of electrons. Electrons are emitted by the cathode, are accelerated by the tube potential through the vacuum to strike the anode. The eV is the energy obtained by an electron after it is accelerated across a potential difference of 1 V. One eV is equal to 1.603×10^{-19} joule (J). An applied x-ray tube potential of 50 kV accelerates electrons to a kinetic energy of 50 keV.

On impact with the target, the kinetic energy of the electrons is converted to other forms of energy. Most interactions, typically greater than 99%, are *collisional* with other electrons in the target material and produce nothing but heat. Electrons that reach the proximity of an atomic nucleus in the target material are decelerated by the positive charge of the nucleus. As discussed in Chapter 3, electrical (Coulombic)

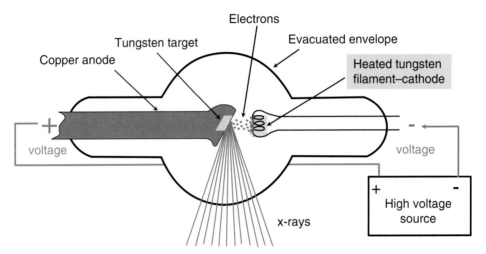

■ **FIGURE 6-1** Minimum requirements for x-ray production include a source and target of electrons, an evacuated envelope, and connection of the electrodes to a high-voltage source.

forces attract and decelerate an electron that changes its direction and velocity, resulting in the radiative emission of an x-ray photon (*i.e.*, bremsstrahlung radiation).

The magnitude of energy lost by an electron is determined by the closest distance between the incident electron and the nucleus, as the Coulombic force is proportional to the inverse square of the distance. At a relatively large distance, Coulombic attraction is weak, resulting in encounters that produce low x-ray energies (Fig. 6-2, electron no. 3). At closer interaction distance, the increased Coulombic force causes a greater electron deceleration and conversion to higher x-ray energies (see Fig. 6-2,

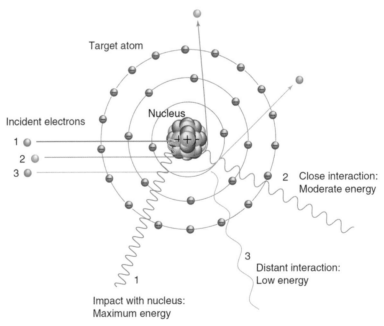

■ **FIGURE 6-2** Bremsstrahlung radiation arises from energetic electron interactions with an atomic nucleus of the target material. In a "close" approach, the positive nucleus attracts the negative electron, causing deceleration and redirection, resulting in a loss of kinetic energy that is converted to an x-ray. The x-ray energy depends on the interaction distance between the electron and the nucleus, and increases as the distance decreases. When the distance is zero (incident electron 1 in the figure), all the kinetic energy of the electron creates the maximum bremsstrahlung photon energy.

electron no. 2). A direct impact with the target nucleus stops an electron and converts all its kinetic energy into an equivalent energy x-ray photon (see Fig. 6-2, electron no. 1), resulting in the highest bremsstrahlung x-ray energy.

The probability of electron interactions that produce x-rays of energy E depends on the radial interaction distance, r, from the nucleus, which defines an annulus of inner diameter 2r, and outer diameter 2(r + dr), where dr is a small fixed radial increment. Increasing the radius in steps of dr from the nucleus defines an incrementally increasing annulus area; thus electron-nucleus interactions generate incrementally larger numbers of x-rays at incrementally decreasing energies. For the closest electron-nucleus interactions (*i.e.*, r = 0), the highest x-ray energy is produced at extremely low probability and small number of x-rays. A *bremsstrahlung spectrum* is the probability distribution of x-ray photon fluence produced as a function of energy, expressed in keV. The *unfiltered* bremsstrahlung spectrum (Fig. 6-3a) shows an inverse linear relationship between the fluence and energy of the x-rays produced, with the highest x-ray energy, x keV, determined by the peak voltage (x kV) applied across the x-ray tube. A typical *filtered* bremsstrahlung spectrum (Fig. 6-3b) has no x-rays present below about 10 keV; the fluence increases to a maximum at about one third to one half the maximal x-ray energy and then drops off to zero at just beyond the peak x-ray energy. Filtration in this context refers to the removal of x-rays by attenuation in materials that are inherent in the x-ray tube (*e.g.*, the glass or metal window of the tube insert), as well as by materials that are intentionally placed in the beam, such as thin aluminum and copper sheets to preferentially attenuate lower energy x-rays and to therefore tune the x-ray spectrum for low-dose imaging (see Beam Filtration in Section 6.5).

Main factors that affect x-ray production efficiency include the kinetic energy of the incident electrons, which is directly related to the tube potential, and the atomic number (Z) of the target material. The approximate ratio of radiative energy loss (bremsstrahlung production) to collisional energy loss (excitation and ionization) within the diagnostic x-ray energy range (over a potential difference of 20 to 150 kV) is expressed as follows:

$$\frac{\text{Radiative energy loss}}{\text{Collisional energy loss}} \cong \frac{E_K Z}{820,000} \quad \text{for } E_K \leq 150 \text{ keV}, \qquad [6\text{-}1]$$

where E_K is the kinetic energy of the incident electrons in keV, and Z is the atomic number of the target electrode material (anode). The most common anode is made

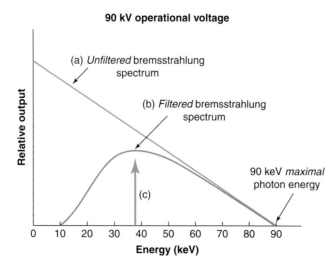

90 kV operational voltage

(a) *Unfiltered* bremsstrahlung spectrum

(b) *Filtered* bremsstrahlung spectrum

90 keV *maximal* photon energy

(c)

Relative output

Energy (keV)

■ **FIGURE 6-3** The bremsstrahlung energy distribution for a 90-kV acceleration potential difference. The unfiltered bremsstrahlung spectrum (a) illustrates the greater probability of low-energy x-ray photon production that is inversely linear with energy up to the maximum energy of 90 keV. The filtered spectrum (b) shows the preferential attenuation of the lowest-energy x-ray photons. The vertical arrow (c) indicates the average energy of the spectrum, which is typically 1/3 to 1/2 the maximal energy, dependent on the amount of added filtration.

TABLE 6-1 ELECTRON BINDING ENERGIES (keV) OF COMMON X-RAY TUBE TARGET MATERIALS

ELECTRON SHELL	TUNGSTEN	MOLYBDENUM	RHODIUM
K	69.5	20.0	23.2
L	12.1/11.5/10.2	2.8/2.6/2.5	3.4/3.1/3.0
M	2.8–1.9	0.5–0.4	0.6–0.2

of tungsten (W, $Z = 74$); in mammography, molybdenum (Mo, $Z = 42$) and rhodium (Rh, $Z = 45$) are also used. As an example, for 100-keV electrons impinging on a tungsten target, the ratio of radiative to collisional losses is $(100 \times 74)/820,000 \cong 0.009 \cong 0.9\%$; at this tube potential of 100 kV, more than 99% of the incident electron energy striking the anode is converted to heat. Due to the low efficiency of x-ray production, x-ray tube design is largely driven by heat dissipation concerns.

6.1.2 Characteristic X-rays

In addition to the continuous bremsstrahlung x-ray spectrum, discrete x-ray energy peaks called "characteristic radiation" are present, with x-ray energies depending on the elemental composition of the anode and the applied x-ray tube voltage. Electrons in an atom are distributed in orbital "shells" and have specific electron binding energies to maintain equilibrium. The innermost shell is designated the K shell and has the highest electron binding energy, followed by the L, M, and N shells, with progressively less binding energy. Table 6-1 lists the common anode target materials and the binding energies of the K, L, and M electron shells that are "characteristic" of the element. When the kinetic energy of an incident electron exceeds the binding energy of an electron shell in a target atom, an interaction can eject an electron from its shell, creating a vacancy. As discussed in Chapter 2, an outer shell electron with less binding energy immediately transitions to fill the vacancy, and a characteristic x-ray is emitted with an energy equal to the difference in the electron binding energies of the two shells (Fig. 6-4).

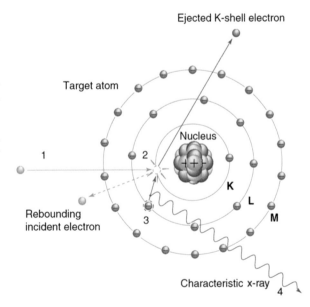

■ **FIGURE 6-4** Generation of a characteristic x-ray in a target atom occurs in the following sequence: (1) The incident electron interacts with the K-shell electron via a repulsive electrical force. (2) The K-shell electron is removed (only if the energy of the incident electron is greater than the K-shell binding energy), leaving a vacancy in the K-shell. (3) An electron from the adjacent L-shell fills the vacancy. (4) A K_α characteristic x-ray photon is emitted with energy equal to the difference between the binding energies of the two shells. In this case, a 59.3-keV photon is emitted.

Ejected K-shell electron

Target atom

Nucleus

Rebounding incident electron

Characteristic x-ray

TABLE 6-2 K-SHELL CHARACTERISTIC X-RAY ENERGIES (keV) OF COMMON X-RAY TUBE TARGET MATERIALS

SHELL TRANSITION	TUNGSTEN	MOLYBDENUM	RHODIUM
$K_{\alpha 1}$	59.32	17.48	20.22
$K_{\alpha 2}$	57.98	17.37	20.07
$K_{\beta 1}$	67.24	19.61	22.72

Note: Only prominent transitions are listed. The subscripts 1 and 2 represent energy levels that exist within each shell.

For tungsten, L-shell electrons have binding energies of 10.2, 11.5, and 12.1 keV. Electrons that transition from the L to an empty K-shell orbital produce discrete characteristic x-rays equal to the difference of 69.5 K-shell binding energy and the respective L-shell binding energies: 59.3, 58, and 57.4 keV. Orbital electrons from outer shells (M, N, ...) with lower binding energy will produce characteristic x-rays of higher energy. For example, a M-shell electron of binding energy of 2.3 keV that fills the K shell vacancy produces a characteristic x-ray of 67.2 keV. Characteristic x-rays are designated by the shell in which the electron vacancy is filled, and a subscript of α or β indicates whether the electron transition is from an adjacent shell (α) or non-adjacent shell (β). For example, K_α refers to an electron transition from the L to the K shell, and K_β refers to an electron transition from the M, N, or O shell to the K shell. It follows that a K_β x-ray is more energetic than a K_α x-ray. Characteristic x-rays other than those generated by K-shell transitions (e.g., M → L) are too low in energy for any human imaging. Table 6-2 lists electron shell binding energies and corresponding K-shell characteristic x-ray energies of W, Mo, and Rh anode targets.

Characteristic K x-rays are produced *only* when the electrons impinging on the target *exceed* the binding energy of a K-shell electron (K_{BE}). X-ray tube potentials must therefore be greater than 69.5 kV for W (K_{BE} = 69.5 keV), 20.0 kV for Mo (K_{BE} = 20.0 keV), and 23.2 kV for Rh (K_{BE} = 23.2 keV) for characteristic x-rays to be produced on these targets. As the x-ray tube voltage increases, the ratio of characteristic to bremsstrahlung x-ray energy fluence also increases. For example, at 80 kV, approximately 5% of the total x-ray energy fluence for a tungsten anode is composed of characteristic radiation, increasing to about 10% at 100 kV. Figure 6-5 illustrates a bremsstrahlung plus characteristic radiation spectrum.

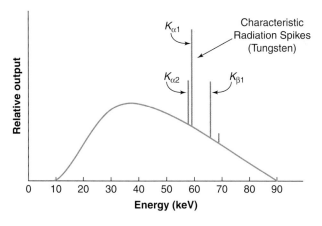

■ **FIGURE 6-5** The filtered spectrum of bremsstrahlung and characteristic radiation from a tungsten target with a potential difference of 90 kV illustrates specific characteristic radiation energies from K_α and K_β transitions. Filtration (the preferential removal of low-energy photons as they traverse matter) is discussed in Section 6.5.

6.2   X-RAY TUBES

The x-ray tube provides an environment to produce bremsstrahlung and characteristic x-rays. Major tube components include the *cathode, anode, rotor/stator, glass or metal envelope, tube port, cable sockets,* and *tube housing,* illustrated in Figure 6-6. An actual x-ray tube showing the x-ray tube insert and a cut-away of the housing is shown in Figure 6-7. The x-ray generator (Section 6.3) supplies the power and permits selection of x-ray tube voltage, tube current, and exposure time. The *x-ray tube voltage* is set to values from 40 to 150 kV for diagnostic imaging, and 25 to 49 kV for mammography, depending on the type of imaging exam and anatomy being imaged. The *x-ray tube current,* measured in milliamperes (mA), represents the number of electrons per second flowing from the cathode to the anode, where 1 mA = 6.24×10^{15} electrons/s. For projection radiography, the tube current typically ranges from 100 to 1,000 mA with exposure times less than 100 ms for most examinations. The kV, mA, and exposure time are the three major selectable parameters on the x-ray generator control panel that determine the x-ray beam characteristics. Often, the product of the tube current and exposure time is considered as one entity, the mAs (milliampere-second). These parameters are discussed further in the following sections.

6.2.1   Cathode

The cathode is the negative electrode in the x-ray tube and is comprised of an electron emitter and *focusing cup* (Fig. 6-8). The emitter is usually a tungsten wire tightly coiled in a filament configuration (often called the filament) electrically connected to the filament circuit in the x-ray generator. Some advanced x-ray tubes have flat surface tungsten emitters (see below). Most x-ray tubes for diagnostic imaging have two filaments of different lengths, each positioned in a slot machined into the focusing cup. Specialized tubes have 2 or 3 filaments of different length for angiography applications, and dental tubes have a single filament. Usually only one filament is energized for an imaging examination, although there are some x-ray tube/generator systems that produce a combined electron distribution by energizing both filaments simultaneously. On many x-ray systems, the small or the large filament can be manually selected, or automatically selected by the x-ray generator, depending on the technique factors (kV and mAs).

■ **FIGURE 6-6** A diagram of the major components of a modern x-ray tube and housing assembly is shown.

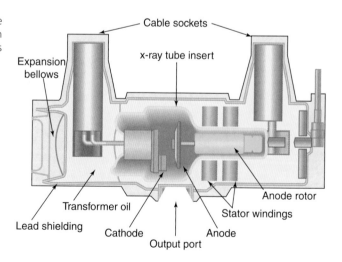

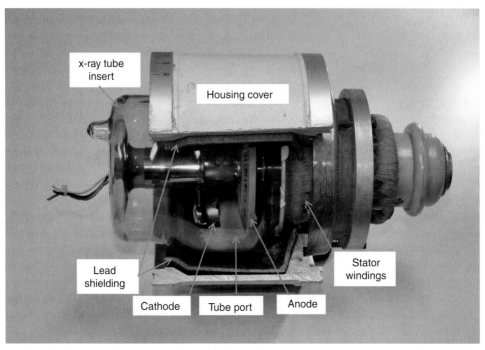

■ FIGURE 6-7 The x-ray tube with various components including the x-ray tube insert and partially cut-away housing. This housing has a lead shielding thickness of 2 mm. The tube port is facing downward (the lucent area between the cathode and anode in the picture).

When energized, the filament circuit is activated to pass current with a potential difference of about 10 V through the filament. Electrical resistance heats the filament to a temperature determined by the amplitude of the current (3 to 7 amperes [A]), resulting in a release of electrons from the filament surface by a process called *thermionic emission*. A static electron cloud "space charge" is formed around the

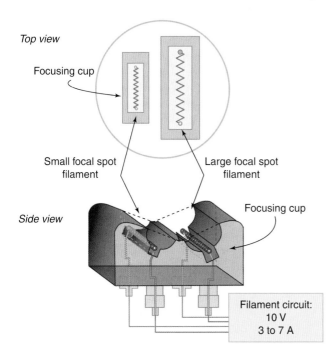

■ FIGURE 6-8 The x-ray tube cathode structure consists of wound tungsten filament emitters positioned within the focusing cup. The filament circuit is activated to heat the selected filament, which emits electrons by thermionic emission at the filament surface.

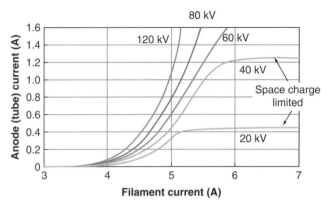

■ **FIGURE 6-9** Relationship of tube current (number of electrons crossing the cathode-anode axis) to filament current for various applied tube kV shows a dependence of approximately $kV^{1.5}$. For high filament current settings, a space charge cloud shields the electric field so that further increases in filament current do not increase the tube current. This is known as "space charge–limited" operation that occurs over a range of kV values, but in particular for lower kVs. For moderate and low filament current, the tube current is in "emission-limited" operation.

filament as the repulsive force of the negative charge of emitted electrons equals the thermionic emission force. When x-ray tube voltage is applied, electrons from the filament are accelerated toward the anode, and represent the x-ray tube current. Note that the x-ray tube current and filament current are not the same but are nonlinearly related, as shown in Figure 6-9. For most diagnostic acquisitions, the x-ray fluence is *emission-limited*, and thus the filament circuit controls the x-ray tube current, which in turn controls the x-ray output. In situations where an already high filament current is needed to produce a higher tube current, the space charge cloud surrounding the filament emitter limits the further emission of electrons from the filament surface. In this case, the tube current cannot be increased by increases in the filament current, particularly at lower kV settings, and x-ray output is *space charge limited.* Higher tube potentials enable larger x-ray tube current for the same filament current; for instance, for the same filament current of 5 A at 80 kV, a tube current of 800 mA is produced, whereas at 120 kV a tube current of about 1,100 mA results.

The focusing cup surrounds the filament emitter with a slotted half-cylindrical structure. Its function is to reduce the spread of electrons during exposure. In most x-ray tubes, the focusing cup is maintained at the same potential difference as the filament relative to the anode, and an electric field exists that repels and shapes the cloud of emitted electrons from the filament surface into a tight distribution. As the tube potential is applied, electrons are accelerated to the anode, striking a small area called the focal spot (Fig. 6-10). Focal spot dimensions are determined by the length of the filament in one direction and the width of the focusing cup in the perpendicular direction.

A *biased* x-ray tube has a focusing cup isolated from the filament and maintained at a more negative voltage (for instance, a bias of −1,000 V), causing the electrons emerging from the filament to be even more tightly distributed by the negative repelling force and to produce a smaller focal spot width (Fig. 6-10, middle). Even greater negative voltage bias of −2,500 to −4,000 V completely stops the flow of electrons, providing a means to rapidly switch the x-ray beam on and off under high x-ray tube voltage (Fig. 6-10, right). A tube with this capability is referred to as a *grid-biased* x-ray tube. Grid-biased x-ray tube switching is used by advanced fluoroscopy systems

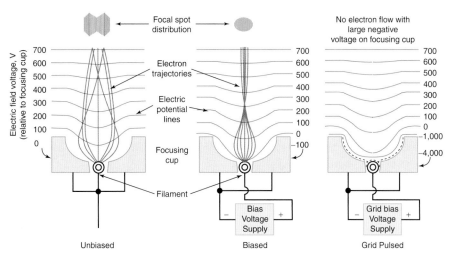

■ **FIGURE 6-10** The focusing cup shapes the electron distribution when it is at the same voltage ("unbiased") as the filament (left). Electrical isolation of the focusing cup from the filament and application of a negative "biased" voltage (~ −100 V) reduces the distribution of emerging electrons by increasing the repelling electric fields surrounding the filament (note the 0 V electric field potential line) and modifying the electron trajectories (middle). At the top are typical electron distributions incident on the target anode (the focal spot) for the unbiased and biased focusing cups. Application of −4,000 V on an electrically isolated focusing cup completely stops electron flow, even with high voltage applied on the tube; this is known as a grid biased or "grid pulsed" tube (right).

for pulsed fluoroscopy and in angiography systems to rapidly and precisely turn on and turn off the x-ray beam. Conventional x-ray generator voltage switching endures a build-up lag to get to peak voltage and a decay lag to return to 0 voltage, chiefly due to capacitance effects in the high-voltage cables. The pulse width is lengthened, and the x-ray beam energy is lowered, which results in extra patient dose and degradation of fast-moving objects in the images.

In computed tomography (CT), x-ray tubes mounted on gantries rotate as fast as 4 revolutions per second and generate high centrifugal forces, which are incompatible with conventional cathode filament emitters. Robust structural integrity is achieved with a flat surface tungsten emitter as shown in Figure 6-11. The tungsten is directly heated to release electrons via thermionic emission at temperatures much lower than a filament emitter, creating an electron distribution that is accelerated toward the anode. This technology combines mechanical and physical robustness and reduces

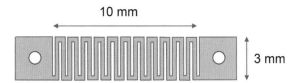

Flat emitting surface cathode

■ **FIGURE 6-11** A flat emitting surface cathode made of tungsten (3 mm × 10 mm active area) is used in many computed tomography x-ray tubes. It can handle the large centrifugal forces occurring at fast rotation speeds of modern CT systems and provide an efficient work function and large surface area for realizing the high tube current requirements of CT and interventional angiography. Magnetic and electrostatic coils are used to focus the electrons along the drift path to the anode, providing the flexibility to position the focal spot distribution on the anode and adjust focal spot size. (Also see Fig. 6-25.)

space charge limitations of conventional cathode emitters, but also requires focusing coils to maintain a tight distribution of electrons when impacting the anode (see Fig. 6-25).

6.2.2 Anode

The anode is a metal target electrode that is maintained at a positive potential difference relative to the cathode. With the cathode filament heated and voltage applied between the electrodes, electrons emitted by the cathode are accelerated toward the anode and deposit most of their energy as heat, with only a small fraction emitted as x-rays. Consequently, the rate of x-ray production, proportional to the tube current, is limited to avoid heat damage to the anode. The anode area impacted by the electrons, the focal spot, also limits the amount of power density (energy per unit time per unit area) that can be deposited. Tungsten is the most widely used anode material because of its high melting point (3,000°C) and high atomic number ($Z = 74$). A tungsten anode can handle substantial heat deposition without cracking or pitting of its surface. An alloy of 10% rhenium and 90% tungsten provides added resistance to surface heat damage. In addition, tungsten provides greater bremsstrahlung production for the same tube current than lower Z elements (Eq. 6-1).

Molybdenum (Mo, $Z = 42$) and rhodium (Rh, $Z = 45$) are used as anode materials in mammographic x-ray tubes. These materials provide useful characteristic x-rays for breast imaging (see Table 6-2). Mammography x-ray tubes and their specialized characteristics are described further in Chapter 8.

6.2.3 Anode Configurations: Stationary and Rotating

A simple x-ray tube design has a stationary anode, consisting of a tungsten insert embedded in a copper block (Fig. 6-12). Copper serves a dual role: it mechanically supports the W insert and efficiently conducts heat from the tungsten target. However, the small area of the focal spot limits the tube current that can be sustained without damage from excessive temperature. Dental x-ray units, low-output mobile x-ray machines, and mobile fluoroscopy systems use fixed-anode x-ray tubes.

Rotating anodes allow higher x-ray output by spreading the heat over a larger area as the anode surface rotates relative to the electron beam. The rotating anode is designed as a beveled disk mounted on a *rotor* assembly supported by bearings in the x-ray tube insert for radiographic x-ray tubes (Fig. 6-13). In many x-ray tube anodes for radiography and fluoroscopy applications, the bulk of the material is molybdenum, with a tungsten target blended with 3% to 10% of rhenium to enhance ductility of ~0.5 mm thickness sintered onto the focal track area. The rotor consists of copper bars arranged around a cylindrical iron shell. A donut-shaped *stator* device, comprised of electromagnet coils, surrounds the rotor and is mounted outside of the

■ **FIGURE 6-12** The anode of a fixed anode x-ray tube consists of a tungsten insert mounted in a copper block. Generated heat is removed from the tungsten target by conduction into the copper block.

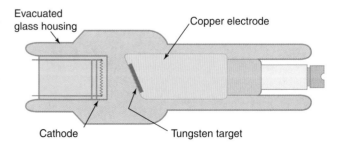

Evacuated glass housing

Copper electrode

Cathode

Tungsten target

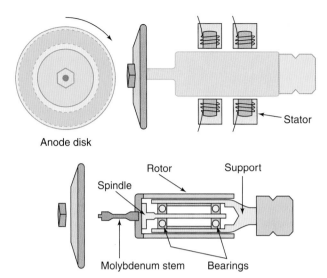

■ **FIGURE 6-13** The anode of a rotating anode x-ray tube is a tungsten disk mounted on a bearing-supported rotor assembly (front view, top left; side view, top right). The rotor consists of a copper and iron laminated core and forms part of an induction motor. The other component is the stator, which exists outside of the insert, top right. A molybdenum shaft (molybdenum is a poor heat conductor) connects the rotor to the anode to reduce heat transfer to the rotor bearings (bottom).

x-ray tube insert. Before an exposure, the stator/rotor induction motor is energized to spin the anode, and after a short delay, rotation speeds of 3,000 to 3,600 (low speed) or 9,000 to 10,000 (high speed) revolutions per minute (rpm) are achieved. X-ray tube-generator systems for general radiography are designed such that the x-ray tube voltage is applied only when the anode is at full speed, causing a short delay (1 to 2 seconds [s]) prior to x-ray exposure when the button is pushed by the technologist.

Rotor bearings are heat sensitive and are often the cause of x-ray tube failure. Bearings require special non-volatile lubricants in the vacuum environment of the x-ray tube insert. Thermal insulation from the hot anode is achieved by using a connector stem to the rotor made of molybdenum, a very poor heat conductor; in fact, most solid anodes are made of molybdenum as the base metal with a tungsten target insert. Most rotating anodes for radiography are cooled by radiative (infrared) emission, transferring heat to the x-ray tube insert and to the surrounding oil bath and tube housing. In imaging situations demanding anodes with higher heat loads and more rapid cooling, sophisticated engineering designs are employed. A tungsten/rhenium (90%–10%) conversion layer of 0.5 to 1 mm thickness and anode support structure made of titanium-zirconium-molybdenum powder-sintered alloy can maintain mechanical integrity at temperatures in excess of 1,200°C. Liquid metal rotor bearings can readily conduct heat for quick cooling with heat exchanger systems using oil or water coolant (see special x-ray tube designs in this section).

The focal track area of the rotating anode is approximately equal to the product of the circumferential track length ($2\pi r$) and the track width (Δr), where r is the radial distance from the axis of the anode to the center of the track (Fig. 6-14). A rotating anode with a 50-mm focal track radius and a 1-mm track width provides a focal track with an annular area 314 times greater than that of a fixed anode with a focal spot area of 1×1 mm. The allowable instantaneous power loading depends on the anode rotation speed and the focal spot area. Faster rotation distributes the heat load over a greater fraction of the focal track area for short exposure times. A larger focal spot distributes energy over a larger anode area and allows much higher output rate to keep exposures short, and should be used in situations where patient motion can be a problem and geometric magnification is small (refer to Chapter 7). Conversely, a small focal spot should be used when magnification is employed, and the likelihood of patient motion is low, because of extended exposure times.

Side view of anode and cathode   Front view of anode

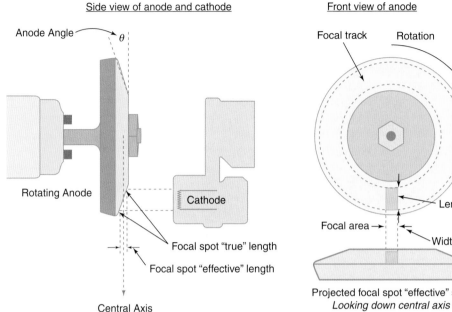
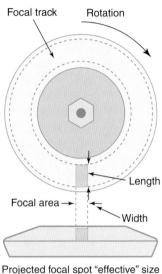

■ **FIGURE 6-14** The anode (target) angle, θ, is defined as the angle of the anode surface in relation to the central axis (left). The focal track represents the total area over which heat is distributed during the x-ray exposure as the anode rotates. The actual focal area is characterized by a length and width (right). The focal spot length, as projected down the central axis, is foreshortened, according to the line focus principle (lower right).

6.2.4 Anode Angle, Field Coverage, and Focal Spot Size

The actual focal spot size is the physical area on the anode that is struck by electrons and is primarily determined by the length of the cathode filament and the width of the focusing cup slot. However, the projected length of the focal spot area at the central ray in the x-ray field is much smaller, because of geometric foreshortening of the projected distribution from the anode surface. The effective and actual focal spot lengths are geometrically related as

$$\text{Effective focal length} = \text{Actual focal length} \times \sin\theta, \qquad [6\text{-}2]$$

where θ is the anode angle. The sin θ term has values from 0.12 for a 7° angle to 0.34 for a 20° angle. The *line focus principle* describes the foreshortening of the focal spot length projected down the central ray, per Equation 6-2.

EXAMPLE: The actual anode focal area for a 15° anode angle is 5 mm (length) by 1.2 mm (width). What is the projected focal spot size at the central axis position?

Answer: Effective length = actual length × sin θ = 5 mm × sin (15°) = 5 mm × 0.26 = 1.29 mm; therefore, the projected focal spot area is 1.29 mm (length) by 1.2 mm (width).

What are the considerations for choosing an anode angle? For x-ray tube designs with a small anode angle, the *effective* focal spot size is smaller for the same *actual* focal area; alternatively, the effective focal spot size remains the same with a longer filament and a larger actual focal area. The first design is beneficial when magnification is employed to reduce geometric blurring; the second design is beneficial when high exposure rate is needed for shortest exposure times using higher mA. However, a small anode angle limits the usable x-ray beam coverage at a given focal spot-to-detector distance, because of beam cutoff on the anode side of the projected x-ray field. In addition, field coverage is smaller for shorter focal spot-to-detector distances (Fig. 6-15). Therefore, the optimal x-ray tube anode angle depends on the clinical imaging application. A small anode angle (~7° to 9°) is desirable for limited field-of-view devices, such as CT scanners with narrow collimation in the A–C dimension, and fluoroscopy C-arm devices where field coverage is determined by the small image receptor diameter (*e.g.*, 23 cm) and focal spot-to-detector distance of 100 cm. Larger anode angles (~12° to 15°) are necessary for general radiographic imaging to achieve large field area coverage (*e.g.*, 43 cm length of a digital detector) at typical focal spot-to-detector distances of 100 cm.

The nominal focal spot size (length and width) is specified at the central ray of the beam. The focal spot length dimension projected toward the anode side of the field becomes smaller, whereas it becomes larger toward the cathode side (Fig. 6-16). The width of the focal spot does not change appreciably with position in the image plane.

Estimating focal spot dimensions can be performed in several ways. Common tools for measuring focal spot size include the pinhole camera, slit camera, star pattern, and resolution bar pattern (Fig. 6-17). In 2005, the International Electrotechnical Commission (IEC) released the International Standard 60336 for measuring focal spots in medical x-ray tubes. Recommendations for detailed measurements and analysis using the first three tools mentioned above are included in that document. The *pinhole camera* uses a tiny circular aperture (10 to 30 μm diameter) in a thin, highly attenuating metal disk to project a magnified image of the focal spot onto an image receptor. Figure 6-17E shows magnified (2×) pinhole pictures of the large (top row)

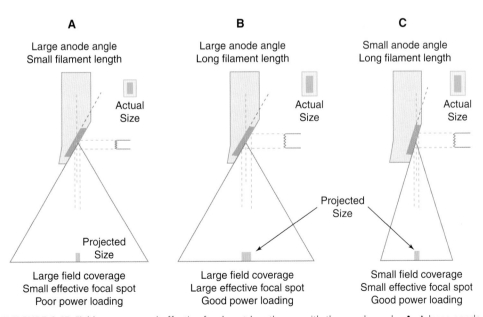

A	B	C
Large anode angle Small filament length	Large anode angle Long filament length	Small anode angle Long filament length
Actual Size	Actual Size	Actual Size
Projected Size	Projected Size	Projected Size
Large field coverage Small effective focal spot Poor power loading	Large field coverage Large effective focal spot Good power loading	Small field coverage Small effective focal spot Good power loading

■ **FIGURE 6-15** Field coverage and effective focal spot length vary with the anode angle. **A.** A large anode angle provides good field coverage at a given distance; however, to achieve a small effective focal spot, a small actual focal area limits power loading. **B.** A large anode angle provides good field coverage, and achievement of high-power loading requires a large focal area; however, geometric blurring and image degradation occur. **C.** A small anode angle limits field coverage at a given distance; however, a small effective focal spot is achieved with a large focal area for high power loading.

■ **FIGURE 6-16** Variation of the effective focal spot size in the image field occurs along the anode-cathode direction. Focal spot distributions are projected as a function of angle, where the central axis bisects the field and the nominal focal spot size is measured. In the field toward the anode side, the focal spot length is shorter, and toward the cathode side it is longer. The width of the focal spot remains the same for projections perpendicular to the anode-cathode axis, although the distribution becomes progressively angled toward the periphery of the field.

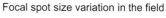
Focal spot size variation in the field

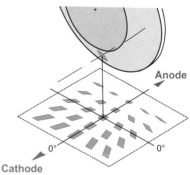

Anode

Cathode

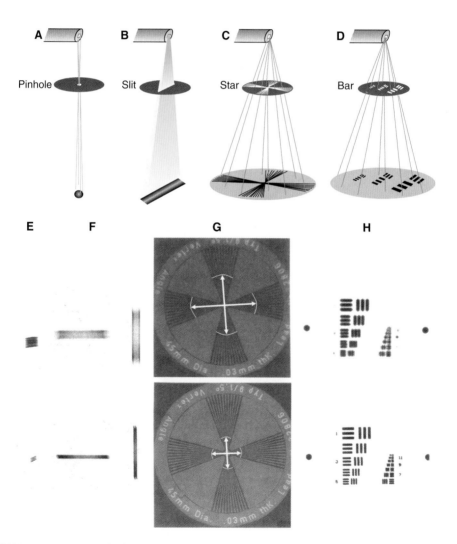

■ **FIGURE 6-17** Various tools allow measurement of the focal spot size, either directly or indirectly. **A and E.** Pinhole camera and images. **B and F.** Slit camera and images. **C and G.** Star pattern and images. **D and H.** Resolution bar pattern and images. For **E–H**, the top row of images represents the measurements of the large focal spot (1.2 mm × 1.2 mm), and the bottom row the small focal spot (0.6 mm × 0.6 mm). The star and bar patterns provide an "equivalent" focal spot dimension based upon the resolvability of the equivalent spatial frequencies.

and small (bottom row) focal spots with a typical "bi-gaussian" intensity distribution. Correcting for the known image magnification allows one to estimate the focal spot dimensions. The *slit camera* consists of a highly attenuating metal plate with an extremely thin slit, typically 10 μm wide, and is the primary method described in the IEC 60336 standard to evaluate focal spot dimensions. Slit images are shown in Figure 6-17F. The *star pattern* test tool (Fig. 6-17G) contains a metal (lead) attenuator radial spoke pattern of diminishing width and spacing on a thin plastic disk. Imaging the star pattern at a known magnification, and measuring the distance between the outermost blur patterns (location of the outermost unresolved spokes as shown by the arrows in Fig. 6-17G) on the image allows the calculation of the effective focal spot dimensions in the directions perpendicular and parallel to the A–C axis. A large focal spot will have a greater blur diameter than a small focal spot, as shown in the figure. For a quick and simple estimate of focal spot size, a *resolution bar pattern* with discrete line pairs can be employed (Fig. 6-17H). Bar pattern images demonstrate the effective resolution parallel and perpendicular to the A–C axis for a given magnification geometry, determined by the bar pattern that can be resolved. If a focal spot dimension is determined to be out of tolerance using this method, one of the methods approved by the IEC standard should be used for more precise evaluation.

For the line spread function (LSF) method, the slit camera is positioned above the image receptor to achieve an enlargement factor of at least 2 for common focal spot nominal values between 0.4 and 1.1 mm, with the center of the slit on the central axis. When the slit camera long axis is oriented perpendicular to the anode-cathode axis, the focal spot length profile image is obtained, and when oriented parallel, the focal spot width profile image is obtained. A line trace of the image values for several rows across each slit image represents the focal spot LSF. The LSF distribution has a peak value that drops to baseline; measuring the width of the LSF at 15% of the peak value and correcting for magnification and pixel dimension calibration for each image yields a measure of the length and width of the focal spot, respectively, as illustrated in Figure 6-18.

Focal spot tolerance limits are listed in Table 6-3 from the IEC 60336 document. Of note are the larger tolerances for the measured focal spot width and length for larger focal spot nominal values. Focal spot "blooming" is an increase in the size of the focal spot resulting from high tube current (mA) caused by electron repulsion and electron beam spreading between the cathode and anode, illustrated in Figure 6-19. It is most pronounced with low tube voltages. Focal spot "thinning" is a slight decrease in the measured focal spot size with increasing kV (electron repulsion and spreading in the x-ray tube is reduced). The IEC 60336 standard requires focal spot measurement to be performed at 75 kV for radiography and fluoroscopy systems using 50% of the maximal rated mA for each focal spot for a 0.1 s acquisition. For CT, the focal spot measurement is performed at 120 kV using 50% of the maximal rated mA for a continuous 4 s acquisition. The exposure time is adjusted for appropriate image quality depending on the focal spot tool used for measurement.

6.2.5 Heel Effect

The *heel effect* refers to a reduction in the x-ray beam fluence on the anode side of the x-ray field (Fig. 6-20). Due to the steep anode angle, x-rays directed toward the anode side of the beam are attenuated by greater path lengths through the anode material than are x-rays directed toward the cathode side of the x-ray field. This reduces x-ray fluence, to the point of complete attenuation and field cutoff. The heel effect is more prominent with a shorter source-to-image distance (SID), for example, for the same

6.2 X-ray Tubes

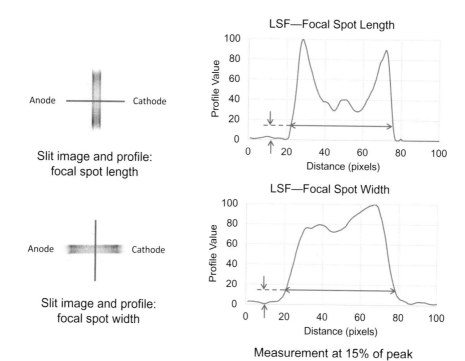

Slit image and profile:
focal spot length

Slit image and profile:
focal spot width

Measurement at 15% of peak

■ **FIGURE 6-18** The focal spot dimensions are determined using a slit camera and measuring the line spread function (LSF) distance at 15% of the peak LSF value of the multi-line profile for the focal spot length and focal spot width. Absolute focal spot size determination requires correction for the magnification factor and the image pixel dimensions. The focal spot dimensions must be less than or equal to the allowed tolerances indicated in Table 6-3.

TABLE 6-3 MAXIMUM PERMISSIBLE DIMENSIONS FOR NOMINAL FOCAL SPOT VALUES

NOMINAL FOCAL SPOT VALUE (mm)	FOCAL SPOT DIMENSIONS: MAXIMUM PERMISSIBLE VALUES AT >15% OF THE PEAK LSF PROFILE	
F	Width—Orthogonal to Tube Axis	Length—Parallel to Tube Axis
0.1	0.15	0.15
0.15	0.23	0.23
0.2	0.30	0.30
0.3	0.45	0.65
0.4	0.60	0.85
0.5	0.75	1.10
0.6	0.90	1.30
0.8	1.20	1.60
1.0	1.40	2.00
1.2	1.70	2.40
1.5	2.00	3.00

Note: Required x-ray tube voltage for radiography is 75 kV and for computed tomography 120 kV, at 50% of the nominal anode input power.

160 mA, 6 ms   **500 mA, 2 ms**   **1,000 mA, 1 ms**

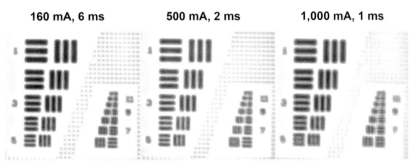

■ **FIGURE 6-19** Focal spot blooming occurs with high tube currents, causing the electron distribution to increase in size, resulting in a larger focal spot and geometric blurring with less resolution as shown in the simple bar pattern focal spot test tool. Shown are three separate acquisitions at 160 mA (1.2 mAs), 500 mA (1 mAs), and 1,000 mA (1 mAs) for a large 1.2 nominal focal spot. The IEC standard 60336 identifies measurement protocols (kV and mA for a specific exposure time) and sets limits on maximum acceptable size (Table 6-3).

detector width, because of beam divergence. Since the x-ray beam fluence is greater on the cathode side of the field, the orientation of the x-ray tube cathode over thicker parts of the patient can result in a better balance of transmitted x-ray photons through the patient and onto the image receptor. For example, the preferred orientation of the x-ray tube for a chest x-ray of a standing patient would be with the A–C axis vertical, and the cathode end of the x-ray tube projected caudally over the diaphragm and the anode end of the x-ray tube projected cranially over the apices of the lungs as illustrated in Figure 6-21.

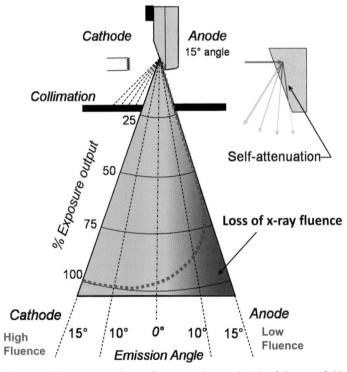

■ **FIGURE 6-20** The heel effect is a loss of x-ray fluence on the anode side of the x-ray field. Electrons interacting at depth within the anode result in the "self attenuation" of x-rays that have a trajectory toward the anode side of the field (upper right).

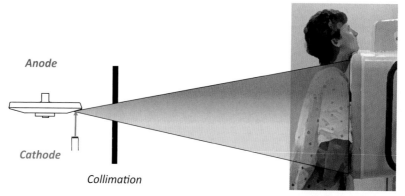

Anode

Cathode

Collimation

■ **FIGURE 6-21** Orientation of the x-ray tube to best compensate for the heel effect are demonstrated for this posterior-anterior chest x-ray acquisition. When possible, the projected anode side of the field should be positioned over the thinner projections (lung apices) and the projected cathode side over the thicker projections (diaphragm) of the patient, so that the transmitted x-ray fluence variations to the detector are reduced.

6.2.6 Off-Focal Radiation

Off-focal radiation results from electrons that elastically rebound from the anode, and accelerate back to the anode, outside of the focal spot. These off-target electrons produce low x-ray fluence over the entire anode surface with a fraction transmitted through the tube port, as shown in Figure 6-22. Off-focal radiation increases quantum noise and reduces contrast in the image, while adding to patient dose. Reducing off-focal radiation is achieved in x-ray tubes designed with a grounded anode, as electrons are just as likely to be attracted to other structures at ground potential. A grounded metal enclosure (hooded anode) in proximity to the focal spot collects rebound electrons in a charge trap and intercepts x-rays produced outside of the focal spot area prior to exiting the tube port.

6.2.7 X-ray Tube Insert

The *x-ray tube insert* contains the cathode, anode, rotor assembly, and support structures sealed in a glass or metal enclosure under a high vacuum. The high vacuum

■ **FIGURE 6-22** Off-focal radiation is produced from back-scattered electrons that are re-accelerated to the anode outside the focal spot. This causes a low-fluence, widespread x-ray radiation distribution pattern demonstrated by the pinhole picture of the anode. Hotspots outside the focal spot indicate areas on the anode where the electrons are more likely to interact.

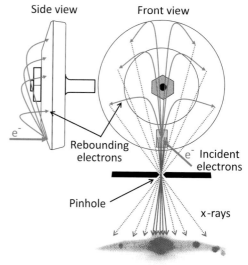

Side view   Front view

Rebounding electrons

Incident electrons

Pinhole

x-rays

Off-focal radiation distribution

prevents electrons from colliding with gas molecules and is necessary in electron beam devices. As x-ray tubes age, molecules can outgas from tube structures and degrade the vacuum. A *"getter"* circuit is used to trap these molecules to maintain the vacuum.

X-rays are emitted in all directions (isotropically) from the focal spot; however, only the x-rays that have trajectories through the *tube port* constitute the useful beam. Except for mammography and special-purpose x-ray tubes, the port is typically made of the same material as the tube enclosure. Mammography tubes use beryllium ($Z = 4$) in the port to minimize absorption of the low-energy x-rays used in mammography, as described in Chapter 8.

6.2.8 X-ray Tube Housing

The x-ray tube housing mechanically supports, electrically and thermally insulates, and protects the x-ray tube insert from the environment. Special oil in the space between the x-ray tube insert and tube housing provides heat conduction and electrical insulation to assist in cooling and protection. In most radiographic x-ray tubes, an expansion bellows accommodates oil expansion as it heats. If the oil heats excessively, a microswitch disables the operation of the x-ray tube until the oil contracts to safe levels. X-ray tubes used in interventional fluoroscopy and CT commonly have heat exchangers that use oil or water coolant to allow prolonged operation at high output.

Lead shielding inside the housing attenuates nearly all x-rays not directed to the tube port (see Fig. 6-7 for the location within the housing). A small fraction of x-rays penetrates the housing and is called *leakage radiation*. Federal regulations (21 CFR 1020.30) require manufacturers to provide enough shielding to limit the leakage radiation exposure rate to 0.88 mGy air kerma per hour (100 mR/h) at 1 m from the focal spot when the x-ray tube is operated at the leakage technique factors. Leakage techniques are the highest tube potential (kV_{max}, typically 125 to 150 kV) at the highest continuous current (typically 3 to 5 mA at kV_{max} for most diagnostic tubes) allowed at that kV. Each x-ray tube housing assembly has a maximal rated tube potential and power rating that must not be exceeded during clinical operation. The x-ray generator has control logic designed to prevent the selection of x-ray technique factors (tube kV, tube current, and exposure time) that could damage the x-ray tube.

6.2.9 X-ray Tube Filtration

Added filtration refers to sheets of metal intentionally placed in the beam typically at the tube port within the collimator assembly. These filters selectively attenuate the low-energy x-rays in the spectrum that have little likelihood of transmission through the patient. Radiation dose to the patient can be substantially reduced by eliminating low energy x-rays that do not contribute to the image formation process.

The total filtration includes both the inherent filtration of the x-ray tube and added metal filters. Inherent filtration includes the thickness (1 to 2 mm) of the glass or metal insert at the x-ray tube port. Glass (primarily silicon dioxide, SiO_2) and aluminum have similar attenuation properties ($Z_{Si} = 14$ and $Z_{Al} = 13$) and effectively attenuate all x-rays in the bremsstrahlung spectrum below about 10 keV. Dedicated mammography tubes, on the other hand, use a thin beryllium ($Z = 4$) tube port to permit the transmission of low-energy x-rays. Inherent filtration also includes attenuation by housing oil and the field light mirror in the collimator assembly.

Aluminum (Al) and copper (Cu) are the most common added filter materials. In mammography, thin filters of Mo, Rh, and silver (Ag) are used to transmit bremsstrahlung x-rays in the intermediate energy range (15 to 25 keV), including characteristic radiation from Mo and Rh anodes, and also to attenuate the lowest and highest x-ray energies in the spectrum (see Chapter 8). The use of rare earth elements, which have K-absorption edges from 39 to 65 keV depending on the element (e.g., erbium Z = 68, K-absorption edge = 57.5 keV) have been advocated for added filtration in radiography to reduce patient dose and improve image contrast, particularly when iodinated contrast agents are used.

Compensation (equalization) filters are used to modify the incident spatial pattern of the x-ray energy fluence to deliver a more uniform transmitted x-ray distribution through the patient to the detector. For example, a trough filter used for chest radiography has a central band of reduced thickness and consequently produces greater x-ray fluence in the middle of the field to compensate for the high attenuation of the mediastinum and to reduce the range of transmitted x-ray fluence through the body. Wedge filters are useful for lateral projections in cervical-thoracic spine imaging, where the incident fluence is increased to match the increased tissue thickness encountered (e.g., to provide a low incident flux to the thin neck area and a high incident flux to the thick shoulders). Wedge filters can also be used with correct orientation to compensate for the anode heel effect (reduced x-ray fluence on the anode side of the projected x-ray beam). "Bow-tie" filters are used in CT to compensate for the thinner tissue thickness at the periphery of the patient. Compensation filters are typically placed close to the x-ray tube port or just external to the collimator assembly.

6.2.10 Collimators

Collimators (x-ray beam apertures) are used to adjust the size and shape of the x-ray field that emerges from the tube port. The collimator assembly typically is attached to the tube housing with a swivel joint. Two pairs of adjustable parallel-opposed lead shutters define a rectangular x-ray field (Fig. 6-23). In the collimator housing,

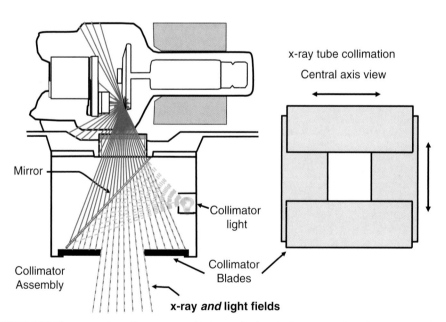

■ **FIGURE 6-23** The x-ray tube collimator assembly is attached to the housing at the tube port, typically on a collar that allows it to be rotated. A light source, positioned at a virtual focal spot location, illuminates the field area from an angled mirror positioned in the x-ray beam path to indicate the x-ray field for patient positioning. The lead collimator blades define the light field and the x-ray field, and annual quality control tests verify their congruence within 2% of the source to image distance on any collimated edge.

a light bulb can be activated to create a light field (reflected by an internal mirror to keep the bulb out of the x-ray field), which defines the x-ray field. Federal regulation (21 CFR 1020.31) requires light field and x-ray field congruence to be within 2% of the SID along either the length or the width of the field. For example, at a SID of 100 cm, the sum of the misalignments between the light field and the x-ray field at the left and right edges must not exceed 2 cm, and the sum of the misalignments at the other two edges also must not exceed 2 cm.

Positive beam limitation (PBL) collimators automatically limit the field size to the useful area of the detector for fixed geometry positions (*e.g.*, chest wall stand). For digital cassette (computed radiography) detectors, mechanical sensors in the cassette holder detect the size and location of the detector and automatically adjust the collimator blades so that the x-ray field matches the cassette dimensions. Adjustment to a smaller field area is possible; however, a field area larger than the detector dimensions requires disabling the PBL circuit.

6.2.11 X-ray Tube Designs

Imaging systems have become specialized with requirements for x-ray sources to meet the dedicated needs with respect to x-ray spectra, mechanical interfaces, and energy throughput. Vendors now supply and service an estimate of more than 500 x-ray tube types that are currently on the market. These include CT, interventional cardiac and vascular x-ray, single exposure and fluoroscopic systems, mammography, and mobile x-ray sources. Characteristics of operation determine the design requirements and power output of x-ray tubes. In Figure 6-24, a broad classification for x-ray tube operation is shown based on typical clinical usage of systems in terms of tube voltage and energy output per exam and exam time. The energy delivered is the product of tube voltage, tube current, and exposure time for the integration period in kilowatt-seconds (kWs). For general radiography, mammography, and CT tubes, exposure time is the x-ray beam on time to image a single patient. For an interventional exam (*e.g.*, cardiovascular imaging) the energy delivered is stated for every 5 minutes (min) of an average procedure

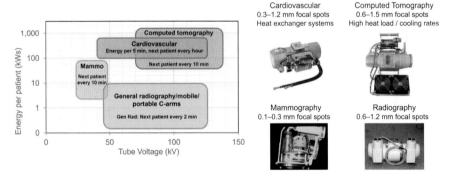

■ **FIGURE 6-24** Classification of the major imaging modalities in terms of kV range (*x*-axis) and typical energy per time period required for x-ray generation (*y*-axis) in most practical clinical cases is illustrated. (Adapted by permission of Taylor and Francis Group, LLC, a Division of Informa PLC. Copyright © 2016 from Behling R. *Modern Diagnostic X-Ray Sources: Technology, Manufacturing, Reliability*.) For CT, mammo (mammography), and general radiography including mobile systems, the integration period is defined as the x-ray on time it takes to image a single patient. For an interventional procedure, the energy value is stated for every 5 min for a typical exam. Application-specific x-ray tubes are designed to meet these criteria in terms of focal spot sizes, x-ray exposure, exposure rate, anode heat loading capacity, and cooling rates (using heat exchangers in cardiovascular and CT modalities) to maintain patient throughput as indicated. On the right are x-ray tube pictures and relevant focal spot size ranges for four categories of x-ray tubes indicated in the figure on the left.

in kWs. Tube designs are specified to meet these x-ray production operational requirements in terms of power output ratings and heat dissipation requirements that are explained in the next section.

Mammography tubes are designed to provide low-energy x-rays necessary to produce optimal mammographic images. The main differences between a dedicated mammography tube and a conventional x-ray tube are the target materials (molybdenum and rhodium) in some systems, the output port (beryllium versus glass or metal insert material), and smaller effective focal spot sizes (typically 0.3 and 0.1 mm nominal sizes) (see Chapter 8).

X-ray tubes for interventional procedures and for CT require high instantaneous x-ray output, high heat loading, and rapid cooling. Furthermore, in CT, with the fast x-ray tube rotation (as low as 0.20 s for a complete rotation about the patient) and the tremendous mechanical forces it places on the CT tube, planar surface cathode emitter and liquid metal bearings for the rotating anode are used. Direct anode cooling is achievable by heat conduction through liquid metal bearings that are in contact with a heat exchanger to remove heat out of the tube housing, thus reducing the overall heat burden on the anode and allowing extended operation at high kV and mA (Fig. 6-25). One manufacturer's CT tube incorporates a design with the cathode and the anode as part of a metal vacuum enclosure. Dynamic steering of the electron beam within the tube is achieved by external electromagnetic deflection coils to direct the electrons to distinct focal spots on the anode (a "flying focal spot"), which can produce slightly different source positions and improve data sampling during CT acquisition (refer to Chapter 10 on CT).

Development of high-resolution CT scanners with larger image matrices and finer sampling of the x-ray projection data necessitates the need for smaller focal spots. One CT system has 6 selectable focal spots, from large to very small, created by selective adjustment of magnetic quadrupole coils in the electron drift tube to focus the electron distribution onto the anode. Achieving the highest capable resolution requires the selection of the smallest focal spot to ensure that the geometric

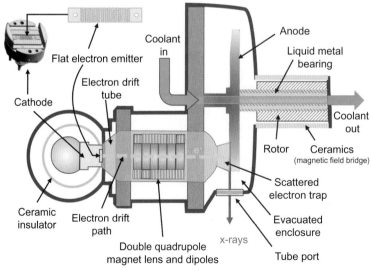

■ **FIGURE 6-25** Diagram of an advanced CT x-ray tube, with a flat surface cathode emitter is illustrated. Electrons are emitted from the cathode in an electron drift tube, focused by magnetic lenses, and accelerated to the anode, which is mounted on a liquid metal bearing assembly with an inner heat exchanger tube. Water coolant flows through the tube inside of the liquid metal bearing assembly and extracts the heat conducted through the bearing. X-rays are emitted from the anode through the tube port, and rebounding electrons are captured by a scattered electron trap mounted near the anode focal area.

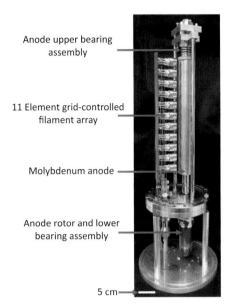

Anode upper bearing assembly

11 Element grid-controlled filament array

Molybdenum anode

Anode rotor and lower bearing assembly

5 cm

■ **FIGURE 6-26** An 11-source x-ray tube assembly is shown—this is the assembly that fits inside a metal housing, which provides the vacuum environment. The array of 11 cathode cups is shown opposite the cylindrical molybdenum anode, which rotates during operation. Each of the cathodes is independently addressable, so each focal spot can be activated in any random or sequential order. Thus, a tomosynthesis acquisition (explained in Chapter 8) can be performed with no moving components, reducing motion blur of the x-ray source and enabling a faster scan. (Courtesy of Paul Schwoebel, PhD, The University of New Mexico.)

blurring is no greater than the digital sampling aperture of the projections. For similar quantum noise in the reconstructed images, this results in a longer acquisition time because power density limitations on the anode require a much lower tube current to achieve the same mAs per rotation.

Single source x-ray tubes must physically move to acquire projections of an object from different angles. A *multiple source x-ray tube* developed by researchers has 11 thermionic cathodes facing a rotating, cylindrical molybdenum anode (Fig. 6-26). This type of x-ray tube may prove to be useful for stationary breast tomosynthesis (see Chapter 8), which would enable much faster acquisitions and reduce patient motion. Since the x-ray tube would be stationary, there is no source motion, and thus would improve the spatial resolution of the scan as well. Each of the sources is individually programmable and allows an electronically controlled sweep of the x-ray beam across the tomographic angle. While several prototype multi-source systems have been developed using field emission technology (cold cathode), this thermionic cathode system allows each source to have its own tube current control, which in turn allows the source array to be pulsed over different x-ray output levels. Dynamic modulation of x-ray beam output has great potential for breast tomosynthesis and other applications.

6.2.12 Recommendations to Maximize X-ray Tube Life

X-ray tubes eventually must be replaced, but a long lifetime can be achieved with appropriate care and use. Several simple rules include:

- Minimize filament boost "prep" time (the first detent of two on the x-ray exposure switch) especially when high mA is used. If applied for too long, filament life will be shortened, unstable operation will occur, and evaporated tungsten will be deposited on the glass envelope.
- Use lower tube current with longer exposure times to produce the desired mAs.
- Avoid extended or repeated operation of the x-ray tube with high technique factors (kV and mAs). If the focal track is damaged, less radiation output and outgassing of the anode structure can result in unstable tube performance.
- Use the manufacturer's recommended warm-up procedure. Do not make high mA exposures on a cold anode, because uneven expansion caused by thermal

stress can cause micro-cracks, which ultimately degrades the performance of the x-ray tube.

• Limit rotor start-and-stop operations, which can generate significant heat within the stator windings; when possible, a 30 to 40 s delay between exposures should be used.

6.3 X-RAY GENERATORS

The principal function of the x-ray generator is to control tube current, high voltage, and exposure time to an x-ray tube. Electric power sources in the clinic or hospital provide from 120 to 480 V, and 50–100 A circuits, while typical x-ray tube operation requires 20 to 150 kV and about 1 A peak tube current. The electrical transformer converts voltage through a process called *electromagnetic induction and* is a principal component of the x-ray generator.

6.3.1 Electromagnetic Induction and Voltage Transformation

Electromagnetic induction occurs when a changing magnetic field induces an electrical potential difference (voltage) in a nearby conductor, or similarly when a conductor is moving through a stationary magnetic field. For example, a bar magnet that moves toward a wire conductor induces an electromotive force and creates a potential difference, resulting in electron flow (Fig. 6-27A). As the magnet moves in the

A Changing magnetic field induces electron flow:

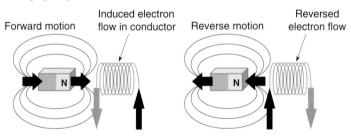

B Current (electron flow) in a conductor creates a magnetic field; its *amplitude and direction* determines magnetic field strength and polarity

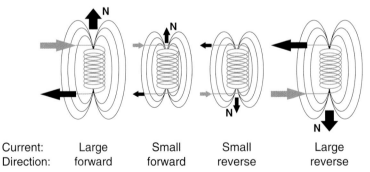

| Current: | Large | Small | Small | Large |
| Direction: | forward | forward | reverse | reverse |

■ **FIGURE 6-27** Principles of electromagnetic induction are illustrated. **A.** Induction of an electrical current in a wire conductor coil by a moving (changing) magnetic field. The direction of the current is dependent on the direction of the magnetic field motion. **B.** Creation of a magnetic field by the current in a conducting coil. The polarity and magnetic field strength are determined by the amplitude and direction of the current.

opposite direction, the polarity of the electromotive force is reversed, and the induced current flows in the opposite direction. The magnitude of the induced potential difference is proportional to the rate of change of the magnetic field strength.

Moving electrical charges (electrons) flowing through a wire produce an associated magnetic field whose magnitude (strength) is proportional to the magnitude of the current (see Fig. 6-27B). A constant (direct) current (DC) is associated with a constant magnetic field. An alternating current (AC) is associated with a changing magnetic field that reverses polarity in synchrony with the reverses in current direction in the wire. In a coiled wire geometry, the magnetic fields from adjacent turns of the wire add to the magnitude of the magnetic field, which is proportional to the number of wire turns. In North America, the standard AC frequency operates at 60 cycles/s (Hz), and in most other areas of the world at 50 Hz. With the AC waveform, the changing electrical current has a corresponding changing magnetic field.

Magnetic fields are unaffected by electrical wire insulation, so a wire conductor carrying AC power will induce a corresponding AC waveform in a nearby conductor via mutual induction through the varying magnetic field component. On the other hand, a DC power source, like that produced by a chemical battery, creates a constant magnetic field and does not result in electromagnetic induction in nearby conductors.

6.3.2   Transformers

Transformers use the principle of electromagnetic induction to change the voltage of an electrical power source. The generic transformer has two distinct, electrically isolated wire coils wrapped about a common iron core (Fig. 6-28). Input AC power to the "primary winding" produces an oscillating magnetic field, where each turn of the wire adds to the magnetic field amplitude that uniformly permeates the iron core. The fluctuating magnetic field then induces a changing voltage on the "secondary winding." The voltage induced on the secondary winding is proportional to the input voltage and the ratio of the number of turns on the primary winding to the number of turns on the secondary winding as stated by the *Law of Transformers:*

$$\frac{V_P}{V_S} = \frac{N_P}{N_S},$$

[6-3]

where N_P is the number of turns in the primary coil, N_S is the number of turns in the secondary coil, V_P is the input voltage on the primary side of the transformer, and V_S is the output voltage on the secondary side.

A transformer can increase, decrease, or isolate input voltage, depending on the ratio of the numbers of turns in the two coils. For $N_S > N_P$, a "step-up" transformer increases the secondary voltage; for $N_S < N_P$, a "step-down" transformer decreases the secondary

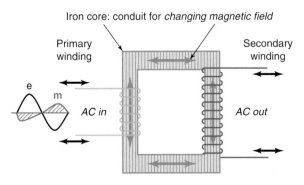

Iron core: conduit for *changing magnetic field*

Primary winding

Secondary winding

e

m

AC in

AC out

■ **FIGURE 6-28** The basic transformer consists of an iron core, a primary winding circuit, and a secondary winding circuit. An AC flowing through the primary winding produces a changing magnetic field, which permeates the core and induces an alternating voltage on the secondary winding. This mutual electromagnetic induction is mediated by the containment of the magnetic field in the iron core and permeability through wire insulation.

■ **FIGURE 6-29** Transformers increase (step up), decrease (step down), or leave unchanged (isolate) the input voltage depending on the ratio of primary to secondary turns, according to the Law of Transformers. In all cases, the input and the output circuits are electrically isolated.

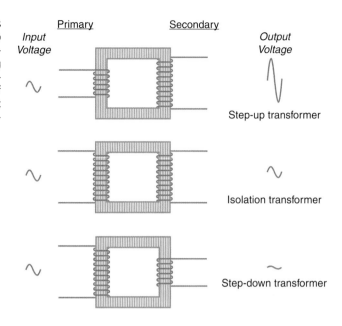

voltage; and for $N_S = N_P$, an "isolation" transformer produces a secondary voltage equal to the primary voltage. Most laptop computers and cell phones have transformers on the power cords that reduce the 120 or 240 V line voltage to 12 V or less. Configurations of these transformers are shown in Figure 6-29. A step-up transformer circuit provides the high voltage necessary (20 to 150 kV) for a diagnostic x-ray generator.

Alternating waveforms in the transformer switch between negative and positive voltage during each half cycle. However, for continuous production of x-rays, the anode must have positive voltage with respect to the cathode, and this occurs only half of the time when the AC waveform is directly attached to the x-ray tube electrodes. A *diode* is an electronic device with two electrodes that allow large current flow in one direction when the voltage polarity on one electrode is positive and negative on the other. However, when the voltage polarity reverses, there is no current flow. Diodes come in all sizes, from large, x-ray tube–sized devices down to microscopic, solid-state components on an integrated circuit board. Clever use of diodes arranged in a *bridge rectifier circuit* can route the electron flow through an AC circuit to a unidirectional movement of electrons in which the voltage polarity does not change at the electrode. Rectification is an important function of the high voltage circuits in an x-ray generator.

Power is the rate of energy production or expenditure per unit time. The SI unit of power is the watt (W), defined as 1 J of energy per second. For electrical devices, power, P, is equal to the product of voltage V, and current, I.

$$P = IV \qquad [6\text{-}4]$$

Because a volt is defined as 1 J per coulomb and an ampere is 1 coulomb per second,

$$1 \text{ watt} = 1 \text{ volt} \times 1 \text{ ampere.}$$

For an ideal transformer, the power output is equal to the power input. Thus, the product of voltage and current in the primary circuit is equal to that in the secondary circuit

$$V_P I_P = V_S I_S, \qquad [6\text{-}5]$$

where I_P is the input current on the primary side and I_S is the output current on the secondary side. Therefore, a decrease in current must accompany an increase in voltage, and vice versa. Equations 6-3 and 6-5 describe ideal transformer performance. Power losses in an actual transformer due to inefficient coupling cause both the voltage and current on the secondary side of the transformer to be less than those predicted by these equations.

EXAMPLE: The ratio of primary to secondary turns is 1:1,000 in a transformer. If an input AC waveform has a peak voltage of 50 V, what is the peak voltage induced in the secondary side?

$$\frac{V_P}{V_S} = \frac{N_P}{N_S}; \quad \frac{50}{V_S} = \frac{1}{1,000}; \quad V_S = 50 \times 1,000 = 50,000 \, V = 50 \, kV$$

What is the secondary current for a primary current of 10 A?

$$V_P I_P = V_S I_S; \quad 50 \, V \times 10 \, A = 50,000 \, V \times I_S; \quad I_S = 0.001 \times 10 \, A = 0.01 \, A = 10 \, mA$$

For x-ray transformers, the center of the secondary winding is usually connected to ground potential ("center tapped to ground"). Ground is the electrical potential of the earth. Center tapping to ground does not affect the maximum potential difference applied between the anode and cathode of the x-ray tube, but it limits the maximum voltage at any point in the circuit relative to ground to one half of the peak voltage applied to the tube. Therefore, the maximum voltage at any point in the circuit for a center-tapped transformer of 150 kV is −75 kV or +75 kV, relative to ground. This reduces electrical insulation requirements and improves electrical safety. In some x-ray tube designs (*e.g.*, mammography and CT), the anode is maintained at ground potential. Even though this places the cathode at peak negative voltage with respect to ground, the low kV (less than 50 kV) used in mammography does not present an electrical insulation problem, while in modern CT systems (up to 140 kV) the x-ray generator is placed adjacent to the x-ray tube in the enclosed gantry.

6.3.3 X-ray Generator Modules

Modular components of the x-ray generator (Fig. 6-30) include the high-voltage power circuit, the stator circuit, the filament circuit, the focal spot selector, and automatic exposure control (AEC) circuit. Generators have circuitry and microprocessors that monitor the selection of potentially damaging overload conditions to protect the x-ray tube. Combinations of kV, mA, and exposure time that would deliver excessive power to the anode are prohibited by system logic. Calculated thermal loading on the x-ray tube anode are based on kV, mA, and exposure time settings for heat input and cooling, which occurs over time. Some x-ray systems are equipped with sensors to measure the temperature of the anode and to protect the x-ray tube and housing from excessive heat buildup by prohibiting exposures until cooling makes it safe to operate. This is particularly important for CT scanners and high-powered interventional fluoroscopy systems.

6.3.4 Operator Console

The parameters that are selected in the operation of a radiographic system include the tube voltage (kV), the tube current (mA), the exposure time (s), or the product of mA and time (mAs), fixed technique versus AEC mode, the AEC sensor

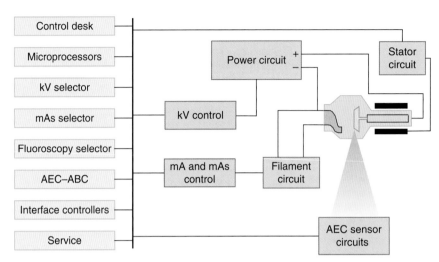

■ **FIGURE 6-30** A modular schematic view shows the basic x-ray generator components. Most systems are now microprocessor controlled and include service support diagnostics.

location to be used, and the focal spot size (large or small). If AEC is used, exposure time is determined during the exposure. The focal spot size (i.e., large or small) is usually determined by the mA setting; low mA selections allow the small focal spot to be used, and higher mA settings require the use of the large focal spot due to anode heating concerns. On many x-ray generators, preprogrammed techniques can be selected for various examinations (e.g., chest; kidneys, ureter and bladder; cervical spine; and extremities). For fluoroscopic procedures, although kV and mA can sometimes be manually selected, the generator's automatic exposure rate control (AERC) circuit, also known as automatic brightness control (ABC), is most commonly activated. The kV and mA are interactively adjusted by feedback signals from a sensor indicating the radiation exposure rate at the image receptor.

6.3.5 High-Frequency X-ray Generator

Several x-ray generator circuit designs are in use, including single-phase, three-phase, constant potential, and high-frequency inverter generators. The high-frequency generator is now the contemporary choice for diagnostic x-ray systems. A high-frequency alternating waveform (up to 40,000 Hz) is generated and used for efficient conversion of low to high voltage by a step-up transformer. Subsequent rectification and voltage smoothing produce a nearly constant voltage between the cathode and anode. These conversion steps are illustrated in Figure 6-31. The operational frequency of the generator is variable, depending on the exposure settings (kV, mA, and time), the charge/discharge characteristics of the high-voltage capacitors on the x-ray tube, and the frequency-to-voltage characteristics of the transformer.

Figure 6-32 shows the circuit diagram of a general-purpose high-frequency inverter generator. Low-frequency, low-voltage input power (50 to 60 cycles/s AC) is converted to a low voltage, DC. An inverter circuit creates a low voltage high-frequency AC waveform as input to the primary coil of the high-voltage transformer. The secondary coil outputs a high-voltage, high-frequency waveform that is rectified and smoothed to supply high-voltage capacitors attached to the x-ray tube electrodes with sufficient accumulated charge to produce the requested kV according to the relationship $V = Q/C$, where V is the voltage (volts), Q is the charge (coulombs), and

Single phase input voltage

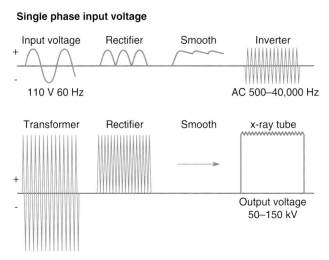

■ **FIGURE 6-31** In a high-frequency inverter generator, a single- or three-phase AC input voltage is rectified and smoothed to create a DC waveform. An inverter circuit produces a high-frequency AC waveform as input to the high-voltage transformer. Rectification and capacitance smoothing provide the resultant high-voltage output waveform, with properties similar to those of a three-phase generator system.

C is the capacitance (farads). Feedback circuits monitor the tube voltage and tube current during operation and continuously supply charge to the capacitors as needed to maintain a nearly constant voltage.

For kV adjustment, a voltage comparator measures the difference between the reference voltage (a calibrated value proportional to the requested kV) and the actual kV measured across the tube by a voltage divider (the kV "sense" circuit). A difference initiates pulses to produce more charge to the high voltage capacitors to maintain the potential difference across the x-ray tube electrodes in a closed-loop voltage regulation circuit.

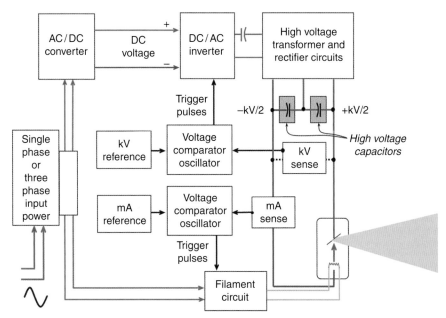

■ **FIGURE 6-32** Modular components and circuits of the high-frequency generator. The selected high voltage across the x-ray tube is created by charging high voltage capacitors to the desired potential difference. During the exposure when the x-ray circuit is energized, tube current is kept constant by the "mA sense" circuit that maintains the proper filament current by sending trigger pulses to the filament circuit, and tube voltage is kept constant by the "kV sense" circuit that sends trigger pulse signals to the DC/AC inverter to maintain the charge on high voltage capacitors.

The tube current (mA) is regulated in an analogous manner to the kV, with a resistor circuit sensing the actual tube current (the voltage across a resistor is proportional to the current) and comparing it with a reference voltage. If the mA is too low, the mA comparator circuit increases the trigger frequency, which boosts the power to the filament to raise its temperature and increase the thermionic emission of electrons. The feedback circuit eliminates the need for electron space charge compensation circuits and corrects for filament ageing effects.

There are several advantages to the high-frequency inverter generator. Single-phase or three-phase input voltage can be used. Closed-loop feedback and regulation circuits ensure reproducible and accurate kV and mA values. Transformers operating at high frequencies are efficient, compact, and less costly to manufacture than older generator designs. Modular, compact design makes equipment installation and repairs relatively easy.

The high-frequency inverter generator is the preferred system for all but a few applications, for example, those requiring extremely high power, extremely fast kV switching, or submillisecond exposure times provided by a *constant-potential* generator, which is both bulky and costly.

6.3.6 Voltage Ripple

Ideally, the voltage applied to an x-ray tube would be constant. However, variations occur in the high voltage produced by an x-ray generator that is applied to the x-ray tube for various types of x-ray generators (including historical single phase and three phase generators) as illustrated in Figure 6-33. For older single-phase generators, which are no longer prominent, there was a substantial difference in the average kV and the peak kV (kVp) by as much as 30%, justifying the use of the kVp descriptor. Voltage ripple is no longer a major issue, as most generators in use today are of high frequency designs. For this reason, the use of kVp has been appropriately replaced with kV throughout this book, as there is little difference (typically less than 5%) between the average and peak kilovoltage with modern x-ray generators.

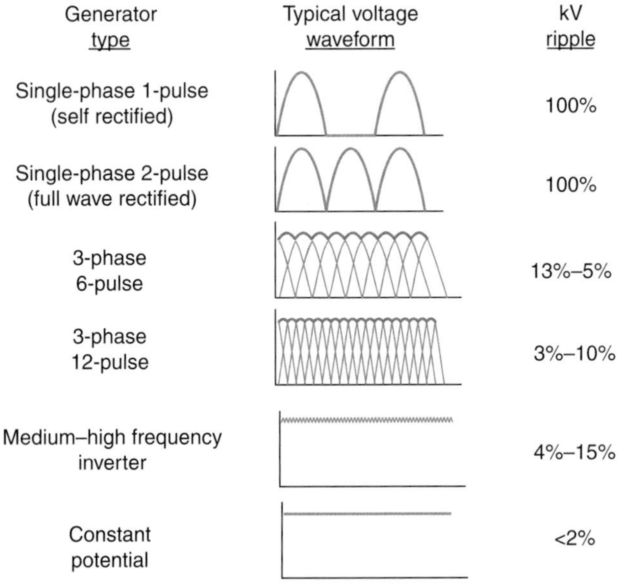

■ **FIGURE 6-33** Typical voltage ripple for various x-ray generators used in diagnostic radiology varies from 100% voltage ripple for a single-phase generator to almost no ripple for a constant-potential generator. Most x-ray generators are high frequency and have voltage ripple from about 3% to 10%.

Generator type	Typical voltage waveform	kV ripple
Single-phase 1-pulse (self rectified)		100%
Single-phase 2-pulse (full wave rectified)		100%
3-phase 6-pulse		13%–5%
3-phase 12-pulse		3%–10%
Medium–high frequency inverter		4%–15%
Constant potential		<2%

6.3.7 Timers

Digital timers have largely replaced electronic timers based on resistor-capacitor circuits and charge-discharge timers in older systems. Digital timer circuits have extremely high reproducibility and microsecond accuracy, but ultimately the precision and accuracy of the x-ray exposure time depends chiefly on the type of switching (low voltage, high voltage, or x-ray tube switching) employed in the x-ray system. A countdown timer, also known as a backup timer, is used as a safety mechanism to terminate a radiographic acquisition in the event of an exposure switch failure.

6.3.8 Switches

The high-frequency inverter generator typically uses electronic switching on the primary side of the high-voltage transformer to initiate and terminate the exposure. The high-frequency waveform allows exposure times as short as 2 ms.

Alternatively, a grid-controlled x-ray tube can be used with any type of generator to switch the exposure on and off by applying a bias voltage (about $\sim -2,000$ to $-4,000$ V) to the focusing cup. This is the fastest switching method, with minimal turn-on–turnoff "lag"; however, there are extra costs for these components and high-voltage insulation issues to be considered.

6.3.9 Automatic Exposure Control

The AEC system is used far more often than manual exposure time settings in radiography. AEC measures the actual amount of radiation incident on the image receptor during the acquisition and terminates x-ray production when the optimal radiation levels are obtained. AEC compensates for patient thickness and other variations in attenuation to produce more consistent exposures than manual techniques. The AEC system consists of one or more radiation detectors, an amplifier, digital signal to noise (SNR) selector that allows the operator to adjust the exposure to accommodate image quality requirements, signal integrator circuit, comparator circuit, termination switch, and backup timer safety shutoff switch (Fig. 6-34). X-rays transmitted through the patient and antiscatter grid, if present, generate signals in one to three selectable ionization chambers positioned in front of the digital detector. An amplifier boosts the signal, which is fed to a voltage comparator and integration circuit. A user-selectable SNR selector on the generator control panel increases or decreases the reference voltage by 10% to 15% per selection step from the neutral position with negative (lower SNR) or positive (higher SNR) steps. When the accumulated signal produces a voltage that equals the selected reference voltage, an output signal terminates the exposure. The AEC sensors are placed in front of the image receptor to measure the transmitted x-ray flux through the patient (see Fig. 6-34). Positioning in front of the image receptor is possible because of the high transparency of the ionization chambers with x-ray beams operated at 50 kV or higher. In the event of an AEC detector or circuit failure, the backup timer safety switch terminates the x-ray exposure after a preset "on" time.

To allow flexibility in imaging different body parts, wall-mounted chest, table cassette stands, and DR image receptors typically have three sensor areas arranged in locations as shown in Figure 6-34 (front view). The technologist can select the AEC detectors activated for each radiographic application. For instance, in posteroanterior chest imaging, the two outside areas are usually selected so that the x-ray beam

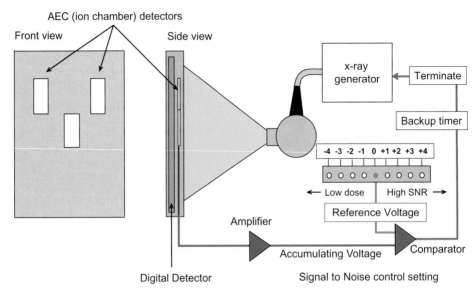

■ **FIGURE 6-34** AEC detectors measure the radiation incident on the detector and terminate the exposure according to a preset calibrated signal-to-noise ratio achieved in the digital image. A front view (left) and side view (middle) of a chest cassette stand and the locations of ionization chamber detectors are shown. The desired signal to the image receptor and thus the signal-to-noise ratio may be selected at the operator's console with respect to a normalized reference voltage.

transmitted through the lungs determines the exposure time. This prevents signal saturation in the lung areas, which can occur when the transmitted x-ray flux is measured under the highly attenuating mediastinum with the center chamber.

6.4 POWER RATINGS, ANODE LOADING, AND COOLING

The *power rating* of an x-ray tube focal spot or x-ray generator is the maximal power that an x-ray tube focal spot can accept, or the generator can deliver under certain conditions. General diagnostic x-ray tubes and x-ray generators use 100 kV and the maximum ampere rating (A_{max}) available for a 0.1 s exposure to benchmark the power, as

$$\text{Power (kW)} = 100 \text{ kV} \times I \text{ (A}_{max}) \text{ for a 0.1 s exposure time.} \qquad [6\text{-}6]$$

For instance, a generator that can deliver 800 mA (0.8 A maximum) tube current at 100 kV for 0.1 s exposure has a power rating of 80 kW according to Equation 6-6. X-ray generator power ratings vary considerably. The highest generator power ratings are specified for interventional radiology and cardiovascular angiography imaging suites, as well as modern multirow detector CT scanners with 80 to 120-kW generators. General radiographic or radiographic/fluoroscopic systems use generators with 30 to 80 kW power ratings. Lower powered generators (5 to 30 kW) are found in mobile radiography and fluoroscopy systems, dental x-ray systems, and other systems that have fixed anode x-ray tubes. The power rating of the generator should be reasonably matched to the power characteristics of the largest focal spot. Generator power that is too low for the large focal spot of the x-ray tube assembly limits x-ray fluence rate and results in longer exposure times, while generator power that is too high for the large focal spot is a waste of capabilities that cannot be realized.

The power rating of the focal spot is determined by several characteristics of the anode including anode angle, diameter, rotation speed, mass, and size of the focal spot. For conventional x-ray tubes, small anode angles, large focal spots ($\geq 1.2 \times 1.2$ mm), large diameter anodes, and fast anode rotation speeds are necessary to achieve 80 to 100 kW power ratings. Most medium focal spot dimensions (0.6 mm $\times$ 0.6 mm) have moderate power ratings (30 to 50 kW), and smaller focal spots (0.3 mm $\times$ 0.3 mm) have low power ratings (5 to 15 kW). For CT x-ray tubes, a shallow anode angle (7°), bearings mounted outside of the x-ray tube vacuum or liquid metal bearings with active heat conduction from the anode allow for extended high-power operation (*e.g.*, continuous operation at 800 mA and 120 kV for 10's of seconds). X-ray generators have circuits or firmware to prohibit combinations of kV, mA, and exposure time that exceed the power deposition tolerance of the focal spot.

6.4.1 Anode Heating and Cooling

Historically, the power characteristics of an x-ray tube were described with anode heating and cooling charts. A premium was placed on the maximum heat loading of the anode so that many exposures could be made without having to wait for anode heat dissipation and tube cooling that occurred by slow radiative emission of the built-up heat. The charts did not serve any real practical use in a clinical situation. In addition, advanced x-ray tubes that use conduction cooling to rapidly dissipate anode heat are not as constrained by anode heat loading. The IEC decided to abandon the historical Maximum Anode Heat Content measure, and in 2010 published IEC standard 60613 and the concept of clinically relevant input power. This is a single value for the x-ray tube that characterizes both heating and cooling, as described by the following:

1. **Nominal radiographic anode input power:** POWER, which can be applied for a single X-RAY TUBE LOAD with a LOADING TIME of 0.1 s and a CYCLE TIME of 1.0 min, for an indefinite number of cycles. The nominal radiographic anode input power is stated as a single value, defining the short time power that the tube can sustain to produce a single exposure of 100 ms length every minute; it characterizes pulse performance as well as cooling capability.

2. **Nominal CT anode input power:** POWER, which can be applied for a single X-RAY TUBE LOAD with a LOADING TIME of 4 s and a CYCLE TIME of 10 min, for an indefinite number of cycles. This simple scalar value characterizes the capability of the CT tube in lieu of heat loading expressed in MHU (see below). Cooling performance is included as the loading is assumed to be repeated in a practical sequence with average patient frequency (10 min cycles) and reflects typical exposure times around 4 s.

   In more complicated situations, an alternative is described as CT scan Power Index. More information on this metric can be found in the IEC standard documentation.

6.4.2 Historical Units: The Heat Unit and the Joule

The heat unit (HU) is a traditional unit that provides a simple way of expressing x-ray tube anode energy deposition and dissipation for a single-phase generator. The number of HU can be calculated from the parameters defining the radiographic technique:

$$\text{Energy (HU)} = \alpha \times \text{peak voltage (kVp)} \times \text{tube current (mA)} \times \text{exposure time (s)}, \quad \text{[6-7]}$$

where α is a multiplicative factor as a function of the kV waveform.

Equation 6-7 is used for single-phase generator waveforms ($\alpha = 1$) with significant voltage ripple, but underestimates the energy deposition of three-phase, high-frequency, and constant-potential generators. A multiplicative factor ($\alpha = 1.35$) compensates for these waveforms. For instance, an exposure of 80 kV, 250 mA, and 100 ms generates 2,000 HU for a single-phase generator ($\alpha = 1.0$), but 2,700 HU for a three-phase or high frequency generator ($\alpha = 1.35$).

For continuous x-ray production (fluoroscopy), the power input rate is defined as follows:

$$HU/s = kV \times mA. \qquad [6\text{-}8]$$

Heat accumulates by energy deposition and simultaneously disperses by anode cooling. The anode cools faster at higher temperatures due to non-linear physics of temperature dissipation, so that for most fluoroscopic and long CT procedures, a steady-state equilibrium exists as shown in Figure 6-35, and Equation 6-8 overestimates the heat energy delivered to the anode. The anode thermal characteristics chart for heat input and heat output curves considers both heating and cooling.

The joule (J) is the SI unit of energy. One joule is deposited by a power of one watt acting for 1 s ($1\,J = 1\,W \times 1\,s$). The energy, in joules, deposited in the anode is calculated as follows:

$$\text{Energy (J)} = \text{RMS voltage (V}_{RMS}) \times \text{Tube current (A)} \times \text{Exposure time (s)}. \qquad [6\text{-}9]$$

The root-mean-square voltage, V_{RMS}, is the constant voltage that would deliver the same power as a varying voltage waveform (*e.g.*, for a single-phase generator $V_{RMS} = 0.71$). Thus, from Equations 6-7 and 6-9 with unit conversions, the relationship between the deposited energy expressed in joules and HU is approximated as

$$\text{Energy (HU)} \cong 1.4 \times \text{Heat input (J)}. \qquad [6\text{-}10]$$

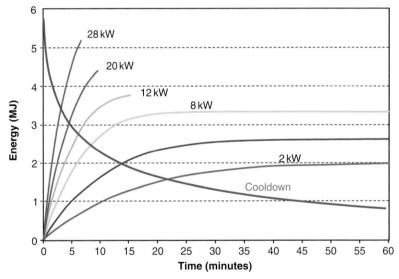

Anode Heating and Cooling Curve: CT Tube

■ **FIGURE 6-35** Anode heating and cooling curve chart for a CT scanner plots *energy* in megajoules (MJ) on the vertical axis and *time* in minutes on the horizontal axis. A series of power input curves from low (2 kW) to high (28 kW) are determined by the kV and mA settings with continuous x-ray tube operation as a function of time. The cooling curve shows the rate of cooling and indicates faster cooling with higher anode heat load (temperature). In this example the maximum capacity is 5.7 MJ. For low power inputs, heating and cooling rates eventually equilibrate and reach a steady state, as shown for the 2, 4, and 8 kW curves.

6.5 FACTORS AFFECTING X-RAY EMISSION

The output of an x-ray tube is often described by the terms *quality*, *quantity*, and *exposure*. *Quality* describes the penetrability of an x-ray beam, with higher energy x-ray photons having a larger half-value layer (HVL) and higher "quality." (The HVL is discussed in Chapter 3.) *Quantity* refers to the number of x-ray photons comprising the beam. *Exposure*, defined in Chapter 3, is proportional to the energy fluence (energy weighted photon number) of the x-ray beam spectrum. X-ray production efficiency, quality, and quantity are dependent on the x-ray tube target (anode) material, tube voltage, tube current, exposure time, beam filtration, and generator waveform.

6.5.1 Anode Target Material

The elemental composition of the **Target** affects the *efficiency* of bremsstrahlung radiation production, where x-ray output is linearly proportional to the target atomic number. Incident electrons are more likely to have radiative interactions in higher-Z materials (see Eq. 6-1). The energies of characteristic x-rays produced in the target depend on the elemental composition of the target. Therefore, the target affects the quantity of bremsstrahlung photons and the quality of the characteristic radiation.

6.5.2 Tube Voltage (kV)

The applied potential difference across the cathode and anode determines the peak energy in the bremsstrahlung spectrum and affects the quality of the output spectrum. The efficiency of x-ray production is related to tube voltage, approximately proportional to the square of the tube potential in the diagnostic energy range.

$$\text{Exposure} \propto \text{kV}^2 \qquad [6\text{-}11]$$

For example, according to Equation 6-11, the relative exposure of a beam generated with 80 kV compared to 60 kV for the same tube current and exposure time is calculated as follows:

$$\left(\frac{80}{60}\right)^2 \cong 1.78,$$

indicating an increase in exposure of approximately 78% (Fig. 6-36). An increase in kV increases the efficiency of x-ray production and *the quantity and quality* of the x-ray beam.

Changes in the kV must be compensated by corresponding changes in mAs to maintain the same exposure. At 80 kV, 1.78 units of exposure occur for every 1 unit of exposure at 60 kV. To achieve the original 1 unit of exposure the mAs must be adjusted to $1/1.78 = 0.56$ times the original mAs, which is a *reduction* of 44%. An additional consideration of technique adjustment concerns the x-ray attenuation characteristics of the patient. To achieve equal transmitted exposure through a typical patient (*e.g.*, 20-cm tissue), the compensatory mAs varies approximately as the fifth power of the kV ratio.

$$\left(\frac{\text{kV}_1}{\text{kV}_2}\right)^5 \times \text{mAs}_1 = \text{mAs}_2 \qquad [6\text{-}12]$$

■ **FIGURE 6-36** X-ray tube output exposure varies as the square of tube voltage (kV). In this example, the same tube current and exposure times (mAs) are compared for 60, 80, 100 and 120 kV. The relative area under each spectrum roughly follows a squared dependence (characteristic radiation is ignored).

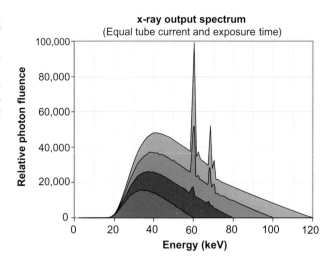

According to Equation 6-12, if a 60-kV exposure requires 40 mAs for a proper transmitted exposure through a typical adult patient, at 80 kV the adjusted mAs is approximately

$$\left(\frac{60}{80}\right)^{5} \times 40 \text{ mAs} \cong 9.5 \text{ mAs},$$

or about one fourth of the original mAs. The value of the exponent (between four and five) depends on the thickness and attenuation characteristics of the patient.

6.5.3   Tube Current (mA)

The number of x-ray photons produced is proportional to the number of electrons flowing from the cathode to the anode per unit time; thus the exposure rate of the beam for a given kV and filtration is proportional to the tube current. In this situation, the quantity of x-rays is directly proportional to the product of tube current and exposure time (mAs), as shown in Figure 6-37.

■ **FIGURE 6-37** X-ray tube exposure is proportional to the mAs (tube current and exposure time). Shown is the result of increasing the mAs from a baseline value (blue spectrum) by a factor of two (purple spectrum) and three (green spectrum), with a proportional change in the number of x-rays produced.

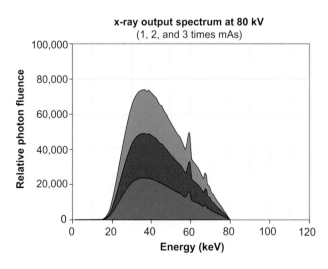

6.5.4 Beam Filtration

Added metal filters modify both the quantity and quality of the x-ray beam by preferentially removing the low-energy photons in the spectrum due to their higher attenuation. This results in a lower quantity of x-rays with a relatively greater number of higher energy photons in the spectrum. The effective energy of the beam (the number of x-ray photons at each energy multiplied by the photon energy) is analogous to beam quality, so increasing beam filtration increases beam quality (Fig. 6-38). For heavily filtered beams, the mAs required to achieve an x-ray exposure output at a fixed kV will be much higher than for lightly filtered beams. It is therefore necessary to know the HVL of the beam and the normalized x-ray tube exposure per mAs (in addition to the geometry) to calculate the incident exposure and radiation dose to the patient. One cannot simply use kV and mAs for determining the "proper technique" or to estimate the dose to the patient without this information. In the United States, x-ray system manufacturers must comply with minimum HVL requirements specified in the Code of Federal Regulations, 21 CFR 1020.30 (Table 6-4), which have been adopted by many state regulatory agencies. A pertinent clinical example of the radiation dose savings achievable with added filtration compared to the minimum filtration is shown in Figure 6-39, comparing the surface entrance radiation dose to the *same signal* generated in the detector for 0 mm Al (minimum filtration), 2 mm Al, 0.1 mm Cu, and 0.2 mm Cu. With more filtration, the dose savings become larger. For instance, as listed in Table 6-5, the comparison of 30 cm polymethylmethacrylate (PMMA) at 100 kV indicates a dose savings of 49% when a 0.2 mm Cu filter is added to the beam. To achieve this requires an increase in mAs of 37%, from 14.5 to 19.8 mAs at 100 kV. Even though the acquisition technique is higher, the entrance dose is lower, with no loss of image quality. Using added filtration of 0.1 to 0.9 mm Cu is common for interventional angiography procedures, determined by the patient size, imaging protocol (*e.g.*, fluoroscopy versus digital subtraction angiography), and selected dose level (low, normal, or contrast emphasis). Using added filtration in a modern radiography system is as simple as pushing the filter selection button on the x-ray collimator or automatically selecting the filter with anatomical programming. It is important to indicate the added filtration in addition to the technique factors in radiography exam protocols.

The x-ray beam *quantity* is approximately proportional to $Z_{target} \times kV^2 \times mAs$. The x-ray beam *quality* depends on the kV, the generator waveform, and the tube filtration. X-ray exposure depends on both the quantity and quality of the x-ray beam.

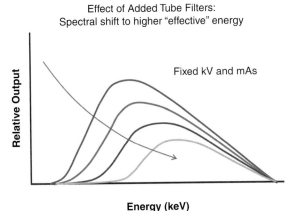

Effect of Added Tube Filters:
Spectral shift to higher "effective" energy

Fixed kV and mAs

Relative Output

Energy (keV)

■ **FIGURE 6-38** X-ray tube exposure decreases and spectral quality (effective energy) increases with increasing thickness of added tube filters. Shown are spectra with added filtration at the same kV and mAs.

TABLE 6-4 MINIMUM HVL REQUIREMENTS FOR X-RAY SYSTEMS IN THE UNITED STATES (21 CFR 1020.30)

DESIGNED OPERATING RANGE	MEASURED X-RAY TUBE VOLTAGE (kV)	MINIMUM HVL (mm ALUMINUM)
<51 kV	30	0.3
	40	0.4
	50	0.5
51–70 kV	51	1.3
	60	1.5
	70	1.8
>70 kV	71	2.5
	80	2.9
	90	3.2
	100	3.6
	110	3.9
	120	4.3
	130	4.7
	140	5.0
	150	5.4

Note: This table refers to systems manufactured after June 2006. It does not include values for dental or mammography systems.

Filters added at the x-ray tube port can significantly lower patient dose by selectively attenuating the low energy x-rays in the bremsstrahlung spectrum, but a compensatory increase in the mAs is required to achieve acceptable tube output.

6.6 SUMMARY

In summary, x-rays are the basic radiologic tool for most medical diagnostic imaging procedures. Knowledge of x-ray production, x-ray generators, and x-ray beam control is important for further understanding of the image formation process and the need to obtain the highest image quality at the lowest possible radiation dose.

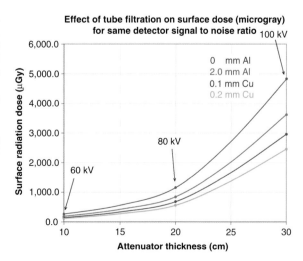

■ **FIGURE 6-39** Added x-ray tube filters can significantly reduce patient dose. Compared are measured entrance doses (air kerma with backscatter) to 10, 20, and 30 cm sheets of PMMA when using phototimed exposures at 60, 80, and 100 kV, respectively. The top curve represents the nominal beam condition, then 2.0 mm Al, 0.1 mm Cu + 1 mm Al, and 0.2 mm Cu + 1 mm Al for the lowest curve. For constant signal-to-noise ratio, the mAs is increased to compensate for added filter attenuation, as listed in Table 6-4.

Effect of tube filtration on surface dose (microgray) for same detector signal to noise ratio

0 mm Al
2.0 mm Al
0.1 mm Cu
0.2 mm Cu

TABLE 6-5 TUBE FILTRATION, MEASURED CHANGES IN REQUIRED mAs, AND MEASURED SURFACE DOSE (μGy) FOR EQUIVALENT SIGNAL IN THE OUTPUT DIGITAL IMAGE

	10 cm PMMA (60 kV)				20 cm PMMA (80 kV)				30 cm PMMA (100 kV)			
	Tube Current		*Dose (μGy)*		*Tube Current*		*Dose (μGy)*		*Tube Current*		*Dose (μGy)*	
FILTRATION	*mAs*	*% Δ*	*Dose*	*% Δ*	*mAs*	*% Δ*	*Dose*	*% Δ*	*mAs*	*% Δ*	*Dose*	*% Δ*
0 mm Al	3.8	0	264	0	6.8	0	1,153	0	14.5	0	4,827	0
2 mm Al	5.0	32	188	−29	8.2	21	839	−27	16.5	14	3,613	−25
0.1 mm Cu + 1 mm Al	6.2	63	150	−43	9.3	37	680	−41	17.6	21	2,960	−39
0.2 mm Cu + 1 mm Al	8.8	132	123	−53	11.2	65	557	−52	19.8	37	2,459	−49

Note: % Δ indicates the percentage change from the *no added filtration* measurement. For mAs, there is an increase in the mAs required to compensate for increased attenuation of the beam by the added filters. For surface dose, there is a decrease in the percentage surface dose change with more added filters for equivalent absorbed signal in the detector because of less attenuation of the beam in the object.

SUGGESTED READING AND REFERENCES

Behling R. *Modern Diagnostic X-ray Sources: Technology, Manufacturing, Reliability*. Boca Raton, FL: CRC Press, Taylor & Francis; 2016.

ICRU Report No. 85a. Fundamental Quantities and Units for Ionizing Radiation (Revised). The International Commission on Radiation Units and Measurements. *J ICRU*. 2011;11(1a).

IEC 60336. *Medical Electrical Equipment—X-ray Tube Assemblies—Characteristics of Focal Spots*. 4th ed. Geneva, Switzerland: International Electrotechnical Commission; 2005.

IEC 60613. *Electrical and Loading Characteristics of X-ray Tube Assemblies for Medical Diagnosis*. 3rd ed. Geneva, Switzerland: International Electrotechnical Commission; 2010.

CHAPTER 7

Radiography

Radiography involves the production of a two-dimensional image from a three-dimensional object, the patient (Fig. 7-1). The procedure projects the x-ray shadows of the patient's anatomy onto the image receptor and is often called *projection radiography*. The source of radiation in the x-ray tube is a small spot, and x-rays that are produced in the x-ray tube diverge as they travel away from this spot. Because of beam divergence, the collimated x-ray beam becomes larger in area and less intense with increasing distance from the source. Consequently, x-ray radiography results in some magnification of the object being radiographed. Radiography is performed with the x-ray source on one side of the patient, and the image receptor is positioned on the other side of the patient. During the exposure, incident x-rays are differentially attenuated by anatomical structures in the patient. A small fraction of the x-ray beam passes unattenuated through the patient and is recorded on the image receptor, forming the latent radiographic image.

Although the principles in this chapter are described in terms of general radiography, they apply to other forms of medical imaging including mammography, fluoroscopy and interventional imaging, and the projection images acquired for planning computed tomographic examinations.

7.1 GEOMETRY OF PROJECTION RADIOGRAPHY

The geometry of projection transmission imaging is described in Figure 7-2. Magnification can be defined simply as

$$M = \frac{L_{\text{image}}}{L_{\text{object}}},$$

[7-1]

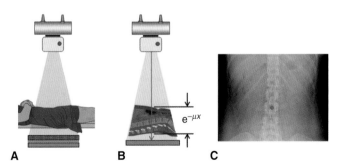

A   **B**   **C**

■ **FIGURE 7-1** The basic geometry of radiographic imaging is illustrated. The patient is positioned between the x-ray tube and the image receptor **(A)**, and the radiograph is acquired. The ion chamber (shown between the grid and image receptor) determines the correct exposure level to the image receptor (automatic exposure control). In transmission imaging **(B)**, the x-rays pass through each point in the patient, and the absorption of all the structures along each ray path combine to produce the primary beam intensity at that location on the image receptor. The signal level at each point in the image **(C)** reflects the degree of x-ray beam attenuation across the image. For example, the gray scale under the red dot on **(C)** corresponds to the total beam attenuation along the red line shown in **(B)**.

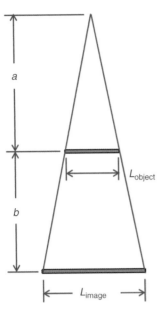

■ **FIGURE 7-2** The geometry of beam divergence is shown. The object is positioned a distance a from the x-ray source, and the image receptor is positioned a distance ($a + b$) from the source. From the principle of similar triangles, the magnification, $M = \dfrac{L_{image}}{L_{object}} = \dfrac{a+b}{a}$.

where L_{image} is the length of the object as seen on the image and L_{object} is the actual length of the object. Due to similar triangles, the object magnification can be computed using the source to object distance (a) and the object to receptor distance (b)

$$M = \frac{a+b}{a}. \qquad [7\text{-}2]$$

The magnification will always be greater than 1.0 but approaches 1.0 when a relatively thin object (such as a hand in radiography) is positioned in contact with the detector, where $b \approx 0$. The magnification factor changes slightly for each plane perpendicular to the x-ray beam axis, also known as the *central ray*, and thus anatomical structures at different depths in the patient are magnified differently. This characteristic means that, especially for thicker body parts, an AP (anterior-posterior) image of a patient will have a subtly different appearance to an experienced viewer than a PA (posterior-anterior) image of the same patient. Knowledge of the magnification in radiography is sometimes required clinically, for example, in angioplasty procedures where the diameter of the vessel must be measured to select the correct size of a stent or angiographic balloon catheter. In these situations, an object of known dimension (*e.g.*, a catheter with notches at known spacing) is placed near the anatomy of interest, so that the magnification can be determined and a correction factor calculated.

Radiographic detectors should be exposed to x-ray intensities within a relatively small range. X-ray technique factors such as the applied tube voltage (kV), tube current (mA), and exposure time will be discussed later, but an important parameter that should be kept consistent is the distance between the x-ray source and the image receptor. For most radiographic examinations, the source-to-image distance (SID) is fixed at 100 cm (40 inches), and there are usually detents in the radiographic equipment that help the technologists to set this distance. Upright chest radiography is an exception, where the SID is typically set to 183 cm (72 inches). The larger SID used for chest radiography reduces the differential magnification in the lung parenchyma. Another consequence of projection of a three-dimensional object on a two-dimensional plane is that anatomic structures distant from the central ray experience differential magnification from those located near the central ray, even when they are at the same depth in the patient. This geometric distortion is more apparent for large body parts and short SID.

The focal spot in the x-ray tube is very small but is not truly a point source, resulting in magnification-dependent loss of resolution. The blurring from a finite x-ray source is dependent upon the geometry of the exam, as shown in Figure 7-3. The length of the *edge gradient* (L_g) is related to the length of the focal spot (L_f) by

$$L_g = L_f \frac{b}{a}, \qquad [7\text{-}3]$$

where b/a represents the magnification of the focal spot. The edge gradient is measured using a highly magnified metal foil with a sharp edge. In most circumstances, higher object magnification increases the width of the edge gradient and reduces the spatial resolution of the image. Consequently, in most cases, the patient should be positioned with the anatomy of interest as close as possible to the image receptor to reduce magnification. For thin objects placed in contact with the image receptor, the magnification is approximately 1.0, and there will be negligible blurring caused by the finite dimensions of the focal spot. In some settings (*e.g.*, mammography), a very small focal spot is used intentionally with magnification. In this case, the small focal spot produces much less magnification-dependent blur, and the projected image is larger as it strikes the image receptor. This intentional application of magnification radiography is used to overcome resolution limitations of the image receptor, and increases spatial resolution.

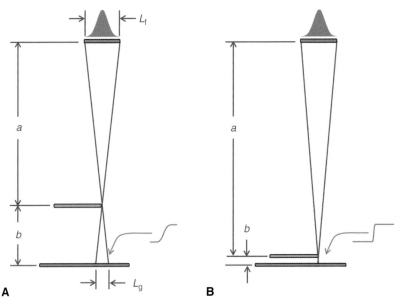

■ FIGURE 7-3 The magnification of a sharp edge in the patient will cause blurring of that structure because the focal spot of the x-ray tube is not truly a point source. For a focal spot with width L_f, the intensity across this distributed source will affect how the edge is projected onto the image plane. The edge will no longer be perfectly sharp as shown in part **B**, but rather its shadow will reflect the source distribution as shown in part **A**. The intensity across the focal spot usually is approximately gaussian in shape, and thus the blurred profile of the edge will also appear gaussian. The length of the blur in the image is related to the width of the focal spot by $L_g = \frac{b}{a} L_f$.

As x-rays pass through the patient's anatomy, they can interact by the fundamental physical processes of the photoelectric effect (PE) or Compton scatter, or they can continue on their way to the image receptor without interacting. X-rays that lose some of their energy through Compton scatter also usually change directions and can reach the image receptor divergent from the central ray. Typical image receptors have no means to discriminate between primary x-rays, which carry the important projection information, and secondary x-rays that tend to obscure the projection information. Therefore, methods are employed to restrict or minimize off-focus radiation from reaching the image receptor.

7.2 SCATTERED RADIATION IN PROJECTION RADIOGRAPHIC IMAGING

The basic principle of projection x-ray imaging is that x-rays travel in straight lines. However, when x-ray scattering events occur in the patient, the resulting scattered x-rays are not aligned with the trajectory of the original primary x-ray, and thus the straight-line assumption is violated (Fig. 7-4). Scattered radiation that does not strike the detector has no effect on the image; however, scattered radiation emanating from the patient is of concern for surrounding personnel due to the associated radiation dose. If scattered radiation is detected by the image receptor, it does have an effect on the image and can be a significant cause of image degradation. Scattered radiation generates image gray scale where it does not belong, and this can significantly reduce contrast. Contrast can be increased in digital images by window/leveling or other adjustment schemes, so for digital radiographic images, scatter acts chiefly as a source of noise, degrading the signal-to-noise ratio (SNR).

The amount of scatter detected in an image is characterized by the *scatter-to-primary ratio* (SPR) or the *scatter fraction* (F). The SPR is defined as the amount of energy deposited in a specific location in the detector by scattered photons, divided by the amount of energy deposited by primary (non-scattered) photons in that same location. Thus,

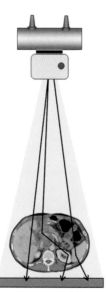

■ **FIGURE 7-4** X-rays scattered in the patient that reach the detector stimulate gray scale production, but since they are displaced on the image, they carry little or no information about the patient's anatomy.

primary x-ray   scattered x-rays

$$SPR = \frac{S}{P} \qquad [7\text{-}4]$$

For an SPR of 1, half of the energy deposited on the detector at that location is from scatter—that is, 50% of the information in the image is largely useless. The scatter fraction is also used to characterize the amount of scatter, defined as

$$F = \frac{S}{P + S}. \qquad [7\text{-}5]$$

The relationship between the SPR and scatter fraction is given by

$$F = \frac{SPR}{SPR + 1}. \qquad [7\text{-}6]$$

The vast majority of x-ray detectors integrate the x-ray energy and do not count photons, which is typical in nuclear medicine imaging. Thus, the terms S and P in this discussion refer to the energies absorbed in the detector from the scattered and primary photons, respectively.

If uncorrected, the amount of scatter on an image can be high (Fig. 7-5). The SPR increases typically as the volume of tissue that is irradiated by the x-ray beam increases. Figure 7-5 illustrates the SPR as a function of the side of a square field of view (FOV), for different patient thicknesses. The SPR increases as the field size increases and as the thickness of the patient increases. For a typical 30×30 abdominal radiograph in a 25-cm-thick patient, the SPR is about 4.5—so 82% (the scatter fraction) of the information in the image is essentially useless, if scatter rejection methods are not used.

7.2.1 The Antiscatter Grid

The *antiscatter grid*, or sometimes just called a scatter grid, is the most widely used technology for reducing scatter in radiography, fluoroscopy, and mammography. The grid is placed between the detector and the patient (Fig. 7-6). Ideally, it would allow all primary radiation incident upon it to pass, while absorbing all of the scattered radiation. The scatter grid has a simple geometric design, in which open interspace regions and alternating x-ray absorbing septa are aligned with the x-ray tube focal

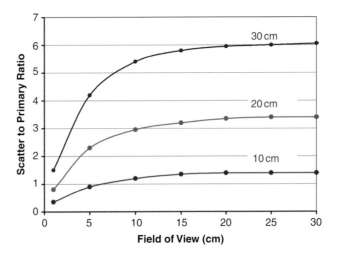

■ FIGURE 7-5 The scatter-to-primary ratio (SPR) is shown as a function of the side dimension of a square field of view, for three different patient thicknesses. For example, the 15-cm point on the *x*-axis refers to a 15 × 15-cm field. The SPR increases with increasing field size and with increasing patient thickness. Thus, scatter is much more of a problem in the abdomen as compared to extremity radiography. Scatter can be reduced by aggressive use of collimation, which reduces the field of view of the x-ray beam.

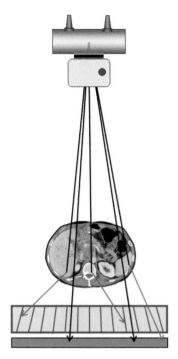

■ **FIGURE 7-6** The antiscatter grid is located between the patient, who is the principal source of scatter, and the image receptor. Grids are geometric devices, and the interspace regions in the grid are aligned with the x-ray focal spot, which is the location from which all primary x-ray photons originate. Scattered photons are more obliquely oriented, and as a result have a higher probability of striking the attenuating septa in the grid. Hence, the grid allows most of the primary radiation to reach the image receptor, but prevents most of the scattered radiation from reaching it.

spot. This alignment allows x-ray photons emanating from the focal spot (primary radiation) to have a high probability of transmission through the grid, thereby reaching the detector, while more obliquely angled photons (scattered x-rays emanating from the interior of the patient) have a higher probability of striking the highly absorbing grid septa (Fig. 7-7). The alignment of the grid with the focal spot is crucial to its efficient operation, and errors in this alignment can reduce grid performance or cause artifacts in the image.

There are several parameters that characterize the antiscatter grid. For practical radiographic imaging in the clinical imaging environment, the following grid parameters are important:

7.2.2 Grid Ratio

The grid ratio is the most fundamental descriptor of the grid's construction. The grid ratio (see Fig. 7-7) is the ratio of the height of the *interspace material* to its width—the septa dimensions do not affect the grid ratio metric. Grid ratios in general diagnostic radiology are most commonly 8, 10, or 12, with 6 or 14 used less often. Grid ratios are lower (~5) in mammography. The grid septa in a grid are typically manufactured from lead ($Z = 82$, $\rho = 11.3$ g/cm^3).

7.2.3 Interspace Material

Ideally, the interspace material would be air; however, the lead septa are very malleable and require support for structural integrity. Therefore, rigid material is placed in the interspace in the typical linear grid used in general radiography to keep the septa aligned. Low-cost grids in diagnostic radiology can have aluminum ($Z = 13$, $\rho = 2.7$ g/cm^3) as the interspace material, but aluminum can absorb an appreciable number of the primary photons, especially at lower x-ray energies. Carbon fiber ($Z = 6$, $\rho = 1.8$ g/cm^3) has high primary transmission due to the low atomic number

■ **FIGURE 7-7** The basic dimensions of a 10:1 antiscatter grid are shown. The grid is comprised of alternating layers of interspace material and septa material. This illustration shows parallel grid septa; however, in a focused grid, the septa and interspace are pointed toward the expected location of the focal spot and thus would be slightly angled.

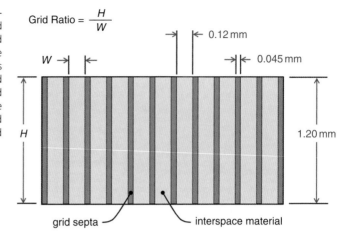

of carbon and its lower density in fiber form, and thus is desirable as interspace material. Consequently, carbon fiber interspaced grids are more common in state-of-the-art imaging systems.

7.2.4   Grid Frequency

The grid frequency is the number of grid septa per centimeter. Looking at the grid depicted in Figure 7-7, the septa are 0.045 mm wide and the interspace is 0.120 mm wide, resulting in a line pattern with 0.165 mm spacing. The corresponding frequency is 1/0.165 mm = 6 lines/mm or 60 lines/cm. Grids with 70 or 80 lines/cm are also available, at greater cost. For imaging systems with discrete detector elements, a stationary high-frequency grid can be used. For example, a 2,048 × 1,680 chest radiographic system has approximately 200 μm detector elements, and thus a grid with 45-μm-wide grid septa (see Fig. 7-7) should ideally be invisible because the grid bars are substantially smaller than the spatial resolution of the detector. Even high-frequency grids can create patterns of non-uniformity in the image due to aliasing of the grid lines and the detector matrix. Unfortunate pairing of grids and detectors can cause pronounced artifacts, as can misalignment.

7.2.5   Grid Type

The grid pictured in Figure 7-7 is a linear grid, which is fabricated as a series of alternating septa and interspace layers. Grids with crossed septa are also available but seldom are used in general radiography applications. Crossed grids are widely used in mammography (Chapter 8).

7.2.6   Focal Length

The interspace regions in the antiscatter grid should be aligned with the x-ray source, and this requires that the grid be focused (see Fig. 7-6). The focal length of a grid is typically 100 cm for most radiographic suites and is 183 cm for most upright chest imaging units. If the x-ray tube is accidentally located at a different distance from the grid, then *grid cutoff* will occur. The focal distance of the grid is more forgiving for lower grid ratio grids, and therefore high grid ratio grids will have more grid cutoff if the source-to-detector distance is not exactly at the focal length. For systems where the SID can vary appreciably during the clinical examination (fluoroscopy), the use of lower grid ratio grids allows greater flexibility and will suffer less from off-focal grid cutoff, but will be slightly less effective in reducing the amount of scattered radiation that reaches the image receptor.

7.2.7 Moving Grids

Grids are located between the patient and the image receptor, and for high-resolution image receptors, the grid bars will be seen on the image if the grid is stationary. Stationary grids were common in upright screen-film chest radiography systems, and the success of this methodology suggests that radiologists are quite adroit at "looking through" the very regularly spaced grid lines on the image. A **Bucky** grid is a grid that moves with a reciprocating motion during the x-ray exposure, causing the grid bars to be blurred by this motion and not visible in the image. The motion is perpendicular to the long axis of the linear septa in the grid.

7.2.8 Bucky Factor

The *Bucky factor*, not to be confused with the moving Bucky grid, describes the relative increase in x-ray intensity or equivalently, mAs, needed when a grid is used, compared to when a grid is not used. The Bucky factor essentially describes the radiation dose penalty of using the grid—and typical values of the Bucky factor for abdominal radiography range from 3 to 8. The Bucky factor was critical for screen-film radiography, but is less germane to digital imaging systems. In screen-film radiography, the use of the grid slightly reduces the amount of detected primary radiation and substantially reduces the amount of scattered radiation detected, and both of these effects reduce the optical density (OD) of the resulting film. Thus, the x-ray technique has to be increased by the Bucky factor to replace this lost radiation, in order to produce films of the same OD. Digital systems, however, have much wider dynamic ranges than screen-film systems in general, and therefore the digital image can be amplified to compensate for the lower detected signal without increasing the x-ray technique. One could argue that the technique does not *have to* be increased to replace the scattered x-ray exposure to the detector, because it has no information content. However, the primary radiation that is blocked by the septa and interspace material would have contributed to the signal so it might be reasonable to increase the technique by the inverse of the *primary transmission factor* of the grid to maintain the SNR in the image. In practice, because screen-film image receptors enjoyed a century of clinical practice before being supplanted by digital imaging systems, the exposure factors used in digital systems largely follow the trends of what was used in the screen-film era. Nevertheless, these considerations suggest that digital radiography (DR) systems may be used to provide lower dose examinations than those in the screen-film radiography.

It is important to note that for thin anatomical structures, there is very little scattered radiation, and an antiscatter grid is unnecessary. For example, for hand or forearm radiography, scatter levels are low and the technologist will usually place the limb to be imaged directly on the detector, without a grid, if it is removable. Likewise, for pediatric patients often the body part thickness is small and scatter removal is unnecessary.

There are other parameters that characterize the performance of the antiscatter grid, which are used primarily in the scientific evaluation of grid performance. These parameters are less important to x-ray technologists and radiologists, but are of interest to those engaged in designing grids or optimizing their performance. These metrics are discussed below.

7.2.9   Primary Transmission Factor

T_p is the fraction of primary photons that are transmitted through the grid, and ideally it would be 1.0. In Figure 7-7, the grid bars cover 27% of the field (0.045/[0.045 + 0.120]) and primary x-rays striking the top of the septa (parallel to their long axis) will be mostly attenuated. For that grid, then, the primary transmission would at most be 73%, and this does not consider the attenuation of the interspace material. Values of T_p typically run from 0.50 to 0.75 with modern grids, and this value is kV-dependent due to the penetration of the interspace material. As mentioned above, this metric may be more germane to clinical radiography using digital image receptors than the Bucky factor.

7.2.10   Scatter Transmission Factor

T_s is the fraction of scattered radiation that penetrates the grid. Ideally, it would be 0. The value of T_s can range substantially depending on the amount of scatter in the field, the x-ray energy, and the grid design. Typical values of T_s range approximately from 0.05 to 0.20 in general diagnostic radiography.

7.2.11   Selectivity

Selectivity (Σ) is simply defined as the ratio between the transmission of primary and scattered radiation, hence,

$$\Sigma = \frac{T_p}{T_s}.$$ [7-7]

7.2.12   Contrast Degradation Factor

The *contrast degradation factor* (CDF) refers to the reduction in contrast due to scattered radiation. It can be shown that contrast is reduced by

$$CDF = \frac{1}{1 + SPR}.$$ [7-8]

However, because digital images can be adjusted to enhance contrast, CDF is less critical in digital radiography than in film-screen radiography. However, this metric indicates the degree to which contrast must be adjusted to compensate for scatter.

7.2.13   Other Methods for Scatter Reduction

While the antiscatter grid is by far the most ubiquitous tool used for scatter reduction, air gaps and slot-scan techniques have been studied for years (Fig. 7-8). The principle of the air gap is that by moving the patient away from the image receptor, less of the scatter emitted from the patient will impinge on the image receptor. The concept is similar to the inverse square law, where radiation intensity decreases as the square of the distance from the source. However, scatter from the patient does not originate from a point, but instead from a large volume, and thus is an extended source of radiation. The scattered x-ray intensity decreases as the air gap distance increases proportional to $1/r$, rather than $1/r^2$. Increasing the air gap distance also increases the magnification of the patient's anatomy (see Fig. 7-2). Practical factors limit the utility

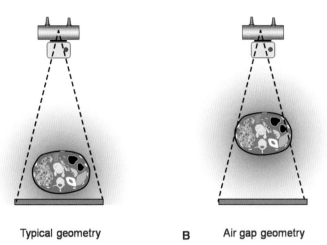

A   **Typical geometry**   B   **Air gap geometry**

■ **FIGURE 7-8** The air gap technique has been used to reduce scattered radiation, and this figure shows the air gap geometry. The scattered radiation that might strike the image receptor in the typical geometry **(A)** has a better probability of not striking the image receptor as the distance between the patient and the image receptor is increased. **B.** While often discussed, the air gap technique suffers from limited field coverage and magnification issues, and is used only rarely in diagnostic radiography.

of the air gap method for scatter reduction—as magnification of the patient anatomy increases, the coverage of a given detector dimension is reduced, there is a loss in spatial resolution due to the increased blurring of the finite focal spot with magnification (see Fig. 7-3), and the exposure technique may need to be increased if the overall SID is lengthened in order to maintain the same exposure level at the image receptor.

The slot-scan system for scatter reduction (Fig. 7-9) is one of the most effective ways of reducing the detection of scattered x-rays, and images produced from scan-slot systems are often noticeably better in appearance due to their excellent contrast and SNR. Slot-scan radiography can be regarded as the gold standard in scatter

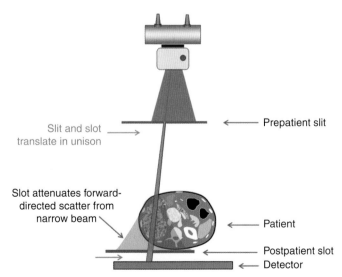

Slit and slot translate in unison →

← Prepatient slit

Slot attenuates forward-directed scatter from narrow beam ↘

← Patient

← Postpatient slot
← Detector

■ **FIGURE 7-9** The scanning slit (or "slot-scan") method for scatter reduction is illustrated. The prepatient slit is aligned with the postpatient slot, and these two apertures scan across the field of view together. The challenge is to keep the slot aligned with the slit, and this can be done electronically or mechanically. This geometry was deployed for an early digital mammography system, but is also commercially available for radiography applications. Excellent scatter reduction can be achieved using this method.

reduction methods. The method works because a very small field is being imaged at any point in time (see Fig. 7-5), most scatter is prevented from reaching the image receptor, and the image is produced by scanning the small slot across the entire FOV. In addition to excellent scatter rejection, slot-scan radiography also does not require a grid and therefore has the potential to be more dose efficient. The dose efficiency of slot-scan systems is related to the geometric precision achieved between the alignment of the prepatient slit and the postpatient slot. If the postpatient slot is collimated too tightly relative to the prepatient slit, primary radiation that has passed through the patient will be attenuated, reducing dose efficiency. If the postpatient slot is too wide relative to the prepatient slit, then more scatter will be detected.

Despite the excellent scatter reduction from these systems, the technology has inherent limitations compared to conventional large FOV radiography. The scanning approach requires significantly longer acquisition times, and the potential for patient motion during the acquisition increases. The narrow aperture for scanning requires a high x-ray tube current and the longer scan time causes significant heat loading of the x-ray tube anode. Alignment of mechanical systems is always a source of concern, and complex mechanical systems invariably require more attention from service personnel. These practical limitations have likely constrained the clinical success of slot-scan systems.

As mentioned above, the primary effect of scatter is to degrade contrast in the image. With digital image receptors, contrast can be modified by digital image processing so long as enough primary x-rays contribute to the image in order to maintain the SNR. Several commercial products have been introduced for substituting image processing for an actual physical antiscatter grid, mainly for bedside radiography. In bedside radiography, the short SID and non-compliant patient amplify the challenges of using an antiscatter grid. Misregistration of the grid with respect to the central ray of the x-ray beam, difficulty maintaining perpendicular alignment, and variability in SID can generate undesired non-uniformity or "grid washout" in the image. Clinically, this can cause one lung to appear dark and the other light, mimicking a pathological condition.

Restoring the contrast lost from scatter is not a simple process. The first step involves estimating the amount of scatter in the image. As noted previously, the amount of scatter produced depends on the volume of tissue in the x-ray beam. The software estimates the amount of scatter based on the output of the x-ray generator and the signal reaching the image receptor. From this information, the thickness of the patient is estimated. After the amount of scatter is estimated, the reduction of scatter expected from an actual physical antiscatter grid is estimated. Next, the proportion of scatter that was calculated to be removed by a physical grid is subtracted from the original image. Subsequent image processing may be applied to reduce noise or further modify contrast.

Although grid simulation appears to have promise for producing exceptional quality images without the dose penalty involved with physical grids, the technology has encountered some skepticism. Scatter is non-uniform across the FOV and depends on collimation and the anatomy included in the FOV, which is variable in bedside radiography. It is unclear how the software compensates for these variables in the scatter estimation step. The second step attempts to estimate the performance of a specific physical grid of the manufacturer's choosing, which may not be similar to the one preferred by the clinical end user. The fundamental uncertainty when subtraction is applied to an image is how the algorithm determines what is noise and what is signal for the subtraction step. The error in this method is likely small for high-contrast features such as bone, but possibly greater for low-contrast soft tissue features. Unfortunately, some manufacturers employ a low kV and radiation dose to the detector that is similar to acquisition with a physical grid, compromising the advantage in patient radiation dose.

7.3 TECHNIQUE FACTORS IN RADIOGRAPHY

The principal x-ray technique factors used for radiography include the tube voltage (the kV), the tube current (mA), the exposure time, and the x-ray source-to-image distance, SID. The SID is standardized to 100 cm typically (Fig. 7-10) and 183 cm for upright chest radiography. In general, lower kV settings will increase the dose to the patient compared to higher kV settings for the same imaging procedure and same body part, but the trade-off is that subject contrast is reduced with higher kV. The kV is usually adjusted according to the examination type—lower kVs are used for bone imaging and when iodine or barium contrast agents are used; however, the kV is also adjusted to accommodate the thickness of the body part. For example, in bone imaging applications, 55 kV can be used for wrist imaging since the forearm is relatively thin, whereas 75 to 90 kV might be used for lumbar spine radiography, depending on the size of the patient's abdomen. The use of the 55-kV beam in abdominal imaging would result in a prohibitively high radiation dose. Lower kVs emphasize contrast due to the photoelectric effect in the patient, which is important for higher atomic number (Z) materials such as bone ($Z_{calcium} = 20$) and contrast agents containing iodine ($Z = 53$) or barium ($Z = 56$). Conversely, for chest radiography, the soft tissues of the cardiac silhouette and pulmonary anatomy are of interest, and the ribs obscure them. In this case, high kV is used (typically 120 kV) in order to decrease the conspicuity of the ribs by reducing photoelectric interactions. While the anatomy of interest in the chest examination is soft tissue, the rib examination for the same FOV, uses lower kV to emphasize contrast of bony structures. Sometimes higher kV technique is selected irrespective of the loss of subject contrast, in order to increase the output of the x-ray tube and achieve a reasonable exposure at the image receptor in a reasonable exposure time to avoid patient motion during the exposure. In the example above, the 55 kV beam would require at least four times as long an exposure as the 75 kV beam at the same mA setting, without considering any differences in attenuation.

With the SID and kV adjusted as described above, the overall x-ray fluence is then adjusted by using the mA and the time (measured in seconds). The product of the mA and time (s) is called the *mAs*, and at the same kV and distance, the x-ray fluence is linearly proportional to the mAs—double the mAs, and the x-ray fluence doubles.

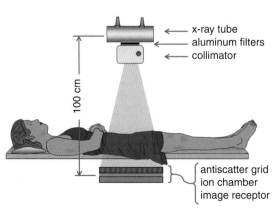

■ FIGURE 7-10 The standard configuration for radiography is illustrated. Most table-based radiographic systems use a SID of 100 cm. The x-ray collimator has a light bulb and mirror assembly in it, and, when activated, casts a light beam onto the patient allowing the technologist to position the x-ray beam with respect to the patient's anatomy. The light beam is congruent with the x-ray beam. X-rays that pass through the patient must also pass through the antiscatter grid and the ion chamber (part of the AEC system) in order to reach the image receptor.

Modern x-ray generators and tubes designed for radiography can operate at relatively high mA (such as 500 to 800 mA), and higher mA settings allow the exposure time to be shorter, which "freezes" patient motion. Some examinations, so-called breathing techniques, employ deliberately long exposure times to allow patient motion to blur anatomic features and emphasize features that would otherwise be obscured by overlying anatomy.

Manual selection of x-ray technique, also called "fixed technique," was used in radiography until the 1970s, whereby the technologist selected the kV and mAs based on experience and in-house "technique charts" (Table 7-1). The technique chart was considered by some to be the radiologist's prescription for radiation exposure for the specified view. The technique chart was used in conjunction with the "protocol book," a document that specifies the number and type of radiographic views that constitute an examination, and details of the FOV and anatomic markers of each view. Most examinations consist of one view where the x-ray beam is perpendicular to the anatomy and another orthogonal view. This is intended to allow the radiologist to visualize the anatomy in three dimensions. Examinations may include views from other angles such as oblique or decubitus views in order to present the anatomy of interest. Many institutions required technologists to use large calipers to measure the thickness of the body part to be imaged, to improve the consistency of the radiographic film OD.

Today, radiography usually relies on *automatic exposure control* (AEC), informally called *phototiming* because of an early device used for the same purpose. The mA is set to a high value such as 500 mA, and the exposure time (and hence the overall mAs) is determined by the AEC system. In general radiography, an air-ionization chamber is located behind the patient and grid, but in front of the x-ray detector (Fig. 7-10). During exposure, the AEC integrates the exposure signal from the ion chamber in real time until a preset exposure level is reached, and then the AEC immediately terminates the exposure. The preset exposure levels are calibrated by the service personnel, and the sensitivity of the radiographic detector is taken into account in the calibration procedure. For screen-film radiography, the AEC was set to deliver proper film darkening. For a digital radiographic system, the AEC is adjusted so that the exposure levels are both in the range of the detector system and produce images with good statistical integrity based on a predetermined SNR. This means that a trade-off between radiation dose to the patient and noise in the digital image should be reached. For some digital imaging systems, the signal from the detector itself can serve as the AEC sensor.

The reliance of technologists on AEC for exposure factor control gives rise to a number of problems, even for modern digital radiographic systems. First, the technique chart still exists; it is embedded in the modern x-ray operator console. It incorporates many assumptions about the size of the patient, usually segregated into six classes, namely large, medium, and small adult and pediatric patients. The technologist must make a determination of the size category of the patient, the default typically being medium adult. Incorrect assessment of patient size has consequences for the technique factors selected and often the postacquisition digital image processing. For example, if the mA setting is appropriate for a large patient, but the patient is actually small, the exposure time may be shorter than the response time of the AEC system (less than 5 ms), resulting in unintended overexposure. Second, most systems allow the technologist to perform the exposure out of the configuration called for by the technique guide, for example, excluding the antiscatter grid or acquiring at a different SID. This has consequences for image quality that may not be immediately obvious. Third, AEC assumes proper positioning of the patient with respect to the

TABLE 7-1 ABBREVIATED TECHNIQUE CHART

ANATOMY	VIEW	SID (cm)	Focal Spot	Grid	SMALL ADULT kV	mA	ms	MEDIUM ADULT kV	mA	ms	LARGE ADULT kV	mA	ms	AEC Active Cells
			THORAX THICKNESS		**21–23 cm**			**23–25 cm**			**25–27 cm**			
Chest	PA	183	Large	Y	125	250	8	125	320	10	125	400	12	RL
Chest	LAT	183	Large	Y	125	320	10	125	400	12	125	500	16	C
Rib	AP UPPER (AP LOWER)	100	Large	Y	65 (70)	400 (500)	62.5 (64)	65 (70)	400 (500)	62.5 (64)	70 (75)	400 (630)	80 (63.5)	C
Rib	AP OBL UPPER (AP OBL LOWER)	100	Large	Y	65 (70)	400 (500)	62.5 (64)	65 (70)	400 (500)	62.5 (64)	70 (75)	400 (630)	80 (63.5)	C
			ABDOMEN THICKNESS		**21–23 cm**			**23–25 cm**			**25–27 cm**			
Abdomen	AP	100	Large	Y	80	400	40	80	500	40	90	500[a]	39.7	C[b]
L-Spine	AP	100	Large	Y	80	400	20	80	500	25	80	630	39.7	C
L-Spine	LAT	100	Large	Y	80	400	20	80	500	25	80	630	39.7	C
Skull	PA	100	Large	Y	75	500	32	75	500	40	75	500	50	C
Skull	LAT	100	Large	Y	70	400	31.3	70	400	40	70	400	50	C
Hand	PA	100	Small	N	50	200	16	50	200	20	55	200	25	Fixed only
Hand	LAT	100	Small	N	55	200	16	55	200	20	60	200	25	Fixed only

BEDSIDE

ANATOMY	VIEW	SID (cm)	Focal Spot	Grid	SMALL PED kV	mAs	MEDIUM PED kV	mAs	LARGE PED kV	mAs	AEC
					14–17 cm		**16–19 cm**		**19–21 cm**		
Chest	AP	100	Large	Y	90	3.2	100	2	105	2	
Abdomen	AP	100	Large	Y	80	8	80	10	80	16	
			THORAX THICKNESS								
Chest	AP	100	Small	N	78	1.2	85	1.2			
Chest	AP	100	Large	Y					90	2.5	RL

[a]630 mA for fixed mode.
[b]RLC for large adult.

AEC sensor. If the dense anatomy such as bone is positioned in front of the active AEC sensor, the exposure time may be much longer than intended. If the AEC sensor is uncovered, that is, outside the shadow of the patient, the exposure time may be much shorter than intended resulting in a noisy, non-diagnostic image. There are usually multiple AEC sensors that can be selected independently or in groups. If the technologist activates the wrong sensors for a particular view, inappropriate exposure may be delivered. Finally, the computerized operator console in one room may not contain the same technique settings as an identical room next door. This causes unintended variability in the appearance of images.

Creation of an appropriate technique chart must consider all aspects of the imaging chain from production of the x-rays to presentation of the image for interpretation. The exposure factors specified must consider the output of the x-ray generator as well as the quality of the beam, and mA/mAs selections that are available on the control console. It should consider SID for the exam and view and the collimated FOV. It should adjust for the thickness of the patient and should account for attenuation by the patient support/table and by the antiscatter grid. It needs to be consistent with the sensitivity of the image receptor, so that enough x-rays reach the detector in order to produce an acceptable SNR in the image. It should also be harmonized with the digital image processing that is applied to the image. The dose to the patient should comply with limits established by regulatory bodies and should be consistent with the standard of care. Default technique settings are provided by medical imaging manufacturers; however, optimization of technique is the responsibility of the local clinical operation.

7.4 SCINTILLATORS AND INTENSIFYING SCREENS

Materials that are convenient for collecting and storing charge tend to be limited in sensitivity to high energy photons such as x-rays. This includes photographic emulsions and electronic devices composed of silicon (Si). Materials that convert x-rays to light are used to increase the sensitivity of these detectors. These materials are known as *scintillators* or *intensifying screens*.

An indirect x-ray detector system uses a scintillator to convert the x-ray fluence incident on the detector into a visible light signal, which is then used to expose the emulsion in screen-film radiography or a photoconductor in digital radiographic systems. Over the long history of screen-film radiography, a number of scintillators were developed. Most intensifying screens are comprised of fine-grain crystalline scintillating powders (also called *phosphors*), formed into a uniformly thick intensifying screen that is held together by a binder. During production, the phosphor power is mixed with the binder material at high temperature, and then this molten mixture is layered onto a metallic sheet, where rollers spread the material into a uniform thickness. The material hardens as it cools, and the intensifying screen is cut to the desired dimensions. The binder is usually a white powder, and intensifying screens appear white to the naked eye. Intensifying screens are considered *turbid* media—they are not strictly transparent to optical light (otherwise they would appear clear), but instead the visible light that is produced in the screen from x-ray interactions undergoes many scattering events as it propagates through the intensifying screen. The light photons have a certain probability of being absorbed as well. Most intensifying screens are amorphous (lack structure), and are comprised of billions of tiny crystals of the scintillator randomly embedded in the inert binder layer. Because the index of refraction of the binder is different than the scintillator crystals, the facets of these tiny crystals are sites where light scattering and absorption occur. Each light photon that is produced by x-ray interaction inside a scintillator crystal propagates in a random direction in the screen, refracting off thousands of small surfaces until it either exits the screen matrix or is absorbed. Consequently, a burst of perhaps 2,000 light photons produced at the point of x-ray interaction propagates inside the screen matrix undergoing many scattering and absorption events, and eventually about 200 photons reach the surface of the screen where they can interact with the photodetector.

In thicker screens, the packet of photons diffuses a greater distance before emerging from the phosphor layer, and this causes more spreading of light that reaches the light detector (see Fig. 7-11). The extent of lateral light spread is also governed by the design of the phosphor screen itself—the relative coefficients of optical scattering and optical absorption affect the amount of blurring, and the overall sensitivity of the screen. Increasing the optical absorption reduces light spread, improving spatial resolution for the same screen thickness, but less light reaches the surface.

Some crystalline scintillators such as CsI form in long columnar crystals, which are tiny natural light pipes, and this structured crystal tends to reduce lateral light spread and preserve spatial resolution for a given screen thickness. CsI is a salt, chemically similar to NaCl, and is hygroscopic (absorbs moisture from the air). It therefore must be sealed to keep out moisture; it may be kept in a vacuum or encapsulated in a plastic layer. CsI is too fragile and expensive for screen-film radiography applications, however it enjoys widespread use in indirect digital radiography and conventional fluoroscopy.

In portal imaging, where high energy photon beams used to treat cancer are also used to verify the therapeutic radiation field, metals such as Cu have been used similarly to convert the high energy photons to lower energies where they are easier to detect.

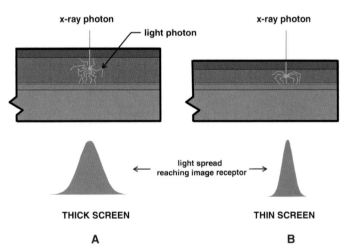

■ **FIGURE 7-11** The indirect detection process is illustrated, with a thick intensifying screen **(A)** and a thin intensifying screen **(B)**. In both cases, incident x-ray photons may interact with the screen and create light photons by scintillation. The light photons diffuse by scattering through the screen matrix until some eventually reach the image receptor. The thicker screen creates a geometry where the light photons can travel farther laterally, and this increases the width of the light distribution reaching the image receptor compared to the thinner screen. Thicker screens absorb more x-ray photons (are more sensitive) but have reduced spatial resolution compared to thinner screens. Not shown in this diagram is the fact that exponentially more x-ray photons are deposited in the surface of the screens, due to the exponential manner in which x-rays are absorbed.

7.5 ABSORPTION EFFICIENCY AND CONVERSION EFFICIENCY

Because of the dynamics of indirect x-ray detection described above, there are two factors that are important in x-ray detectors. The first is the absorption efficiency in the phosphor layer, which is determined by the phosphor composition, that is, its effective Z and density (ρ), and the conversion layer thickness. The absorption efficiency is also dependent on the x-ray beam energy. The term *quantum detection efficiency* is used to describe how well x-ray detectors capture the incident x-ray photon beam; however, this metric does not consider x-ray fluorescence, where a considerable fraction of the detected photon energy is re-emitted by the detector. The *energy absorption efficiency* is perhaps a better metric, given that most x-ray detectors are *energy integrators*, not *photon counters*. Thicker, denser phosphor layers absorb more of the incident x-ray beam (Fig. 7-12), and increased absorption efficiency is always desirable. However, increasing the conversion layer thickness has to be balanced with the concomitant increase in blurring and loss of spatial resolution that results in a thicker conversion layer.

A second factor describes how efficiently the optical signal is transferred from the scintillator to the silicon photodetector, and then how it is amplified and converted to signal in the image, that is, gray scale value or digital number. *Conversion efficiency* (CE) includes x-ray-to-light-photon energy transfer in scintillators, light-to-charge CE for photodiodes, light-to-OD in film, geometry and lens efficiency for optically coupled detectors, and the electronic gain in a digital detector (see Fig. 7-12). CE has a direct effect on the radiation dose necessary to generate a desired signal level in the image. If CE is increased by a factor G (where $G > 1$) the x-ray fluence must be reduced by a factor of G to produce the same signal level. Assuming that absorption

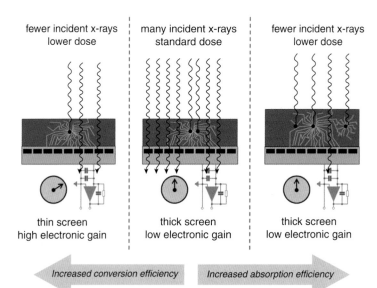

■ **FIGURE 7-12** The center panel represents a higher exposure level indicated by the larger number of x-ray photons incident on the detector system. Using a thicker screen (right panel) increases the absorption efficiency so that a smaller number of incident x-rays will yield the same number absorbed in the detector, producing the same signal level with the low electronic gain. Achieving the same signal level using fewer incident x-rays by increasing the conversion efficiency (left panel) with a higher electronic gain increases the relative noise in the image because the number of x-rays absorbed in the detector is less.

efficiency is unchanged, only $1/G$ of the photons would be absorbed in the detector, and hence relative quantum noise would increase by a factor of $\sqrt{G}$.

If, on the other hand, the absorption efficiency is increased by the factor G, the x-ray fluence can be decreased by the same factor. The increase in absorption is balanced by the reduction in x-ray fluence, saving dose, while producing the same signal level. In this case, the same number of x-rays are absorbed by the detector (*i.e.*, $G \times 1/G = 1$), and the quantum noise therefore is unchanged. So, for the case where *the same signal levels in the image are being compared*, increasing the speed of the detector, and lowering the radiation dose, by increasing CE *increases* image noise, whereas increasing absorption efficiency can reduce dose but has no detrimental effect on quantum noise in the image.

7.6 COMPUTED RADIOGRAPHY

Computed radiography (CR) refers to photostimulable phosphor (PSP) image receptor systems, which typically enclose a *PSP screen* in a cassette with dimensions similar to a screen-film cassette. Traditional scintillators, such as Gd_2O_2S and cesium iodide (CsI), emit light promptly (nearly instantaneously, by *fluorescence*) when irradiated by an x-ray beam. When x-rays are absorbed by PSP screens, some light is also emitted promptly, but a fraction of the absorbed x-ray energy is trapped in the PSP screen and can be released later using laser light (*photostimulated luminescence*, or PSL). For this reason, PSP screens are also called *storage phosphors*. CR was introduced in the 1970s, saw increasing use in the late 1980s, and was in wide use at the turn of the century as many departments installed PACS.

Most PSP screens are composed of a mixture of BaFBr and other halide-based phosphors, often referred to as barium fluorohalide. A PSP screen, or *imaging plate*, is typically a flexible screen that is enclosed in a light-tight cassette. The CR cassette is exposed to x-rays during the radiographic examination and is subsequently placed in a CR reader. Once placed in the CR reader, the following steps take place:

1. The cassette is moved into the reader unit, and the imaging plate is mechanically removed from the cassette.
2. The imaging plate is translated vertically in the (y) direction by rollers across a moving stage and is scanned horizontally in the (x) direction by a laser beam of approximately 700 nm wavelength. The laser is deflected across the imaging plate by a multifaceted rotating mirror. This method of reading the plate is called the "*flying spot*."
3. Red laser light stimulates the emission of trapped energy in a tiny area (x, y location) of the imaging plate, and indigo visible light is emitted from the storage phosphor as energetic electrons drop down to their ground state.
4. The light emitted through PSL is collected by a fiber optic light guide and strikes a photomultiplier tube (PMT), where it produces an electronic signal.
5. The electronic signal is digitized and stored as a pixel value. For every spatial location (x, y) on the imaging plate, a corresponding gray scale value is determined that is proportional to the locally absorbed x-ray energy.
6. The imaging plate is exposed to bright white light to erase any residual trapped energy.
7. The imaging plate is returned to the cassette and is ready for reuse.

The digital image that is generated by the CR reader is stored temporarily on a local hard disk. Once acquired, the digital radiographic image undergoes image

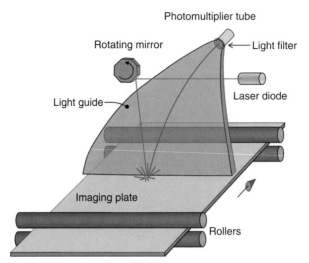

■ FIGURE 7-13 The readout mechanics of a CR system are shown. The imaging plate is translated through the mechanism by a series of rollers, and a laser beam scans horizontally across the plate. The rotating multi-faceted mirror causes the laser beam to scan the imaging plate in a raster fashion. The light released by laser stimulation is collected by the light guide and produces a signal in the PMT. The red light from the laser is filtered out before reaching the PMT.

processing by the CR reader. The image is then typically sent to a PACS for interpretation by a radiologist and long-term archiving.

The imaging plate itself is a completely analog device, but it is read out by analog and digital electronic techniques, as shown in Figure 7-13.

The light that is released from the imaging plate is a different color than the stimulating laser light (Fig. 7-14). Indeed, the *indigo*[1] light that is emitted from the imaging plate has shorter wavelength and higher energy per photon than the stimulating red light. This is energetically feasible only because the energy associated with the emitted indigo light was actually stored in the screen from the absorption of very energetic x-ray photons, and the red light serves only to release this energy from the storage phosphor. To eliminate detection of the scattered excitation laser light by the PMT, an optical filter that is positioned in front of the PMT transmits the indigo light and attenuates the red laser light.

The actual underlying mechanism of PSL is still somewhat controversial. Figure 7-15 illustrates PSL according to the Biomolecular Recombination Model (or Takahashi model). A small mass of screen material is shown being exposed to x-rays. Typical imaging plates are composed of about 85% BaFBr and 15% BaFI, activated with a small quantity of europium. The PSP layer of the imaging plate is amorphous (lacks structure); the barium fluorohalide crystals are small and are held together by an inert, optically transparent binder. The nomenclature BaFBr:Eu indicates that the BaFBr phosphor is activated by europium. This activation procedure, also called *doping*, creates defects in the BaFBr crystals that allow electrons to be trapped more efficiently. The defects in the crystalline lattice caused by the europium dopant give rise to so-called *F-centers* or color centers.

---

[1]Is "indigo" really a color? Indigo is one of the original seven colors identified in the visible light spectrum by Isaac Newton. Indigo, named for the color of a plant dye, is shorter wavelength than blue and longer wavelength than violet. Some regard it to be deep blue or blue violet.

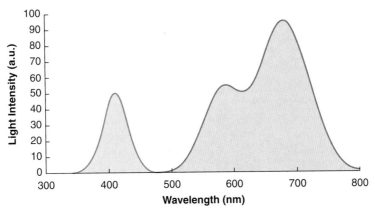

■ **FIGURE 7-14** The red laser light (600 to 700 nm) is used to stimulate the emission of indigo light (400 to 450 nm); the intensity of the indigo light is proportional to the x-ray exposure to the region of the detector illuminated by the laser light.

When x-ray energy is absorbed by the BaFBr phosphor, some of the energy excites electrons associated with the europium atoms, oxidizing divalent europium atoms (Eu^{+2}) to their trivalent state (Eu^{+3}). The excited electrons become mobile, and a fraction of them interact with F-centers. The F-centers trap these electrons in a higher-energy, metastable state, where they can remain for minutes to weeks, with only slight fading over time. The latent image that is encoded on the imaging plate after x-ray exposure, but before readout, exists as billions of electrons trapped in F-centers. The number of trapped excited electrons per unit area of the imaging plate is proportional to the intensity of x-rays incident at each location of the imaging plate during the x-ray exposure.

When the red laser light scans the exposed imaging plate, some energy is absorbed at the F-center and transferred to the electrons. A proportional fraction of electrons gains enough energy to reach the conduction band, become mobile, and then drop to the ground energy state, and thus Eu^{+3} is converted back to Eu^{+2}. A portion of the emitted indigo light is captured by a light guide and channeled to the PMT (Fig. 7-15).

Contrary to the Takahashi model, it seems that the Eu^{+2} captures the hole created by x-ray absorption without forming Eu^{+3}. Also, PSL occurs even at very low temperatures that should dramatically affect electrons in the conduction band. The Photostimulable Luminescence Complex Model (or von Seggern model) shown in Figure 7-16 attempts to address these discrepancies. The von Seggern model invokes *tunneling* as the mechanism for the stimulated electrons to return to the Eu atom without entering the conduction band.

The first readout of the imaging plate does not release all of the trapped electrons that form the latent image; indeed, a plate can be read out a second time and a third time with only slight degradation. To erase the latent image so that the imaging plate can be reused for another exposure without ghosting, the plate is exposed to a very bright light source, which flushes almost all of the metastable electrons to their ground state, emptying most of the F-centers.

It is important to note that CR was the technology that enabled the totally digital radiology department and enjoyed widespread clinical use for two decades, and is still economical in settings where the volume of radiography is somewhat limited. CR technology has always been limited by the inherent need for diligent active quality assurance and maintenance. Recently, the Centers for Medicare and Medicaid

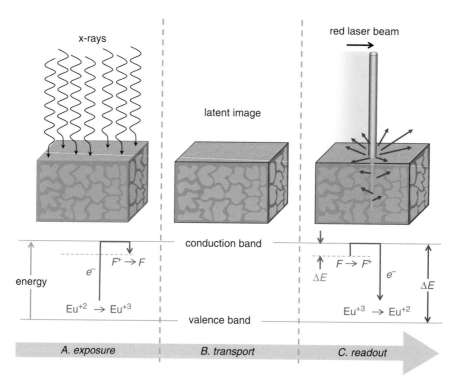

■ **FIGURE 7-15** Takahashi model for photostimulated luminescence (PSL). **A.** During exposure, x-rays are absorbed in the storage phosphor and some of the electrons reach the conduction band, where they may interact with an *F*-center, causing the reduction of europium (Eu) ions. **B.** Electrons trapped in this high-energy, metastable state can remain there for minutes to months. **C.** During readout, the phosphor is scanned by a red laser, which provides the trapped electrons enough energy to be excited into the conduction band. Here, some fraction of electrons will drop down to the valence band, emitting indigo light during the transition. When the *F*-center releases a trapped electron, the trivalent europium (Eu^{+3}) is converted back to its divalent state (Eu^{+2}).

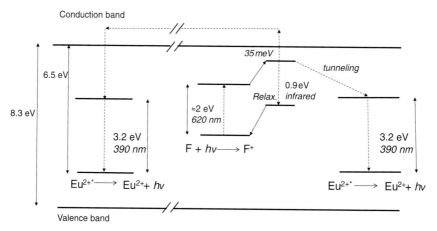

■ **FIGURE 7-16** von Seggern model for PSL. Electrons excited by x-irradiation are trapped in the *F*-center. The electrons can follow three different paths from the *F*-center. First, they can de-excite by relaxation and emission of an infrared photon. Second, they can escape into the conduction band with only a tiny amount of energy (35 MeV). From the conduction band, the electron can migrate to a distant Eu hole center and de-excite by prompt fluorescence. Third, the electron can tunnel to a nearby Eu hole center and de-excite generating PSL.

Services (CMS) began reducing reimbursement for CR imaging, as an incentive for healthcare operations to move to more advanced imaging technologies. It is possible that CR will continue to have a role in radiography outside the United States, as long as manufacturers are willing to produce and maintain these systems.

7.7 CHARGE-COUPLED DEVICE AND COMPLEMENTARY METAL-OXIDE SEMICONDUCTOR DETECTORS

Charge-coupled device (CCD) detectors form images from visible light (Fig. 7-17A). CCD detectors are used in commercial-grade television cameras and in scientific applications such as astronomy. The CCD chip itself is an integrated circuit made of crystalline silicon, as is the central processing unit of a computer. A CCD chip has an array of discrete detector electronics etched into its surface. Linear arrays are configured with single or multiple rows in a wide selection, such as $1 \times 2,048$ detector elements (dexels), or $96 \times 4,096$ dexels in a rectangular format for line scan detection (*e.g.*, movement of a slot-scan detector with a narrow fan-beam collimation). Area arrays have a 2.5×2.5-cm dimension with $1,024 \times 1,024$ or $2,048 \times 2,048$ detector elements on their surface. Larger chips and larger matrices spanning 6×6 cm are available, but are very expensive, and ultimately the size is limited by the dimensions of crystalline silicon wafers. Another limitation is the requirement for a small dexel (*e.g.*, 20 μm dimension and smaller) to achieve charge transfer efficiency of 99.99% to keep additive electronic noise low. The silicon surface of a CCD chip is photosensitive—as visible light falls on each dexel, electrons are liberated and build

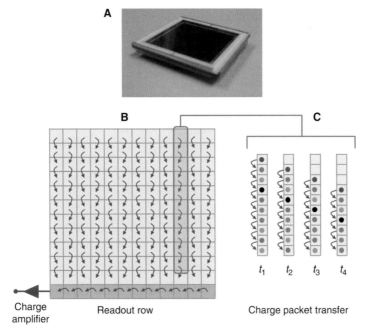

■ **FIGURE 7-17 A.** A photograph of a high-resolution CCD chip is shown. **B.** The readout procedure in a CCD chip is illustrated. After exposure, electrodes in the chip shift the charge packets for each detector element by switching voltages, allowing the charge packets to move down by one detector element at a time. Charge from the bottom element of each column spills onto the readout row, which is rapidly read out horizontally. This process repeats itself until all rows in each column are read out. **C.** This illustration shows the shift of a given pattern of exposure down one column in a CCD chip in four (t_1–t_4) successive clock cycles.

up in the dexel. More electrons are produced in dexels that receive more intense light. The electrons are confined to each dexel because there are electronic barriers (voltage) on each side of the dexel during exposure.

Once the CCD chip has been exposed, the electrical charge that resides in each dexel is read out. The readout process is akin to a bucket brigade (Fig. 7-17B). Along one column of the CCD chip, the electronic charge is shifted dexel by dexel by appropriate control of voltage levels at the boundaries of each dexel. The charge packet from each dexel in the entire column is shifted simultaneously, in parallel. For a two-dimensional CCD detector, the charges on each column are shifted onto the bottom row of electronics, that entire row is read out horizontally, then the charge packets from all columns are shifted down one detector element (Fig. 7-17C), and so on.

CCD detectors are small, whereas the FOV in most medical imaging applications is large. Unfortunately, it is impossible to focus the light emitted from a large scintillation screen (~43 × 43 cm) onto the surface of the CCD chip (~4 × 4 cm) without losing a large fraction of light photons due to optical lens coupling inefficiency. The amount of light transferred to the CCD is determined by the directionality of light emitted by the scintillator, the lens characteristics (f number, the ratio of the focal length of a lens to its effective diameter), and the demagnification factor, m, required to focus the image from the screen onto the CCD array. For a typical scintillator material (so-called Lambertian emitter), the amount of light recorded is inversely proportional to the square of the f number times the square of the demagnification factor. Even with an excellent lens (*e.g.*, f number = 1) and a demagnification of 10, less than 1% of the light produced by x-ray interactions will reach the CCD array (Fig. 7-18A).

Many x-ray imaging systems are multi-stage, where the signal is converted from stage to stage. For example, in a CCD system, x-rays are converted to visible light in the scintillator, and then the light is converted to electrons in the CCD chip. X-ray photons, visible photons, and electrons are all forms of *quanta*. The *quantum sink* refers to the stage where the number of quanta is the lowest and therefore where the statistical integrity of the signal is the worst. Ideally, in a radiographic image, the quantum sink should be at the stage where the x-ray photons are absorbed in the converter (scintillator or solid-state detector). This is referred to as an *x-ray quantum limited detector*. However, if there is a subsequent stage where the number of quanta is less than the number of absorbed x-rays, the image statistics and consequently the image noise will be dominated by this stage, and a secondary quantum sink will occur. Although an image can be produced, an x-ray detector system with a secondary quantum sink will have image quality that is not commensurate with the x-ray dose used to make the image. Large FOV CCD-based radiographic detectors have a secondary quantum sink due to the very low coupling efficiency of the lens system. Despite this, higher doses can be used to create acceptable quality images. These systems are relatively cost-effective and are sold commercially as entry-level digital radiographic systems. Higher end area CCD radiography systems typically make use of CsI input screens with improved x-ray detection efficiency and light capture efficiency, while less costly systems use Gd_2O_2S screens. For a typical 43 × 43 cm FOV, 3,000 × 3,000-pixel CCD camera (4 × 4 cm area with ~13 μm dexels) and ~10:1 demagnification, the pixel dimensions in the resulting images are approximately 140 to 150 μm.

Linear CCD arrays optically coupled to an x-ray scintillator by fiberoptic channel plates (a light guide made of individual light conducting fibers), often with a de-magnification taper of 2:1 to 3:1, are used in *slot-scan* x-ray systems. These systems operate using a narrow x-ray fan beam with pre- and post-patient collimators, acquiring an image by scanning the beam over the anatomy for several seconds. An advantage

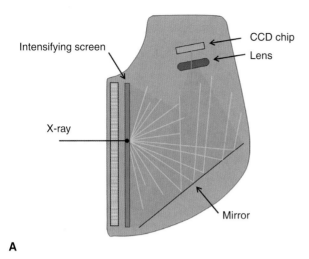

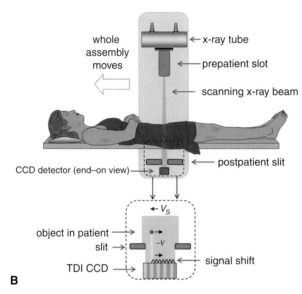

■ **FIGURE 7-18 A.** A CCD-based DR system is shown. The x-ray is converted to visible light in the intensifying screen, which propagates through the light-tight enclosure. A small fraction of the light photons will strike the mirror and be redirected to the lens to ultimately be detected in the CCD chip. **B.** A CCD-based time delay and integration (TDI) system is shown. As the x-ray tube/slit-slot/detector assembly moves at velocity V (to the left in this figure), the CCD chip is read out at a velocity $-V$ (to the right). By synchronizing the velocity of the readout with the scanning motion, the signal region under an object in the patient travels across the entire field of view of the detector, and its contrast signal is built up across all of the dexels in the TDI CCD chip.

of this geometry is the excellent scatter rejection achieved, allowing the elimination of the antiscatter grid and the associated dose penalty (see Section 7.2 in this chapter). Coupling of the scintillator to the linear CCD array requires less demagnification than with a two-dimensional CCD system, reducing the secondary quantum sink problem. A readout process known as time-delay and integration (TDI) can deliver high dose efficiency and good signal to noise ratio. TDI readout is a method that electronically integrates signal information from the stationary patient anatomy by compensating for the velocity V of the x-ray/detector assembly by reading out the CCD in the opposite direction at a velocity $-V$ (Fig. 7-18B). The transmitted x-ray beam passes through the same object path during the dwell time of the scan over the area. Disadvantages of slot-scan systems include the longer exposure time required for the scan, increasing the potential for motion artifacts, and substantially increased x-ray tube loading. Imaging systems using slot-scan acquisition have shown excellent clinical usefulness in x-ray examinations of the chest and in full-body trauma imaging.

Complementary metal-oxide semiconductor (CMOS) light sensitive arrays are an alternative to the CCD arrays discussed above. Based upon a crystalline silicon matrix, these arrays are essentially random access memory "chips" with built-in photo-sensitive detectors, storage capacitors, and active readout electronics, operating at low voltage (3 to 5 V). Inherent in the CMOS design is the ability to randomly address any detector element on the chip in a read or read and erase mode, enabling unique opportunities for built-in AEC capabilities that are not easily performed with a CCD photo detector. A major issue with CMOS has been electronic noise from both acquisition (storage) and readout/reset noise sources. Correlated sampling methods can reduce the electronic reset noise common to multiple measurements. Construction of a large area detector is a hurdle, because the maximum dexel size currently achievable is on the order of 50 µm. CMOS detector applications for radiography are currently limited to small FOV (10 × 15 cm) applications such as specimen tissue imaging of surgery samples.

7.8 FLAT PANEL THIN-FILM-TRANSISTOR ARRAY DETECTORS

Flat panel thin-film-transistor (TFT) array detectors (Fig. 7-19) exploit technology similar to that used in flat panel displays, to simplify the wiring otherwise required for a huge number of individual display elements. Instead of producing individual electrical connections to each one of the elements in a flat panel display, a series of horizontal and vertical electrical lines is used that, when combined with appropriate readout logic, can address each individual display element. This signal modulates light transmittance from a backlit liquid crystal display element in the flat panel display. With this approach, only 2,000 connections between the display and the electronics are required for a 1,000 × 1,000 display, instead of 1,000,000 individual connections. For a flat panel display, the wiring is used to send signals from the computer graphics card to each display element, whereas in an x-ray detector the wiring is used to measure the signal generated in each detector element.

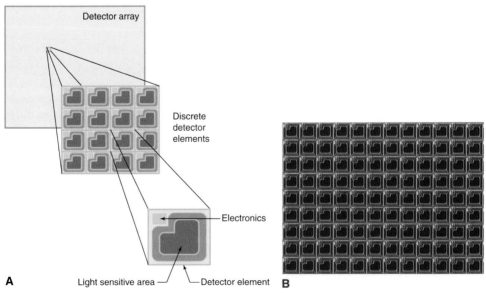

■ **FIGURE 7-19 A.** Flat panel detector systems are pixelated discrete detector systems. The detector array is comprised of a large number of individual detector elements (dexels). Each dexel has a light-sensitive region and a light-insensitive area where the electronic components are located. **B.** A photomicrograph of an actual TFT system is shown. The electronics component can be seen in the upper left corner of each dexel. (Image courtesy John Sabol and Bill Hennessy, GE Healthcare.)

Flat-panel TFT arrays are made of amorphous silicon (*a*-Si), where lithographic etching techniques are used to deposit electronic components and connections needed for x-ray detector operation. The large area TFT array is divided into individual detector elements (dexels), arranged in a row and column matrix. Electronic components within each dexel include a TFT, a charge collection electrode, and a storage capacitor. The TFT is an electronic switch that is comprised of three connections: gate, source, and drain. Gate and drain lines connect the source and drain of the TFTs along the row and columns, respectively.

The gate is the transistor's "on/off" switch, and is attached to the gate conductor line along each row of the array. The source is attached to the storage capacitor, and the drain is attached to the drain conductor line running along each column of the array. The charge collection electrode captures the charge produced by incident x-ray energy deposited over the area of the dexel (by either indirect or direct conversion, as discussed below), and the storage capacitor stores it. During x-ray exposure, the TFT switch is closed, allowing charge in each dexel to be accumulated and stored. After the exposure is completed, sequential activation of the TFT array occurs one row at a time, by sequentially turning on the gate line to every dexel in the row (Fig. 7-20). This allows the accumulated charge in each dexel capacitor to flow through the transistor to the drain line, and subsequently to the connected charge amplifier. The charge amplifiers are positioned outside of the panel active area. They amplify the charge, convert it to a proportional voltage, and digitize the voltage level, resulting in a gray scale value for each dexel in the row. This sequence is repeated row by row, to fully read out the array. The speed of the detector readout is governed by the intrinsic electronic characteristics of the x-ray converter material and the TFT array electronics.

In practice, the architecture of TFT arrays is more complicated. A constellation of array readout chips (ARC) and line driver chips control limited regions of the TFT array. The complete FOV is a composite of the readout from the individual regions. The specific architecture varies among manufacturers. For example, one detector is comprised of 480 blocks (20 × 24), each controlling 128 × 128 dexels, while another is comprised of 64 blocks (8 × 8), each controlling 256 × 256 dexels. The specific architecture can affect the manifestation of problems that arise in the detectors, such as non-uniform sensitivity calibration or component failure.

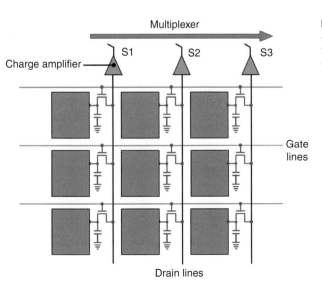

■ **FIGURE 7-20** This diagram shows circuitry for a TFT flat panel detector system. The readout process is described in the text.

7.8.1   Indirect Detection TFT Arrays

Indirect x-ray conversion TFT arrays use a scintillator to convert x-rays to light with optical coupling of the scintillator to the active matrix. The scintillator is layered on the front surface of the flat panel array. Thus the light emanating from the *back* of the scintillator layer strikes the flat panel and, because x-ray interactions are more likely to occur toward the front of the scintillator layer, the light that is released in the scintillation layer has to propagate relatively large distances, which can result in appreciable "blurring" and a loss of spatial resolution (Fig. 7-21A). To improve this situation, most flat panel detector systems for general radiography use a CsI scintillator instead of Gd_2O_2S. CsI is grown in columnar crystals, and the columns act as light pipes that reduce the lateral spread of light. The reduction of the lateral propagation of light helps to preserve spatial resolution.

Because the electronics occupy a certain amount of area of the dexel, the entire surface area is not photosensitive. This reduces the geometrical efficiency of light collection of each dexel to less than 100%. The *fill factor* refers to the percent of the area of each dexel that is photosensitive. The fill factor is typically about 80% for dexel dimensions of 200 μm $\times$ 200 μm, and much less (40% to 50%) for smaller dexel dimensions. The space occupied by the electronics limits the practical minimum size of dexels in a TFT array, and currently the smallest indirect detector dexel size is about 100 μm. Technological advances are now overcoming fill factor penalties by stacking the electrical components of each dexel in lithographic layers under the photosensitive layer.

7.8.2   Direct Detection TFT Arrays

Direct x-ray conversion TFT arrays use a semiconductor material that produces electron-hole pairs in proportion to the incident x-ray intensity. Absorbed x-ray energy is directly converted into charge in the detector—there is no intermediate step involving the production of visible light photons. Amorphous selenium (*a*-Se) is the semiconductor most widely used, and is layered between two surface-area electrodes connected to the bias voltage and a dielectric layer. The dielectric layer prevents overcharging dexels, which could damage the TFT array. Ion pairs are collected under applied voltage across the solid-state converter (10–50 V/μm of thickness). This electric field in the converter almost completely eliminates lateral spreading of

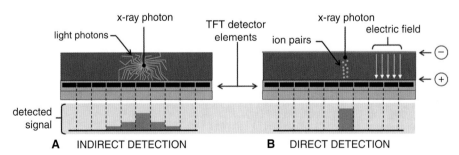

■ **FIGURE 7-21** Indirect and direct detector TFT–based x-ray detectors are shown. **A.** Photons in the indirect system propagate laterally, compromising resolution. The detected signal shown for the indirect detector shows this lateral spread in the signal from one x-ray photons interaction. **B.** For the direct detector system, the ion pairs liberated by x-ray interaction follow the electric field lines (electron holes travel upwards, electrons travel downwards) and have negligible lateral spread. Here, the detected electronic signal from one x-ray photon interaction is collected almost entirely in one detector element, and therefore better spatial resolution is achieved.

the charges during transit through the semiconductor, resulting in high spatial resolution (Fig. 7-21B). Even though Se has a relatively low atomic number and consequently low absorption efficiency, the Se layer can be made thick (0.5 to 1.0 mm) to improve detection efficiency and still maintain excellent spatial resolution. Fill factor penalties are not as significant with direct conversion TFT systems compared to indirect conversion TFT arrays. This is because the electrical potential field lines are designed to bend and thereby direct charge carriers to the collection electrode, avoiding the insensitive regions of the dexel. In addition to selenium, other materials such as mercuric iodide (HgI_2), lead iodide (PbI_2), and cadmium telluride (CdTe) are being studied for use in direct detection flat panel systems.

7.9 OTHER CONSIDERATIONS WHEN CHOOSING A DIGITAL DETECTOR SYSTEM

The choice of a digital detector system requires a careful assessment of the needs of the facility. CR is often the first digital radiographic system installed in a hospital, because it can directly replace screen-film cassettes in existing radiography units and in bedside examinations, where the cost of retakes in both technologist time and money is high. A benefit of CR over TFT-based digital radiographic technology is that the relatively expensive CR reader is stationary, but because the CR imaging plates themselves are relatively inexpensive, several dozen plates may be used in different radiographic rooms simultaneously. The number of rooms that one CR reader can serve depends on the types of rooms, workload, and proximity. Typically, one multi-cassette CR reader can handle the workload of three radiographic rooms. The cost of an individual flat panel detector is high, and it can only be in one place at one time. The obvious use for flat panel detectors or other solid-state digital radiographic systems is for radiographic suites that have high patient throughput, such as a dedicated chest room. Because no cassette handling is required and the images are rapidly available for technologist approval, the throughput in a single room using flat panel detectors can be much higher than for CR systems, where manual cassette handling is required. Recent introduction of portable TFT flat panel cassettes using wireless technology is an alternative to the portable CR detectors that have historically been used in bedside radiography; however, the consequences of the technologist dropping the fragile flat panel cassette can be expensive.

7.10 RADIOGRAPHIC DETECTORS, PATIENT DOSE, AND EXPOSURE INDEX

In traditional screen-film radiography, film OD serves as an exposure indicator, and direct feedback is obtained by simple visual inspection of the processed film image (Fig. 7-22, left). CR and DR detectors have wide exposure latitude and with image postprocessing, these systems produce consistent image gray scale even with underexposed and overexposed images (Fig. 7-22, right). Automatic adjustment of the gray scale on digital radiographic images disables the traditional method of exposure factor control provided to the technologist from the immediate feedback of film density. Underexposed DR images use fewer absorbed x-rays, which can be recognized by increased image noise, but overexposed images can easily go unnoticed, resulting in unnecessary exposure to the patient. Furthermore, underexposed images are likely to be criticized by radiologists for excessive image noise, whereas overexposed

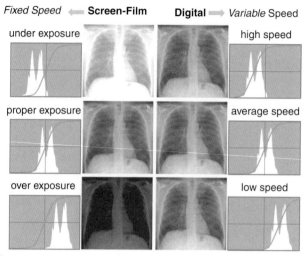

Fixed Speed ⟸ **Screen-Film**   **Digital** ⟹ Variable Speed

under exposure   high speed

proper exposure   average speed

over exposure   low speed

Exposure distribution   Resultant Images   Histogram distribution

■ **FIGURE 7-22** Response of a screen-film system with fixed radiographic speed and a digital system with variable radiographic speed to underexposure, correct exposure, and overexposure are shown. For screen film, to the left of each radiograph is a distribution representing the x-ray exposure absorbed by the screen and converted to OD on the film. Note that the characteristic curve translating exposure to OD is fixed on the exposure axis. For digital systems, to the right of each radiograph is a distribution representing the frequency of digital values (a histogram) linear with exposure absorbed by the image receptor and converted to a digital value. Note that the look-up table curve translating the digital values to brightness and contrast on a display monitor is variable and adjusts to the histogram to achieve optimal rendering of the image contrast.

images will likely be of high quality. This contributes to a phenomenon known as "dose creep," whereby technologists tend to use unnecessarily high exposures. Dose creep is most likely to occur in examinations such as bedside radiography in which AEC is not feasible and manual technique factors must be chosen.

In most digital radiographic systems, image-processing algorithms are used to align measured histogram values (after exposure) with a predetermined lookup table, to make gray scale of the digital image appear similar to screen-film images. The measured histogram distribution on each radiograph is used to determine the incident radiation exposure to the detector, and to provide an "exposure index" value. Anatomically relevant areas of the radiograph are automatically segmented into parts of the image without patient attenuation (high exposure regions), regions outside the collimated FOV (low exposure regions), and the remaining region of interest. The segmentation process is known as "exposure recognition." A histogram is generated from the relevant image area, and is compared to an examination-specific (e.g., chest, forearm, head, etc.) histogram shape. The gray scale values of the raw image are then digitally transformed using a look-up table (LUT) to provide desirable image contrast in the "for presentation" image. Adjustment of the image by histogram analysis accomplishes four specific tasks: *exposure compensation*, *latitude compensation*, *contrast maximization* for the values of interest (VOI), and *calculation of the exposure index*.

The median value of the histogram is used in many systems to determine a proprietary exposure index (EI) value, which is dependent on each manufacturer's algorithm and image receptor calibration method. This EI indicates the amount of radiation reaching the image receptor and is not a *direct* indicator of dose to the patient. Unfortunately, widely different methods to calculate the EI value have evolved, as shown in Table 7-2.

An international standard for an EI for digital radiographic systems has been published by the International Electrotechnical Commission (IEC), IEC 62494-1.

TABLE 7-2 MANUFACTURER, CORRESPONDING SYMBOL FOR EI, AND CALCULATED EI FOR THREE INCIDENT EXPOSURES TO THE DETECTOR

MANUFACTURER	SYMBOL	5 µGy	10 µGy	20 µGy
Canon (Brightness = 16, contrast = 10)	REX	50	100	200
Fuji, Konica	S	400	200	100
Kodak (CR, STD)	EI	1,700	2,000	2,300
IDC (ST = 200)	F#	−1	0	1
Philips	EI	200	100	50
Siemens	EI	500	1,000	2,000

This standard describes "Exposure Indices" and "Deviation Indices," along with a method for placing these values in the DICOM header of each radiographic image. The manufacturer's responsibility is to calibrate the imaging detector according to a detector-specific procedure, to provide methods to segment pertinent anatomical information in the relevant image region, and to generate an EI from histogram data that is proportional to detector exposure.

This dose index standard for radiography requires staff to establish *target exposure index* (EI_T) values for each digital radiographic system and for each type of exam; for instance, the EI_T for a skull radiograph will, in general, differ from that of a chest radiograph. Feedback to the user on whether an "appropriate" exposure has been achieved is given by the *deviation index (DI)*, calculated as

$$DI = 10 \log_{10}(EI/EI_T). \qquad [7\text{-}9]$$

The *DI* provides feedback to the operator with a value that is equal to 0 (zero) when the intended exposure to the detector is achieved (*i.e.*, $EI = EI_T$), a positive number when an overexposure has occurred, and a negative number when an underexposure has occurred. A *DI* of +1 indicates an overexposure of about 26%; a value of −1 indicates an underexposure of 20% less than desired. When the *DI* is in the desired range, the radiographic system is considered to be working well and is able to deliver the EI_T values set up by the institution. Tracking *DI* values with respect to equipment and technologist can be useful in maintaining high image quality for radiography at an institution.

Initial recommendations for the acceptable range of *DI* values were not well thought out. They were too strict (from +1 to −1) and "did not accurately reflect clinical practice," especially bedside radiography, where the combination of the severity of the patient's illness and the challenges of the imaging environment leads to wide variation in exposure factor control. Further study of actual clinical data has led to a revision of recommendations to accept a wider range of *DI* values based on statistical variation of clinical *DI* data. For operational purposes, a range of ±3 represents a doubling or halving of exposure and is a reasonable action level for suspicion of inappropriate exposure factor control. The *DI* between ±1.5 represents a total exposure range of two, which should be achievable in most cases when compared to the limited exposure latitude of screen-film systems.

The value of *DI* depends on many factors including proper calibration and configuration of DR systems, proper selection of the EI_T values, compliance of technologists with technique guidance, proper calibration of AEC, correct selection of the examination and view by the technologist, and appropriate collimation of the radiation field, which has a major effect on image segmentation. It is important to note that the *EI* reports the exposure to the detector for a standard x-ray beam that may not represent the beam exiting the patient in a clinical examination. Regardless of the *DI* or *EI* value reported, the ultimate question of whether the image is adequate must be addressed by the radiologist: *does the image have sufficient quality to answer the clinical question?*

7.11 ARTIFACTS IN DIGITAL RADIOGRAPHY

Artifacts are undesired features in an image that mimic or mask clinical features. Artifacts may be serious or merely cosmetic in nature depending on their magnitude, location in the FOV, and pattern. For example, an artifact in the periphery of the FOV may not jeopardize the clinical value of the image. A periodic artifact, such as prominent grid lines, may pose only a distraction to the radiologist. Other artifacts, such as a wispy shadow from long hair that reaches down to the level of the lung apices, can mimic the appearance of a pneumothorax, a significant clinical finding.

In digital radiography, artifacts arise from a variety of sources, and the visual appearance of an artifact may not provide an unambiguous clue to its underlying cause. Consider the ideal conditions of projection radiography described above: anything that interferes with these ideal conditions can produce an artifact. This includes high-Z particles in the x-ray tube and collimator assembly; defects in prepatient filters; clothing, jewelry, and bedding material; metallic implants in the patient; lead aprons and shielding blankets; lead markers used to indicate laterality, physical defects in the patient support or antiscatter grid; misalignment of the antiscatter grid; improper calibration of the digital image receptor; defects in the x-ray conversion layer; defective dexels; errors in automatic segmentation of the digital image; and incorrect digital image processing. In a bedside setting, backscatter can produce the image of electronic or structural components superimposed on the projected image. Some of these non-ideal conditions are under the direct control of the radiologic technologist; however, some are non-obvious to the operator and may go unnoticed without ongoing active quality control and critical feedback from radiologists. Some artifacts are unavoidable because of the patient's medical condition and the setting in which imaging must be conducted, such as the intensive care unit. Positioning of lines and tubes to minimize their interference is a challenging task for the radiologic technologist.

In an ideal world, all dexels would have identical sensitivity to radiation. In practical reality, individual dexels have different gain and some are completely defective, providing no signal whatsoever. The gain and offset of pixelated detectors must be calibrated in order to correct for differences and to compensate for non-functional dexels (Fig. 7-23). Over time, the performance of the dexels change and additional dexels fail giving rise to artifacts, so calibration must be repeated periodically. Calibration may not correct non-uniformity, in which case the detector or other components, such as the antiscatter grid or patient support, may need replacement (Fig. 7-24).

Similarly, in CR the collection efficiency across the imaging plate is not uniform. CR scanners must be calibrated to correct for this non-uniformity. Unlike DR systems, the CR calibration is only in one dimension of the image receptor; however, because imaging plates of different sizes may be scanned in different orientations, artifacts can appear along different directions in the FOV. Dust and dirt inside the scanner or on the surface of the imaging plate can interfere with the collection of PSL. Periodic cleaning with a lint-free cloth or the appropriate solvent is necessary. Imaging plates are subject to mechanical and chemical degradation causing artifacts

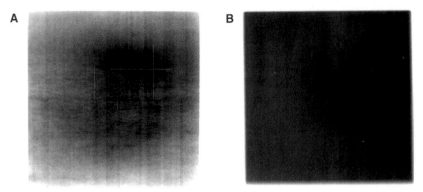

■ FIGURE 7-23 Calibration compensates for non-uniform gain and defective detector elements. **A.** Raw image of uniform x-ray field before calibration. **B.** Image of uniform x-ray field after calibration.

and may need to be replaced. Mechanical forces can damage the protective layer of the imaging plate, exposing the PSP to humidity. Water can cause oxidation of the iodine in the PSP to iodate, which is yellow-colored, resulting in blotchy artifacts where the protective layer is compromised.

Calibration of the image receptor is accomplished by exposing it to a uniform field of x-rays. As described in Chapter 6, the exposure from an x-ray tube varies in intensity across the FOV along the anode-cathode (A-C) axis because of the heel effect. Calibration of the image receptor compensates for exposure non-uniformity simultaneously with gain compensation. Unfortunately, if the image receptor is exposed in an orientation opposite to the calibration condition with respect to the A-C axis, the non-uniformity from the heel effect is doubled. The magnitude of the heel effect decreases with SID, so calibrations are usually performed at large SID. Some manufacturers perform individual gain calibrations at various SID and orientations for radiographic rooms; however, this may not properly compensate for cross table exposures where the A-C axis changes from the table exposure orientation. Multiple calibration orientations do not appear practical for bedside systems.

Another note about gain calibration: the shadow of anything in the x-ray path at the time of calibration will be compensated by the gain calibration resulting in an inverse (positive) image present in all subsequent images. This includes the effect from residual phosphorescence in the x-ray conversion layer, caused by repeated high exposures.

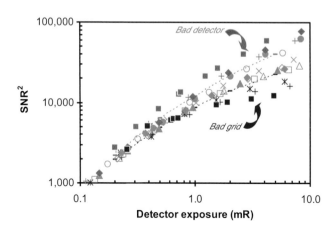

■ FIGURE 7-24 Variation in exposure-dependent SNR is improved by gain and offset calibration. SNR at the central axis of the image of a phantom is shown for 14 identical DR systems. After calibration, 12 systems performed within confidence limits. One discrepant system required detector replacement. One discrepant system required replacement of its antiscatter grid. SNR^2 is a surrogate for noise equivalent quanta.

The x-ray conversion layer is subject to degradation over time. As mentioned above, CsI is hygroscopic (tends to absorb water). When exposed to ambient humidity, the crystalline structure breaks down losing its ability to restrict lateral spread of light. This leads to a generalized loss of spatial resolution, but can also create artifacts when the crystalline structure is disrupted in local regions. Damage to the x-ray conversion layer will require replacement of the image receptor.

7.12 SPECIAL CONSIDERATIONS FOR PEDIATRIC DIGITAL RADIOGRAPHY

Radiography of children poses special challenges. Children vary from neonate to adult-sized patients. Smaller children are often non-compliant and may not be able to stand unassisted, and the small size of their body parts is not consistent with the size of AEC ion chambers. For these reasons, children are often radiographed using shorter SID than adults, in AP orientation on tables of radiographic rooms, rather than using the upright exposure station, and using manual technique selection, rather than AEC. Their small body parts create less scatter to the extent that antiscatter grids are often unnecessary. Children are more sensitive to ionizing radiation than adults, and usually have more years of life remaining to develop late effects. Special attention to appropriate practices that limit radiation exposure to children is necessary in radiography.

A common misconception is that radiographic generators with less power are appropriate for pediatric imaging, because the patients are smaller. On the contrary, high powered generators that are capable of producing exposures at high mA stations are necessary to minimize exposure time and the associated motion artifacts from non-compliant patients. The small focal spot should be used for pediatric radiography to minimize focal spot blur with the typically short SID. Any delay between exposure actuation and x-ray production confounds the radiologic technologist's attempts to capture full inspiration for chest radiographs. Restriction of the x-ray field is critical in pediatric radiography, not only for reducing unnecessary exposure to tissue surrounding the anatomy of interest but also for enabling proper segmentation of the digital image. Inclusion of unwanted anatomy, such as the mandible, in the FOV of a chest radiograph can compromise contrast in the lungs. Therefore, convergence of collimation and the light field indicating the field are critical.

Traditionally, lead blankets and gonadal shields have been employed to limit exposure in pediatric radiology. Recent studies show limited benefit to this type of shielding and often cause interference with image segmentation, Routine use of post-acquisition digital "shutters" leads to careless attention to the collimated x-ray field. The routine appearance of digital markers for orientation instead of the image of lead markers is a clue that digital shutters may also be used.

The necessity for manual technique in pediatric radiology means that the technique chart needs particular attention, by the radiology technologists who need to follow it and the medical physicists who should monitor the design of the chart, and compliance with its instructions.

The smaller thickness of pediatric anatomy translates into a smaller range of exposures in the projected anatomy. This suggests that digital image processing for pediatric radiography is likely different from processing that is appropriate for adults, even for the same radiographic view.

The *Image Gently* ® alliance is a campaign to promote the judicious use of ionizing radiation for pediatric imaging. This includes best practice in radiography, fluoroscopy, computed tomography, and nuclear medicine imaging. The campaign was so successful that it inspired a similar effort for adult radiology called *Image Wisely* ®.

7.13 DUAL-ENERGY SUBTRACTION RADIOGRAPHY

As mentioned in Chapter 4, anatomical noise can contribute to a loss of conspicuity in radiological imaging. Dual-energy subtraction radiographic techniques have been developed, which can in some instances reduce anatomical noise and thereby produce an image that has better information content. Dual-energy subtraction chest radiography is a good example of this and will be used to illustrate the concept.

Figure 7-25A shows the attenuation characteristics of iodine, bone, and soft tissue as a function of x-ray photon energy. The curves have different shapes, and thus the energy dependencies of bone, iodine, and soft tissue attenuation are different. The reason for these differences is that higher atomic number materials (*i.e.*, bone, with effective $Z \approx 13$, or iodine, with $Z = 53$) have higher photoelectric absorption levels than lower atomic materials such as soft tissue (effective $Z \approx 7.6$). The photoelectric interaction component of the linear attenuation coefficient has an energy dependency of E^{-3}, as opposed to very little energy dependency for the Compton scattering component in the x-ray energy range used for diagnostic imaging.

The different energy dependencies in tissue types allow either the bone component or the soft tissue component in the image to be removed by digital image processing of radiographic images acquired at two very different effective energies (*i.e.*, different kVs). The general algorithm for computing dual-energy subtracted images on each pixel (x, y) is

$$\mathrm{DE}(x, y) = \alpha + \beta \left[\ln\{I_{\mathrm{HI}}(x, y)\} - R \ln\{I_{\mathrm{LO}}(x, y)\} \right], \qquad [7\text{-}10]$$

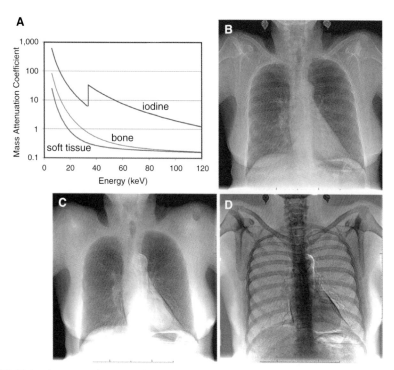

■ **FIGURE 7-25** Dual-energy subtraction chest radiography is illustrated. **A.** The linear attenuation coefficients for soft tissue, bone, and iodine are shown. **B.** The single-energy (120 kV) radiograph is shown. **C.** The bone-subtracted, soft tissue–only image is illustrated. This image shows the lung parenchyma and mediastinum, which are the principal organs of interest on most chest radiographs. **D.** The soft tissue–subtracted, bone-only image is illustrated. Note that the earrings, which are made of metal and are more similar to bone than soft tissue in terms of composition, show up on the bone-only image.

where DE(x, y) is the gray scale value in the dual-energy image, $I_{HI}(x, y)$ is the corresponding gray scale value in the acquired high-energy image, and $I_{LO}(x, y)$ is the corresponding gray scale value in the acquired low-energy image. The value of R is selected to isolate bone, iodine, or soft tissue in the subtraction, and α and β scale the output image for brightness and contrast for optimal display. Equation 7-10 represents *weighted logarithmic subtraction.*

Figure 7-25B shows a standard single-energy chest radiograph for comparison, and Figure 7-25C and D illustrate the soft tissue and bone-only images, respectively. Notice on the tissue-only image (Fig. 7-25C), the ribs are eliminated and the soft tissue parenchyma of the lungs and mediastinum are less obscured by the ribs. On the bone-only image, bones are of course better depicted. Interestingly, one can also see the metallic earrings on this patient, whereas they are not visible on the soft tissue–only image. The metal earrings have attenuation properties more like bone than soft tissue. The white area along the border of the heart and aortic arch in the soft tissue–only image is caused by cardiac motion between the first (low energy) exposure and the second (high energy) exposure. Misregistration of the two images is also often observed along the diaphragm, even with breath-holding by the patient.

An alternative to dual energy subtraction is to use a specialized image processing algorithm on the single high energy image. The software recognizes ribs and other bony structures and subtracts them from the original image to produce a soft tissue–only image without the dose penalty of the second low energy exposure and absent of misregistration artifacts. The method produces remarkable images; however, it also may introduce artifacts that mimic pathology.

SUGGESTED READING AND REFERENCES

Alvarez RE, Seibert JA, Thompson SK. Comparison of dual energy detector system performance. *Med Phys.* 2004;31:556-565.

Amis ES, Butler PF, Applegate KE, et al. American College of Radiology White paper on radiation dose in medicine. *J Am Coll Radiol.* 2007;4:272-284.

Chan H-P, Doi K. Investigation of the performance of antiscatter grids: Monte Carlo simulation studies. *Phys Med Biol.* 1982;27:785-803.

Chan H-P, Higashida Y, Doi K. Performance of antiscatter grids in diagnostic radiology: experimental measurements and Monte Carlo simulations studies. *Med Phys.* 1985;12:449-454.

International Electrotechnical Commission, Report IEC 62424-1. 2008.

Li G, Greene TC, Nishino TK, Willis CE. Evaluation of cassette-based digital radiography detectors using standardized image quality metrics: AAPM TG-150 Draft Image Detector Tests. *J Appl Clin Med Phys.* 2016;17:391-417.

Rowlands JA. The physics of computed radiography. *Phys Med Biol.* 2002;47:R123.

Shepard SJ, Wang J, Flynn M, et al. An exposure indicator for digital radiography: AAPM Task Group 116 (Executive Summary). *Med Phys.* 2009;36:2989-2914.

von Seggern H. Photostimulable x-ray storage phosphors: a review of present understanding. *Braz J Phys.* 1999;29:254-268.

Willis CE, Vinogradskiy YY, Lofton BK, White RA. Gain and offset calibration reduces variation in exposure-dependent SNR among systems with identical digital flat panel detectors. *Med Phys.* 2011; 38:4422-4429.

CHAPTER 8

Breast Imaging: Mammography

Mammography is a radiographic examination that is optimized for detecting breast cancer. Breast cancer screening with mammography can catch cancers at an earlier, more treatable stage. Technological advances over the last several decades have greatly improved the diagnostic sensitivity of mammography. Early x-ray mammography was performed with direct exposure film, required high radiation doses, and produced images of low contrast and poor diagnostic quality. Mammography using the xeroradiographic process was very popular in the 1970s to early 1980s, and featured high spatial resolution and edge-enhanced images; however, poor sensitivity for mass lesions and higher radiation dose compared to screen-film mammography led to its demise in the late 1980s. Screen-film mammography was widely used until full-field digital mammography technology matured in terms of reliability and image quality as verified by the Digital Mammography Imaging Screening Trial (DMIST; Pisano et al., 2005). More recently, digital breast tomosynthesis (DBT) systems using limited angle acquisition introduced in 2011 have rapidly augmented digital mammography with pseudo-3D images that reduce tissue overlap, with improved sensitivity and specificity. Dedicated breast CT is a true three-dimensional modality that promises to also have a role in breast screening and diagnosis (Fig. 8-1). The move from 2D to pseudo 3D to true 3D breast imaging is not without challenges, as the number of images increases and places a greater demand on image interpretation time for the radiologist. One way to meet these challenges is through the application of artificial intelligence (AI) and deep learning algorithms to augment the radiologist in the interpretation of these larger image data sets, but significant work remains to determine how this might come about.

The American College of Radiology (ACR) mammography accreditation program changed the practice of mammography in the mid-1980s, with recommendations for minimum standards of practice and quality control (QC) that led to improvements in image quality. The federal Mammography Quality Standards Act (MQSA) was enacted in 1992; the law and associated federal regulations (Title 21 of the Code of Federal Regulations, Part 900) issued by the US Food and Drug Administration (FDA), made many of the quality assurance (QA) procedures of the accreditation program mandatory, making mammography the only federally regulated imaging modality in the United States. For digital mammography systems, the performance evaluation requires following and adhering to the manufacturer's QC procedures. An optional alternative has been FDA-approved as a harmonized, manufacturer-independent QC program for digital mammography and DBT by the ACR, as published in the 2018 ACR Digital Mammography Quality Control Manual.

Breast cancer screening programs depend on x-ray mammography because it is a low-cost, low–radiation dose procedure that has the sensitivity to detect early-stage breast cancer. Mammographic features characteristic of breast cancer include masses, particularly ones with irregular or "spiculated" margins; clusters of microcalcifications; and architectural distortions of breast structures. In screening mammography as practiced in the United States, two x-ray images of each breast, in the

2D Mammo   2D Synthetic Mammo   Tomosynthesis   Dedicated breast CT

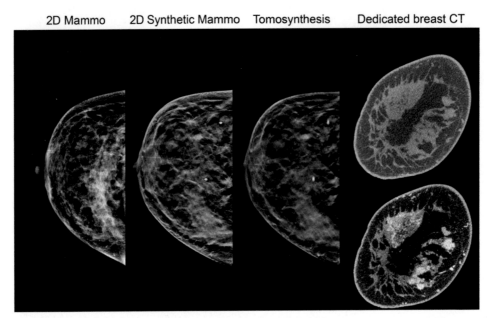

■ **FIGURE 8-1** Improvements in mammography and breast x-ray imaging. Images of a cranial-caudal view and coronal tomographic slice of the breast are shown. On the left is a 2-dimensional (2D) full-field digital mammogram (acquired after tomosynthesis study). On the middle left is a 2D synthetic mammogram created from the digital breast tomosynthesis exam on the middle right; shown is a 1-mm focal plane image of ~60 images depicting several lesions made more conspicuous. On the right are reconstructed coronal slices of the breast (of about 500) positioned at the site of the lesions from pre- and postcontrast injection acquisitions using a dedicated breast CT scanner. The contrast enhanced image (bottom) shows significant uptake in glandular tissues as a biomarker for malignancy. This illustrates the power of full 3D tomography and the benefits of no tissue overlap provided by dedicated breast CT.

mediolateral oblique and craniocaudal views, are acquired. Whereas *screening mammography* attempts to detect breast cancer in the asymptomatic population, *diagnostic mammography* procedures are performed to assess and delineate lesions identified by screening mammography. The diagnostic mammographic examination may include additional x-ray projections, magnification views, spot compression views, tomosynthesis, ultrasound, magnetic resonance imaging (MRI), mammoscintigraphy, or breast CT.

Ultrasound (Chapter 14) is often used to differentiate cysts (typically benign) from solid masses (often cancerous) using anatomic appearance or elastography evaluation, or for biopsy needle guidance. Automated breast ultrasound systems are used as supplemental screening options for women with dense breast tissue. MRI (Chapters 12 and 13) has excellent tissue contrast sensitivity and can differentiate benign from malignant tumors with contrast enhancement by evaluating signal intensity-time curves. MRI is used for diagnosis, staging, and biopsy guidance, and for screening of high-risk women. Mammoscintigraphy with Tc-99m sestamibi as the radiotracer is used to evaluate suspected breast cancer in patients for whom mammography is non-diagnostic. It is also used to assist in identifying multicentric and multifocal carcinomas in patients already diagnosed with breast cancer.

The specific requirements of breast cancer imaging, including the differentiation of normal and cancer tissues and visualization of microcalcifications require the use of x-ray equipment specifically designed for breast imaging. As shown in Figure 8-2A, the difference in attenuation between normal and cancer tissue is extremely small. Subject contrast, shown in Figure 8-2B, is highest at low x-ray energies (10 to 15 keV)

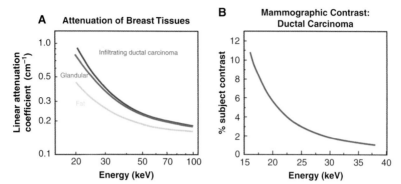

■ **FIGURE 8-2 A.** Attenuation of breast tissues as a function of energy, showing fat, glandular, and ductal carcinoma linear attenuation coefficients. Comparison of the three tissues shows a very small difference between the glandular and the cancerous tissues. **B.** Calculated percentage contrast of the ductal carcinoma relative to the glandular tissue declines rapidly with energy; contrast is optimized using a low energy, nearly monochromatic x-ray spectrum. (Adapted from Yaffe MJ. Digital mammography. In: Haus AG, Yaffe MJ, eds. *Syllabus: A Categorical Course in Physics: Technical Aspects of Breast Imaging.* Oak Brook, IL: RSNA; 1994:275-286. Copyright © Radiological Society of North America.)

and decreases with higher energies. Low x-ray energies provide the best differential attenuation between breast tissues; however, the high absorption at these low energies results in higher radiation doses. Detection of microcalcifications in the breast is also important because they are often early markers of breast cancer. The need to visualize microcalcifications requires x-ray tubes with small focal spots and very high-resolution detectors. Enhancing contrast sensitivity, reducing dose, and providing the spatial resolution necessary to depict microcalcifications impose challenging requirements on mammographic equipment and detectors. Therefore, dedicated x-ray equipment design, specialized x-ray tubes, breast compression devices, antiscatter grids, digital x-ray detectors, and automatic exposure control (AEC) subsystems are essential for mammography (Fig. 8-3).

Strict QC procedures to verify optimal system performance and assure communication teamwork by the technologist, radiologist, and medical physicist are necessary to ensure high-quality breast imaging at a facility. The technical and physical considerations of mammographic x-ray imaging are discussed in this chapter. Many

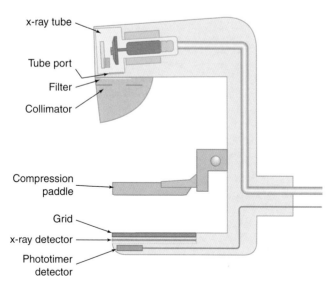

x-ray tube

Tube port

Filter

Collimator

Compression paddle

Grid

x-ray detector

Phototimer detector

■ **FIGURE 8-3** A dedicated mammography system has many unique attributes, including K-edge filtration, collimation, and compression. Automatic Exposure Control (AEC) has an external or internal sensor for digital detectors and can be positioned by the user. Major components of a typical system, excluding the generator and user console, are shown.

of the basic concepts regarding image quality, x-ray production, and radiography are presented in Chapters 4, 6, and 7, respectively. The applications of these concepts to mammography, together with many new topics specific to mammography, are presented here.

8.1   X-RAY TUBE COMPONENTS, STRUCTURES, AND OPERATION

This section compares and contrasts the differences between mammography and general radiography x-ray tubes.

8.1.1   Cathode

The mammography x-ray tube is configured with dual filaments in the focusing cup to produce 0.3- and 0.1-mm focal spot sizes, with the latter used for magnification studies to reduce geometric blurring. An important distinction between mammography and conventional x-ray tube operation is the low operating tube potential, below 40 kV. The tube current is also limited to 100–200 mA for the large (0.3 mm) focal spot and 25–50 mA for the small (0.1 mm) focal spot depending on the target material.

8.1.2   Anode

Molybdenum (Mo) ($Z = 42$) is a common anode target material used in mammography x-ray tubes by some manufacturers, and one manufacturer also has a rhodium (Rh) ($Z = 45$) target material. K-shell characteristic x-rays are generated with energies of 17.5 and 19.6 keV for Mo and 20.2 and 22.7 keV for Rh, within the optimal energy range for thin to thick compressed breast tissues. Tungsten (W) is also a common anode material because of its increased x-ray production efficiency due to its high atomic number ($Z = 74$) and high heat loading capability. However, because of unwanted low-energy (8–10 keV) L-shell characteristic x-ray emission, thicker x-ray tube filtration is required, which reduces some of the output advantages of tungsten. Digital detectors enable postacquisition image processing, which can enhance contrast. Thus, the characteristic radiation from Mo or Rh is not as important in digital mammography as it was for contrast-limited screen-film mammography.

Mammography x-ray tubes have rotating anodes, with anode angles ranging from 0° to 16°, depending on the manufacturer. The tubes are typically positioned at a source-to-image distance (SID) of 65–70 cm. In order to achieve adequate field coverage on the anterior (nipple) side of the field, the x-ray tube must be physically tilted so that the *effective anode angle* (the actual anode angle plus the physical tube tilt) is at least 22° for coverage of a common 24 × 30-cm field area at the SID. Details of the tube field coverage are illustrated in Figure 8-4.

The intensity of the x-rays emitted from the focal spot varies across the field of view (FOV), with the highest x-ray fluence on the cathode side of the field and the lowest x-ray fluence on the anode side, a consequence of the *heel effect* (Chapter 6). Positioning the x-ray tube such that the cathode-anode axis runs posterior to anterior achieves better uniformity of the x-rays *transmitted* through the compressed breast (Fig. 8-5), as the compressed breast is thicker near the chest wall (posterior) and thinner towards the nipple (anterior). Orientation of the tube in this way also decreases the equipment bulk near the patient's face. For a "uniform" exposure on the detector,

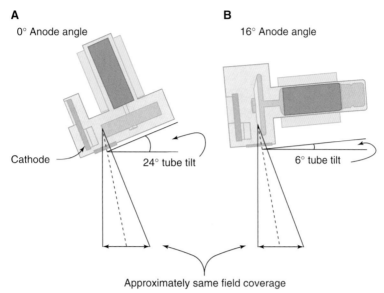

A
0° Anode angle

B
16° Anode angle

Cathode

24° tube tilt

6° tube tilt

Approximately same field coverage

■ **FIGURE 8-4** Design of a dedicated mammography system includes unique geometry and x-ray tube design. A collimated "half-field" geometry projects the x-ray beam central axis perpendicular to the plane of the image receptor at the chest wall, and centered horizontally. Full-area x-ray beam coverage at 60- to 70-cm SID and 24 cm depth (posterior to anterior) requires a tube tilt of about 20° to 24° to avoid cutoff on the anode side of the field. **A.** An anode angle of 0° requires a tube tilt of 24°. **B.** An anode angle of 16° requires a tube tilt of about 6°.

digital values on the anterior (anode) side of the field will be consistently less. For fixed, non-removable digital flat-panel detectors, the reduced fluence on the anode side of the field can be corrected with "flat-fielding" procedures to adjust the digital number uniformity across the FOV (see Section 8.5). However, the quantum noise (and thus the standard deviation of the digital numbers) will be higher in this area due to reduced x-ray fluence.

8.1.3 Focal Spot

Focal spot dimensions are small compared to general radiography tubes. Sizes of 0.3 to 0.4 mm for contact mammography and 0.10 to 0.15 mm for magnification exams are necessary to limit geometric blurring onto the detector so that fine detail microcalcifications can be resolved in the images. By convention, the *nominal* focal spot size is measured at a *reference axis,* which bisects the x-ray field along the chest wall—anterior direction (Fig. 8-6A), since all mammography systems utilize a "half-field" x-ray beam geometry where the central axis of the x-ray beam (the "central ray") is positioned at the chest wall edge of the detector and perpendicular to the image detector surface. Nominal focal spot size and tolerance limits for the width and length are listed in Table 8-1. As a consequence of the effective focal spot size variation in the field (the line focus principle, see Chapter 6, Fig. 6-16), sharper image detail is rendered on the anode (anterior) side of the field toward the nipple and is more evident with magnification examinations, as described in Section 8.3.

System resolution is a combination of geometric (focal spot) and detector resolution, measured with a high-resolution bar pattern with frequencies from 4 to 20-line pairs/mm. For contact breast imaging, the bar pattern is placed 4.5 cm above the breast support platform near the chest wall edge, corresponding to the entrance surface of the average breast. For magnification imaging, the pattern is placed 4.5 cm

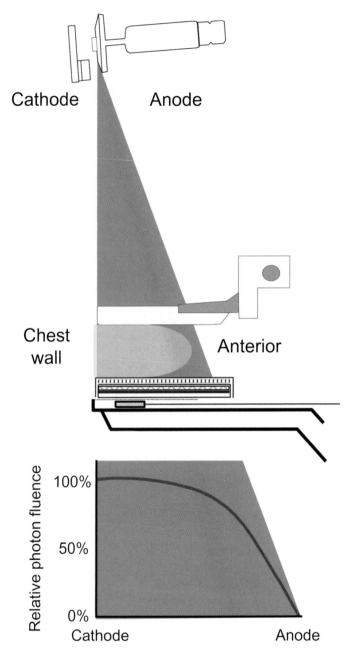

■ **FIGURE 8-5** The x-ray tube is oriented with the cathode over the chest wall side and the anode over the anterior side of the breast. X-ray fluence is reduced on the anode side of the field, a result of self-filtration of x-rays by the anode known as the heel effect. The thickest part of the breast (at the chest wall) is positioned below the cathode, which helps equalize the transmitted x-ray fluence reaching the image receptor. The bottom illustration shows the reduction in fluence to zero, from the projection parallel to the anode surface. Note that with magnification (moving the breast towards the focal spot), the heel effect becomes more prominent over the imaged breast.

above the magnification platform. Orientation of the bar pattern parallel and perpendicular to the cathode-anode direction of the x-ray tube yields measurements of overall *effective* resolution including the focal spot length and width dimensions, the acquisition geometry, and the detector sampling characteristics. Orientation at a 45° angle yields a resolution measurement up to a factor of 1.4 times higher, resulting

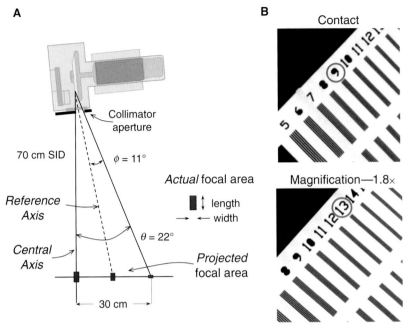

■ **FIGURE 8-6** Focal spot size and image resolution. **A.** The actual focal spot size is determined by the electron distribution area incident on the anode (width × length). The nominal focal spot size is specified on a *reference axis* bisecting the field from the cathode to the anode, with 0.3- and 0.1-mm sizes typical. The *projected* focal spot length increases towards the chest wall and decreases towards the anterior side of the breast according the line focus principle. **B.** A resolution bar pattern measures overall system resolution, including detector sampling and geometric magnification. For contact mammography using a 0.3-mm focal spot with the pattern 6 cm above the detector plane (1.09× magnification), a resolution of 9 lp/mm is resolved. For magnification using a 0.1-mm focal spot with the pattern 35 cm above the detector plane (2.0× magnification), a resolution of 13 lp/mm is resolved. These measurements are for a source-image distance (SID) of 70 cm, 0.07 mm detector element size, and bar pattern at 45° to the detector array.

from the increased physical distance between bars of the bar pattern relative to the detector element sampling array and when the focal spot does not limit resolution. Without correction for bar pattern spacing at an angle, the reported resolution can exceed the theoretical maximum resolution of a detector defined by the Nyquist sampling criterion (see Chapter 4). A resolution bar pattern is shown in Figure 8-6B for contact and magnification images using 0.3- and 0.1-mm focal spots, respectively. The resolving capability of the imaging system is limited by the component that

TABLE 8-1 NOMINAL FOCAL SPOT SIZE AND MEASURED TOLERANCE LIMITS OF MAMMOGRAPHY X-RAY TUBES SPECIFIED BY IEC STANDARDS

NOMINAL FOCAL SPOT SIZE (mm)	WIDTH (mm)	LENGTH (mm)
0.10	0.15	0.15
0.15	0.23	0.23
0.20	0.30	0.30
0.30	0.45	0.65
0.40	0.60	0.85
0.60	0.90	1.30

Data from International Electrotechnical Commission. Medical Electrical Equipment—X-Ray Tube Assemblies for *Medical Diagnosis—Characteristics of Focal Spots*. 4th ed. IEC 60336;2005. www.iec.ch.

causes the most blurring. In magnification mammography, this is generally the focal spot, whereas in contact mammography, it may be the detector element size. In clinical breast imaging, patient motion can be the limiting factor.

8.1.4   Tube Port, Tube Filtration, and Beam Quality

The tube port and added tube filters play an important role in shaping the mammography x-ray photon spectrum. The x-ray tube port window is made of beryllium (Be). The low atomic number ($Z = 4$) of Be and the thin window (0.5 to 1 mm) allow the transmission of all but the lowest energy (5 keV and less) bremsstrahlung x-rays. In addition, Mo and Rh targets produce beneficial K-characteristic x-ray peaks at 17.5 and 19.6 keV (Mo) and 20.2 and 22.7 keV (Rh) (see Chapter 6, Table 6-2), whereas W targets produce a large fraction of undesirable L-characteristic x-rays at 8 to 10 keV that will deliver dose with little or no contribution to image formation. Figure 8-7 illustrates the contributions of the bremsstrahlung and characteristic radiation to the unfiltered composite x-ray spectrum generated by an x-ray tube operated at 30 kV with a Mo target and Be tube port window.

Added x-ray tube filtration helps to optimize the energy distribution of the mammography output spectrum by selectively removing the lowest *and* highest energy x-rays from the x-ray beam, while transmitting a band of x-ray energies that produces acceptable image quality at reasonable dose. This is accomplished by using

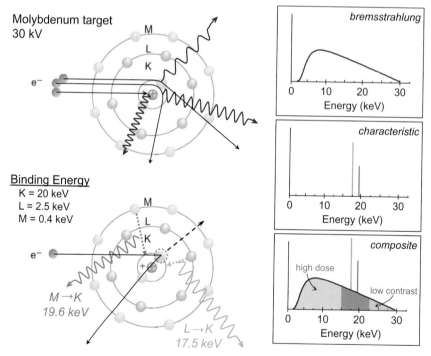

■ **FIGURE 8-7** The x-ray spectrum of a mammography x-ray tube is composed of bremsstrahlung (with a continuous photon energy fluence) and characteristic (discrete energy) radiation (see Chapter 6 for more details). A Mo anode tube operated at 30 kV creates the continuous spectrum (upper right) as well as characteristic radiation with photon energies of 17.5 and 19.6 keV (middle right). On the lower right, the "unfiltered" composite spectrum transmitted through 1 mm of Be (tube port material) has a large fraction of low-energy x-rays that deposits high dose without contributing to the image, and a substantial fraction of high-energy x-rays that reduces subject contrast of the breast tissues. The ideal spectral energy range (shaded in green) is from ~15 to ~25 keV, depending on breast tissue composition and thickness.

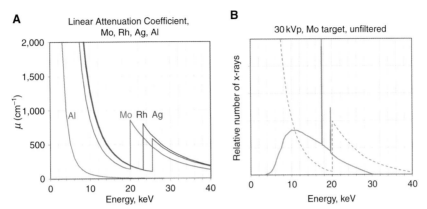

■ **FIGURE 8-8 A.** The linear attenuation coefficients of Al, Mo, Rh, and Ag are plotted as a function of energy. A low-attenuation "transmission window" exists below the K-absorption edge energy for the higher Z elements. **B.** An unfiltered Mo target spectrum generated at 30 kV shows a large fraction of low- and high-energy photons. Superimposed on the same energy scale is a dashed line illustrating Mo filter attenuation as a function of energy (attenuation values from Fig. A).

thin, uniform sheets of pure metal comprised of elements with a K-absorption edge energy (Chapter 3) between 20 and 26 keV, including Mo (20.0 keV), Rh (23.2 keV), and Ag (25.5 keV). At the lowest x-ray energies in the spectrum, the beam attenuation by these filters is very high. The attenuation decreases as the x-ray energy increases up to the K-edge of the element constituting the filter. For x-ray energy just above the K-edge, photoelectric absorption by interaction with the K-shell electron creates a step increase of ~6× in attenuation, and then decreases with higher x-ray energies (Fig. 8-8A). Selective transmission of x-rays in a narrow band from about 15 keV up to the K-absorption edge energy of the filter is achieved with the added filter. In Figure 8-8B, an unfiltered Mo target spectrum and a superimposed attenuation curve for a Mo filter are shown. Note: the characteristic x-ray energies produced by the Mo target occur at the lowest attenuation by the filter in this energy range.

The spectral output of a Mo target and 0.030-mm-thick Mo filter is shown in Figure 8-9A, illustrating the selective transmission of Mo characteristic radiation and significant attenuation of the lowest and highest x-rays in the transmitted spectrum. The Mo target/Mo filter is used for thin and adipose-replaced breasts, with lower (25–30) kV settings. For thicker and more glandular compressed breasts, a 0.025-mm-thick Rh filter produces a higher effective energy beam by transmitting higher energy bremsstrahlung x-rays above 20 keV as shown in Figure 8-9B, with higher (28–32) kV settings.

For systems using the Rh target of a dual Mo and Rh anode, the benefit achieved is the production of Rh characteristic x-ray energies at 20.2 and 22.7 keV. With a 0.025 mm Rh filter, higher effective energy for a set kV can be achieved (Fig. 8-10A) compared to a Mo target. An incompatible combination is a Mo filter with a Rh target, because characteristic x-rays from Rh are significantly attenuated by the Mo filter (Fig. 8-10B). The use of a silver (Ag) filter of 0.025 mm thickness can produce another step up in effective energy when used with a Rh target spectrum by transmitting bremsstrahlung x-rays up to the K-edge energy of Ag (25.5 keV).

W targets are used for many digital mammography systems due to higher bremsstrahlung production efficiency and higher anode heat loading capacity compared to Mo and Rh targets, but the very large fraction of L characteristic x-rays in the 8- to 12-keV range (Fig. 8-11A) must be removed to negligible levels, requiring a thicker filter. Selectable K-edge filters of Rh or Ag are used to shape the output x-ray energies within a narrow continuous spectral range, with minimum filter thickness of

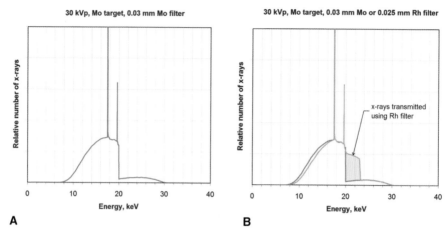

FIGURE 8-9 A. A filtered output spectrum is shown for a Mo target and 0.030-mm Mo filter for a 30-kV tube voltage, with prominent characteristic peaks at 17.5 and 19.6 keV. This spectrum is selected for less dense and thinner breast tissues, particularly with lower operating tube voltages (25 to 30 kV). **B.** A filtered output spectrum is shown for a Mo target and 0.025-mm Rh filter, superimposed on the Mo/Mo spectrum in **(A)**, indicating the transmission of higher energy bremsstrahlung x-rays up to the K absorption edge of Rh at 23.2 keV. The spectrum, including the Mo characteristic x-rays, has a higher effective energy and is preferable for imaging thicker and denser breast tissues.

0.05 mm, as shown in Figure 8-11B. Consequently, the output fluence rate of a W target is lower than Mo or Rh targets mainly because of the doubled filter thickness (0.05 mm compared to 0.025 mm). Higher fluence rate for a W target is achieved by using an Al filter of 0.5–0.7 mm thickness to sufficiently attenuate the L x-rays of lower energy and permit a larger fraction of higher energy x-rays in the transmitted spectrum. In breast tomosynthesis implemented by one vendor, requirements for rapid image capture are satisfied by the W/Al selection, and the loss of tissue subject contrast by the higher energy spectrum is offset by image reconstruction processing with reduced superimposition of tissues in the tomographic images, as well as digital contrast enhancement (see Section 8.5).

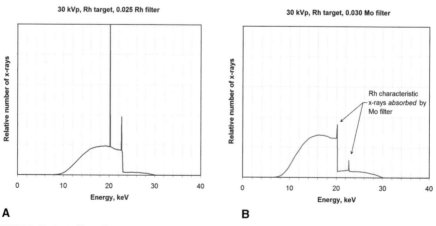

FIGURE 8-10 A. A filtered output spectrum is shown for a Rh target and 0.025-mm Rh filter for a 30-kV tube voltage, with prominent Rh characteristic x-rays at 20.2 and 22.7 keV. This spectrum provides a higher effective energy than a Mo target—Rh filter x-ray beam at the same kV, due to the presence of higher energy characteristic x-rays. **B.** A combination of a Rh target and Mo filter is inappropriate, as the Rh characteristic x-rays are strongly attenuated by the Mo filter at the energies of the Rh characteristic x-rays, as shown.

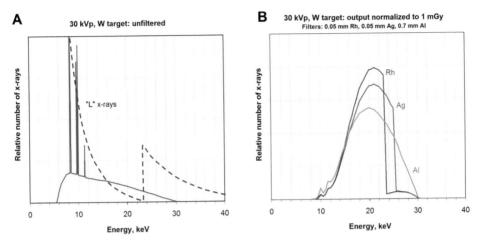

■ **FIGURE 8-11 A.** An unfiltered W target spectrum generated at 30 kV shows a large fraction of lower energy L-characteristic x-rays from 8 to 11.5 keV. Superimposed at the same energy scale is a dashed line illustrating the relative attenuation characteristics of a Rh filter. **B.** Filtered W-target x-ray spectra by Rh (0.05 mm), Ag (0.05 mm), and Al (0.7 mm) are normalized to the same exposure output. The L x-rays are reduced to negligible levels by using the indicated thicknesses.

8.1.5 Half-Value Layer

The half-value layer (HVL) of a mammography x-ray beam is the thickness of an attenuator (usually Al) required to reduce the incident x-ray beam air kerma by one half. HVL depends on kV, target material (Mo, Rh, W), filter material (Mo, Rh, Ag, Al), and filter thicknesses typically used in mammography, and ranges between 0.3 and 0.7 mm Al (Fig. 8-12). Measurement of HVL is performed with the compression paddle well above the breast platform and collimation in a narrow beam configuration (see Chapter 3) with the radiation dosimeter placed in the beam on the breast platform. At a fixed kV and mAs, repeated measurements of air kerma are made, first with no added filter (other than the compression paddle), then with sequential 0.1 mm sheets of 0.999 purity Al added near the tube port, until the air kerma value drops below one half of the first measurement. The HVL is determined by identifying the nearest added thicknesses corresponding to air kerma values below and above the 50% air kerma value and then using mathematical or graphical interpolation to determine the Al thickness that corresponds to the 50% air kerma value.

An x-ray beam with a Mo target, 0.03-mm Mo filter, and 1.5 mm Lexan compression paddle at 28 kV has an HVL of about 0.35-mm Al, whereas a W target and 0.05-mm Rh filter with the same kV and compression paddle has an HVL of about 0.53-mm Al. HVLs of mammography beams for a set kV and target/filter combination vary from machine to machine because of slight variations in actual filter thicknesses, compression paddles, and kV accuracy.

The minimum HVL in mm Al of an x-ray beam per MQSA regulations must be greater than or equal to kV/100. For example, a mammography system operated at 30 kV must have an HVL ≥ 0.3 mm Al. Under this HVL condition, a large fraction of very low energy x-rays is removed by inherent and added filters in the bremsstrahlung spectrum incident on the breast. Maximum HVL limits have been suggested in earlier accreditation guidelines but are not enforced. An x-ray beam that is "harder" than optimal indicates a problem such as a pitted anode or aged tube and can result in reduced output and poor image quality. Estimates of the radiation dose to the breast glandular tissues require accurate assessment of the HVL (see Section 8.6).

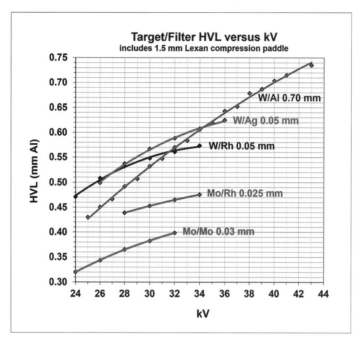

■ FIGURE 8-12 The HVL (including the Lexan compression paddle attenuation) versus kV is plotted for Mo targets with Mo and Rh filters, and for W targets with Rh, Ag, and Al filters. HVL measurements are representative of an average of several evaluations on various mammography systems at UC Davis Health. The solid lines represent a second-order polynomial fit to the data.

The HVL of breast tissue is highly dependent on tissue composition (glandular, fibrous, or fatty) and the HVL of the incident x-ray beam. Typically, the HVL expressed as breast tissue thickness is from 1 to 3 cm.

8.1.6 Tube Output and Tube Output Rate

While the energy fluence of the x-ray beam best describes output, the air kerma is easily measured and is a practical measure of output. Air kerma is typically normalized to 100 mAs, at a specified distance from the source (focal spot). In this chapter, the x-ray tube output is expressed in units of mGy/100 mAs at 50 cm from the source. The kV, anode target, filter material, filter thickness, and focal spot size must also be specified. X-ray tube output curves for Mo and W targets are shown for several filters and thicknesses as a function of kV in Figure 8-13. Even though W targets are more efficient at producing x-rays, thicker added filters result in lower x-ray tube output rate compared to a Mo target. However, W spectra have higher HVLs and greater beam penetrability (*i.e.*, more of the incident x-ray beam on the breast reaches the detector), and with higher possible maximum tube current, exposure times are comparable to a Mo target/filter for a similar breast thickness.

Calibrated output values of an x-ray tube X mGy (per 100 mAs at 50 cm) for a specific target/filter combination and kV (Fig. 8-13) are necessary for calculating the free-in-air incident air kerma, Z mGy, to the breast for an acquisition requiring Y mAs at a source-to-breast surface distance, D, according to Equation 8-1:

$$Z \, \text{mGy} = X \, \text{mGy} \ (\text{per } 100 \ \text{mAs}) \times \frac{Y \, \text{mAs}}{100} \times \left(\frac{50 \ \text{cm}}{D \ \text{cm}} \right)^2. \qquad [8\text{-}1]$$

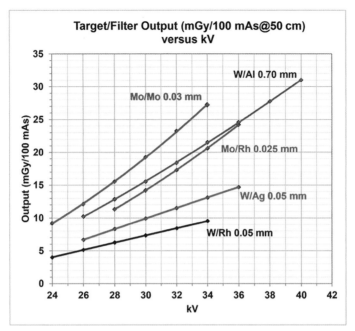

■ **FIGURE 8-13** Tube output (mGy/100 mAs at 50-cm distance from the source with compression paddle in the beam) for two clinical mammography units is measured at 2-kV intervals. A Mo target with 0.03-mm Mo and 0.025-mm Rh filter, and a W target with filter thicknesses of 0.05-mm Rh, 0.05-mm Ag, and 0.70-mm Al are plotted.

The source-to-breast surface distance, D, is determined from the compressed breast thickness, the source to image (detector) distance (SID), and the breast platform to detector distance. Entrance surface air kerma to the breast is adjusted by the inverse square law relative to the output calibration distance $(50 \text{ cm}/D \text{ cm})^2$.

EXAMPLE: Calculate the entrance surface breast air kerma for the following acquisition: W target and Rh filter, technique of 30 kV and 200 mAs, SID of 70 cm, compressed breast thickness of 6 cm, breast platform to detector distance of 2 cm.

Answer: The source to breast surface is 62 cm (SID [70 cm] – breast thickness [6 cm] – space between platform and detector [2 cm]). From Figure 8-13, the tube output for W/Rh at 30 kV is 7.2 mGy/100 mAs at 50 cm. Calculation of incident air kerma considers tube output, the mAs used, and inverse square law correction from 50 cm (calibration point) to 62 cm (breast surface distance), using Equation 8-1:

$$7.2 \text{ mGy (per 100 mAs)} \times \frac{200 \text{ mAs}}{100 \text{ mAs}} \times \left(\frac{50 \text{ cm}}{62 \text{ cm}}\right)^2 = 9.4 \text{ mGy}.$$

Calculation of the mean glandular dose (MGD) to the breast is determined from the measured incident breast surface air kerma value and other parameters as discussed in Section 8.6.

Tube output rate is the air kerma rate at a specified distance from the x-ray focal spot and is a function of the tube current achievable for an extended exposure time (typically ~300 mAs for an exposure time greater than 3 seconds). Legacy systems are required to be capable of producing an air kerma rate of at least 7.0 mGy/s, when operating at 28 kV in the standard (Mo/Mo) mammography mode, at any SID for which the system is designed to operate. With the introduction of W targets and lower output rates, each manufacturer has set a lower acceptable output rate limit for a designated kV and filter for this test.

8.1.7 X-ray Tube Alignment and Beam Collimation

The x-ray tube and collimation alignment with respect to the light field, active detector area, and compression paddle ensure that the x-ray beam central axis is perpendicular to and intercepts the center of the chest wall edge of the image receptor. This protects the patient from unnecessary radiation dose to the lungs and includes as much breast tissue as possible in the image. Figure 8-14 shows the projected light field and x-ray field for a 24 × 29 cm detector area, and the corresponding detected x-ray image. Congruence is verified for the light and x-ray fields, and by matching the edges of the coins with the x-ray field edges, the x-ray field projects beyond the active detector area in the worst case by about 5 mm, or about 0.7% for a 70 cm SID. Also, the chest wall edge alignment with the compression paddle edge (5 mm) is within the allowable tolerance of 1% of the SID, or 7 mm. Details on the tolerance limits for light field/x-ray field congruence and requirements for x-ray field alignment with the active detector and compression paddle edge are described in the MQSA program requirements (FDA, 2020). See also Section 8.7.

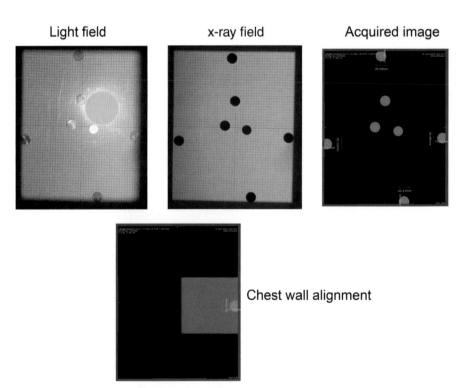

■ **FIGURE 8-14** Light field to x-ray field and x-ray field to detector congruence and alignment evaluations. Upper left: The light field is projected onto phosphor plate with coins placed at light field edges. Upper middle: X-ray field generates green luminescence, indicating the coin positions and demonstrating good light-field–x-ray field congruence. Upper right: Acquired image of coins and measurement of coin to field edge distance to determine x-ray field to active detector congruence. Lower: Compressed 40 mm attenuator thickness and coin placed at the edge of the compression paddle to evaluate paddle edge alignment and missed tissue at the chest wall in the acquired x-ray image.

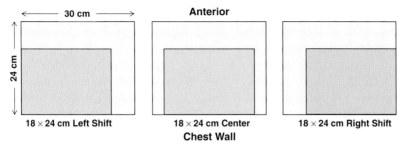

■ **FIGURE 8-15** The large field of view area digital detector size is typically 24 cm × 30 cm, for imaging a large breast. For small breast size, the field of view is reduced to 18 cm × 24 cm with adjustment of the collimator and reduction of the digital image matrix. For cranial-caudal views, the active detector area is centered, as shown in the middle diagram. A shift of the field to the left and right edges of the large area detector provides improved patient positioning of the shoulder and arm for the medial-lateral oblique projections.

Two detector sizes are commonly used in mammography: 24 cm × 30 cm to accommodate larger breasts and 18 cm × 24 cm for the remainder. For flat-panel digital detectors, adjustable collimator blades direct the x-ray beam to the active detector area. When operating with the small field area, one of three active acquisition areas is used: center for the cranial-caudal (CC) views; left shift and right shift for the medial-lateral oblique (MLO) views. This requires the collimator assembly to restrict the x-ray field to the corresponding active detector areas. Shifts to the left and right edges of the receptor are used for optimizing the oblique projections for subjects with smaller breasts to accommodate positioning of the arm and shoulder (Fig. 8-15).

8.2 MAMMOGRAPHY X-RAY GENERATOR

A dedicated mammography x-ray generator is like a conventional x-ray generator in design and function. Lower voltages supplied to the x-ray tube are used, and space charge compensation is more of a concern. In most cases, AEC is employed for mammography screening and diagnostic examinations, although there are instances when the technologist will use manual controls to set the tube current–exposure time product (mAs). Like most contemporary x-ray imaging systems, high-frequency generators are used for mammography due to low voltage ripple, fast response, easy calibration, long-term stability, and compact size. There are sensors that prohibit x-ray exposures if the setup is incomplete (*e.g.*, insufficient compression, cassette not in the tunnel for computed radiography [CR] detectors, or the digital detector array is not ready to capture an image).

8.2.1 Automatic Exposure Control

The AEC circuit employs one or more radiation sensors, a charge to voltage amplifier, a voltage comparator, and a reference voltage selector to control the exposure (Fig. 8-16A). For cassette-based CR image receptors, the dosimeter sensor is located *underneath* the cassette, and consists of a single ionization chamber or an array of three or more semiconductor diodes that can be physically positioned by the technologist. For flat panel detectors (FPDs), the AEC signal is generated by the detector, and the sensor area is selected by the user at the generator console as a choice of several (~5) discrete small square areas spaced equally from the central axis at the chest wall edge to about the middle of the detector. In "auto AEC" mode, the sensor

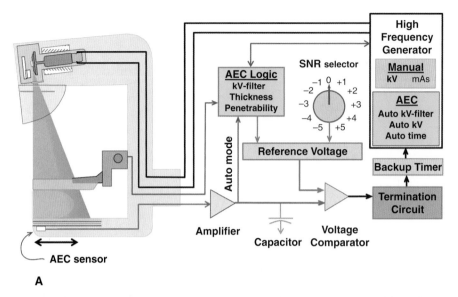

A

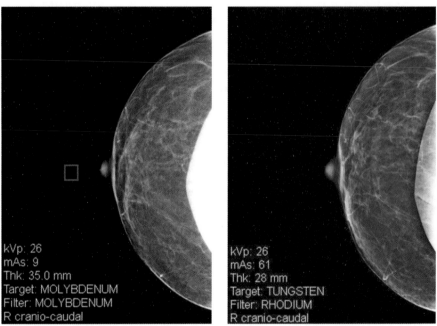

kVp: 26
mAs: 9
Thk: 35.0 mm
Target: MOLYBDENUM
Filter: MOLYBDENUM
R cranio-caudal

kVp: 26
mAs: 61
Thk: 28 mm
Target: TUNGSTEN
Filter: RHODIUM
R cranio-caudal

B

■ **FIGURE 8-16 A.** Automatic exposure control (AEC) circuits use several selectable algorithms to determine the optimal exposure to the breast. The basic AEC operation uses the signal measured by the AEC sensor during the exposure in an operator positioned region that is transmitted to a comparator circuit to match a predetermined level that sends a signal to the generator to terminate the exposure. This is commonly known as "Auto-time." More sophisticated modes are also available, as explained in the text. **B.** Left: Image is an implant displaced view of the breast. The square in the open field represents the position of the AEC sensor, which was set in the open field from the previous acquisition, causing an underexposure and significant noise. Right: Patient returns for repeat study on a different unit using AEC "auto" mode that determines the attenuation characteristics of the breast and achieves a proper exposure. Note the technique factors for each acquisition.

area is defined by the lowest signal region (highest attenuation) over the active digital detector area. The AEC sensor is wired to a charge to voltage amplifier that produces voltage in proportion to the accumulated x-ray exposure. The voltage comparator circuit has a calibrated reference voltage as one input, and the AEC sensor voltage as the other input. During an exposure, the sensor voltage increases from zero volts to a voltage equal to the reference voltage, which triggers the comparator circuit to terminate the exposure. The reference voltage produces a known incident x-ray fluence to the detector and thus determines the radiation exposure to the breast, as well as the quantum mottle in the digital image.

AEC algorithms use several inputs to achieve a consistent detected x-ray fluence, including compressed breast thickness, AEC control selector settings on the generator console, kV, tube anode selection (if available), and tube filter. The operator typically has two or three options for AEC settings:

- A fully automatic AEC mode that sets the optimal kV and filtration (and target material on some systems) from a short test exposure of approximately 100 ms to determine the penetrability of the breast.
- Automatic kV selection with a short test exposure, with user-selected target and filter values.
- Automatic time of exposure using manually set target, filter, and kV values.

For most patient imaging, the fully automatic mode is used.

At the generator control panel, an exposure selector control modifies the AEC reference voltage to the comparator circuit to permit adjustments for unusual imaging circumstances such as imaging breasts with implants, magnification, or for radiologist preference in overall digital image signal to noise ratio (SNR) in the output image. Depending on the manufacturer, several steps (*e.g.*, -3 to 0 [neutral] to $+4$) are available to increase or decrease exposure by adjusting the AEC input level to the comparator circuit. Each step provides a difference of 10% to 15% positive (greater exposure) or negative (lesser exposure) per step from the baseline neutral (0) setting.

An x-ray exposure under AEC control that exceeds a preset time (*e.g.*, greater than 5 s) is terminated by a *backup timer*. This can occur if there is a malfunction of the AEC sensor or amplifiers, or if the kV is set too low with insufficient x-ray transmission through the breast. In the latter situation, the operator must select a higher kV to achieve greater beam penetrability and a shorter exposure time to correct the problem.

Inaccurate phototimer response resulting in an under- or overexposed digital image can be caused by breast tissue composition (adipose versus glandular) heterogeneity, compressed thickness beyond the calibration range (too thin or too thick), a faulty radiation sensor, or an inappropriate kV setting. For extremely thin or fatty breasts, the AEC circuit and x-ray generator response can be too slow in terminating the exposure, causing overexposure. In situations where the exposure is terminated too quickly, gridline artifacts can appear in the image due to lack of complete grid motion during the short exposure.

The position of the AEC detector (*e.g.*, under dense or fatty breast tissue) will change the detected fluence and affect the image SNR. Images from a previous exam can aid the technologist in positioning the AEC detector to achieve an exposure that will deliver the desired image SNR for glandular areas of the breast. Most systems allow positioning from the chest wall to anterior direction, while some newer systems also allow side-to-side positioning under the breast to provide flexibility for unusual anatomy. In modern AEC systems, an "auto" selection evaluates the entire exposed area of the detector and identifies the signal under the most attenuating region of the breast to measure an adequate detected fluence for that region prior to terminating the exposure. In situations such as imaging breast implants, however, the "auto" selection should not be used, except for implant displaced views. An example of a sensor position inadvertently set in the open field (Fig. 8-16B left image) results in an unacceptably noisy image. The patient returns to a different unit for a repeat study performed under "auto" mode (Fig. 8-16B right image) with appropriate image quality.

8.2.2 Technique Charts

Technique charts are useful guides to help determine the appropriate kV and target-filter combinations for specific imaging tasks, based on breast thickness and breast composition (fatty versus glandular tissue fractions) where AEC might not be able to provide consistent results. The proper choice of kV is essential for a reasonable exposure time for systems that have a fixed tube current, defined as a range from approximately 0.5 to 4 s to achieve the desired SNR (the longest times occur with magnification and use of the small focal spot). An exposure that is too short can cause visible grid lines to appear on the image, whereas an exposure that is too long can result in breast motion, either of which degrades the quality of the image. Digital postprocessing allows flexibility for rendering image contrast and allows a wide range of kV settings. A technique chart example for an amorphous selenium (Se) FPD system using a Mo target with Mo or Rh filtration, a W target with Rh or Ag filtration, or a W target with Al filtration and no grid for digital tomosynthesis is listed in Table 8-2.

8.3 COMPRESSION, SCATTERED RADIATION, AND MAGNIFICATION

8.3.1 Compression

Breast compression is an important part of the mammography examination. Firm compression reduces overlapping anatomy, decreases tissue thickness, and reduces inadvertent motion of the breast (Fig. 8-17A). Less geometric blurring of anatomic structures and lower radiation dose to the breast tissues are also benefits. A uniform compressed breast thickness reduces detector dynamic range requirements and allows more flexibility in image processing enhancement of the digital image.

Compression is achieved with a compression paddle, a Lexan plate attached to a mechanical assembly (Fig. 8-17B). The full area compression paddle matches the

TABLE 8-2 TECHNIQUE CHART FOR A DIGITAL MAMMOGRAPHY SYSTEM WITH SELENIUM DETECTOR FOR 50% GLANDULAR 50% ADIPOSE COMPOSITION

THICKNESS (cm)	DIGITAL, Mo TARGET, CELLULAR GRID			DIGITAL, W TARGET, CELLULAR GRID			DIGITAL TOMOSYNTHESIS, W TARGET, NO GRID		
	Filter	kV	mAs	Filter	kV	mAs	Filter	kV	mAs
<3	Mo 30 μm	24	35	Rh 50 μm	25	40	Al 700 μm	26	35
3–5	Mo 30 μm	27	75	Rh 50 μm	28	80	Al 700 μm	29	50
5–7	Mo 30 μm	31	100	Rh 50 μm	31	150	Al 700 μm	33	65
>7	Rh 25 μm	33	150	Ag 50 μm	32	200	Al 700 μm	38	85

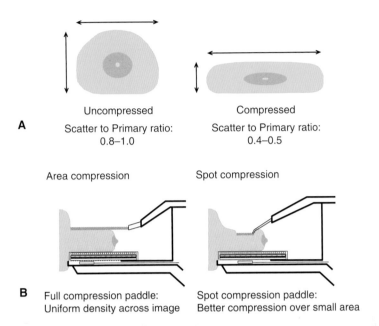

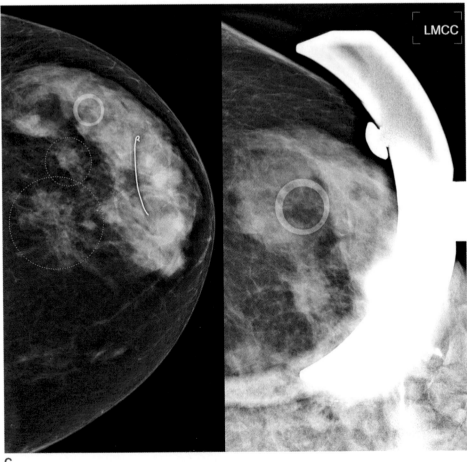

C

■ **FIGURE 8-17** **A.** Compression is essential for mammographic studies to reduce breast thickness (less scatter, reduced radiation dose, and shorter exposure time) and to spread out superimposed anatomy. **B.** Suspicious areas often require "spot" compression to eliminate superimposed anatomy by further spreading the breast tissues over a localized area. **C.** Example of image with suspicious finding (left). Corresponding spot compression (digitally magnified) illustrates less tissue overlap (right).

size of the image receptor (18 × 24 cm or 24 × 30 cm) and is flat and parallel to the breast support table. The compression paddle has a right-angle edge at the chest wall to produce a flat, uniform breast thickness when an adequate force of 111 to 200 newtons (25 to 44 lb) is applied. A smaller "spot" compression paddle (~7-cm diameter) produces more compression over a specific region where the tissue surrounding the paddle bulges out, allowing more aggressive compression over a limited FOV (Fig. 8-17C). Alternatives to the flat compression paddle include a "flex" paddle that is spring-loaded on the anterior side to tilt and accommodate variations in breast thickness from the chest wall to the nipple, and a curved paddle, providing a more comfortable yet adequate compression of the breast.

A hands-free (*e.g.*, foot-pedal operated), motor-driven compression paddle is used, which is operable from both sides of the patient allowing the technologist to position the breast tissue for optimal compression. In addition, a mechanical adjustment knob near the paddle holder allows fine manual adjustments of compression. While firm compression is not comfortable for the patient, it is necessary for a high-quality mammogram.

8.3.2 Scattered Radiation and Antiscatter Grids

The x-ray beam that exits the breast just above the detector contains primary and scattered radiation. Primary x-rays are those that have passed through the breast unattenuated, and scattered x-rays are x-rays that have experienced one or more scattering events. The collection of primary x-rays striking each detector element carry information regarding the spatially dependent attenuation characteristics of the breast and deliver subject contrast to the detector. Scattered radiation is an additive, gradually varying radiation distribution that degrades subject contrast and adds quantum noise. If the maximum subject contrast without scatter is C_0 and the maximum contrast with scatter is C_s, then the contrast degradation factor (CDF) is approximated as

$$\text{CDF} = \frac{C_s}{C_0} = \frac{1}{1 + \text{SPR}},$$ [8-2]

where SPR is the scatter-to-primary ratio (Chapter 7). X-ray scatter increases with increasing breast thickness and breast area, with typical SPR values shown in Figure 8-18. A breast of 6-cm compressed thickness will have an SPR of approximately 0.6 and a calculated CDF of $(1/(1 + 0.6)) = 0.625 = 62.5\%$ according to Equation 8-2. Without some form of scatter rejection, therefore, only a fraction of the inherent subject contrast can be acquired. The main adverse effect of scatter in digital mammography is that scattered photons add x-ray quantum noise, degrading the image SNR.

Scattered radiation reaching the image receptor can be greatly reduced by using an *antiscatter grid* or *air gap*. (Antiscatter grids are described in Chapter 7.) For contact mammography, an antiscatter grid is located between the breast and the detector. Mammography grids transmit about 60% to 70% of primary x-rays and absorb 75% to 85% of the scattered radiation. Linear focused grids with grid ratios (height of the lead septa divided by the interspace distance) of 4:1 to 5:1 are common (*e.g.*, 1.5 mm height, 0.30-mm distance between septa, 0.016-mm septa thickness), with carbon fiber interspace materials (Fig. 8-19A). Grid frequencies (number of lead septa per cm) of 30/cm to 45/cm are typical. To avoid the appearance of gridlines, the grid must oscillate over approximately 20 lines perpendicular to the direction of the gridlines during the exposure. Excessively short exposures are the cause of most gridline artifacts because of insufficient grid motion.

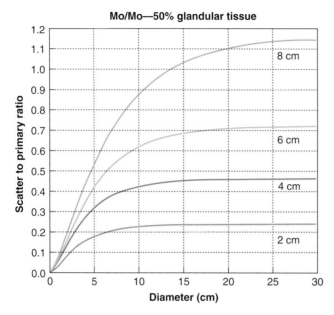

Mo/Mo—50% glandular tissue

■ FIGURE 8-18 X-ray scatter reduces the radiographic contrast of the breast image. Scatter is chiefly dependent on breast thickness and x-ray field area. The scatter-to-primary ratio is plotted as a function of the diameter of a semicircular field area aligned to the chest wall edge, for several breast thicknesses of 50% glandular tissue.

A cellular grid, made of thin copper septa, provides scatter rejection in two dimensions (Fig. 8-19B). Typical specifications of this design include a septal height of 2.4 mm, 0.64-mm distance between septa (3.8 ratio), a septal thickness of 0.03 mm, and 15 cells/cm. The metal honeycomb structure of the cellular grid provides structural rigidity and hence air is used as the interspace material. During image acquisition, grid motion in both the x- and y-axis directions is necessary for complete blurring of the grid structure, so specific exposure time increments are necessary, which are determined by evaluation of the first 100 ms of the exposure by AEC logic circuits. With two-dimensional scatter rejection and low attenuation air interspaces, the cellular grid attenuates more of the scattered radiation that would otherwise reach the detector compared to a 5:1 ratio linear grid.

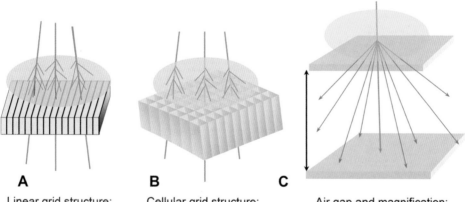

A
Linear grid structure:
1D scatter rejection

B
Cellular grid structure:
2D scatter rejection

C
Air gap and magnification:
geometric scatter rejection

■ FIGURE 8-19 Antiscatter devices commonly employed in mammography include **(A)** the linear grid of approximately 5:1 grid ratio and carbon fiber interspace material, **(B)** a cellular crosshatch grid structure made of copper sheet of approximately 3.8 grid ratio with air interspaces and scatter rejection in two dimensions, and **(C)** the air gap intrinsic to the magnification procedure. *Note:* while the illustration depicts 100% scatter rejection by the grid, approximately 15% of scattered x-rays are transmitted.

Grids impose a dose penalty to compensate for loss of primary radiation by attenuation of grid septa. Increased exposure to the breast by a factor of ~2 is typical when using an antiscatter grid to achieve a desired SNR.

An air gap reduces scatter by increasing the distance of the breast from the detector by moving closer to the source on a magnification stand, so that a large fraction of scattered radiation misses the detector (Fig. 8-19C). The consequences of using an air gap, however, are that the FOV is reduced, the magnification of the breast is increased, and the dose to the breast is increased due to the reduced source to object distance. However, use of a sufficiently large air gap makes the antiscatter grid unnecessary, thus allowing a lower acquisition technique factor (*e.g.*, mAs) such that the dose to the breast is like that of the contact mammography acquisition.

The loss of image contrast that occurs when a grid is not used in contact mammography can be recovered to a high degree by digital image processing techniques for compressed breast thicknesses less than 6 cm. Several manufacturers have optional "no-grid" acquisition techniques that use scatter reduction image postprocessing. This involves characterization of the scatter point spread function, which is dependent on compressed breast thickness and local anatomy, to generate an image-specific scatter image. The subtraction of the scatter image from the original (primary + scatter) image produces the scatter-corrected image. Because a significant fraction of the original image is comprised of signal due to scatter, the amount of radiation dose reduction by not using a grid is typically only about 20% to ~30% less than that for a grid acquisition to ensure an adequate SNR in the scatter corrected image.

8.3.3 Magnification Techniques

Geometric magnification of the breast is used to improve overall mammography system resolution, and this is useful when the detector element size is the limiting factor for detection and discrimination of microcalcifications. Object magnification is achieved by placing a breast support platform (a magnification stand) that allows the breast to be positioned well above the detector. In addition to geometrical changes, other parameters include selecting the small (0.1 mm) focal spot, removing the antiscatter grid, and using a compression paddle specifically for magnification (Fig. 8-20). Most dedicated mammographic units offer geometric magnifications of 1.5×, 1.8×, or 2.0×.

There are several advantages of magnification:

- Increased spatial resolution—Geometric magnification of the x-ray pattern onto the surface of the detector enlarges the object with respect to detector element size. This improves overall resolution when the size of the projected focal spot penumbra (geometric blurring) onto the detector is less than the detector element pitch, and typically occurs with the 0.1-mm focal spot.
- Reduction of quantum noise relative to the objects being rendered—Since there are more x-rays passing through a given object in the breast in a magnified image, the quantum noise is reduced compared to the standard contact image.
- Reduction of scattered radiation—The large air gap between the surface of the magnification breast support stand and the image receptor lowers the amount of scattered radiation reaching the image receptor, thus improving image contrast, reducing quantum noise, and making the use of an antiscatter grid unnecessary.

Magnification has several limitations, the most significant being geometric blurring caused by the finite focal spot. Spatial resolution is reduced on the cathode side of the x-ray field (toward the chest wall), where the effective focal spot size is largest. The 0.1-mm focal spot has a tube current limit of about 25–35 mA, so a 100-mAs

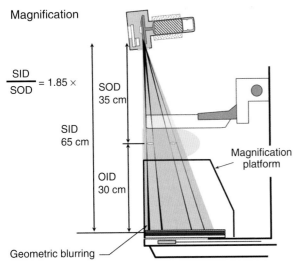

Magnification

$$\frac{SID}{SOD} = 1.85 \times$$

SOD
35 cm

SID
65 cm

OID
30 cm

Magnification platform

Geometric blurring

■ FIGURE 8-20 Geometric magnification. A support platform positions the breast closer to the source focal spot, resulting in 1.5× to 2.0× image magnification. A small focal spot (0.1 to 0.15 mm nominal size) reduces geometric blurring. Effective focal spot size varies along the cathode-anode axis (large to small effective size) and is accentuated with magnification. Best spatial resolution and detail in the image exist on the anode side of the field. SID, source to image distance; SOD, source to object (midplane) distance; OID, object to image distance.

acquisition can require up to 3–4 s. Even slight breast motion will result in image blurring, which is exacerbated by the magnification.

Regarding breast dose, the elimination of the grid reduces the necessary technique factors (dose) by a factor of ~2, but the shorter distance between the x-ray focal spot and the breast increases dose by about the same factor due to the inverse square law. In addition, the smaller FOV reduces the volume of the breast that is exposed to primary radiation. As a result, the breast dose is about the same for magnification and contact imaging.

8.4 DIGITAL ACQUISITION SYSTEMS

Digital acquisition devices for mammography became available in the 1990s as small field-of-view digital biopsy systems. Several full-field digital mammography systems were introduced in the early 2000s, and at the same time an international investigation, the DMIST (discussed in the introduction), compared the capabilities of full-field digital mammography with the (then) gold-standard screen-film detector systems. Results of the large trial demonstrated non-inferiority in general with superior performance for dense breasts, leading to the almost complete replacement of screen-film detectors with digital detectors by 2015 in the United States. Many digital mammography systems have been approved by the FDA in the United States over the past decade, including digital tomosynthesis and dedicated breast CT systems described in the following sections of this chapter.

8.4.1 Full-Field Digital Mammography

There are compelling advantages to digital mammography, the most important of which is the ability to overcome the exposure latitude (dynamic range) limitations of screen-film detectors and to produce better image quality at lower doses. Other reasons include increased technologist productivity by eliminating film processing steps with reduced patient waiting time. The ability to manipulate the (digital) image post-acquisition is an underappreciated but important factor that improves image quality and lesion detectability through digital image processing.

FPD arrays became clinically available in the late 1990s for general radiography (see Chapter 7), and in the mid 2000s for mammography. FPDs are now the major detector in use for full-field digital mammography, and are comprised of an active matrix, thin film transistor (TFT) array with millions of detector elements interconnected by rows of "gate" lines and columns of "drain" lines. Electronic components in each detector element include a charge collection electrode, a storage capacitor, and a transistor. The transistor is an electronic semiconductor with three terminals—one connected to the charge capacitor, one connected to the drain line, and a controlling terminal connected to the gate line. It acts as an electronic switch to allow charge to flow from the capacitor to the drain line. During x-ray acquisition, all transistors are in the "off" position, a proportional charge in each detector element is captured by the charge collection electrode in proportion to the local transmitted x-ray fluence, and is stored in the local capacitor. Immediately after the exposure, detector readout occurs by activating each gate line, one row at a time, to turn on the transistors along each row, allowing charge transfer from the capacitors via the drain lines along each column in parallel to a series of charge amplifiers and digitizers. Digital data are stored in computer memory at the corresponding row position. The image is produced sequentially using the row by row readout scheme (Fig. 8-21). In some "fast" flat panel designs, readout of the whole array is performed in hundreds of milliseconds, often by reading quadrants of the detector element panels in parallel, allowing near "real-time" acquisition of data for applications such as digital tomosynthesis.

Common to all flat panel TFT arrays is the amorphous silicon circuit layer (Fig. 8-22A). At present, approved digital mammography systems are based on three major technologies. The first is an indirect x-ray conversion TFT flat panel array receptor with 100-μm sampling pitch and 18 × 23-cm or 24 × 31-cm FOV (Fig. 8-22B). A structured cesium iodide (CsI) phosphor converts x-rays into light; the light is emitted onto a photodiode in each detector element, from which the charge is generated and stored in a local capacitor. *Indirect conversion* describes absorption of x-rays in the CsI, the production of secondary light photons that ultimately strike a photodiode, and the generation of charge, which is stored on the storage capacitor in that detector element.

A second technology is based on a direct x-ray conversion TFT detector with 70 or 85 μm sampling pitch (depending on manufacturer) and 24 × 30-cm FOV (Fig. 8-22C). A semiconductor x-ray converter, Se, is uniformly deposited between

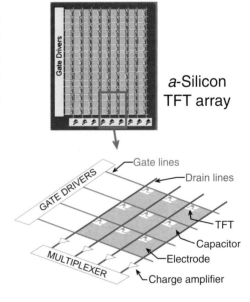

■ **FIGURE 8-21** The flat panel array is a two-dimensional matrix of detector elements lithographed on an amorphous silicon substrate. Each detector element is comprised of an electronic switch (the TFT), a charge collection electrode, and a storage capacitor. The gate and drain lines provide the mechanism to extract the locally stored charge by activating gate lines row by row and collecting charge down each column. Charge amplifier and digitizers convert the signals to corresponding digital values for transfer to the digital image matrix.

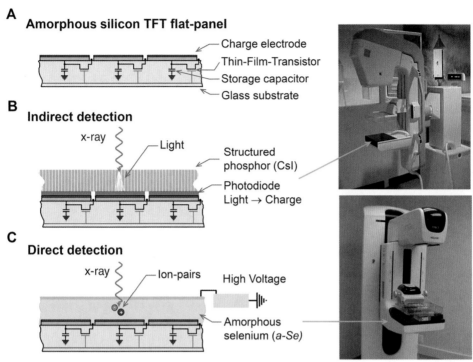

A Amorphous silicon TFT flat-panel

Charge electrode
Thin-Film-Transistor
Storage capacitor
Glass substrate

B Indirect detection

x-ray
Light
Structured phosphor (CsI)
Photodiode
Light → Charge

C Direct detection

x-ray
Ion-pairs
High Voltage
Amorphous selenium (a-Se)

■ **FIGURE 8-22 A.** TFT flat panel arrays have a common underlying amorphous silicon structure. There are two classifications of TFT detectors, determined by the conversion of the x-rays into electrical signals. **B.** "Indirect x-ray conversion" TFT arrays have an additional photodiode layer placed on the charge collection electrode of each detector element. The photodiodes are optically coupled to a layer of a phosphor, such as CsI, that produces light when irradiated by x-rays. The light produced by x-ray absorption in the phosphor in turn creates mobile electric charge in the photodiode. The charge is collected by the electrode and stored in the capacitor. **C.** A "Direct x-ray conversion" TFT array has a semiconductor layer of approximately 0.5 mm thickness between the surface electrode extending over the detector area and each detector element electrode, under a potential difference of approximately 10 V/μm. As hole-electron pairs are created in the semiconductor layer by x-rays, the electrons and holes migrate to the positive and negative electrodes, with minimal lateral spread. A proportional charge is stored on the capacitor. The outward appearances of the indirect and direct detectors are similar, shown by the pictures on the right.

two electrodes, with a large voltage (about 10 V per μm thickness—*e.g.*, for a 200-μm thickness the bias voltage is 2,000 V) placed across the Se layer. X-rays from a mammography exposure interact in the Se directly to produce electron-hole pairs; the applied voltage causes the electrons to migrate to one electrode and the holes to the opposite electrode. The local storage capacitor captures the charge from the collection electrode. *Direct conversion* refers to the direct production and capture of ions produced by x-ray ionization in the converter, without using light emission (scintillation) as an intermediate step.

A third technology uses Complementary Metal-Oxide Semiconductor (CMOS) arrays that are manufactured from crystalline silicon wafers with lithography production methods similar to the fabrication of dynamic random-access memory (DRAM). The detector uses a scintillator (typically CsI structured phosphor) to convert incident x-rays into light. A photodiode produces charge from light in each detector element; a charge-to-voltage converter produces a corresponding output voltage (Fig. 8-23). These on-chip components and a process called "double correlated sampling" produce a readout scheme with very low electronic noise, resulting in high detective quantum efficiency at low radiation doses. CMOS detectors are often referred to as

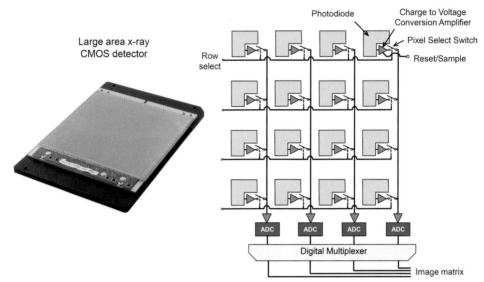

FIGURE 8-23 A large-area CMOS detector shown on the left is created on a crystalline silicon substrate, using a lithography process like dynamic memory (DRAM) to build up the electronic components and switches in layers. On the right is a schematic of the underlying electronics. Each "active pixel" element is comprised of a photodiode to collect x-ray induced light photons and create a proportional charge, an active charge to voltage conversion amplifier, and a sample/reset switch to direct the voltage signal along the readout columns to a massive array of analog to digital converters connected to a digital multiplexer, and digital output to the corresponding image matrix location. For x-ray imaging, detector element dimensions of 50 to 100 μm are typical, and detector dimensions are as large as 30 cm × 30 cm.

active pixel arrays, as the detector elements are directly addressable and their content can be sampled or reset, similar to DRAM. In operation, readout of the CMOS array occurs like a TFT array by activating rows one at a time and collecting signal down columns in parallel. In many CMOS detectors, conversion of the voltage to a digital value occurs at each column with an analog to digital converter, and a digital multiplexer synchronizes the output into the corresponding image matrix position. The historic challenge for CMOS x-ray detector systems has been the manufacture of large area arrays with detector elements of 50 × 50 μm or larger. Limitations also include the availability and cost of crystalline silicon wafers needed to manufacture large area detectors suitable for x-ray applications. Developing CMOS wafers with three "buttable" sides allows manufacturers to produce detector mosaics up to 30 cm × 30 cm. Compared to amorphous silicon TFT array technology, advantages of the CMOS detector are lower electronic noise, flexibility of data readout, and the ability to incorporate amplification and voltage conversion electronics at each detector element within the array. Double correlated sampling and feedback loops result in electronic readout noise that is much lower than a TFT array. CMOS large area detectors are currently being used for full-field digital mammography, DBT, and dedicated breast CT applications.

A legacy technology approved for full-field digital mammography is a cassette-based, CR imaging plate detector and reader system (see Chapter 7 for a description of CR data acquisition details) with 18 × 24 cm and 24 × 30 cm imaging plates as a direct replacement for screen-film cassettes and film processing. However, due to lower x-ray detection efficiency compared to flat-panel detectors, labor-intensive handling, and longer readout and processing time, CR has largely been replaced by flat-panel detectors, and the use of CR as a mammography detector has been diminishing.

All current full-field digital mammography detectors have similar attributes with respect to exposure latitude. In terms of spatial resolution, the direct conversion detector achieves the best intrinsic spatial resolution due to active charge collection and minimal signal spread in the semiconductor material, with typical detector element dimensions of ~70 to ~85 μm. The indirect conversion detector uses the CsI-structured phosphor to limit the spread of light onto the detector array, which has a typical detector element dimension of 100 μm. In terms of detective quantum efficiency (DQE—defined in Chapter 4), the indirect acquisition array has better performance at low to intermediate spatial frequencies, and the direct acquisition array has better performance at higher spatial frequencies. For cassette-based CR mammography detectors, the image quality and DQE at a given incident radiation exposure to the detector is lower than that of the electronic array detectors, and breast doses are typically higher.

8.4.2 Digital Breast Tomosynthesis

Being a true 2D modality, conventional mammography suffers from overlying and underlying anatomical superimposition, obscuring the detection of a cancer if a cancer is present (reduced sensitivity). DBT uses x-ray tube motion over a limited angle to acquire an image dataset that can be reconstructed into planar images throughout the breast, which reduces tissue overlap and has been demonstrated in multiple studies to aid in the sensitivity and specificity of breast cancer detection. Acquisition parameters for DBT go beyond the combinations of tube voltage, tube current, exposure time, anode target, and filter combinations of digital mammography to additionally include angular range, tube motion, and number of projections. DBT system designs are listed in Table 8-3. In Figure 8-24, DBT acquisition of x-ray projection images with x-ray tube angle is illustrated, and the reconstruction of in-focus image planes throughout the breast from the projection images is demonstrated by a simple "shift and add" algorithm.

Image resolution in DBT is described by in-plane and out-of-plane resolution. The in-plane resolution is the detail achieved in the x–y axis, with resolution cells ranging from 70 to 280 μm. Many systems for DBT operate in a detector element "binning" mode, where adjacent elements in the rows and columns are configured in 2×2 blocks to increase detector readout speed and to improve SNR at a cost of losing some in-plane resolution.

Out-of-plane (z-axis) resolution is a function of the overall tomographic angle, which ranges from 15° to 50° ($\pm 7.5°$ to $\pm 25°$), depending on the manufacturer. During acquisition, the x-ray tube moves in a symmetric arc around the center position of the detector. Larger angles provide better z-axis resolution (Fig. 8-25) but longer acquisition time is required (up to 25 s) and some peripheral breast tissue is not completely imaged at extreme angles, especially for larger and thicker compressed breasts. Systems with smaller tomographic angles have reduced z-axis resolution, which can be a problem for detection of masses; but the acquisitions are faster (about 4 s) and the in-plane (x–y) microcalcification visualization is better.

X-ray tube motion in DBT is either continuous or step and shoot. With continuous acquisition, the x-ray tube sweeps in an arc during gantry rotation, where a limited number of projections are acquired with short exposure times and fast readout of the detector. Faster image acquisition is possible, but a disadvantage is focal spot motion during image acquisition that adds geometric blurring to the projection images. In step and shoot acquisitions, the gantry comes to a complete stop for each

TABLE 8-3 DESIGN AND ACQUISITION CHARACTERISTICS OF DIGITAL BREAST TOMOSYNTHESIS SYSTEMS

PARAMETER	VENDOR A	VENDOR B	VENDOR C	VENDOR D
X-ray Tube				
Anode target	W	Mo/Rh	W	W
Filter(s)	W (700 µm)	Mo (30 µm); Rh (25 µm)	Rh (50 µm)	Al (700 µm); Rh (50 µm)
Tube motion	Continuous	Step and shoot	Continuous	Continuous
Flat Panel Detector				
Conversion	Direct—a-Se	Indirect—CsI	Direct—a-Se	Direct—a-Se
Pixel size (µm)	140 (2 × 2 bin)	100	85	150 (2 × 1 bin); 100 (HR)
Grid	No	Yes	No	No
Acquisition				
Tube arc (°)	15	25	50	15 (ST); 40 (HR)
# Projections	15	9	25	15
Scan time (s)	3.7	10	25	7 (ST); 9 (HR)

Notes: Vendor A: Hologic; B: General Electric; C: Siemens; D: Fujifilm; Al, aluminum; CsI, cesium iodide; FBP, filtered backprojection; HR, high resolution; Mo, molybdenum; Rh, rhodium; Se, selenium; ST, standard mode; W, tungsten.
Reprinted with permission from Tirada N, Li G, Dreizin D, Robinson L, et al. Digital Breast Tomosynthesis: Physics, Artifacts, and Quality Control Considerations. *Radiographics* 2019;39:413-426. Copyright © Radiological Society of North America. doi:10.1148/rg.2019180046..

projection to avoid motion blur, but a longer examination time increases the likelihood of blurring due to patient motion.

A larger number of projections, in general, will result in improved image quality from in-plane resolution and reduced blurring artifacts from high-density objects; however, there is a constraint on radiation dose, which must be kept to levels similar to mammography. Increasing the number of projections while keeping the dose/projection the same will cause an increase in radiation dose; but if the dose is reduced per projection so that the overall procedure dose is kept the same, the electronic noise will increase. Each manufacturer uses a fixed number of projections based on the tomographic angle, acquisition parameters, and processing techniques in an attempt to optimize the relationship between noise, dose, and image quality.

Full 3D tomographic reconstruction in DBT is not possible due to the limited tomographic angle. The limited angle acquisition geometry degrades resolution in the slice-thickness (z-axis) direction, which can be improved by increasing the tomographic angle. Simple back projection (Fig. 8-24) creates a tomographic image that is blurred in the process. Filtered back projection (FBP) applies a high-pass convolution filter to each image projection to improve image sharpness in the reconstructed images but results in higher noise and is prone to enhancing streak artifacts from metal surgical and biopsy clips. Iterative reconstruction (IR) is often applied in conjunction with the FBP reconstruction, where image quality is improved by using adaptive noise suppression techniques. Advanced IR algorithms require longer reconstruction times but provide enhancement by further reducing out-of-plane anatomical structures.

The reconstructed images are typically viewed in stack mode with in-focus planes located at 0.5 to 1.0 mm spacing parallel to the detector plane. While

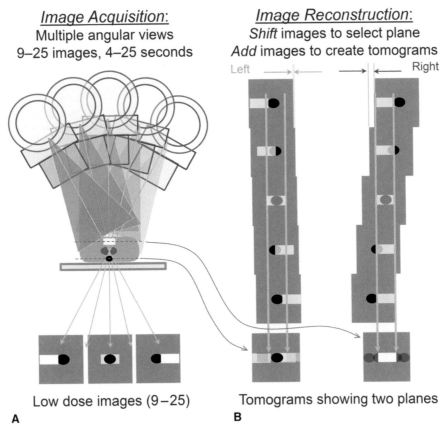

Image Acquisition:
Multiple angular views
9–25 images, 4–25 seconds

Image Reconstruction:
Shift images to select plane
Add images to create tomograms

Left → ←   → ← Right

Low dose images (9–25)

Tomograms showing two planes

A

B

■ **FIGURE 8-24 A.** Digital Breast Tomosynthesis (DBT) images are acquired using low-dose techniques over a limited projection angle, from ±7.5° up to ±25°, with 9 to 25 images constituting the dataset depending on manufacturer. A block and spherical object are illustrated at two depths within the breast. **B.** A simple "shift and add" of the acquired images illustrates the ability to synthesize tomograms with in-focus planes at various depths and blurred underlying and overlying signals. In practice, filtered back projection algorithms reconstruct planes incrementally at 1-mm depths throughout the breast.

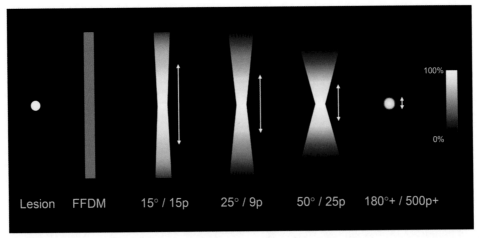

Lesion   FFDM   15° / 15p   25° / 9p   50° / 25p   180°+ / 500p+

100%

0%

■ **FIGURE 8-25** DBT *z*-axis resolution is dependent on the x-ray tube angle and determines the amount of overlying and underlying contributions to the in-focus plane for the tomosynthesis images. A projection image has 100% anatomical overlap. Shown are several manufacturers' implementations for progressively larger sweep angles up to 50° and number of projections (p), with less tissue overlap and improved z-axis resolution. On the right is 180°+ tube rotation with dedicated breast CT, demonstrating no overlap of tissues.

tomosynthesis images may be reconstructed at 1-mm locations in z, this does not mean that the depth resolution of the tomosynthesis dataset is 1 mm. For 1-mm reconstructions, the number of images is slightly greater than the compressed breast thickness (*e.g.*, for a 5-cm compressed breast thickness there will be about 55 images in the stack). Thick slabs can be created by the summation of many individual sections to provide better visualization and delineation of microcalcification distributions.

For one vendor's implementation, 15 projection images of the compressed breast are acquired over a range of 15° (1 image per degree) in 4 s (270 ms per image), using a W target with 0.7-mm Al filtered x-ray beam, 32 to 38 kV, with no antiscatter grid, and 2 × 2 pixel binning of the digital detector array (140-μm sampling). Technology enhancements now provide a high resolution (no binning) mode. MGD (see Section 8.6) for 15 image acquisitions is ~1.5 mGy for a 4.5-cm breast of 50% glandular and 50% adipose tissue (*e.g.*, the ACR accreditation phantom). As with conventional 2D mammography, larger breast thicknesses for tomosynthesis require higher doses. Overall, the dose in tomosynthesis is slightly higher but roughly equivalent to a single-view mammogram at the same compressed breast thickness (see Fig. 8-34).

Early deployment of DBT involved both 2D mammography and tomosynthesis image acquisitions for the CC and MLO projections, resulting in a doubling of the breast dose. Most systems now offer a synthethic 2D image reconstructed from the tomosynthesis data, which is a replacement for a 2D image mammogram of the breast (Ratanaprasatporn et al., 2017). Therefore, the dose in a screening tomosynthesis acquisition is similar to a 2D conventional screening acquisition. Because the synthetic 2D image presents the anatomy and microcalcifications with slightly reduced resolution, adoption of the synthetic mammogram in lieu of the physically acquired 2D mammogram is a local practice decision and not universal.

In Figure 8-26A, four images from ~70 tomograms reconstructed from a patient imaged in the left CC projection are selected, at the entrance and exit points of the x-ray beam and at two intermediate depths. Rapid "stack mode" viewing helps the perception of anatomical findings. Comparison of the 2D projection image obtained conventionally and the tomosynthesis-derived synthetic image is shown in Figure 8-26B. The spatial resolution of the 2D digital image is superior to the 2D synthesized image; however, image processing and calcification enhancement create a similar presentation.

Artifacts specific to DBT are chiefly related to the incomplete blurring of high-density anatomy and objects, due to the limited tomographic angle. These arise from the incomplete suppression of out-of-plane anatomic signals. Most obvious artifacts are seen adjacent to large calcifications and metal biopsy clips, where "halo" (dark and bright bands around the object) artifacts are common. Outside of the focal plane in adjacent slices, the anatomy appears slightly larger due to blurring, and slowly fades with distance from the current in-focus plane. Truncation artifacts occur when the breast tissue at the periphery of the detector does not fall within the entire reconstructed volume or results in non-uniform contribution due to a longer x-ray path through the breast tissues, resulting in a "stair-step" appearance. Anatomical objects far outside of the breast such as a partial projection of the shoulder or a biopsy needle can also result in stair-step artifacts. Patient motion, dead detector elements, and reconstruction errors also contribute to the artifacts in DBT images.

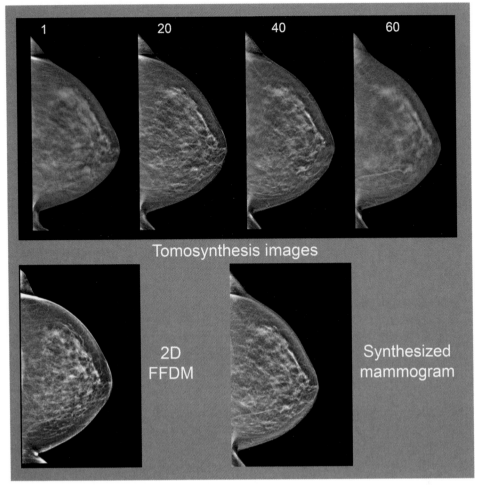

■ **FIGURE 8-26** Top row: Tomosynthesis images are shown for the left cranial-caudal projection at 4 depths (in mm) from the support platform. The overall breast dose is slightly higher than a single projection mammogram. Lower left: 2D full field digital mammogram (FFDM). Lower right: Synthesized mammogram (from tomosynthesis image acquisition) taken at a different time. This 2D image is often used in lieu of the 2D FFDM acquisition, and radiation dose to the breast can be reduced by about 50% compared to the combination.

8.4.3 Breast CT

Breast CT systems generally use cone beam CT geometry with a woman lying prone, with the single breast to be imaged hanging through a hole in the support table in "pendant geometry" (Fig. 8-27, left). Cone beam CT uses an FPD coupled with an x-ray tube in a horizontal orientation on a gantry, and low-dose projection images are acquired as the gantry rotates around the breast. The hundreds of projection images are used to reconstruct true 3D volume data sets of the breast anatomy. Breast compression is not used for breast CT, because the preferred geometry for CT of the breast is circular and not flat. Radiation dose levels are kept reasonable by using much higher x-ray beam energies than those typically used in digital mammography.

Breast CT produces true 3D volume data sets of the breast, which are less susceptible to superposition issues that can reduce cancer detection performance in 2D images (Fig. 8-27, right). When combined with the injection of an iodinated contrast agent (see Fig. 8-1), breast CT is thought to be largely equivalent to breast

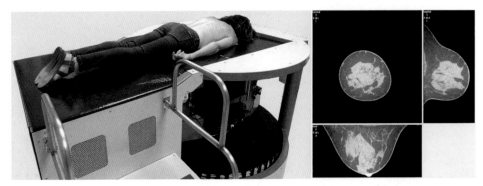

■ **FIGURE 8-27** Dedicated breast CT. Left: Patient is on the scanner in the prone position with one breast placed at the center of the gantry; about 500 projection images are acquired during a 360° rotation of the x-ray tube and detector about the breast. Right: CT tomographic slices are reconstructed in the coronal plane (upper left), with multiplanar reformatting to produce the sagittal (right) and axial (lower left) image planes.

MRI, which almost always uses (Gd) contrast injection. Compared to breast MRI, breast CT produces substantially higher spatial resolution images, can be used in women with metallic implants, is less likely to cause claustrophobia, and is far less expensive than breast MRI. Furthermore, breast CT systems can be located in the breast imaging clinic and operated by the principally female technologists in that setting.

8.4.4 Stereotactic Breast Biopsy

Stereotactic breast biopsy systems provide the ability to localize breast lesions in three dimensions and physically sample them with a targeted biopsy instrument. Generally, these systems are used for biopsy of microcalcification based lesions, whereas biopsy of masses is performed either with ultrasound guidance or with MRI. There are two stereotactic biopsy system configurations—one uses a horizontal table with the patient lying prone, with the breast to be biopsied hanging through a table port with the breast in pendant orientation. The other uses a standard digital mammography upright system and biopsy add-on device with the patient sitting or standing upright. Figure 8-28A shows a prone-geometry stereotactic biopsy system. One manufacturer's contemporary biopsy system uses a detector area of 14 cm × 12 cm and 70 μm detector element size with an amorphous selenium TFT array detector.

For biopsy, the breast is aligned and compressed with a paddle that has open apertures for needle access. After verification with a scout image, two images of the breast are acquired, at +15° and −15° from the normal (0°) position, causing the lesion projections to shift on the detector and in the acquired images, as shown in Figure 8-29. Manufacturers have specific methods of calculation. In the example shown in the figure, the shift distance in the x-direction of the lesion is measured in the stereo image pairs. This represents the opposite side of two right triangles with a common adjacent side, each at a 15° angle (30° total). The adjacent side represents the lesion distance from the detector. From trigonometry of right triangles, the lengths of the opposite ($X/2$) and adjacent (Z) sides are related to the angle as: Opposite/Adjacent = $\tan(\theta)$, where $\theta = 15°$. The equation is $\tan(15°) = (X/2)/Z$, and the solution is $Z = X/(2 \tan(15°)) = 1.866 \times X$ (mm). Trajectory information is determined by the position of the marked points in the images correlated with the frame of reference of the detector and the biopsy device, which is positioned under computer guidance algorithms. The radiologist verifies the positions, inserts the needle, and

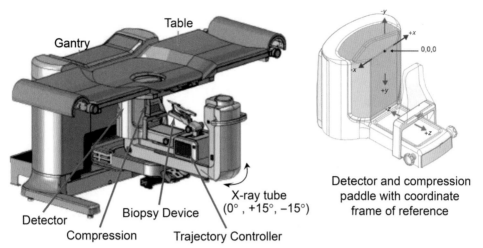

Detector and compression paddle with coordinate frame of reference

Gantry   **Table**

X-ray tube
(0°, +15°, −15°)

Detector
Compression   **Biopsy Device**   **Trajectory Controller**

■ **FIGURE 8-28** A stereotactic biopsy system with a prone positioning system is shown. The breast is positioned through the hole onto the detector platform and compressed by an open-access paddle (close-up shown on the right, with the *x, y, z* coordinate directions indicated). The x-ray tube pivots horizontally about a fulcrum point to acquire digital images at +15°, and −15° projections.

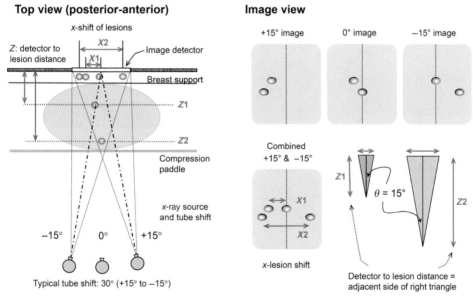

■ **FIGURE 8-29** Stereotactic breast biopsy geometry and lesion targeting are shown. Depicted on the left is a view looking from posterior to anterior of a breast slab and the x-ray beam angles used for acquiring stereo pairs. A lesion positioned closer to the detector (green, distance $Z1$) shifts less than a lesion further from the detector (red, distance $Z2$) in the +15° and −15° projections ($X1$ and $X2$, respectively). On the right are the corresponding image views (including the 0° image), illustrating the amount of shift for each lesion in the combined image. The x-shift distance gives solution for Z (distance to the detector, which is the adjacent side of a right triangle), where tan θ = opposite/adjacent sides, and $\frac{1}{2}X$ is the adjacent side distance. Thus, $\tan(15°) = (X/2)/Z$, and $Z = X/2 \tan(15°)$. From the x, y image locations and calculated z distance to the detector, the biopsy needle trajectory controller provides the three-dimensional coordinate targeting to the lesion.

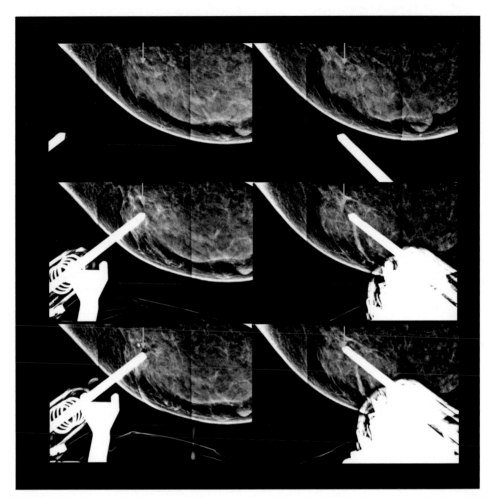

■ **FIGURE 8-30** Stereotactic biopsy images are acquired at −15° and +15° from the normal projection. Upper row is the stereo image pair from which the targeting coordinates and shift of the lesions are determined. Middle row is the "prefire" biopsy needle inserted into the breast a distance from the target. Bottom row shows the biopsy needle at the intended location in the "postfire" stereo image pair. The orange arrows point at the same location in all three image pairs, and the compression paddle square open area is indicated by the vertical and horizontal lines in the images.

activates the biopsy mechanism to capture the tissue samples under suction through a side port in biopsy needle device. Example image pairs and the biopsy needle placement are shown in Figure 8-30.

8.5 PROCESSING, VIEWING, AND ANALYZING IMAGES

8.5.1 Image Preprocessing and Detector Corrections

Even the best digital detectors have malfunctioning detector elements, column and line defects, and variation in gain across the detector area. Without correction, these artifacts would result in unacceptable image quality and interfere with the diagnostic interpretation. Manufacturers use "preprocessing" algorithms to correct these defects. First, the locations of inoperative detector elements and line defects are determined,

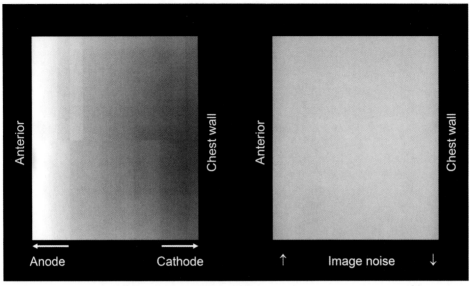

■ **FIGURE 8-31** Gain correction for flat-panel detectors—this example is for a tungsten target and rhodium filter. Left: Uncorrected flat-field image acquired with uniform x-ray field and 4 cm Lucite phantom on the breast platform. Note the detector modules and variable gain of this inverted grayscale image, where brighter grayscale indicates less x-ray fluence (signal). Right: Gain-corrected image of the Lucite phantom showing uniform response. Image noise (standard deviation of digital values) is higher on the anterior side of the uniform x-ray image from less x-ray exposure due to the anode heel effect.

and these data are interpolated from nearest-neighbor pixels. Next, a uniform beam of x-rays exposes the detector and generates an image, showing the variable gain from the detector submodule electronics as well as systematic variations such as the anode heel effect. Multiple images are averaged together to create a *flat-field* correction image, which is normalized and inverted as an inverse-gain map. When applied to an uncorrected image on a pixel-by-pixel basis, the gain variations are normalized, and the corrected "raw" image is uniform without major deviations (Fig. 8-31). In practice, flat-field gain maps for various acquisition conditions are measured, stored on the system, and applied to each clinical image that is acquired under similar conditions.

8.5.2 Image Postprocessing

Digital detectors have exposure dynamic range (the minimum to maximum x-ray intensities that can be incorporated into a useful signal) greater than 1,000:1 in comparison to that of screen-film of about 25:1 for mammography. The unprocessed raw data that have been corrected for detector flaws (bad detector elements and gain variation) are contained in the DICOM *For Processing* image shown in Figure 8-32A. This image type has wide latitude, has digital signals that are proportional to the detector exposure or the logarithm of exposure, and is therefore quantitatively consistent from manufacturer to manufacturer. While not useful for diagnosis by the radiologist, this is the preferred image for *Computer-Assisted Detection* (CADe) and AI/Deep Learning programs because of its quantitative nature, which use computer algorithms to identify image features that may indicate the presence of breast cancer. Contrast enhancement of the *For Processing* image is shown in Figure 8-32B, which looks similar to a screen-film image. Non-linear postprocessing algorithms applied to the *For Processing* image data identify the skin line of the mammogram, modify the local-area pixel

■ **FIGURE 8-32 A.** The DICOM *For Processing* images of the right and left cranial-caudal breast projection images have detector and gain map corrections applied with unity radiographic contrast. **B.** Linear contrast and brightness adjustments are applied—the skin line is not visible. **C.** Non-linear processing identifies the breast skin line and densest parts of the image, to equalize the response of the processed image with contrast and spatial resolution enhancement.

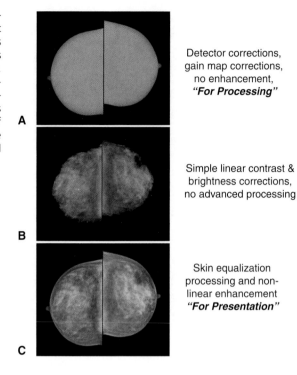

Detector corrections, gain map corrections, no enhancement, **"For Processing"**

Simple linear contrast & brightness corrections, no advanced processing

Skin equalization processing and non-linear enhancement **"For Presentation"**

values, and equalize the response in the high-signal, low-attenuation skin area to the other areas of the breast. Contrast and spatial resolution enhancements are then applied to create the *For-Presentation* image for viewing and diagnosis (Fig. 8-32C). Each manufacturer has proprietary methods of image processing. For consistency, the radiologist must adopt a particular "look" for viewing current and prior digital mammograms, making it a challenge when images from different manufacturers are compared in prior and current images to identify clinically relevant changes. Example images from two manufacturers demonstrate the differences of non-linear image processing algorithms in Figure 8-33.

8.5.3 Image Size Considerations

Because of the high spatial resolution characteristics of digital mammography, images are quite large. A digital mammography system with a 0.07-mm pixel, 2 bytes per pixel, and a 24 × 29-cm active detector area produces a 27-MB image. One screening study (4 images) will therefore contain 108 MB of data and, if 3 years of prior images are reviewed, 432 MB of data will be required per patient reading session. The network overhead and storage required for the picture archiving and communications system are very large and even larger with the increased number of images in a diagnostic exam. In addition, if *For Processing* images are stored, another factor of two in data size is incurred. Typical digital image sizes for 2D mammography systems are listed in Table 8-4.

For DBT, the amount of data is significantly increased with the number of projection images (9 to 25 images) in addition to the number of 1-mm reconstructed tomographic slices equal to the compressed breast thickness in mm plus a few extra (*e.g.*, for 60 mm, a total of about 65 images are reconstructed). Each manufacturer has slightly different acquisition and processing schemes, with storage requirements for the projection images (9 to 25 images) and tomosynthesis slices (1 mm through the compressed thickness) listed in Table 8-5.

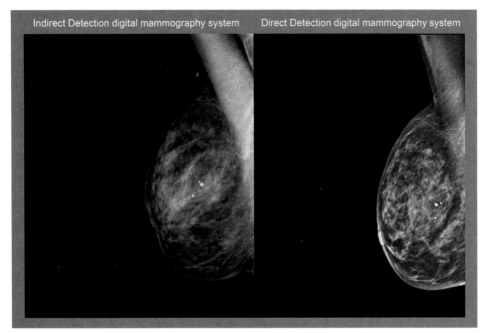

Indirect Detection digital mammography system   Direct Detection digital mammography system

■ **FIGURE 8-33** Manufacturers use different processing algorithms to distinguish their products and take advantage of the beneficial characteristics of the detector. On the left is an image from an indirect conversion detector, and on the right from a direct conversion detector. An issue is the consistency of appearance when evaluating longitudinal studies acquired on different systems and the ability to adapt to the unique characteristics of the images.

Many specific considerations for handling, viewing, and storing mammography and DBT images (image compression, storage retention) are described in the ACR practice guideline, "Determinants of Image Quality in Digital Mammography" (ACR, 2017) and the Integrating the Healthcare Enterprise (IHE) profiles (IHE, 2007, 2016).

8.5.4 **Image Display Considerations**

Diagnostic interpretation of digital mammograms should be performed on display monitors approved by the FDA for mammography having a minimum of 5 million pixels (5 MP), a portrait display of ~53 cm diagonal with a pixel pitch of ~160 μm (2,560 × 2,048 matrix) and a calibrated, sustained luminance of at least 450 cd/m^2 (per ACR guidelines for digital mammography). Monitors of

TABLE 8-4 DIGITAL IMAGE SIZE FOR MAMMOGRAPHY SCREENING EXAMS

DETECTOR TYPE	FOV (cm)	PIXEL SIZE (mm)	IMAGE SIZE (MB)	EXAM SIZE (MB)	+3 Y PRIORS (MB)
Indirect TFT	19 × 23	0.100	9	35	140
Indirect TFT	24 × 31	0.100	15	60	240
Direct TFT	18 × 24	0.085	12	48	192
Direct TFT	24 × 30	0.085	20	80	320
Direct TFT	18 × 24	0.070	18	70	280
Direct TFT	24 × 29	0.070	27	108	432

TABLE 8-5 DIGITAL BREAST TOMOSYNTHESIS IMAGE STORAGE REQUIREMENTS—60 cm COMPRESSED BREAST THICKNESS, 24 × 30 cm FIELD SIZE—THREE MANUFACTURER IMPLEMENTATIONS

DBT	INDIRECT DETECTOR, 0.100 mm		DIRECT DETECTOR, 0.085 mm		DIRECT DETECTOR, 0.070 mm	
Acquisition	Matrix	# Images	Size (MB)	Matrix	# Images	Size (MB)	Matrix	# Images	Size (MB)
Projections	2,394 × 2,850	9	120	2,816 × 3,584	26	507	2,560 × 4,096	15	315
Planes	2,394 × 2,850	145	1,900	2,816 × 3,584	61	821	2,560 × 3,328	66	1,120

Note: Detector element binning (2 × 2) is used by some manufacturers in the acquisition of the planar images, with reconstruction of the tomosynthesis planes at a smaller pixel pitch (e.g., 140 to 100 μm).

Data rom Tirada N, Li G, Dreizin D, et al. Digital breast tomosynthesis: physics, artifacts, and quality control considerations. *Radiographics.* 2019;39:413-426. doi: 10.1148/rg.2019180046.

lower luminance make reading conditions more susceptible to poor illuminance conditions (background lighting) in the reading room area. A typical workstation configuration has two 5 MP monitors side by side, with alternatives of a single 10 or 12 MP monitor of 76–80 cm diagonal to create two virtual seamless display areas of at least 5 MP. A lower resolution, smaller format "navigation" monitor is used for patient lists and operating system access. All monitors should be calibrated to conform to the DICOM Grayscale Standard Display Function (GSDF), as described in Chapter 5, to ensure image grayscale range and anatomic contrast is consistently and optimally displayed.

To optimize the workflow of the radiologist, mammography workstations should provide automated *mammography-specific hanging protocols* that present the images in a useful and sequential way for review and diagnosis according to view, laterality, magnification, tomosynthesis series, and prior examination comparisons.

8.5.5 IHE Mammography Image and Digital Breast Tomosynthesis Profiles

Implementation of full field digital mammography over the past two decades has resulted in several differences in image acquisition, processing, and display attributes, creating an issue for interoperability of sites reviewing mammography images on Picture Archiving and Communications Systems (PACS). The IHE initiative (see Chapter 5) defines Integration Profiles that use established standards (*e.g.*, DICOM) to integrate systems from multiple vendors to address issues of incompatibility and inconsistency for efficient workflow and patient care. The IHE Mammography Image Profile (IHE, 2007), is designed to provide complete storage and retrieval of mammography data with sufficient display functionality to allow adequate review of current and prior images and CAD results (see next subsection) for the purpose of primary interpretation by radiologists. This profile specifies the way to generate correct digital mammography image content to ensure optimal presentation of images at a mammography review workstation, including:

- Necessary data for identifying patients, technique acquisition parameters
- Scaling of images from the same patient regardless of detector and detector element dimensions, to display at the same size during interpretation
- Orienting and justifying images correctly for proper interpretation
- Providing a clear definition of breast tissue and background air to maintain background blackness during contrast adjustments for optimal viewing of the breast structures

With the introduction of newer pertinent DICOM objects, such as the breast tomonsynthesis object (BTO) and breast projection x-ray image object (BPO), the IHE has published the Digital Breast Tomosynthesis Extension (DBT Extension) Profile (IHE, 2016), which specifies the creation, exchange and use of DBT images. It defines basic display capabilities that image displays are expected to provide for simultaneous review of DBT, conventional 2D and synthesized (generated 2D) mammography images.

8.5.6 Computer-Aided Detection and Artificial Intelligence

A computer-aided detection (CADe) system is a computer-based set of algorithms that incorporates pattern recognition and uses sophisticated matching and similarity rules to flag possible findings on a digital mammogram. The computer software searches for abnormal areas of density, mass, calcifications, and/or structural patterns (*e.g.*, spiculated masses, architectural distortion) that may indicate the presence of cancer. The CADe system then marks these areas on the images, alerting the radiologist for further analysis. For digital mammograms, the CADe algorithms require the use of linear, *For Processing* images for analysis, as the algorithms are trained on these images.

Computer-assisted diagnosis (CADx) devices include software that provides information beyond identifying suspicious findings; this additional information includes an assessment of identified features in terms of the likelihood of the presence or absence of disease, or disease type. For instance, a CADx system for mammography will not only identify clusters of microcalcifications and masses on digital mammograms but also provide a probability of malignancy score to the radiologist for each identified "lesion."

CAD systems using heuristic rules are being supplanted by AI and machine learning algorithms that use algorithms that mimic the human brain and learning process. "Convolutional neural networks" (CNN) (see Chapter 5) AI algorithms require a large training set of annotated and curated images associated with known outputs, including malignant and benign lesions. Training is applied on thousands of input images. Once trained, the AI algorithm has "knowledge by node weighting" and can be applied to unknown cases to produce detection cues. The future of AI is expanding and will likely be a major component in assisting the radiologist in diagnosis of mammograms and associated breast imaging modalities moving forward.

8.6 RADIATION DOSIMETRY

X-ray mammography is the technique of choice for detecting non-palpable breast cancers in a screening environment. However, the risk of carcinogenesis from the radiation dose to the breast is of concern because of the very large number of women undergoing repeated screening exams. Thus, the optimization of breast dose is important and dose monitoring of the mammography equipment is required annually by the MQSA regulations.

The glandular tissue is the tissue of concern in the breast, and thus the established dose metric is the *mean glandular dose* (MGD) (also called the average glandular dose). Because the glandular tissues receive different doses due to spatial heterogeneity, estimating the dose is not trivial. For mammography accreditation, a phantom with a 50% glandular, 50% adipose tissue composition is used for the measurement of dose.

8.6.1 Mean Glandular Dose

In one method of estimating MGD, the following formula is used:

$$D_g = X_{ESAK} \times D_{gN}, \qquad [8\text{-}3]$$

where D_g is the MGD, X_{ESAK} is the entrance surface (skin) air kerma (ESAK) to the breast in mGy, and D_{gN} is a conversion factor specified as mGy glandular dose per mGy entrance surface air kerma.

X_{ESAK} is determined in two steps:

1. The technique factors (target/filter combination, kV, HVL, and mAs) and known x-ray tube output at the calibration distance give the air kerma at 50 cm from the focal spot (see Fig. 8-13).

2. The breast compression thickness and distance from the breast support platform to the image plane (with the known SID) give the distance from the focal spot to the surface of the breast. Calculation of the air kerma to the surface of the breast is determined with inverse square law adjustment of the two distances (see Eq. 8-1). This is conceptually similar to what is done in radiography dose assessment as well (see Eq. 11-11).

The conversion factor D_{gN} in Equation 8-3 is determined by Monte Carlo computer simulation methods to track radiation dose to the glandular tissues. The algorithms consider tube target material, filter material, kV, HVL, x-ray breast thickness, and glandular/adipose tissue composition percentages to arrive at D_{gN} values included in many tables (Boone, 1999). Monte Carlo derived D_{gN} values are listed in Table 8-6 for a W target/0.05 mm Rh filter x-ray spectrum over a range of kV and HVL inputs for various breast thicknesses of 50% glandular tissue composition. Using the example calculation in Section 8.1 (tube output and output rate) for a 6-cm compressed breast at 30 kV for a W/Rh target/filter combination and 200 mAs, X_{ESAK} = 9.4 mGy. The corresponding D_{gN} (from Table 8-6) is 0.230 mGy MGD/mGy ESAK, and therefore the MGD is calculated as 9.4 × 0.230 = 2.16 mGy. D_{gN} values decrease with an increase in breast thickness for constant beam quality and breast composition, because the glandular tissues furthest from the entrance beam receive much less dose in the thicker breast due to attenuation (e.g., D_{gN} = 0.327 for 4 cm versus 0.173 for 8 cm compressed breast thickness using a W target and Rh filtration at the same kV). However, the lower D_{gN} values for thicker breasts are more than offset by a large increase in the ESAK necessary to achieve the desired image quality (SNR) in a digital image. Measured MGDs for 50% glandular/50% adipose tissue of 2- to 8-cm tissue thicknesses using a W/Rh spectrum and AEC in auto-filter mode are shown in Figure 8-34 for a digital system using 2D and DBT acquisitions.

Another breast dosimetry method adopted by the 2018 ACR QC program and some manufacturers uses the following equation:

$$MGD = Kgcs \qquad [8\text{-}4]$$

TABLE 8-6 CONVERSION FACTOR D_{gN} (mGy MEAN GLANDULAR DOSE PER mGy ENTRANCE SURFACE AIR KERMA TO THE BREAST) FOR W TARGET AND Rh FILTER, 2, 4, 6, 8 cm BREAST THICKNESSES OF 50% GLANDULAR AND 50% ADIPOSE TISSUE COMPOSITION

		D_{gN} (mGy MGD/mGy ENTRANCE SURFACE AIR KERMA)			
	HVL	Compressed Breast Thickness			
kV	(mm Al)	2 cm	4 cm	6 cm	8 cm
27	0.489	0.491	0.307	0.215	0.161
28	0.500	0.499	0.314	0.220	0.165
29	0.509	0.506	0.321	0.225	0.169
30	0.518	0.513	0.327	0.230	0.173
31	0.527	0.519	0.332	0.234	0.177
32	0.535	0.525	0.338	0.239	0.181

Note that HVL is determined from the Monte Carlo simulation, and does not include the attenuation of the compression paddle, which increases the HVL to slightly higher values than indicated, and will thus represent a slight underestimate of the D_{gN} factor for a given kV. Expanded tables include a range of HVL for each kV.
Adapted with permission from Boone JM. Glandular breast dose for monoenergetic and high-energy x-ray beams: Monte Carlo assessment. *Radiology*. 1999;213(1):23-37. Copyright © Radiological Society of North America. doi: 10.1148/radiology.213.1.r99oc3923.

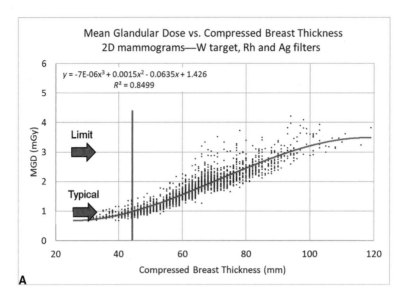

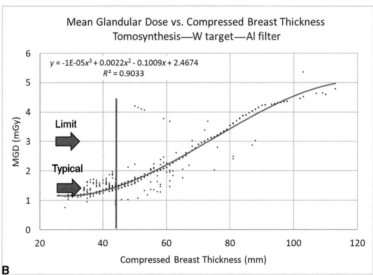

■ **FIGURE 8-34** Mean Glandular Dose for 2D mammograms and digital breast tomosynthesis exams—sample of one month of data at UC Davis Health Mammography Clinic. **A.** MGD versus compressed breast thickness for examinations for screening mammograms using automatic exposure control (selection of kV and filter) for a system with a tungsten target and rhodium/silver filters of 0.05 mm thickness. **B.** MGD versus compressed breast thickness for digital breast tomosynthesis screening examinations using automatic exposure control (selection of kV and filter) for a system with a tungsten target and aluminum filter of 0.7 mm thickness. In both graphs a least square fit of the data to a 3rd order polynomial is shown.

In Equation 8-4, MGD is equal to the product of the entrance surface air kerma, K (the same as X_{ESAK} as previously described) and three Monte Carlo derived conversion factors. The factor g is the fraction of K that is absorbed by the glandular tissue, for a breast of 50% glandular and 50% adipose composition calculated for a range of beam qualities (HVL) and breast thicknesses. As there is a wide heterogeneity in breast tissue composition, the factor c corrects for those differences in glandularity from 50%, and like g, is also a function of beam quality and breast thickness. The factor s accounts for the characteristics of the x-ray spectrum based on the target and filter combination for other than a Mo target and Mo filter. Further details and expanded tables are available (Dance et al., 2000, 2009).

These two methods provide a similar estimate of MGD based upon the entrance surface air kerma, and one or the other is used by the manufacturers to report the values with the acquired images. The method expressed in Equation 8-3 requires separate tables for each target and filter combination and percent glandular tissue composition, while the method expressed in Equation 8-4 uses correction factors to adjust for target and filter spectral differences.

MGD for DBT exams has a dependence on x-ray tube projection angle, where the dose is lower as the angle increases from the 0° projection (the reference dose) by up to 10% at steeper angles for current systems. The relative glandular dose (RGD) as described by the AAPM Report 223 (Sechopoulos et al., 2014) for the D_{gN} method (Eq. 8-3) and the T factors as described as an added factor to the United Kingdom and European protocols (Dance et al., 2011) for the MGD method (Eq. 8-4) are ways to improve the accuracy of the dose delivered to the breast in the tomosynthesis acquisition.

The overall MGD estimates have been based on assumptions of a homogeneous glandular tissue distribution in the breast. More recent work from breast CT researchers demonstrates a heterogenous distribution of glandular tissues, with a larger fraction located near the center of the breast as shown in Figure 8-35 (Hernandez et al., 2015). Glandular tissue in this instance is thus shielded by a more superficial layer of adipose tissue, and consequently the historical D_{gN} (or K) values are about 30% less when this more accurate model of breast tissue is considered. It will, however, take some time before these new values are incorporated into official MQSA dose estimates.

8.6.2 Factors Affecting Breast Dose

Breast dose in mammography varies considerably and depends on several technical and physical considerations.

Detector characteristics and detective quantum efficiency (DQE): Detector element size, method of x-ray conversion (direct or indirect), thickness of the converter, and electronic/digitization noise affect DQE, a measure of information transfer efficiency (see Chapter 4). DQE is measured as a function of spatial frequency, DQE(f), and ranges from 100% (all information recorded) to 0% (no information recorded). In general, the radiation dose needed to achieve a level of SNR in a digital image is inversely related to the detector DQE at zero spatial frequency, DQE(0)$^{-1}$.

Acquisition technique factors: Target, filter, and kV affect x-ray beam HVL and thus beam penetrability. A higher HVL x-ray beam will be more penetrable, thus requiring less incident exposure to the breast to achieve enough transmitted fluence to the detector; this lowers the MGD, but also decreases subject contrast.

Antiscatter grids: Grids reject scattered radiation to improve subject contrast but also absorb a fraction of primary radiation and increase radiation dose, typically by a factor of 2 or more, to compensate for lost primary photons and statistical image characteristics. Most mammography systems use an antiscatter grid for contact mammography but not for magnification exams.

Breast thickness and tissue composition: Compressed breast thickness is the most impactful factor on breast dose, as x-rays are exponentially attenuated. A similar exponential compensation in the incident radiation fluence is needed to ensure an adequate number of transmitted photons to the detector to achieve an appropriate SNR.

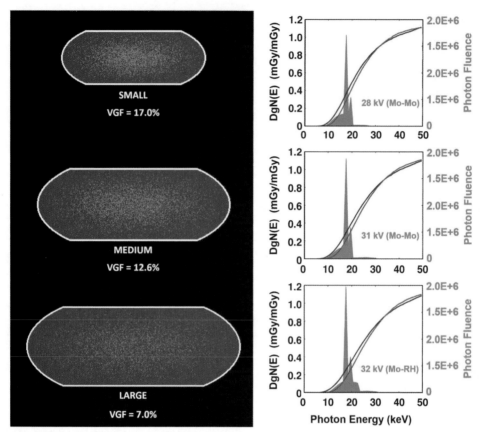

■ **FIGURE 8-35** Glandular tissue is not homogeneously distributed in the breast (Hernandez et al., 2015). Left column: Small, medium, and large breast cross sections show typical glandular tissue distribution and volume glandular fractions from analysis of breast CT data. Right column: Monte Carlo derived D_{gN} values as a function of photon energy, and the corresponding spectra used for imaging the breasts show the D_{gN} values for a homogeneous glandular/adipose mixture (blue curves) and the D_{gN} values assuming a heterogenous glandular/adipose distribution (red curves). On average, about a 30% lower breast MGD estimate occurs when considering the effect of shielding by the adipose tissue. (Courtesy of Andrew M. Hernandez, PhD, UC Davis Health.)

The MQSA regulations limit the MGD for a compressed breast thickness of 4.2 cm and a breast composition of 50% glandular and 50% adipose tissue (the MQSA-approved mammography phantom) to 3 mGy per mammogram. The same dose limit applies for DBT. If the MGD exceeds 3 mGy, the mammography system must be taken out of service until it is calibrated and is within compliance. The MGD typically ranges from less than 1 mGy to about 1.8 mGy per view for flat-panel detectors when imaging the accreditation phantom for mammography and DBT acquisitions.

8.7 REGULATORY REQUIREMENTS

Regulations mandated by the MQSA of 1992 specify operational and technical requirements that are required to perform mammography in the United States. These regulations are contained in Title 21 of the Code of Federal Regulations, Part 900.

8.7.1 Accreditation and Certification

Accreditation and certification are two separate processes. For a facility to perform mammography legally under MQSA, it must be accredited and certified. To begin the process, the facility must first apply for accreditation from an accreditation body (the ACR or one of several states if located in one of those states). The accreditation body verifies that the mammography facility meets standards set forth by the MQSA to ensure safe, high-quality mammography through annual inspections conducted by federally trained and certified personnel. The scope of the accreditation process includes assessment of the initial qualifications and continuing medical education of interpreting physicians, technologists, and physicists involved in the mammography program. An active QC program is required. *Certification* is the approval of a facility by the US FDA to provide mammography services and is granted when accreditation is achieved.

8.7.2   Quality Assurance and Quality Control

QA in mammography comprises all management practices implemented by the Lead Interpreting Radiologist in charge of the program to ensure the appropriateness of every imaging procedure, that the images are correctly interpreted with results made available in a timely manner, and that the examination has the lowest possible radiation dose, cost, and inconvenience to the patient. The QA program includes efficacy studies, continuing education, QC, preventive maintenance, and calibration of equipment. With an enhanced focus on image quality, the FDA launched the Enhancing Quality Using the Inspection Program (EQUIP) on January 1, 2017, under the auspices of the Division of Mammography Quality Standards (DMQS) to emphasize the responsibilities of the Lead Interpreting Radiologist in the clinical image quality process, where previously there was greater emphasis to the technical aspects of the QC program. The EQUIP process requires that mechanisms are put in place to provide ongoing feedback by the Interpreting Radiologists on image quality, for documenting corrective action and effectiveness of corrective action taken, engaging in regular reviews of image quality for technologists, documenting the review process, and having a system in place for the Lead Interpreting Radiologist review of all required performance tests, with corrective actions taken. Ultimate responsibility for mammography QA rests with the radiologist in charge of the mammography practice, who must ensure that all interpreting radiologists, mammography technologists, and medical physicists meet the initial qualifications and maintain the continuing education and experience required by the MQSA regulations.

Mammography is a very demanding imaging procedure in terms of equipment performance, with strict QC procedures in place to ensure reproducible, consistent, and safe operation. Achieving the full potential of mammography requires careful optimization of acquisition protocols, equipment, and associated components of the imaging chain. Even a small change in performance or image-viewing conditions can decrease the sensitivity and specificity of interpretation of the exam. Thus, many of the MQSA requirements are technical regarding the operation of the mammography and peripheral equipment. Essentially all mammography systems in the United States now have digital detectors, and QC entails following the manufacturer's specific FDA-approved QC procedures for digital mammography systems in terms of scope and frequency of required tests. After many years of stakeholder meetings at the ACR, a testing procedure for *all* digital mammography and DBT systems has been developed. This "unified" QC program (ACR, 2018a) is FDA-approved as an alternate, optional way to meet accreditation requirements and annual physics evaluations, including the use of an updated and required accreditation phantom described in the next section. For multi-vendor mammography clinics, in which specific QC tests can vary significantly from vendor to vendor, adoption of this alternate QC program could be useful by providing consistent tests for equipment performance verification, as well as unified display monitor evaluation for both technologist and radiologist workstations.

8.7.3 Accreditation Phantoms, QC Tests, and Performance Requirements

The purpose of the mammography accreditation phantom is to simulate the radiographic attenuation of an average-size compressed breast with structures that model very basic image characteristics of breast parenchyma and cancer. Its role is to help determine the adequacy of the overall imaging system including digital postprocessing in terms of detection of subtle radiographic findings in DICOM "For Presentation" images. It is also used to assess the quantitative SNR and CNR reproducibility over time in DICOM "For Processing" images.

There are now two accreditation phantoms: the legacy phantom (Fig. 8-36), and an updated digital phantom (Fig. 8-37), the latter being required for the ACR QC program alternative standard including DBT QC procedures. Both are similar in terms of objects embedded within a wax phantom insert and representing a 4.2-cm breast of 50% glandular, 50% adipose tissue content. The updated phantom provides a more challenging test for visualizing smaller objects of strict composition and size in the phantom wax insert, a block of PMMA to totally cover the digital detector area, and a shallow uniform depth hole drilled into the PMMA above the wax insert in lieu of an external attached disk for measuring the contrast signal. Identification of the smallest objects of each type that are visible in the phantom image with no obvious artifacts indicates system performance. MQSA image quality standards require a minimum number of visualized objects of each type (fibers, calcifications, masses) at an MGD of less than 3 mGy.

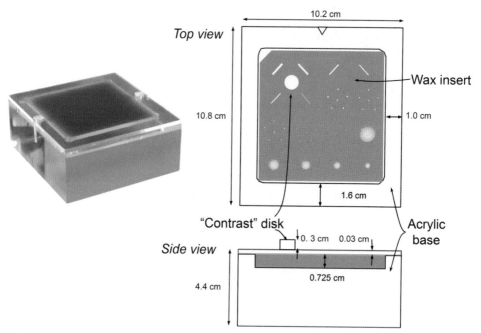

■ **FIGURE 8-36** The legacy mammography accreditation phantom contains a wax insert, which has six nylon fibers, five aluminum oxide speck groups (six specks in each group), and five disks simulating masses. The wax insert is placed into a cutout in a clear acrylic phantom. The phantom is intended to mimic the attenuation characteristics of a "standard breast" of 4.2-cm compressed breast thickness of 50% adipose and 50% glandular tissue composition, where the smallest object of each type is identified in the acquired image. Note the "contrast disk" on top of the phantom, which generates a signal for evaluation of contrast required for some system manufacturers.

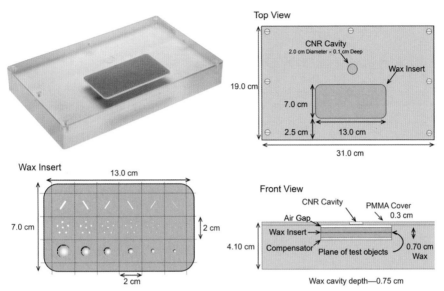

■ **FIGURE 8-37** ACR full-field digital mammography phantom contains a wax insert embedded in a large area (19 cm × 31 cm × 4.1 cm) acrylic block. The wax insert has fibers, specks, and masses of diminishing size from left to right in rows as shown in the lower left schematic, where the smallest object along each row is identified in the acquired image.

For digital mammography, each manufacturer has set the criteria for meeting an acceptable performance level in terms of qualitative visibility of the objects in the legacy accreditation phantom in DICOM "For Presentation" images, as well as specific tests using the quantitative evaluation of regions of interest (ROIs) to calculate SNR and CNR in DICOM "For Processing" images. Minimum standards require visualizing 4 fibers, 3 speck groups, and 3 masses. Quantitative evaluation for one manufacturer includes the evaluation of the signal under the added acrylic disk and in the background using ROIs of a specified size and locations, while another uses the largest mass in the legacy accreditation phantom and an adjacent background location. The SNR is calculated as the average signal in the background ROI divided by its standard deviation. The CNR is determined as the difference of the average signals from the object and background, divided by the standard deviation in the background ROI. Each manufacturer requires the mammography site technologist to measure the SNR and CNR weekly using the accreditation phantom, and to verify that the calculated values are within the manufacturer's established limits. When found out of tolerance, the system may not be used clinically until the causes of the failures are determined and the corrections are implemented and verified with subsequent tests.

In Table 8-7 the "harmonized" tests for all digital mammography and DBT equipment (excluding manufacturer required calibrations such as detector correction and flat-fielding procedures) are listed. For this program, the updated accreditation phantom (Fig. 8-37) must be used. Visualization of ≥2 fibers, ≥3 calcification groups, and ≥2 masses is the minimum requirement for 2D mammography and digital tomosynthesis acquisitions. In addition, no obvious artifacts should be visible in the acquired images. Figure 8-38 shows a comparison of the images from the two phantoms.

Federal regulations specify three different categories of QC tests (*A, B, C*) and action levels that must occur for digital mammography systems.

Category A QC tests are specific to the digital acquisition system and, when outside of the prescribed action limits, the source of the problem must be identified, and corrective action taken before any patient imaging can be performed. These tests

TABLE 8-7 DIGITAL MAMMOGRAPHY (2D and DBT) QUALITY CONTROL TESTS—ACR 2018 QUALITY CONTROL MANUAL

Technologist Tests		
1. ACR DM Phantom Image Quality	Weekly	Before clinical use
2. Computed Radiography Cassette Erasure *(if applicable)*	Weekly	Before clinical use
3. Compression Thickness Indicator	Monthly	Within 30 days
4. Visual Checklist	Monthly	Critical items: before clinical use; less critical items: within 30 days
5. Acquisition Workstation Monitor QC	Monthly	Within 30 days; before clinical use for severe defects
6. Radiologist Workstation Monitor QC	Monthly	Within 30 days; before clinical use for severe defects
7. Film Printer QC *(if applicable)*	Monthly	Before clinical use
8. Viewbox Cleanliness *(if applicable)*	Monthly	Before clinical use
9. Facility QC Review	Quarterly	Not applicable
10. Compression Force	Semiannual	Before clinical use
11. Manufacturer Calibrations *(if applicable)*	Mfr. Recommendation	Before clinical use
Optional—Repeat Analysis	As Needed	Within 30 days after analysis
Optional—System QC for Radiologist	As Needed	Within 30 days; before clinical use for severe artifacts
Optional—Radiologist Image Quality Feedback	As Needed	Not applicable
Medical Physicist Tests		
1. Mammography Equipment Evaluation (MEE)—MQSA Requirements	MEE	Before clinical use
2. ACR DM Phantom Image Quality	MEE and Annual	Before clinical use
3. DBT Z Resolution	MEE and Annual	Within 30 days
4. Spatial Resolution	MEE and Annual	Within 30 days
5. DBT Volume Coverage	MEE and Annual	Before clinical use
6. Automatic Exposure Control System Performance	MEE and Annual	Within 30 days
7. Average (Mean) Glandular Dose	MEE and Annual	Before clinical use
8. Unit Checklist	MEE and Annual	Critical items: before clinical use; less critical items: within 30 days
9. Computed Radiography *(if applicable)*	MEE and Annual	Before clinical use
10. Acquisition Workstation Monitor QC	MEE and Annual	Within 30 days; before clinical use for severe defects
11. Radiologist Workstation Monitor QC	MEE and Annual	Within 30 days; before clinical use for severe defects
12. Film Printer QC *(if applicable)*	MEE and Annual	Before clinical use

TABLE 8-7 DIGITAL MAMMOGRAPHY (2D and DBT) QUALITY CONTROL TESTS—ACR 2018 QUALITY CONTROL MANUAL (*Continued*)

13. Evaluation of Site's Technologist QC Program	Annual	Within 30 days
14. Evaluation of Display Device Technologist QC Program	Annual	Within 30 days
15. Manufacturer Calibrations (*if applicable*)	Mfr. Recommendation	Before clinical use
16. Collimation Assessment	MEE or Troubleshooting Annual (DBT only)	Within 30 days
MEE or Troubleshooting—Beam Quality (Half-Value Layer) Assessment	MEE or Troubleshooting	Before clinical use
MEE or Troubleshooting—kVp Accuracy and Reproducibility	MEE or Troubleshooting	MEE: before clinical use; troubleshooting: within 30 days
Troubleshooting—Ghost Image Evaluation	Troubleshooting	Before clinical use
Troubleshooting—Viewbox Luminance	Troubleshooting	Not applicable

Reproduced with permission from Digital Mammography (2D and DBT) Quality Control Tests, from ACR. *Digital Mammography Quality Control Manual.* Reston, VA: American College of Radiology; 2018..

include system resolution, breast dose, accreditation phantom image quality evaluation, SNR/CNR, flat-field calibration, and compression paddle operation.

Category B QC tests are specific to the performance of a diagnostic device used for mammographic interpretation, including the review workstation and laser film printer. When tests produce results that fall outside of the action limits specified by the manufacturer, the source of the problem shall be identified and corrective action taken before that specific device can be used for interpretation. Image acquisition can continue, if there are alternate approved diagnostic devices available for interpretation.

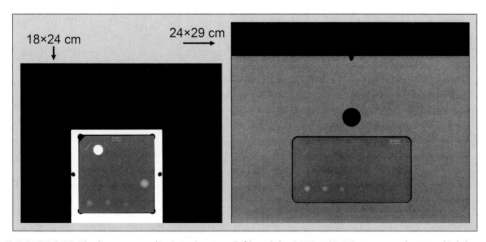

■ **FIGURE 8-38** The legacy accreditation phantom (left) and the 2018 ACR QC program phantom (right) are shown for a FFDM system. The large block phantom represents a more challenging detection task, as the objects have progressively smaller dimensions than the legacy phantom and are more stringent in their size specifications. Object specifications and sizes are detailed in the 1999 and 2018 ACR quality control manuals and in Figure 8-37. Images are DICOM "For Processing" with linear window width and window level enhancement. (Large phantom image provided by Steven M. LaFontaine, TherapyPhysics, Inc., Signal Hill, CA.).

Category C QC tests evaluate performance of components other than the digital image receptor or diagnostic devices for interpretation. When test results are outside the action limits specified by the manufacturer, the source of the problem shall be identified, and corrective action shall be taken within 30 days of the test date. Clinical imaging and mammographic image interpretation can continue during this period. Applicable QC tests include collimation assessment, field luminance evaluation, kV accuracy, HVL assessment, AEC performance and reproducibility, radiation output rate, and compression thickness indicator accuracy.

8.8 SUMMARY

Mammography breast imaging has unique requirements to ensure an optimal x-ray imaging exam at the lowest possible MGD for screening of women and for diagnostic workup of positive findings. There are many physics issues to be considered for achieving these goals. While the physics doesn't change, the technology continues to advance with equipment, information technology, and standards updates that must be considered. In addition, the personnel involved in breast imaging must also meet stringent requirements to maintain optimal quality through training and continuous education. The technologist performs the examinations, that is, patient positioning, compression, image acquisition, and evaluation of digital image quality. The technologist also performs the daily, weekly, monthly, and semiannual QC tests, including an analysis of retake rates. The medical physicist is responsible for equipment performance measurements before first clinical use, annually thereafter, following major repairs, and for oversight of the QC program performed by the technologist. Ultimate responsibility rests with the radiologist in charge of the mammography practice, who must ensure that all interpreting radiologists, mammography technologists, and medical physicists meet the initial qualifications and maintain the continuing education and experience required by MQSA regulations.

SUGGESTED READING AND REFERENCES

ACR. *Digital Mammography Quality Control Manual*. Reston, VA: American College of Radiology; 2018a.

ACR. *Practice Parameter for the Performance of Screening and Diagnostic Mammography*. Reston, VA: American College of Radiology; 2018b. https://www.acr.org/Files Practice-Parameters/Screen-Diag-Mammo

ACR–AAPM–SIIM. *Practice Parameter for Determinants of Image Quality in Digital Mammography*. Reston, VA: American College of Radiology; 2017. https://www.acr.org/-/media/ACR/Files/Practice-Parameters/Dig-Mamo.pdf

Boone JM. Glandular breast dose for monoenergetic and high-energy x-ray beams: Monte Carlo assessment. *Radiology*. 1999:213;23-37.

Dance DR, Skinner CL, Young KC, Beckett JR, Kotre CJ. Additional factors for the estimation of mean glandular breast dose using the UK mammography dosimetry protocol. *Phys Med Biol*. 2000;45:801-813.

Dance DR, Young KC, vanEngen RE. Further factors for the estimation of mean glandular dose using the United Kingdom, European and IAEA breast dosimetry protocols. *Phys Med Biol*. 2009;54:4361–4372.

Dance DR, Young KC, vanEngen RE. Estimation of mean glandular dose for breast tomosynthesis: factors for use with the UK, European and IAEA breast dosimetry protocols. *Phys Med Biol*. 2011;56:453-471.

FDA. Mammography Quality Standards Act (MQSA). 2020. The MQSA regulations and other documentation are available on the Web at http://www.fda.gov/cdrh/mammography

Hernandez AM, Seibert JA, Boone JM. Breast dose in mammography is about 30% lower when realistic heterogeneous glandular distributions are considered. *Med Phys*. 2015;42:6337-6348.

IEC. *Medical Electrical Equipment—X-Ray Tube Assemblies—Characteristics of Focal Spots, 60336*. 4th ed. Geneva, Switzerland: International Electrotechnical Commission; 2005.

IHE. *Radiology Mammography User's Handbook. Integrating the Healthcare Enterprise*. 2007. https://www.ihe.net/resources/user_handbooks/

IHE. Digital Breast Tomoynthesis Profile. Integrating the Healthcare Enterprise. 2016. https://www.ihe.net/uploadedFiles/Documents/Radiology/IHE_RAD_Suppl_DBT_Rev1.3_TI_2016-09-09.pdf

Pisano ED, Gasonis C, Hendrick E, et al. Diagnostic performance of digital versus film mammography for breast-cancer screening. *N Engl J Med*. 2005;353:1773-1783.

Ratanaprasatporn L, Chikarmane SA, Giess CS. Strengths and weaknesses of synthetic mammography in screening. *Radiographics*. 2017;37:1913-1927.

Sechopoulos I, Sabol JM, Berglund J, et al. Radiation dosimetry in digital breast tomosynthesis: report of AAPM Tomosynthesis Subcommittee Task Group 223. *Med Phys*. 2014;41:091501.

Tirada N, Li G, Dreizin D, et al. Digital breast tomosynthesis: physics, artifacts, and quality control considerations. *Radiographics*. 2019;39:413-426.

CHAPTER 9

Fluoroscopy

Fluoroscopy systems provide real-time or near real-time x-ray imaging of patients. Fluoroscopy systems provide the temporal resolution necessary for the operator to use image guidance for the placement of medical devices (*e.g.*, catheters, stents, etc.) or to observe temporal physiological phenomena. Common uses for fluoroscopy include upper and lower gastrointestinal studies, where the radiologist may manipulate barium or air contrast around the GI tract, in order to observe bowel obstruction, anatomical abnormalities, or polyps. The fluoroscopy imaging system is also a crucial tool in the placement of catheters and devices for vascular imaging and interventions, such as for abdominal, cerebral, or cardiac procedures. Other uses of fluoroscopy include percutaneous needle biopsy, swallowing studies, hardware placement and positioning during surgery, etc.

There are two basic modes of operation for fluoroscopic systems: (1) fluoroscopy, which provides real-time imaging for positioning, which is generally not recorded and is relatively low in radiation dose, and (2) fluorography, which essentially uses the fluoroscopic imaging chain in a pulsed radiographic mode to record and document clinically relevant temporal sequences such as blood flow through vessels (angiography), mechanical motion of joints, etc., with higher levels of radiation consistent with radiography.

Image intensifiers were the central technology enabling low-dose fluoroscopy since the early 1960s. These earlier fluoroscopy systems used continuous x-ray sources with 30 frames per second (FPS) acquisition rates, analog TV cameras for fluoroscopic viewing, and film-based devices for recording. Modern fluoroscopic systems make use of pixelated flat-panel detectors (FPDs) with large, multiple fields of view (FOVs), numerous modes of operation, a pulsed x-ray beam to reduce vascular motion, flexible frame rates, and numerous image processing techniques such as digital subtraction angiography (DSA) and road-mapping, and some systems even have cone beam CT acquisition capabilities.

The radiation dose rate for fluoroscopy has been reduced substantially with improvements in x-ray tube technology, replacing minimally filtered (Al) high tube potential (90 kV) imaging of the past with highly filtered (Cu), low x-ray tube potential (*e.g.*, 60 kV) imaging. With these improvements in the x-ray spectra used in fluoroscopy, not only have the dose rates been reduced considerably, but image quality has improved as well. More complicated fluoroscopic suites include numerous methods for radiation safety of the staff, including ceiling-hung clear x-ray shields for protecting the upper body of the operator, along with numerous other devices deployed for reducing the scattered radiation received by staff.

The modern fluoroscopy system embraces both fluoroscopy viewing and fluorography recording and many imaging protocols designed for specific imaging applications. All modern systems embrace sophisticated computer interfaces, large ceiling-hung display monitors, and tableside controls enabling dozens of operational modes. All these features challenge the physician operator to become familiar with the increasing complexity of these systems and learn the most appropriate protocol

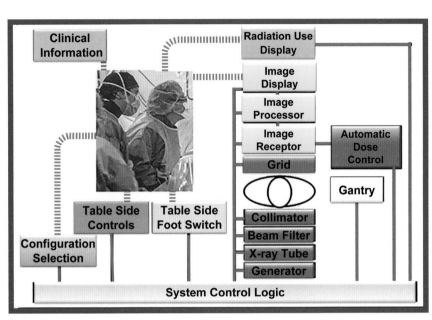

■ **FIGURE 9-1** Block diagram of an interventional fluoroscope. Key components and control loops are shown. The operator is a key control element with the ability to select and modify radiation factors, imaging geometry, image processing, etc. (© Stephen Balter.)

for optimizing the acquisition of patient information while reducing radiation dose levels to both the patient and staff.

Fluoroscopic systems are flexible general-purpose devices that are configurable to meet the requirements of a wide range of clinical procedures. Most fluoroscopes have hundreds of preprogrammed imaging protocols intended to optimize many more procedures than might be obvious from the system's "type." Image acquisition and display controls include x-ray generator settings including automatic exposure rate control (AERC), image-receptor FOV, image processing methods, and image display adjustments. Clinically appropriate combinations are combined into "Examination Protocol Selection Buttons" (EPSB). Operators should understand these controls as well as the other aspects of the imaging system as they are a central node in the fluoroscope's control loops (Fig. 9-1).

9.1 FLUOROSCOPIC IMAGING CHAIN OVERVIEW

The principal feature of the imaging chain that distinguishes fluoroscopy from radiography is the fluoroscope's ability to acquire acceptable real-time x-ray images with potentially high frame rates and lower dose per image. An up-to-date fluoroscopic imaging chain is shown in Figure 9-2. Its key component is the solid-state image receptor, commonly called a flat panel detector (FPD). This device converts the x-ray signal into a series of digital images.

Digital radiography (DR) systems use a similar image receptor. Older DR systems acquired single images, and current advanced systems can acquire low frame-rate sequences. The underlying technologies are close to convergence, and future systems with tunable gain capabilities may provide both fluoroscopy and radiography with the same hardware.

The x-ray tube in an angiography system with substantial copper beam filtration combined with low kV allows angiography systems to achieve lower patient radiation

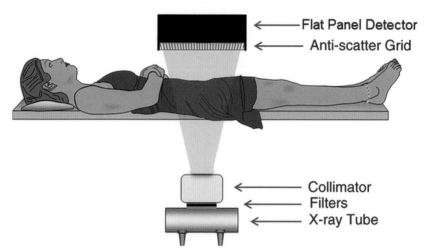

■ **FIGURE 9-2** Diagram of a fluoroscopic system. The fluoroscopic imaging chain is illustrated, with the patient in the supine position. This figure includes a flat panel detector system. The x-ray system includes a collimator with motorized blades that automatically adjust to conform to the current field of view (FOV) and source-to-image-receptor distance (SID).

dose compared to older systems, while still delivering high iodine image contrast for angiographic applications. A collimator changes the size of the x-ray beam in response to the operator limiting the active FOV to a clinically relevant area, to adjust for changes in the source-to-image-receptor distance (SID) or when the overall FOV of the image-receptor is changed, commonly due to the operator changing the magnification mode.

The basic product of a fluoroscopic imaging system is a projection x-ray image similar to a radiograph; however, a 20-min "on time" interventional fluoroscopic procedure, conducted at 15 FPS, produces a total of 18,000 individual fluoroscopic images, in addition to a potentially large number of fluorographic (*e.g.*, digital angiography [DA], DSA, cine) images. Due to the large number of images (also referred to as frames), fluoroscopic systems must produce each frame with much less dose than a comparable radiograph.

Fluoroscopes use sensitive, low noise detectors. Standard fluoroscopy typically uses a 10–100 nGy detector dose per image, the amount often dependent on frame rate. Fluorographic images use 100–1,000 nGy per image. DR systems operate at 1,000–5,000 nGy air kerma to detector per image, and computed-radiography detectors use a range from 3,000–10,000 nGy per image.

9.2 IMAGING CHAIN COMPONENTS

9.2.1 X-ray Image Intensifier

The x-ray image intensifier (II) was the key component of a fluoroscopy system from approximately 1960 to 2010. As some II based systems remain in clinical use, their characteristics will be discussed below. A diagram of an II is shown in Figure 9-3.

There are four principal components in an image intensifier: (1) an input screen that absorbs incident x-rays and converts the image to an electron pattern, (2) the electron optics, which accelerates the electrons and minifies the electron image,

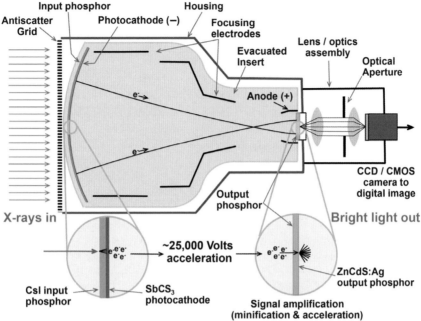

■ FIGURE 9-3 Diagram of an image intensifier. The image intensifier: x-rays pass through the input window of the vacuum element and strike the input screen, producing light that stimulates the photocathode to emit electrons, which are ejected into the electronic lens system. The electronic lens system adds energy to the image carrying electrons, while minifying the image onto a small output screen. The electron image is finally converted back to light at the output screen. These conversion steps are sketched on the bottom of the figure. The combination of energy input and minification in the electron optics yields an image 5–10 thousand times as bright as the image emerging from the input screen.

(3) an output screen, which converts the accelerated electrons into a visible light image, and (4) a housing that maintains a vacuum, contains the other components, and provides an unimpeded path for the electrons that carry the image.

Input Screen

The input screen includes a cesium-iodide (CsI) scintillator that converts the x-ray image into a visible light image and a photocathode that converts the light image into an electron image. The photocathode chemically degrades over time, which reduces the gain of the system. The input screen is curved to meet the needs of the II's electron optics. This curvature results in pincushion distortion of the image.

The II's CsI scintillator is like those found in most FPDs. Thus, the x-ray conversion properties of IIs and FPDs are similar. However, there are two differences:

1. The II's input screen is inside the vacuum housing; a modest fraction of the x-ray beam is attenuated by the housing.
2. The FPD does not have a chemical photocathode and thus does not lose gain over time.

Electron Optics

Several electrodes in the II create an electrical field when appropriate voltages are applied to:

1. add energy to the electrons emitted by the photocathode under a potential difference of 25-40 kV between the photocathode and the output-screen/anode.

2. focus the electrons generated in the active area of the input onto the fixed size output-screen.

Multi-mode image intensifiers have additional sets of electrodes for each input field size.

Output Screen

The output screen of an image intensifier consists of a layer of silver doped zinc cadmium sulfide (ZnCdS) coated onto either a glass or fiber optic output layer. This phosphor produces green light. Its composition was initially chosen when image intensifier outputs were directly viewed by the human eye because the eye is most sensitive to green light.

The output screen produces an image of fixed phosphor dimension, typically 2.5 cm, irrespective of the size of the active input layer. Even though the ZnCdS grains are very small, they limit the spatial resolution of the image intensifier. The limiting resolution of an image intensifier is inversely proportional to the input screen's diameter. (As discussed below, this is not true for flat-panel detectors.)

One effect of the electron optics is the concentration of all the signal intensity produced at the input screen onto the substantially smaller output screen. The gain in light intensity produced by minifying the image is proportional to the ratios of the areas of the input and output screens.

Maintaining the constant light output required by the video system requires a higher x-ray flux for magnified modes (active area of the input screen smaller than its full size) relative to the flux needed for operation at the full-size setting. For a constant output light level, the input dose level for an image intensifier is inversely proportional to the area of the input screen (also expressed as $1/d^2$ where d is the diameter of the active input area).

The brightness gain of an image intensifier is the ratio of the light intensity produced by fluorescence in the CsI input layer to the light intensity exiting the image intensifier. Its two components are electronic gain produced by the voltage applied between the photocathode and anode (output screen) and minification gain provided by focusing the large input area onto the small output area. A metric called the conversion factor is the light intensity exiting the II divided by the exposure rate at the input that measures overall performance and takes into account the brightness gain. The conversion factor decreases with degradation of the input phosphor/photocathode, and is one of the factors that contribute to image intensifier failure.

$$\text{Brightness Gain} = \text{Electronic Gain} \times \text{Minification Gain} \qquad [9\text{-}1]$$

Vacuum Envelope

The purposes of the vacuum include providing an unimpeded path for the electrons from the photocathode to the output screen and avoiding artifacts caused by accelerating residual gas ions onto the output screen. Either or both effects will degrade image quality, eventually to the point where the tube is not clinically acceptable. The useful life of an image intensifier is prolonged by outgassing of its components during manufacturing and by active sequestration of internal gas during its service life.

The downside of the vacuum envelope is that it must be mechanically strong enough to handle atmospheric pressure without distorting. Thus, in early tubes, the input window was made of several mm of glass. X-ray absorption and scattering in the glass degraded the tube's detective quantum efficiency (DQE—see

Chapter 4). Over time, improved glass-metal seals allowed replacement of glass with aluminum or titanium. This reduced input x-ray flux losses and improved the DQE.

Optical Distributor

The II is coupled to a video camera either by an optical lens system or by a fiber optic plate. Analog video cameras only function within a limited range of light intensity. They rely on adjustable apertures in an optical chain to maintain an appropriate light level during different modes of operation of the fluoroscope and to compensate for deterioration of the image intensifier's photocathode over time. Many fluoroscopes with analog video used beam splitters to deliver the higher-brightness image needed for film-based fluorography (no longer used) while permitting simultaneous video visualization.

Figure 9-4A and B illustrate distributors with digital fluorography and an analog video camera tube. Fluorographic images require more radiation to reduce quantum noise to a clinically acceptable level. The open optical aperture permits all the light to reach the camera during fluoroscopy. Closing the aperture drives the system to produce more radiation, thus decreasing quantum noise. CCD cameras have enough dynamic range to accommodate the x-ray intensities required for both digital fluoroscopy and digital fluorography. Beam splitters and lenses are not required, resulting in simpler optics (Fig. 9-4C).

Video Cameras

Charge coupled device (CCD) and complementary metal oxide semiconductor (CMOS) photosensitive cameras are solid-state electronic arrays that convert an optical image into a digital image and then into a video signal. Such a device has a rectangular array of photodiode semiconductor detector elements that convert incident light intensity into corresponding electronic charge (electrons), and locally store the charge for electronic readout. Both CCD and CMOS cameras have small dexel dimensions, on the order of 10–20 μm, incorporated into a 2.5 × 2.5 cm area. The typical matrix comprises 1,000 × 1,000 or 2,000 × 2,000 detector elements, but there is a wide selection of sizes that a manufacturer might choose to include in a system. CCD and CMOS cameras have linear responses over a very wide

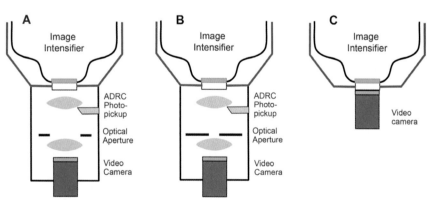

■ **FIGURE 9-4** Optical components used to manage an Image Intensifier's output images. **A.** The video pickup is used for both fluoroscopy and video-fluorography. Here the optical aperture is open to permit all the light emerging from the II to enter the camera during fluoroscopy. **B.** The optical aperture has been closed to restrict the amount of light reaching the video pickup during fluorography. **C.** A video pickup with very wide dynamic range allows operation at both fluoroscopic and fluorographic dose rates. Because there is no need to control light intensity, the pickup is directly coupled to the image intensifier.

brightness range. In either camera (CCD or CMOS), a digital image is produced, processed, stored in the fluoroscope, and then converted to a video signal displayed on one or more monitors in the fluoroscopy suite. For study transfer to a Picture Archiving and Communications System (PACS), the appropriate DICOM image and patient demographics metadata are attached to each of the digital image files or video sequences (see Chapter 5 for information on PACS).

9.2.2 Flat-Panel Detectors

The flat panel image receptor replaces the image intensifier tube, optical system, and cameras by directly converting the x-ray images into a digital form. Because FPDs do not operate in a vacuum, they are mechanically protected by carbon fiber covers instead of the stronger metallic input surface of an image intensifier. This reduces x-ray attenuation and improves the quantum detection efficiency compared to the II. FPDs are comprised of thin film transistor (TFT) arrays of individual detector elements (dexels) that are packaged in a square or rectangular area (Fig. 9-5A). Both indirect and direct x-ray conversion modes are used with TFT panels for fluoroscopy (Fig. 9-5B). In both types of systems, each dexel has a capacitor, which accumulates and stores the signal as an electrical charge, and a transistor that serves as a switch. Indirect detection TFT systems have a phosphor layer that absorbs the x-rays and converts a fraction of their energy into light; each dexel has a transistor and a capacitor, in addition to a photodiode that converts the x-ray induced light from the phosphor into a corresponding charge (Fig. 9-5C). For direct detection fluoroscopy detectors, a semiconductor (selenium) produces x-ray induced charge directly, which is collected under an applied voltage to ensure that the signal is captured within the same dexel as the x-ray absorption event. In either detector type, while a frame (image) is being acquired, the electrical charge proportional to the x-ray flux incident on that dexel is accumulated and stored by the capacitor. Readout of the FPD is performed by electronically switching a gate line "on," which opens all transistor gates for a given row. The charge stored in each dexel flows through its transistor's drain line to a charge amplifier, and then the amplified signal is digitized. The gate line is then switched "off," and readout progresses to the next gate line on the panel. Reading the array discharges the capacitors and readies them for acquiring the next frame. This is performed row by row until the entire frame is read. Even in continuous fluoroscopic acquisitions, the charge continues to be stored in each capacitor in a steady-state situation so that x-ray information is always collected as the flat-panel image receptor provides real-time fluoroscopic presentation of image data.

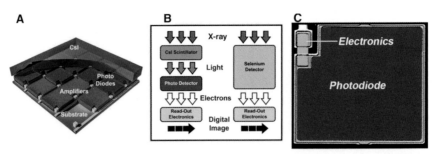

■ **FIGURE 9-5** Flat-panel detectors (FPD). **A.** Components in an indirect FPD. Note that the CsI layer is continuous and that there is space between individual dexels. The dexels in a direct x-ray system are also separated (not shown). **B.** Information flow through indirect and direct FPDs. **C.** The photodiode, and some of the electronics in a single indirect dexel. (© Stephen Balter.)

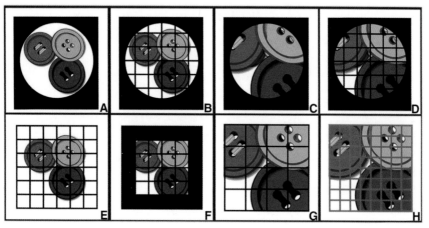

■ **FIGURE 9-6** Pixel size and magnification mode—image intensifier and flat-panel detector. **A–D.** Image Intensifier—Analog and digital camera outputs. The full pixel array of the digital camera captures the output of the II at any magnification mode. **E–G.** Flat-panel detector with a fixed dexel array (*e.g.*, Table 9-1 small detector). The same dexel covers the same portion of the patient irrespective of magnification mode **(E,F)**. Resolution does not change when the image is digitally magnified. **H.** Flat-panel detector with unbundled dexels (*e.g.*, Table 9-1 large detector, small FOV). Resolution is improved if the FPD can unbundle dexels when using a small FOV. (© Stephen Balter.)

Dexel Arrays

The effects of reducing the FOV on spatial resolution are fundamentally different for an image intensifier and a flat panel. As noted above, the FOV of an image intensifier is reduced by electro-optically focusing a smaller portion of its input screen onto the fixed size output screen. This provides a fixed image size (image-matrix size) for the camera and image processor. The FOV is reduced by selecting a sub-array of dexels in a FPD. Its image processing pipeline handles larger numbers of dexels for large FOVs and smaller numbers of dexels for small FOVs. This difference is illustrated in Figure 9-6.

Processing Dexels into Pixels

Large FPDs have more dexels than the number of pixels in the image matrix. This affords a large enough dexel matrix to provide adequate spatial resolution in the detector's smallest FOV. An image processing pipeline bins dexels to fit the active pixel matrix into the image matrix. Some processing occurs within the FPD itself, the remainder in downstream devices. Processor bandwidth limitations may require additional binning to accommodate very high frame rates. Table 9-1 provides an example of this effect. The effects of binning on spatial resolution, image noise, and radiation usage are discussed below.

Although the rectangular format, compact design, and digital output attributes of flat panel systems enhance functionality, the electron optics in the image intensifier produces images with very little added electronic noise. The cameras receive enough light at fluoroscopic dose rates to overcome video camera noise. Flat panel systems, however, have amplifier systems that work at the very limit of what digital electronics can deliver, and consequently, there is appreciably more electronic noise in most flat panel fluoroscopy systems when they are used for fluoroscopy. Thus, flat panel fluoroscopy detectors use slightly higher exposures per frame than image intensifiers. Electronic noise is far less of an issue for FPDs in fluorographic and radiographic acquisition modes, and thus, the exposure per frame is similar to that of the image intensifier.

TABLE 9-1 DEXELS, PIXELS, AND FIELD OF VIEW

	FIXED DEXEL = 0.18						BINNABLE DEXEL = 0.15				
Active Dexels		Fluoro/Cine		Digital Angio		Active Dexels		Fluoro/Cine		Digital Angio	
FOV	DEXELs	PIXELS 6–30 FPS	Psize	PIXELS >6 FPS	Psize	FOV	DEXELs	PIXELS 6–30 FPS	Psize	PIXELS >6 FPS	Psize
26 (18)	1,000	1,000	0.18	1,000	0.18	42 (30)	2,000	1,000	0.30	2,000	0.15
20 (14)	800	800	0.18	800	0.18	30 (20)	1,400	700	0.30	1,400	0.15
13 (9)	500	500	0.18	500	0.18	21 (15)	1,000	1,000	0.15	1,000	0.15
						15 (10)	700	700	0.15	700	0.15

9.3 FLUOROSCOPIC X-RAY SOURCE ASSEMBLY

9.3.1 X-ray Tube

The general construction of all x-ray tubes is similar. However, due to the nature of the procedures, fluoroscopic x-ray tubes are commonly used in a more continuous manner than radiographic tubes. These tubes also operate at radiographic power levels during fluorography. Fluoroscopic tubes have higher heat-storage capacity and faster cooling rates than radiographic tubes. Traditionally, the small focal spot is used for fluoroscopy and the large focal spot for fluorography. Thus, spatial resolution is likely to decrease when going from fluoroscopy to fluorography. Some tubes also have an additional micro-focus focal spot intended for geometrically magnified procedures. Newer systems select the smallest available focal spot that can accommodate the immediate x-ray power level for all modes of operation. This will result in similar spatial resolution for thin body parts and lower resolution for fluorography of thick parts.

9.3.2 Collimator

Fluoroscopic collimators are designed to dynamically adjust the overall x-ray field size in response to a combination of inputs from both the operator and the system. The intention is to confine the x-ray beam to the smallest area within the active area of the image receptor that is consistent with immediate clinical requirements. Many systems also have additional, operator controlled, x-ray translucent elements (sometimes called wedge filters) that are used to equalize image receptor inputs when anatomical structures providing very different attenuation(e.g., lung and mediastinum) are simultaneously in the beam.

Portions of the x-ray beam that are not seen by the imaging chain do not supply any clinical information. Such irradiation unnecessarily increases both patient and staff radiation risk. Scatter from these areas also degrades image quality in the useful image.

Confinement of the beam to the active FOV is a system function. For both the image intensifier and the flat panel, the x-ray collimator automatically adjusts to limit the x-ray beam to the active FOV whenever the FOV is changed and to accommodate changes in the source-to-image-receptor-distance (SID). Ideally, the system should be set so that an unirradiated area is always seen around the edges of the image.

Collimation of the beam within the active FOV is the operator's responsibility. Smaller beams produced by collimator adjustment by the operator reduce total irradiation, thus improving both safety and image quality. The goal is to only irradiate the region of immediate clinical interest. Obtaining a smaller FOV by selection of a magnification mode does reduce the beam size and magnifies the displayed image; however, most fluoroscopes increase the dose-rate when the FOV is reduced by this method. Depending on programming, this increase may diminish or even negate the radiation saving effects of collimation within the FOV. Image magnification of a collimated area within a larger FOV can also be offered by the image processor through pixel replication and interpolation, or by simply viewing the image on a larger monitor. If the resulting image is clinically acceptable, this can reduce radiation dose relative to the use of magnification mode.

9.3.3 X-ray Spectral Shaping Filters

By 1990, the DQE of the image intensifier was near 50% and x-ray quantum noise was the major noise source in fluoroscopy. There was only a factor of two available for reducing patient irradiation by improving the efficiency of the image receptor. Radiation levels can also be reduced when the radiological conspicuity of clinically important items, such as contrast media and guidewires, is increased.

One way of improving the conspicuity of higher atomic number (Z) elements is to increase the fraction of x-ray photons in the beam with energies slightly above the K absorption edge of the material of interest (*e.g.*, iodine at 33.2 keV). Spectral shaping can be accomplished by adding a copper filter (0.1–1.0 mm) and simultaneously restricting the x-ray tube's operating kV (Fig. 9-7). Adding copper reduces the number of photons in the beam below the iodine edge. Reducing the kV limits the number of higher energy photons. For a given amount of electrical power consumed by the tube, such kV-filter combinations decrease the photon fluence available to form the image. Adequate fluence using spectrally shaped beams became feasible when x-ray tubes were developed with high power ratings.

Most modern fluoroscopic systems include variable thickness copper filters in the collimator assembly. The thickness of copper used at any given moment is automatically controlled by the AERC and operator selection of settings. In some systems, the acquisition selection (*e.g.*, low-dose-rate fluoro, standard-dose-rate fluoro) determines the filter thickness. In other systems, the AERC further controls filter thickness

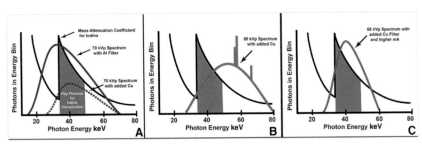

■ **FIGURE 9-7** Shaping the spectrum of the x-ray beam. **A.** The x-ray spectrum emerging from the tube is modified by a copper layer. The overall intensity of the beam is reduced, and the resultant spectrum has shifted to higher average energy. This figure shows the original spectrum, the attenuation coefficient of iodine as a function of energy, and the resultant modified spectrum with a higher fraction of photons above the iodine K edge. **B.** Increasing kV shifts the spectrum further, but most of the higher energy photons are far from the iodine K edge and do not contribute very much to iodine visualization. Tungsten K characteristic photons are seen here as well. **C.** Reducing kV moves more of the spectrum toward the iodine K edge. There are fewer low energy photons that would contribute to skin dose but not to the image. The photons, with energies above 60 kV shown in **B** are not produced. X-ray tubes need to have high power capabilities so that they can provide adequate x-ray flux without increasing kV. (© Stephen Balter.)

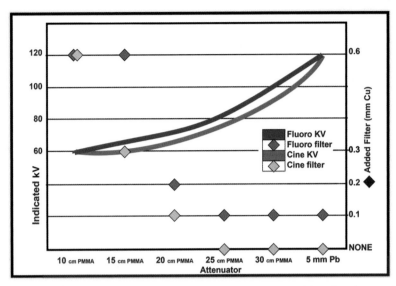

■ FIGURE 9-8 AERC controlled Cu spectral shaping filter thickness. Measured data from interventional fluoroscope installed in 2010. Layers of poly methyl methacrylate (PMMA) and lead were used to simulate different patient sizes. The AERC selected a kV and filter thickness based on the image-receptor signal. Separate algorithms were used for fluoroscopy and fluorography (cine). Note that although the kV was similar at every step, the filter used for cine declined much more rapidly than for fluoro. The removal of copper is the reason for a higher cine HVL at 80 kV than 90 kV. (© Stephen Balter.)

along with the usual x-ray factors. In some cases, for increasing patient thickness or acquisition mode changes, the limits of the x-ray tube power output require the filter thickness to decrease and the kV to increase. In such settings, at the same kV, the half value layer (HVL) will differ between fluoroscopy and fluorography; and the HVL may decrease with an increase in kV if there is a simultaneous decrease in copper thickness. Figure 9-8 illustrates this behavior for a typical interventional fluoroscope.

9.4 CONTROLS

9.4.1 Automatic Exposure Rate Control

Fluoroscopes offer at least two fluoroscopic and one fluorographic sub-modes. Often, systems offer literally dozens to hundreds of sub-modes to accommodate a wide range of operator preferences and clinical requirements. Most of these use an AERC system. The purpose of AERC is to deliver a constant x-ray intensity to the image receptor irrespective of tissue thickness in the beam path. This results in a reasonably constant detector SNR over its working range. In a FPD, the AERC collects detected x-ray intensity information observed by a predetermined subset of dexels. Depending on clinical configuration, the subset ranges from dexels in a relatively small central area to all dexels within the collimated beam. If the average signal is too low, the AERC commands the generator to increase x-ray output. Similarly, too high a signal initiates a command to reduce radiation output. AERCs commonly further adjust outputs when the FOV or frame rate is changed. These adjustments stabilize the image noise perceived by the fluoroscopist when these factors vary.

For large patients or steep projection angles, the x-ray air kerma rate may reach the normal fluoroscopy regulatory limit (88 mGy/min). The resulting x-ray flux reaching the image receptor (II or FP) is lower than desired, and x-ray quantum noise is higher than desired. Necessary additional electronic amplification may add additional noise. The noise in the resulting image may be too high for some clinical purposes. Some fluoroscopes have a specially activated high-level control (HLC), which enables a higher limit (176 mGy/min) to reduce noise. The high-level mode should be only used when clinically necessary.

Under AERC, the system changes the x-ray factors (kV, mA, pulse width), focal spot, and beam filtration in a predetermined manner that varies between systems. As noted above, the same system usually offers user-selectable options with markedly different behaviors. These selections are part of the toolkit used to select the balance between patient dose and image quality appropriate to different types of examinations, and in some cases different operator imaging requirements. The change in output, and the maximum output dose rate when changing from "low" to "normal" to "high-level" at any patient thickness is also included in the system's configuration. Image processing parameters may also be controlled by the AERC. These changes further influence image presentation to the operator.

Figure 9-9 illustrates some possibilities with a hypothetical system equipped with three fluoroscopic modes, each with a different regulatory exposure-rate limit. In Figure 9-9A, the output is the same until the mode's limit is exceeded. All three modes produce the same radiation output for thin to medium size patients. The "low" mode is limited to an air kerma rate (for C-arm gantries, at 30 cm from the image receptor assembly) of 44 mGy/min; in this mode all thicker patients receive the limiting dose rate while image quality decreases as patient thickness increases. Similar behavior is seen for the "normal" and "high-level" modes when their limits are reached. Figure 9-9B illustrates a system with three fluoroscopic modes. The lower two fluoroscopic modes converge near the regulatory limit. The high-dose-rate mode is higher for all patient thicknesses and has double the usual regulatory limit.

Figure 9-9C illustrates that the relationship between patient thickness and patient dose for any mode and dose rate limit is programmable. The upper curve is intended to maximize the visibility of iodinated contrast media as much as possible. The generator is programmed to keep the kV low and adjust mA and/or pulse width to provide an appropriate detector signal. The lowest curve is intended to minimize patient irradiation at the possible expense of iodine visualization. It does so by rapidly increasing kV with increasing patient thickness. One or more additional intermediate curves may be provided on a given system.

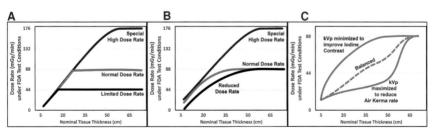

■ **FIGURE 9-9** Output dose rates as a function of patient size are programmable. **A.** Example of a system with three maximum fluoroscopic dose-rate modes. In this system, the dose rate is identical for all modes until the individual mode limit is exceeded. **B.** A system with three fluoroscopic modes. The lower two fluoroscopic modes converge near the regulatory limit. The high-dose-rate mode is higher for all patient thicknesses and has double the usual regulatory limit. **C.** Hypothetical trajectories. Keeping the kV low for as long as possible improves Iodine contrast at the expense of higher skin dose for heavy patients (upper curve). Raising the kV quickly minimizes patient dose at the expense of Iodine contrast for many patients (lowest curve). The balanced curve represents a possible trade-off between dose and Iodine visibility. (© Stephen Balter.)

The shapes of the curves themselves may also vary when different body parts are selected for the procedure. The actual curves are included in each protocol selection setting. It is the operator's responsibility to select the correct protocol, and corresponding sub-settings, to meet the clinical needs of the current patient.

9.4.2 Field of View and Magnification Modes

Image intensifiers and FPDs are available with maximal input fields-of-view ranging from 20 to 50 cm. Larger image receptors are needed to image large anatomical areas such as the entire abdomen. Some fluoroscopes have small image receptors suitable for imaging smaller organs, such as the heart; an advantage of such image receptors is that they permit the gantry to be positioned at larger angulations without colliding with the patient.

The size and shape of the largest FOV is determined by the physical size of the image receptor. Most fluoroscopes offer one or more smaller FOVs, achieved by selecting a magnification mode. The active FOV of an image intensifier is established by focusing a portion of its input screen onto the full area of the output screen. This results in an increase in image magnification as the FOV decreases. FPDs reduce the size of the active FOV by accepting information from a smaller area of the image receptor. The subsequent image is digitally resized to fill the fluoroscope's display. This was illustrated in Figure 9-6.

Spatial resolution and radiation dose changes with FOV differ between the II and the FPD. This section compares an image intensifier with the large and small format FPDs shown in Table 9-1. All FOVs are zoomed to fill the display monitor area. This is accomplished using electronic zoom within the II and by digital processing in the FPD image chain.

As discussed previously, the brightness gain (and hence the overall gain) of the II decreases as the magnification increases. The AERC circuitry compensates for the lower signal by boosting the x-ray exposure rate. The increase in the exposure rate is commonly equal to the inverse of the square of the diameter ratio (the inverse ratio of FOV areas), although the user can deviate from this algorithm to lower the radiation dose to the patient at the expense of greater quantum noise in the image.

Flat panel fluoroscopy systems can provide similar exposure rate adjustment as a function of field size as is needed for image intensifiers; however, the exposure rate is controlled by system logic and is explicitly calibrated into the fluoroscopy system. In principle, the exposure rate need only be changed when the final pixel size changes. In practice, quantum noise is more visible to the operators in zoomed modes. Additional exposure rate increases are often applied to meet perceptual requirements. As a first approximation, exposure rate for FPD increases inversely with the size of the FPD's active diagonal dimension (not as quickly as for IIs—inversely with active FOV diameter squared).

9.5 MODES OF OPERATION

Modern x-ray generators and imaging systems are controlled by computers, resulting in a great deal of flexibility regarding operational modes and their configurations. Brief descriptions of fluoroscopy (intended for real-time viewing) and fluorography (intended for storage and individual image review) modes are given below.

9.5.1 Continuous Fluoroscopy

The continuous fluoroscopy mode produces an uninterrupted x-ray beam with its intensity driven by a combination of patient size, system settings selected by the operator, and system technical requirements. The mode is the most basic approach to fluoroscopy and was used up until the 1990s. Some simple mobile fluoroscopes still operate in this mode. The image stream is partitioned into discrete frames by the video system. The typical frame rate was 30 FPS, corresponding to US video standards. Quantum noise and anatomical motion occurring in a single frame (1/30 s) is averaged and can be blurred using image processing. A second stage of averaging (1/5 s) occurs in the observer's eye. When a single frame is frozen and viewed on a monitor it will appear nosier and sharper than a real-time sequence because observer eye averaging no longer affects perception.

9.5.2 Pulsed Fluoroscopy and Fluorography

In pulsed fluoroscopy, the x-ray generator produces a series of short pulses, one per frame, each with an on-time smaller than the frame-time (Fig. 9-10A). Short pulses (*e.g.*, 3–10 ms) reduce blurring from anatomical motion (*e.g.*, pulsatile vessels and cardiac motion) and other moving objects in individual images in comparison to continuous fluoroscopy. The overall appearance of a moving object when viewed dynamically is dependent on the interactions of object motion, frame rate, processing of gap-filling display frames, and temporal filtering. The image of a slowly moving object will partially overlap on adjacent frames and will appear to be blurred. The image of a rapidly moving object will appear in different regions on adjacent frames and will appear to be multiple sharp objects. The object will often appear sharper when a single image is viewed because of the lack of the influence of the image processor and the human visual system caused by temporally close images. Temporal averaging in the observer's eye still contributes to perceived blur. In addition, the video system provides an output frame rate high enough to avoid the perception of image flicker (above the observer's critical flicker frequency [CFF]). Each image may be shown multiple times when low acquisition frame rates are used (Fig. 9-10B).

   At 30 FPS, the average dose for a single video frame is roughly similar for continuous and pulsed fluoroscopy because enough flux per frame is needed to reduce x-ray quantum noise to an acceptable value. Pulsed imaging can reduce radiation because the acquisition frame rate is decoupled from the display frame rate. These systems will save radiation when they are operated at low fluorographic or fluoroscopic frame rates. Because fluorographic images are intended to be viewed individually, the same dose per pulse needs to be delivered at any frame rate. Fluoroscopic images are intended to be viewed dynamically. Image integration by the eye affects quantum noise perception. Images will appear noisier if the same dose per pulse is used for all frame rates. Increasing the dose per pulse by about $\sqrt{2}$ when the FPS is halved maintains constant noise perception at the expense of less dose saving by reducing frame rate (Fig. 9-10C).

9.5.3 Fluorography (Unsubtracted)

Fluorographic images, also known as digital angiography (DA) images, or cine, should only be obtained if the intent is to store them for later review either individually or as a sequence. This requires enough dose per image to reduce

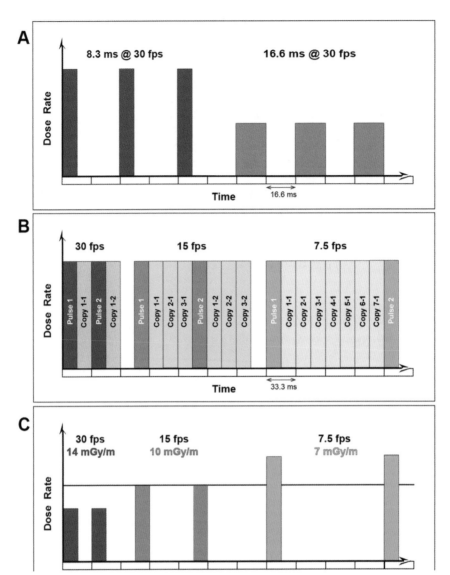

■ **FIGURE 9-10** Pulse widths, frame rates, and dose rates. **A.** The same dose per pulse can be delivered using a high dose rate for a short time or a lower dose rate for a longer time. Short pulses minimize individual frame motion blur. **B.** The imaging system eliminates flicker at any frame rate by providing copies to fill the gaps at an appropriate rate. **C.** Some fluoroscopes adjust the dose rate to produce equal perceived noise at different frame rates. (© Stephen Balter.)

quantum noise to an acceptable value without relying on temporal resolution in the observer's eye. Typically, a single fluorographic frame will require about ten times the radiation needed for a comparable fluoroscopic frame. Figure 9-11 illustrates single fluoroscopic and fluorographic frames. Historically, "fluorographs" were obtained either singly (as in spot-films) or at rates up to a few per second.

9.5.4   Digital Subtraction Angiography

Digital subtraction angiography (DSA) is used to subtract out static anatomy and in doing so reduces the anatomical noise in the image—so the physician can focus solely on the vascular anatomy. DSA is performed by placing a catheter

A   **B**

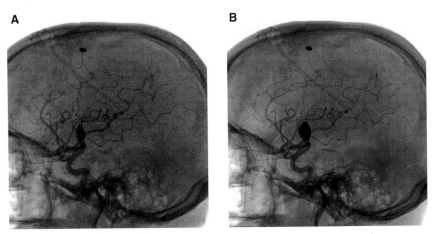

■ **FIGURE 9-11** Fluoroscopic and fluorographic images. These two images were taken a few seconds apart. The fluorographic DA image **(B)** from a DSA series required approximately 50 times the dose needed for the single fluoroscopic frame **(A)**. Note the increased quantum noise in image **A**. (© Stephen Balter.)

intravascularly using fluoroscopic visualization, and then a series of DA images (*e.g.*, 1 to 6 images per second) is acquired while a contrast agent (*e.g.*, Iodine or CO_2) is injected through the catheter. Figure 9-12 illustrates DSA images with iodine and CO_2 as contrast agents. The first few images contain no contrast agent, and one of these anatomy-only images is selected as the mask image. The contrast agent moves through the vessels in the angiographic FOV, and images acquired during this phase of the study contain both anatomy and contrast-enhanced vessels. The mask image is subtracted (pixel by pixel) from the iodinated images, resulting in the subtraction of the anatomical background. In the absence of patient motion, DSA images depict only the vascular anatomy, unobscured by overlying anatomy. Software tools permit automatic or manual reregistration of the mask and live image to minimize motion artifacts. The elimination of the anatomical background in DSA allows the physician to concentrate on the patient's vascular anatomy. Also, the iodinated contrast agent injected dose for a DSA exam can be reduced compared to an unsubtracted DA image because of the increased conspicuity of the vasculature.

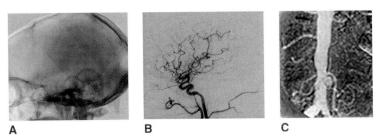

A   **B**   **C**

■ **FIGURE 9-12** Image subtraction. **A.** Mask image: This image will be subtracted from a later image in the series (not shown) in which iodine is present in the patient's arterial tree. **B.** Result of the subtraction: Structures common to both images have been removed. X-ray quantum noise from both images is present. The contrast of the image has been increased to improve the conspicuity of the vessels. It is necessary to use high radiation doses when acquiring the images to reduce the visibility of quantum noise. **C.** CO_2 subtraction image of the abdominal aorta. The CO_2 bubble does not fill the entire aorta at any one time. This image is reconstructed by subtracting the mask from a sequence of CO_2 containing images and then combining them to reconstruct the vascular tree. (© Stephen Balter.)

DSA using CO_2 as the contrast agent (available since the 1980s) can be of clinical benefit. Images are recorded while a CO_2 gas injection displaces blood. The optimum technique uses a higher kV to reduce unwanted photoelectric attenuation in the patient's tissues, and image stitching to produce a composite image or image series of the entire artery by following the CO_2 bubble through the patient's arteries over time. CO_2 is rarely used in the present era of low toxicity iodine-based contrast agents.

DSA removes fixed information found in both the mask and live image. All x-ray images contain stochastic quantum noise with the point-to-point noise intensity proportional to the square root of the local signal intensity. Random noise does not subtract but adds and produces more noise in the difference image than in either initial image. The final step in DSA is to greatly increase the contrast of the display to improve visibility of blood vessels or other moving structures by using window width and window level adjustments. This increases the visibility of quantum noise in the image. Suppressing quantum noise requires the use of more radiation in both the mask and live images. Nominally, up to ten times the dose is needed for a single DSA frame than for a comparable unsubtracted fluorographic (DA) image. Fortunately, DSA images are usually acquired at low frame rates so that the total radiation dose is acceptable. Many systems have DSA modes with variable frame rates. These can be programmed on a run by run basis to match the temporal behavior of contrast flow in the vessels. Using low frame rates where practicable reduces radiation.

9.5.5 Cine Fluorography (Analog and Digital)

Coronary procedures require fluorographic capture, storage, and replay using frame rates high enough to visualize small portions of the nominal one-second cardiac cycle.

Digital cine-fluorography systems were introduced around the year 2000 when CCD video cameras became available. This digital image chain supported fluoroscopy, DSA, and cine. Imaging modes are changed by appropriately configuring the x-ray generator and imaging system.

Pulsed x-ray sources and digital image displays also became widely available at this time. The two major gains were as follows: (1) x-rays could be emitted for a fraction of the frame time, reducing the blur caused by anatomical motion; and (2) image display could be provided at a frame rate high enough to eliminate flicker at any image acquisition rate. The transition from image intensifiers to flat-panels led to band-width limitations in the FPS (Table 9-1): (1) Full, unbinned FPD resolution could only be achieved at a few FPS, and (2) further restrictions on output matrix size were needed at high (60 FPS) rates.

In most cases, the only remaining technical differences between fluoroscopy, DSA, and cine-fluorography are the dose requirements for each frame in these different classes of images, and image processing/display parameters optimized for each mode. (Recursive filtering—a method of temporal image averaging—is desirable to reduce noise impressions in fluoroscopy; it is not needed for DA, DSA, or cine because the noise is low enough already.)

Cine frame rates can be set to conform to procedure specific anatomical requirements. In many cases, they can be lower than the rates needed for fluoroscopic guidance of device placements. Certainly, any reduction in cine frame rate produces a major reduction in patient dose.

Also, because the imaging channel is identical, retrospectively stored fluoroscopy (if of adequate quality) can be substituted for cine in the clinical image stream. This further saves radiation, and can also reduce the volume of contrast media used in a procedure.

9.5.6 Last-Image-Hold, Last-Sequence-Display

Modern fluoroscopic systems are required to continuously display the last fluoroscopic frame acquired when operator stops irradiation (LIH). This mode provides the operator with an image useful for planning the next step in the procedure without unnecessary beam-on time. LIH images may be processed to improve their appearance. Unless deliberately stored, this image vanishes at the start of the next irradiation.

Systems may also offer the option of retrospectively reviewing the last 10–30 s of fluoroscopy acquired before the sequence was stopped. Sequence capture is usually initiated by the operator by a tableside control. The stored sequence is dynamically displayed to the operator as soon as capture is complete with the same image processing that was applied during acquisition or with fluorographic postprocessing. Stored fluoroscopic sequences may contain enough clinical information to avoid a subsequent fluorographic acquisition. Both radiation and contrast media (dye) use are avoided when this happens.

9.6 IMAGE PROCESSING

Modern fluoroscopic systems include fast image processors in their imaging chains. These can be programmed to perform several tasks in real time as well as many additional postprocessing tasks. Processing can either be uniform across an entire image or differentially in different portions of the same image. For didactic purposes, the first portions of this section presume uniform processing across the entire image. Local image processing is discussed in Section 9.6.4. The effects of image quality and the effects of image processing on image quality are discussed in Section 9.7.

Image processing is used to optimize the coupling of information extracted from the patient into the operator's brain. Processing can reduce radiation dose if the images are adequate to meet the operator's clinical needs for the procedure being currently performed. Evaluating and optimizing fluoroscopic processing using technical tests alone is not sufficient to meet this requirement because of patient and operator factors.

9.6.1 Single Image Processing

Single images can be processed using a wide variety of algorithms. Older digital fluoroscopes only used the few algorithms that were compatible with the combination of image frame rates and computer power at the time that they were designed. This section discusses blurring and unsharp masking, two algorithms that are still commonly found in newer systems. Both are applied uniformly across the entire image. Newer algorithms, discussed in Section 9.6.6, use local spatial and temporal processing to enhance the visibility of different clinical objects in different parts of the same image.

Images are spatially blurred to suppress the visibility of quantum noise. They do this by replacing an initial pixel value with the average value observed in that pixel and its neighbors. The number of neighbors included in the average, and the way that each neighbor is weighted as it contributes to the average are both programmable. Figure 9-13 is an example. The "original" image on the left is a 1 k × 1 k gray scale representation of a color photograph. Two intensities of gaussian noise were digitally added to the original (rows). Each pair of images was then blurred using a gaussian blur function of a given size. The size of the blur function increases from left to right. A larger blur function reduces the appearance of noise relative to a smaller blur function. However, the visibility of object details decreases as the size of the blur function increases. Typically, fluorographic images have less noise than fluoroscopic images. Smaller blur sizes yield clinically acceptable noise in fluorography. Therefore, fluorographic images appear to be sharper than corresponding fluoroscopic images.

Images can be visually sharpened using a variety of processes such as unsharp masking. This technique combines sharp and blurred versions of the same image. A similar process occurs in the retina by interactions at a neural level. The results of the process are Mach bands outlining the edges of recorded or visualized objects. Here again, the magnitude of the effect in the digital domain can be configured at tableside. Figure 9-14 illustrates this process. The first column contains three different blurred representations of the lighthouse. Weighted combinations of the original and blurred images are combined to produce the final image. Each of the three right-hand columns uses a different weighting factor. The effects of these combinations are seen. Note that combinations of larger blurred representation and higher weighting of the blurred versions increases the presence of the digital equivalent of Mach bands.

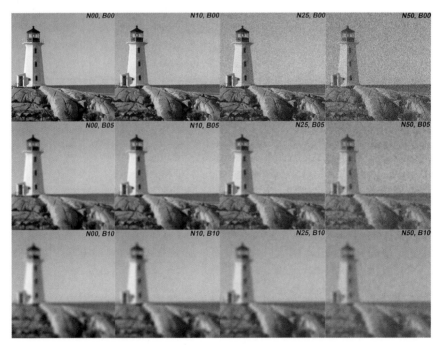

■ **FIGURE 9-13** Image blurring to reduce the visibility of noise. Gaussian noise (N) was added to the original image (512 × 512 pixels, 8-bit gray scale) at 3 levels (5%, 25%, 50%). The resultant images were then blurred using gaussian blurring (B) using radii of 5 and 10 pixels. The original (no added noise) image is in the upper left corner. (© Stephen Balter.)

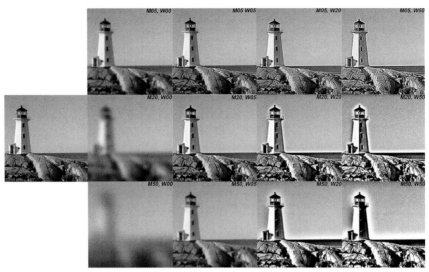

■ **FIGURE 9-14** Effects of unsharp masking parameters. The original image is on the left. Each row has constant gaussian blur radius M of 5, 20, or 50 pixels. The first column is the mask before inversion. Subsequent columns have weighting factors W of 50%, 200%, or 500%. (© Stephen Balter.)

9.6.2 Temporal Image Processing (Multi-Frame)

Fluoroscopy is intended to visualize motion in real time. The temporal resolution of every run must be high enough to fulfill its clinical purpose. For safety reasons, there are limits on the amount of irradiation that can be used. The resulting individual fluoroscopic images are relatively noisy, with their noise patterns statistically changing from frame to frame. However, the underlying anatomical information remains coherent. Appropriately combining several fluoroscopic frames will improve the perceived SNR while maintaining the system's inherent spatial resolution at a potential cost of blurring moving objects. Similar processing is seldom needed during fluorography (*e.g.*, cine) because the higher dose per frame in this mode has already reduced noise perception.

The human eye has this capability. Images presented to the retina at low light levels are integrated by the rods over a nominal running time interval of around 200 ms. Fluoroscopic systems have had the capability of supplementing retinal processing since the introduction of video-fluoroscopy. Analog video pickup tubes inherently integrate light at their photo pickup layers. The degree of integration differs for different technologies. The only way to change the lag of an analog system is to change the camera type. One manufacturer replaced the vidicon (noticeable lag, the word for integration at the time) with a low lag plumbicon in a GI fluoroscopic system. Even though patient dose rates were identical, many radiologists were uncomfortable with the increased noise observed with the plumbicon.

With the advent of digital fluoroscopy and fluorographic systems, temporal filtering can be applied using recursive filtering.

In recursive filtering, the displayed image (DI) is calculated using a fraction (α) of the just acquired image (NI) is added to the previously displayed image (PDI) using

$$\text{Displayed Image (DI)} = \alpha \text{NI} + (1 - \alpha)\text{PDI}. \qquad [9\text{-}2]$$

The parameter α ranges from 0 to 1; as α is reduced, the contribution of the current image (NI) is reduced, the contribution of the previous displayed image (PDI) is enhanced, and the amount of lag is increased. As α is increased, the amount of lag is reduced, and at $\alpha = 1$, no lag occurs. The current displayed image (DI) becomes the PDI for the next frame, and the weighted image data from an entire sequence of images (not just two images) is included (Fig. 9-15).

As noted above, increasing lag increases the blurring of moving objects. The nature of this blur is related to the selection of the pulse sequence, the blurring algorithm, as well as to the motion itself. Additional information is provided in Section 9.7. Newer image processors are no longer limited to identical processing across the entire image but provide the capability of different local processing depending on the contents of different portions of the same image. Some aspects of this rapidly evolving field are discussed in Section 9.6.4.

9.6.3 Look Up Tables

The relationship between the x-ray intensity illuminating an image receptor dexel and the brightness of the corresponding area on the display is determined by the image processor, a look-up table (LUT), also known as a display transform function, the characteristics of the display device, and ambient illumination. These are key factors in determining the transfer of anatomical information into the observer's cognitive system. The intents of the LUT include compensation for display and ambient effects.

The LUT is a look-up table that converts the image processor's output pixel levels into the corresponding display pixel levels. The actual LUT is arbitrary. A simple example is the familiar window-level control found on a CT scanner. Most

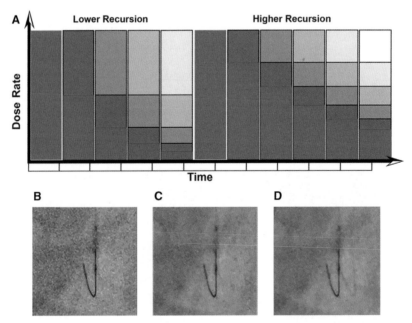

■ **FIGURE 9-15** Global temporal recursive filtering. **A.** Contribution of previous images to the current single frame: Increased recursion (decreased α) increases contribution of any one image to the series. **B–D.** Visual noise decreases and ghosts of moving objects increase with increased recursion **B** = no recursion, **C** = low recursion, **D** = High recursion. (Image **A**, © Stephen Balter. Images **B–D**, © Siemens Healthineers 2019. Used with permission.)

fluoroscopes have several LUTs intended for different imaging tasks. In many fluoroscopes, the appropriate LUT is one of the factors chosen when a clinical task (*e.g.*, abdominal DSA) is selected. Different operators have different visual needs and benefit from "bespoke" LUTs. Operators can immediately tune these selections using accessible display controls (*e.g.*, brightness, contrast, window, level) on the fluoroscope.

LUT selection can have a profound effect on clinical performance and procedural radiation utilization. Less than optimal image display during a clinical procedure can lead to longer fluoro time to provide the operator with relevant information. Some operators will use higher fluoroscopic dose rates or substitute fluorography as a means of achieving the image quality that they need. These effects cannot be predicted by quality testing of dose-rate settings, physical test-object visibility, or technical monitor performance values.

9.6.4 Local and Adaptive Image Processing

Image processing algorithms were initially applied to entire digital images, as illustrated in Figures 9-13–9-15. Faster image processing hardware now allows the use of different algorithms in different regions of the same image. Automatically optimizing local image processing in each region relies on a combination of a-priori knowledge of the purpose of the procedure and feature extraction within an image or a sequence of images.

Figure 9-16 illustrates the image of a small portion of a static test object used for daily quality assurance in an interventional laboratory. The image was acquired fluoroscopically and incorporates the image processing appropriate to angiography. The image processor interpreted high contrast structures as contrast filled arteries. It also interpreted the periphery of the image as to have nothing of clinical interest. Recursive filtering was only applied in the periphery to suppress quantum noise. The system saw that the "artery" was of high contrast and might move during fluo-

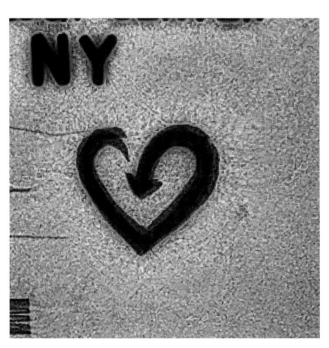

■ **FIGURE 9-16** Example of locally adaptive image processing. The image processor interpreted the lettering, lead-wire heart, guidewires, and stent as vessels and assumed that it might move during a fluoroscopic sequence. It therefore reduced the amount of temporal filtering in its vicinity resulting in increased local noise visibility. Compare this region with the heavily filtered region in the lower right corner of the image. (Fluoroscopic single frame image of daily QA test object—Enhanced for publication.) (© Stephen Balter.)

roscopy. It therefore locally disabled recursive filtering in that region of the image as well as applying an edge-enhancement filter. The sharp borders of the "artery" and the increased noise in its region result from these actions.

Adaptive image processing can be as simple as turning off recursive filtering when the fluoroscope or table are in motion as a means of reducing motion blur. There are many additional adaptations that can be applied based on combinations of a-priori knowledge and computerized image interpretation.

9.6.5   Image Displays

Viewing monitors and the human eye are the links in the imaging chain that transfer information extracted from the patient into the observer's brain. For photopic vision, the eye's relative contrast sensitivity peaks around 1 min of visual angle (Fig. 9-17A). The effect of viewing distance is shown in Figure 9-17B. The lesson from this figure is that the observer should be further from the image when trying to detect large objects. Morgan's comments at the time that his paper was published (1966) is that the radiologist's chair in a film reading room should be on wheels so that a greater distance can easily be achieved when looking for non-calcified nodules in a chest radiograph.

Operators often adjust their position depending on the clinical procedure and monitor size. Figure 9-17C illustrates an angiographer at work using a 20-inch display monitor. Note that he leans forward to maximize his ability to see the opacified vessels. Figure 9-17D shows an angiographer using a 55-inch monitor while examining similar size vessels. He is seen standing back and away from the beam

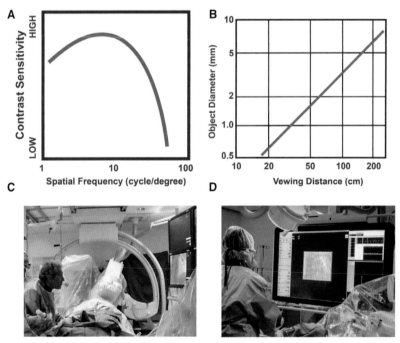

■ **FIGURE 9-17** Perception, viewing distance, and monitor size. **A.** Relative contrast sensitivity of the eye expressed in terms of visual angle. **B.** Optimum viewing distance for detection of an object depends on its size. **C.** The operator has leaned toward a small monitor to see objects of interest. **D.** The operator can see similar objects of interest on a large monitor while standing further away from the patient. (© Stephen Balter.)

to maximize his viewing ability. Thus, large format monitors yielded two increases in operator safety: (1) Increased distance decreases the intensity of the scatter field where he is standing. (2) Standing upright, instead of leaning over, decreases his orthopedic load and will help to reduce the injurious effects of wearing heavy personal protective equipment (PPE).

Because of differences in clinically important object sizes, shapes, and the presence of noise, in-room fluoroscopy monitors can seldom be meaningfully tested using mammography monitor protocols or other primary diagnostic monitor testing protocols. Key points include sufficient monitor luminance to allow room lights to be on as well as good contrast differentiation in both the blacks and whites. Specular and diffuse reflection of objects in the room can impede visibility. A simple test is to verify that the 0%–5% and 95%–100% steps in the SMPTE pattern are simultaneously visible from the operator's working position under clinical room lighting (see Chapter 5—display monitors).

9.7   IMAGE QUALITY IN FLUOROSCOPY

The purpose of each fluoroscopic or fluorographic run is the performance of a clinical task. Clinically useable image quality also involves the observer's imaging preferences, the observer's general medical knowledge, and a-priori information regarding the patient. Detailed discussion of such human factor concerns is beyond the scope of this chapter. Nevertheless, the resulting images should be good enough to not objectively or subjectively interfere with clinical goals. Images that are much better than required are often realized at the cost of unnecessary irradiation of both patients and staff.

Before 2010, image quality was mainly determined by the x-ray parameters and the hardware characteristics of the image receptor chain. In the past decade, improved image computer capabilities have enabled additional functionality including adaptively changing x-ray and display parameters using real-time image content and knowledge of devices deployed in the patient as considerations. Image processing has evolved from global spatial and temporal techniques to regional processing around local features in individual images (single image processing) and across time (multiple image processing). The resultant images facilitate clinical performance at lower radiation levels than required in the past. A full evaluation of these effects is beyond the scope of this chapter because it involves analysis of total radiation utilization and clinical outcomes.

Appropriate hardware-level image quality is an essential input to adaptive image processing. Figure 9-18 illustrates the image processing pipeline. There is a key point between the image receptor hardware and the final image processor. At this point, the images are in a "For Processing" state. Images displayed to the operator or archived when the system is in clinical mode are called "For Presentation." Technical image evaluation should be performed on images at or close to the "For Processing" state, as these images are corrected for detector imperfections and variable offset gain of the digital detector components, and represent a linear response to radiation fluence. Non-linear processing, including contrast and spatial resolution enhancement, characterizes the "For Presentation" images as discussed in Section 9.6. This section discusses key image quality parameters assuming that that the processing is uniform across an entire image.

Performance Evaluation: Component testing (*e.g.*, x-ray tube focal spot, intrinsic image receptor spatial resolution) are beyond the scope of this chapter. System image

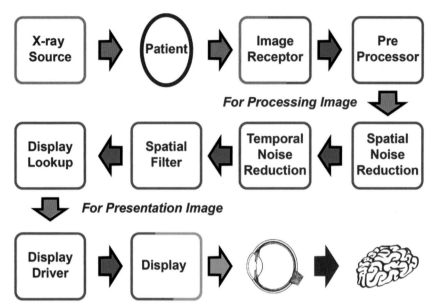

■ **FIGURE 9-18** Information flow. Upper: The primary x-ray beam is modulated by the patient, captured by the image receptor, and adjusted, where necessary by a pre-processor. The result is a "For Processing" image. Middle: Images are processed to reduce noise, manage sharpness, and optimize display conspicuity into a "For Presentation" image. Lower: The accessibility of patient information in the image is further influenced by the display and finally processed by the observer's eye-brain system before being used clinically. (© Stephen Balter.)

quality testing should be performed using a geometrical setup similar to performing clinical procedures on that fluoroscope. The results include the effects of focal-spot size and geometric magnification as well as the x-ray parameters and image receptor characteristics. Representative tools for measuring radiation output, spatial resolution, and low contrast performance are shown in Figure 9-19. An experimental small fluoroscopic contrast-detail test object, designed for local measurement, is also shown in the figure.

To avoid single frame noise effects, fluoroscopic images should be evaluated either when the beam is on or by viewing dynamic replays provided that the image processing of the replay is identical to that of the live image. Fluorographic images (cine, DA, DSA) are intended to be reviewed as individual frames. Therefore, they should be evaluated as single frames.

9.7.1 Spatial Resolution

Routine visual assessment spatial resolution is usually conducted using a relatively high-contrast bar pattern together with an attenuator simulating a thin patient (Fig. 9-19B). The system should be allowed to use its AERC to set its parameters based on the most common clinical use for that system. Low dose fluoroscopic modes may have a different observed resolution because of quantum noise effects. Imaging geometry (geometric magnification) and selected focal-spot size affect limiting resolution and need to be considered while testing. Without objective digital analysis of spatial resolution, observers should evaluate images under conditions where their own eyes do not limit resolution.

The absolute limiting resolution of an II is determined by its output screen and subsequent imaging chain. Magnification within an II is accomplished by projecting

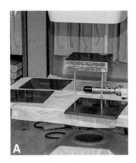
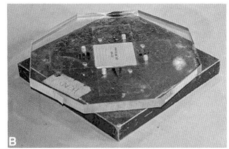
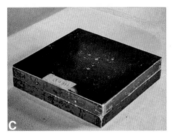
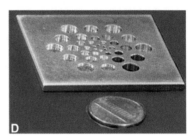

■ **FIGURE 9-19** QA tools. **A.** Fluoroscopic exposure rates using FDA test geometry. The system is set to minimum SID, the dosimeter is 30 cm from the image receptor, and attenuators used to drive the AERC are midway between the dosimeter and receptor to reduce scatter effects. **B.** High contrast bar target placed at the same location as the dosimeter in **A.** The bars are oriented at 45° to the image matrix to avoid moire effects. This plate also includes contrast-detail targets of different sizes and with different concentrations of iodine (base 19 mm Al). **C.** Low contrast detectability target at the same location. This setup provides four different object sizes with a single contrast step (1 mm Al on top of a 38-mm Al base). **D.** Research contrast-detail target. This 3-mm-thick plate has six sets of holes (1–6 mm) and provides contrast steps of 3 to 0.5 mm in 0.5-mm increments. It is used with an appropriate thickness base. (© Stephen Balter.)

a smaller portion of the input screen onto the fixed size output screen. Increases in limiting resolution occur as the magnification is increased. In some cases, regulatory requirements for limiting resolution are based on testing using a prescribed FOV but are vague on imaging geometry and focal spot size (Fig. 9-20).

The absolute limiting resolution of an FPD is determined by the pitch of its dexels (Table 9-1). Secondary limits are often imposed with a large active FOV and/or high frame rate. Physically small FPDs (*e.g.*, 20 cm) typically have a nominal dexel matrix

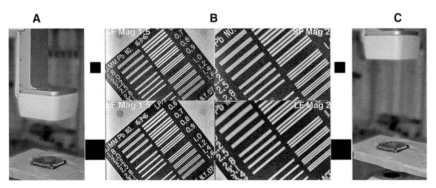

■ **FIGURE 9-20** Spatial resolution: geometry and focal spot size. **A.** This fluoroscope is at its minimum SSD (90 cm). The test plate is 60 cm from the focal-spot (magnification = 1.5). **B.** Spatial resolution with the small focal spot improves with magnification—system resolution is image receptor limited. Spatial resolution with the large focal spot degrades with magnification—system resolution is focal spot size limited. **C.** SSD has been increased to maximum SSD (120 cm). Constant 60 cm from the test plate to the focal-spot (magnification = 2.0). (© Stephen Balter.)

of $1,000 \times 1,000$. This corresponds to the nominal $1,000 \times 1,000$ pixel matrix of the final digital image. Fewer pixels are irradiated using a small FOV or a collimated beam than with an open beam large FOV. For this detector size, the limiting spatial resolution does not change as FOVs change. Physically large FPDs (*e.g.*, 40 cm) have dexel matrices that exceed the size of the down-stream digital display pixel matrices. At large FOVs binning dexels is needed to map the FPD to the image display. This also reduces dose requirements because visual noise is influenced by the total number of x-ray photons contributing to a single image pixel. At a certain magnification point, the FPD dexel matrix is the same as the image matrix. Most systems unbundle the FPD dexels at that point. A consequent increase in limiting resolution can be observed. However, dexels may remain bundled at relatively small FOVs when high image frame rates are used. This is done to limit the bandwidth needed to move the images. In such systems, a change in limiting resolution will be observed when the frame rate is changed across this threshold. Beyond these considerations, there is no physical reason for the limiting spatial resolution to change with FOV. The change in limiting resolution in proportion to the reciprocal of FOV as for IIs is incorrect in FPDs.

The x-ray tube's focal spot affects resolution as well. Chapter 6 reviews the effects of focal-spot size and geometric magnification on resolution. When the intrinsic limiting resolution of the image receptor is too low, the resolution of objects in the patient might be improved by using a small or micro focal-spot and geometric magnification. This arrangement is typically used for intercranial angiography.

9.7.2 Noise Limited Imaging

The perception of key clinical objects in an image is influenced by image noise. In a fluoroscopic image, visual noise can be grouped into two categories: The first is the noise produced by statistical variations in the numbers of x-ray photons converted into light (or charge) by the fluoroscopic detector (quantum noise). The second category is the combination of all other noise sources in the imaging chain and the observer's eye-brain system (system noise). Quantum noise is dependent on the local x-ray dose. System noise is independent of x-ray dose but may be dependent on factors such as electronic noise and illumination level. The amount of noise in an image changes with dose only when quantum noise is dominant.

Ideally fluoroscopic dose should always be reduced to a value just above the level where x-ray quantum noise interferes with the conduct of the examination. The limiting contrast resolution of fluoroscopy is low compared to radiography due to this image noise. When higher exposure rates are used, limiting contrast resolution improves, but dose to the patient also increases. The use of exposure rates consistent with the image quality needs of the fluoroscopic examination is an appropriate guiding principle. Fluoroscopic systems with different dose settings (selectable at the console) allow the user flexibility from patient to patient to adjust the compromise between contrast resolution and patient dose.

Invasive fluoroscopic procedures involve the use of contrast media and/or devices. The mass attenuation coefficients are substantially different than tissue. Their differential attenuation coefficients are strongly influenced by the x-ray spectrum used to form the images. An object's contrast to noise ratio (CNR) is improved when the x-ray energy spectrum is matched to the inserted materials. Standard angiographic techniques presume that the object of interest contains iodine ($Z = 53$) or materials of similar atomic number (*e.g.*, barium, $Z = 56$). Devices containing high Z materials (*e.g.*, Pt, Z = 78; Au, Z = 79) will do better with a corresponding higher energy spectrum. Automatically keeping the fluoroscope aware of what devices are in the patient at a given moment is an interesting engineering challenge.

Limiting contrast resolution is usually subjectively measured by viewing contrast-detail phantoms (Fig. 9-19C and D). Most of these phantoms are made of a single material (*e.g.*, Al). The x-ray energy spectra imaging the targets and their background are essentially identical. The measurements are thus effectively SNR versus object size and dose. Such measurements do not completely predict the results expected for most clinical fluoroscopic scenarios (*e.g.*, iodine contrast against a soft-tissue background). Additional direct measurements of CNR with test objects that replicate the clinical situation may prove to be a more reliable tool for predicting clinical utility for many fluoroscopic tasks.

9.7.3 Temporal Resolution

The primary purpose of fluoroscopy (and associated fluorography) is to observe and document motion. This requires temporal resolution appropriate to the clinical task. Clinical temporal resolution includes the behavior of the observer's eye. Two important factors are image averaging in the eye (approximately 200 ms) and the eye's sensitivity to images provided at low frame rates (CFF approximately 30 FPS).

Digital viewing systems typically refresh their images at rates well above 100 Hz (100 new images drawn and displayed per second). This is well above the CFF and provides a visually constant image. Displays accommodate images provided at low frequencies by displaying the same image multiple times. The history of commercial motion pictures provides some insight. Early film cameras ran at relatively low frame rates; their images were projected at the acquisition frame rate, and had distinctive flicker (one of the nicknames of motion-pictures is "flicks") The Hollywood standard acquisition rate in the camera was 24 FPS, below the CFF for many. Commercial film projectors doubled the display rate by mechanically displaying each frame twice before advancing the film. This rate (48 images per second) is high enough to suppress the impression of flicker for most people.

Analog video in the USA was recorded at 30 FPS for synchrony with the 60 Hz AC power frequency. These images were composed of two interlaced fields yielding an effective rate of 60 FPS, partially as a means of reducing flicker.

Eye integration does not apply when a single image is continuously displayed. Perceived noise is limited by the x-ray dose used to acquire that image. Fluoroscopic images are acquired at relatively low dose per frame. A single fluoroscopic image will appear noisier than when the same scene is viewed as a sequence. Fluorographic images are intended to be viewed one-by-one. This is the principal reason for using more radiation for fluorography than fluoroscopy.

Global temporal averaging (lag) is an inherent characteristic of analog video tubes. The lack of lag in newer camera types increased the appearance of noise, including x-ray quantum noise. The noise content of a single fluoroscopic image can be reduced by recursive filtering. This process simulates eye physiology by adding a running average of previous frames to the current frame. Figure 9-15 illustrates the effects of recursive filtering. The original images were acquired using pulsed fluoroscopy with short pulses. There is minimum motion blur of the rapidly moving guidewire in the original images (it is in a different position in each image). The number of older images contributing to the current image increases with increased recursion. This results in ghosting of previous guidewire positions.

■ **FIGURE 9-21** Recursive filter ghost images and motion unsharpness. This is a single frame of a fluoroscopic sequence of the NEMA XR-21 rotating disk tool. It includes the effects of the recursive filtering applied when this image was captured. The disk has five uniform wires of different diameters and two lead dots near the #5 wire. The direction of rotation is shown. Local linear velocity increases toward the periphery. Motion blur causes tapering of the wire images. Recursive filtering produces ghost images of the wires, dots, and numbers. (© Stephen Balter.)

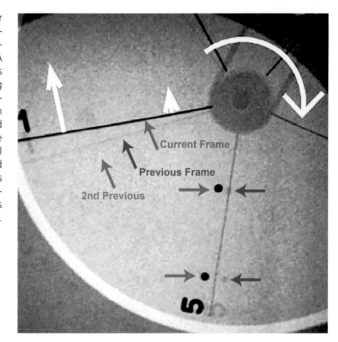

Figure 9-21 illustrates both motion unsharpness due to individual fluoroscopic frame pulse-width and recursive filtering caused by summing multiple frames (Section 9.6.2).

Some new fluoroscopes automatically adjust the recursion coefficient on a pixel by pixel basis as a means of reducing motion blur. For example, if the image processor expects iodine filled moving vessels in an image, it can locally reduce recursive filtering in that area. This minimizes the blurring that occurs if a moving vessel is averaged over several frames. The increased noise around a structure that an image processor interpreted as a vessel is shown in Figure 9-16.

9.7.4 Dose Rates

Regulatory compliance, and the functional behavior of any specific operating mode can be measured in the hospital. The test setup, shown in Figure 9-19A is representative for a system where the x-ray beam always passes through the tabletop. All removable attenuators between the x-ray tube and measuring point should be removed from the beam. The system is set to its minimum SID. The radiation detector is 30 cm from the image receptor (at the FDA dose regulatory point for this C-arm fluoroscope). To minimize backscatter, the attenuators are 10 cm from the radiation detector. Figure 9-19C illustrates a low contrast detectability tool on the tabletop. This tool provides a single contrast step (1 mm Al with a 38-mm base) with a series of target sizes. Other available tools provide a series of contrast steps and target sizes. Such tools are intended to provide data for a contrast-detail plot.

Attenuator thicknesses (as shown in Fig 9-19A) should cover the range of patient sizes examined on the fluoroscope under test. Water or plexiglass of appropriate thickness may be used if desired. Metallic attenuators are lighter and easier to transport but may cause small oscillations in output because the AERC expects to see water. A typical metallic set includes 19 mm Al (pediatric patient), 38 mm Al (small adult), 38 mm Al + 0.5 mm Cu (average adult), and 38 mm Al + 2.0 mm Cu (heavy adult). An additional attenuator, such as 3 mm lead or 10 mm Cu, is needed to drive the fluoroscope to its maximum output in all modes of operation. Measurements are taken using the most common clinical fluoroscopic and acquisition modes used by that system.

Changing the frame rates and magnification modes provides additional information. It is also important to test the effect of SID variation on maximum output by leaving the detector in place and moving the image receptor from minimum to maximum SID.

9.8 PATIENT RADIATION MANAGEMENT

The primary task for any medical procedure is to produce the intended result without exposing the patient to unnecessary risks. Fluoroscopic procedures provide potential benefits to the patient while exposing both patients and staff to radiation and non-radiation risks. Operators should be aware of radiation levels as a procedure proceeds because there are no regulatory limits on radiation use.

The fluoroscope's AERC adjusts radiation output to accommodate differences in patient anatomy and SID. It also accommodates operator selections such as the dose-rate family associated with a specific clinical mode, operator selectable choices between normal and low dose-rate fluoroscopy, etc. In many cases, the AERC program limits maximum outputs to values well below regulatory limits.

Regulatory limitations on the maximal permitted fluoroscopic dose rate is an old tool used for radiation management. There are no regulatory limitations on any acquisition mode (*e.g.*, cine, digital angiography, DSA) included in a fluoroscopic system. In addition, there are no regulatory limitations on the irradiation time used for a fluoroscopic procedure.

In the United States, federal regulations limit the maximum permissible fluoroscopic air kerma rate for a C-arm fluoroscope to 88 mGy/min at 30 cm from the entrance surface of the image receptor at any source to image receptor distance (SID). Under clinical conditions, actual maximum patient entrance air kerma rate is usually higher for C-arms when the image receptor is more than 30 cm from the tabletop. Different regulatory measurement points are prescribed for other types of fluoroscopes. For example, the measurement point for a GI fluoroscope with an under-table x-ray tube is 1 cm above the tabletop at any SID.

Operators are a key control element in radiation management (Fig. 9-1). Pragmatic radiation management points that should be known to the operator and staff are shown in Table 9-2.

9.8.1 Patient Dose Metrics

Fluoroscopic Time (5 Min Timer)

Recording fluoroscopic time does not provide useful information on patient irradiation for the simple reason that it does not include any contribution from fluorography. Currently, about half of the patient's total irradiation in interventional procedures is attributable to fluorography. Historically, fluoro-time, and the accompanying 5-min fluoro-time buzzer were introduced in the era before digital-fluorography. (Clinical documentation was obtained by acquiring spot-films using radiographic cassettes.) Fluoro-time therefore supplies little useful information on either potential patient tissue reactions or stochastic risk to patients or staff.

TABLE 9-2 SUMMARY OF OPERATIONAL FACTORS THAT AFFECT IMAGE QUALITY AND RADIATION DOSE TO THE PATIENT AND STAFF

	EFFECT ON IMAGE QUALITY & RADIATION DOSE		
OPERATIONAL CHANGE	*Image Quality*	*Radiation Dose to the Patient*	*Radiation Dose to the Staff*
Increase in patient size	Worse (increased scatter fraction)	Higher	Higher
Increase in tube current (mA) with constant kV (*i.e.*, AERC off)	Better (lower image noise)	Higher	Higher
Increase in tube potential (kV) with AERC active	Soft tissue: Better (lower noise) Bone and contrast material: Worse: (decreased subject contrast)	Lower	Lower
Increase in tube filtration from 0.2 to 9.4 mm Cu with AERC active	Little change	Lower	Lower
Increase in source to skin distance	Slightly better	Lower	Little change
Increase in skin to image receptor distance (fixed source-skin distance)	Slightly better (less scatter) excluding x-ray tube focal spot size effects)	Higher	Higher
Increase in Image Receptor Magnification Factor	May be better (improved spatial resolution)	Higher	Higher
Increase in collimator opening	Worse (increased scatter fraction)	Little change (however higher integral and effective dose)	Higher
Increase beam on time	No effect	Higher	Higher
Increase in pulsed fluoroscopy frame rate	Better (improved temporal resolution)	Higher	Higher
Grid is used	Better (decreased scatter fraction)	Higher	Higher
Image recording modes (cine, DSA, radiographic)	Better (lower noise, higher resolution)	Higher	Higher

Kerma-Area Product (KAP, DAP)

Kerma-area product (KAP) (or dose area product—DAP), also referred to as P_{KA}, is a radiation dose metric that is commonly tracked in many parts of the world. KAP is the same at any location between the x-ray tube and the patient. Historically, KAP was measured by placing a transmission detector in the x-ray tube's collimator assembly. More recently, KAP is computed from irradiation parameters (kV, mA, exposure time, collimation blade settings). KAP does not provide a direct indicator of the possibility of skin reactions because a procedure producing the same KAP can deliver low skin dose to a large surface with large field sizes or a high skin dose to a small surface with a small field. KAP does provide useful information in terms of x-ray energy imparted to the patient and therefore is useful for estimating stochastic risk to both patients and staff.

Reference Air Kerma

All fluoroscopes installed in the United States after 2006 are required to provide real-time information to the operator on the total air kerma (without backscatter) delivered to a reference point on the system ($K_{a,r}$). The reference point on an interventional fluoroscope is on the central ray of the x-ray beam and 15 cm from isocenter toward the x-ray tube. Thus, the reference point moves with the gantry and is seldom exactly on the patient's skin (Fig. 9-22). Different reference points are defined for different types of fluoroscopic systems.

For interventional C-arms, the reference air kerma is not a direct measure of the patient's skin dose. However, it has proven to be of great utility in managing patient irradiation during procedures as well as for later quality management processes.

The $K_{a,r}$ value reported on the fluoroscope is not the peak skin dose (PSD) received by the patient. Its reference point is fixed relative to the fluoroscope's mechanical construction. Therefore, the reference point moves relative to the patient whenever the fluoroscopic table or gantry is moved. Increased motion decreases the correlation between $K_{a,r}$ and PSD. The reference point may be inside the patient, on the patient's skin, or outside the patient during any irradiation (Fig. 9-22). This can lead to an under- or overestimation of the local entrance skin kerma (ESK) during that irradiation. Obtaining local skin dose requires both a geometric calculation and the addition of back scatter (typically 30%–40%) to the $K_{a,r}$ for that irradiation. It is also important to note that the reference point is not usually the FDA dose-rate compliance point, which is defined relative to the image receptor.

Skin Dose Maps

Newer interventional fluoroscopes offer real-time skin dose maps. These systems combine the $K_{a,r}$ from a single irradiation event (*e.g.*, foot-peddle actuation), a backscatter factor, collimator settings, gantry angle, and table position to model the distribution of dose on the surface of a mathematical-model patient. Dose distributions add in the same area if there is no beam motion between irradiations. Distributions are mapped to different regions on the model when motion occurs. Radiation is additive between irradiations in regions of overlap. The PSD is simply the highest dose mapped to any portion of the model. In-room displays provide the map to operators as a resource for their ongoing clinical benefit/risk assessment. Displays often include additional information such as the current size and location of the x-ray beam. This facilitates repositioning the beam if possible when surface dose is of concern. Figure 9-23 is an example of such a real-time map.

Many off-line fluoroscopic dose tracking systems also provide surface dose reconstruction and organ dose estimation. The radiation dose structured report (RDSR)

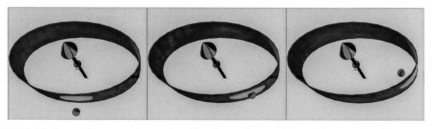

■ **FIGURE 9-22** Dose reference point motion. The dose reference is located at a point that is separately defined for different types of fluoroscopic systems. For interventional C-arms, its location is 15 cm from isocenter toward the x-ray tube and moves in space as the gantry is rotated. In this example, with an arbitrary elliptical patient model, the reference point is outside the patient for the PA projection, on the patient's skin at 45°, and inside the patient near the Lateral. The actual location will vary depending on patient size and table height. (© Stephen Balter.)

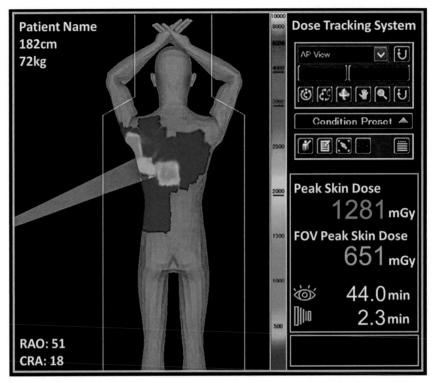

■ FIGURE 9-23 Real-time skin dose map. The fluoroscope uses its geometric and dosimetric data to "paint" the distribution of radiation on a mathematically modeled patient's skin in real time. This capability will be provided on all new interventional fluoroscopes in the early 2020s. The map shows the total distribution of radiation using a color code. The peak skin dose is indicated numerically. It also shows the current location of the x-ray beam. In this case, the current beam location does not correspond to PSD. Operators can use these displays as part of ongoing patient benefit-risk evaluations. (Used with permission from Canon Medical Systems USA, Inc.)

produced by the fluoroscope at the end of the case is the starting point for the necessary calculations.

9.8.2 Patient Radiation Documentation and Follow-Up

Records of doses to the patient from each procedure should be kept for quality assurance purposes. Data should be entered into both the individual patient's medical record and departmental QA systems. If the estimated skin doses are large enough to cause skin injury, arrangements should be made for clinical follow-up of the patient. Such large skin doses are most likely to be imparted by prolonged fluoroscopically guided interventional procedures, or multiple procedures performed in the same anatomical area within months.

The Joint Commission (JC) requires recording of the dose delivered by procedures in a retrievable format as well as a process for tracking patients receiving doses above a facility determined threshold. Alerts should be appropriately triggered at the end of the procedure before the patient leaves the room. Dose archives can be established and maintained by a variety of means ranging from manually recording the in-room displays at the end of the procedure to fully automated dose management servers. Key demographic (*e.g.*, height, weight) and procedural (*e.g.*, room, operator, CPT code, contrast use) should also be captured to facilitate analysis. A well-constructed database furnishes the information needed for radiation quality management (*e.g.*, comparison with DRLs). Beyond alerts, data should be periodically analyzed as part of the department's quality management system. Two examples of such analysis are as follows: What are the differences in radiation use when similar procedures (*e.g.*, diagnostic carotid angiography) performed on different systems? Are there differences when the same procedure is performed by different operators on the same fluoroscope?

Many systems provide a DICOM RDSR at the end of the procedure. The RDSR provided by interventional fluoroscopes contains the information needed for radiation documentation purposes and can also be used to construct a postprocedure skin-dose map.

Displayed radiation data ($K_{a,r}$, P_{KA}) are calculated values obtained when the beam is on from the factors (kV, mA, pulse width, pulse rate, filtration, field-size, etc.) used to generate x-rays. US and international standards allow an uncertainty of ±35%. Most systems are substantially more precise than this limit. The RDSR includes a field for reporting the correction factor. Its value should be determined by the medical physicist as part of routine QA, and then inserted into the fluoroscope for inclusion in the RDSR.

Installed fluoroscopes use different units of measure to display $K_{a,r}$ (*e.g.*, mGy, R) and P_{KA} (*e.g.*, Rcm^2, Gym^2, cGycm^2, mGycm^2, μGym^2) their measurements. The use of different units has the potential for confusion when an operator uses different makes and models of fluoroscopes. Knowing which units are used by an individual fluoroscope is essential to using the data for patient management. Fortunately, most interventional fluoroscopes display $K_{a,r}$ in units of mGy. Newer model fluoroscopes of all makes are converging to the use of Gy-cm^2 for $P_{KA.}$

9.9 OPERATOR AND STAFF RADIATION SAFETY

Occupational exposures of physicians, nurses, technologists, and other personnel who routinely work in fluoroscopic suites is often unavoidable. To reduce radiation exposure in fluoroscopy, everyone in the fluoroscopy suite should always wear radiation attenuating aprons and thyroid shields. Leaded eyewear (with side protection) is appropriate for individuals who are routinely close to the patient while the beam is on. The use of ceiling-mounted and table-mounted radiation shields can substantially reduce the radiation doses to personnel. Movable lead shields should be available for additional protection to other staff members participating in the procedure. The dose to personnel is reduced when the dose to the patient is reduced, so patient dose reduction measures are beneficial to everyone.

Situational awareness by operators and all other staff members is important. Individuals need to be aware of the location of the primary and scattered radiation fields so that they can minimize unnecessary irradiation. Images of the operator's hands in the beam are not infrequent and seldom medically justified. Real-time personnel monitoring is currently available with combinations of audible and visible feedback means. These tools are excellent in a training situation, but often are distracting, ignored, or both after they have been deployed for a while. Several research groups have recently demonstrated the ability to compute the spatial distribution of scatter in real time while tracking the position of individuals in these radiation fields.

Stray radiation in the fluoroscopic environment is mainly attributable to scatter from the patient, with a small additional contribution from x-ray tube leakage. Most of the scatter in the room is produced where the primary beam enters the patient. Scatter levels on the exit side of the patient are typically a factor of ten lower than those encountered on the patient's entrance side.

A great deal of specific scatter information is provided by manufacturers of IEC compliant fluoroscopes in the system users' manuals. Figure 9-24A is a good example of the data available for a mobile C-arm at the operator's position. Figures 9-24 B-D are examples supplied with fixed interventional systems. Data is supplied for representative beam angles (vertical, horizontal), often as horizontal plots at different heights (100–150 cm) above the floor.

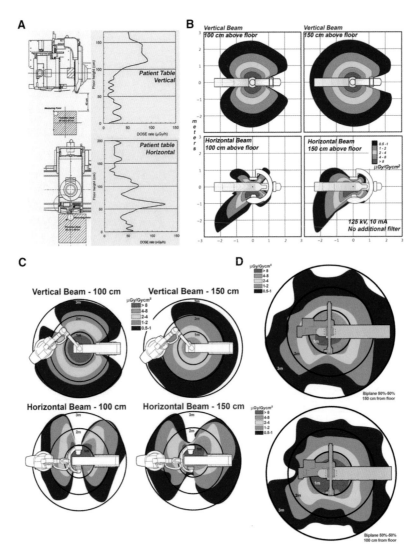

■ **FIGURE 9-24** Scatter Radiation Maps provided in system user manuals. **A.** Zone of significant occupancy (where the operator usually stands) for a general purpose R/F system. **B and C.** Area around two different single-plane interventional systems. Horizontal plots at 100, 150 cm above floor for horizontal and vertical beam orientations. Portions of the gantry and x-ray tube attenuate the scatter resulting in a low scatter field behind them. In both **B and C** (lateral at 100 cm) it is seen that there is no stray radiation field behind the x-ray tube assembly that also indicates that there is minimal tube-leakage contribution to the stray field. The asymmetry in scatter from the patient can be seen in the lateral plots. In the absence of protective devices, an operator standing near the x-ray tube would be exposed to 1–10 mGy/h; on the image receptor side the value is reduced by an order of magnitude. **D.** Area around a biplane interventional system. Both planes are operating simultaneously. Each plane supplies 50% of the KAP and thus contributes to the scatter field. At any point, however, the fraction of scatter supplied by each plane differs. Plots **B–D** are scaled in KAP; lower dose rates and better collimation will reduce operator dose: Adapted with permission from Canon Medical Systems, Philips, Siemens Healthineers, and GE Healthcare.

9.9.1 Worker Dose Monitoring and Tracking

Fluoroscopic procedures usually result in the irradiation of one or more staff members. Specialized fluoroscopes (*e.g.*, "remote control systems") facilitate the performance of procedures with all staff protected by structural radiation barriers. However, it is prudent to assume that the entire fluoroscopic team (physicians, nurses, technicians) is occupationally irradiated.

The scatter fields produced by fluoroscopy vary in time and space during procedures. These fields are further modified by radioprotective devices (*e.g.*, face shields, table-mounted drapes). Staff move within these fields as they perform their duties. Because of this variability, radiation monitors worn by every person working in a fluoroscopic room are currently the only practicable means of assessing individual irradiation levels.

The dose delivered to a fluoroscopist's organs from a single procedure varies by several orders of magnitude. Factors include the physical distribution of scatter in the room, the fluoroscopist's posture relative to the field, the use of radiation PPE, and shielding of deeper organs by superficial tissues.

However, radiation monitors report irradiation at the point that they are worn; thus, they give no direct information about the dose received elsewhere in the body. The goals of every radiation monitoring program are to assure individuals that they are working at a safe level and to detect unexpected changes in either the radiation environment or in the individual's working methods.

Two common methods are a single monitor worn outside radiation PPE at collar level, and the collar monitor plus a second monitor worn inside the PPE at chest level. Additional monitors are used to measure eye, hand, and fetal irradiation. Monitoring configurations, and the interpretation of the results are discussed in the Radiation Protection chapter (Section 21.2.6).

Different facilities have different policies regarding monitor placement. When assigned monitors are consistently worn in their designated locations, their readings can be used to calculate the worker's effective dose with an accuracy that is acceptable for radiation protection surveillance. However, if they are inappropriately worn (*e.g.*, reversing collar and chest monitors) they can overestimate dose by orders of magnitude. This can be of individual and regulatory concern.

9.10 LOOKING AHEAD

Fluoroscopic x-ray tubes and image receptors have not changed in any fundamental manner since the 2010s. The job of the image acquisition elements of the fluoroscopic system is to deliver technically adequate images to the system's digital image processor. These images are then processed, and the results delivered to the observer. Increased image processing power has had a substantial impact on both improving clinical conspicuity and reducing radiation use in the same time interval.

Presentation images usually undergo non-linear transformations, that are configured based on presumed clinical content. Many fluoroscopes delivered after 2010 have enough computational resources to provide different algorithms in different regions of the same image. These algorithms rely on a-priori knowledge of the examination in progress. Such information is currently supplied by the operator. A future fluoroscope might improve performance by collecting information on current activities (*e.g.*, implanted devices in the patient, etc.), and by analysis of the patient's current and historical images.

Fluoroscopy is one means of imaging during clinical procedures. The use of live fluoroscopy and fluorography can be safely reduced by using other real-time modalities (*e.g.*, ultrasound) and/or historical data (*e.g.*, volumetric CT data sets). Appropriate information can always be presented to the fluoroscopist on parallel image displays. Fusing multi-modality data into a single composite image is of value. Thus, the deployment and use of image-fusion technology is likely to increase.

SUGGESTED READING AND REFERENCES

AAPM. *Functionality and Operation of Fluoroscopic Automatic Brightness Control/Automatic Dose Rate Control Logic in Modern Cardiovascular and Interventional Angiography Systems. A Report of AAPM Task Group 125.* 2012.

ACR–AAPM. Technical standard for management of the use of radiation in fluoroscopic procedures. 2018. https://www.acr.org/-/media/ACR/Files/Practice Parameters/MgmtFluoroProc.pdf. Accessed May 8, 2020.

Balter S. Fluoroscopic technology from 1895 to 2019 drivers: physics and physiology. *Med Phys Int J* (Special Issue, History of Medical Physics). 2019;2.

ICRP. Radiological protection in fluoroscopically guided procedures outside the imaging department. ICRP Publication 117. *Ann ICRP.* 2010;40(6):1-102.

ICRP. Occupational radiological protection in interventional procedures. ICRP Publication 139. *Ann ICRP.* 2018;47(2):1-118.

Image Wisely, Fluoroscopy. https://www.imagewisely.org/Imaging-Modalities/Fluoroscopy. Accessed May 8, 2020.

International Atomic Energy Agency. Chapter 8: Fluoroscopic imaging systems. *Diagnostic Radiology Physics: A Handbook for Teachers and Students*, 2014. RPOP.IAEA.ORG

Morgan RH. Visual perception in fluoroscopy and radioqraphy. *Radiology.* 1966;86:403-416.

NCRP. *Radiation Dose Management for Fluoroscopically-Guided Interventional Procedures.* NCRP Report No. 168. Bethesda, MD: National Council on Radiation Protection and Measurement; 2010.

Nickoloff EL. AAPM/RSNA physics tutorial for residents: physics of flat-panel fluoroscopy systems. *RadioGraphics.* 2011;31(2):591-602.

CHAPTER 10

Computed Tomography

Computed tomography (CT) has experienced enormous growth in clinical use over the past three decades (Fig. 10-1) primarily due to significant advances in image quality and a dramatic (1,000 fold) reduction in acquisition time as the technology has advanced. Image quality has increased as a result of better detector sampling along the long axis (z-dimension) of the patient when multiple detector array systems were developed. CT reconstruction has also advanced from filtered backprojection (FBP) to different generations of iterative reconstruction, and now deep learning (DL)-based adjuncts to the CT reconstruction process have led to lower noise images at lower radiation dose levels. Many other subtle technologies, discussed in this chapter, have also led to better spatial resolution and contrast resolution in CT. CT acquisition times have plummeted with the advent of helical scanning (continuous table movement), combined with multiple detector array CT systems that allow 40 mm (or greater) sections of the patient to be imaged in one rotation of the gantry. With half-second gantry rotation (or shorter), 80 mm of patient length can be acquired in 1 second (s), and hence 400 mm of patient length can be scanned in 5 s. The speed of the CT examination is one of the factors that has driven its clinical use as shown in Figure 10-1.

These technical advances have allowed CT imaging to gain widespread use across many clinical applications, and the medley of CT images illustrated in Figure 10-2 shows the broad application of CT technology to abdominal, thoracic, head, musculoskeletal, and many other imaging applications. High temporal resolution CT can allow CT angiography (CTA) or organ specific CT perfusion. Dual energy CT allows 3D reconstruction and segmentation of bone structures from soft tissue, with accurate assessment of iodinated contrast agent concentration over time in three dimensions. Dual energy CT also allows physicians to characterize gout, and is used in radiation therapy treatment planning for assessment of electron density.

Conventional CT scanners scan along the z-dimension (long axis) of the patient's body or head with a gantry rotating rapidly around the patient. This acquisition geometry leads to a reconstruction plane in the axial plane of the patient. A single abdominal CT image is shown in Figure 10-3, and the axial plane corresponds to the principal reconstruction plane of most CT scanners—coronal and sagittal CT images are typically synthesized from the reconstructed (thin section) axial CT images. The two-dimensional image shown is comprised of individual pixel elements (pixels), and typically each pixel has equal dimensions in the horizontal (x) and the vertical (y) dimensions. The two-dimensional CT image corresponds to a volumetric section of the patient's body, which has a given thickness (Δz) depending upon acquisition and reconstruction parameters. Hence, each pixel in the image corresponds to a volume element or voxel in the patient's body. For normal resolution (NR) CT scanner, the dimensions of each voxel can be on the order of 0.60 mm (Δx and Δy) by 0.50 mm (Δz)—corresponding to 0.18 mg of unit-density tissue. Hence, a 75-kg person can be imaged using over 400 million voxels using CT.

Because of the small in-plane pixel dimensions (Δx, Δy) and the correspondingly small slice thickness (Δz), the volume data set of axial CT images are routinely

■ **FIGURE 10-1** The number of CTs performed annually in the United States is illustrated for almost 3 decades. The dramatic increase in the use of CT demonstrates both the clinical utility of the modality, as well as increases in technical performance, such as better image quality and shorter acquisition times. The fluctuation in the curve from 2012 onward is the result of some concerns over radiation dose, but primarily is due to changes in reimbursement related to exam bundling (and hence how CT examinations are counted).

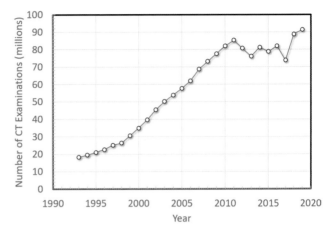

reformatted from the original (axial) reconstruction plane into both coronal and sagittal images (Fig. 10-4), allowing the radiologist to view truly orthogonal images, which provide a more intuitive impression of patient anatomy. The ability to routinely visualize both coronal and sagittal CT images provides important additional information to the interpreting physician, including spinal alignment, orientation of pathology and normal anatomy including identifying feeding vessels, gastrointestinal tract topography, abdominal organ placement and orientation, trauma, and other factors.

10.1 BASIC CONCEPTS

X-ray CT scanners typically run at 120 kV for routine scanning; however, the x-ray tube voltage can be varied to optimize the trade-off between image quality and radiation dose for different clinical imaging applications and different patient sizes. This

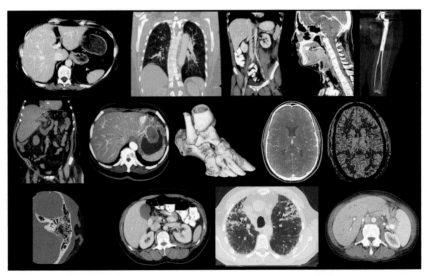

■ **FIGURE 10-2** The high spatial resolution and excellent contrast resolution of modern CT systems, as illustrated on this medley of images, have contributed to the clinical demand for CT imaging. While the primary forte of CT imaging is fundamental three-dimensional anatomical imaging, with the addition of iodinated contrast, functional imaging including enhancement and perfusion metrics can be assessed quickly, accurately, and quantitatively.

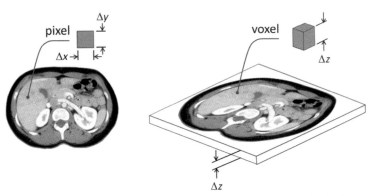

■ **FIGURE 10-3** Individual CT images (with axial images shown here) are comprised of a two-dimensional matrix of picture elements, referred to as *pixels*. For most CT images, Δx and Δy are identical due to the nature of the reconstruction. While the individual CT image is typically a two-dimensional presentation, each pixel in the image corresponds to a volume element or *voxel* in the patient. The Δz dimension of a voxel typically is slightly different from the Δx or Δy dimension, because of differences in the geometry of CT acquisition.

allows the development of protocols that are very patient-specific. The high kV combined with the added filtration in the x-ray tube leads to a relatively "hard" x-ray spectrum—one with relatively high effective energy. The tube voltage options in CT depend on the vendor; however, 80-, 100-, 120-, and 140-kV spectra are typical (but not exclusive) in the industry (Fig. 10-5). The high x-ray energy used in CT is important for understanding what physical properties of tissue are being displayed on CT images. The effective energies of the four spectra illustrated in Figure 10-5 range from about 43 to 70 keV, and this region is overlaid on the mass attenuation coefficients for soft tissue in Figure 10-6. In this region, it is seen that Rayleigh scattering and photoelectric effect have the lowest interaction probability and the Compton scatter interaction has the highest interaction probability. Also visible from the figure, it is seen that the Compton scattering interaction is 10-fold more likely than the photoelectric effect *in soft tissue* (the atomic number dependent photoelectric effect does

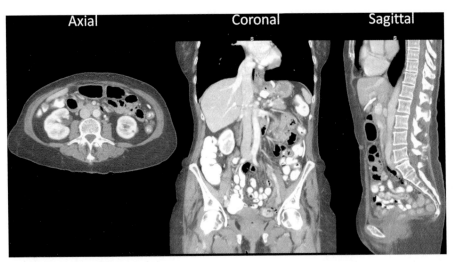

■ **FIGURE 10-4** In the earlier days of CT technology, the slice thickness of the images (Δz in Fig. 10-3) was typically much larger than the in-plane (Δx or Δy) voxel dimensions, and this limited the majority of image interpretation to the axial image presentation. With modern CT systems, dimensions of Δz can be smaller than the in-plane voxel dimensions, and consequently the presentation of both coronal and sagittal images (along with axial images) is typical in modern viewing environments.

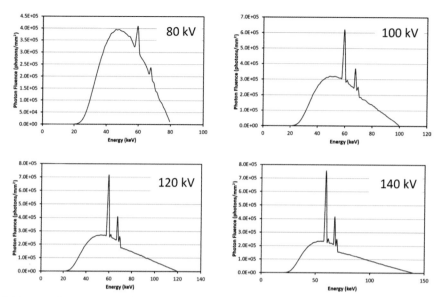

■ **FIGURE 10-5** The x-ray spectra for computed tomography are shown for 80, 100, 120, and 140 kV—each spectrum is filtered with 10 mm of aluminum, which approximates the typical amount of filtration at the center of the beam for most CT scanner models. The high tube potentials along with the large filtration thicknesses lead to x-ray beams with high effective energy.

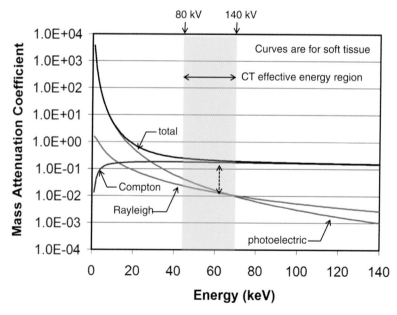

■ **FIGURE 10-6** What physical parameter does the grayscale in a CT image correspond to? The mass attenuation coefficient of soft tissue is shown as a function of x-ray energy in this graph. The curves correspond to the attenuation coefficients for the photoelectric effect, Rayleigh and Compton scattering. The effective energy in CT is outlined by the vertical band. In this region, it is seen that the Compton cross section is approximately tenfold that of the Rayleigh or photoelectric cross sections, meaning that the gray scale (Hounsfield Unit) in CT for soft tissue is primarily determined by the physical dependency of Compton scattering—electron density.

play a larger role in x-ray photon attenuation in bone, metal implants, and iodinated contrast agent). For soft tissue, the CT image grayscale (also known as CT number or Hounsfield Unit) represents the physical property for which Compton scattering is most dependent on, which is electron density. As discussed in Chapter 3, the Compton scatter linear attenuation coefficient, $\mu_{Compton}$, is proportional to

$$\mu_{Compton} \propto \rho N \frac{Z}{A},$$ [10-1]

where ρ is the mass density of the tissue in a voxel, N is Avogadro's number (6.023×10^{23}), Z is the atomic number, and A is the atomic mass. The primary constituents of soft tissue are carbon, hydrogen, oxygen, and nitrogen, and the Z/A ratio for most of these elements is ½. For hydrogen, however, the Z/A ratio is 1. While this would imply that hydrogenous tissues such as adipose tissue would have a higher $\mu_{Compton}$, in reality, hydrogen content in tissues is small and the lower density of adipose ($\rho \approx 0.94$ g/cm³) relative to soft tissue ($\rho \approx 1$) tends to dominate Equation 10-1 when it comes to the difference between soft tissue and hydrogen-rich adipose tissues. Consequently, adipose tissue appears darker (has a lower $\mu_{Compton}$) than soft tissues such as liver or other organ parenchyma (see Fig. 10-4).

While radiographic modalities tend to demonstrate the exponential attenuation properties of tissues, the preprocessing steps and subsequent reconstruction used in CT lead to grayscale in CT, which is a linear function of the linear attenuation coefficient. Indeed, the grayscale in CT is given a special name Hounsfield Unit (or HU) after one of the principal developers of the technology, Sir Godfrey Hounsfield. The Hounsfield Unit is scaled as described in Equation 10-2:

$$HU_K \equiv 1{,}000 \left[\frac{\mu_K - \mu_w}{\mu_w - \mu_{air}} \right] \simeq 1{,}000 \left[\frac{\mu_K - \mu_w}{\mu_w} \right].$$ [10-2]

For a given voxel K in the image, which contains tissue with an average linear attenuation coefficient μ_K, the Hounsfield Unit is scaled relative to the linear attenuation coefficient of water, μ_w. The linear attenuation coefficient of water, μ_{air}, is also used in the definition; however this value is so small that it is negligible (as the rightmost term in Eq. 10-2 shows). The scaling shown in Equation 10-2 defines the HU range at two physically meaning points: it can be seen that if voxel K contained only pure water, then $\mu_K = \mu_w$, and thence $HU_K = 0$. If voxel K contained only air, then $\mu_K \approx 0$, and $HU_K = -1{,}000$.

The linear attenuation coefficient has relatively strong dependencies on the x-ray beam energy (Fig. 10-6), and so could be written as $\mu_w(E)$. Equation 10-2 avoids this notation by inferring that the linear attenuation coefficients in the equation represent the *effective* linear attenuation coefficient, μ_{eff}. With this in mind, it should be noted that the calibration of the Hounsfield Unit is different for each x-ray tube potential used in CT, and thus the value of $\mu_{w\text{-}eff}$ changes (slightly) for 80 kV, 100 kV, etc. While for water, HU = 0, always; other tissues such as liver and bone will have slightly different HU values at different tube potentials.

The ideal for each CT scanner is that $HU_w = 0$; however the impact of many other factors (calibration, scattered radiation, quantum noise, beam hardening, etc.) mean that water will in fact have a range of HU values, for example $HU_w \approx \pm 5$. It is also true in principle that for air, $HU_{air} = -1{,}000$; however air is relatively unique in CT. For example, the bowel will often contain large pockets of air, but during CT acquisition x-ray scatter from surrounding tissues will be detected in the same detector elements where the shadow of air should be recorded. This leads to an increase in HU_{air}, which can often be in the −800 to −900 range for air voxels in the bowel.

In the early days of single detector array CT, the x-ray beam was typically collimated to 5 mm at the isocenter of the scanner, and this narrow-beam geometry allowed for excellent scatter rejection. Today, in the era of multiple detector array CT, the collimated x-ray beam can be 40 mm wide, or even greater. This means that modern CT scanners don't have the same scanner rejection properties as the earlier scanners, and scattered radiation that is recorded by the detectors can lead to substantial imprecision in HU values.

10.2 CT SYSTEM DESIGNS

10.2.1 The Gantry—Geometry and Detector Configuration

Most clinical CT scanners have detector arrays that are arranged in an arc across from the x-ray tube, as shown in Figure 10-7. This arc is efficient from several standpoints—firstly, by mounting the detector modules on a support structure that is aligned along a radius of curvature emanating from the x-ray source, there is very little difference in fluence to the detectors due to the inverse square law. Very importantly, the primary x-rays strike the detector elements in a nearly normal manner, and so there is effectively no x-ray beam parallax that can reduce spatial resolution. Figure 10-7 also defines a *fan beam* projection. The individual rays in this geometry each define a line integral that extends between the x-ray source and each individual x-ray detector along the detector array. A collection of these rays across all the detector elements constitutes a view (or *projection*) that is specific to the view angle at which the data are acquired and which changes as the gantry rotates around the patient. Rays and views make up the fundamental raw data collected during CT acquisition.

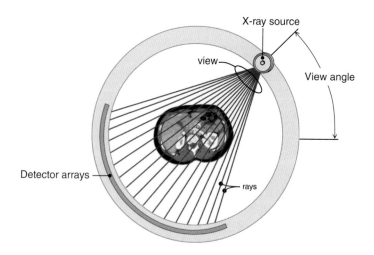

The fan beam projection

■ **FIGURE 10-7** The general configuration of a CT scanner is illustrated in cross section. The x-ray tube is mounted on a rotating gantry, onto which the x-ray detector arrays are also mounted, in the typical rotate-rotate (third generation) geometry of all modern CT scanners. The x-ray tube and detector arrays rotate together in a fixed geometrical orientation. The x-ray source fan projects a beam of x-rays, which, after transmission through the patient, reach the detector and record the raw acquired signal. The line between the x-ray source and each individual detector element (dexel) corresponds to the fundamental measurement in CT, a *ray*. The group of rays corresponding to one fan-beam projection is called a *view*. Rays and views are the fundamental data in CT imaging.

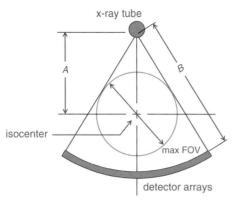

x-ray tube

A

B

isocenter

max FOV

detector arrays

■ **FIGURE 10-8** Some of the basic geometrical dimensions of a modern rotate-rotate CT scanner are shown. The detector arrays are located on a radius-of-curvature positioned a distance *B* from the x-ray source. The source-to-isocenter distance is given by a distance *A*, and hence the magnification factor (*M*) of objects at isocenter are given by the ratio *M* = *B*/*A*. For most modern CT scanners, the fan angle is about 50°–60°, and combined with the other geometric parameters this defines the maximum field-of-view (FOV).

Figure 10-8 illustrates some basic geometry pertinent to CT scanners. The *isocenter* is the center of rotation of the CT gantry, and in most cases (but not all), the isocenter is also the center of the reconstructed CT image—that is, pixel (256, 256) on the 512 × 512 reconstructed CT image. The source-to-isocenter distance is illustrated as *A* in Figure 10-8, and the source-to-detector distance is labeled *B*. The magnification factor *M* from the isocenter to the detectors is then given by *M* = *B*/*A*. By convention in the industry, detector width and length and the collimated beam width are quoted at the isocenter. For example, if the (minimum) nominal CT detector thickness is quoted on a scanner as 0.50 mm, the physical detector width is larger by the magnification factor *M*. Thus, for this 0.50-mm nominal detector with *B* ≈ 95 cm and *A* ≈ 50 cm, then the *M* = 1.9 and the physical width of the detector array is *M* × 0.50 mm = 0.95 mm. Most whole body CT systems make use of the gantry system with a fan angle on the order of 50°–60°. The fan angle, combined with the source-to-isocenter and source-to-detector distances, defines the maximum field of view (FOV) obtainable by the CT system. Some CT systems are designed to have larger fields of view, for example for bariatric imaging or treatment planning in radiation therapy, where it is typical to have the patient's arms positioned along their side which creates the need for a larger FOV. In diagnostic imaging of the torso, if they are able to, the patients typically raise their arms above their head, which reduces artifacts and reduces the FOV requirements.

Figure 10-9 illustrates gantry components on a modern multidetector array CT scanner (MDCT). A single detector array CT scanner has only one detector array which spans the fan angle—and that technology was the dominant configuration from the 1970s until the mid-1990s. Most modern CT systems use MDCT geometry, where 16, 64, 128, or more detector *arrays* are aligned next to each other along the fan angle. Because multiple detector arrays are abutted next to each other on the gantry, extending the total width of the detector assembly, a divergent x-ray beam in the *z*-axis giving rise to the *cone angle* (Fig. 10-9) results. For a 64 detector array CT scanner with 0.625 mm individual detector width, the thickness (along *z*) of the entire detector array measures 40 mm (defined at isocenter), since 64 × 0.625 mm = 40 mm. A newly introduced high-resolution CT scanner uses 160 detector arrays that are 0.25 mm in width, also spanning 40 mm (160 × 0.25 mm = 40 mm).

While a given CT scanner may have *n* detector arrays (*e.g.*, *n* can be 64), most systems allow a configuration that "bins" the signals from adjacent detector arrays to produce lower *z*-axis resolution CT images (e.g., *n*/2). Using the high-resolution CT system mentioned above as an example, the system has acquisition modes including 160 × 0.25 mm and 80 × 0.5 mm, with progressively reduced resolution in *z* as the effective detector width increases. One may ask why any imaging system would

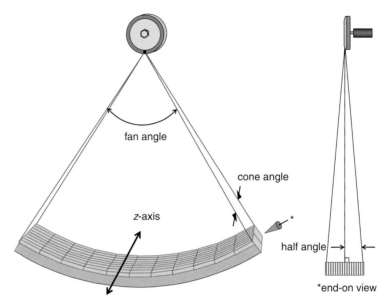

FIGURE 10-9 This figure defines the angles associated with a modern rotate-rotate CT scanner using multidetector arrays. The fan angle is defined between the x-ray source and the extent of the detector arrays in-plane. All modern multiple detector array CT scanners (MDCT) can be considered cone beam CT systems, with full cone angles of 4.2° for a 40-mm detector width at isocenter, and 17.2° for a 160-mm detector width. This cone angle is fully considered in the reconstruction algorithm used to convert the raw acquired data into the final CT volume data set.

intentionally acquire data in a lower resolution mode. In CT, the finer detector spacing leads to larger data sets, which increases reconstruction time and can increase the number of CT images produced for a given FOV, which increases requirements on bandwidth for transfer as well as computer storage issues. Also, there are many clinical protocols where high resolution simply is not required for the diagnostic task at hand. But one of the most important reasons why some CT scanners allow detector binning modes is that the electronic noise can be reduced. This is because, using the high resolution CT scanner (HRCT) example above, when the signal from two adjacent 0.25 mm detector arrays is added to form an effective detector array width of 0.50 mm, *electronic noise* is reduced (relative to the signal) prior to the gain stages in the electronics that ultimately lead to the final digitization of the signal. This effect is over and above the issue of x-ray *quantum noise* versus slice thickness, which will be discussed later.

With MDCT, the reconstructed slice thickness and collimated x-ray beam width are separate parameters—acknowledging some practical clinical constraints, they are largely decoupled. This was not the case in the era of a single detector array CT, where the slice thickness in the reconstructed images was essentially equal to the collimated beam width. A thinner slice thickness improves resolution but required long scan times in these scanners, while wider beam widths make for faster scanning but offered decreased resolution. Thus, a significant compromise was necessary in the single detector array CT era between scan time and z-axis spatial resolution. By almost completely decoupling these parameters with MDCT, the slice thickness is primarily determined by the detector array configuration, and the x-ray beam width is determined by the collimator (along with the total width of the detector arrays). This leads to thinner slices and faster scans, a noteworthy combination made possible by multiple detector array CT. Examples will be given to illustrate this.

Faster Scans

In the standard terminology of CT, the detector thickness is T (measured at isocenter) and the number of detector arrays is n. For one manufacturer's 64 slice (n) scanner, $T = 0.625$ mm and so the collimated x-ray beam width is $nT = 40$ mm. For contiguous images, the scan for a 320-mm length (along z) of a patient's abdomen could be acquired in just 4 s (e.g., 40 mm beam width, ½ s gantry rotation, helical pitch = 1.0), since 80 mm of patient length along z can be scanned in 1 s. In practice, the scan would take perhaps 4.5 s due to over-ranging, which will be described later.

Thinner CT Images (Improved *z*-Axis Resolution)

For an NR scanner, the 40-mm beam width discussed in the above section can produce 0.625 mm thick images. For the 320-mm section of the abdomen discussed above, this would lead to 512 images. It should be noted that it is not always desirable to reconstruct the thinnest slice possible, due to the increase in quantum noise that is associated with thinner slices. More about this will be discussed later.

10.2.2   Wide Beam (Cone Beam) CT Systems

All top of the line ($\geq$64 detector channels) whole body CT systems are technically cone beam CT systems, as the reconstruction algorithm used for synthesizing the raw data into CT images takes into account the cone angle. However, most conventional (~64 slice) CT systems still make use of only slight cone angles on the order of ~2° (cone beam half-angle). Some vendors, however, have developed what could be called true cone beam CT scanners—where the half cone angle approaches 9°. For example, some vendors have developed multiple-detector array systems with z-axis coverage (nT) of 16 cm. There are of course benefits and trade-offs with such wide cone beam designs. The challenges of wide cone beam imaging include increased x-ray scatter and increased cone beam artifacts. The benefit of this design, however, is that whole organ imaging can be achieved without table motion—so for CTA or CT perfusion studies, the anatomical coverage is sufficient for most organs (e.g., head, kidneys, heart, etc.) to be imaged in a single rotation. Hence, with these systems whole-organ perfusion imaging with high temporal resolution is possible.

Some niche CT scanners make use of flat panel detectors for the detector array, and an example of this (for breast CT) is shown in Figure 10-10. This geometry represents a full cone beam geometry, where the cone angle is almost as large as the fan angle. The use of the planar flat panel detector system leads to a fully two-dimensional bank of detectors, which have no curvature, and so a slightly different reconstruction geometry is required. This means that techniques (such as flat-fielding) are needed to correct for the inverse square law and heel effect–based spatial differences in fluence to the detector. There is also some parallax (non-normal x-ray incidence onto the detector) that occurs in this geometry, which cannot be corrected for.

Flat panel detectors have on the order of 3 million pixels, and hence the read out rate is much slower than purpose-built CT detector arrays. Because of this, most cone beam CT systems use a pulsed x-ray tube output to improve spatial resolution. In contrast, most whole body CT systems use continuously-on (non-pulsed) x-ray tube control.

The cone angle that exists with some flat panel based cone beam scanners can be appreciable; for example, using a standard 30 × 40 cm flat panel detector at a source-to-detector distance of 90 cm, the full fan angle spans about 25° and the full cone angle spans about 19°. Flat panel detectors are used for cone beam systems in dental and maxillofacial CT, breast CT, orthopaedic, angiographic, and radiation therapy imaging applications.

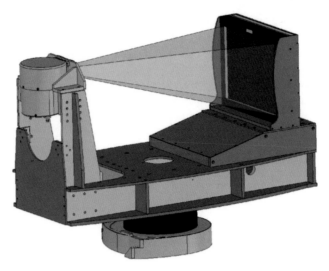

■ **FIGURE 10-10** While modern whole-body CT systems are rightly considered as (small cone angle) cone beam systems, more traditional specialty application cone beam CT systems typically use a flat panel detector opposed to an x-ray source in a rotate-rotate (third generation) cone beam geometry, as illustrated. The system in this diagram is designed for pendant-geometry breast imaging and rotates in the horizontal plane. Flat panel based cone beam CT systems enable dedicated CT applications in orthopedic, dental, breast, radiation therapy positioning, and angiographic applications, and typically provide higher spatial resolution images albeit with greater artifact potential.

10.2.3 The Slip Ring

Figure 10-11 shows a diagram of a modern slipring used in virtually all state-of-the-art CT scanners. The slipring itself interfaces with the rotating gantry, and it has a number of large brass tracks that carry electrical current at high voltage from a gliding contactor. The contactor is similar to the *brushes* that are used in an automobile generator. The large tracks on the slipring are used to maintain electrical contact with, and conduct electrical power from, the stationary frame to the rotating gantry. There are also numerous small tracks of the slipring that are used to conduct low-power (digital) signal data off of the rotating gantry to the stationary frame.

The use of the slipring in CT scanner design enables the gantry to rotate continuously in one direction. Prior to the use of sliprings, the rotating frame of the CT system was connected to the stationary frame using cables that extended and retracted on cable spools. Both thick power cables and thin ribbon cables for signal conduction were used. This mechanical linkage allowed about 720° of rotation. With these cables, the gantry was accelerated before acquisition, the source was energized for a 360° acquisition, and the gantry was then electronically braked, came to a stop, and then rotated in the other direction for the next scan, after table indexing. The 720° allowed enough rotation for gantry acceleration and deceleration, along with the 360° axial scan. A typical 360° rotation time for axial CT acquisition with cable-connected gantries was 2.0–3.0 s. With modern slipring technology, the CT gantry can ramp up to faster rotation velocities, and current 360° rotation periods can be as short as 0.28–0.35 s, and prototype air bearing gantries may someday allow rotation periods approaching 0.20 s, that is, 300 RPM.

It should be obvious that helical (spiral) CT scanning would not be possible without the slipring geometry. Another consequence of slipring-based CT systems is that with these fast rotational velocities, the g-forces at the periphery of the rotating gantry can be impressive—exceeding 20 *g*'s. This calls for special design considerations for

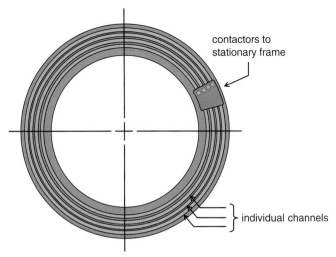

contactors to
stationary frame

individual channels

■ **FIGURE 10-11** A CT scanner involves a rotating frame (the gantry), as well as stationary frame that includes mechanical and electrical components. To convey power onto the rotating gantry from the stationary frame, as well as to conduct signal data from the rotating gantry to the stationary frame, a slipring is used. A slipring uses gliding contacts to allow communication and power transfer between the stationary and rotating frames without the use of wires, and this enables the gantry to rotate continuously in a single direction. Previous generations of CT systems did not use sliprings, and were bound by mechanical cable-based connections, substantially limiting gantry rotation rates. Sliprings have enabled gantry rotation periods to move from 3.0 s (when cables were used) to modern CT rotation periods of as little as 0.25 s. The power transfer components of the slipring may involve the conductance of ~50 A at ~400 V—so accidental contact would be deadly.

all the hardware located on the rotating gantry, recognizing that the g-forces increase from the center to the periphery of the rotating gantry.

10.2.4 The Patient Table (or Couch)

The patient table is an important and highly integrated component of the CT scanner. The CT computer controls table motion using precision motors with telemetric feedback, for patient positioning and CT scanning. This is critically important in helical scanning where the coordination of tube rotation and table movement is essential. The patient table (or *couch*) can be retracted from the bore of the CT gantry and lowered to sitting height to allow the patient to comfortably get on the table, usually in the supine position as shown in Figure 10-12. Under the CT technologist's control, the system then moves the table upward and inserts the table with the patient into the

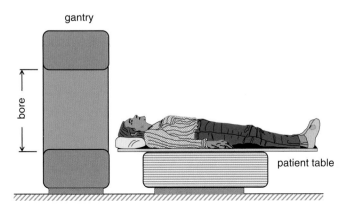

gantry

bore

patient table

■ **FIGURE 10-12** The patient table is a perfunctory but surprisingly high-tech component of a CT scanner. The patient table lowers to sitting height to allow patients—including the elderly and physically impaired—to sit on the table and reposition to a prone or supine position, with help from the attending technologist.

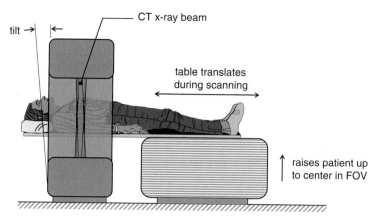

■ **FIGURE 10-13** Once the table is raised to the appropriate height (which involves centering the patient verti-cally with the isocenter), the table becomes the essential linkage between the translation of the patient along the z-dimension during acquisition and the position of the resulting CT image data set. Hence, the translational accuracy of the table is an essential component of quality control procedures. The table involves significant cantilever with potentially heavy patients, which could result in vertical vibration. Hence, as CT scanners have moved to higher resolution capabilities, the rigidity of the table is a key component in the design of state-of-the-art high-resolution CT systems.

bore of the scanner (Fig. 10-13). A series of laser lights provide references in multiple directions to allow the patient to be centered in the bore (both laterally and in terms of table height) and to adjust the patient longitudinally.

The CT table on modern systems plays an important part in image quality and accuracy. The table is cantilevered into the bore of the gantry, and can flex with the weight of a patient. Newer table designs address this with a more rigid bearing sys-tem, to reduce vibration (motion) during imaging, which is essential for preserving spatial resolution. In addition, the accuracy of anatomic positioning along the z-axis in the CT images is directly related to the accuracy of the position sensors in the table. Given that CT image data are used for targeting interventions (*e.g.*, radiation ther-apy, needle biopsy, surgical planning, *etc.*), anatomical accuracy is clearly essential. Hence, table positioning accuracy is an important parameter that is evaluated during routine CT scanner consistency testing.

The cranial-caudal axis of the patient is parallel to the z-axis of the CT scanner (Fig. 10-14). Most CT scanners allow both head-first and feet-first positioning of the patient, depending upon the type of scan to be performed. All CT scanners have a detachable head holder, which inserts into the end of the table closest to the gantry. The head holders are typically fabricated from carbon fiber, which is very transpar-ent to x-rays, and they also conform better to the shape of the head, which provides excellent motion reduction for head CT.

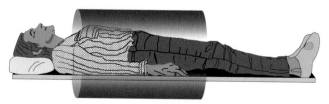

■ **FIGURE 10-14** The rotational nature of the CT gantry means that the field-of-view in the axial plane is a circle. Combined with the translational nature of the table, the field-of-view in computed tomography is a cylinder, as illustrated in this figure. It should be noted that the acquisition field-of-view is typically large, while the display field-of-view is a consequence of decisions made by the CT technologists as they set up the examination.

The scanner FOV is a circle in the *x-y* plane but can extend considerably along the *z*-axis, essentially forming a cylindrical FOV, which envelopes the patient (Fig. 10-14).

10.2.5 The X-ray Tube Housing

X-ray tubes for CT scanners have much more power than tubes used for radiography or fluoroscopy, and consequently, they are large and quite expensive. It is not unusual to replace an x-ray tube every 9 to 12 months on CT systems. CT x-ray tubes have a power rating from about 5 to 7 megajoule (MJ), whereas a standard radiographic room may use a 0.3 to 0.5 MJ x-ray tube. There were many advancements in x-ray tube power development during the decade of the 1990s, which took x-ray tube design up to the limits imposed by physics. While powerful tubes are still important in CT, the advent of multiple detector array CT scanners make more efficient use of the x-ray tube output, by opening up the collimation. For example, in changing from a 10-mm collimated beam width to a 40-mm beam width, a fourfold increase (400%) in usable x-ray beam output results.

As CT gantry rotation speeds approach 5 rotations per second (0.20 s rotation time), the demand for increased tube output has risen proportionally. That is, to maintain the same scanner output (tube current × time, or mAs) with shorter rotation times means the instantaneous tube current (mA) values must increase. Therefore, these faster gantry rotations require accompanying increases in x-ray tube power.

In addition, as gantry rotation speeds increase, the resulting high angular velocities create enormous g-forces on the components that rotate, as noted earlier. The x-ray tube is mounted onto the gantry such that the plane of the anode disk is parallel to the plane of gantry rotation (Fig. 10-15), which is necessary to reduce gyroscopic

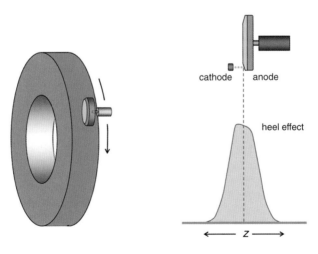

A tube position relative to gantry   **B** x-ray beam profile

■ **FIGURE 10-15 A.** The plane of the x-ray tube anode is parallel with the rotation of the x-ray tube around the gantry, as illustrated. The high rotational velocity and the large mass of the x-ray tube anode creates large gyroscopic forces, and when considered with the high rotational velocity of the gantry, the only practical mechanical orientation of the x-ray tube is to have the rotational planes of the anode and the gantry be parallel. **B.** With the orientation of the x-ray tube and the gantry as defined in **(A)**, this means that the anode-cathode direction is aligned with the *z*-axis of the CT scanner. Hence, the heel effect (which is always parallel to the anode-cathode axis) runs along the *z*-dimension of the scanner, which is also the dimension of table/patient travel corresponding to the vertical dimension of coronal and sagittal CT images.

■ **FIGURE 10-16** The juxtaposition of the x-ray tube anode within the context of the orthogonal dimensions of CT acquisition is displayed. **A.** The x-ray beam plane emanating from the plane of the anode constitutes the fan beam, which spreads laterally across the fan angle (see also Fig. 10-9), **(B)** the beam thickness dimension, which extends across the anode-cathode plane, corresponds to the cone angle of the scanner.

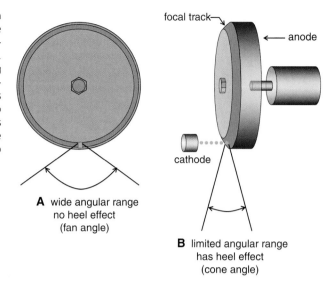

A wide angular range
no heel effect
(fan angle)

B limited angular range
has heel effect
(cone angle)

effects that would add significant torque to the rotating anode if configured otherwise. Furthermore, this configuration means that the anode-cathode axis and thus the heel effect run parallel to the z-axis of the scanner. The angular x-ray output from an x-ray tube can be very wide in the dimension parallel to the anode disk but is quite limited in the anode-cathode dimension (Fig. 10-16) due to the heel effect, and so this x-ray tube orientation is necessary given the approximately 60° fan beam of current scanners.

Most modern CT scanners use a continuous output x-ray source; the x-ray beam is generally not pulsed during the scan (some exceptions are described later). The detector array sampling time in effect becomes the acquisition interval for each CT projection that is acquired, and the sampling dwell times typically run between 0.2 and 0.5 ms, meaning that between 1,000 and 3,000 projections are acquired per 360° rotation for a ½-s gantry rotation period. For a typical CT system with about a 60-cm diameter FOV, the circumference of the FOV is about 1,885 mm. Thus, with (for example) 2,000 samples around 360°, each sample represents a distance of ~0.94 mm of gantry motion at the periphery of the FOV. This circumferential (and angular) displacement of the x-ray source over the time it takes to acquire one projection leads to motion blurring and a loss of spatial resolution at the periphery of the field.

To compensate for this, some scanners use an x-ray tube with a magnetic steering system for the electrons as they leave the cathode and strike the anode. With clockwise rotation of the x-ray tube in the gantry (Fig. 10-17A), the electron beam striking the anode is steered counterclockwise in synchrony with the detector acquisition interval (Fig. 10-17C), and this stops the apparent motion of the x-ray source and helps to preserve spatial resolution. Notice that given the 1- to 2-mm overall dimensions of an x-ray focal spot in a CT scanner x-ray tube, steering the spot a distance of ~1 mm is realistic in consideration of the physical dimensions of the anode and cathode structures. While this can effectively stop the motion artifact caused by the motion of the x-ray source, the detector array is still moving.

Some CT manufacturers use a focal spot steering approach to provide oversampling in the z-dimension of the scan as well. This x-ray tube design provides the ability to stagger the z-axis position of the x-ray focal spot inside the x-ray tube, using magnetic fields produced by steering coils. Due to the steep anode angle on these tubes, modulating the electron beam landing location on the focal track causes an

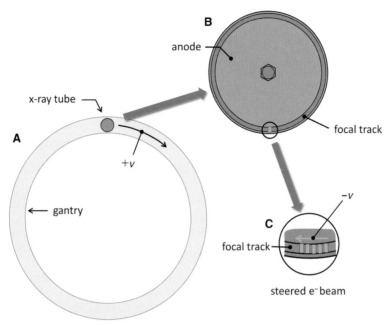

■ **FIGURE 10-17** Patient motion during acquisition is always a problem in medical imaging, but even with a stationary patient, the rotating CT gantry **(A)** produces motion blur (rotational velocity of $+v$). **(B)** To partially address this, some CT systems steer the focal spot (by steering the electron beam between the cathode and anode) in the opposite direction ($-v$) of gantry motion **(C)**.

apparent shift in the source position along the z-axis of the scanner. For helical (spiral) scans, this approach leads to an oversampling in the z-dimension, which leads to Nyquist-appropriate sampling in z (see Chapter 4).

While it is true that most modern CT systems use a continuously-on x-ray source, at least one vendor pulses the x-ray tube *potential* to enable dual energy CT image acquisition (see Section 10.3.8). In this technique, the x-ray tube potential (kV) is rapidly switched, allowing alternate CT projections to be acquired at different effective x-ray energies. It should be noted that most examples of pulsed x-ray sources (*e.g.*, commonly used for flat panel cone beam scanners) modulate tube current, not the x-ray tube potential as with this dual energy example.

Figure 10-7 illustrates the rotation of the x-ray source around the circular FOV. Virtually all modern CT scanners have a design where both the x-ray tube and detector are attached to the rotating gantry, and this leads to a so-called rotate-rotate (third generation) geometry. Thus, as the gantry rotates, the x-ray tube and detector arrays stay in fixed, rigid alignment with each other. This fixed geometry allows the use of a two dimensional anti-scatter grid in the detector array, as shown in Figure 10-18. The grid septa are aligned with the dead spaces between individual detectors, in an effort to preserve the geometrical detection efficiency of the system. As the width of the x-ray beam has increased with multidetector array CT (to 40, 80 mm, and larger), there is greater need for more aggressive scatter suppression. The use of a two dimensional grid is now common on modern multidetector array CT systems.

With a minor exception discussed later, all modern multidetector array CT scanners use indirect (scintillator based) solid-state detectors. Intensifying screens used for radiography are composed of rare earth crystals (such as Gd_2O_2S) packed into a binder, which holds the screen together. To improve the detection efficiency of the scintillator material for CT imaging, the scintillator crystals (Gd_2O_2S and other

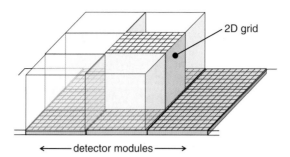

■ **FIGURE 10-18** As the collimated beam width of modern CT systems has increased with the advent of multiple detector CT systems, the amount of scattered radiation striking the x-ray detector has dramatically increased. X-ray scatter reduces the validity of the Lambert-Beers law (Eq. 10-6), leading to inaccurate computation of the Hounsfield unit in a high scatter environment. To address this, modern multiple detector CT systems use a two-dimensional high grid ratio system to reduce the amount of detected scattered radiation. To reduce the impact of the primary attenuation of the anti-scatter grid, the grid septa are aligned with the dead spaces in the detector array.

materials as well) are *sintered* to increase physical density, x-ray detection efficiency, and light output. The process of sintering involves heating the phosphor crystals to just below their melting point for relatively long periods of time (h), with repeated steps of compression. In the end, densification occurs, and the initial scintillating powder is converted into a high-density ceramic. The ceramic phosphor is then scored with a high resolution cutting tool to create a number of individual detector elements in a detector module, for example, 64 × 64 detector elements. An opaque filler is pressed into the space between detector elements to reduce optical cross talk between detectors. The entire fabrication includes a photodiode in contact with the ceramic detector (Fig. 10-19A). CT detectors are so-called pixelated detector elements, because of their discrete design.

The detectors sit on top of a large stack of electronic modules, which provides power to the detector array and receives the electronic signals from each photodiode (Fig. 10-19B). The electronics module has gain channels for each detector in the module and also contains the analog-to-digital converter, which converts the amplified electronic signal into a digital number. The detector array modules are mounted

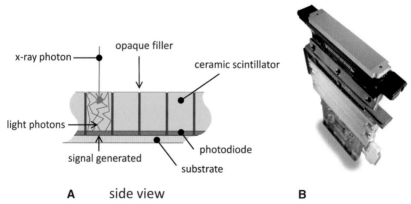

A   side view   **B**

■ **FIGURE 10-19 A.** A cross section of a modern CT detector is illustrated. A ceramic wafer comprised of an x-ray scintillator (*e.g.*, Gd_2O_2S) is layered onto a photodiode and corresponding substrate. Small kerf cutting tools are used to generate slits between individual detector elements (dexels), and these slits are subsequently filled with an opaque material to eliminate optical cross-talk between dexels. **B.** A picture of a modern CT detector module is shown, with the scintillator on top, corresponding electronics, amplification circuits, digitizer and heatsink shown in the figure.

onto a rigid frame on the mechanical gantry assembly. They are modular to allow rapid swap out when the occasional detector failure occurs.

The exception to scintillator based detectors in CT relates to an emerging technology of energy-discriminating photon counting detectors for CT. This technology is proprietary (*i.e.*, details are unavailable), but uses direct solid-state detector technology (no scintillator). Instead of integrating the energy from a detected x-ray photon as with traditional CT detectors, photon counting detectors count x-ray photons and assign them into different energy bins, much like gamma cameras do in nuclear medicine. Photon counting with energy discrimination may be the future of CT detector technology, and would allow multispectral imaging (including dual energy) without multiple scans at different tube potentials. One of the technical challenges of building photon counting detector-based systems relates to the high bandwidth requirements of the electronics, since the detectors in CT receive very high photon flux.

10.2.6 Over Beaming and Geometrical Efficiency

Figure 10-20 illustrates a cross section of the x-ray beam as it emanates from the x-ray tube anode, passes through the collimator, and then strikes the detector arrays. The orientation of this figure is illustrated in the inset, and the horizontal dimension on the figure corresponds to the *z*-axis in the CT scanner. What this figure explicitly illustrates is that the x-ray beam is collimated such that the periphery of the x-ray beam (left and right edges in this figure) extends a bit past the detector arrays on the edges—and this is called *over beaming*. The slice sensitivity profile (SSP) will

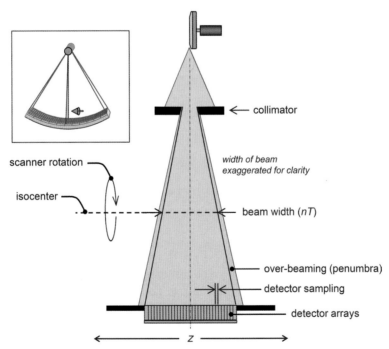

■ **FIGURE 10-20** The inset shows the viewing position of the remaining figure. The x-ray beam emanates from the x-ray source, is confined by the x-ray collimator, passes through the isocenter (where the patient is, not shown in this figure) and then strikes the x-ray detector arrays. The innovation of multidetector CT systems (MDCT) is that the beam width is much larger than the width (in *z*) of an individual detector array. With this configuration, the detector width determines the spatial resolution in the *z*-dimension, while the beam width determines the coverage of the CT system as it acquires data along the *z*-axis of the patient. In the earlier era of single detector array CT, the CT beam width and detector sampling in *z* were both governed by the collimator, forcing a compromise between *z*-axis resolution and the speed of the CT acquisition.

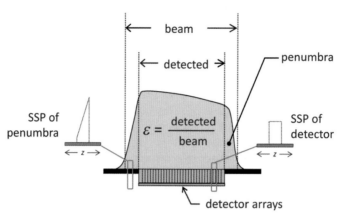

■ FIGURE 10-21 With the advent of MDCT systems, the x-ray beam striking the detector array needs to be loosely collimated so that the penumbra of the x-ray beam is positioned outside the active detector array. This leads to higher dose levels to the patient. The shape of the slice sensitivity profile (SSP) for each detector array is approximately a rectangle function; however, the SSP of the penumbra is dramatically anisotropic. Hence to match the SSPs of all detector elements in the array, including the edge arrays, the penumbra is positioned just off the active detector arrays.

be discussed in more detail later; however, it represents the distribution (along the z-axis) of the x-ray beam profile. For a 64-slice MDCT system, all of the central detector arrays (e.g., detector arrays 3–62) have SSPs that are rectangular in shape, due to the homogeneous x-ray beam incident upon each detector and the uniform response of the detector elements along the z-axis. However, if the edge of the x-ray beam was collimated tightly to the edge detectors (e.g., such that the penumbra of the x-ray beam landed on detectors 1 and 2, and 63 and 64), the SSPs for these detector arrays would have very skewed SSP distributions due to the penumbra at the edges of the beam, relative to the more central detector arrays (Fig. 10-21). The penumbra is the blurry edge of the x-ray beam and is a result of the finite-sized focal spot being collimated by the sharp, highly magnified collimator blades.

A dramatically different SSP at the edge detector arrays (compared to the more central detector arrays) would result in significant artifacts. Realize that for helical acquisition (when pitch ≤1.0), all of the detector arrays contribute to the raw data for each reconstructed CT image. Hence, to avoid artifacts in MDCT systems, the penumbra of the x-ray beam is "parked" off of the active detector array. This reduces the dose efficiency of the CT scanner, because the x-ray beam in the penumbra has passed through the patient contributing radiation dose but is not detected. In the early days of MDCT systems, when the number of detector arrays was small (e.g., 4 or 8), the dose due to over beaming was a considerable fraction of the total dose (up to 30%). As the number of detector arrays increased to 64 and above, with a concomitant increase in the physical width of the active detector area, the fraction of the x-ray beam represented by the over beaming is much smaller, and so the dose efficiency of modern 64+ MDCT systems is approaching 95%.

10.2.7 Adapting Data Acquisition to Patient Anatomy: Noise Propagation in CT Images

Since CT images are reconstructed from many (1,000–2,000) projection data acquired around the patient, the image noise at a given pixel in the CT image is the consequence of the noise from all of the projection data that intersect that pixel. The noise variance (σ^2) at a point in the CT image results from the propagation of noise variance from the individual projections (p1, p2, …, pN). A simplified mathematical description of the noise propagation is given by

$$\sigma^2_{\text{CT image}} = \sigma^2_{\text{p1}} + \sigma^2_{\text{p2}} + \sigma^2_{\text{p3}} + \cdots + \sigma^2_{\text{pN}}, \qquad [10\text{-}3]$$

where the total noise in the CT image is the square root of $\sigma^2_{\text{CT image}}$, and this form of noise propagation is called "adding in quadrature." The consequence of the total noise adding in this way is that larger subcomponents of noise contribute significantly (since they are squared) to the final CT image noise. Therefore, methods that can reduce large subcomponents of noise in the projection image data are especially useful. Examples of these methods include those that reduce unnecessary radiation exposure to the patient without impacting image noise properties such as the use of a bow tie filter, as well as tube current modulation. Both of these are discussed in the following.

10.2.8 Beam Shaping Filters

The majority of CT scans are either of the head or of the torso, and the torso is typically broken up into the chest, abdomen, and pelvis. These exams represent over ¾ of all CT procedures in a typical institution. All of these body parts are either circular or approximately circular in shape. Figure 10-22A shows a typical scan geometry where a circular body part is being scanned. The shape of the attenuated (primary) x-ray beam, which reaches the detectors after attenuation in the patient, is shown in this figure as well, and this x-ray beam profile is due to the attenuation of the patient when no corrective measures are taken. Figure 10-22B shows how the x-ray beam striking the detector array is made more uniform when a beam shaping filter is used. The beam shaping filter, often called a *bow tie filter* due to its shape, reduces the intensity of the incident x-ray beam in the periphery of the x-ray field where the attenuation path through the patient is generally thinner. This tends to equalize or flatten the x-ray fluence that reaches the detector array. Because the beam intensity is reduced for thinner patient projections at the periphery, the dose at the periphery is reduced with no appreciable loss in image quality due to the quadrature noise addition described in Section 10.2.7.

The bow tie filter has consequences both on patient dose and on image quality. When the dose distribution from an entire rotation of the x-ray tube around the patient is considered, when no bow tie filter is used, increased radiation dose at the periphery of the patient results, as shown in Figure 10-23A. An ideal bow tie filter equalizes dose to the patient perfectly, as shown in Figure 10-23B. If the bow tie filter has too much peripheral beam attenuation, then it will concentrate the radiation toward the center of the patient and lead to higher central doses as in Figure 10-23C. While this is not common, the situation shown in Figure 10-23C could occur if a head bow tie filter were used for body imaging.

The standard adult head is about 17 cm in diameter, whereas the standard adult torso ranges from 24 up to 45 cm or greater, with an average diameter ranging between 26 and 30 cm. Because of these large differences, all commercial CT scanners make use of a minimum of two bow tie filters—a head and a body bow tie. The head bow tie filter is also used in pediatric body imaging on some scanners.

In the absence of a bow tie filter, the higher dose that is delivered to the periphery of the patient is essentially wasted and does not contribute to better image quality (*i.e.*, lower noise). Hence, the bow tie filter is a very useful tool because it reduces patient dose with little to no loss of image quality—a win-win proposition that must

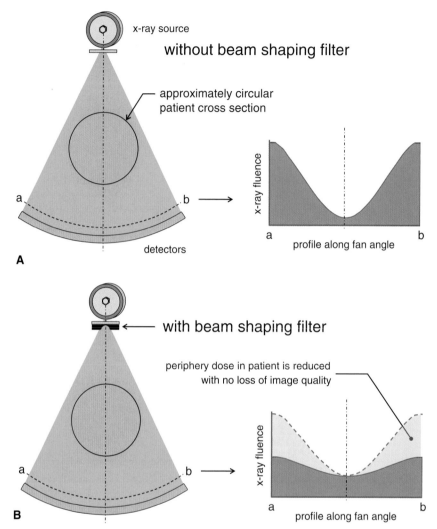

■ **FIGURE 10-22** This figure shows the standard fan-beam geometry in CT, with the x-ray beam emitted from the x-ray source and then striking the detector. **A.** The cross section of most patients tends to be circular (bodies and heads), and in the absence of a beam shaping filter this would lead to the distribution of x-ray fluence as illustrated—with high fluence levels striking the detector at the periphery, but low fluence levels striking the detector under the center of the patient. **B.** A beam shaping filter, often called a *bow tie filter*, is positioned near the x-ray source and shapes the x-ray beam to reduce the high x-ray fluence levels at the periphery of the fan beam. The bow tie filter reduces the imbalance of signal levels received at the center and periphery of the detector, and in doing so provides considerable radiation dose reduction to the periphery of the patient—with no loss in image quality.

be implemented in CT imaging. Indeed, the bow tie filter is used in all commercial whole body CT scanners and in all patient CT acquisition scenarios.

10.2.9   View Sampling

The bandwidth of the data acquisition chain is intrinsic to the design of a CT scanner. The *view sampling* of the scanner is related to both the rotation period of the gantry around 360°, and the number of samples that the detector system can acquire in this period of time (*i.e.*, *frames per second*, FPS). Recalling that for most whole-body CT scanners, the x-ray tube is not pulsed, this means that the frame rate of the detector

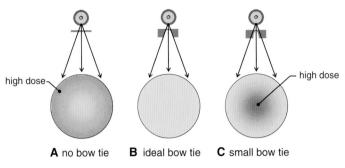

A no bow tie   **B** ideal bow tie   **C** small bow tie

Dose distributions in a circular patient

■ **FIGURE 10-23** This figure illustrates the relative dose distributions between a CT system with **(A)** no bow tie, **(B)** a well-designed bow tie filter, and **(C)** a bow tie filter that is too centrally focused. The primary role of the bow tie filter is to reduce dose to the periphery of the patient.

system is a fundamental limitation to view sampling. Figure 10-24A illustrates view sampling. To illustrate the consequences of view sampling, let's assume a simple example where the gantry rotation period is 0.5 s, and the data acquisition is 2,000 FPS. This combination of acquisition parameters results in a view sampling angle (dr) of 0.36° (1,000 views around 360°). Figure 10-24B shows that for a given view sampling angle, the width of the sampling sector increases from the center of the FOV to the periphery, as $r\,dr$. For example, for the sampling conditions described above, the width of the sampling sector is 0.31, 0.63, 0.94, and 1.26 mm at radii of 50, 100, 150, and 200 mm, respectively. The dimensions of a typical pixel in CT reconstruction with a 512 matrix range from about 0.5 to 0.7 mm for body imaging. Notice that the blurring caused by view sampling (which increases with radius in the FOV) is greater than the pixel dimensions for radii greater than 100 mm (*i.e.*, a FOV diameter of 200 mm). While the use of x-ray focal spot dithering (Fig. 10-17) can essentially freeze the motion of the focal spot during gantry rotation, the detector array is still rotating.

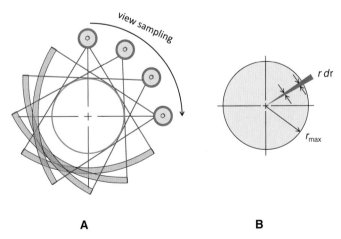

A   **B**

■ **FIGURE 10-24** **A.** Most CT scanners operate the x-ray tube in continuously-on mode during CT acquisition, that is, the x-ray source is not pulsed. View sampling is defined by the data acquisition system associated with the detector arrays, which operate with relatively high bandwidth. For example, to acquire 1,000 views over 360° rotation of the gantry in 0.35 s, each detector needs to be sampled at almost 3,000 samples per second. **B.** This figure shows that for a given view sampling width/angle, the width of the sampling sector increases from the center of the field-of-view to the periphery, as $r\,dr$.

10.2.10 High Resolution CT Scanners

HRCTs have been developed for specialty applications for many years, particularly for small animal and specimen imaging. Some specialty micro-CT scanners deliver voxel dimensions on the order of 10 μm, but require ~30 min scans. Cone beam CT scanners have higher spatial resolution than conventional CT systems, due to the smaller detector element dimensions on flat panel detectors. A new class of whole-body CT scanners has been designed for high spatial resolution imaging in humans.

The major impediments to high resolution in whole body CT are the detector element size and the relatively large focal spots on x-ray tubes designed for CT imaging. One vendor has combined smaller detector elements (0.25 × 0.25 mm versus 0.50 × 0.50 mm) with a cathode assembly capable of delivering 6 different focal spot sizes—from small to large. In addition to the traditional 512^2 CT image matrix, the HRCT scanner can reconstruct $1,024^2$ and $2,048^2$ CT images, with 250 μm section thickness. While high-resolution CT may introduce new clinical applications for CT imaging, at the same dose levels, HRCT will theoretically be noisier than normal resolution CT. However, innovative reconstruction algorithms will likely address this in time. Thus, it is likely that HRCT will have an important role to play in thoracic, MSK, extremity, neuro, and many other imaging applications. Indeed, for these applications, the 3D resolution of HRCT is equivalent to or better than the 2D resolution of digital radiography. As a CT scan of the abdomen includes high contrast high-resolution structures in the spine and in bowel where the contrast to noise ratio is naturally large, high-resolution CT imaging may improve CT diagnostic accuracy across an array of clinical applications.

10.3 ACQUISITION MODES

10.3.1 The CT Scan Radiograph

Once the patient is on the table and the table is moved into the gantry bore, the technologist performs a preliminary scan called the scanned projection radiograph. This image is also called the scout view, topogram, scanogram, or localizer; however, some of these terms are copyrighted to specific vendors. The scanned projection radiograph is acquired with the CT x-ray tube and detector arrays stationary (no gantry rotation), the patient is translated through the gantry, and a digital radiographic image is generated from this line-scan data. CT systems can scan anterior-posterior (AP), posterior-anterior (PA), or lateral. With the advent of tube current modulation discussed below, the use of two orthogonal localizers is now common practice (as discussed later). The PA CT radiograph is preferred over the AP to reduce breast dose in women and girls.

Using the scanned projection radiograph, the CT technologist uses the software on the CT console to plan the CT scan locations (Fig. 10-25). The process for doing this is specific to each vendor's CT scanner; however, a common theme is to define the beginning and end of each CT scan. It is at this point in the scanning procedure that all the CT scan parameters are set, usually using preset protocols. For a basic CT scan, these parameters include kV, mA, gantry rotation time, type of scan (helical or axial), direction of scan (craniocaudal or caudal-cranial), pitch, focal spot size,

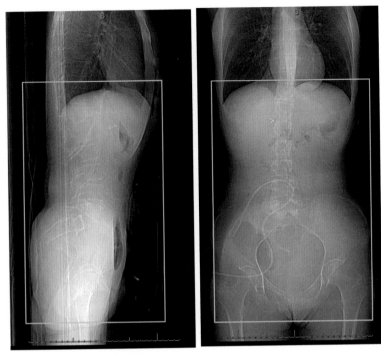

lateral localizer   AP localizer

■ **FIGURE 10-25** Most CT examinations start with the acquisition of the localizer, also known as the *scan projection radiograph*. This figure shows both the AP and lateral localizer images, which require separate scans. These images are acquired by keeping the gantry stationary (no rotation), while translating the patient on the table through the gantry. The scan projection radiograph is used by the technologists to define the position of the CT scan with respect to the patient's anatomy, including stop and start points in z, and to adjust different regions of the scan for different acquisition parameters or post-acquisition parameters.

detector configuration, reconstruction kernel(s), reconstruction mode, mA modulation parameters, if used, and so on. Complexity increases for more advanced scanning protocols.

10.3.2 Axial (Sequential) Acquisition

The axial (also called sequential) CT scan is the basic step-and-shoot mode of a CT scanner (Fig. 10-26), available since the earliest days of CT. The gantry rotates at typical rotation speeds of 0.5 s or so, but the x-ray tube is not turned on all the time. The table is stationary during the axial data acquisition sequences. The system acquires 360° of projection data with the x-ray tube on, then the x-ray tube is turned off, the table is moved with the x-ray beam off, another scan is acquired, and so on. This process is repeated until the desired anatomical area is covered. Because the table and patient are stationary during an axial scan, the x-ray focal spot trajectory defines a circle around the patient. Due to the table's start/stop sequence, axial CT requires more acquisition time than helical scanning (described below). With the advent of MDCT, it is common to acquire multiple *contiguous* CT images during an axial acquisition. This implies that between each axial acquisition, the table moves a distance D, which is essentially equal to the width of the detector arrays at isocenter (nT). This results in a series of images in the CT volume data set, which are contiguous and evenly spaced along the z-direction. In practice, the x-ray beam width is slightly wider than the distance nT due to over beaming and so the series of axial scans results in some x-ray beam overlap between axial acquisitions.

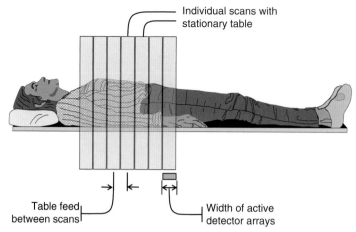

Individual scans with
stationary table

Table feed
between scans

Width of active
detector arrays

■ **FIGURE 10-26** This figure illustrates axial (or sequential) CT acquisition, the original step-and-shoot mode for CT acquisition. The patient is positioned, the scanner performs a one rotation acquisition with the table stationary, the patient is translated to the next position with x-rays off, the gantry scans again, and so on. Typically, contiguous image data sets are acquired, so the translation distance between axial scans is equivalent to the collimated slice thickness.

10.3.3 Helical (Spiral) Acquisition

With helical (also called spiral) scanning, the table moves at a constant speed while the gantry continuously rotates around the patient. This geometry results in the x-ray source following a helical path around the patient, as shown in Figure 10-27. The advantage of helical scanning is speed—by eliminating the start/stop motion of the table as in axial CT, there are no inertial constraints to the procedure and the overall CT exam can therefore be shorter in duration. Similar to the threads on a screw, the *pitch* describes the relative advancement of the CT table per rotation of the gantry. The pitch of the helical scan is defined as

$$\text{pitch} = \frac{F_{\text{table}}}{nT}, \qquad \text{[10-4]}$$

where F_{table} is the table feed distance per 360° rotation of the gantry, and nT is the nominal collimated beam width. For example, for a 40-mm (nT) detector width in

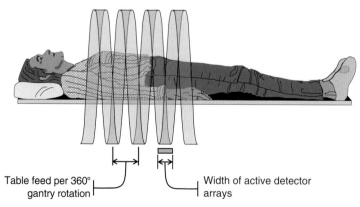

Table feed per 360°
gantry rotation

Width of active detector
arrays

■ **FIGURE 10-27** Helical (or spiral) CT is performed with continuous rotation of the gantry *while* the table is moving. Helical CT was made possible when slip rings were introduced to CT. With the gantry rotating, once the table is up to speed, helical CT scans proceed with no inertial impediment until the scan is completed.

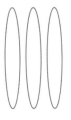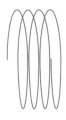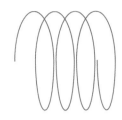

■ **FIGURE 10-28** The trajectory of the x-ray source around the patient is shown for **(A)** axial (sequential) imaging, **(B)** low pitch helical (spiral) imaging, and **(C)** high pitch helical imaging.

A axial/sequential   **B** low pitch helical/spiral   **C** high pitch helical/spiral

z and a 0.5-s rotation time for the gantry, a pitch of 1.0 would be obtained if the table moved 80 mm/s (*i.e.*, 360° in 0.5 s). For most CT scanning, the pitch ranges between 0.75 and 1.5; however, some vendors give more flexibility in (lower values of) pitch selection than others. A pitch of 1.0 corresponds in principle to contiguous axial CT (Fig. 10-28A). A pitch lower than 1.0 (Fig. 10-28B) results in over scanning the patient and hence higher radiation dose to the patient than a pitch of 1.0, if all other factors are held constant. A pitch greater than 1.0 represents under scanning (Fig. 10-28C), and results in lower radiation dose to the patient (all other things held constant). The relationship between relative dose and pitch is given by (again if all other factors are held constant):

$$\text{dose} \propto \frac{1}{\text{pitch}}. \qquad [10\text{-}5]$$

Pitch settings near 1.5 allow for faster scanning and are used for pediatric CT scanning where speed is important to reduce scan time and avoid patient motion. Low pitch values are used in cardiac imaging, or when a very large patient is to be scanned and the other technique factors (kV and mAs) are already maximized.

Because the table is moving along the z-axis during helical acquisition, there is a motion artifact that reduces the spatial resolution very slightly. However, this concern is generally balanced by the speed of the helical CT scan and the corresponding reduction in patient motion blurring that may result. This is especially important in the torso, where the beating heart and slow intestinal motion (peristalsis) cannot be voluntarily stopped in even the most compliant of patients.

The acquired data at the very beginning and end of a helical scan do not have sufficient angular coverage to reconstruct artifact-free CT images. Consequently, along the z-direction, helical scans start about $\frac{1}{2}nT$ before an axial scan would start, and stop about $\frac{1}{2}nT$ after an axial scan would end. For example, for a scan where $nT = 20$ mm and there is a desired scan length of 200 mm, an axial scan would scan only the desired 200 mm, but a helical scan would require 220 mm of acquisition to reconstruct that same 200 mm of image data. Thus, in this example, 10% of the radiation dose to the patient is essentially wasted. Newer helical systems, however, have adaptive beam collimation (various trade names exist) as shown in Figure 10-29. With this shielding, most of the wasted dose at the outer edges of a helical scan is collimated out. The amount of dose that is saved as a percentage of the overall dose increases for scans of smaller scan length, and for CT scanners with larger collimated beam widths (nT). Some manufacturers achieve adaptive beam collimation using an additional set of motorized collimators in the x-ray tube head assembly, while others use a cam-shaped collimator, which can rotate to achieve the same effect.

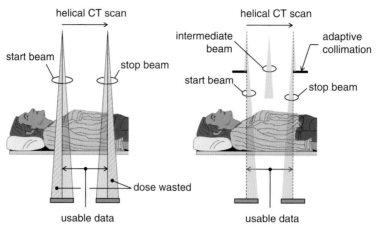

A no adaptive beam collimation **B** adaptive beam collimation

■ **FIGURE 10-29** This figure illustrates the benefits of adaptive beam collimation. **A.** For helical CT scanning, a minimum of 180° of acquisition data is necessary to reconstruct image data, and so as the scan starts with the table moving, there is a region of the patient that is irradiated but no images are produced. This is called *over ranging*. This also occurs at the end of the helical scan, where part of the patient is irradiated but no images are produced there. **B.** Adaptive beam collimation can reduce (but not completely eliminate) the over ranging problem by narrowing the collimated beam width at both the beginning and the end of the helical CT scan. Over ranging does not occur in axial scanning mode.

10.3.4 Selection of CT Slice Width

With multiple detector CT systems, the collimator adjusts the overall beam width (nT) and the minimum slice thickness is governed by the width of an individual detector array (T). For a state-of-the-art scanner (typically ≥64 detector channels), each detector array has its own data channel and all of the detector array signals are recorded during a CT scan. Let's use the example of a 64-slice scanner with 0.5-mm-wide detector arrays (at isocenter). The data from each detector array are recorded, and so the system can be instructed to reconstruct 64×0.50 mm, 32×1.0 mm, 16×2.0 mm, 8×4.0 mm (*etc.*) section thicknesses. Any combination of signals from adjacent detector arrays is possible, although the actual selections on commercial scanners are limited to standard, usable combinations. So, assuming that the acquired raw data exist[1] on the CT scanner console computer, one can go back later and re-reconstruct CT images with different section thicknesses. It is typical to reconstruct 2.5-mm axial slices for radiologist interpretation, and 0.50–0.625-mm axial slices to be used for reformatting to coronal or sagittal data sets, and for viewing thin-section images to rule out partial volume issues when necessary.

There is a compromise required in terms of reconstructed CT section thickness; while the thinnest slices (*e.g.*, 0.625 mm) provide maximal resolution along the z-axis, they are also the noisiest. By reconstructing thicker slices (*e.g.*, 5 mm thick), the CT images have lower noise at the same radiation dose levels (Fig. 10-30). Thicker image reconstruction also requires the radiologist to view fewer images for the same section of anatomy. The signal-to-noise ratio (SNR) is related to the number of x-ray photons used to form an image. For example, a 5-mm section is 8 times thicker than a

---

[1]In practice, the raw projection data is saved on the CT scanner until that storage space is needed for subsequent scan data. Raw projection data may only reside on the scanner for a day or two on a busy scanner, following a data management scheme called "FIFO"—first in, first out.

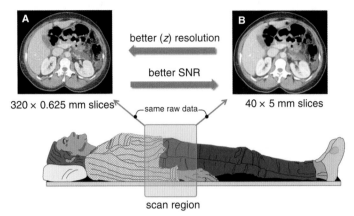

FIGURE 10-30 Modern multidetector CT systems allow the acquisition of thin slice data but provide the option of reconstructing images that are thin, medium, or thick sections. **Image A** shows 0.625 mm thick images, while **image B** shows 5-mm slice images, both data sets derived from the same CT scan (meaning no additional radiation dose to the patient). The thin images **(A)** have better z-axis spatial resolution but are noisier, and while the 5 mm thick images have reduced z-axis spatial resolution they do have much better signal-to-noise ratio (SNR).

0.625-mm CT section, and therefore 8 times more photons interrogate this section of tissue. Hence, the SNR is $\sqrt{8}$ times higher (a factor of 2.8). The selection of the most optimal slice thickness(es) to reconstruct is a key element in CT protocol development.

10.3.5 X-ray Tube Current Modulation

Some body regions in the patient are more circular than other regions. An elliptical cross section of a patient is shown in Figure 10-31A. With fixed x-ray tube current and hence constant x-ray flux, the CT detectors will receive more primary x-rays when the gantry is in position a compared to gantry position b, due to the increased attenuation path in position b. However, as we have already seen in the context of Equation 10-3, the noise variance in the projection data propagates into the reconstructed CT image in a manner that is more optimal when the projection data variance levels are nearly matched. Hence, the higher signal levels (higher dose and lower signal variance) in position a are essentially wasted when combined with those in position b during CT image reconstruction. Thus, the radiation dose to the patient in position a can be reduced with little or no loss in image quality when the x-ray flux (mA) is modulated to provide relative constant x-ray signal levels at the detector. Thus, the mA is reduced in position a compared to position b as shown in Figure 10-31B.

The mA modulation scheme shown in Figure 10-31 occurs as the x-ray gantry rotates once around the patient. However, as the patient translates through the gantry along the z-dimension (for instance in a helical scan), the shape, size, and attenuation of the patient's body can change appreciably. Thus, tube current modulation is also applied along the z-axis of the patient. The average mAs values (average mA × gantry rotation time) are shown as a function of position along a patient's torso in Figure 10-32. The angular modulation as a function of gantry rotation is semi-sinusoidal in elliptical body parts and constant in round body regions, and these fluctuations occur over relatively shorter distances as highlighted in Figure 10-32. The impact of mA modulation is illustrated on CT images in Figure 10-33, where the average mAs per CT image is indicated.

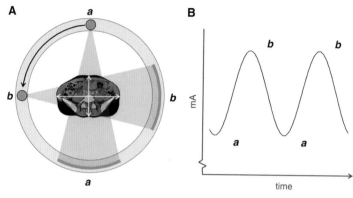

Tube rotation around oval patient   mA modulation

■ **FIGURE 10-31** X-ray tube current modulation is demonstrated. **A.** Some cross sections of some patients depart substantially from circularity. In this figure the patient is wider laterally than she is in the AP direction, and with constant tube current during gantry rotation, the detector in the **b** position would receive less dose compared to the **a** position—due to the greater attenuation path along **b**. Because of the way noise propagates during CT reconstruction (Eq. 11-3), the extra dose received by the detectors in the **a** position will essentially be wasted. **B.** To accommodate for this, the scanner can use *x-ray tube current modulation* to reduce the tube current when the gantry is in the **a** position, and then increase the current at the **b** position.

The methods of controlling tube current modulation are different for different CT vendors. One manufacturer uses the real time attenuation measured by the detectors near the central ray in the scanner to adjust the target mA for 180° later in the scan, where approximately the same tissue path length will be realized again. Virtually all manufacturers use the attenuation data measured during the acquisition of the scanned projection radiograph to plan the mA modulation scheme for each patient, and many times both AP and lateral CT radiographs are preferred to achieve more optimal mA modulation plans.

X-ray attenuation increases exponentially as a function of tissue path length; consequently the mA required to achieve similar dose levels to the detectors (essentially the goal of tube current modulation) needs to increase exponentially to accommodate this (Fig. 10-34). X-ray tube current is adjusted using the x-ray filament current (Chapter 6), and it should be realized that thermal inertia of the filament (or emitter) plays a role in how quickly mA modulation can be realized.

■ **FIGURE 10-32** The performance of x-ray tube current modulation is illustrated for a specific patient. The overall impact of mA modulation (yellow) is illustrated, showing high mA at the start of the exam (over the shoulder region of the patient) on the left, with substantial reduction in mA while scanning through the lungs, some increase over the abdomen, and a larger increase in mA over the pelvis. The orange curve illustrates the mA modulation, which happens during gantry rotation, and the modulation here reflects the difference between the AP and lateral dimensions of the patient.

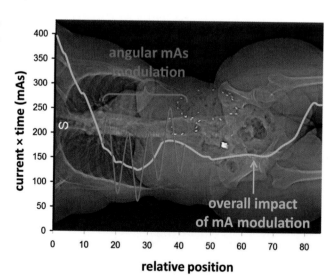

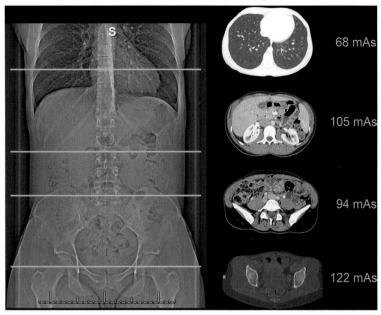

FIGURE 10-33 When x-ray tube current modulation is on, the mA can be continuously fluctuating as the gantry rotates and as the table increments along *z* during a helical CT examination, but the total mAs is tallied for each reconstructed image. This figure illustrates the different overall technique (*i.e.*, mAs) factors for various images along the length of the patient—the fact that the mAs is changing along the length of the patient is evidence that mA modulation was used.

X-ray tube modulation not only adjusts the mA up or down to accommodate the different tissue path lengths during the rotation of the gantry around the patient and the translation of the patient through the gantry, but the x-ray tube current modulation settings also determine the *overall radiation dose levels* used for the scan. Hence, the role of tube current modulation in CT is analogous to that of automatic exposure control (AEC) in radiography and automatic exposure rate control in fluoroscopy. With this in mind, it is also very important to understand the very different use of CT AEC settings for the selection of the overall dose levels between CT vendors.

One vendor's approach is to set a parameter related to the actual noise level (*i.e.*, the standard deviation in HU values) in the reconstructed CT image, and this value is used to guide the overall dose levels (by adjusting the mA levels used). With this approach, when *lower* noise levels are selected, the mA values and resulting radiation doses are *higher—much higher*, because radiation dose varies as the square of the

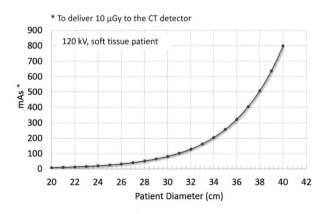

FIGURE 10-34 The necessary technique (product of tube current and rotation time, mAs) to deliver a constant dose to the detector is plotted as a function of patient diameter, assuming a 120-kV tube potential and a soft tissue–only patient. This plot is a direct consequence of the exponential attenuation of x-rays, but it also illustrates the dynamic range of mA values that are required for the operation of x-ray tube current modulation.

image noise. A different vendor's approach to mA modulation is to set a nominal mA level for a "standard" sized patient, that the system then uses as guidance for patients of different size. In this situation, *higher* nominal mA values result in higher mA settings and *higher* radiation dose to the patient.

When used correctly, AEC in CT and the resulting mA modulation techniques produce excellent CT images at near-optimal radiation dose levels. X-ray tube current modulation allows CT radiation dose reduction with little or no loss in image quality, due to the noise propagation issues described above in Section 10.2.7. Therefore, it is an important feature of modern CT scanners that should be used in most clinical settings. However, when the responsibility of adjusting something as important as the overall radiation dose in CT is turned over to the CT's control system, it is important that the operators (technologists, radiologists, medical physicists) understand the role of specific AEC parameters, which control dose for each CT manufacturer.

10.3.6 Acquisition Modes Focused on Temporal Aspects: CT Angiography and CT Perfusion Imaging

Computed tomography is often described as an anatomical imaging modality, and that of course is true. However, when an iodine-based contrast agent is injected into the vasculature (typically the venous vasculature), functional image data can be obtained. In the case of blood vessels, CTA can depict arteries and other vascular components that may be constricted or stenotic from disease or damaged due to blunt or penetrating trauma. Examples of cerebral CTA are shown in Figure 10-35. The use of iodine-based vascular contrast agents also can help physicians determine the level of perfusion for organs including brain, liver, kidney, and heart (etc.). In many cases the timing of the CT examination—relative to the time of injection—will determine which functional characteristics are best highlighted in the images. For example, arterial phase imaging is performed rather quickly after injection, while venous phase imaging is performed with slightly longer delays.

While iodine-based contrast agents are most utilized by far for vascular imaging, CO_2 has also been used as a negative contrast agent for vascular imaging. The use of gold nanoparticle contrast agent has been studied; however, use in humans has not been widely reported.

Beyond CTA, CT perfusion imaging is used to quantitatively evaluate vascular perfusion and other physiological parameters related to blood flow to a specific organ. While most often used to evaluate stroke or vasospasm in the brain, CT perfusion is

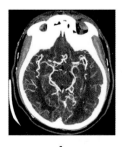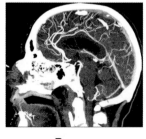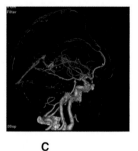

| A | B | C |

■ **FIGURE 10-35** CT angiography (CTA) of the head is illustrated, with an **(A)** axial, **(B)** sagittal, and **(C)** rendered view of the iodine contrast in the cerebral arteries of the head. In addition to the exquisite anatomical information, the functional viability of the cerebral vascular system is also depicted in this example of CTA.

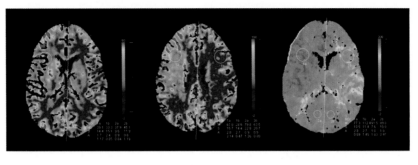

blood volume   perfusion   time to peak
                                          enhancement

■ **FIGURE 10-36** CT perfusion imaging involves following the inflow and outflow of iodine contrast as it perfuses the organ, in this example showing CT perfusion of the head. The kinetics of each voxel in the CT image data set are evaluated over the time course of the CT perfusion study, and from this temporal-spatial information pertaining to the 3D map of blood volume, perfusion, and time to peak enhancement can be determined using sophisticated software.

also used for abdominal organ imaging, especially in the oncologic setting. CT perfusion can be a relatively high radiation dose study—the CT scanner acquires images of an organ repeatedly in real time to quantify the in-flow and out-flow of iodine-based contrast agent through that organ. Typical head CT perfusion protocols call for the acquisition of about 20–40 CT images, each using a ~1 s acquisition, resulting in about 30–50 s of scanning in the same area of tissue (Fig. 10-36). CT perfusion takes advantage of the wide collimated beam width (20 to 160 mm) of top of the line scanners to image a volume of tissue in the same region of the body, repeatedly. The CT scan starts prior to the intravenous injection of contrast, and hence the scanner produces several CT image data sets prior to the arrival of the contrast bolus to the organ of interest. This is necessary because the mathematical models (Patlak, etc.) that are used to compute the parametric maps require an input function before the arrival of the contrast bolus. From this data set of temporal CT scans, and with physician outlining of the location of the input function, parametric maps are computed with high resolution. In addition to the raw grayscale CT images, most commercial perfusion software packages compute several three-dimensional parametric anatomical maps using pseudo-colored images, showing for example blood volume, tissue perfusion, and time to peak enhancement (Fig. 10-36). Perfusion CT is an example of where the well-appreciated anatomical capabilities of CT are combined with the high temporal resolution capabilities of the modality to produce quantitative, physiologically meaningful functional images.

10.3.7 Acquisition Modes to Account for Motion: Cardiac CT

Imaging the heart is challenging due to both cardiac motion, as well as the CT scanner FOV along the z-direction. With a typical heart rate of 60 beats per minute, one cardiac cycle is about 1 s. Therefore, to "freeze" cardiac motion, an image acquisition time window of 100 ms or less is required. To image the entire heart using modern rotate-rotate (third-generation) CT scanners, which have gantry rotation periods in the 0.25–0.35 s time frame, *cardiac gating* techniques are required. With cardiac gating methods, the image data for CT reconstruction are acquired over several cardiac cycles. Gating methods are made more challenging if the cardiac motion changes from cycle to cycle, and thus patients with a regular heartbeat are the ideal candidates for cardiac CT. To steady the heart rate of patients with an irregular heartbeat, beta-blockers can be administered prior to imaging, and this has been found to produce higher quality cardiac CT images in many settings.

When third-generation (rotate-rotate) CT scanners were first introduced with cardiac gating capabilities, it was common to use retrospective gating techniques (Fig. 10-37A). With this approach, the heart was imaged continuously with the rapidly rotating CT scanner, and the electrocardiogram (ECG) data were recorded in synchrony with the CT data acquisition. Because the heart is longer in the z-dimension than what many MDCT scanners can image (nT), the procedure for imaging the heart requires data acquisition at several table positions, so that the entire length of the heart is imaged. As long as the cardiac cycle is not in perfect synchrony with the scanner's gantry rotation speed, after several cardiac cycles, enough data are acquired over several consecutive phases of the cardiac cycle to reconstruct CT images of the heart (section by section in z). With retrospective reconstruction, projection data are acquired over the entire cardiac cycle, for several (5–10) cardiac cycles. Therefore, CT images can be synthesized using the ECG gating information over the entire cardiac cycle (split into for example 10 temporal regions of the ECG trace), and in addition to the typical thin slice CT image data set, a 3D rendered "beating heart" image could be produced. In clinical practice, however, most of the interest in cardiac CT imaging is in identifying blockages in the coronary arteries, as these represent the greatest risk to the patient. For the evaluation of coronary stenoses, a temporal depiction of the heart is not necessary and only the end-diastole images are necessary. While the dynamic information achieved from retrospective cardiac imaging is

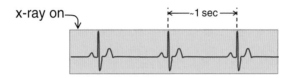

A retrospective cardiac gating

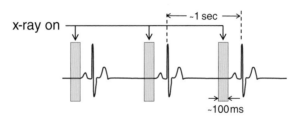

B prospective cardiac gating

■ **FIGURE 10-37 A.** Retrospective gating: Retrospective gating for cardiac imaging is illustrated, where the x-ray beam is on throughout the entire cardiac cycle, over many cardiac cycles to acquire the gated data necessary for the 3D reconstruction data set. This type of study can be used to portray the "beating heart" in three dimensions; however, the temporal information provided by retrospective gating is not considered necessary for evaluation of coronary artery patency. The downside of retrospective gating is that the x-ray tube is activated during the entire procedure, leading to high radiation dose levels to the heart, thorax, and breasts. **B.** Prospective gating: Prospective cardiac gating involves the use of the ECG signal to actively pulse the x-ray tube in the CT scanner to acquire data in a narrow window of the cardiac cycle, end diastole. The data set acquired in prospective cardiac gating is sufficient to produce 3D volume sets of the heart to enable diagnosticians to evaluate the patency of the coronary arteries, which supply blood to the heart muscle. While only one snapshot in time is available with prospective gating, the data set delivered to this technique is adequate enough to diagnose the most common form of cardiac disease. As illustrated in this figure, the beam is on for a much shorter period in prospective gating, making it a much lower dose technique than retrospective gating.

visually dramatic, it represents a high-dose procedure, with five or more seconds of CT scanning continuously at the same location in the thorax.

Most cardiac CT systems have advanced so that *prospective gating* techniques are used (Fig. 10-37B). With prospective gating, the ECG signal is used to actively trigger the x-ray tube such that beam is pulsed on and off so that the raw CT projection data are acquired only during the (most stationary) period of the cardiac cycle, end-diastole. The benefit of prospective cardiac CT is that the radiation dose to the patient is significantly reduced compared to retrospective gating. One downside of prospective gating is that if the patient's heartbeat is irregular during the scan, the acquisition may lead to an incomplete CT data set, which may not be recoverable.

For CT scanners with 40 mm detector width (nT), perhaps 4 acquisitions at different locations along the z-axis are required to image the entire heart, and these 3D volume sets will then be stitched together in software. For scanners with 160 mm FOV along z, one table position is all that is needed to image the entire heart.

One CT vendor has taken a more distinctive approach toward building a cardiac CT scanner, by building a dual source CT (DSCT) system that has two entire imaging systems on it (Fig. 10-38). There is a large FOV imaging system comprising an x-ray tube (Tube A) and associated detector arrays, and a second imaging system with another x-ray tube (Tube B) and a smaller detector array is mounted almost orthogonal to the other (A) tube and detectors. The B imaging system has a smaller FOV because of space limitations on the gantry. However, the FOV required for imaging

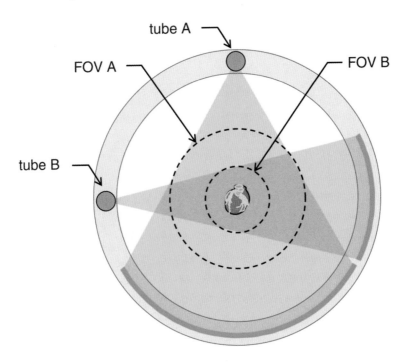

dual source CT

■ **Figure 10-38** One CT vendor's approach to cardiac imaging was to develop a CT scanner with 2 complete imaging chains (x-ray source and detector array) on the same rotating gantry. By arranging the imaging systems approximately 90° apart, 90° rotation of the gantry delivers 180° of information (by combining the information from both imaging chains), which is the minimum necessary for reconstructing data near the center of the field of view. With this arrangement, cardiac imaging can be performed with imaging times of less than 100 ms, which is considered adequate to suppress motion when synchronized with the heart's quiescent phase in the cardiac cycle, end-diastole.

the relatively small heart does not have to be as large as the standard FOV required for imaging the body.

True CT reconstruction requires only 180° plus the fan angle, and due to the small dimensions of the heart, the fan angle is small as well. The full 360° gantry rotation of the DSCT system is 0.33 s, and so a 180° rotation requires ½ × 0.33 s = 166 ms. With two redundant x-ray systems configured approximately 90° with respect to each other, a quarter of a rotation of the gantry results in a full 180° acquisition data set when the projection data from both imaging chains are combined. The 90° rotation of the gantry requires just ¼ × 330 ms = 83 ms. Hence, with the two redundant x-ray imaging systems, the DSCT scanner can acquire data fast enough during cardiac end-diastole to freeze the motion of the heart and provide excellent cardiac CT images.

It is noted that cardiac CT requires only an intravenous injection of contrast agent, while the competing technology coronary angiography requires intra-arterial contrast injection, a far more invasive procedure. For *diagnostic* cardiac procedures, CT techniques offer the patient and their physician a less invasive diagnostic procedure. However, for cardiac *interventional* procedures involving balloon angioplasty with or without the placement of coronary stents, coronary angiography is still required.

10.3.8 Acquisition Modes to Acquire Dual Energy CT Data

In his original notes on CT, Godfrey Hounsfield predicted the use of CT for dual energy decomposition methods to separate physical density from the elemental composition of materials. The initial experimental work on dual energy x-ray imaging was performed on a CT scanner in the mid-1970s, as this was the only platform at that time that could conveniently produce digital images. Dual energy CT is similar conceptually to dual energy projection imaging discussed in Chapter 7.

The concept of using CT for dual energy imaging has been known in the research arena for decades, but the dual source cardiac CT scanner described above for cardiac imaging launched the most recent clinical interest in dual energy CT. The DSCT scanner was designed primarily for cardiac imaging; however, the availability of two complete x-ray systems on the same gantry clearly lends itself to the acquisition of a low and high kV data set during the same CT acquisition. On single source CT systems, other manufacturers have developed the ability to rapidly switch the kV to achieve dual energy acquisition in a single acquisition. Other vendors have developed two-layer detectors, where the top layer absorbs the lower energy photons and the bottom layer absorbs the higher energy photons in the spectrum. Still another vendor uses a beam hardening filter that is located at the x-ray tube, but it only covers half of the width of the detector array. For example, for a 40 mm wide detector array, 20 mm of the detectors would have this additional filter. Thus, during helical CT acquisition (with lower pitch factors than usual), data are acquired at each position in the data set with both the filtered and unfiltered x-ray beam, thereby acquiring the data necessary for dual energy imaging.

As discussed above, there are multiple CT scanner designs that allow the acquisition of both low and high effective energy x-ray beams for each location in the CT scanner FOV. These various technologies enable various degrees of separation between the effective energies of the low and high x-ray spectra, and this energy separation affects the quality of the dual energy reconstructions.

There are two approaches to reconstructing dual energy CT images—the raw dual energy image data sets for each projection angle can be subjected to logarithmic weighted subtraction techniques, similar to those used in projection radiography, and then the dual energy subtracted projection data can be used to reconstruct CT images with different x-ray energy ranges. As an alternative to this, the low kV and high kV data sets can be reconstructed separately using standard reconstruction techniques, and algorithmic methods (in the CT image domain) or other digital image manipulation can be used to extract dual energy images. In clinical practice, the latter technique is most widely used. Note that the HU values in CT are already linear with respect to the linear attenuation coefficient (discussed later), and so no additional logarithms are necessary. Ultimately, the data necessary for producing dual energy images are two image data sets acquired of the same anatomy at approximately the same time, using low- and high-energy x-ray beams. Figure 10-39 illustrates the mapping of HU values between the 80- and 140-kV images for various elements and compounds.

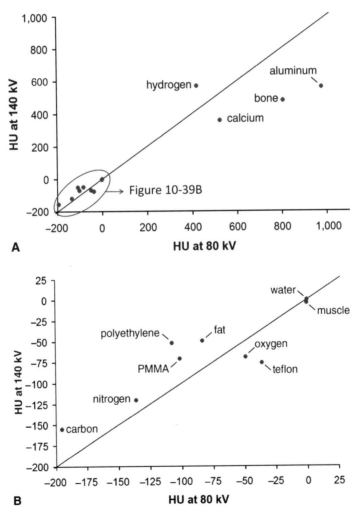

■ **FIGURE 10-39** Dual energy CT allows discrimination between high density and high atomic number, both of which increase the numerical value of the Hounsfield unit. This plot shows the HU values at 140 kV, as a function of HU values at 80 kV. In **A**, it can be seen that higher atomic number materials are below the line of identity, while lighter materials are above the line of identity. In **B**, a blowup of the cluster of materials between −200 and 0 HU is illustrated. Dual energy CT algorithms use tables such as that shown here to identify specific materials on a voxel by voxel basis.

10.4 Reconstruction

■ **FIGURE 10-40** Probably the best clinical application of dual energy CT is the identification of gout, as illustrated in this figure. The bony foot is illustrated in this pseudo-3D rendering, with regions of uric acid crystals (the manifestation of gout) shown color-coded in purple.

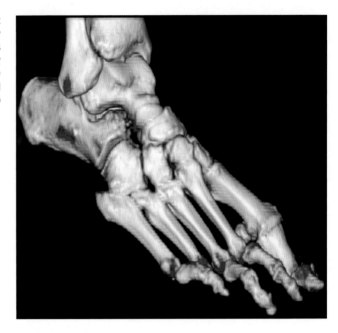

The dual energy 3D data set is produced by mapping combinations of HU (low energy) and HU (high energy) to typically a false color image, which would for example make bone, soft tissue, iodine, and gout to have different assigned colors. Subsequent 3D rendering methods are then applied to the dual energy data set to allow pseudo-3D depiction of the anatomy (Fig. 10-40).

10.4 RECONSTRUCTION

10.4.1 CT Protocols

A typical CT scanner may have 100 to 300 different pre-set protocols loaded onto it, some come with the scanner, some are entered by the CT applications personnel when the scanner is delivered, and some are designed and entered by radiologists and CT technologists. The CT operator usually starts a patient scan procedure by selecting the CT protocol appropriate to the scan for that patient. The CT protocol encompasses a wide variety of parameters, which can be set by the user, including CT acquisition parameters such as type of scan (axial, helical, etc.), kV, mA (or automatic exposure control/tube current modulation parameters), rotation time, slice thickness, pitch, scan FOV, display FOV, the type of scanned projection radiograph (AP, lateral, etc.), contrast delay, voice commands to the patient (on/off, and language), and so on. The reconstruction parameters designed for the protocol are also either pre-set or can be reset, including reconstruction algorithms used (many can be specified), including filtered backprojection (with associated parameters such as kernel), iterative resolution (with associated parameters such as type and strength), artificial intelligence reconstruction using convolutional neural networks (CNNs), or other algorithms. The reconstructed views can be set as well, including axial, sagittal, and coronal, or combinations thereof. The reconstruction parameters all include additional parameters that can often be set, including reconstructed slice thickness, window/level settings for initial display, and so on. It should be emphasized that once the CT raw data are acquired, virtually all reconstruction techniques could be applied with no additional dose to the patient. It is also possible to go back to the scanner, and reconstruct image data sets with new parameters, as long as the raw data remain on the scanner.

The protocol is the starting point in the scanning procedure, and once the patient is on the table and the CT scan is about to commence, it is the role of the experienced CT technologist to modify the protocol in some cases. For example, for very large patients, the mAs (or maximum mAs for dose modulation schemes) need to be increased to produce a diagnostic quality CT examination. For a fussy child, the technologist may increase the pitch and the mAs (to compensate for the increase in pitch) to perform the scan faster, in the hopes of reducing patient motion artifacts.

10.4.2 Preprocessing

There are a number of preprocessing procedures that are applied to the actual acquired projection data prior to CT image reconstruction. The details of these steps are proprietary to each vendor and unknown to users; however, some general observations can be made. During routine calibration of the CT scanner, the influence of the bow tie filter is characterized by performing air scans. The air scans also characterize differences in individual detector response, which may be due to differences in individual amplifier gain. The measured projection data for a given CT scan to be reconstructed are normalized by the calibration scans, and this procedure corrects for previously identified inhomogeneities in the field. In some scanners, a small fraction of the detector elements may be inoperable, and these are routinely identified using software for this purpose. A "dead pixel" correction algorithm is applied, which replaces dead pixel data with interpolated data from surrounding pixels. Scatter correction algorithms, if used, generally need to be applied before the logarithm of the projection data is applied. Some adaptive noise filtration methods can also be applied; for example, the scanner can invoke algorithms, which identify regions in the projection data that correspond to low signal areas, and these areas will correspond to locations of higher noise on the CT images. To reduce the impact of noise, some algorithms identify these low signal areas and then apply smoothing or other data processing steps to reduce the noise in these areas.

The projection data undergo normalization and logarithmic transformation, in order to correct for the exponential attenuation characteristics of x-ray interaction. Each projection measurement (*i.e.*, each ray) through the patient corresponds to a discrete measurement of I_j at detector element j, where

$$S_j = k_j I_o e^{-(\mu_1 t + \mu_2 t + \mu_3 t + \cdots + \mu_n t)}, \qquad [10\text{-}6]$$

and where I_o is the energy fluence of the x-ray beam and k_j is a scalar constant accounting for various gain values, bow tie filter attenuation, inverse square law, *etc.*, for detector element j. The signal in a reference detector S_r located outside the FOV of the patient (sometimes near the x-ray tube assembly as shown in Fig. 10-41) is also measured during the CT scan:

$$S_r = k_r I_o, \qquad [10\text{-}7]$$

where I_o is the energy fluence striking the reference detector and k_r represents scalar constants, as before. The calibration scans performed routinely (*e.g.*, daily) behind the scenes are performed to essentially measure the constants k_j and k_r, and these are

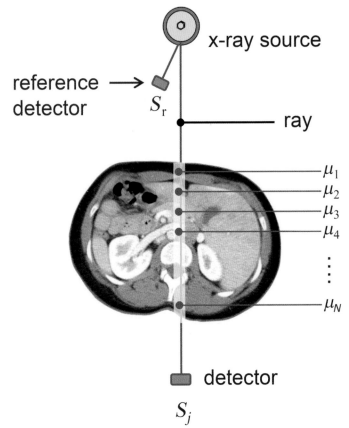

■ **FIGURE 10-41** This figure illustrates a common strategy in CT technology, where the reference signal (S_r) is measured with the detector near the x-ray to tube, and the projection image data for a given detector (S_j) are simultaneously measured. This figure illustrates just one data point S_j; however, 70,000 to 280,000 are measured on a modern MDCT system. Equation 10-8 describes the preprocessing measures necessary to compute the sum of the linear attenuation coefficients (μ_1, μ_2, μ_3, ...) for each individual ray.

stored on the scanner's computer. The projection value for detector element j, P_j is then calculated:

$$P_j = \ln\left\{\frac{\alpha S_r}{S_j}\right\} = t(\mu_1 + \mu_2 + \mu_3 + \cdots + \mu_n),\qquad [10\text{-}8]$$

where $\alpha = k_j/k_r$ and other factors. From Equation 10-8, we see that the projection measurements, P_j, after preprocessing and logarithmic conversion, correspond to linear sums of the linear attenuation coefficients through the patient and along the path of the ray, and this is illustrated in Figure 10-41 as well. Some systems may correct for beam hardening by using $P_j' = f(P)P_j$ where $f(P)$ is computed from the x-ray spectrum and other measurements. After the preprocessing steps described above, the data representing a raw sinogram are developed (Fig. 10-42) for a given CT scan. The sinogram is represented by $P(j, \theta)$, where j corresponds to each detector (i.e., each ray) and θ represents the view angle (Fig. 10-7) the data set was acquired at.

10.4.3 Simple Backprojection

To start the discussion as to how the CT image is computed from the projection data sets, let's examine a simplified but realistic example of the problem (Fig. 10-43). As discussed above, the logarithm converts the exponential nature of x-ray absorption

object scanned

raw sinogram data

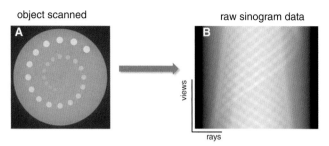

■ **FIGURE 10-42** This figure shows the object scanned **(A)**, and the resulting sinogram data produced from the CT scan of this object **(B)** for one plane in the object using axial scanning. The purpose of CT reconstruction is to use the data from the raw sinogram data to reconstruct an image of the scanned object. Notice that the circles in the object form a track with a sinusoidal pattern in the sinogram data, and the more peripheral circles generate a sinusoidal path with larger amplitude.

into a linear problem, and we will therefore deal with this example as a linear problem. The 3 × 3 grid of numbers in the central boxes in Figure 10-43 are the data of interest—these numbers represent the object, and the image of the object. Four projections through this "patient" are shown, *a–d*. It can be seen that the projected value through each *line integral* passing through the patient is the linear sum of the voxel values that each ray intersects. Creating the projections from the central data is called forward projection, and that is what the CT scanner hardware does physically. Mathematical forward projection is used in iterative reconstruction techniques and many other reconstruction processes as well. The problem that is posed by Figure 10-43 is, if you erase the values in the 3 × 3 box, can you figure out what they are from the

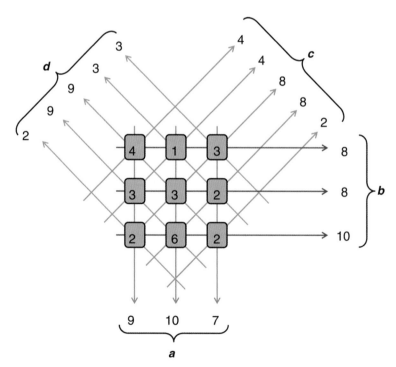

■ **FIGURE 10-43** A simplified version of CT reconstruction is described here, in a process very similar to that of a sudoku puzzle. There are four projections through the 3 × 3 image, labeled a, b, c, and d. If you remove the numbers corresponding to the rectangles in the object space, the reconstruction challenge is then to use the projection data to reconstruct the values in the 3 × 3 pixel image. While "guess and check" can work with the simple 3 × 3 object in this figure, for realistic CT images (512² or 1,024²) computer algorithms are required.

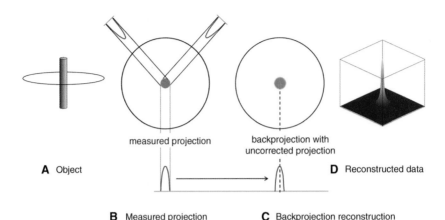

A Object

measured projection

backprojection with
uncorrected projection

D Reconstructed data

B Measured projection   **C** Backprojection reconstruction

■ **FIGURE 10-44** This figure illustrates simple backprojection, where an object (**A**, a simple cylinder placed at the center of the field-of-view) is scanned producing a measured projection (**B**), and these measurements are made repeatedly over 360° (only 3 are shown in the figure), and these hundreds or thousands of measured projections are backprojected onto an empty matrix (**C**). The reconstructed data suffers from a 1/r blurring as seen in the isometric plot (**D**).

projection data? This looks very much like a sudoku problem at this point, and given the simplicity of the 3 × 3 problem, it can be solved by trial and error. However, in a CT scanner, the matrix is typically 512 × 512 (or 1,024 × 1,024 for newer scanners), and the task of reconstructing this many values in the image from the projection values is more formidable.

Figure 10-44 shows an example of forward projection of a simple circular object at the center of the field (Fig. 10-44A), and because of the symmetrical position of the object the projections at each angle are identical (Fig. 10-44B). The projection of a circle is a parabola, and that is seen in Figure 10-44B. If that same (uncorrected) projection shape was used to backproject the CT image from all projection angles (Fig. 10-44C), the resulting image would have a characteristic blurring as shown in the isometric plot in Figure 10-44D. The take-home message is this: Using *simple* backprojection as described above, the reconstructed image has a characteristic 1/r blurring that results from the geometry of backprojection. To correct for this, a mathematical filtering operation is required, and that leads to the discussion of *convolution or filtered backprojection* in the next sections.

10.4.4 Convolution Backprojection

In the case of simple backprojection, the process of summing projections from a large number of angles around 360° results in the 1/r blur function as seen graphically in Figure 10-45A. The mathematical function 1/r is illustrated in Figure 10-45B. It is possible to correct for the impact of the 1/r function using image processing procedures. The mathematical operation of *convolution* describes such a procedure, and convolution is discussed in more detail in Chapter 4, and in Appendix G. When "undoing" an effect caused by convolution, *deconvolution* is used. Deconvolution is mathematically identical to convolution, except that the deconvolution kernel is (by definition) designed to *undo* a specific effect. The convolution process is defined mathematically as

$$p'(x) = \int_{x'=-\infty}^{\infty} p(x')\ h(x-x')\mathrm{d}x' = p(x) \otimes h(x),$$

[10-9]

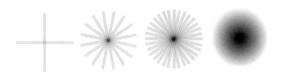

A   backprojection causes a 1/r blur

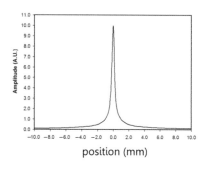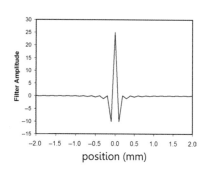

B   1/r blur function   **C**   deconvolution kernel

■ **FIGURE 10-45** A graphical representation of how backprojection leads to more concentrated energy in the center than in the periphery is shown **(A)**. The 1/r blur function which results from simple backprojection is illustrated **(B)**. The convolution kernel shown in **(C)** can correct for the 1/r blurring. In convolution-backprojection, the projection image data is mathematically convolved prior to backprojection.

where $p(\cdot)$ is each measured projection, $h(\cdot)$ is the deconvolution kernel, and $p'(x)$ is the corrected projection value, which is used in filtered backprojection. The right-hand side of Equation 10-9 shows the short-hand notion for convolution, where $\otimes$ is the mathematical symbol for convolution. The deconvolution kernel that is designed to undo the 1/r blurring shown in Figure 10-45B is shown in Figure 10-45C. The oscillatory nature of the deconvolution kernel in Figure 10-45B is a result of the discrete nature of the operation, as applied in a computer. As mentioned in Chapter 4, when a convolution kernel has negative values such as that shown in Figure 10-45C, in general it "sharpens" an image. The kernel in Figure 10-45C is a 1-dimensional function, and it is used to deconvolve the measured 1D projection values prior to backprojection, as illustrated in Figure 10-46. In this figure it is seen that when all of the measured projections of the object are deconvolved with the appropriate kernel, subsequent backprojection results in a faithful representation of the object. Hence, the isotropic portrayal of the CT image (Fig. 10-46C) is an accurate depiction of the object scanned (Fig. 10-44A). Convolution backprojection as described in Equation 10-9 can be considered to be a specific implementation of filtered backprojection.

10.4.5   Fourier-Based Filtered Reconstruction

Convolution as described in Equation 10-9 can be performed faster in a computer using properties of the Fourier transform. Specifically, Equation 10-9 can be recast as

$$p'(x) = FT^{-1}\{FT[p(x)] \times FT[h(x)]\},\qquad [10\text{-}10]$$

where $FT[\cdot]$ refers to the Fourier transform operation and $FT^{-1}[\cdot]$ is the inverse Fourier transform. Equation 10-10 is mathematically equivalent to Equation 10-9; however, the Fourier transform approach can be performed faster in a computer. Therefore, the Fourier approach is used in commercial scanners more often than the

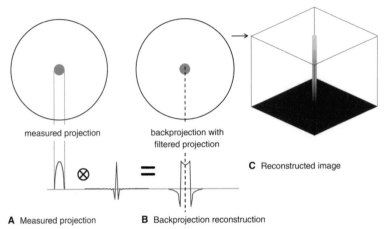

measured projection

backprojection with
filtered projection

C Reconstructed image

A Measured projection

B Backprojection reconstruction

■ **FIGURE 10-46** The process of filtered backprojection is shown. The "filter" in filtered backprojection refers to the mathematical operation, as depicted in this figure. The measured projection **(A)** is convolved with an appropriate convolution kernel resulting in an edge-enhanced projection data set, which is then backprojected (full 360° backprojected image is shown) **(B)**. The use of this mathematical filtering eliminates the 1/*r* blurring, and so the resulting image **(C)** accurately describes the input object (Fig. 10-44A).

convolution approach. Notice that the Fourier transform of the convolution kernel $h(x)$ is performed in Equation 10-10; however, because $h(x)$ does not change for a given CT reconstruction, its Fourier transform is precomputed. Because of the routine use of Fourier-based filtered backprojection (FBP), it is very common in the CT vernacular to refer to FT[$h(x)$] more so than to $h(x)$, and it is also common nomenclature to refer to FT[$h(x)$] as $H(f)$. The Fourier transform of the deconvolution kernel (Fig. 10-45C) is illustrated as the "ramp" filter in Figure 10-47. The ramp filter is the starting point for the filters used in FBP, as will be described in more detail below.

But why is the ramp filter *the* filter that we start with in filtered backprojection? Figure 10-45A shows the 1/*r* blurring effect that results from simple backprojection, and it turns out that this is a 1/*f* effect in the frequency domain. So, if you have an

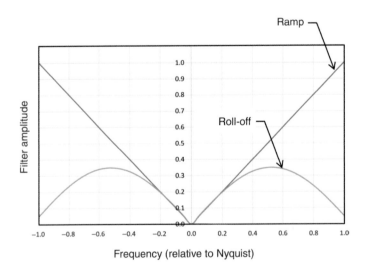

■ **FIGURE 10-47** The convolution kernel shown in Figure 10-45C is a spatial domain convolution kernel. Historically, the filtering in filtered backprojection has been implemented in the frequency domain, where (after the Fourier transform) the shape of the convolution kernel becomes a ramp as shown in this figure. A ramp filter, however, amplifies linearly as a function of frequency, so small structures (especially quantum noise) are amplified. Therefore, some form of apodization or roll-off is applied to the ramp filter.

image in the frequency domain (or Fourier domain) that has a $1/f$ dependency that you want to correct for, the correction process would involve multiplying that image by a function that has an f dependency, which is described mathematically as

$$H(f) = \alpha \times f, \qquad [10\text{-}11]$$

where α is a scaling factor. This correction process results in $f \times (1/f) = 1$, which eliminates any frequency dependency. It should be recognized that Equation 10-11 defines the ramp filter seen in Figure 10-47. For advanced readers, it should be noted that the value of $H(f)$ has a slight taper to it as $f \to 0$ to maintain HU value accuracy (hence $H(0) > 0$), and thus Equation 10-11 has some subtle complexities to it.

As mentioned above, the ramp function $H(f)$ shown in Figure 10-47 is the *starting point* in designing the shape of the filter in filtered backprojection. It would work well in the case of an image where there was very little quantum noise in the projection image data sets (the measured data during CT reconstruction). However, because the radiation dose levels in CT are kept to a minimum to enable diagnosis, the measured data in fact contain a large amount of *quantum* noise (see Chapter 4 for more on this). Notice the shape of the ramp filter in Figure 10-47; it has high values at high spatial frequencies, and therefore it amplifies the signals with high spatial frequencies in the projection data—and this high frequency region is also where quantum noise tends to dominate. Consequently, if one were to use the ramp filter directly for filtered backprojection, the reconstructed CT image would in most cases be unacceptably noisy. Therefore, it is customary to apply an *apodization* function that "rolls off" the amplitude of the reconstruction filter at high spatial frequencies, as shown in Figure 10-47. The roll-off reduces the high frequency component of the reconstructed image, and reduces high frequency noise as a result. All commercial CT scanners allow a choice of apodization filters that can be selected for a given type of exam (discussed later).

Figure 10-48 illustrates the Fourier filtering of the raw sinogram data. Figure 10-48A shows the raw sinogram data, which has a low-frequency or "blurry"

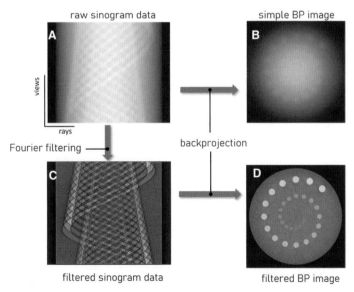

■ **FIGURE 10-48** Fourier-based filtered backprojection reconstruction is illustrated. If the raw sinogram data **(A)** are backprojected directly to produce an image **(B)**, it will be blurred with the $1/r$ problem described previously. Instead, the raw sinogram data are Fourier transformed filtered and then multiplied by a filter **(C)** and then backprojected to perform the filtered backprojection image **(D),** which has eliminated the $1/r$ problem.

appearance to it. After Fourier filtering, using for example the roll-off filter shown in Figure 10-47, the filtered sinogram data (Fig. 10-48C) shows much higher spatial frequencies—for example, the DC or constant levels of the raw sinogram data are suppressed, and the edges are enhanced. Edges are high frequency, and the constant (or DC) levels of an image are near zero frequency.

The specific roll-off function varies for the specific application in CT. In the mathematical reconstruction literature, the names of specific roll-off filters include Shepp-Logan, Hamming, cosine, *etc.* Some commercial CT manufacturers give these mathematical filters application-specific names such as soft tissue, bone, or lung filters. Other companies use numerical designations for their filters, such as H47 or H50 for head filters and B40 or B70 for body filters.

For a given CT scan, the interpreting radiologist is interested in all aspects of the anatomy, including (for example) lung tissue, soft tissue, and bone tissues for a thoracic CT scan. Hence, it is common to reconstruct the same acquired data using several different kernels, each of which best depicts the various tissues within the FOV of the scan. This does not increase the radiation dose levels of the examination; however, it does increase the interpretation time on the part of the radiologist.

10.4.6 Cone Beam Reconstruction

Cone beam scanners typically use a detector that is large enough to enable the entire object of interest to be scanned in one 360° rotation of the gantry, and with no table motion. This is accomplished using (most commonly) flat-panel detectors that have a physical height (*e.g.*, 30 cm) that is comparable to their width (*e.g.*, 40 cm), as seen in Figure 10-9.

Cone beam reconstruction algorithms are similar to standard fan beam reconstruction algorithms, but these algorithms also take into consideration the beam divergence (cone angle) in the z-direction (Fig. 10-9). Filtered backprojection occurs as described above; however, the algorithm backprojects the individual rays including angles in both the fan and the cone angles. Referring back to Section 10.4.2, this means that the fan beam geometry sinogram data $P(j, \theta)$ in Figure 10-48A needs to also consider the cone angle, hence these data become $P(j, \Phi, \theta)$, where j is the detector location that defines the fan angle, Φ defines the cone angle, and θ defines the view angle.

The basic cone beam reconstruction process, referred to as the Feldkamp, Davis and Kress algorithm, or FDK, reconstructs the entire volume data set (a series of CT images of a given section thickness) simultaneously. Cone beam reconstruction violates mathematical requirements for sampling Fourier space, and for extreme cone beam geometries used in flat panel detectors (as in Fig. 10-10) or other very wide cone beam CT systems, this can lead to cone beam artifacts (discussed later).

10.4.7 Iterative Reconstruction in CT

Iterative reconstruction is numerically intensive and has been used in the clinical environment for many years for smaller data sets (such as with single photon emission computed tomography, SPECT). As a result of the computational complexity of iterative reconstruction algorithms, filtered backprojection was the primary method for reconstructing CT images for many decades due to time constraints. However, advancements in algorithm design coupled with modern (faster) computer hardware have led to clinically useful iterative reconstruction algorithms for CT images, even given their large data sets.

The fundamental problem in CT image reconstruction is shown in Figure 10-49, where projection data sets are shown with a CT image. The projection data are what is

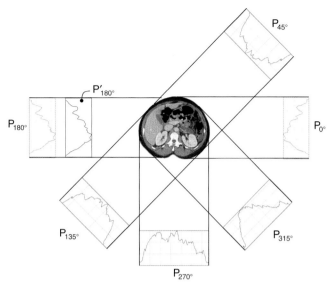

■ **FIGURE 10-49** This figure shows measured projections for a few of the angles around 360°. In filtered back-projection, these projection data are backprojected to form the reconstructed CT images. Iterative reconstruction methods make use of the same data set, but generate the reconstructed image in a series of iterations where the measured data (such as P_{180}) are compared with forward-projected images (such as P'_{180}) that are generated mathematically from the current iteration of the image-in-progress. After the measured and forward projected images are compared (e.g., $P_{180} – P'_{180}$), the iterative algorithm updates the image based upon that comparison, until some stopping criteria are met and the final image is produced.

known, and the CT image is the *unknown* and therefore needs to be reconstructed. The projection data sets are used to reconstruct the CT image as illustrated in Figure 10-49, but if the CT image (or an approximation of it) is known, then the projection data can be computed using forward projection (as shown for p'_{180}). Note that in Figure 10-49 only six projection data sets are illustrated, but in clinical CT, a large number of projection data are acquired around 360° (900–1,200 or more projections).

To put the CT reconstruction problem into perspective, a typical 400-mm abdomen-pelvis scan using 0.5 mm detector dimensions (at isocenter) acquires on the order of 720 million rays of raw data (assuming 1,000 view angles around 360°), and the reconstructed data set includes 82 million voxels (400 1-mm-thick images)—that represents a ratio of 8.8 raw data points (rays) per reconstructed voxel.

Statistical Iterative Reconstruction

Iterative reconstruction techniques go through a series of iterations in the process of CT reconstruction, as illustrated in Figure 10-50. In many implementations of CT

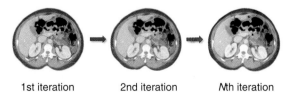

1st iteration   2nd iteration   *N*th iteration

■ **FIGURE 10-50** Traditional nuclear medicine iterative reconstruction would sometimes start with a blurry image guess and iterate towards a sharper image. In CT, in part to reduce computation time, some iterative approaches start with a filtered backprojection image (1st iteration) and then use subsequent iterations to apply denoising or other adaptive filtering methods to reduce noise while attempting to preserve spatial resolution in the final (*N*th) iteration.

iterative reconstruction (IR), the initial image is computed using FBP. Subsequent iterations use statistical methods to adaptively reduce noise in the images using iterative techniques—and there are scores of variations in the details of IR implementation. Figure 10-50 illustrates a first iteration (*e.g.*, FBP), a second iteration with some noise abatement, and then finally after N iterations, the final IR image is produced. Figure 10-49 outlines a general approach to IR reconstruction—a forward projection ($P'_{180°}$) is generated from the current image, and this is compared (by subtraction or other means) to the measured projection ($P_{180°}$) at that angle, and the differences determined from all angles are then used to update the next iteration of the image.

Model Based Iterative Reconstruction

The challenge of IR is to achieve a balance between accurately depicting anatomical information with excellent detail (spatial resolution) while suppressing the noise in the image. Second generation IR methods in CT go beyond purely statistical methods and *model* many of the physical parameters of the CT scanner that filtered backprojection cannot, such as the shape of the x-ray spectrum, the blurring of the focal spot, the detection properties of the detector arrays, the influence of scattered radiation, etc. These are called model-based iterative reconstruction (MBIR). In principle, both statistical and model-based iterative algorithms make better use of the acquired data—they produce images with higher SNR at the same dose, or they can produce images of similar SNR (as FBP) at lower doses. Figure 10-51 illustrates comparisons between images reconstructed using filtered backprojection images and iterative methods, and the iteratively reconstructed images clearly show a distinct advantage. Many IR algorithms do not explicitly use Fourier filtering methods

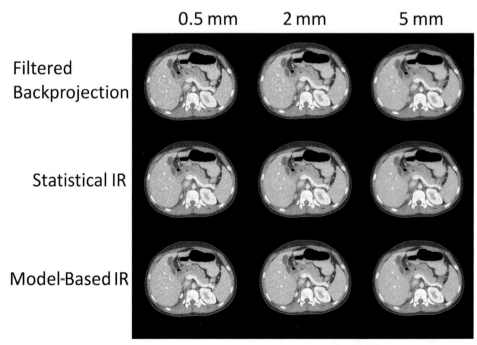

■ **FIGURE 10-51** In this figure, filtered backprojection, statistical iterative reconstruction (first generation IR), and model-based iterative reconstruction (second-generation IR) are illustrated for images of varying section thickness. The thinner the images, the more visible the noise, as expected. The more sophisticated the iterative reconstruction algorithm is, the greater the reduction in noise. (Used with permission from Canon Medical Systems USA, Inc.)

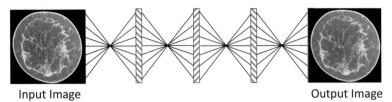

Input Image   Output Image

■ **FIGURE 10-52** Artificial intelligence–based convolutional neural networks (CNN) are challenging the most sophisticated of model-based iterative reconstruction techniques for suppressing noise while maintaining signal amplitude and spatial resolution. While methods vary, a common approach to the application of CNN-based reconstruction is to start with a reconstructed CT image (using filtered backprojection, for example) and then apply the CNN to this image to produce a CT image with greater noise suppression and signal enhancement, as implied in this figure.

as described above, and consequently the noise *texture* in the images can be quite different than with filtered backprojection images. Noise texture will be discussed later.

10.4.8 Deep Learning and Convolutional Neural Network Reconstruction

The most recent class of reconstruction algorithms to enter the market is based on artificial intelligence or DL methods. The concept is illustrated in Figure 10-52, where there are many layers with full interconnections between the input image and the output image. The interconnections between layers (shown as lines in the figure) represent weighting factors, with non-linear operators at each layer. This type of algorithm is *trained* using a large number of cases, for example a training set consisting of 1,000 pairs of input and output images, with each image representing (for example) a $1,024^2$ CT image. During training, an algorithm iteratively adjusts the individual connection weights and threshold values on the non-linear operators, in order to attempt to compute the output image from the corresponding input image. In the end, once the iterative learning algorithm has completed its task, the use of this *convolutional neural network* (CNN) amounts to a huge filtering operation with built-in intelligence for the task it was trained to perform.

A typical example of the data set used to train a CNN as described above would be N pairs of identical CT images (N was stated to be 1,000 in the above paragraph), with the input image being a very low dose (and noisy) CT scan of the patient, and the output image being a very high dose (and low noise) CT scan of the patient at the same anatomical location. The training algorithm is essentially teaching the CNN to perform de-noising on the low dose input image to produce the low noise output image, and the large number of pairs of images allows the algorithm to generalize this de-noising process. After training (which can take hours or days), the weights and thresholds of the CNN are defined and can be used to operate on low dose input images that are not a part of the training set, to achieve a general de-noising effect for these types of images. This calculation (using the trained algorithm with its static weights to convert the input image to the output image) can be performed very quickly. While this type of mathematical operation is often criticized as a "black box," the fact is that they generally work well and have been shown to achieve superior levels of de-noising compared to iterative reconstruction algorithms with substantially less computation time. Figure 10-53 illustrates the same CT image data from a commercial CT scanner, reconstructed with FBP, statistical IR, model-based IR, and DL reconstruction, for comparisons.

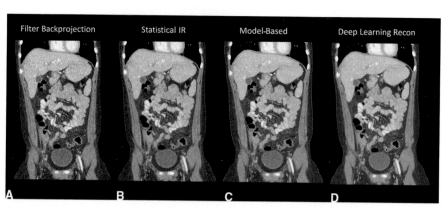

■ **FIGURE 10-53** For the same acquired data set, 4 reconstruction methods are demonstrated including **(A)** filtered backprojection, **(B)** statistical iterative reconstruction, **(C)** model-based iterative reconstruction, and **(D)** deep learning reconstruction using a CNN. (Used with permission from Canon Medical Systems USA, Inc.)

10.5 IMAGE QUALITY IN CT

10.5.1 Spatial Resolution

Spatial resolution in CT results from the fundamental resolution properties of the image acquisition, as well as the resolution characteristics of the reconstruction filter that is used. Factors that determine the physical limitations related to resolution include the focal spot size and distribution, the detector dimensions, the magnification factor, whether or not gantry motion is compensated for, patient motion, etc. Because CT images are the result of an elaborate mathematical reconstruction process (with many different reconstruction algorithms and parameters), CT resolution is also very dependent on the characteristics of the reconstruction algorithm and associated parameters selected for that algorithm.

Spatial Resolution in the Reconstruction (*x, y*) Plane

The in-plane CT image is a direct product of the CT reconstruction, and by far most clinical CT images are acquired and then natively reconstructed in the axial plane. Some variations in patient positioning (*e.g.*, bent neck with head tilted forward) lead to occasional exceptions to this. Spatial resolution has historically been measured in the clinical environment in CT using bar patterns, as illustrated in Figure 10-54. These images were acquired using the American College of Radiology (ACR) accreditation phantom, which has eight different bar pattern modules around the periphery of the 20-cm diameter phantom. The bar phantom has modules corresponding to spatial frequencies of 0.4, 0.5, 0.6, 0.7, 0.8, 0.9, 1.0, and 1.2 line pairs per mm (lp/mm). Note that in most of the commercial CT literature, the resolution is quoted in *line pairs per cm* instead of the *line pairs per mm* as is typical in the rest of x-ray imaging. Here, we use lp/mm for consistency, recognizing that lp/cm = 10 × lp/mm—thus, 12 lp/cm = 1.2 lp/mm.

The images shown in Figure 10-54A and B were generated from the same CT acquisition, and the differences in spatial resolution are the result of the reconstruction filter used. For the soft tissue image (Fig. 10-54A), three of the bar patterns can be easily resolved corresponding to a limiting spatial resolution of 0.6 lp/mm. The CT image reconstructed with the bone kernel (Fig. 10-54B) allows six of the modules to be resolved, for a limiting spatial resolution of 0.9 lp/mm. Figure 10-54C shows the

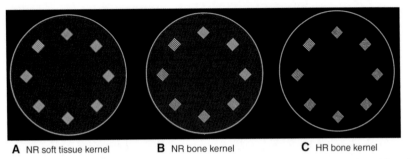

A NR soft tissue kernel   **B** NR bone kernel   **C** HR bone kernel

■ **FIGURE 10-54** Traditional line pair phantoms are used for in-the-field measurements of spatial resolution in computed tomography. These images show the American College of Radiology phantom reconstructed with **(A)** a soft tissue kernel, and **(B)** a bone kernel, for a normal resolution CT scanner. The higher spatial frequency characteristics of the bone kernel are apparent by observing the higher frequency line pair modules. **(C)** The same phantom is shown imaged on a high resolution CT scanner, with all of the line pair modules resolved.

same ACR phantom imaged on a high resolution CT system with a $1,024^2$ matrix, and here the maximum 1.2 lp/mm resolution module on the phantom is seen.

The modulation transfer function (MTF) is a more rigorous measure of the spatial resolution characteristics of an imaging system, as discussed in Chapter 4. The MTF can be measured using a wire or plane of metal foil scanned on a CT scanner, and the MTF(f) is computed by taking the Fourier transform of the measured line spread function, LSF(x), with some normalization as well. Five MTF(f) curves are shown in Figure 10-55, corresponding to a specific manufacturer's reconstruction filters, as indicated. It is noted that the limiting resolution of each kernel is approximately at the 10% MTF level, which range from 0.59 to 0.97 mm^{-1}.

HRCTs have now entered the market, with better resolution performance due to a detector array with much smaller detector elements, along with several focal spot dimensions that can be managed to accommodate the trade-off between high spatial resolution (small focal spots) and fast acquisition (large focal spots). The high-resolution CT scanner can also be operated in NR mode, and the measured MTFs for both NR and HR are shown in Figure 10-56. The NR MTF reflects an apodization kernel with mid-frequency enhancement (where MTF > 1.0), and the super high-resolution (SHR) mode shows resolution performance out to approximately 2.0 mm^{-1} compared to the limiting resolution of about 1.0 mm^{-1} for the NR mode. To put this in terms of physical dimensions, the NR mode of this scanner is capable of faithfully imaging objects down to about 0.50 mm, while the SHR mode

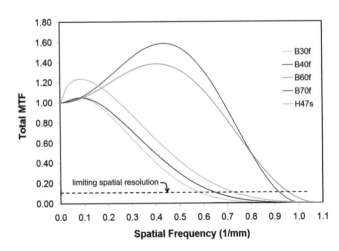

■ **FIGURE 10-55** The modulation transfer function (MTF) is a more complete measure of the spatial resolution characteristics of an imaging system, especially in computed tomography. Because CT images are reconstructed, some apodization kernels can produce an MTF that exceeds unity, as shown in this figure. Kernels can be selected which smooth (e.g., B30f) or sharpen (e.g., B70f) the image. (© Siemens Healthineers 2019. Used with permission.)

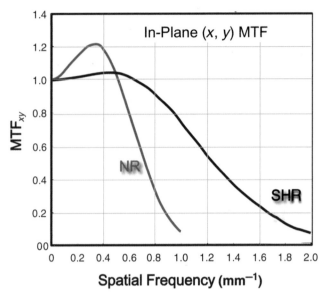

■ FIGURE 10-56 Next-generation CT systems which employ finer detector spacing and smaller focal spots can produce higher spatial resolution images, typically reconstructed to a $1,024^2$ matrix in comparison to the traditional 512^2 matrix for CT. The measured MTF's shown in this figure illustrate the normal resolution (NR) and the high-resolution (SHR) modes of a high-resolution CT system. Not only does the spatial frequency content extend to 2.0 mm^{-1} (corresponding to object sizes on the order of 0.25 mm) for the high-resolution system, the contrast transfer at 1.0 mm^{-1} has much higher amplitude, meaning that objects with sizes on the order of 0.50 mm will be better seen in the high-resolution CT image.

can faithfully image objects down to about 0.25 mm. These MTFs also suggest that an object with dimensions of about 0.625 mm ($f \approx 0.8$ mm^{-1}) would be imaged with about 40% of its contrast in the NR mode, but with 100% of its contrast with the SHR mode. In other words, the high-resolution mode is not only capable of showing smaller objects, it shows mid-sized objects with much better fidelity, as these MTFs demonstrate.

Spatial Resolution along the z-axis

Historically, the spatial resolution along the z-axis of the CT data set (the slice thickness direction) has been measured using the *slice sensitivity profile* (SSP—Fig. 10-57A). The SSP is defined as the shape of the system contrast from a point input in the z-dimension. In the ACR phantom, there are a series of high contrast rods spaced 0.5 mm apart in the z-dimension (Fig. 10-57A). Counting the number of visible "lines" on a CT scan of this test module and multiplying by 0.5 mm results in a field measurement of the slice thickness. Images were reconstructed on the scanner at nominal slice thicknesses of 5 mm (Fig. 10-57B) and 2.5 mm (Fig. 10-57C), and the ACR test suggests that these slice thicknesses are accurate.

The typical reconstructed slice thickness in the mid-1990s was 5–7 mm, and the SSP was routinely used in that era to characterize the "slice thickness." Today it is routine to reconstruct images with 0.5- to 0.625-mm slice thicknesses (0.25 mm for HRCT), rivaling the dimensions of the voxel in the (x, y) plane. Since the SSP is essentially the LSF along the z-dimension in the CT scanner, we can use the MTF metric to characterize the spatial resolution in the z-dimension as illustrated in Figure 10-58. For image data sets that are reconstructed into thicker sections (*e.g.*, $T = 2.5$ mm), the MTF(f) degrades as expected. It is noted that the z-dimension in an axially acquired CT data set can routinely have higher spatial resolution compared

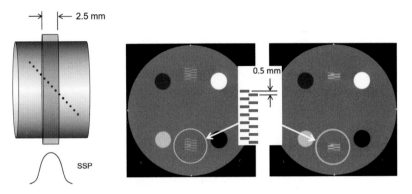

A measurement concept   **B** 5 mm slice thickness   **C** 2.5 mm slice thickness

■ **FIGURE 10-57** Resolution measurement along the z-axis of the CT scanner has, up until recently, been performed using the so-called slice sensitivity profile (SSP, **A**). The SSP shows the contrast of a small object as a function of its position in the field along the z-axis. A module from the American College of Radiology CT phantom is illustrated **(B)** for a 5-mm reconstruction section thickness and **(C)** a 2.5-mm section thickness. The phantom contains small rods staggered at 0.5 mm intervals along the z-dimension. Section thickness is estimated by counting the number of visible rods (the side view of the rods are shown in the axial image) and multiplying by 0.5 mm.

to the (x, y) axial in-plane geometry. In part this is because the apodization kernel affects the resolution in the (x, y) plane but not in the z-dimension. For this reason, coronal and sagittal CT images have the potential for better spatial resolution than axial CT images.

Figures 10-56 and 10-58 illustrate that conventional methods (slit → LSF → Fourier Transform → MTF) can be used to measure the MTF in CT in both the xy- and z-dimensions. It is also possible to use a slanted edge, hemisphere, or spherical test object to measure both the MTF_{xy} and MTF_z in the same image acquisition, with subsequent analysis of the three-dimensional image data. Figure 10-59 shows the three-dimensional MTF as an isometric plot. Projections of the "3D" curve reveal the individual MTF_{xy} and MTF_z curves. As tomographic imaging in CT and other modalities redefine the field of radiological imaging, it is only natural that the metrics used to characterize these 3D image data sets also take on three-dimensional properties.

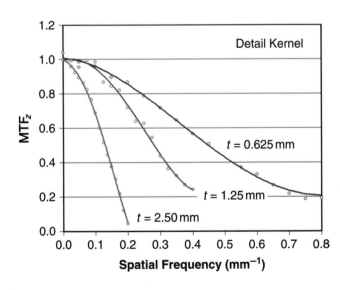

■ **FIGURE 10-58** Recognizing that the slice sensitivity profile is similar conceptually to the line spread function in the z-dimension, it is straightforward to compute the modulation transfer function in the z-dimension for CT. Here, the MTFs for different slice thickness (as indicated) are shown. Of course, the smaller the section thickness, the better the MTF. Because the apodization kernel is typically not applied in the z-dimension, the z-dimension of modern CT scanners can have superior resolution compared to the in-plane (x, y) images.

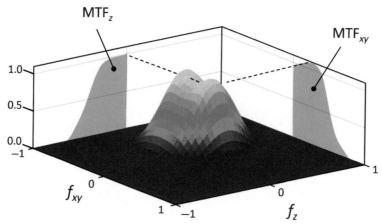

■ **FIGURE 10-59** The 3D modulation transfer function can be computed from three-dimensional CT data sets, using appropriate phantoms or spherical objects placed within a homogeneous medium. The three-dimensional modulation transfer function gives a full description of the spatial resolution properties of the CT system, and resolution properties will have some location dependence that can be well characterized using the 3D MTF metric.

10.5.2 Noise Assessment in CT

Contrast Detectability Phantom: Visual Assessment

The traditional method for quantifying *contrast resolution* in CT is to visually assess a contrast detail phantom, as shown in Figure 10-60. These images were produced from the ACR phantom. The image on the left was produced using four times the radiation levels as the image on the right, and the number of visible test objects (low-contrast rods) is far greater. The test objects in this phantom are designed to have 6 HU greater density (0.6%), than the background and they also vary in diameter. The smaller circular test objects have lower SNR and therefore are theoretically and experimentally more difficult to see. This visual assessment of the low contrast resolution of a CT scanner is a subjective measure of the noise characteristics of a CT scanner—national and international accreditation standards (which are hard to change) tend to perpetuate these subjective methods for characterizing the low contrast performance of CT scanners. However, more quantitative methods are moving into the mainstream, as described below.

Image Noise in CT: The Standard Deviation σ

The CT image of a region of the phantom that is homogeneous in composition can be used to quantify the noise directly, using software available on virtually any CT scanner or PACS system. The standard deviation σ, the direct measurement of "noise," is computed using the root mean square method:

$$\sigma = \sqrt{\frac{\sum_{i=1}^{N}(\mathrm{HU}_i - \overline{\mathrm{HU}})^2}{N-1}}. \qquad [10\text{-}12]$$

Consistent with the Poisson noise distribution, the noise estimated using Equation 10-12 in the right image (using 71 mAs) is about twice that of the left image (using 285 mAs) since the radiation levels were reduced by a factor of 4 (Fig. 10-60). This underscores the relationship in quantum limited imaging where the noise (σ) is proportional to the square root of the dose—for example, double the dose and the

ACR phantom—low contrast detectability section

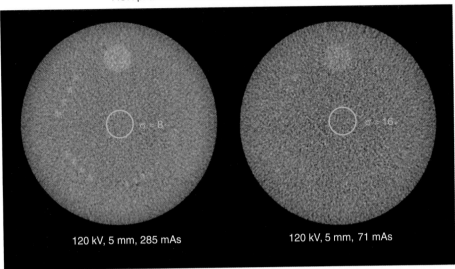

120 kV, 5 mm, 285 mAs   120 kV, 5 mm, 71 mAs

■ **FIGURE 10-60** Traditional estimation of the noise in computed tomography images make use of a so-called low contrast phantom, which is comprised of a homogeneous material with cylindrical inserts of different diameter and different contrast level. This figure shows the low contrast phantom section of the American College of Radiology phantom, imaged at different dose levels that vary by a factor of four. It can be seen that the high dose image on the left shows a measured standard deviation that is about half that of the low dose image on the right, which is to be expected. Furthermore, more of the objects embedded in the phantom are visible on the high dose image (left) compared to the low dose image on the right. This is a classic demonstration of *contrast resolution*.

noise decreases to 71%, use 4× the dose and the noise decreases to 50% (reduced by a factor of 2). The two images in Figure 10-60 illustrate this relationship qualitatively. While scalar quantitative measurements (such as σ) of noise are very useful, a full description of the noise characteristics in CT can be developed when the frequency-dependent characteristics of the noise in the image are measured. The frequency dependence of noise in CT and other images is referred to as noise *texture*. Because CT images are increasingly subject to new reconstruction methods and a variety of different task-dependent kernels with FBP, characterizing the noise texture goes a long way towards better understanding image quality in CT, and can help greatly in developing more optimal CT protocols.

Noise Texture in CT: The Noise Power Spectrum

The MTF(f) described previously characterizes how *signal* propagates through an imaging system, while the noise power spectrum (NPS) describes how the *noise* propagates through an imaging system. The NPS(f) is a mathematical metric that describes both the overall noise amplitude (σ^2) and the noise *texture*—a term referring to the frequency dependence of the noise in an image. The NPS describes how the noise at one point in the image is *correlated* to the noise in the surrounding points of the image. Noise correlation occurs for a variety of reasons, but the point spread function of the imaging system tends to be a primary culprit in causing noise correlation. The NPS in CT is computed by taking the Fourier transform of a 2D region of interest (2D NPS) or a 3D volume of interest of CT image data (3D NPS), where these ROIs or VOIs are simply patches of noise (with the mean of each patch subtracted) in an otherwise featureless part of a phantom. Typically, many dozens of NPS (either 2D or 3D) are averaged together to reduce noise in the measurement. In most situations using filtered backprojection reconstruction (which has linear mathematical properties), the NPS has the same characteristics in the x- and y-dimensions of an axial CT image. Hence, it is common to combine these using:

$$f_{xy} = \sqrt{f_x^2 + f_y^2}.$$

[10-13]

Figure 10-61A shows patches of white (uncorrelated) noise as well as correlated noise. The patch of correlated noise was made by convolving the white noise image with a gaussian point spread function. Figure 10-61B shows the influence of the apodization kernel on the noise texture, with the NPS illustrated for both body and lung kernels. Figure 10-55 illustrates how various kernels impact the MTF (signal modulation), and the NPS (noise modulation) has a similar but not identical impact on the noise properties of an image. Figure 10-61C illustrates the NPS for two different radiation dose levels for image acquisition, but reconstructed using the same (lung) kernel and filtered backprojection. Notice that the frequency dependence (shape) of these two curves is identical, only the amplitude is different. This is because the integral (area under the curve) of the NPS is equal to the noise variance—σ^2, and the noise variance of the 17.1-mGy curve is about 3.5 times less than the 4.9-mGy curve (17.1/4.9 = 3.5) Finally, Figure 10-61D illustrates the NPS for the same acquired

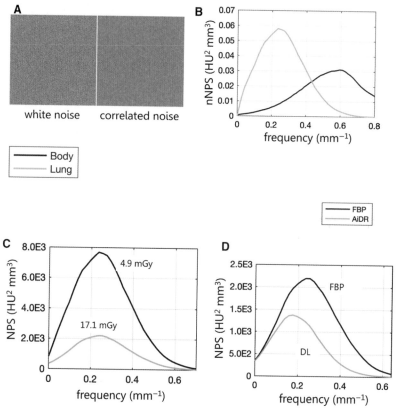

■ **FIGURE 10-61** While in the field measurements of low contrast inserts are still commonplace, the more quantitative measurement of the noise in CT includes not only characterizing the noise amplitude (which the σ levels capture in Fig. 10-60), but also the noise texture. The noise texture is demonstrated by the frequency dependence of the noise amplitude, as characterized by the noise power spectrum (NPS). **A.** Examples of white noise and correlated noise are shown. **B.** The normalized NPS for different reconstruction kernels is illustrated. **C.** The NPS for different radiation dose levels (CTDIvol values are shown) are illustrated, and the lower dose image data demonstrates more noise. **D.** This NPS shows the difference between standard filtered backprojection and a deep learning algorithm approach towards reconstruction, for the same acquired data set.

data set reconstructed using FBP and a DL reconstruction algorithm. It can be seen that the DL algorithm produces some low-pass filtering (the peak frequency is shifted left), but the overall amplitude (area under the curve) of the noise variance is reduced considerably, demonstrating the de-noising that it was trained to deliver.

10.6 CT IMAGE ARTIFACTS

10.6.1 Beam Hardening

Beam hardening refers to the increase in effective energy of the x-ray beam as the poly-energetic spectrum passes through increasing thicknesses of tissue. Due to the higher attenuation of bone (or iodine or metal) compared to soft tissue, beam hardening occurs more dramatically for those rays that pass through these more attenuating materials (Fig. 10-62). Beam hardening occurs in all x-ray imaging modalities; however, the consequences of beam hardening are more visible in CT because of the backprojection process. For a given voxel to be reconstructed in the middle of the region of soft tissue, CT rays are backprojected through that voxel from many different angles. Some of those rays may have passed through thick regions of bone, while other rays at different angles may have only traversed soft tissue. This means that the amount of beam hardening that occurred between these two rays can be quite different, and this leads to the formation of so-called beam hardening artifacts. The image inset in Figure 10-62 shows classic beam hardening artifacts in head CT, where the dense petrous bones cause significant beam hardening that is not matched at the other angles in the backprojection process, creating a discontinuity in the soft tissue region. Note that the harder x-ray beam has higher effective energy, which means that the linear attenuation coefficient for tissue (or bone) is lower. Hence, beam hardening manifests as low density (darker) streaks that typically run between two high density regions. Figure 10-63 shows beam hardening

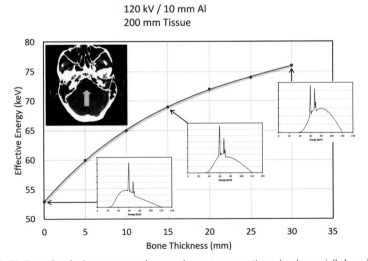

■ **FIGURE 10-62** Beam hardening occurs as the x-ray beam traverses tissue (and especially bone) through the patient. Because CT images are reconstructed from different projection angles, and the spectral changes that result from beam hardening are different for different projections, this can cause the appearance of a streaking artifact between objects with high attenuation, as indicated by the yellow arrow on the head CT image. The plot shows the effective energy as a function of bone thickness, for a 120-kV x-ray beam (with 10 mm Al and 200 mm soft tissue filtration). The shape of the spectrum changes with increasing bone thickness, gradually being depleted of low energy components in the spectrum at greater thicknesses.

■ **FIGURE 10-63** A body CT image is shown that includes spinal hardware in the field-of-view. The metallic implants cause significant beam hardening artifacts, which is manifest as low density (dark) rays emanating from the very bright metal implants.

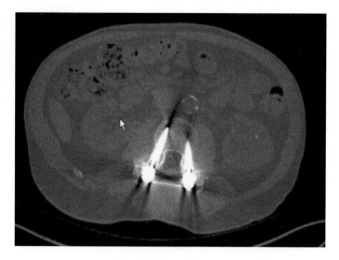

associated with implanted spinal hardware, and the dark streaks emanating from the metal artifact are clearly seen.

Beam hardening only occurs in the presence of a polyenergetic x-ray spectrum—when a monoenergetic x-ray beam is used for CT imaging, no beam hardening artifacts are produced. While most x-ray spectra in clinical radiology are polyenergetic, exotic x-ray sources such as synchrotrons can produce monoenergetic x-ray beams that have been studied in the research environment. To reduce beam hardening artifacts in CT, the x-ray beam is filtered by relatively thick sheets of metal such as aluminum or titanium. Whereas a radiographic x-ray beam may be filtered with 3 mm of aluminum, the average CT x-ray spectrum is filtered with 10 mm or more of aluminum. Hence, the x-ray beams used in CT are "pre-hardened" to reduce beam hardening artifacts, to the extent possible.

10.6.2 Streak Artifacts

Streak artifacts have several origins. Objects that appear bright (high HU values) on the CT image correspond to highly attenuating objects in the patient, which in turn correspond to low signal areas reaching the detector arrays in the shadow of these objects. Often this occurs with metallic implants or dental fillings (Fig. 10-64). The large discontinuity in the signal levels near these areas can challenge the linearity of the detector system, leading to streak artifacts. Streak artifacts are exacerbated when a dense object has slight movement, as in the case of dental fillings—where the patient may inadvertently be moving the jaw during the scan as a nervous reaction to the procedure. Even slight movement of a dental filling can cause dramatic streak artifacts due to the high attenuation of older fillings, which contain a mercury-based amalgam (the atomic number of mercury is 80 with density $\approx$ 14 g/cm^3).

Metal artifact reduction algorithms are present on many CT systems, and these can reduce the presence of streak artifacts. There is a well-defined mapping between a given voxel in the CT volume data set and the raw projection data acquired by the scanner. Algorithms that essentially go back and forth between the reconstructed image and the raw data can iteratively adjust the raw data to reduce streak artifacts.

10.6.3 View Aliasing

The raw data set for CT is comprised of rays and views, as seen on Figure 10-42. In CT images that have high frequency content (e.g., sharp edges), in some cases the

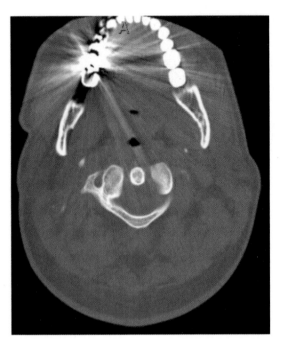

■ **FIGURE 10-64** A head CT image is shown, with the classic streak artifacts radiating from a dental filling. Streak artifacts are exacerbated by slight motion of highly attenuating structures. The amalgam in dental fillings contains mercury, a highly attenuating metal.

number of views required is not sufficient to convey these edges during backprojection. This can cause so-called *view aliasing*, where the number of views acquired is insufficient to properly reconstruct the high-frequency detail in the CT image (Fig. 10-65). View aliasing artifacts are often exacerbated by linear structures in the object or patient being imaged.

10.6.4 Ring Artifacts

Ring artifacts are a characteristic of third-generation (rotate-rotate) CT geometry, where the detector arrays are mounted on the same rotating gantry as the x-ray tube. Figure 10-66A demonstrates the geometric nature of ring artifacts, where a bad detector can cause a ring artifact because each detector has a strong role to play in the projection data set for a given annulus in the image. Figure 10-66B illustrates a clinical image where three detectors were out of calibration in the same scan (with rings highlighted), and Figure 10-66C shows the same image without the rings overlaid. In the early days of CT, when detector technology and computer

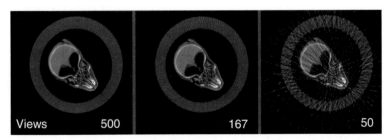

| Views | 500 | 167 | 50 |

■ **FIGURE 10-65** View aliasing is illustrated in the CT images of a mouse skull, acquired on a micro CT scanner. While little to no view aliasing is illustrated when 500 views are used in the reconstruction, some view aliasing is seen for 167 views, and significant view aliasing (as well as image noise) is seen with only fifty views used in the reconstruction.

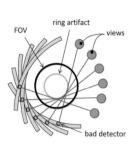 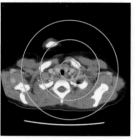 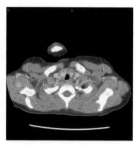

A description   **B** rings highlighted   **C** ring artifacts

■ **FIGURE 10-66** The cause of ring artifacts is illustrated graphically in **(A)**. In third-generation CT, a given detector has significant influence for a given annulus in the reconstructed image, and any mis-calibration of that detector may result in a ring artifact. **B.** A body CT images illustrated, and the three ring artifacts are highlighted with the overlaid graphics. **C.** The CT image is displayed without the overlaid graphics, showing three ring artifacts.

algorithms were relatively crude by today's standards, ring artifacts posed more problems than with the sophisticated detectors and algorithms available today. Ring artifacts are considered particularly troublesome because in some cases—given the circular profile of some patients—they could confuse the diagnosis if not recognized as artifacts.

Figure 10-66 shows ring artifacts for an axial CT of the body. When a mis-calibrated detector is present during a *helical* CT scan, a series of partial ring artifacts can be seen in subsequent images along the z-dimension as shown in Figure 10-67.

■ **FIGURE 10-67** With a multiple detector array CT combined with helical acquisition, a mis-calibrated detector may occur in only one detector of the many (*e.g.*, 64) detector arrays. For helical acquisition with a pitch of one, all 64 detector arrays contribute to the image data for every reconstructed CT image—and so a bad detector will only show up for certain sectors of the image. This series of 4 images shows streak artifacts for subsequent images (along the z-axis), with the position of the artifact located at different regions in the image.

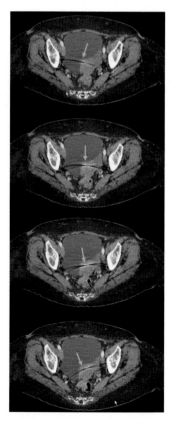

5-mm section thickness   1.25-mm section thickness

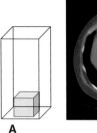 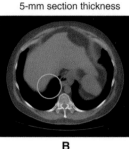 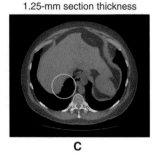 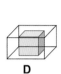

A   **B**   **C**   **D**

■ **FIGURE 10-68** These images illustrate partial volume artifacts. For the 5 mm section thickness **(B)**, a small calcification is barely seen because the length of the voxel is much longer than the calcification (as shown in **A**), and thus the average linear attenuation coefficient (which scales to the Hounsfield Unit) is low. For the 1.25 mm section thickness **(C)**, the high attenuation of the calcification is less diluted in the volume (see graphic in **D**), resulting in a higher linear attenuation coefficient (and HU values) in the image with significantly better detectability.

10.6.5 Partial Volume

Partial volume artifacts occur (Fig. 10-68) when the CT voxels are large and encompass several types of tissue, such as a combination of soft tissue and calcium. The attenuation of a given voxel in the patient will be weighted by the amount of soft tissue and calcium in that voxel. In Figure 10-68A, a cube of calcium occupies a relatively thick voxel, and this leads to a reduction in contrast as seen on the associated thick section (5 mm) image (Fig. 10-68B). Figure 10-68D shows the same cube of calcium, but now in a voxel that is four times smaller in volume than before—consequently, the voxel is brighter and therefore depicts the calcification better in the thinner (1.25 mm) section image Figure 10-68C.

10.6.6 Cone Beam Artifacts

Cone beam acquisition geometry can lead to undersampling in the cone angle dimension, and this can cause a well-known cone beam artifact (Fig. 10-69). The Defrise phantom, which is a stack of attenuating disks separated by low density material

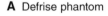
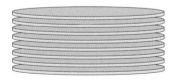

A Defrise phantom

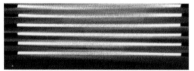

B Some cone beam artifacts

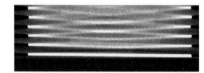

C Pronounced cone beam artifacts

■ **FIGURE 10-69** Cone beam artifacts occur when the ray sampling along the cone angle is insufficient to obey Tuy's condition. **A.** The DeFrise phantom—a stack of plastic discs with air in between—illustrates cone beam artifacts very well. **B.** This coronal image is illustrated with the phantom located at a slight distance from the central x-ray beam (small cone angles), and **(C)** this image shows pronounced cone beam artifacts image at a high cone angle.

(Fig. 10-69A), can be used to evaluate cone beam artifacts. In a well-sampled environment, cone beam artifacts can be kept to a minimum (Fig. 10-69B); however, the use of large cone angles can lead to considerable artifacts (Fig. 10-69C). Cone beam artifacts are a result of fundamental deficits in the acquired data, and the most obvious solution for these artifacts is to acquire a more complete data set.

SUGGESTED READING AND REFERENCES

Boone JM. Determination of the pre-sampled MTF in computed tomography. *Med Phys.* 2001;28:356-360.

Defrise M, Townsend D, Geissbuhler A. Implementation of three-dimensional image reconstruction for multi-ring positron tomographs. *Phys Med Biol.* 1990;35(10):1361-1372.

Feldkamp LA, Davis LC, Kress JW. Practical Cone-beam algorithm. *JOSA A.* 1984;1:612-619.

Jacobson FL, Jaklitsch MT. Computed tomography scanning for early detection of lung cancer. *Annu Rev Med.* 2018;69:235-245.

Joseph PM, Spital RD. A method for correcting bone induced artifacts in computed tomography scanners. *J Comput Assist Tomogr.* 1978;2(1):100-108.

Kalender WA. *Computed Tomography: Fundamentals, System Technology, Image Quality, Applications.* 3rd ed. Erlangen, Germany: Publics Publishing; 2011.

Kalender WA, Seissler W, Klotz E, Vock P. Spiral volumetric CT with single-breath-hold technique, continuous transport, and continuous scanner rotation. *Radiology.* 1990;176(1):181-183.

Krause B. Dual energy computed tomography: technology and challenges. *Radiol Clin.* 2018;56(4): 497-506.

Seeram E. Computed tomography, a technical review. *Radiol Technol.* 2019;91:161CT-180CT.

Seidensticker PR, Hofmann LK. *Dual Source CT Imaging.* Heidelberg, Germany: Springer; 2008.

Yang K, Kwan AL, Huang S-Y, Packard NJ, Boone JM. Noise power properties of a cone-beam CT system for breast cancer detection. *Med Phys.* 2008;35(12):5317-5327.

CHAPTER 11

X-ray Dosimetry in Projection Imaging and Computed Tomography

Radiation dosimetry is a field of study that encompasses the measurement and calculation of ionizing radiation energy deposition into matter. Dosimetric quantities and units are used in estimating radiation dose to patients, workers, and members of the public. Dosimetric quantities and units were discussed in Chapter 3. Some of these quantities, such as absorbed dose and kerma, are defined entirely in terms of other physical quantities, particularly energy and mass. Other quantities, equivalent dose, effective dose equivalent, and effective dose, are intended for use in radiation protection and involve the use of weighting factors chosen by expert bodies to account for the detriment from the biological effects of ionizing radiation. This chapter addresses the application of dosimetry to x-ray projection imaging and x-ray computed tomography.

11.1 X-RAY TRANSMISSION

Understanding x-ray dosimetry starts with an understanding of the factors in an x-ray system that lead to a specific x-ray spectrum that is incident upon the patient. This spectrum interacts with the patient's tissues by several mechanisms that lead to radiation dose deposition in those tissues. The details of x-ray production are described in Chapter 6. A typical x-ray spectrum used in diagnostic radiology shows x-ray photon fluence as a function of x-ray energy for a tube potential of 100 kV and 3 mm inherent aluminum filtration (Fig. 11-1). The spectrum consists of bremsstrahlung radiation and tungsten characteristic radiation peaks at ~58 and ~67 keV and is commonly referred to as *polyenergetic*, indicating a range of x-ray energies.

As described in Chapter 3, x-ray interactions within the tissues of the patient have energy dependencies that must be considered for accurate radiation dosimetry. Indeed, the dose deposited by primary photons (those emitted by the x-ray tube) at a specific depth (x) within the patient is computed for each photon energy (E), and then the total dose at that depth is summed (integrated) over the entire x-ray spectrum:

$$D(x) = \int_{E_{min}}^{E_{max}} \left\{ \frac{\mu_{en}(E)}{\rho} \right\} E\phi(E)e^{-\mu(E)x}\, dE, \qquad [11\text{-}1]$$

where $\phi(E)$ is the photon fluence (photons/cm²), $[\mu_{en}(E)/\rho]$ is the mass-energy absorption coefficient for photons of energy E, ρ is the density of the tissue, and $\mu(E)$ is the linear attenuation coefficient for photons of energy E. As is mentioned below, this equation does not account for energy deposition by scattered photons and so severely underestimates actual doses.

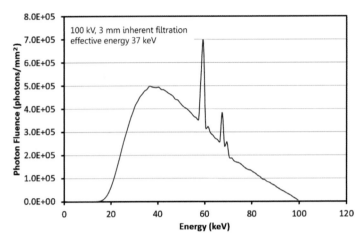

■ **FIGURE 11-1** A typical x-ray spectrum used in radiography, fluoroscopy, and other x-ray imaging systems is illustrated. This is a 100-kV spectrum with 3 mm of inherent aluminum filtration. The area of the spectrum is normalized to 1 mGy air kerma, and the half-value layer is 3.8 mm of aluminum. The average energy is 50 keV, and the effective energy is 37 keV.

If this operation is performed for the x-ray spectrum [$\phi(E)$] shown in Figure 11-1, using the energy-dependent linear attenuation coefficients for tissue [$\mu(E)$], the curve marked "transmitted" is generated as shown in Figure 11-2. This curve describes the transmission of primary radiation (scatter is not included here) to the depths of a patient's soft tissues, and the shape of the curve is due to the exponential in Equation 11-1. The curve labeled "attenuated" in Figure 11-2 illustrates the fraction of the incident beam that is attenuated (removed from the transmitted beam) due to photoelectric, Rayleigh, and Compton scattering interactions.

In most situations, the transmission of the polyenergetic x-ray spectrum through tissue can be accurately calculated using a monoenergetic approximation, as shown by the solid circles for given depths, x, in Figure 11-2. These data were computed as a single exponential:

$$D(x) = D_o e^{-\mu_{eff} x}, \qquad [11\text{-}2]$$

where a 37 keV monoenergetic x-ray beam was found to match the attenuation characteristics (μ_{eff}) of the 100 kV x-ray spectrum reasonably well.

As the incident x-ray beam is attenuated with depth in the patient, the diverging beam also decreases the beam intensity through the inverse square law, as illustrated in Figure 11-3. The inset on this figure demonstrates the nature of the inverse square law, with the same number of unattenuated photons passing through two different planes. The number of *photons per unit area*, the photon fluence, is reduced in the more distant plane because it has a larger area. Since the area increases as the square of the distance from the source, a corresponding reduction of the primary x-ray beam intensity occurs as a function of depth as shown by the curve. The x-ray dose is therefore the product of the transmission curve shown in Figure 11-2 and the inverse square law curve shown in Figure 11-3. If the beam is not divergent, which would be called a "parallel beam," then the inverse square law is not at play. Hence, the transmission curve shown in Figure 11-2 is that of a parallel beam geometry, a common way of depiction that does not depend on a specific geometry, such as the x-ray source-to-object distance.

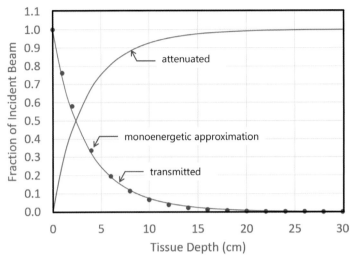

■ **FIGURE 11-2** The *transmitted* x-ray beam shows the approximately exponential transmission versus tissue depth for the x-ray spectrum illustrated in Figure 11-1. The corresponding symbols demonstrate the transmission of a monoenergetic x-ray beam comprised of 37-keV x-ray photons, showing the *monoenergetic approximation* to the attenuation curve of the 100-kV polyenergetic spectrum. As a beam of photons passes through tissue, attenuation processes including the photoelectric effect, Rayleigh scatter, and Compton scatter occur, and these photons that have been eliminated from the primary beam are shown as the *attenuated* curve. The data in this curve show only the attenuation of the primary x-ray beam, assuming a parallel beam geometry. While the transmission curve appears to reach zero at about 25 cm of tissue depth, a logarithmic vertical axis would show penetration to 0.1%, 0.01%, or greater.

The transmission curve shown in Figure 11-2 only describes the passage of the primary beam through the tissues of the patient and does not include any tissue heterogeneity such as bones or gas pockets. In addition, when a primary x-ray photon experiences a scattering interaction, it is considered a *scattered* photon, and there is no simple equation to describe the actual composition of the primary and scattered photons as a function of depth. The generation of x-ray scatter and the complex geometry of the trajectory of scatter requires the use of computer-based Monte Carlo

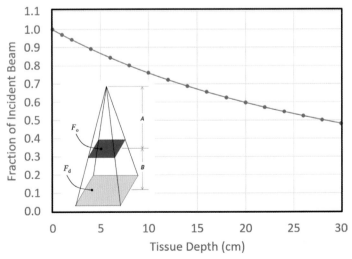

■ **FIGURE 11-3** Because the x-ray beam is emitted from essentially a point source, the *inverse square law* also reduces the intensity of the beam as a function of tissue depth, even if there was no tissue present. This curve assumes a specific x-ray beam geometry, where A = SSD = 68 cm, and B = 30 cm (see inset).

techniques, as described in the next section, to accurately track the passage of both primary and scattered photons through the patient's tissues.

11.2 MONTE CARLO SIMULATION

All modern x-ray dosimetry relies extensively on Monte Carlo simulation. Monte Carlo simulation requires a sophisticated computer program that tracks simulated x-ray photons as they are incident onto the patient, photon-by-photon, which potentially interact with tissue, and in some cases pass through the patient undergoing no interactions—these latter ones being the primary photons that are detected and used to form the image. However, for dosimetry, we are interested in the vast majority of photons (99.0%–99.9%) in the x-ray beam that *do* interact in the patient, and deposit dose through interactions including the photoelectric effect and Compton scattering.

Monte Carlo simulations are often described as computing the random walk of a photon as it interacts with the patient's tissues, similar to that shown in Figure 11-4. Typically, this involves tracing the path of billions of x-ray photons through the object, using the computer to keep track of where energy is deposited. While this walk is stochastic in nature, it is not truly random because virtually all of the interactions between x-ray photons in the tissues in the body are described statistically, including the photoelectric effect, Rayleigh scatter, and Compton scatter. In order to include the statistical properties of x-ray scattering, all Monte Carlo routines use

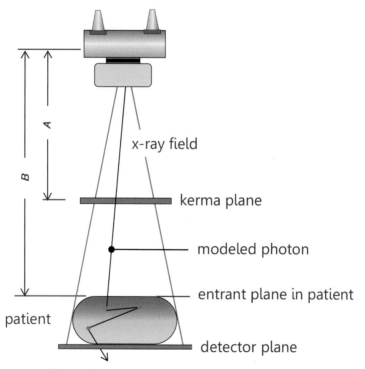

■ **FIGURE 11-4** A typical design for Monte Carlo simulation of dose deposition is illustrated. The simulated (virtual) x-ray beam is emitted from a point source and is collimated onto a detector plane. X-ray interactions are computed in a virtual patient, where the dose deposition and its distribution are tallied. The air kerma passing through the kerma plane is recorded, and the radiation dose in the patient is also tallied. This geometry can then be used to define a coefficient, which is the ratio of patient dose to incident air kerma. More specific anatomical geometry can also tally dose to specific organs, and other interaction sites of interest.

random number generators. A random number generator is the equivalent of a dice roll for a computer, but uses a subroutine that returns random numbers, typically in the interval from 0 to 1; these are then used with some additional mathematics to accurately compute the stochastic physical processes that underlie the Monte Carlo simulation. Most Monte Carlo simulations include both the attenuation processes (Fig. 11-2) as well as the geometry-dependent inverse square law (Fig. 11-3). As discussed in Section 3.4, the quantity absorbed dose is defined as *energy deposited by ionizing radiation per unit mass.*

$$D_{absorbed} = \frac{dE}{dm}.$$ [11-3]

The probabilities of these interactions depend on the x-ray photon energy and the specific tissue in the patient, including soft tissue, adipose tissue, bone, *etc.* When an x-ray photon interacts via the photoelectric effect in tissue, all of the energy of that photon is deposited locally and therefore contributes to radiation dose. For high Z attenuators (iodine contrast material and metal implants are examples in the patient), x-ray fluorescence (*i.e.*, characteristic radiation) is typically produced after a photoelectric interaction; these x-rays then carry energy away from the interaction site. However, for the low Z elements that comprise soft tissue (*e.g.*, C, H, O, N), the fluorescent yield is essentially zero; hence the photoelectric effect results in essentially total local absorption for most soft tissues. When an x-ray photon interacts via the Rayleigh scattering mechanism, the scattered photon carries with it the same amount of energy as the incident photon, so there is no deposition of energy. Consequently, while Rayleigh scattering redirects x-ray photons, it is a zero-dose event. This does not mean, however, that a photon that was Rayleigh scattered could not undergo a subsequent interaction that does deposit energy and hence dose. Therefore, it is necessary to track Rayleigh scattered photons during a Monte Carlo simulation to accurately calculate the radiation dose distribution. When an x-ray photon experiences Compton scattering in tissue, a fraction of its energy is deposited at the interaction site contributing to the accumulation of dose, and a larger fraction of the energy remains as a scattered photon, with a deflected trajectory. The deflection angle of x-ray scatter depends on the x-ray's energy and the effective Z of the tissue where the interaction took place, both of which are defined in probability tables developed for this purpose.

A complete Monte Carlo simulation for a specific application, such as computing the dose of an abdominal radiograph, includes looping over the range of energies (*e.g.*, in 1 keV steps) that are present in the simulated x-ray spectrum. For example, the 100-kV x-ray spectrum illustrated in Figure 11-1 contains photons ranging from 17 to 100 keV, so each of these photon energies is simulated using millions to billions of x-rays at each (monoenergetic) energy (*i.e.*, 84 different runs). These intermediate results are then weighted by the photon distribution in the spectrum. While Monte Carlo simulations may use many billions (10^9) of virtual photons in the calculation, this is far fewer than the number of x-ray photons used in an actual x-ray imaging exam. For example, an abdominal radiograph may use the 100 kV x-ray spectrum (Fig. 11-1) and 220 mAs, and would expose an image receptor of approximately 300 $\times$ 300 mm—such an examination would require about 4×10^{13} x-ray photons. If 10^6 photons required ½ minute to run in the computer for the simulations, the full simulation (4×10^{13}) would require 38 years. Because Monte Carlo simulations are so computationally expensive, it is not practical to perform them for individual patients undergoing a common imaging procedure. Instead, published tables produced from Monte Carlo simulations are commonly used. To correct for the fact that fewer x-ray photons are used during Monte Carlo dose simulations, the simulation geometry (Fig. 11-4) is set up to calculate both the air kerma that is incident upon the simulated patient, as well as the corresponding radiation dose deposited in the patient. In this way, coefficients can be produced that relate the radiation dose absorbed in the patient to the air kerma incident upon the patient. These coefficients can then be used with incident kerma levels measured in the real world, in order to estimate a specific patient's absorbed dose. For radiographic and fluoroscopic procedures, the entrance air kerma at the surface of the patient is used as a normalization point. For computed tomography procedures, the air kerma at the center of rotation (isocenter) of the gantry is used as a normalization point. While the kerma plane is placed well above the "patient" in Figure 11-4, the inverse square law can be used to compute the kerma at any location in the field.

In the early days of Monte Carlo simulations, mathematical phantoms comprised of simple geometrical shapes were used to simulate the geometry of the human body (Fig. 11-5A). More recently, whole-body CT images have been used to model the geometry of the human body (Fig. 11-5B). Typically, these whole-body CT scans (often produced from cadavers) are segmented into relatively large (*e.g.*, 2 × 2 × 2 mm, 5 × 5 × 5 mm, *etc.*) voxels for use in Monte Carlo simulations. Once a mathematical model of the patient is developed, specific radiographic projections or other imaging geometries need to be defined so that the radiation dose coefficients can be computed for specific clinical examinations, such as PA chest radiography, lateral head radiography, abdominal CT with helical acquisition, *etc.* The geometry of a PA abdominal radiograph is demonstrated in Figure 11-5A, corresponding to a 300 mm × 300 mm field of view projected onto a mathematical anthropomorphic phantom.

11.3 THE PHYSICS OF X-RAY DOSE DEPOSITION

X-rays deposit energy (and hence dose) through interactions with electrons. Both the photoelectric effect and Compton scattering interactions ionize an atom or molecule at the site of interaction, resulting in the ejection of an energetic electron. These

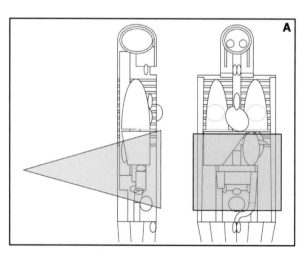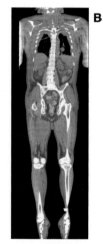

■ **FIGURE 11-5 A.** Historically, Monte Carlo studies made use of anatomical models defined by simple geometrical shapes; here the Medical Internal Radiation Dose (MIRD) phantom is illustrated. **B.** The power of modern computers combined with the availability of high-resolution anatomical data from CT scans have allowed Monte Carlo simulations to be performed with very detailed anatomical models.

energetic electrons interact with tissue, depositing most of their energy in a very small volume. Indeed, the initial electron ejected from an x-ray interaction will collide with many other electrons in atoms and molecules before it comes to rest, causing subsequent ionization events along its path. These secondary energetic electrons (called "delta rays") impart much of the radiation energy near the initial ionization event. This energy deposition causes chemical changes that damage molecules of biological importance. The ultimate health impact of this molecular damage will depend on which molecules have been damaged, the extent of the damage, the subsequent fidelity of repair processes, as well as many other factors discussed in greater detail in Chapter 20. DNA is, of course, a critical molecule, and radiation-induced DNA base damage and double-strand breaks followed by base excision repair and non-homologous end-joining, respectively, are well-known examples of these ubiquitous damage and repair processes occurring throughout life.

Figure 11-6 illustrates the concept of air kerma. "Kerma" stands for *Kinetic Energy Released in Matter* and was discussed in Chapter 3. X-ray photons entering a small volume of air interact with the air molecules, whereby each interaction produces an ion pair—an energetic electron and the positively charged atom or molecule that it came from. Normally the accurate measurement of radiation assumes that within the measurement volume of air, the energy carried out of the volume by electrons leaving the volume is equal to the energy carried into the volume by electrons produced outside of the volume—so-called electron equilibrium. Kinetic energy is the energy of motion, and it is these energetic electrons (primarily) that ultimately produce absorbed dose. Kerma (K) is defined as a "point quantity," although the energy considered is transferred to electrons in a very small mass of material. The sum of this kinetic energy (in joules), divided by the mass (in kilograms) of air in the measurement volume is the air kerma, with the typical unit of milligray (mGy) in diagnostic radiology.

Energetic electrons can graze an air molecule (*e.g.*, O_2 or N_2) and experience the nuclear charge of an atom, causing the electron to be decelerated. As described in Chapter 6, when electrons bombard a target inside the x-ray tube,

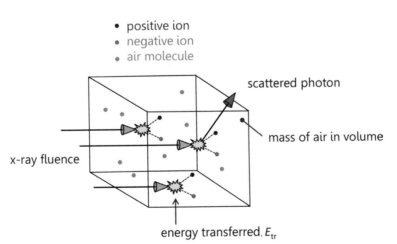

- positive ion
- negative ion
- air molecule

scattered photon

mass of air in volume

x-ray fluence

energy transferred, E_{tr}

■ **FIGURE 11-6** The basic concept of air kerma is illustrated. X-rays are incident upon a small volume of air and ionize air atoms producing ion pairs as defined in the figure. With these interactions, x-ray photons transfer their energy to the ion pair, resulting in kinetic energy of these charged particles. When a Compton scattering event takes place, the scattered photon leaves the volume of interest. The air kerma (kinetic energy released in matter) is the energy transferred to charged particles, divided by the mass of the air in the measurement volume.

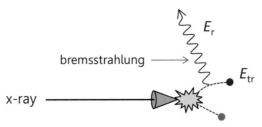

■ **FIGURE 11-7** When an x-ray interacts with an atom or molecule that transfers energy to an ion pair (E_{tr}), subsequent interactions between an energetic electron and other atoms in the interaction volume can result in deceleration of the electron, producing bremsstrahlung radiation (E_r: radiated energy). When the bremsstrahlung x-ray leaves the measurement volume, the absorbed energy (E_{en}) is given by: $E_{en} = E_{tr} - E_r$.

they are decelerated and produce bremsstrahlung radiation. The same interaction can occur in the volume of air, generating a bremsstrahlung x-ray that then leaves the volume of air, taking with it some of the kinetic energy (E_r, r = radiative) that was originally transferred to the electron (Fig. 11-7). The remaining absorbed energy (E_{en}) in the volume of air is the difference between the initial energy transferred to electron motion (E_{tr}, tr = transferred), subtracting the loss of energy through radiative emission:

$$E_{en} = E_{tr} - E_r. \qquad [11\text{-}4]$$

It is the absorbed energy E_{en} (in joules) per unit mass of the volume (in kilograms) that gives rise to the absorbed dose. Figure 11-8 illustrates the absorbed dose, and if in a volume of air, this would be the air dose. The amount of bremsstrahlung radiation released (Fig. 11-7) in the diagnostic x-ray energy region is very low—almost to the point of being negligible. However, for x-rays with higher energies (>250 keV) the radiative emission (E_r) can be a larger fraction of E_{tr}. So in the diagnostic energy region, $E_r \to 0$, and thus $E_{tr} \approx E_{en}$, meaning that air kerma is about equal to air dose in diagnostic radiology.

It was stated above that the volume shown in Figure 11-8 could be air, but this volume could just as well be tissue—the mechanisms of radiation dose deposition that occur in a volume of low-density air are the same that occur in a small volume of near unit-density tissue. The description above discusses the physics of dose deposition, and also describes some of the elements that a Monte Carlo simulation program must take into consideration in order to perform a radiation dose calculation (in silico).

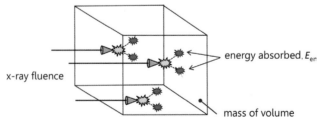

■ **FIGURE 11-8** When x-ray photons (x-ray fluence) are incident upon the measurement volume, initially energy is transferred (E_{tr}), some energy may be radiated away (as shown in Fig. 11-7), and the energy that remains E_{en}, divided by the mass of that volume, represents the absorbed dose. The volume of interest in this figure could be filled with air, and hence the dose would be the air dose; however, this can also be a small volume of tissue, corresponding to the absorbed dose in tissue.

11.4 DOSE METRICS

The concept of radiation dose has evolved considerably as our understanding of the effects of ionizing radiation has advanced; consequently, there are a number of metrics that describe radiation dose in different ways. Each of these metrics has utility in describing and understanding radiation dose from x-ray diagnostic medical imaging procedures. Radiation dose in nuclear medicine procedures is described in Chapter 16. It is important to note that, as we review different quantities that describe radiation dose, in some cases (but not all) the unit associated with a quantity may change. It is very important to understand the differences between the quantities and the units and to make sure that the proper unit is used when discussing the associated quantity.

11.4.1 Entrance Skin Air Kerma

The entrance skin air kerma (ESAK) simply describes the amount of radiation incident upon the surface of the patient (formerly the quantity *entrance skin exposure* was used). For radiographic procedures using x-ray beams with similar energy spectra, ESAK is roughly proportional to the surface dose in the patient and so can be used to compare procedures from a dosimetric perspective. ESAK is an appropriate metric for radiographic (including mammographic) and fluoroscopic procedures, but not for computed tomography. The ESAK is typically estimated free-in-air, (*i.e.*, neglecting scatter from the patient) and can be determined from the known output characteristics of the x-ray system in association with the geometry of the radiographic procedure (discussed below).

Imagine a radiographic procedure of a patient's abdomen, where the surface of the patient's abdomen is located 70 cm from the x-ray source. By measuring the output of the system at 70 cm from the x-ray source using a radiation meter and ionization chamber with no other object in the field of view, the air kerma "free-in-air" is determined. However, if the patient (or more likely a phantom) is positioned at 70.1 cm from the x-ray source and the ionization chamber is positioned just in front of the phantom with the same x-ray exposure settings (*i.e.*, kV, mA, exposure time), the radiation meter will record a larger value of air kerma by about 15%–20%, because scattered radiation coming back from the phantom will be detected, in addition to the primary radiation emanating from the x-ray tube. So, when ESAK is used as a dose metric unless otherwise stipulated, this measurement is made in the absence of a phantom and therefore in the absence of backscattered radiation, in the geometry known as "free-in-air." For air kerma measured at the entrant surface of the skin, the common unit for this measurement value is mGy.

11.4.2 Entrance Skin Dose

As the x-ray beam enters the first microscopic layers of the skin, the radiation dose imparted to that layer of skin is referred to as the entrance skin dose. Recall that from Figure 11-8, in diagnostic radiology the air kerma is essentially equal to the air dose, and thus the air dose just above the layer of skin is equivalent numerically (both typically in the units of mGy) to the air kerma, as $D_{air} \cong K_{air}$. When considering only the dose to a microscopic layer of skin or tissue at the surface of the patient, two things are intentionally neglected: (1) the attenuation that occurs at depth in the tissue, and

(2) backscattered radiation that would contribute to the dose at the entrant surface. With this understanding, the dose to the entrance skin (tissue) is computed as:

$$D_{\text{tissue}} = D_{\text{air}} \frac{\left\{\dfrac{\mu_{\text{en}}}{\rho}\right\}_{\text{tissue}}}{\left\{\dfrac{\mu_{\text{en}}}{\rho}\right\}_{\text{air}}}, \qquad [11\text{-}5]$$

where the ratio of the mass-energy attenuation coefficients (tissue over air) is used to convert the air dose to the entrance surface to tissue dose. Except for bone, the ratio of mass-energy attenuation coefficients for soft tissues in Equation 11-5 is approximately 1.09.

11.4.3 Absorbed Dose

The quantity *absorbed dose* embodies the fundamental concept of radiation dose, with its strengths and weaknesses. Fundamentally, absorbed dose is defined as $D_{\text{absorbed}} = \dfrac{dE}{dm}$, *i.e.,* energy per unit mass (Eq. 11-3). When the energy is expressed in joules, and the mass is expressed in kilograms, the absorbed dose takes on the unit gray. Strictly speaking, absorbed dose is defined at a specific point, and the dose nearly always varies with location in a phantom or patient. For x-ray beams used in diagnostic and interventional imaging, the dose is higher in the tissues closer to the source than those deeper in the body. The average (mean) absorbed dose is what is often referred to when the simple term "dose" is used. Given this definition, the quantity absorbed dose in the context of biological risk is all too often open to misinterpretation, due to a number of factors including the volume of tissue that received the dose, and the specific tissue that received the dose. For example, which is more concerning from a radiation risk perspective? (1) An average dose of 10 Gy to your finger, or (2) an average dose of 10 mGy to your abdomen? Example 1 results in a total energy imparted of 0.2 joules (J) deposited in a 20-g finger, and example 2 results in 0.2 J deposited in a 20-kg abdomen. So, without specifying the total mass of tissue that receives a given absorbed dose value, the associated radiation risk is hard to assess. In addition, the organ or tissue in which the dose is deposited also affects the risk.

To add to the complication of using dose to convey risk, when a patient has had multiple diagnostic medical imaging procedures, for example after trauma, there is no single number that conveys risk. If a patient received 70 mGy to the head, 1.2 mGy to the knee, and 10 mGy to the abdomen after an automobile injury, there is no simple way to use absorbed dose as a metric to quantify this. That said, absorbed dose—or just "dose"—is the gold standard measurement describing one or more radiation exposure events.

11.4.4 Mean Glandular Dose

While the absorbed dose is the most appropriate metric for describing the magnitude of radiation exposure to a patient's organs, radiation exposure to the breast has a unique metric. The breast is comprised of several tissues, including fibroglandular tissue, adipose tissue (fat), and skin. However, the radiosensitivity of the glandular tissue for future cancer is far greater than that of the skin or adipose tissue. Indeed, *breast cancer* refers to cancers of the glandular tissues in the breast, not the adipose or skin tissues. Consequently, and specific to breast imaging, the mean glandular dose (MGD, also referred to as the mean fibroglandular dose) is the preferred metric for estimating radiation dose in the breast. Hence, the Monte Carlo routines that are used for computing dosimetry in breast imaging specifically tabulate the radiation dose delivered to the glandular tissue. The unique dosimetry used for mammography is discussed in Chapter 8.

11.4.5 Organ Dose

Metrics

The metric commonly used for evaluating the dose to an organ or tissue with regard to possible stochastic effects is the average (mean) absorbed dose delivered to the specific organ or tissue. It may be calculated as the quotient E/m, where E is the total energy imparted in the organ or tissue and m is the mass of the organ or tissue. The volume of interest in which the imparted energy (E) and mass (m) are computed is defined by the organ boundaries. For paired organs such as breasts and kidneys, the organ volume includes both organs. Calculating mean organ doses is the first (and likely most important) step in estimating risk of stochastic effects such as cancer from medical imaging procedures using ionizing radiation. Mean organ doses are unique because the mass of the entire organ is used in the calculation (m), even if only a fraction of the organ was exposed to radiation. For example, for a 10-kg liver, if 40% of the liver volume experienced an x-ray imaging procedure (such as a lesion-targeted CT scan) that deposited a total of 0.10 J in the liver, the mean organ dose to the liver would be 0.10 J/10 kg = 0.01 Gy or 10 mGy. Had the entire liver been exposed at the same radiation levels, the energy deposited would have been 0.25 J and the mean organ dose would have been 25 mGy. If a targeted radiographic procedure exposed the left kidney to 0.20 mGy, and the right kidney received no appreciable radiation, the mean kidney organ dose would be 0.10 mGy. The implicit assumption in the methodology just described is that at low dose, the stochastic risk (*e.g.*, future cancer in the exposed organ) is the same whether one half of the organ receives all of the radiation or if the exposure was evenly distributed throughout the entire organ.

Anthropomorphic Phantoms

With well-defined patient anatomy in the form of an anthropomorphic phantom incorporated into computer code, the organ doses resulting from x-ray exposure can be estimated using Monte Carlo techniques. The original anthropomorphic phantoms used with Monte Carlo programs to calculate radiation dose in the late 1950s and early 1960s employed rather elementary shapes like cylinders, spheres, ellipsoids, and prolate spheroids due to the lack of computational power available to the scientists of that era. Stylized computational phantoms have had a long history of development. In the 1960s much of the effort was tied to the need to estimate the absorbed dose to organs in patients who had been administered radiopharmaceuticals in the rapidly developing field of nuclear medicine and to radiation workers who may have become internally contaminated with radioactive material. Figure 11-9A shows organ doses (as different colors) using a 1980s era anthropomorphic phantom for a typical x-ray imaging procedure of the upper abdomen and thorax, with the different colors representing different organ doses. The organ and body contours of these stylized phantoms were defined by 3D mathematical surface equations. Further refinements led to CT based voxel Monte Carlo simulations of phantoms in which organs and body tissues were defined by groupings of 3-D cuboids or voxels

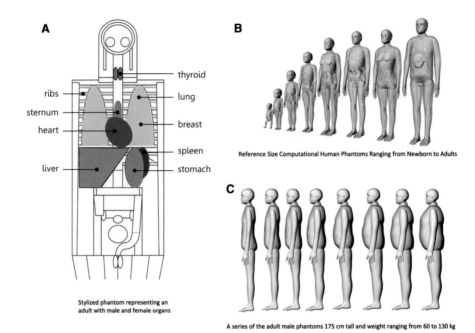

Stylized phantom representing an
adult with male and female organs

Reference Size Computational Human Phantoms Ranging from Newborn to Adults

A series of the adult male phantoms 175 cm tall and weight ranging from 60 to 130 kg

■ **FIGURE 11-9** The x-ray interactions illustrated in Figures 11-6 to 11-8 show fundamental interactions that take place physically, but in Monte Carlo modeling these interactions are calculated mathematically, with the statistically known x-ray cross sections, attenuation coefficients, and scattering angles within an anthropomorphic phantom to estimate absorbed dose. **(A)** represents a 1980s stylized anthropomorphic phantom developed at Oak Ridge National Laboratory representing adult with male and female anatomy while **(B)** is an example of state-of-the-art (2020) hybrid phantoms from the National Cancer Institute's library of computational human phantoms showing their reference size computational human phantoms ranging from newborn to male and female adults and **(C)** their series of the adult male phantoms 175 cm tall of varying body habitus with weight ranging from 60 to 130 kg. (**B:** Reprinted with permission from the National Cancer Institute: Division of Cancer Epidemiology and Genetics. https://ncidose.cancer.gov/#phantoms. Accessed July 6, 2020. **C:** Reproduced with permission from Chang LA, Borrego D, Lee C. Body-weight dependent dose coefficients for adults exposed to idealised external photon fields. *J Radiol Prot.* 2018;38(4):1441. © IOP Publishing. All rights reserved.)

to define the anatomical structures based on segmentation of patient medical images. While these phantoms were anatomically very accurate, they were not very flexible (with regard to adjustments for desired changes in resolution or age or body habitus of the phantom) and were computationally intensive. The optimal balance between accuracy and simulation efficiency came in the form of hybrid modeling. The hybrid modeling of the imaging processes combines the analytical and Monte Carlo simulation methods as well as the ability to integrate different Monte Carlo packages. Modern computational phantoms are typically constructed by the hybrid method defining surfaces or meshes based on the segmentation of 3-D patient imaging data (*e.g.*, MRI and CT). The PHANTOMS library developed from CT images of patients shown in Figure 11-9B is an example of employing the hybrid method and was the product of a collaboration between the University of Florida and the National Cancer Institute (Geyer et al., 2014; Lee et al., 2010). Best quality anatomical reference CT images were selected from an archive of 1,000+ patients. More than 100 organs and tissues were manually segmented and reviewed by practicing radiologists. The original PHANTOMS library consisted of a series of reference male and female anatomies (newborn, 1-, 5[1]-, 10-, 15-year-old, and adult). This library was later extended to 370 phantoms representing children and adults of both genders and various heights and weights, Figure 11-9C. NCI researchers also added anatomical details such as

[1]See footnote in Chapter 3, page 67.

lymphatic nodes, substructures of the heart (*e.g.*, atria, ventricles, arteries), and substructures of the brain (*e.g.*, gray and white matter, cerebellum, brain stem). The PHANTOMS library was carefully adjusted to match several international reference data including reference person height and weight, organ mass, tissue elemental composition, and dimensions of gastrointestinal structures. The pediatric phantoms have been adopted by the International Commission on Radiological Protection (ICRP) as an international reference (ICRP, 2020[q]).

No One Dose Metric Can Do It All

It is often said that a tally of organ doses represents the most comprehensive assessment of radiation dose from medical imaging procedures; however, there is no single metric that quantifies this. This is because the detriment of radiation exposure to the different organs has been studied in detail. Early classical cell survival studies demonstrated that for a given absorbed dose to the same type of cells in culture, some forms of radiation (like doubly charged alpha particles that produce dense ionization tracks) produced more cell death than sparsely ionizing forms of radiation (like x- and γ-ray and beta particles). Furthermore, based on the studies of radiation exposures to large populations (primarily the Japanese A-bomb survivors), it is known that different organs demonstrate different radiosensitivity with respect to developing radiogenic cancers. The ICRP developed the quantities *equivalent dose (H)* and *effective dose (E)* to take these and other factors (discussed in Chapter 21), relevant to the potential of future risks to a population exposed to low dose radiation.

Equivalent Dose

As mentioned in Chapter 3, the ICRP established the radiation weighting factors (w_R) to account for the greater effectiveness of higher Linear Energy Transfer (LET) radiations for producing biologic damage compared to low LET radiation (x-rays, γ rays, and energetic electrons). Low LET radiation is assigned a w_R value of 1. Higher LET radiations, such as protons and alpha particles, are assigned w_R values greater than 1 (*e.g.*, alpha $w_R = 20$) reflecting the fact that the damage caused by the dense ionization tracks of this type of radiation are more difficult to repair per unit dose than the more sparsely ionizing low LET radiations. When the absorbed dose is multiplied by the appropriate radiation weighting factor, it is transformed from a physical quantity (*i.e.*, energy per unit mass) to a radiation protection quantity *equivalent dose (H)*:

$$H = Dw_R. \qquad [11\text{-}6]$$

While the equivalent dose is *numerically* equal to the absorbed dose for x-rays, since $w_R = 1$, it should be kept in mind that the equivalent dose is a different *quantity* (with the unit of a sievert, Sv) than the absorbed dose (with the unit of Gy).

11.4.6 Effective Dose

The first thing to know about effective dose is that, like the equivalent dose, it is not a dose in the true sense of the word. Rather, the effective dose is a radiation protection quantity that incorporates a rough approximation of the relative biological variations in tissue sensitivities by assigning particular organs and tissue (T) the proportion of the detriment (harm) from stochastic effects (*e.g.*, cancer, hereditary and other effects discussed further in Chapter 20) resulting from irradiation of that tissue compared to uniform whole-body irradiation. The proportion of the total (*i.e.*, 1.0) assigned to a particular organ/tissue is referred to as the *tissue weighting factor* (w_t). Tissue weighting factors range from $w_t = 0.01$ for radioresistant tissues (*e.g.*, brain), to $w_t = 0.12$ for

TABLE 11-1 TISSUE WEIGHTING FACTORS (W_t) FOR VARIOUS TISSUES AND ORGANS (ICRP 103)

TISSUE	W_t
Gonads	0.08
Bone marrow	0.12
Colon	0.12
Lung	0.12
Stomach	0.12
Bladder	0.04
Breast	0.12
Liver	0.04
Esophagus	0.04
Thyroid	0.04
Skin	0.01
Bone surface	0.01
Brain	0.01
Salivary glands	0.01
Remainder	0.12
Total	1.00

W_t values are unitless and convert equivalent dose (in Sv) to effective dose (in Sv).

more radiosensitive tissues such as the intestines, lung, breast, stomach, and bone marrow (Table 11-1). In assigning the tissue weighting factors, the ICRP relied primarily on the results of epidemiological studies on large human populations exposed to radiation with long-term follow-up, to assess the relative risk of radiation-induced cancer (and other less frequent bioeffects) for each organ or tissue type.

In quantifying organ dose for the computation of effective dose, the radiation weighting factor w_R is applied to convert absorbed dose to equivalent dose. For x-ray radiation, $w_R = 1$, so an absorbed dose of X (mGy) results in an equivalent dose of X (mSv). If the entire body of an individual were exposed to a uniform absorbed dose of 5 mGy (and hence an equivalent dose of 5 mSv, whole-body), the effective dose would be 5 mSv. This is a consequence of all the tissue weighting factors (w_t) summing to 1.0. When multiple organs and tissues receive different doses, the sum of the products of the mean equivalent dose to each organ or tissue irradiated (H_T) and the corresponding tissue weighting factor (w_T) for that organ or tissue is calculated to obtain the effective dose (E).

$$E(\text{Sv}) = \sum_T \left[w_T \times H_T(\text{Sv}) \right]. \qquad [11\text{-}7]$$

The effective dose is expressed in the same units as the equivalent dose (Sv).

The reason why there are so many different dose metrics pertinent to radiation levels in diagnostic imaging is that each one has its strengths and weaknesses. The **strengths** of the effective dose metric include the following: (1) it takes into consideration partial body exposure, which occurs during diagnostic medical imaging procedures; (2) it provides a method to include the internal dose from radiopharmaceuticals used in nuclear medicine imaging procedures (see Chapter 16); (3) it provides a single-value metric that has been used to represent the long-term potential for harm (detriment) to a population, for multiple exposures to different areas in the body (including x-ray and nuclear medicine procedures); and (4) because background radiation can also be expressed in terms of an annual per capita effective dose, it can be used to make numerical comparisons to radiation doses associated with medical imaging procedures in a more understandable context for patients and healthcare providers who are not radiation experts. For example, few patients can relate to the 3-mSv effective dose received from a single head CT examination; however, when they learn that the annual background radiation in coastal California is 3.1 mSv, and in Colorado, it is 5.2 mSv, they have a better understanding of the relative risk of their imaging procedure.

The **weaknesses** of the metric effective dose are as follows: (1) As defined by the ICRP, the effective dose, was *never* meant, and should not be used, as a risk-related metric for a specific person or for a population that significantly differs from the population for which the radiation and tissue weighting factors were intended. The cancer risk uncertainties in the low-dose range and the underlying approximations, simplifications, and sex- and age-averaging used in generating E make it unsuitable for these purposes. However, in practice, medical imaging professionals and authors of peer-reviewed medical publications have frequently and incorrectly used E as a surrogate for whole-body dose to calculate cancer risk estimates for specific patients or patient populations. This frequent misuse has popularized E for uses for which it was neither designed nor intended (Bushberg, 2019). (2) As a risk metric pertinent to medical imaging, effective dose does not take into consideration patient-specific factors such as the health status and clinical indication for the procedure, the relative risk of not having the procedure or alternative imaging procedures, the patient sex, and age at the time of the exam, all of which are factors that must be considered when evaluating the potential risks against the benefits of any particular imaging procedure. For example, take two different patients who have had imaging procedures that lead to the same effective dose, where patient Julian is a 15-year-old healthy boy who had a head CT scan because of a sports injury, and patient Edna is an 83-year-old woman who had a head CT scan for follow-up after radiation therapy to treat her glioblastoma. This example shows the perils of using the quantity of effective dose as a risk factor when the patient's individual situation is not considered—clearly the risk of radiation exposure (while still low) is greater for the younger, healthy boy than that of the older woman with serious health conditions. This is because the evaluation of radiation risk to an individual includes, among other things, their life expectancy relative to the typical latent period for radiation-induced cancers of concern and any sex differences in radiosensitivity of the tissues exposed. That said, the effective dose is a very useful metric in comparing different imaging protocols (*e.g.*, CT versus radiography) to the same patient population.

Additional information on the ICRP system of radiation protection and their dose metrics is provided in Chapter 3 and Appendix H. Potential risks associated with radiation exposure are discussed in detail in Radiation Biology, Chapter 20.

11.5 RADIATION DOSE IN PROJECTION RADIOGRAPHY

Projection radiography is by far the most prevalent radiological imaging examination performed and is a remarkably low dose and cost-effective diagnostic procedure. In order to provide reasonably accurate estimates of the radiation dose associated with radiographic examinations, data describing the measurable radiation output levels of the x-ray system used to perform the examination are required. An example is shown

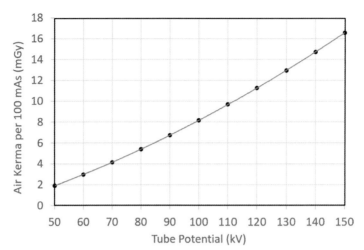

■ **FIGURE 11-10** When modeling radiation dose to patients in the real-world setting, the radiation levels produced by the equipment used for the exam need to be well understood. Medical physicists often make measures of air kerma for given x-ray tube potentials (kV) for various tube current-time products (mAs) as a part of annual consistency testing, as shown in this figure. These data were computed to a distance of 100 cm from the x-ray source. Notice the slight curvature of the data, indicating a $(kV)^n$ dependency on x-ray output, where $n > 1$. While air kerma does describe the x-ray tube output in a useful manner, these measurement data are also dependent upon the mass-energy attenuation coefficient of air, $(\mu_{en}/\rho)_{air}$.

in Figure 11-10, which shows the air kerma (in the units of mGy) per 100 mAs measured at a distance of 100 cm from the x-ray source as a function of x-ray tube potential. This type of information is required to be evaluated as part of the annual testing of radiographic rooms by many states in the United States. Figure 11-10 is an example of the measurable output (*e.g.*, air kerma) characteristics of a specific x-ray room in a facility; it should not be used for dosimetric calculations, as every x-ray room has slightly different x-ray output characteristics. As discussed in Chapter 6, the *radiation output* of an x-ray system is best characterized by the energy fluence at a given technique, for example for specific tube potential (kV), tube current (mA), and exposure time (s) settings, and this is shown in Figure 11-11 for the same x-ray

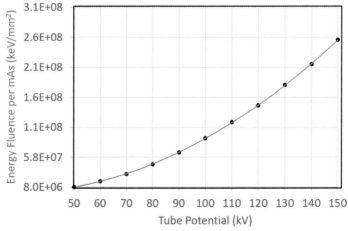

■ **FIGURE 11-11** The most fundamental metric of x-ray tube output is the energy fluence, which is described in this figure. The energy fluence is that physical parameter that imparts radiation dose to the patient and is also a fundamental parameter creating signal in the typical energy-integrating detector. With proper characterization of the x-ray spectrum, the energy fluence can be readily computed.

system that is described by the air kerma output in Figure 11-10. While air kerma (related to the older quantity of *exposure*) is the quantity that medical physicists use to describe the measurable output characteristics of a specific x-ray system, the energy fluence (joules/mm^2) is a better descriptor of x-ray tube output because it has a more direct relationship with the x-ray dose to the patient (*e.g.*, Eq. 11-1).

Figure 11-10 describes the air kerma for a given x-ray tube potential at a given distance in an x-ray room. To compute the patient's dose from a radiographic procedure using this information, the first step is to use the inverse square law to compute a correction factor (C_1) to relate the measured air kerma (from Fig. 11-10) to the surface of the patient's body:

$$C_1 = \left[\frac{100 \text{ cm}}{SSD}\right]^2, \tag{11-8}$$

where the source-to-skin distance (SSD) is specific to the patient's examination (Fig. 11-12). The next step is to adjust the entrance air kerma to the tube current (mA) and exposure time (s) used in the specific examination (Fig. 11-10), where the product of tube current and exposure time is described as the "mAs."

$$C_2 = \frac{x \text{ mAs}}{100 \text{ mAs}}. \tag{11-9}$$

In Equation 11-9, "x" is the mAs used for the patient's radiographic examination, as opposed to the 100 mAs for which the raw data in Figure 11-10 were measured (Table 11-2). Because Figure 11-10 represents the air kerma as a function of tube potential, AK (kV), estimating the entrance skin air kerma (ESAK) is given by:

$$ESAK = C_1 C_2 AK(kV). \tag{11-10}$$

Figure 11-12 illustrates a typical geometry for an anterior-posterior rib radiograph, with the patient lying on the table. The typical source-to-image distance (SID)

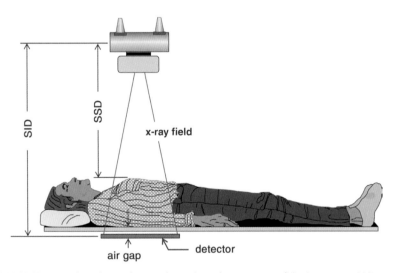

■ **FIGURE 11-12** To properly estimate dose to the patient, the geometry of the image acquisition needs to be well defined. This figure shows the imaging geometry for an AP rib radiograph. For most tabletop radiographic imaging protocols, the source-to-image distance (SID) is typically 100 cm. The air gap between the bottom of the patient and the top of the detector can be estimated and is typically between 2 to 5 cm. Estimating the thickness of the patient (*e.g.*, from a lateral radiograph) then allows the source-to-skin distance (SSD) to be estimated.

11.5 Radiation Dose in Projection Radiography

TABLE 11-2 HALF-VALUE LAYER AND OUTPUT LEVELS AS A FUNCTION OF kV FOR A TYPICAL GENERAL DIAGNOSTIC X-RAY SYSTEM

kV	HVL (mm Al)	OUTPUT (mGy per 100 mAs)
40	1.15	1.1
45	1.36	1.7
50	1.57	2.3
55	1.79	2.9
60	2.00	3.5
65	2.22	4.3
70	2.43	5.0
75	2.65	5.8
80	2.86	6.7
85	3.08	7.5
90	3.29	8.5
95	3.50	9.5
100	3.71	10.5
105	3.92	11.6
110	4.12	12.7
115	4.32	13.9
120	4.51	15.1
125	4.71	16.4
130	4.89	17.8
135	5.08	19.2
140	5.25	20.6

Output was measured free-in-air at a distance of 100 cm from the x-ray source, along the central beam. Multiply output column by 1.145 to get mR/mAs.

for most radiographic procedures is 100 cm, with the major exception being the upright chest radiograph. In order to compute the ESAK, an estimate of the SSD is needed for Equation 11-8. In many cases when the lateral examination is available, the thickness of the patient can be estimated, and the SSD is computed as: SSD = SID − [(air gap) + patient thickness]. The technical factors for the examination (kV, mAs) are usually provided in the DICOM header information.

Once the ESAK is estimated for typical radiographic examination, the radiation dose can be estimated using widely available tabular data. Tables are available for computing organ doses as well as effective doses, and an example is shown in Table 11-3 (for upright chest radiography). These tables are produced using Monte Carlo techniques and report radiation dose (organ dose or effective dose) as a function of ESAK. Older tables report dose levels in older units, such as in rads per entrance skin exposure.

State-of-the-art radiography systems with flat-panel detectors calculate kerma area product (KAP)—also known as dose area product (DAP) from the acquisition technique factors (tube potential, mAs, filtration) and geometry (collimator settings) and put the information in the DICOM header of the acquired image. This information is often displayed on the overlay of the image (Fig. 11-13). The indicated KAP value is equal to the product of the cross-sectional area of the x-ray beam and air

TABLE 11-3 EFFECTIVE DOSE PER ENTRANCE SURFACE DOSE (mSv/mGy) FOR CHEST RADIOGRAPHY AT 183 cm SOURCE-TO-DETECTOR DISTANCE AS A FUNCTION OF kV AND FILTRATION FOR THREE PROJECTIONS

X-RAY POTENTIAL (kV)	FILTRATION (mm OF Al)	ANTEROPOSTERIOR (mSv/mGy)	POSTEROANTERIOR (mSv/mGy)	LATERAL (mSv/mGy)
90	2	0.176	0.116	0.074
90	3	0.196	0.131	0.084
90	4	0.210	0.143	0.091
100	2	0.190	0.128	0.081
100	3	0.208	0.143	0.091
100	4	0.222	0.155	0.098
110	2	0.201	0.139	0.088
110	3	0.219	0.154	0.097
110	4	0.232	0.165	0.104
120	2	0.211	0.149	0.094
120	3	0.228	0.163	0.103
120	4	0.240	0.174	0.110

Note: The kV and filtration levels allow adjustment for different x-ray technique factors used for the procedure. Source: Estimation of effective dose in diagnostic radiology from entrance surface dose and dose-area product measurements. From Hart D, Jones DG, Wall BF. *Estimation of Effective Dose in Diagnostic Radiology from Entrance Surface Dose and Dose-Area Product Measurements.* Chilton, England: National Radiological Protection Board; 1994. © Crown copyright. Reproduced with permission of Public Health England.

kerma exiting the collimator assembly for the exposure with units of mGy-cm². As the beam diverges, the KAP remains constant—therefore, one can determine the incident air kerma for a given field size by dividing the KAP by the area of the beam at any point between the source and the detector. The beam area projected onto the patient, the anatomy, and the digital detector is known; thus the total imparted energy is proportional to the KAP and effective dose. Personal computer–based software PCXMC (Tapiovaara et al., 1997) is a Monte Carlo–based software program for calculating patient effective dose by matching x-ray beam technique factors and the entrance surface beam area dimensions to the patient, and simulating photon transport in the corresponding anthropomorphic phantom with estimates of absorbed dose to the organs. Effective dose is calculated as described in Section 11.4.6 using Equation 11-7 for the anatomical projection (*e.g.*, anterior-posterior radiograph of the abdomen) and the estimated organ doses. A correspondence of KAP to effective dose is determined from evaluating multiple patient images of different size and technique factors. By using linear regression to the data points, a conversion equation can be derived that allows the estimation of effective dose based upon KAP as shown in the graph of Figure 11-13 (Chen et al., 2020). Conversion equations to estimate effective dose from KAP do not currently exist for most radiographic exams; however, relative comparisons regarding the radiation dose burden to the patient population can be made with KAP values for similar radiographic projections.

11.6 RADIATION DOSE IN FLUOROSCOPY

Radiation dose assessment in fluoroscopy is conceptually similar to that in radiography, as they both are planar projection imaging procedures. However, there are several considerations that make dose assessment in fluoroscopy more complicated: (1)

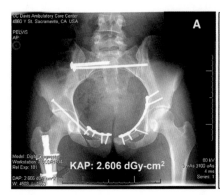
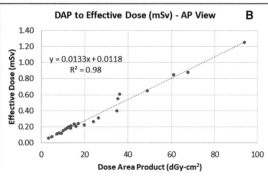

■ **FIGURE 11-13** The Kerma Area Product (KAP), also referred to as the Dose Area Product (DAP) in the DICOM header, is a metric available on modern digital radiography systems. **A.** an Anterior-posterior (AP) projection of the pelvis in a thin patient, with a measured KAP of 2.61 dGy-cm². (Note, dGy-cm² is the standard DICOM unit for KAP, not the more commonly used mGy-cm² unit.). **B.** Plot of the calculated Effective Dose versus indicated KAP for a range of patient sizes using x-ray acquisitions using automatic exposure control. The linear regression fit gives the slope (mSv/dGy-cm²) and offset, that is used to estimate effective dose directly from the KAP for any similar exam. For the patient radiograph shown in A, the effective dose is estimated to be 0.046 mSv (0.0118 + 0.0133 × 2.606).

Instead of dealing with the product of tube current and exposure time together (mAs) as in radiography, in fluoroscopy the tube current can vary over an extended time interval, so tube current (mA) is often considered separately from the fluoroscopic time (s). (2) Fluoroscopic projections are more complicated geometrically than radiographic projections. In radiography, the alignment of a given projection is performed by an x-ray technologist who has been extensively trained in consistent patient alignment, which gives rise to the use of standard tables for computing dose metrics from ESAK. In fluoroscopy, positioning of the imaging system is typically performed by a physician who is responding in real time to the requirements of the examination, without consideration of standardized projections. (3) Furthermore, the fluoroscopy system allows the use of several different magnification modes, which change both the air kerma rate and the field of view of the x-ray beam incident upon the patient. (4) The location where the x-ray beam intercepts the patient and the angle of the beam may be changed by the operator during a procedure. (5) The x-ray source to patient's skin distance can change during a procedure if the operator adjusts the height of the table holding the patient or if the operator rotates the gantry to change the incidence angle of the x-ray beam. (6) The x-ray source-to-detector distance (SID) can change during fluoroscopy as the fluoroscopist seeks to keep the image receptor as close to the patient is possible. (7) Finally, fluoroscopic fields of view can be square, rectangular, or circular, depending upon the technology of the fluoroscopy system and the clinical application.

In addition to the challenges of reconstructing the radiation dose from a complicated fluoroscopy procedure, for procedures that run long—for example in the cardiac catheterization laboratory or the interventional neuroradiology suite, the possibility of a radiation skin injury, with erythema and epilation, and at very large skin doses, even desquamation, ulceration, and skin necrosis, exists. While erythema is seen infrequently, and severe injuries very rarely, for long procedures it is essential to monitor the localized skin dose to attempt to avoid injury and to ensure proper patient management, post-procedure. Such radiation-induced skin injuries are discussed in Chapter 20, Section 20.4.

As discussed in Chapter 9, most modern fluoroscopy procedures are performed with automatic kerma rate control activated, whereby the tube potential (kV) and average tube current (mA) are automatically controlled to produce an acceptable image. Hence, characterization of the radiation output of the fluoroscopic system, and subsequent dose evaluation, need to use a methodology that embraces the automatic kerma rate control systems. Figure 11-14 illustrates the air kerma rate as a function of the detector field of view, for three thicknesses of polymethyl methacrylate (PMMA), a common plastic surrogate for tissue used in dosimetry. The experimental setup for measuring the air kerma rate is shown in the inset, where different phantom thicknesses (10, 20, 30 cm shown here) are used to stimulate the automatic air kerma rate circuitry in the fluoroscopic system. The active volume of the ion chamber is placed to measure the "tabletop" exposure levels just under the phantom material. Since the fluoroscopic system is designed to deliver uniform image quality as a function of patient thickness and magnification factor, the feedback system circuitry increases the air kerma rate with increasing phantom thickness and decreasing field of view (*i.e.*, increasing magnification factor). In this measurement geometry, backscatter (scattered radiation coming from the phantom) contributes significantly to the measurement.

In a simple example of a short fluoroscopic examination performed with the patient supine without substantial movement of the imaging chain, the graphical data illustrated in Figure 11-14 can be used to estimate the ESAK, and the skin dose can be estimated from that (Eq. 11-5). As discussed in Chapter 9, most modern fluoroscopy systems also record the air kerma at a reference point and dose calculations can be based on that as well. Subsequent assessment of organ dose can be made as described previously if the appropriate tables are available. It is seen in Figure 11-14 that the increase in air kerma rate between the 20- and 30-cm phantom is far greater than that between the 10- and 20-cm phantom curves, which is simply the manifestation of exponential x-ray absorption. Thus, using an estimate of the patient's thickness and the known detector field of view that was used for the fluoroscopic study, exponential interpolation can be used with the data in the plot to accurately approximate the air kerma rate used for that patient. Fluoroscopic doses can be reconstructed from complicated examinations, essentially by summing calculations for each touch of the fluoroscopic pedal. Many interventional angiographic systems incorporate geometric tracking along with the recorded x-ray techniques in the DICOM header or DICOM Radiation

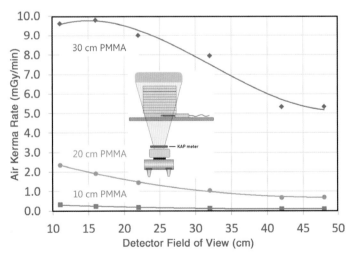

■ **FIGURE 11-14** Virtually all modern fluoroscopic systems only work in automatic exposure rate control mode, and therefore characterization of the output of the system needs to embrace this. The air kerma rate is shown as a function of the detector field of view, for three thicknesses of polymethyl methacrylate (PMMA), a tissue surrogate. For calculation of patient dose in fluoroscopy using the data shown in the figure, the medical physicist also needs to know (for each touch of the fluoroscopic peddle), what the patient thickness was and what the detector field of view was. For patient thicknesses that are substantially different from the three shown (10, 20, and 30 cm), exponential interpolation can be used at each detector field-of-view setting.

Dose Structured Report (RDSR) to allow precise computation of the fluoroscopic radiation dose to the patient. Associated software can assist in such calculations. For a long fluoroscopic study, tracking the geometry of the imaging chain around the stationary patient is essential for accurately estimating skin dose, to assure that erythema levels have not been reached (see peak skin dose mapping capabilities described in Chapter 9). Experienced interventional radiologists and cardiologists know to vary the geometry of the fluoroscopic system during the fluoroscopic study when possible to distribute the entrance skin dose across a larger surface area, in the attempt to reduce hot spots.

Similar to radiographic systems (Figure 11-13), some fluoroscopic systems employ kerma-area-product (KAP) meters. For older systems, the KAP meter is mounted between the x-ray source and the patient (Fig. 11-14, inset). Many newer fluoroscopy systems calculate the KAP value using the tube potential, current, and filtration settings from look-up tables stored during machine calibration. If radiographic images are acquired during a fluoroscopy examination, the doses from these are also included in the KAP value. The value of KAP is the product of the total air kerma exiting the x-ray tube housing and the cross-sectional area of the x-ray beam, and hence the units are mGy-cm². The KAP is essentially constant, regardless of the point in the x-ray beam where the air kerma and cross-sectional area are measured. A calibration procedure can be performed to convert the KAP value into an estimate of ESAK.

Fluoroscopy systems also are required to provide the "air kerma at a defined reference point in the center of the beam axis." The location of this reference point is specified in the regulations of the US Food and Drug Administration and is intended to be near the location where the x-ray beam intercepts the patient's skin. This value can be used directly to estimate the entrance skin dose:

$$D_{skin} = K_{a,r} \cdot \left(\frac{d_{source\text{-}ref\,pt}}{SSD} \right)^2 \cdot BSF \cdot \frac{(\mu_{en}/\rho)_{tissue}}{(\mu_{en}/\rho)_{air}}, \qquad [11\text{-}11]$$

where $K_{a,r}$ is the air kerma at the reference point while the x-ray beam is incident on a particular area on the skin, $d_{source\text{-}ref\,pt}$ is the distance from the source in the x-ray tube to the reference point, SSD is the source-to-skin distance, BSF is the backscatter factor (which accounts for dose from backscattered x-rays), and the last term conforms to Equation 11-5 above. The backscatter factor increases with the cross-sectional area of the x-ray beam and typically ranges from about 1.2 to 1.5 (ICRU Report 74).

11.7 RADIATION DOSE IN COMPUTED TOMOGRAPHY

Accurate assessment of the radiation dose to a patient from a medical imaging procedure requires an understanding of the output characteristics of the specific system used for imaging. For radiography and fluoroscopy discussed above, the x-ray output is measured at the entrant surface of the patient. However, in computed tomography, the x-ray tube rotates around the patient, so there is no well-defined entrance surface. Consequently, in CT the measurements made for computing dose are performed at the center of rotation ("isocenter") of the scanner. Another important difference between CT dosimetry and x-ray projection imaging is that the x-ray beam produced by CT scanner is spatially dependent due to the beam-shaping filters used in CT. Consequently, a measurement in air will vary considerably depending on the placement of the ion chamber position across the field.

Because of these considerations, a benchmark metric has been defined that is related to the output of the CT scanner; the volume computed tomography dose index, $CTDI_{vol}$. The $CTDI_{vol}$ was never meant to be a surrogate metric for patient dose; indeed it does not even consider the size of the patient. However, the $CTDI_{vol}$ does provide a reasonable metric characterizing the radiation output of the CT scanner. The $CTDI_{vol}$ metric is comprised of CTDI-100 measurements, which are used to compute $CTDI_{vol}$, as described in the next section.

11.7.1 Computed Tomography Dose Index, $CTDI_{100}$

The basic $CTDI_{100}$ measurement involves the use of a 100-mm-long cylindrical ("pencil") ion chamber, approximately 9 mm in diameter, inserted into either the center or a peripheral hole of a PMMA phantom. The chamber has a uniform response to radiation along its length, and angle of exposure (around 360°). PMMA is not an ideal water or tissue surrogate, but it is readily available and easy to machine. The density of PMMA is about 1.19 g/cm³, so that needs to be considered in some settings. There are two standard PMMA dosimetry phantoms; the body phantom is 32 cm in diameter and 15 cm long, and the head phantom is 16 cm in diameter and 15 cm long (Fig. 11-15). The head phantom can also serve as a pediatric torso phantom.

Each PMMA phantom has several parallel holes for insertion of the pencil chamber. Normally, the physicist making these measurements has only one pencil chamber, so a series of axial CT scans (at the same technique settings) is necessary to obtain all the raw data. The ion chamber is placed either in the central hole or one of the peripheral holes, and PMMA rods are used to plug all the remaining holes in the phantom. A dose measurement is obtained for one rotation of the gantry and typically repeated 3 times with the data averaged. After measurements are made with the ion chamber in one position (*e.g.*, the center position), the ion cham-

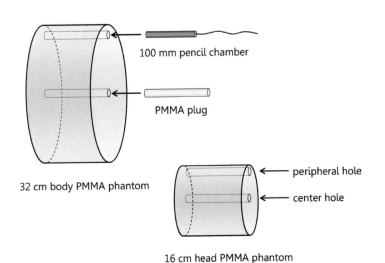

■ **FIGURE 11-15** The 32-cm-diameter body phantom and 16-cm-diameter head phantom used for dosimetry in computed tomography are shown. A 100-mm-long pencil chamber, placed serially in the center and peripheral holes of the phantom, allows for measurement of the $CTDI_{100, center}$, and $CTDI_{100, periphery}$ values that are used to compute the $CTDI_{vol}$ of the CT scanner.

ber is then moved to one of the peripheral positions, with PMMA rods replacing all voids, and subsequent measurements are made. Most of these phantoms have at least four peripheral holes (at 12, 3, 6, and 9 o'clock positions), and it is typical to make $CTDI_{100}$ measurements in each of them—even with the center of the phantom aligned with the center of rotation of the CT scanner, the radiation dose levels at the peripheral holes differ slightly due to the presence of the patient table, which the phantom is resting on. While all 4 peripheral probe locations record radiation, the largest fraction of that measurement is made when the x-ray tube is nearest the x-ray probe—because that is where the phantom attenuation is the least and the inverse square law has its largest effect. For example, with the probe in the 12 o'clock position, no table attenuation occurs as the x-ray tube passes through 12 o'clock, and when the probe is at the 6 o'clock position, the table is in the beam as the x-ray source passes through the 6 o'clock position. For the two lateral positions (3 and 9 o'clock), there is also no table in the beam as the x-ray tube passes by those locations during gantry rotation.

The phantom is positioned so that its central hole is parallel to and approximately on the CT scanner's axis of rotation, and the 100-millimeter pencil chamber is placed at the central hole in the PMMA phantom. Because the phantom is 15 cm long, with the 10-cm-long pencil chamber centered in the hole along its length, there is approximately 2.5 cm on either side of the pencil chamber. Once the ion chamber is properly positioned, the phantom is aligned so that an axial CT scan (i.e., no table motion) is acquired at the center of the phantom along the z-axis (and hence at the center of the pencil chamber as well, Fig. 11-16). These narrowly collimated x-ray beams expose only the center of the 100-mm pencil chamber, but scattered radiation from the phantom exposes its entire length. A thorough characterization of CT scanner output would require making these measurements for each of the collimated x-ray beam widths (e.g., 5, 10, 20, 40 mm) used clinically by the scanner. For some scanners capable of producing collimated x-ray beam widths ranging from 80 mm up to 160 mm, alternate measurement procedures are required, as discussed later.

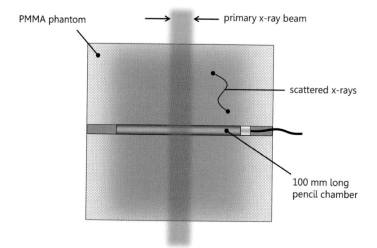

■ **FIGURE 11-16** This figure shows the 100-mm pencil chamber positioned at the center of a CT dose phantom (in z), with the axial primary x-ray beam exposing the center (with 360° rotation of the x-ray tube) and the scattered radiation extending well beyond the extent of the primary beam. Indeed, the dose at the center of the body phantom is less than 10% from the primary beam, with the majority of the dose imparted by scattered radiation.

An ionization chamber can only produce an accurate dose estimate if its entire sensitive volume is irradiated by the x-ray beam. Therefore, for the partially irradiated 100-mm CT pencil chamber used in CT measurements, the nominal beam width (i.e., the collimated x-ray beam width as indicated on the CT console) is used to correct the chamber reading for the partial volume exposure. The correction for partial volume is essential and is calculated using

$$K_{corrected} = \frac{100 \text{ mm}}{B} K_{measured},$$ [11-12]

where B is the nominal beam width as reported by the scanner (in mm) for a single axial scan. The value of B is the product of the z-axis collimation (T) and the number of data channels n. T is the width of the tomographic section along the z-axis imaged by one data channel, where several detector elements may be grouped together to form one data channel and n is the number of active data channels used in a single scan. For example, on a 64-slice CT scanner where $T = 0.625$ mm and $n = 32$ data channels, $B = 32 \times 0.625$ mm $= 20$ mm. The measured air kerma reading ($K_{measured}$) is corrected by the partial volume factor, as described in Equation 11-12, to yield $K_{corrected}$.

The classical CTDI$_{vol}$ measurement performed on the phantoms illustrated in Figure 11-15 and in the geometry shown in Figure 11-16 essentially fail when the collimated beam width approaches or exceeds the 100 mm length of the pencil chamber. This is true for several commercially available whole-body CT scanners with 160 mm collimated beam widths at isocenter, and for other cone-beam scanners in which the collimated beam thicknesses at isocenter exceeds 100 mm. In this case, the preferred measurement geometry is to use a small thimble chamber (10–20 mm active chamber length) as shown in Figure 11-17. With this measurement geometry, the ion chamber is completely exposed to the primary (and scatter) beam, so no partial volume correction factor as described in Equation 11-12 is necessary.

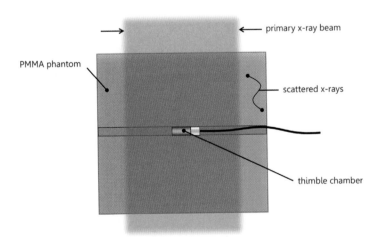

■ **FIGURE 11-17** For cone beam CT geometry, including whole-body systems with 160 mm collimated beamwidth and more traditional cone beam systems, the 100-mm pencil chamber is not the right tool for assessing dose within the phantom. Instead, a thimble chamber with an active length of 10–20 mm is used, with no partial beam correction needed.

11.7.2 Weighted CTDI (CTDI$_w$), and volume CTDI (CTDI$_{vol}$)

With a general discussion of the measurement geometry and procedure for estimating dose through the CTDI$_{100}$ discussed above, we can now focus on some of the details. The CTDI$_{100}$ is defined as

$$CTDI_{100} = \frac{1}{nT} \int_{L=-50\text{ mm}}^{+50\text{ mm}} D(z)\,dz. \qquad [11\text{-}13]$$

The CTDI$_{100}$ in the above equation describes the measurement of the dose distribution, $D(z)$, along the z-axis, from a single circular (axial or sequential) rotation of the scanner with a nominal (collimated) x-ray beamwidth of nT, defined at the isocenter. The primary and scattered radiation are measured over a 100-mm length, from -50 to $+50$ mm, where the center of the x-ray beam is positioned at $z = 0$. The nominal beam width refers to the beam width as reported by the scanner, not the actual measured beamwidth, which is generally a bit wider. As mentioned previously, CTDI$_{100}$ measurements are made for both the center (CTDI$_{100,center}$) and periphery (CTDI$_{100,periphery}$). The CTDI$_{100,periphery}$ value is typically computed as the average of the four measurements performed at the 12, 3, 6 and 9 o'clock positions. Combining the center and peripheral measurements using a ⅓ and ⅔ weighting scheme provides a good estimate of the average dose to the phantom (at the central CT slice along z), giving rise to the weighted CTDI, CTDI$_w$:

$$CTDI_w = \frac{1}{3}\,CTDI_{100,center} + \frac{2}{3}CTDI_{100,periphery}. \qquad [11\text{-}14]$$

In helical (also called spiral) CT scanning, the CT dose is inversely proportional to the helical pitch used, that is,

$$\text{dose} \propto \frac{1}{\text{pitch}}, \qquad [11\text{-}15]$$

where the pitch is defined as the table translation distance (mm) during a full rotation (360°) of the gantry, divided by the nominal beam width nT (in mm). Thus, for a 20-mm nominal beam width, and a 15-mm table translation per gantry rotation, the pitch would be 0.75 (*i.e.*, 15 mm/20 mm), and for a 40-mm nominal beam width and a 60-mm table travel per gantry rotation, the pitch would be 1.5 (60 mm/40 mm).

Because of the dependency of dose on pitch, the CTDI$_w$ is converted to the volume CTDI (CTDI$_{vol}$) using

$$CTDI_{vol} = \frac{CTDI_w}{\text{pitch}}. \qquad [11\text{-}16]$$

Modern CT scanners are required to display the CTDI$_{vol}$ on the CT scanner console *prior* to the actual scan. The value can be displayed because the CT manufacturer has measured CTDI$_{vol}$ in the factory over the range of kV values for that model of scanner, and then that stored value, scaled appropriately by the mAs and pitch (and other factors), is displayed on the console.

There are two different CTDI$_{vol}$ metrics, one for the 16-cm-diameter head phantom and another for the 32-cm-diameter body phantom. It is essential that when stating the CTDI$_{vol}$, the phantom in which it was measured be stated as well.

The product of the $CTDI_{vol}$ and the length of the CT scan along the z-axis of the patient, L, is the dose length product (DLP):

$$DLP = CTDI_{vol} \times L. \qquad [11\text{-}17]$$

The DLP is an interesting metric, which is in general more related to the patient's radiation risk than the $CTDI_{vol}$. Given that dose = energy/mass, we can rearrange this equation to energy = dose × mass. Realizing that for the PMMA phantoms illustrated in Figure 11-15, the mass scales linearly with length. A length of 1 cm of the 16-cm-diameter phantom has a mass of 0.23 kg and the mass of a 1-cm-long section of the 32-cm-diameter phantom is 0.95 kg. In each case, double the length, and the mass will double as well. Thus, for a given diameter phantom, the DLP is linearly proportional to the energy imparted. It has been shown that the DLP (approximately energy imparted) is proportional to the effective dose (E) for specific body regions, and this will be discussed later. Just like the $CTDI_{vol}$, the DLP should be reported with the phantom (head or body) in which it was measured.

Example values of $CTDI_{100,center}$, and $CTDI_{100,peripheral}$, are shown for the 16-cm-diameter PMMA head and the 32-cm-diameter body phantoms in Figure 11-18. The corresponding $CTDI_{vol}$ values are also shown, for pitch = 1. For the same CT technique factors (kV, mA, rotation time, and pitch), the head $CTDI_{vol}$ is greater than the body $CTDI_{vol}$ because the smaller phantom has less attenuation. It is also seen from Figure 11-18 that the peripheral measurements for both body and head phantoms are greater than the center measurement, and this is due to several reasons: (1) when the x-ray tube is on the same side of the phantom where the peripheral measurement is being made, the thickness of the phantom material is less than a centimeter so only modest attenuation occurs, resulting in a high reading for the peripheral measurement, and (2) when the x-ray tube is on the same side of the phantom where the peripheral measurement is being made, the x-ray tube is closer to the ionization chamber, so the inverse square law increases the peripheral measurement as well.

The main purpose of the 100-mm-long pencil chamber is, in addition to capturing the dose from the primary x-ray beam, the dose from the scattered x-ray beam along the length of the pencil chamber is measured also (Fig. 11-16). The x-ray beams used in CT (e.g., 120 kV, 10 mm aluminum filtration) are very "hard" (are primarily composed of high-energy x-ray photons), and so the primary interaction

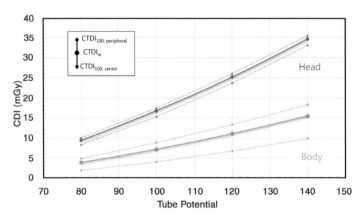

■ FIGURE 11-18 The CTDI values (both $CTDI_{100}$ and $CTDI_w$) measured from a whole-body clinical CT system are shown for both the head and body phantom. The dotted lines correspond to the $CTDI_{100}$ measurements, while solid lines show the data for the $CTDI_w$ computations from the $CTDI_{100,peripheral}$, and $CTDI_{100,center}$ measurements. For both head and body phantoms, the peripheral measurements are higher than the center measurements for reasons discussed in the text.

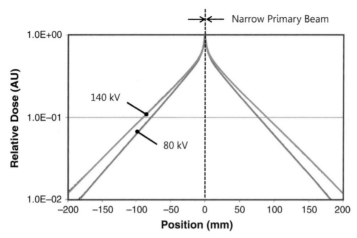

■ **FIGURE 11-19** These data are derived from Monte Carlo studies and demonstrate the longitudinal spread of scattered radiation from a very thin (0.1 mm) primary CT beam. The vertical axis is logarithmic, with a linear horizontal axis. For 140 kV, more than 2% of the dose from scattered radiation is deposited 200 mm from the primary beam (more than 1% on each side). Due to the lower energy of the scattered radiation, the longitudinal spread of the 80 kV beam is slightly less.

in tissue (or the PMMA phantom) is by Compton scattering. Hence, a very large component of radiation dose internal to the patient (or phantom) is the dose from scattered radiation, which tends to extend far out longitudinal from the primary beam. The 100-mm pencil chamber captures the most proximal scattered dose (±50 mm) along the longitudinal (z) axis of the patient. Data from Monte Carlo studies demonstrate that the radiation dose from scattered radiation extends well beyond the center (±50 mm) surrounding the primary x-ray beam, as illustrated in Figure 11-19.

11.7.3 CT Dose Consideration for Different Scan Lengths

As mentioned previously, scattered radiation deposits the majority of the radiation dose to the patient during CT scanning, especially towards the center of the patient. With the high energies of the x-ray photons used in CT scanning, the scattered photons can travel considerably in the longitudinal dimension (along the z-axis). Figure 11-19 illustrates the lateral range of scatter radiation on a semi-logarithmic plot. For a very narrow (e.g., 0.1 mm) 140-kV primary beam incident upon a phantom at a position corresponding to 0 mm on the graph (80-kV beam is also shown), more than 2% of the x-ray beam propagates laterally and is deposited more than 200 mm away from the center of the beam (i.e., 1% to the left, 1% to the right). These values can build up when the primary beam width is considerably wider than the 0.1-mm beam width used to compute the data in Figure 11-19. To illustrate this in a different manner the relative dose at the center of the phantom (or patient) builds up as the scan length increases, as illustrated in Figure 11-20. This figure illustrates that the dose to the patient at the center of the CT scan increases as the scan length increases, for the same exact primary beam intensity (a function of kV, mA, gantry rotation time, and pitch). The asymptotic increase in dose at the center of the field of view along z (Fig. 11-20) has been dubbed "The rise to equilibrium curve" in AAPM Report 111.

When a complete dose distribution is plotted along the z-axis for different scan lengths, we can better appreciate the fact that the doses are highest towards the center of the field, and taper off at the edges of the field in the +z and −z directions, as illustrated in Figure 11-21. It is important to realize that the data points corresponding to the circular symbols shown in Figure 11-21 correspond to the data

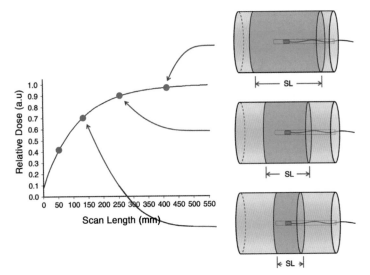

■ **FIGURE 11-20** The relative dose at the center of the phantom (in arbitrary units) is shown as a function of scan length, for scan lengths ranging from 50 to >400 mm. The exposure conditions are shown graphically. As the scan length increases, the dose at the center of the scan also increases due to the scattered radiation that extends to the center from peripheral exposure by the primary beam. This figure illustrates the practical influence on dose measurements in CT from the long-ranged scatter tails illustrated in Figure 11-19.

points along the rise to the equilibrium curve illustrated in Figure 11-20—these are two different graphical representations of the same measurements.

11.7.4 The Size-Specific Dose Estimate, SSDE

It has long been recognized that the $CTDI_{vol}$ dose metric determined from the 32 cm diameter PMMA adult body phantom *underestimates* the radiation dose received from computed tomography for all but the largest of patients. The 32-cm-diameter PMMA phantom, due to its high 1.19 g/cm^3 density, is more like a 38-cm-diameter patient,

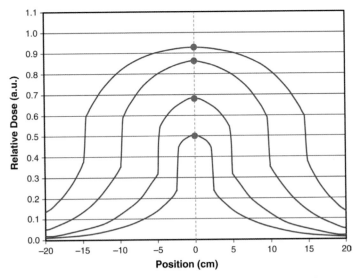

■ **FIGURE 11-21** Dose profiles along the z dimension are shown for scan lengths of 50, 100, 200, and 300 mm, where the primary beam exposure is the same. This figure shows how the radiation dose builds up at the center of the scan (and beyond) as the scan length gets wider due to scattered radiation. The data points at the center of these profiles correspond in principle to those shown in Figure 11-19. These data were derived from Monte Carlo simulations.

corresponding to a 109-cm or 43-inch circumference (*i.e.*, belt size). Because dose is related to energy per unit mass, when the mass is large (as it is with the 32-cm-diameter PMMA phantom), for a given set of CT technique factors, the dose ($CTDI_{vol}$) is relatively low. For smaller patients (with lower mass), therefore, for the same technique factors (kV, mA, rotation time, pitch), the radiation dose will be higher. Recognizing this, groups in the AAPM have studied these relationships and have produced AAPM Report 204 for the torso and AAPM Report 293 for the head. The resulting size-specific dose estimate (SSDE) uses the scanner's $CTDI_{vol}$ and corrects that for the size of the patient's body part being scanned. The $CTDI_{vol}$ is displayed on the CT console before and after the CT scan, and it is also recorded in the DICOM header, so these AAPM reports embrace the availability of the $CTDI_{vol}$ as a scanner output metric and then apply a patient size–dependent correction. The conversion factors in these reports can be used to scale the reported $CTDI_{vol}$ values to produce more accurate estimates of absorbed dose at the center (in z) along the scan, for patients of differing sizes.

The water-equivalent diameter (D_w) is the diameter of a circular cross section of water that has the same overall attenuation properties as the patient's cross section. The first step in computing the SSDE is to estimate the water-equivalent diameter (D_w) of the patient. Because the CT image data set contains accurate size information, the CT images themselves are used to determine D_w, where:

$$A = \sum_x \sum_y \Delta \left[\frac{HU(x,y) + 1{,}000}{1{,}000} \right]$$ [11-18]

$$D_w = 2\sqrt{\frac{A}{\pi}},$$

and where A is the area of the tissue (excluding air in and around the patient), Δ is the area of a single pixel, $HU(x, y)$ is a given image in the (x, y) plane, and D_w is the water-equivalent diameter. The term in the square brackets corrects for the water equivalence of the pixel at location (x, y). Note that, in principle, the term in the brackets becomes 0 when $HU(x, y) = -1{,}000$, for air. Equation 11-18 weighs denser pixels (*e.g.*, bone) more, and less dense pixels (*e.g.*, lung) less, resulting in approximating a water-equivalent cross section of the patient. The inset in Figure 11-22 illustrates the water-equivalent diameter for an axial abdominal CT scan. This method is accurate as long as all the patient's anatomy is visible on the CT image. For CT images that have anatomical cutoff, CT vendors have developed vendor-specific methods to estimate D_w using the raw data acquired during the localizer scan along the z-axis of the patient.

Once D_w is estimated, the curves shown in Figure 11-22 are used to compute the normalized dose coefficients. These curves are fit to Equation 11-19:

$$f = ae^{-bD_w},$$ [11-19]

where (in Fig. 11-22) for the body $a = 3.7043$ and $b = 0.03672$ cm^{-1} and for the head $a = 1.9852$ and $b = 0.0486$ cm^{-1}.

$$D_{abs}^{z=0} = f CTDI_{vol}.$$ [11-20]

Figure 11-22 shows graphs for both the body and head f conversion factors, which can be used to convert the $CTDI_{vol}$ to the estimated absorbed dose at the center (along z) of the CT scan ($D_{abs}^{z=0}$) using Equation 11-20. The concept of SSDE has recently been included in the standards for CT scanners, and SSDE will be part of the information provided on all modern CT scanners in the future.

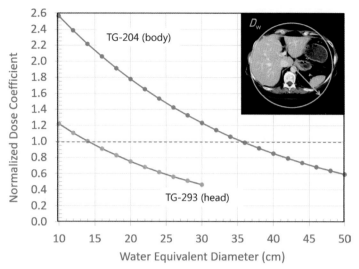

FIGURE 11-22 The normalized dose coefficients as a function of water-equivalent diameter are shown for both the head and body phantoms. These coefficients are used to estimate the size-specific dose estimate (SSDE), where the results are described in AAPM Report 204 (body) and Report 293 (head). The computer fits from a comprehensive mix of measured data (both physical measurements and Monte Carlo simulation data) from several groups are shown.

11.7.5 Effective Dose Estimates in CT

An interactive tool called "ImPACT" produced by the United Kingdom's National Health Service was built from extensive Monte Carlo calculations and allowed users to input various CT parameters (model of scanner, region on the body scan, kV, mAs, pitch, etc.), and it estimates $CTDI_{vol}$, DLP, and, using organ dose data, effective dose. This tool was used by scientists in the European Union to study the relationship between DLP and effective dose. They found excellent correlation between these parameters, and linear regression showed an essentially zero intercept. Consequently, the slope term derived from linear regression forms a proportionality between effective dose and DLP,

$$E = k \times DLP, \qquad [11\text{-}21]$$

where E is the effective dose (in mSv), DLP is the dose length product (in mGy-cm), and the slope k is in the unit mSv/(mGy-cm). With the same concerns about the applicability of the effective dose to specific patients as expressed in Section 11.4.6, Equation 11-21 can be used with the k-factors provided in Table 11-4 for various CT exam types to estimate effective dose.

TABLE 11-4 CONVERSION FACTORS ("k FACTORS") FOR ESTIMATION OF EFFECTIVE DOSE (mSv) FROM DOSE-LENGTH PRODUCT (mGy-cm), FOR VARIOUS CT EXAMINATION TYPES (FROM AAPM REPORT 96)

CT EXAM TYPE	k FACTOR (mSv/[mGy-cm])
Head	0.0021
Chest	0.017
Abdomen	0.015
Abdomen-pelvis	0.015
Pelvis	0.015

11.8 DOSE REPORTING SOFTWARE AND DOSE REGISTRIES

In the 2008–2012 time frame, there were several accidents involving CT in the State of California and other states that led to patient overexposures. While the scanners operated without malfunction, the advent of tube current modulation, that is, automatic exposure control, with different AEC parameters for specific scanner types, led to sophisticated performance but also complicated the use of these systems. Unfortunately, for patients undergoing evaluation for stroke, CT perfusion studies of the head—already a high dose procedure—used erroneously high dose settings that led to epilation in hundreds of patients. As a result, California legislators developed regulations that took effect in 2012, which required the CTDIvol and DLP to be reported in the physician's interpretive report. Subsequent to these events in California, The Joint Commission codified requirements into their accreditation process, essentially creating a nationwide mandate for the documentation of dose information from individual CT examinations.

With this as a backdrop, several vendors and software companies have developed automatic dose reporting software, which inserts the $CTDI_{vol}$ and DLP metrics into the interpretive report, saving physician time and preserving the accuracy of the data by eliminating human error. The automatic nature of this software led naturally to the formation of databases that have allowed institutions to monitor these dose metrics for the CT scans performed at their institution. These datasets have been a gold mine for better understanding the relative dose metrics that are produced across CT protocols. For example, Figure 11-23 shows the median $CTDI_{vol}$ as a function of water-equivalent diameter, and the increase in the curve is a result of the tube current modulation used by this CT scanner. Similar data can be used to compare (and then tune) scanner performance between scanners, within a hospital, or across national norms.

As discussed in Chapter 5, the DICOM RDSR provides a standard for transferring dose information from individual examinations and contains a great deal of information. Furthermore, at a large hospital or clinic, thousands of dose values for various imaging procedures on individual patients can be recorded automatically from the DICOM header in a short period of time, as the images move electronically through the institution. The automatic assessment of dose information across many x-ray imaging

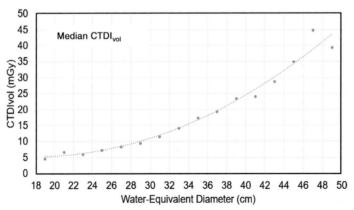

■ **FIGURE 11-23** Dose reporting in CT became required in California in 2012 and has spread across the United States through Joint Commission regulations. While the immediate requirement of the legislation was to record the patient $CTDI_{vol}$ and DLP data in the physician's interpretive report, this led to the development of databases that can now be used for comprehensive protocol assessment for CT scanners at the same institution, and across the country. The data in this figure show the median $CTDI_{vol}$ for abdomen CT scans as a function of water-equivalent diameter, for a CT scanner that routinely uses x-ray tube current modulation.

modalities has led to wider use of the Diagnostic Reference Levels (DRLs) as a quality assurance measure. Although setting up the infrastructure for automatic assessment of DRL data (and other dose metrics) requires initial resources and ongoing maintenance, the use of DRLs has been embraced both nationally and internationally.

Given this availability of the radiation dose metrics from x-ray examinations, the American College of Radiology and other organizations have developed a dose index registry, which compiles CT dose metrics from registered institutions, for the purposes of comparing the dose levels between institutions. Dose statistics (such as mean $CTDI_{vol}$ for an abdominal CT) are compiled at each subscribing institution and are compared against regional and national norms. This exercise permits radiology managers to better understand how their x-ray techniques compare with other institutions.

11.9 DIAGNOSTIC REFERENCE LEVELS AND ACHIEVABLE DOSES

A DRL represents the 75 percentile of the dose distribution for an imaging examination from a sample across institutions. There is an assumption that those radiology practices that are in the top quartile ($>75\%$) should consider revising protocols to reduce their dose levels. The achievable dose is the 50 percentile (median) of the dose distribution and is a potential target for those facilities in the top quartile. As an example (Kanal et al., 2017), for abdomen CT the DRL was reported as a $CTDI_{vol}$ of 20 mGy and a DLP of 1,004 mGy-cm, whereas the achievable dose levels were a $CTDI_{vol}$ of 13 mGy and a DLP of 657 mGy-cm (over the all size category). For head CT, the DRL was $CTDI_{vol}$ of 57 mGy and the DLP was 1,011 mGy-cm, whereas the achievable dose values were 49 mGy ($CTDI_{vol}$) and 849 mGy-cm (DLP). The use of DRLs and achievable doses as part of an overall program of radiation protection for patients and staff is discussed in Chapter 21.

11.10 SUMMARY

It is important that radiology and imaging science professionals understand the different aspects of radiation dosimetry, and that they use the proper quantities with the proper units in the proper settings. Air kerma is the most commonly measured parameter in the x-ray imaging environment, and such measurements then are used to inform specific dose calculations. The absorbed dose corresponds to the fundamental notion of "dose"; however, when different body parts are exposed as is common in a trauma setting (*etc.*), it is not possible to fully characterize the absorbed dose across different exposed regions with a single dose metric. Absorbed doses to *different* body parts *cannot be added*. The conversion of absorbed dose (units: mGy) to equivalent dose (units: mSv) is perfunctory in x-ray imaging because $w_r = 1.0$; however it is a necessary bookkeeping step. The product of the organ tissue weighting factors w_T and the equivalent organ doses (units: mSv) is summed to compute the effective dose (units: mSv) to get a single numeric descriptor of a parameter that is related to the patient's radiation risk. In this way, effective doses computed from exposure to different body parts *can be added*. However, the quantity effective dose should not be used to characterize risk for individual patients. A list of typical effective doses for various radiological procedures is given in Table 11-5, and some familiarity with the range of doses that are received in radiological imaging is useful. DRLs and achievable doses are useful in assessing imaging protocols, to optimize the balance between possible radiation risk to the patient and achieving the clinical goal of a diagnostic examination or image-guided intervention.

TABLE 11-5 TYPICAL EFFECTIVE DOSES FOR VARIOUS RADIOGRAPHIC PROCEDURES

PROCEDURE	AVERAGE EFFECTIVE DOSE (mSv)
Radiographic Procedures	
Skull	0.14
Cervical spine	0.36
Thoracic spine	1.0
Lumbar spine	1.4
PA and lateral chest	0.10
Mammography	0.36
Abdomen	0.6
Pelvis	0.6
Hip	0.4
Shoulder	0.006
Knee	0.003
Upper GI series[a]	6.0
Barium enema[a]	6.0
CT Procedures	
Head	1.6
Calcium scouring	1.7
Chest	6.2
Abdomen & pelvis	7.7
Three-phase liver	15
Spine	8.8
CT colonography	10

[a]Includes dose from fluoroscopy.

Adapted with permission from National Council on Radiation Protection and Measurements (NCRP). *Report No. 184 Medical Radiation Exposure of Patients in the United States*. 2019. http://NCRPonline.org.

SUGGESTED READING AND REFERENCES

Bauhs JA, Vrieze TJ, Primak AN, et al. CT dosimetry: comparison of measurement techniques and devices. *Radiographics*. 2008;28(1):245-253. Review.

Boone JM. The trouble with CTDI$_{100}$. *Med Phys*. 2007;34(4):1364-1371.

Boone JM. Dose spread functions in computed tomography: a Monte Carlo study. *Med Phys*. 2009;36(10):4547-4554.

Boone JM, Buonocore MH, Cooper VN III. Monte Carlo validation in diagnostic radiological imaging. *Med Phys*. 2000;27:1294-1304.

Boone JM, Hendee WR, McNitt-Gray MF, Seltzer SE. Radiation exposure from CT scans: how to close our knowledge gaps, monitor and safeguard exposure—proceedings and recommendations of the Radiation Dose Summit, sponsored by NIBIB, February 24–25, 2011. *Radiology*. 2012;265(2):544-554.

Boone JM, Strauss KJ, Cody DD, McCollough CH, McNitt-Gray MF, Toth TL. AAPM Report 204: size specific dose estimates (SSDE) in pediatric and adult body CT examinations. 2011.

Boone JM, Strauss KJ, Hernandez AM, et al. AAPM Report 293: size specific dose estimate (SSDE) for head CT. 2019.

Bushberg JT. Uses of effective dose: the good, the bad, and the future. *Health Phys*. 2019;116(2):129-134.

Chen DS, Escobedo EM, Eastman JG, Bloomstein JD, Taylor SL, Seibert JA. Dose area product to effective dose conversion coefficients for pelvic radiography using a Monte Carlo program. *Am J Roentgenol*. 2020;13:1-6.

DeMarco JJ, Cagnon CH, Cody DD, et al. A Monte Carlo based method to estimate radiation dose from multi-detector CT (MDCT): cylindrical and anthropomorphic phantoms. *Phys Med Biol.* 2005;50(17):3989-4004.

DeMarco JJ, Cagnon CH, Cody DD, et al. Estimating radiation doses from multidetector CT using Monte Carlo simulations: effects of different size voxelized patient models on magnitudes of organ and effective dose. *Phys Med Biol.* 2007;52(9):2583-2597.

Dixon RL. A new look at CT dose measurement: beyond CTDI. *Med Phys.* 2003;30(6):1272-1280.

Dixon RL, Anderson JA, Bakalyar DM, et al. AAPM Report 111: comprehensive methodology for the evaluation of radiation dose in x-ray computed tomography. 2010.

Dixon RL, Boone JM. Cone beam CT dosimetry: a unified and self-consistent approach including all scan modalities—with or without phantom motion. *Med Phys.* 2010;37(6):2703-2718.

Dixon RL, Boone JM. Stationary table CT dosimetry and anomalous scanner-reported values of CTDIvol. *Med Phys.* 2014;41(1):011907.

Dixon RL, Boone JM. Analytical equations for CT dose profiles derived using a scatter kernel of Monte Carlo parentage with broad applicability to CT dosimetry problems. *Med Phys.* 2011;38(7):4251-4264.

Dixon RL, Boone JM, Kraft RA. Dose equations for shift-variant CT acquisition modes using variable pitch, tube current, and aperture, and the meaning of their associated CTDIvol. *Med Phys.* 2014;41(11):1906.

Dixon RL, Boone JM. Dose equations for tube current modulation in CT scanning and the interpretation of the associated CTDIvol. *Med Phys.* 2013;40(11):111920.

Geyer AM, O'Reilly S, Lee C, Long DJ, Bolch WE. The UF/NCI family of hybrid computational phantoms representing the current US population of male and female children, adolescents, and adults—application to CT dosimetry. *Phys Med Biol.* 2014;59(18):5225-5242.

International Atomic Energy Agency. Guidance on Diagnostic Reference Levels (DRLs). https://www.iaea.org/resources/rpop/health-professionals/radiology/diagnostic-reference-levels

International Commission on Radiation Units and Measurements. ICRU Report No. 74: patient dosimetry for x rays used in medical imaging. *J ICRU.* 2005;5(2):1-113.

International Commission on Radiation Units and Measurements. ICRU Report No. 87: radiation dose and image-quality assessment in computed tomography. *J ICRU.* 2012;12(1):1-149. doi: 10.1093/jicru/ndt007. PMID: 24158924.

Kanal KM, Butler PF, Sengupta D, Bhargavan-Chatfield M, Coombs LP, Morin RL. US diagnostic reference levels and achievable doses for 10 Adult CT examinations. *Radiology.* 2017;284:120-133.

Khursheed A, Hillier MC, Shrimpton PC, et al. Influence of patient age on normalized effective doses calculated for CT examinations. *Br J Radiol.* 2002;75:819-830.

Lee C, Lodwick D, Hurtado J, Pafundi D, Williams JL, Bolch WE. The UF family of reference hybrid phantoms for computational radiation dosimetry. *Phys Med Biol.* 2010;55(2):339-363.

McCollough CH, Leng S, Yu L, Cody DD, Boone JM, McNitt-Gray MF. CT dose index and patient dose: they are not the same thing. *Radiology.* 2011;259(2):311-316.

McCollough CH, Bruesewitz MR, Kofler JM Jr. CT dose reduction and dose management tools: overview of available options. *Radiographics.* 2006;26(2):503-512. Review.

McCollough CH, Primak AN, Braun N, et al. Strategies for reducing radiation dose in CT. *Radiol Clin North Am.* 2009;47(1):27-40. Review.

Menke J. Comparison of different body size parameters for individual dose adaptation in body CT of adults. *Radiology.* 2005;236:565-571.

Mettler FA Jr, Wiest PW, Locken JA, et al. CT scanning: patterns of use and dose. *J Radiol Prot.* 2000;20(4):353-359.

Mettler, et al. Effective doses in radiology and diagnostic nuclear medicine: a catalog. *Radiology.* 2008;248:254-263.

Seibert JA, Boone JM, Wootton-Gorges SL, Lamba R. Dose is not always what it seems: where very misleading values can result from volume CT dose index and dose length product. *J Am Coll Radiol.* 2014;11(3):233-237.

Shope T, Gagne R, Johnson G. A method for describing the doses delivered by transmission x-ray computed tomography. *Med Phys.* 1981;8:488-495.

Tapiovaara M, Lakkisto M, Servomaa A. *PCXMC. A PC-Based Monte Carlo Program for Calculating Patient Doses in Medical X-Ray Examinations.* Helsinki, Finland: Finnish Centre for Radiation and Nuclear Safety (STUK); 1997.

Zhou H, Boone JM. Monte Carlo evaluation of CTDI (infinity) in infinitely long cylinders of water, polyethylene, and PMMA with diameters from 10 mm to 500 mm. *Med Phys.* 2008;35:2424-2431.

Magnetic Resonance Basics: Magnetic Fields, Nuclear Magnetic Characteristics, Tissue Contrast, Image Acquisition

Nuclear magnetic resonance (NMR) is the spectroscopic study of the magnetic properties of the *nucleus* of the atom. The protons and neutrons of the nucleus have a *magnetic* field associated with their nuclear spin and charge distribution. *Resonance* is an energy coupling that causes the individual nuclei, when placed in a strong external magnetic field, to selectively absorb, and later release, energy unique to those nuclei and their surrounding environment. The detection and analysis of the NMR signal has been extensively studied since the 1940s as an analytic tool in chemistry and biochemistry research. NMR is not an imaging technique but rather a method to provide spectroscopic data concerning a sample placed in a small volume, high field strength magnetic device. In the early 1970s, it was realized that magnetic field gradients could be used to localize the NMR signal and to generate images that display magnetic properties of the proton, reflecting clinically relevant information, coupled with technological advances and development of "body-size" magnets. As clinical imaging applications increased in the mid-1980s, the "nuclear" connotation was dropped, and magnetic resonance imaging (MRI), with a plethora of associated acronyms, became commonly accepted in the medical community.

MR applications continue to expand clinical relevance with higher field strength magnets, improvements in anatomic and physiologic data acquisition/analysis, and advances in spectroscopy for accurate electronic tissue biopsies. The high contrast sensitivity to soft tissue differences and the inherent safety to the patient resulting from the use of non-ionizing radiation have been key reasons why MRI has supplanted many CT and projection radiography methods. With continuous improvements in image quality, acquisition methods, and equipment design, MRI is often the modality of choice to examine anatomic and physiologic properties of the patient. There are drawbacks, however, including high equipment and siting costs, scan acquisition complexity, relatively long imaging times, significant image artifacts, patient claustrophobia, and MR safety concerns.

This chapter reviews the basic properties of magnetism, concepts of resonance, tissue magnetization and relaxation events, generation of image contrast, and basic methods of acquiring image data. Advanced pulse sequences, illustration of image characteristics/artifacts, MR spectroscopy (MRS), MR safety, and biologic effects are discussed in Chapter 13.

12.1 MAGNETISM, MAGNETIC FIELDS, AND MAGNETIC PROPERTIES OF MATERIALS

12.1.1 Magnetism

Magnetism is a fundamental property of matter; it is generated by moving charges, usually electrons. Magnetic properties of materials result from the organization and motion of the electrons in either a random or a nonrandom alignment of magnetic "domains," which are the smallest entities of magnetism. Atoms and molecules have electron orbitals that can be paired (an even number of electrons cancels the magnetic field) or unpaired (the magnetic field is present). Most materials do not exhibit overt magnetic properties, but one notable exception is the permanent magnet, in which the individual magnetic domains are aligned in one direction.

Unlike the monopole electric charges from which they are derived, magnetic fields exist as dipoles, where the north pole is the origin of the magnetic field lines and the south pole is the return (Fig. 12-1A). One pole cannot exist without the other. As with electric charges, "like" magnetic poles repel and "opposite" poles attract. *Magnetic field strength*, **B** (also called the magnetic flux density), can be conceptualized as the number of magnetic lines of force per unit area, which decreases roughly as the inverse square of the distance from the source. The SI unit for **B** is the Tesla (T). As a benchmark, the earth's magnetic field is about 1/20,000 = 0.00005 T = 0.05 mT. An alternate (historical) unit is the gauss (G), where 1 T = 10,000 G.

12.1.2 Magnetic Fields

Magnetic fields can be induced by a moving charge in a wire (*e.g.*, see the section on transformers in Chapter 6). The direction of the magnetic field depends on the sign and the direction of the charge in the wire, as described by the "right hand rule": The fingers point in the direction of the magnetic field when the thumb points in the direction of a moving positive charge (*i.e.*, opposite to the direction of electron movement). Wrapping the current-carrying wire many times in a coil causes a superimposition of the magnetic fields, augmenting the overall strength of the magnetic field

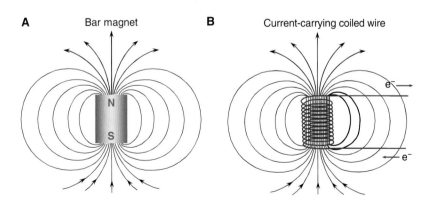

Dipole magnetic field

■ **FIGURE 12-1 A.** The magnetic field has two poles with magnetic field lines emerging from the north pole (N), and returning to the south pole (S), as illustrated by a simple bar magnet. **B.** A coiled wire carrying an electric current produces a magnetic field with characteristics similar to a bar magnet. Magnetic field strength and field density are dependent on the amplitude of the current and the number of coil turns.

inside the coil, with a rapid falloff of field strength outside the coil (see Fig. 12-1B). Amplitude of the current in the coil determines the overall magnitude of the magnetic field strength. The magnetic field lines extending beyond the concentrated field are known as fringe fields.

12.1.3 Magnetic Properties of Materials

Magnetic *susceptibility* describes the extent to which a material becomes magnetized when placed in a magnetic field. In some materials, induced internal magnetization opposes the external magnetic field and lowers the local magnetic field surrounding the material. On the other hand, the internal magnetization can form in the same direction as the applied magnetic field and increase the local magnetic field. Three categories of susceptibility are defined: *diamagnetic*, *paramagnetic*, and *ferromagnetic*, based upon the arrangement of electrons in the atomic or molecular structure. Diamagnetic elements and materials have slightly negative susceptibility and oppose the applied magnetic field, because of paired electrons in the surrounding electron orbitals. Examples of diamagnetic materials are calcium, water, and most organic materials (chiefly owing to the diamagnetic characteristics of carbon and hydrogen molecules). Paramagnetic materials, with unpaired electrons, have slightly positive susceptibility and enhance the local magnetic field, but they have no measurable self-magnetism. Examples of paramagnetic materials are molecular oxygen (O_2), deoxyhemoglobin, some blood degradation products such as methemoglobin, and *gadolinium-based* contrast agents. Locally, these diamagnetic and paramagnetic agents will deplete or augment the local magnetic field (Fig. 12-2), affecting MR images in known, unknown, and sometimes unexpected ways. Ferromagnetic materials are "superparamagnetic"—that is, they augment the external magnetic field substantially. These materials, containing iron, cobalt, and nickel, exhibit "self-magnetism" in many cases, and can significantly distort the acquired signals.

12.1.4 Magnetic Characteristics of the Nucleus

The nucleus, comprising protons and neutrons with characteristics listed in Table 12-1, exhibits magnetic characteristics on a much smaller scale than for atoms/molecules and their associated electron distributions. Magnetic properties are influenced by spin and charge distributions intrinsic to the proton and neutron. A mag-

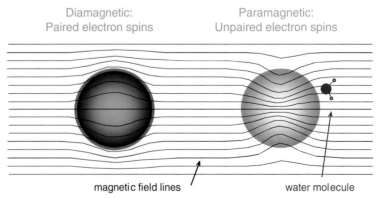

Diamagnetic:
Paired electron spins

Paramagnetic:
Unpaired electron spins

magnetic field lines

water molecule

■ **FIGURE 12-2** The local magnetic field can be changed in the presence of diamagnetic (depletion) and paramagnetic (augmentation) materials, with an impact on the signals generated from nearby signal sources such as the hydrogen atoms in water molecules.

TABLE 12-1 PROPERTIES OF THE NEUTRON AND PROTON

CHARACTERISTIC	NEUTRON	PROTON
Mass (kg)	1.674×10^{-27}	1.672×10^{-27}
Charge (coulomb)	0	1.602×10^{-19}
Spin quantum number	½	½
Magnetic moment (J/T)	-9.66×10^{-27}	1.41×10^{-26}
Magnetic moment (nuclear magneton)	-1.91	2.79

netic dipole is created for the proton, with a positive charge equal to the electron charge but of opposite sign, due to nuclear "spin." Overall, the neutron is electrically uncharged, but subnuclear charge inhomogeneities and an associated nuclear spin result in a magnetic field of opposite direction and approximately the same strength as the proton. Magnetic characteristics of the nucleus are described by the *nuclear magnetic moment*, represented as a vector indicating magnitude and direction. For a given nucleus, the nuclear magnetic moment is determined through the pairing of the constituent protons and neutrons. If the sum of the number of protons (P) and number of neutrons (N) in the nucleus is even, the nuclear magnetic moment is essentially zero. However, if N is even and P is odd, or N is odd and P is even, the resultant non-integer nuclear spin generates a nuclear magnetic moment. A single nucleus does not generate a large enough nuclear magnetic moment to be observable, but the conglomeration of large numbers of nuclei ($\sim10^{15}$) arranged in a non-random orientation generates an observable nuclear magnetic moment of the sample, from which the MRI signals are derived.

12.1.5 Nuclear Magnetic Characteristics of the Elements

Biologically relevant elements that are candidates for producing MR signals are listed in Table 12-2. Key features include the strength of the nuclear magnetic moment, the physiologic concentration, and the isotopic abundance. Hydrogen, having the largest magnetic moment and greatest abundance, chiefly in water and fat, is by far the best element for general clinical utility. Other elements are orders of magnitude less sensitive. Of these, ^{23}Na and ^{31}P have been used for imaging in limited situations, despite their relatively low sensitivity. Therefore, the nucleus of the hydrogen atom, the proton, is the principal focus for generating MR signals.

12.1.6 Magnetic Characteristics of the Proton

The spinning proton or "*spin*" (spin and proton are used synonymously herein) is classically considered to be a tiny bar magnet with north and south poles, even though the magnetic moment of a single proton is undetectable. Large numbers of unbound hydrogen atoms in water and fat, those unconstrained by molecular bonds in complex macromolecules within tissues, have a random orientation of their protons (nuclear magnetic moments) due to thermal energy. As a result, there is no observable magnetization of the sample (Fig. 12-3A). However, when placed in a strong static magnetic field, B_0, magnetic forces cause the protons to realign with the applied field in parallel and antiparallel directions with an excess of a few more oriented parallel to the B_0 field (Fig. 12-3B). At 1.0 T, the number of excess protons in the parallel (low-energy state) is approximately 3 protons per million (3×10^{-6}) at physiologic temperatures. Although this number seems insignificant, for a typical voxel volume in MRI, there

12.1 Magnetism, Magnetic Fields, and Magnetic Properties of Materials

TABLE 12-2 **MAGNETIC RESONANCE PROPERTIES OF MEDICALLY USEFUL NUCLEI**

NUCLEUS	SPIN QUANTUM NUMBER	% ISOTOPIC ABUNDANCE	MAGNETIC MOMENT[a]	% RELATIVE ELEMENTAL ABUNDANCE[b]	RELATIVE SENSITIVITY	GYRO-MAGNETIC RATIO, $\gamma/2\pi$ (MHz/T)
^{1}H	$\frac{1}{2}$	99.98	2.79	10	1	42.58
^{3}He	$\frac{1}{2}$	0.00014	−2.13	0	—	32.43
^{13}C	$-\frac{1}{2}$	0.011	0.70	18	—	10.71
^{17}O	$\frac{5}{2}$	0.04	−1.89	65	9×10^{-6}	5.77
^{19}F	$\frac{1}{2}$	100	2.63	<0.01	3×10^{-8}	40.05
^{23}Na	$\frac{3}{2}$	100	2.22	0.1	1×10^{-4}	11.26
^{31}P	$\frac{1}{2}$	100	1.13	1.2	6×10^{-5}	17.24

[a]Moment in nuclear magneton units = 5.05×10^{-27} J/T.
[b]Note: by mass in the human body (all isotopes).

A No magnetic field   **B** External magnetic field

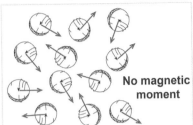
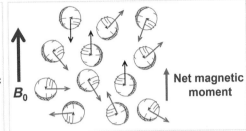

No magnetic moment

B_0

Net magnetic moment

■ **FIGURE 12-3** Simplified distributions of "free" protons without and with an external magnetic field are shown. **A.** Without an external magnetic field, a group of protons assumes a random orientation of magnetic moments, producing an overall magnetic moment of zero. **B.** Under the influence of an external magnetic field, some protons (blue vectors) in the tissue occupy two spin states: parallel or antiparallel to B_0. The difference in number of spins between these two states is a few per million. A slightly greater number exist in the parallel direction at equilibrium, resulting in a measurable net magnetic moment of the tissue sample in the direction of B_0.

are about 10^{21} protons, so there are approximately $3 \times 10^{-6} \times 10^{21}$, or 3×10^{15}, more protons in the parallel direction! This number of excess protons produces an observable "sample" nuclear magnetic moment, initially aligned with the direction of the applied magnetic field. The classical description deals with a single net magnetization of an ensemble of nuclei.

The magnetic moment of spins rotates around the static magnetic field, called *precession*, much in the same way that a spinning top wobbles due to the force of gravity (Fig. 12-4). The precession occurs at an angular frequency (number of rotations/s about an axis of rotation) that is proportional to the magnetic field strength B_0. The *Larmor equation* describes the dependence between the magnetic field, B_0, and the angular precessional frequency, ω_0:

$$\omega_0 = \gamma B_0,$$

where γ is the gyromagnetic ratio unique to each nucleus. This is expressed in terms of linear frequency, where $\omega = 2\pi f$ and $\gamma/2\pi$ is the *gyromagnetic ratio*, with values expressed in millions of cycles per second (MHz) per Tesla, or MHz/T.

$$f_0 = \frac{\gamma}{2\pi} B_0$$

Each nucleus with a non-zero nuclear magnetic moment has a unique gyromagnetic ratio, as listed in Table 12-2 (right column).

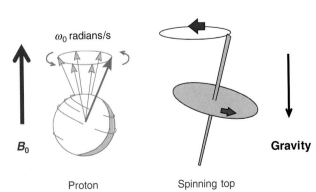

ω_0 radians/s

B_0

Gravity

Proton   Spinning top

Precessional frequency

■ **FIGURE 12-4** A single proton precesses about its axis at an angular frequency, ω, proportional to the externally applied magnetic field strength, according to the Larmor equation. A well-known example of precession is the motion a spinning top makes as it interacts with the force of gravity as it slows.

Typical magnetic field strengths for clinical MR systems range from 0.3 to 7.0 T. For protons, the precessional frequency is 42.58 MHz/T, and increases or decreases with an increase or decrease in magnetic field strength, as calculated in the example below. Accuracy of the precessional frequency is necessary to ensure that the RF energy will be absorbed by the magnetized protons. Precision of the precessional frequency must be on the order of cycles/s (Hz) out of millions of cycles/s (MHz) in order to identify the location and spatial position of the emerging signals, as is described in Section 12.6.

EXAMPLE: What is the frequency of precession of ^1H and ^{31}P at 0.5 T? 1.5 T? 3.0 T? The Larmor frequency is calculated as $f_0 = (\gamma/2\pi)B_0$.

NUCLEUS	FIELD STRENGTH		
	0.5 T	1.5 T	3.0 T
^1H	42.58 × 0.5 = 21.29 MHz	42.58 × 1.5 = 63.87 MHz	42.58 × 3.0 = 127.74 MHz
^{31}P	17.2 × 0.5 = 8.6 MHz	17.2 × 1.5 = 25.8 MHz	17.2 × 3 = 51.6 MHz

The differences in the gyromagnetic ratios and corresponding precessional frequencies allow the selective excitation of one element from another in the same magnetic field strength.

12.2 MR SYSTEM

The MR system is composed of several components including a magnet, magnetic field gradient coil, and radiofrequency (RF) coils, orchestrated by many processors and control subsystems, as shown in Figure 12-5. Details of the individual components, methods of acquiring the MR signals, and reconstruction of images are described in the following sections.

12.2.1 Magnets

The magnet is the heart of the MR system. For any magnet type, performance criteria include field strength, temporal stability, and field homogeneity. These parameters are affected by the magnet design. Air core magnets are made of wire-wrapped cylinders of approximately 1-m diameter and greater, over a cylindrical length of 2 to 3 m, where the magnetic field is produced by an electric current in the wires. When the wires are energized, the magnetic field produced is parallel to the long axis of the cylinder. In most clinically designed systems, the magnetic field is horizontal and runs along the cranial-caudal axis of the patient lying supine (Fig. 12-6A). Solid core magnets are constructed from permanent magnets, a wire-wrapped iron core "electromagnet," or a hybrid combination. In these solid core designs, the magnetic field runs between the poles of the magnet, most often in a vertical direction (Fig. 12-6B). Magnetic fringe fields extend well beyond the volume of the cylinder in air core designs. Fringe fields are a potential hazard and are discussed further in Chapter 13.

To achieve a high magnetic field strength (greater than 1 T) requires the electromagnet core wires to be superconductive. Superconductivity is a characteristic of certain metals (*e.g.*, niobium-titanium alloys) that when maintained at extremely low temperatures (liquid helium; less than 4 K) exhibit no resistance to electric current. Superconductivity allows the closed-circuit electromagnet to be energized and

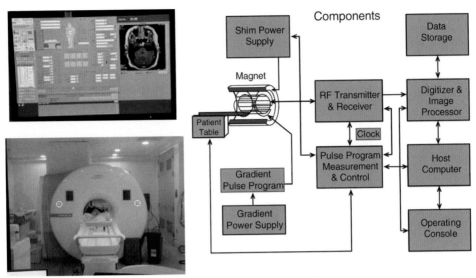

Components

■ **FIGURE 12-5** The MR system is shown (lower left), the operators display (upper left), and the various subsystems that generate, detect, and capture the MR signals used for imaging and spectroscopy.

ramped up to the desired current and magnetic field strength by an external electric source. Replenishment of the liquid helium must occur continuously, because if the temperature rises above a critical value, the loss of superconductivity will occur and resistance heating of the wires will boil the helium, resulting in a "quench." Superconductive magnets with field strengths of 1.5 to 3 T are common for clinical systems.

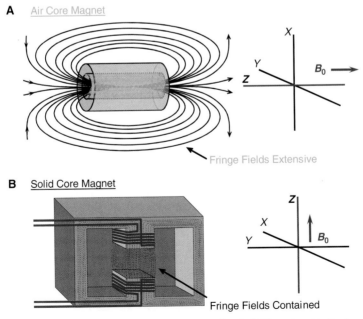

A Air Core Magnet

Fringe Fields Extensive

B Solid Core Magnet

Fringe Fields Contained

■ **FIGURE 12-6 A.** Air core magnets typically have a horizontal main field produced in the bore of the electrical windings, with the z-axis (B_0) along the bore axis. Fringe fields for the air core systems are extensive and are increased for larger bore diameters and higher field strengths. **B.** The solid core magnet has a vertical field, produced between the metal poles of a permanent or wire-wrapped electromagnet. Fringe fields are confined with this design. In both types, the main field is parallel to the z-axis of the Cartesian coordinate system.

12.2.2 Magnetic Field Gradients

A magnetic field gradient is obtained by superimposing the magnetic fields of two or more coils carrying a direct current of specific amplitude and direction with a precisely defined geometry (Fig. 12-7). The bipolar gradient field varies over a predefined field of view (FOV), and when superimposed upon B_0, a small, continuous variation in the field strength occurs from the center to the periphery with distance from the center point (the "null"). Interacting with the much, much stronger main magnetic field, the subtle linear variations are on the order of 0.004 T/m (4 mT/m) and are essential for localizing signals generated during the operation of the MR system.

Inside the magnet bore, three sets of gradients reside along the logical coordinate axes—x, y, and z—and produce a magnetic field variation determined by the magnitude of the applied current in each coil set (Fig. 12-8). When independently energized, the three coils (x, y, z) can produce a linearly variable magnetic field in any arbitrary direction, where the net gradient is equal to $\sqrt{G_x^2 + G_y^2 + G_z^2}$. Gradient polarity reversals (positive to negative and negative to positive changes in magnetic field strength) are achieved by reversing the current direction in the gradient coils.

Two important properties of magnetic gradients are as follows: (1) The *gradient field strength* is determined by its peak amplitude and slope (change over distance), and typically ranges from 1 to 50 mT/m. (2) The *slew rate* is the time to achieve the peak magnetic field amplitude. Typical slew rates of gradient fields are from 5 to 250 mT/m/ms. As the gradient field is turned on, *eddy currents* are induced in nearby conductors such as adjacent RF coils and the patient, which produce magnetic fields that oppose the gradient field and limit the achievable slew rate. Actively shielded gradient coils and compensation circuits can reduce problems caused by eddy currents.

In a gradient magnetic field, protons maintain precessional frequencies corresponding to local magnetic field strength. At the middle of the gradient, called the gradient isocenter, there is no change in the field strength or precessional frequency. With a linear gradient, the magnetic field increases and decreases linearly in addition to the static magnetic field, as does the precessional frequency. The angular precessional frequency at a location within a linear gradient, ω, is

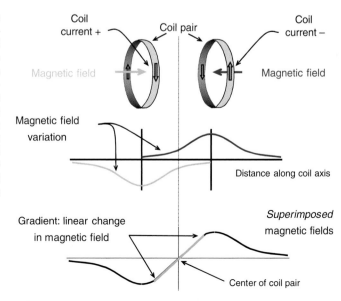

■ **FIGURE 12-7** Gradients are produced inside the main magnet with coil pairs. Individual conducting wire coils are separately energized with currents of opposite direction to produce magnetic fields of opposite polarity. Magnetic field strength decreases with distance from the center of each coil. When combined, the magnetic field variations form a linear change between the coils, producing a linear magnetic field gradient, as shown in the lower graph.

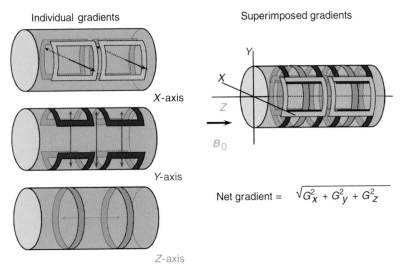

Individual gradients   Superimposed gradients

X-axis

Y-axis

Z-axis

$$\text{Net gradient} = \sqrt{G_x^2 + G_y^2 + G_z^2}$$

■ **FIGURE 12-8** Within the large stationary magnetic field, field gradients are produced by three separate coil pairs placed within the central core of the magnet, along the x, y, or z directions. In modern systems, the current loops are distributed across the cylinders for the x-, y-, and z-gradients, which generates a lower, but more uniform gradient field. Magnetic field gradients of arbitrary direction are produced by the vector addition of the individual gradients turned on simultaneously. Any gradient direction is possible by superimposition of magnetic fields generated by the three-axis gradient system.

$$\omega = \gamma \left(B_0 + G_{net} \cdot d \right),$$

where G_{net} is the net gradient and d is the distance from the gradient isocenter.

EXAMPLE: What is the precession frequency of proton placed 20 cm from the gradient isocenter if the net gradient is 2 G/cm and the field strength is 1.5 T?
The B_0 field strength is 1.5 T and the gradient adds a magnetic field of 40 G or 0.004 T (2 G/cm × 20 cm). The effective magnetic field strength at the location is 1.504 T. The Larmor frequency of proton at 1.504 T is 64.04 MHz (42.58 × 1.504). The Larmor frequency of proton increases by 0.17 MHz due to the gradient field.

12.2.3 Radiofrequency Coils

RF transmitter coils create an oscillating secondary magnetic field formed by passing an alternating current through a loop of wire. Irradiating the sample with an electromagnetic RF energy pulse tuned to the Larmor frequency induces the resonance of the magnetization within the sample. The magnetization along the direction of the static magnetic field, B_0, shrinks with a simultaneous phase coherence that creates a perpendicular magnetization rotating at the Larmor frequency. This phenomenon is called *excitation*. To accomplish excitation and resonance, the created secondary field, called B_1, must be arranged at right angles to the main magnetic field, B_0. In an air core design with a horizontal field, the RF coil secondary field should be in the transverse or vertical axes, as the B_1 field is created perpendicular to the transmit coils themselves. **RF transmitter coils** are therefore oriented above, below, or at the sides of the patient, and are usually cylindrical. In most systems, the body coil contained within the bore of the magnet is most frequently used, but also transmitter coils for the head, extremity, and some breast coils are coupled to a receiver coil.

The transverse magnetization within the sample returns to equilibrium conditions and releases detectable RF energy at the same frequency. While in phase coherence, the rotating magnetization vector generates a signal that is detected by highly sensitive antennas (**RF receiver coils**) to capture the basic MR signal. All **RF receiver coils** must resonate and efficiently store energy at the Larmor frequency. This is determined by the inductance and capacitance properties of the coil. RF transmit and receive coils need to be tuned prior to each acquisition and matched to accommodate the different magnetic inductance of each patient. Receiver coils must be properly placed to adequately detect the MR signal.

Very often, transmit and receive functions are separated to handle the variety of imaging situations that arise, and to maximize the SNR for an imaging sequence. Proximity RF coils include volume or bird-cage coils, the design of choice for brain imaging, the single-turn solenoid for imaging the extremities and the breasts, and the saddle coil. These coils are typically operated as both a transmitter and receiver of RF energy (Fig. 12-9A). *Volume coils* encompass the total area of the anatomy of interest and yield uniform excitation and SNR over the entire imaging volume. However, because of their relatively large size, images are produced with lower SNR than other types of coils. Enhanced performance is obtained with a process known as quadrature excitation and detection, which enables the energy to be transmitted and the signals to be received by two pairs of coils oriented at right angles, either electronically or physically. This detector manages two simultaneous channels known as the real (records MR information in phase with a reference signal) and the imaginary (records MR information 90° out of phase with the reference signal) channels, and increases

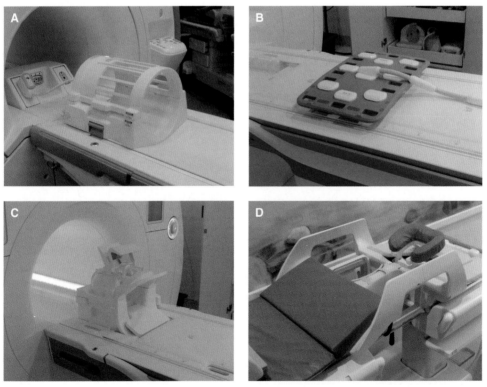

■ **FIGURE 12-9** Radiofrequency surface coils improve image quality and SNR for specific examinations. **A.** A transmit/receive head coil. **B.** A flexible body coil and a spine coil imbedded on the table. **C.** A 64-channel phased array head and neck coil. **D.** A coil and a table dedicated for breast imaging and biopsy.

the SNR up to a factor of $\sqrt{2}$. If imbalances in the offset or gain of these detectors occur, then artifacts will be manifested, such as a "center point" artifact.

Phased array coils consisting of multiple coils and receivers are made of several overlapping loops, which extend the imaging FOV in one direction (Fig. 12-9B–D). The small FOV of each individual coil provides excellent SNR and resolution, and each is combined to produce a composite image with the advantages of the local surface coil, so that all data can be acquired in a single sequence. Phased array coils for the spine, pelvis, breast, cardiac, and temporomandibular joint applications are commonly purchased with an MR system for optimal image quality.

Surface coils are used to achieve high SNR and high resolution when imaging anatomy near the surface of the patient. They are typically receive-only designs and are usually small and shaped for a specific imaging exam and for patient comfort. The received signal sensitivity, however, is limited to the volume located around the coil at a depth into the patient equal to the radius of the coil, which causes a loss of signal with depth. There are now intracavitary coils for endorectal, endovascular, endovaginal, esophageal, and urethral local imaging, and they can be used to receive signals from deep within the patient. In general, a body coil is used to transmit the RF energy and the local coil is used to receive the MR signal.

12.2.4 MR System Subcomponents

The control interfaces, RF source, detector, and amplifier, analog to digital converter (digitizer), pulse programmer, computer system, gradient power supplies, and image display are crucial components of the MR system. They integrate and synchronize the tasks necessary to produce the MR image (Fig. 12-5).

The operator interface and computer systems vary with the manufacturer, but most consist of a computer system, dedicated processor for Fourier transformation, image processor to form the image, disk drives for storage of raw data and pulse sequence parameters, and a power distribution system to distribute and filter the direct and alternating current. The operator's console is located outside of the scan room and provides the interface to the hardware and software for data acquisition (DAQ).

A cross section of the internal superconducting magnet components shows integral parts of the magnet system including the wire coils and cryogenic liquid containment vessel (Fig. 12-10). In addition to the main magnet system, other components are also necessary. Shim coils interact with the main magnetic field to improve homogeneity (minimal variation of the magnetic flux density) over the volume used for patient imaging. RF coils exist within the main bore of the magnet to transmit energy to the patient as well as to receive returning signals. Gradient coils are contained within the main bore to produce a linear variation of magnetic field strength across the useful magnet volume.

12.3 MAGNETIC RESONANCE SIGNAL

Application of RF energy synchronized to the precessional frequency of the protons causes absorption of energy and displacement of the sample magnetic moment from equilibrium conditions. The return to equilibrium results in the emission of energy proportional to the number of excited protons in the volume. This occurs at a rate that depends on the structural and magnetic characteristics of the sample. Excitation, detection, and acquisition of the signals constitute the basic information necessary for MRI and MRS.

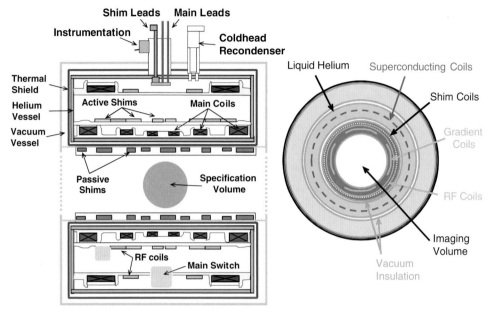

■ **FIGURE 12-10** Internal components of a superconducting air-core magnet are shown. On the left is a cross section through the long axis of the magnet illustrating relative locations of the components, and on the right is a simplified cross section across the diameter.

12.3.1 Orientation, Frame of Reference, and Magnetization Vectors

By convention, the applied magnetic field $\mathbf{B}_0$ is directed parallel to the z-axis of the three-dimensional Cartesian coordinate axis system and perpendicular to the x- and y-axes. For convenience, two frames of reference are used: the *laboratory frame* and the *rotating frame*. The laboratory frame (Fig. 12-11A) is a stationary reference frame from the observer's point of view. The sample magnetic moment vector precesses about the z-axis in a circular geometry about the x–y plane. The rotating frame (Fig. 12-11B) is a *spinning* axis system, whereby the x'–y' axes rotate at an angular frequency equal to the Larmor frequency. In this frame, the sample magnetic moment vector appears to be stationary when rotating at the resonance frequency. A slightly higher precessional frequency is observed as a slow clockwise rotation, while a slightly lower precessional frequency is observed as a slow counterclockwise rotation. The magnetic interactions between precessional frequencies of the magnetic moments of the protons with the externally applied RF (depicted as a rotating magnetic field) can be described more clearly using the rotating frame of reference, while the observed returning signal and its frequency content is explained using the laboratory (stationary) frame of reference.

The net magnetization vector of the sample, M, is described by three components. *Longitudinal magnetization*, M_z, along the z direction, is the component of the magnetic moment parallel to the applied magnetic field, $\mathbf{B}_0$. At equilibrium, the longitudinal magnetization is maximal and is denoted as M_0, the *equilibrium magnetization*. The component of the magnetic moment perpendicular to $\mathbf{B}_0$, M_{xy}, in the x–y plane, is *transverse magnetization*. At equilibrium, M_{xy} is zero. When the protons in the magnetized sample absorb energy, phase coherence of the spins generates a rotating vector in the transverse plane, M_{xy}, generating the all-important MR signal. Figure 12-12 illustrates this geometry.

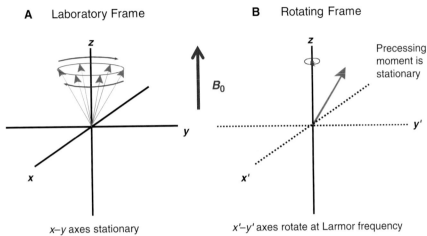

A   Laboratory Frame

B   Rotating Frame

Precessing moment is stationary

B_0

x–y axes stationary

x′–y′ axes rotate at Larmor frequency

■ **FIGURE 12-11** **A.** The *laboratory frame of reference* uses stationary three-dimensional Cartesian coordinates: x, y, z. The magnetic moment of the proton precesses around the z-axis at the Larmor frequency as the illustration attempts to convey. **B.** The *rotating frame of reference* uses rotating Cartesian coordinate axes that *rotate about the z-axis* at the Larmor precessional frequency, and the other axes are denoted: $x′$ and $y′$. When precessing at the Larmor frequency, the proton magnetic moment is stationary.

12.3.2 Resonance and Excitation

When a bar magnet continuously moves back and forth at the same (resonance) frequency of nearby magnetic spins pointing upward, the magnetic interaction causes the spins to tip downward to the perpendicular plane (Fig. 12-13A). Similarly, displacement of the equilibrium magnetization occurs when the magnetic component of the RF excitation pulse, known as the B_1 field, is precisely matched to the precessional frequency of the protons (Fig. 12-13B). In the rotating frame, the B_1 field continuously applies torque on the equilibrium magnetization when it is applied, causing displacement (Fig. 12-13C). If the B_1 field is not applied at the precessional (Larmor) frequency, the B_1 field will not interact with M_z (Fig 12-13D).

12.3.3 Flip Angles

Flip angles represent the degree of M_z rotation by the B_1 field as it is applied along the $x′$-axis (or the $y′$-axis) perpendicular to M_z. A torque is applied on M_z, rotating it from the longitudinal direction into the transverse plane. The rate of rotation

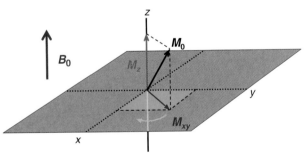

■ **FIGURE 12-12** *Longitudinal magnetization, M_z,* is the vector component of the magnetic moment in the z direction. *Transverse magnetization, M_{xy},* is the vector component of the magnetic moment in the x–y plane. *Equilibrium magnetization, M_0,* is the maximum longitudinal magnetization of the sample, and is shown displaced from the z-axis in this illustration.

M_z: Longitudinal Magnetization: in z-axis direction

M_{xy}: Transverse Magnetization: in x-y plane

M_0: Equilibrium Magnetization: maximum magnetization

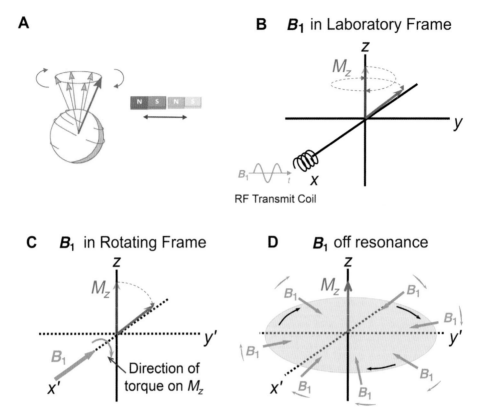

A

B B_1 **in Laboratory Frame**

M_z

z

y

B_1

x

RF Transmit Coil

C B_1 **in Rotating Frame**

z

M_z

y'

B_1

x'

Direction of torque on M_z

D B_1 **off resonance**

z

B_1 M_z B_1

B_1

B_1 y'

B_1

x' B_1 B_1

■ **FIGURE 12-13** An intuitive description of magnetic resonance. **A.** A small magnet near a magnetic dipole moving back and forth at the resonance frequency increases the energy in the dipole and induces larger oscillation, an "excited" state. **B.** In the *laboratory frame*, sinusoidal magnetic fields generated by a coil in the *x*-axis excites the magnetic moment in the *z*-axis into the *x–y* plane. **C.** In the *rotating frame*, the RF pulse (**B_1** field) is applied at the Larmor frequency and is stationary in the *x'–y'* plane. The **B_1** field interacts at 90° to the sample magnetic moment and produces a torque that displaces the magnetic vector away from equilibrium. **D.** The **B_1** field is not tuned to the Larmor frequency and is not stationary in the rotating frame. No interaction with the sample magnetic moment occurs.

occurs at an angular frequency equal to $\omega_1 = \gamma B_1$ as per the Larmor equation. Thus, for an RF pulse (**B_1** field) applied over a time t, the magnetization vector displacement angle, θ, is determined as $\theta = \omega_1 t = \gamma B_1 t$, and the product of the pulse time and **B_1** amplitude determines the displacement of M_z. This is illustrated in Figure 12-14.

Common flip angles are 90° ($\pi/2$) and 180° (π), although a variety of smaller and larger angles are chosen to enhance tissue contrast in various ways. A 90° angle provides the largest possible M_{xy} and detectable MR signal and requires a known **B_1** strength and time (on the order of a few to hundreds of μs). The displacement angle of the sample magnetic moment is linearly related to the product of **B_1** field strength and time: For a fixed **B_1** field strength, a 90° displacement takes half the time of a 180° displacement. With flip angles smaller than 90°, less time is needed to displace M_z, and a larger transverse magnetization per unit excitation time is achieved. For instance, a 45° flip takes half the time of a 90° flip yet creates 70% of the signal, as the magnitude of M_{xy} is equal to the sine of 45°, or 0.707. With fast MRI techniques, small displacement angles of 10° and less are often used.

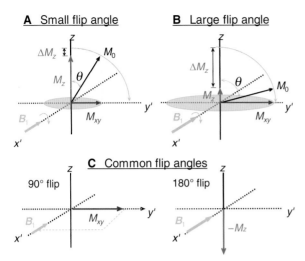

A Small flip angle   **B** Large flip angle

C Common flip angles

90° flip   180° flip

■ **FIGURE 12-14** Flip angles describe the angular displacement of the longitudinal magnetization vector from the equilibrium position. The rotation angle of the magnetic moment vector is dependent on the duration and amplitude of the B_1 field at the Larmor frequency. Flip angles describe the rotation of M_z away from the z-axis. Small flip angles (less than 45°) **(A)** and large flip angles (75° to 90°) **(B)** produce small and large transverse magnetization, respectively. **C.** Common flip angles are 90°, which produce the maximum transverse magnetization, and 180°, which invert the existing longitudinal magnetization to $-M_z$.

12.4 MAGNETIZATION PROPERTIES OF TISSUES

12.4.1 Free Induction Decay: T2 and T2* Relaxation

After a 90° RF pulse is applied to a magnetized sample at the Larmor frequency, an initial phase coherence of the individual protons is established and maximum M_{xy} is achieved. Rotating at the Larmor frequency, the transverse magnetic field of the excited sample induces signal in the receiver antenna coil (in the laboratory frame of reference). A damped sinusoidal electronic signal, known as the *free induction decay* (FID), is produced (Fig. 12-15).

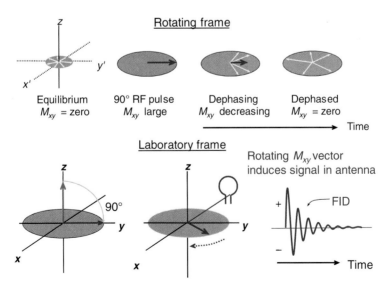

Rotating frame

Equilibrium   90° RF pulse   Dephasing   Dephased
M_{xy} = zero M_{xy} large M_{xy} decreasing M_{xy} = zero

Time

Laboratory frame

Rotating M_{xy} vector induces signal in antenna

90°

FID

Time

■ **FIGURE 12-15** Top: Conversion of longitudinal magnetization, M_z, into transverse magnetization, M_{xy}, results in an initial phase coherence of the individual spins of the sample. The magnetic moment vector precesses at the Larmor frequency (stationary in the rotating frame), and dephases with time. Bottom: In the laboratory frame, M_{xy} precesses and induces a signal in an antenna receiver sensitive to transverse magnetization. An FID signal is produced with positive and negative variations oscillating at the Larmor frequency, and decaying with time due to the loss of phase coherence.

The FID amplitude decay is caused by loss of M_{xy} phase coherence due to intrinsic micromagnetic inhomogeneities in the sample's structure, whereby individual protons in the bulk water and hydration layer coupled to macromolecules precess at incrementally different frequencies arising from the slight changes in local magnetic field strength. Phase coherence is lost over time as an exponential decay. Elapsed time between the peak transverse signal (*e.g.*, directly after a 90° RF pulse) and 37% of the peak level (1/e) is the T2 relaxation time (Fig. 12-16A). Mathematically, this is expressed as

$$M_{xy}(t) = M_0 e^{-t/T2},$$

where $M_{xy}(t)$ is the transverse magnetic moment at time t for a sample that has M_0 transverse magnetization at $t = 0$. When $t = T2$, then $e^{-1} = 0.37$ and $M_{xy} = 0.37 M_0$.

The molecular structure of the magnetized sample and characteristics of the bound water protons strongly affects its T2 decay value. Amorphous structures (*e.g.*, cerebral spinal fluid [CSF] or highly edematous tissues) contain mobile molecules with fast and rapid molecular motion. Without structural constraint (*e.g.*, lack of a hydration layer), these tissues do not support intrinsic magnetic field inhomogeneities, and thus exhibit long T2 values. As molecular size increases for specific tissues, constrained molecular motion and the presence of the hydration layer produce magnetic field domains within the structure and increase spin dephasing that causes more rapid decay with the result of shorter T2 values. For large, non-moving structures, stationary magnetic inhomogeneities in the hydration layer result in these types of tissues (*e.g.*, bone) having a very short T2.

Extrinsic magnetic inhomogeneities, such as the imperfect main magnetic field, B_0, or susceptibility agents in the tissues (*e.g.*, MR contrast materials, paramagnetic or ferromagnetic objects), add to the loss of phase coherence from intrinsic inhomogeneities and further reduce the decay constant, known as T2* under these conditions (Fig. 12-16B).

12.4.2 Return to Equilibrium: T1 Relaxation

Longitudinal magnetization begins to recover immediately after the B_1 excitation pulse, simultaneous with transverse decay; however, the return to equilibrium

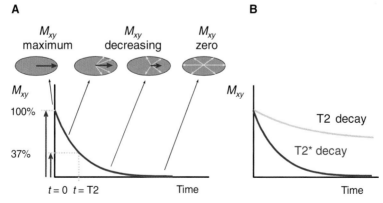

■ **FIGURE 12-16 A.** The loss of M_{xy} phase coherence occurs exponentially caused by intrinsic spin-spin interactions in the tissues and extrinsic magnetic field inhomogeneities. The exponential decay constant, T2, is the time over which the signal decays to 37% of the initial transverse magnetization (*e.g.*, after a 90° pulse). **B.** T2 is the decay time resulting from *intrinsic* magnetic properties of the sample. T2* is the decay time resulting from *both intrinsic and extrinsic magnetic field variations*. T2 is always longer than T2*.

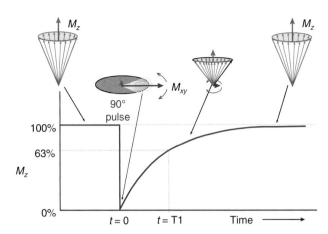

■ **FIGURE 12-17** After a 90° pulse, M_z is converted from a maximum value at equilibrium to $M_z = 0$. Return of M_z to equilibrium occurs exponentially and is characterized by the spin-lattice T1 relaxation constant. After an elapsed time equal to T1, 63% of the longitudinal magnetization is recovered. Spin-lattice recovery takes longer than spin-spin decay (T2).

conditions occurs over a longer time period. *Spin-lattice relaxation* is the term describing the release of energy back to the *lattice* (the molecular arrangement and structure of the hydration layer), and the regrowth of M_z. This occurs exponentially as

$$M_z(t) = M_0 \, (1 - e^{-t/T1}),$$

where $M_z(t)$ is the longitudinal magnetization at time t and T1 is the time needed for the recovery of 63% of M_z after a 90° pulse (at $t = 0$, $M_z = 0$, and at $t = T1$, $M_z = 0.63M_0$), as shown in Figure 12-17. When $t = 3 \times T1$, then $M_z = 0.95M_0$, and for $t > 5 \times T1$, then $M_z \approx M_0$, and full longitudinal magnetization equilibrium is reestablished.

Since M_z does not generate an MR signal directly, determination of T1 for a specific tissue requires a specific "sequence," as shown in Figure 12-18. At equilibrium, a 90° pulse sets $M_z = 0$. After a delay time, ΔT, the recovered M_z component is converted to M_{xy} by a second 90° pulse, and the resulting peak amplitude is recorded. By repeating the sequence from equilibrium conditions with different delay times, ΔT between 90° pulses, data points that lie on the recovery curve are fitted to an exponential equation and T1 is estimated.

The T1 relaxation time depends on the rate of energy dissipation into the surrounding molecular lattice and hydration layer and varies substantially for different tissue structures and pathologies. Gadolinium chelated with complex

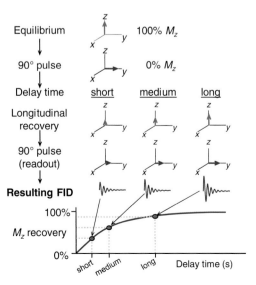

■ **FIGURE 12-18** Spin-lattice relaxation for a sample can be measured by using various delay times between two 90° RF pulses. After an initial 90° pulse, $M_z = 0$, another 90° pulse separated by a known delay is applied, and the longitudinal magnetization that has recovered during the delay is converted to transverse magnetization. The maximum amplitude of the resultant FID is recorded as a function of delay times between initial pulse and readout (three different delay time experiments are shown in this example), and the points are fit to an exponential recovery function to determine T1.

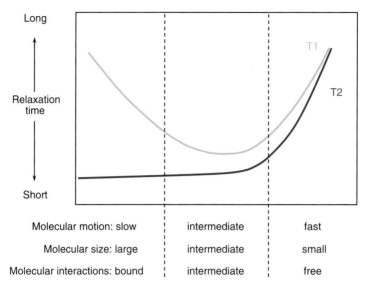

■ **FIGURE 12-19** Factors affecting T1 and T2 relaxation times of different tissues are generally based on molecular motion, size, and interactions that have an impact on the local magnetic field variations (T2 decay) and structure with intrinsic tumbling frequencies coupling to the Larmor frequency (T1 recovery). The relaxation time scale values (vertical axis) are different for T1 and T2.

macromolecules is effective in decreasing T1 relaxation time of local tissues by creating a hydration layer that forms a spin-lattice energy sink and results in a rapid return to equilibrium.

12.4.3 Comparison of T1 and T2

T1 is on the order of 5 to 10 times longer than T2. Molecular motion, size, and interactions influence T1 and T2 relaxation (Fig. 12-19). Because most tissues of interest for clinical MR applications are intermediate to small-sized molecules, tissues with a longer T1 usually have a longer T2, and those with a shorter T1 usually have a shorter T2. In Table 12-3, a comparison of T1 and T2 values for various tissues is listed. Depending on the main magnetic field strength, measurement methods, and biological variation, these relaxation values vary widely. Agents that disrupt the local magnetic field environment, such as paramagnetic blood degradation products, elements with unpaired electron spins (*e.g.*, gadolinium), or any ferromagnetic materials, cause a significant decrease in T2*. In situations where a macromolecule binds free water into a hydration layer, T1 is also significantly decreased.

TABLE 12-3 T1 AND T2 RELAXATION CONSTANTS FOR SEVERAL TISSUES[a]

TISSUE	T1, 0.5 T (ms)	T1, 1.5 T (ms)	T2 (ms)
Fat	210	260	80
Liver	350	500	40
Muscle	550	870	45
White matter	500	780	90
Gray matter	650	900	100
Cerebrospinal fluid	1,800	2,400	160

[a]Estimates only, as reported values for T1 and T2 span a wide range.

To summarize, T1 > T2 > T2*, and the specific relaxation times are a characteristic of the tissues. T1 values are longer for higher field strength magnets, while T2 values are unaffected. Thus, the T1, T2, and T2* decay constants, as well as proton density are fundamental properties of tissues, and can be exploited by machine-dependent acquisition techniques in MRI and MRS to aid in the diagnosis of pathologic conditions such as cancer, multiple sclerosis, or hematoma.

12.5 BASIC ACQUISITION PARAMETERS

Emphasizing the differences of T1 and T2, relaxation time constants, and proton density of the tissues is the key to the exquisite contrast sensitivity of MR images, but at the same time, the need to spatially localize the tissues is also required. First, basic machine-based parameters are described.

12.5.1 Time of Repetition

Acquiring an MR image relies on the repetition of a sequence of events in order to sample the volume of interest and periodically build the complete dataset over time. The time of repetition (TR) is the period between B_1 excitation pulses. During the TR interval, T2 decay and T1 recovery occur in the tissues. TR values range from extremely short (millisecond) to extremely long (10,000 ms) time periods, determined by the type of sequence employed.

12.5.2 Time of Echo

Excitation of protons with the B_1 RF pulse creates the M_{xy} FID signal. To separate the RF energy deposition and returning signal, an "echo" is induced to appear at a later time, with the application of a 180° RF inversion pulse. This can also be achieved with a gradient field and subsequent polarity reversal. The time of echo (TE) is the time between the excitation pulse and the appearance of the peak amplitude of an induced echo, which is determined by applying a 180° RF inversion pulse or gradient polarity reversal at a time equal to TE/2.

12.5.3 Time of Inversion

The TI is the time between an initial inversion/excitation (180°) RF pulse that produces negative maximum magnetization, and a 90° readout pulse. During the TI, M_z recovery occurs. The readout pulse converts the recovered M_z into M_{xy}, which is then measured with the formation of an echo at a time equal to TE as discussed above.

12.5.4 Partial Saturation

Saturation is a state of tissue magnetization less than equilibrium conditions. At equilibrium, the protons in a material are *unsaturated*, with full M_z amplitude. When multiple excitations occur over multiple TRs, the first excitation (B_1) pulse in the sequence produces the largest transverse magnetization, and recovery of the longitudinal magnetization occurs at the T1 time constant over the TR interval. However, because the TR is less than at least five times the T1 of the sample, M_z recovery is incomplete. Consequently, less M_{xy} amplitude is generated in the second excitation pulse. After the third pulse, a "steady-state" equilibrium is reached, where the amount

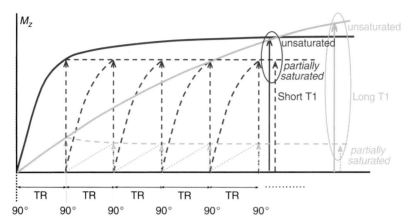

■ **FIGURE 12-20** Partial saturation of tissues occurs because the repetition time between excitation pulses does not allow for full return to equilibrium, and the M_z amplitude for the next RF pulse is reduced. After the third excitation pulse, a steady-state equilibrium is reached, where the amount of longitudinal magnetization is the same from pulse to pulse, as is the transverse magnetization for a tissue with a specific T1 decay constant. Tissues with long T1 experience a greater partial saturation than do tissues with short T1 as shown above. Partial saturation is important in understanding contrast mechanisms and signal from unsaturated and saturated tissues.

of M_z recovery and M_{xy} signal amplitude are constant, and the tissues achieve a state of *partial saturation* (Fig. 12-20). Tissues with short T1 have relatively less saturation than tissues with long T1. Partial saturation has an impact on tissue contrast and explains certain findings such as unsaturated protons in blood outside of the volume moving into the volume and generating a bright vascular signal on entry slices into the volume.

12.6 BASIC PULSE SEQUENCES

Three major pulse sequences perform the bulk of DAQ for imaging: spin echo (SE), inversion recovery (IR), and gradient echo (GRE). When used in conjunction with spatial localization methods, "contrast-weighted" images are obtained. In the following sections, the salient points and considerations of generating tissue contrast are discussed.

12.6.1 Spin Echo

SE describes the excitation of the magnetized protons in a sample with a 90° RF pulse and production of an FID, followed by a refocusing 180° RF pulse to produce an echo. The 90° pulse converts M_z into M_{xy} and creates the largest phase coherent transverse magnetization that immediately begins to decay at a rate described by T2* relaxation. The 180° RF pulse, applied at TE/2, inverts the spin system and induces phase coherence at TE, as depicted in the rotating frame in Figure 12-21. Inversion of the spin system causes the protons to experience external magnetic field variations opposite of that prior to the 180° RF pulse, resulting in the cancellation of the extrinsic inhomogeneities and associated dephasing effects. In the rotating frame of reference, the echo magnetization vector reforms in the opposite direction from the initial transverse magnetization vector.

Subsequent 180° RF pulses during the TR interval (Fig. 12-22) produce corresponding echoes with peak amplitudes that are reduced by intrinsic T2 decay of the

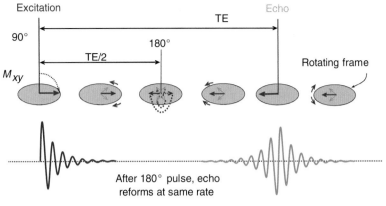

■ **FIGURE 12-21** The SE pulse sequence starts with a 90° pulse and produces an FID that decays according to T2* relaxation. After a delay time TE/2, a 180° RF pulse inverts the spins that re-establishes phase coherence and produces an echo at a time TE. Inhomogeneities of external magnetic fields are canceled, and the peak amplitude of the echo is determined by T2 decay. The rotating frame shows the evolution of the echo vector in the opposite direction of the FID. The sequence is repeated for each repetition period, TR.

tissues and are immune from extrinsic inhomogeneities. Digital sampling and acquisition of the signal occurs in a time window symmetric about TE, during the evolution and decay of each echo.

Spin Echo Contrast Weighting

Contrast is proportional to the difference in signal intensity between adjacent pixels in an image, corresponding to different voxels in the patient. The details of signal localization and image acquisition in MRI are discussed in Section 12.7. Here, the signal intensity variations for different tissues based upon TR and TE settings are described without consideration of spatial localization.

Ignoring the signal due to moving protons (*e.g.*, blood flow), the signal intensity produced by an MR system for a specific tissue using an SE sequence is

$$S \propto \rho_{\mathrm{H}}\left[1 - e^{\mathrm{TR/T1}}\right]e^{-\mathrm{TE/T2}},$$

where ρ_{H} is the proton density, T1 and T2 are physical properties of tissue, and TR and TE are pulse sequence timing parameters. For the same pulse sequence, different

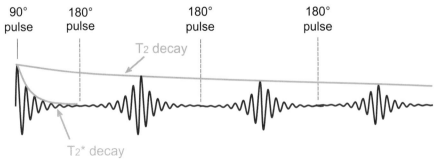

■ **FIGURE 12-22** "True" T2 decay is determined from multiple 180° refocusing pulses acquired during the repetition period. While the FID envelope decays with the T2* decay constant, the peak amplitudes of subsequent echoes decay exponentially according to the T2 decay constant, as extrinsic magnetic field inhomogeneities are cancelled.

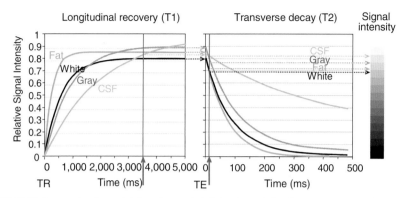

■ **FIGURE 12-23** Proton density weighting: Proton (spin) density weighted contrast requires the use of a long TR (*e.g.*, greater than 2,000 ms) to reduce T1 effects, and a short TE (*e.g.*, less than 35 ms) to reduce T2 influence in the acquired signals. Note that the average overall signal intensity is higher.

values of T1, T2, and ρ_H change the signal intensity S, and generate contrast amongst different tissues. Importantly, by changing the pulse sequence parameters TR and TE, the contrast dependence can be weighted toward T1, proton density, or T2 characteristics of the tissues.

Proton Density Weighting

Proton density contrast weighting relies mainly on differences in the number of magnetized protons per unit volume of tissue. At equilibrium, tissues with a large proton density, such as lipids, fats, and CSF, have a corresponding large M_z compared to other soft tissues. Contrast based on proton density differences is achieved by reducing the contributions of T1 recovery and T2 decay. T1 differences are reduced by selecting a long TR value to allow substantial recovery of M_z. T2 differences of the tissues are reduced by selecting a short TE value. Longitudinal recovery and transverse decay graphs for proton density weighting, using a long TR and a short TE, are illustrated in Figure 12-23. Contrast is generated from variations in proton density (CSF > fat > gray matter > white matter). Figure 12-24 shows a proton density-weighted image with TR = 2,400 ms and TE = 30 ms. Fat and CSF display as a relatively bright signal, and a slight contrast difference between white and gray matter

■ **FIGURE 12-24** Proton density contrast weighting, TR = 2,400 ms, TE = 30 ms. Long TR minimizes T1 relaxation differences of the tissues. Signals with large proton density have higher signal intensity (CSF). Short TE preserves the proton density differences without allowing significant T2 decay. This sequence produces a high peak SNR, even though the contrast differences are less than a T2-weighted image.

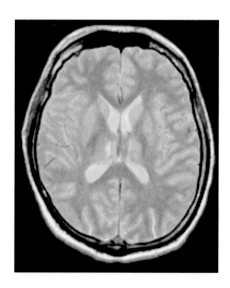

TABLE 12-4 SE PULSE SEQUENCE CONTRAST WEIGHTING PARAMETERS

PARAMETER	T1 CONTRAST	PROTON DENSITY CONTRAST[a]	T2 CONTRAST
TR (ms)	400–600	2,000–4,000	2,000–4,000
TE (ms)	5–30	5–30	60–150

[a]Strictly speaking, SE images with TR less than 3,000 ms are not proton density with respect to the CSF; because of its long T1, only 70% of the CSF magnetization recovery will have occurred and will not appear as bright as for a true PD image. True PD image intensities can be obtained with fast spin echo methods (Chapter 13) with longer TR (*e.g.*, 8,000 ms).
TE, time of echo; TR, time of repetition.

occurs. A typical proton density-weighted image has a TR between 2,000 and 4,000 ms (see footnote in Table 12-4) and a TE between 3 and 30 ms. The proton density SE sequence achieves the highest overall signal intensity and the largest signal-to-noise ratio (SNR); however, the image contrast is relatively low, and therefore the contrast-to-noise ratio is not necessarily larger than achievable with T1 or T2 contrast weighting.

T2 Weighting

T2 contrast weighting follows directly from the proton density-weighting sequence: reduce T1 differences in tissues with a long TR and emphasize T2 differences with a *long* TE. T2 contrast differences are manifested by allowing M_{xy} signal decay as shown in Figure 12-25.

A T2-weighted image (Fig. 12-26) demonstrates high tissue contrast, and the signal intensity in an image is proportional to the T2 values of tissue types (CSF > gray matter > white matter). As TE is increased, more T2-weighted contrast is achieved, but at the expense of less M_{xy} signal and greater image noise. However, even with low signal amplitudes, image processing with *window width* and *window level* adjustments can remap the signals over the full range of the display, so that the overall average brightness is similar for all images. The typical T2-weighted sequence uses a TR of approximately 2,000 to 4,000 ms and a TE of 80 to 120 ms.

T1 Weighting

A "T1-weighted" SE sequence is designed to produce contrast chiefly based on the T1 characteristics of tissues, with de-emphasis of T2 and proton density contributions to

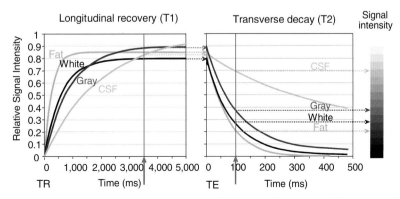

■ **FIGURE 12-25** T2-weighted contrast requires the use of a long TR (*e.g.*, greater than 2,000 ms) to reduce T1 influences, and a long TE (*e.g.*, greater than 80 ms) to allow for T2 decay to evolve. Compared to the proton density weighting, the difference is with longer TE.

■ **FIGURE 12-26** T2 contrast weighting. Long TR minimizes T1 relaxation differences of the tissues. Long TE allows T2 decay differences to be manifested. A second echo provides time for T2 decay to occur, so a T2W image is typically acquired in concert with a PDW image. While this sequence has high contrast, the signal decay reduces the overall signal and therefore the SNR.

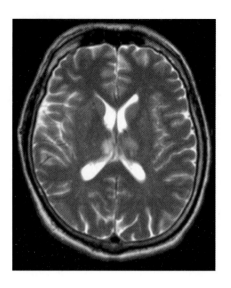

the signal. This is achieved by using a relatively short TR to maximize the differences in longitudinal magnetization recovery during the return to equilibrium, and a short TE to minimize T2 decay during signal acquisition. In Figure 12-27, on the left is the graph of longitudinal recovery in steady-state partial saturation after a 90° RF excitation at time $t = 0$, depicting four tissues (CSF, gray matter, white matter, and fat). The next 90° RF pulse occurs at the selected TR interval, chosen to create the largest signal difference between the tissues based upon their respective T1 recovery values, which is shown to be about 600 ms (the red vertical line). At this instant in time, all M_z recovered for each tissue is converted to M_{xy}, with respective signal amplitudes projected over to the transverse magnetization graph on the right. Decay immediately occurs, $t = 0$, at a rate based upon respective T2 values of the tissues. To minimize T2 decay and to maintain the differences in signal amplitude due to T1 recovery, the TE time is kept short (red vertical line). Horizontal projections from the TE intersection with each of the curves graphically illustrate the relative signal amplitudes acquired according to tissue type. Fat, with a short T1, has a large signal, because there is greater recovery of the M_z vector over the TR period. White matter and gray matter have intermediate T1 values with intermediate signal amplitude, and CSF, with a long

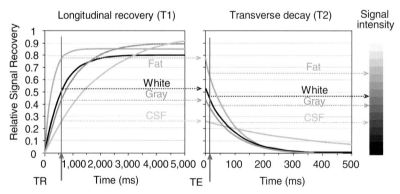

■ **FIGURE 12-27** T1-weighted contrast: Longitudinal recovery (left) and transverse decay (right) diagrams (note the values of the *x*-axis time scales) show four brain tissues and T1 and T2 relaxation constants. T1-weighted contrast requires the selection of a TR that emphasizes the differences in the T1 characteristics of the tissues (*e.g.*, TR = ~500 ms), and reduces the T2 characteristics by using a short TE so that transverse decay is reduced (*e.g.*, TE ≤ 15 ms).

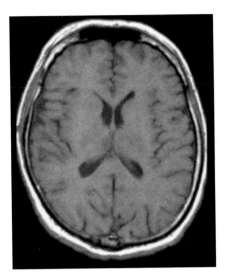

■ **FIGURE 12-28** T1 contrast weighting, TR = 500 ms, TE = 8 ms. Short TR (400 to 600 ms) generates T1 relaxation-dependent signals. Signals with short T1 have high signal intensity (fat and white matter), while signals with long T1 have low signal intensity (CSF). Short TE (less than 15 ms) preserves the T1 tissue differences by not allowing significant T2 decay to occur.

T1, has the lowest signal amplitude. A short TE preserves the T1 signal differences by not allowing any significant transverse (T2) decay.

T1-weighted SE contrast therefore requires a short TR and a short TE. A T1-weighted axial image of the brain acquired with TR = 500 ms and TE = 8 ms is illustrated in Figure 12-28. Fat is the most intense signal, followed by white matter, gray matter, and CSF. Typical SE T1-weighting machine parameters are TR = 400 to 600 ms and TE = 3 to 10 ms.

Spin Echo Parameters

Table 12-4 lists typical contrast-weighting values of TR and TE for SE imaging. For conventional SE sequences, both proton density and T2-weighted contrast signals can be acquired during a single TR by acquiring two echoes with a short TE and a long TE (Fig. 12-29).

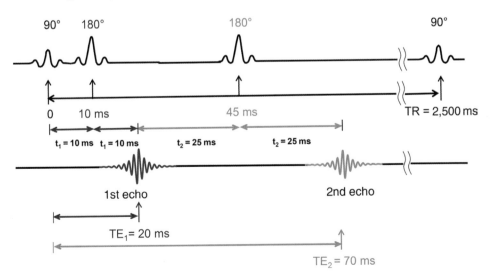

■ **FIGURE 12-29** SE with two 180° refocusing pulses after the initial 90° excitation pulse. The early echo contains information related to proton density of the tissues, and the longer echo provides T2 weighting. This double echo method is used for providing proton density content and T2 weighted content independently during the same TR interval, and used to fill two separate *k*-space repositories that are used in producing the final proton density and T2 weighted images.

Inversion Recovery

IR emphasizes T1 relaxation times of the tissues by extending the amplitude of the longitudinal recovery by a factor of two. An initial 180° RF pulse inverts M_z to $-M_z$. After a programmed delay, the time of inversion—TI, a 90° RF (readout) pulse rotates the recovered fraction of M_z into the transverse plane to generate the FID. A second 180° pulse (or gradient polarity reversal, see next section, GRE) at TE/2 produces an echo at TE (Fig. 12-30); in this situation, the sequence is called *inversion recovery spin echo* (IR SE). The TR for IR is the time between 180° initiation pulses. Partial saturation of the protons and steady-state equilibrium of the longitudinal magnetization is achieved after the first three excitations in the sequence. The echo amplitude associated with a given tissue depends on TI, TE, TR, and magnitude (positive or negative) of M_z.

The signal intensity at a location (x, y) in the image matrix for an IR SE acquisition with non-moving anatomy is approximated as

$$S \propto \rho_H (1 - 2e^{-TI/T1})(1 - e^{-(TR-TI)/T1})(e^{-TE/T2}),$$

where the factor of 2 in the first part of the equation arises from the longitudinal magnetization recovery from $-M_z$ to M_z during TI and turned into the transverse magnetization right after the 90° RF pulse, the second term is the recovery of the longitudinal magnetization from the 90° RF pulse to the next inversion RF pulse, and the last term is T2 decay during TE. For the TI to control contrast between tissues, it follows that TR must be relatively long and TE short. The RF sequence is shown in Figure 12-30 and signal recovery diagram is in Figure 12-31 in case of a long TR for simplicity.

The IR sequence produces "negative" longitudinal magnetization that results in negative (in phase) or positive (out of phase) transverse magnetization when short TI is used. The actual signals are acquired as magnitude (absolute values) such that M_z values are positive. Inversion recovery is used to increase the contrast between tissue types or suppress unwanted tissues, such as fat or fluid. The applications of tissue suppression are described in a later section of this chapter.

Summary, Spin Echo Sequences

MR contrast schemes for clinical imaging use the SE or an IR variant of the SE pulse sequences for many examinations. SE and IR SE sequences are less sensitive

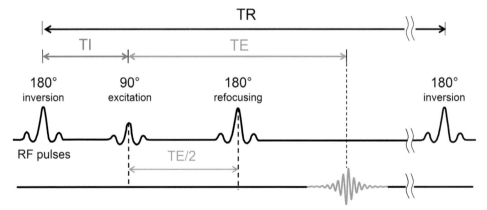

■ **FIGURE 12-30** Inversion-recovery SE sequence is shown. The initial 180° inversion pulse inverts the longitudinal magnetization, and thus requires a factor of two times recovery of the longitudinal magnetization over time. The "inversion time" (TI) is the delay between the inversion pulse and conversion to transverse magnetization of the recovered longitudinal magnetization. Subsequently, a second 180° pulse is applied at TE/2, which refocuses the transverse magnetization as an echo at time TE. The signal strength is chiefly a function of the T1 characteristics of the tissues, as the TE values are kept short.

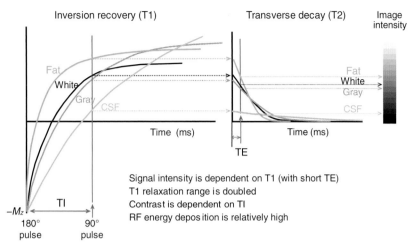

Inversion recovery (T1)   Transverse decay (T2)   Image intensity

Fat
White
Gray
CSF

Time (ms)

TE

Time (ms)

Fat
White
Gray
CSF

Signal intensity is dependent on T1 (with short TE)
T1 relaxation range is doubled
Contrast is dependent on TI
RF energy deposition is relatively high

$-M_z$
180° pulse   TI   90° pulse

■ **FIGURE 12-31** The IR longitudinal recovery diagram shows the $2 \times M_z$ range provided by the 180° excitation pulse. A 90° readout pulse at a time TI and a 180° refocusing pulse at a time TE/2 from the readout pulse forms the echo at time TE. The time scale is not explicitly indicated on the x-axis. A short TE is used to reduce T2 contrast characteristics.

to magnetic field inhomogeneities and magnetic susceptibilities, and generally give high SNR and CNR. The downsides are the relatively long TR and corresponding long acquisition times.

12.6.2 Gradient Echo

The *GRE* technique uses a magnetic field gradient applied in one direction and then reversed to induce the formation of an echo, instead of the 180° inversion pulse. For an FID signal generated under a linear gradient, the transverse magnetization dephases rapidly as the gradient is applied. After a predetermined time, the nearly instantaneous reversal of the GRE polarity will rephase the protons and produce a *GRE* that occurs when the opposite gradient polarity of equal strength has been applied for the same time as the initial gradient. The induced GRE signal is acquired just before and after the peak amplitude, as illustrated in Figure 12-32.

The GRE is not a true SE but a purposeful dephasing and rephasing of the FID used for spatial encoding of signals. Magnetic field (B_0) inhomogeneities and tissue susceptibilities caused by paramagnetic or diamagnetic tissues or contrast agents are emphasized in GRE imaging. This is because the dephasing and rephasing of the FID signals occur based on the spin location in the applied gradient direction, not based on the extrinsic magnetic inhomogeneities. In this situation, unlike a 180° refocusing RF pulse, the external magnetic field variations are not cancelled. Comparing Figures 12-21 and 12-32, the spin dephasing in SE due to the extrinsic magnetic inhomogeneities is compensated after a 180° refocusing RF pulse while the spins are dephased and rephased only due to the applied gradient field in GRE. Significant sensitivity to field non-uniformity and magnetic susceptibility agents thus occurs, as M_{xy} decay is a strong function of T2*, which is much shorter than the "true" T2 achieved in SE sequences. Timing of the GRE is controlled either by inserting a time delay between the negative and positive gradients or by reducing the amplitude of the reversed gradient, thereby extending the time for the rephasing process to occur.

A major variable determining tissue contrast in GRE sequences is the flip angle. Depending on the desired image contrast, flip angles of a few degrees to more than 90° are used, a majority of which are small angles much less than 60°. In the realm

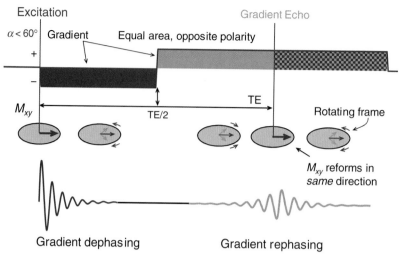

■ **FIGURE 12-32** A magnetic field gradient induces the formation of an "echo" (instead of a 180° RF pulse). Transverse magnetization spins are dephased with an applied gradient of one polarity and rephased with the gradient reversed in polarity; this produces a "gradient echo." Note that the rotating frame depicts the magnetic moment vector of the echo in the *same direction* as the FID relative to the main magnetic field, and therefore extrinsic inhomogeneities are not cancelled.

of very short TR, smaller flip angles require less time and create larger steady-state transverse magnetization compared to larger flip angles. A plot of M_{xy} signal amplitude versus TR as a function of flip angle (Fig. 12-33) shows that smaller flip angles produce more M_{xy} signal than larger flip angles when TR is less than 200 ms. Ultimately, tissue contrast in GRE pulse sequences depends on TR, TE, and flip angle along with specialized manipulation of the acquisition sequence.

Gradient Echo Sequences with Long TR

For GRE sequences with "long" TR (greater than 200 ms) and flip angles greater than 45°, contrast behavior, such as proton density, T1-weighted and T2-weighted, is similar to that of SE sequences. The major difference is image contrast that is based on T2* rather than T2, because external magnetic field inhomogeneities are not cancelled. As for clinical interpretation, the mechanisms of contrast based on T2* are

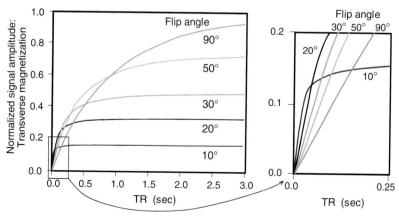

■ **FIGURE 12-33** Transverse magnetization as a function of TR and the flip angle is shown. For small flip angles and very short TR, the transverse magnetization is higher for small flip angles compared to larger flip angles. Detail is shown on the right.

different from those based on T2, particularly for MRI contrast agents. A relatively long TE tends to emphasize the differences between T2* and T2, rather than improve T2 contrast, as would be expected in an SE sequence. T1 weighting is achieved with a short TE (5 to 10 ms). In most situations, however, GRE imaging is not useful with long TR, except when contrast is produced by magnetic susceptibility differences.

Gradient Echo Sequences with Short TR, Less Than 50 ms

Reducing the repetition period below 50 ms (or 2 TR ≪ T2* of tissue) does not allow for transverse decay (T2*) to fully occur, and a steady-state equilibrium of longitudinal and transverse magnetization from pulse to pulse exists. The persistent transverse magnetization is produced from previous RF excitations, and multiple signals are generated: (1) the FID signal generated immediately after the current RF pulse contains T2* or T1 information depending on the TE; (2) a stimulated echo generated from the previous RF pulse acting on the persistent transverse magnetization accruing from the RF pulse twice displaced. The stimulated echo contains T2 and T2* weighting. This is schematically shown in Figure 12-34 for a train of RF pulses and the generated signals.

Given the nature of the overlapping signals, there are generic GRE acquisitions termed coherent, incoherent, and steady-state free precession (SSFP) that provide differential tissue contrast weighting.

Coherent GRE

In GRE sequences with short TR (less than 50 ms) and fixed (flip angle and phase) RF pulses, the measurable spins form coherent signal, the combination of FID and

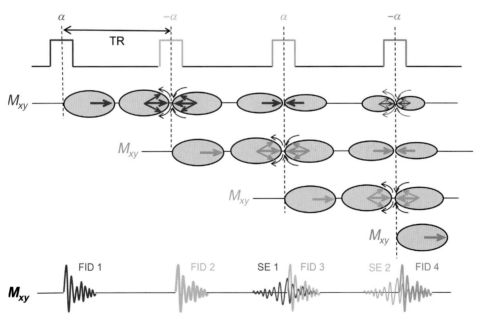

■ **FIGURE 12-34** GRE acquisition with short TR less than 50 ms and flip angles up to 45° produces two signals: (1) the FID from the current RF pulse and (2) stimulated echo from the previous RF pulse resulting from persistent transverse magnetization. These signals overlap, but are shown as distinct in the illustration for clarity. Resultant image contrast is due to the ratio of T1 to T2 in a tissue because of the mixed signals generated by the combined FID (chiefly T1 and T2* contrast) and SE (chiefly T2 and T2* contrast) in the digitized signal. With the train of RF excitation pulses, the second RF pulse stimulates the echo formation of the FID produced from the first RF pulse, which appears during the third RF pulse and superimposes on the current FID. While this is a conceptual illustration, in fact, the actual situation is much more complicated, as there are many higher order stimulated and gradient echoes that contribute to the observed signal.

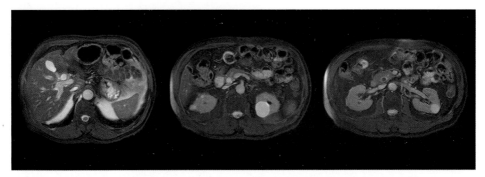

■ **FIGURE 12-35** Three abdominal post gadolinium contrast axial images are part of a breath-hold dataset using a "balanced SSFP" acquisition, which simultaneously accumulates the FID and the stimulated echo with contrast varying according to the T2/T1 ratio (TR: 3.34 ms, TE: 1.2 ms, flip angle 70°, matrix size 192 × 320). Each image is acquired in approximately 700 ms, making this sequence useful for reducing voluntary and involuntary patient motion in contrast enhanced abdominal and cardiac imaging.

stimulated echo signals. A **"Balanced" SSFP** (bSSFP) sequence generates accumulated gradient echo (FID) and stimulated echo signals with the use of symmetrical gradients in 3 spatial directions ("balanced" refers the symmetrical gradients). To effectively generate the stimulated echo signal, the phases of RF pulse are alternating (Fig. 12-35). While it has mainly T2 contrast from the stimulated echo, the fast regrowth of short T1 component contributes more in the coherent echo formation and FID. Therefore, balanced SSFP provides T2/T1 contrast. Because of its high speed, it is particularly useful for cardiac imaging or dynamic imaging. The common acronyms of this technique are TrueFISP and FIESTA. Because the spin refocusing is induced not by 180° inversion but by a small flip angle (30°~60°), the exact phase synchronization between RF pluses and spins is critical and acquired signals have variations due to off-resonance effects. On the affected region that yields a 180° phase error, signal drop-outs are manifested, and are referred to as banding artifacts.

Gradient Spoiling

The signal variations of bSSFP can be avoided using a spoiling gradient, which spreads spin phases within a voxel and removes the transverse magnetization. The spoiler gradient can be applied in any gradient direction or in a combination. Depending on the location of a spoiling gradient, FID or SE can be selectively acquired as shown

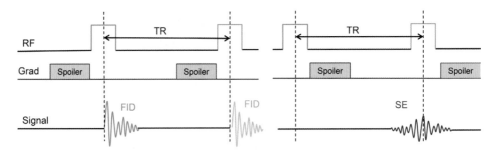

Gradient Recalled Echo   **Steady-State Free Precession**

■ **FIGURE 12-36** Coherent GRE with gradient spoiling: Left, a spoiler gradient is applied before the next RF pulse (after obtaining the echo signal). While FID signal is maintained, the stimulated echo signals from the previous RF pulse are diminished. Right, a spoiler gradient is applied right after an excitation RF pulse to remove the FID signal in order to obtain only the simulated echo signal; this shows T2 weighted contrast.

in Figure 12-36. When a spoiler gradient is applied before the next RF pulse, the stimulated echo signals from the previous RF pulse is diminished and the spin coherence is not perfect any longer (although signals with long T2 still form spin coherence over many TRs). With moderate flip angles of 30° to 60°, the differences in tissue contrast are primarily based upon T2/T1 ratios like bSSFP but with much less SE signals. Since most tissues with a long T2 also have a long T1 and vice versa, there is very little tissue contrast generated. In certain applications such as MR angiography, this is a good outcome because anatomical contrast differences would otherwise compete with the bright blood and reduce the image quality when displayed by image processing techniques (described in Chapter 13). This acquisition technique is described by the acronyms, GRASS (gradient recalled acquisition in the steady state), FISP (*fast imaging with steady-state precession*), FAST (*Fourier acquired steady state*), and other acronyms coined by MRI equipment manufacturers. A GRASS/FISP sequence using TR = 35 ms, TE = 3 ms, and flip angle = 20° shows unremarkable contrast, but in-flowing blood signals show up bright (Fig. 12-37). This technique enhances vascular contrast, from which MR angiography sequences can be reconstructed.

Steady-state free precession (SSFP) sequence emphasizes acquisition of only the stimulated echo, which arises from the previous RF pulse and appears during the next RF pulse at a time equal to 2 × TR (see Fig. 12-36). Although the application of an SSFP sequence is limited, SSFP is often used for 3D volumetric joint imaging because of its true T2-contrast weighting and fast acquisition speed.

Incoherent, "Spoiled" Gradient Echo Techniques

With very short TR steady-state acquisitions, T1 weighting *cannot* be achieved to any great extent, owing to either a small difference in longitudinal magnetization with small flip angles or dominance of the T2* effects for larger flip angles produced by persistent residual transverse magnetization created by stimulated echoes. The T2* influence can be reduced by using a long TR (usually not an option), or by "spoiling" the steady-state transverse magnetization by introducing incoherent phase differences from pulse to pulse. The latter is achieved by adding a phase shift to successive RF pulses during the excitation of protons (called "RF spoiling"). Both the RF transmitter and RF receiver are

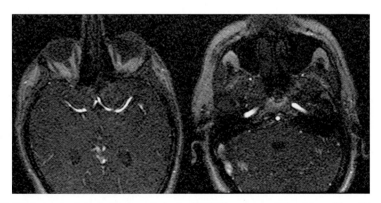

■ **FIGURE 12-37** A *steady-state* gradient recalled echo (GRASS) sequence (TR = 24 ms, TE = 4.7 ms, flip angle = 50°) of two slices out of a volume acquisition is shown. Contrast is unremarkable for white and gray matter because of a T2-/T1-weighting dependence. Blood flow appears as a relatively bright signal. MR angiography (see Chapter 13) depends on pulse sequences such as these to reduce the contrast of the anatomy relative to the vasculature.

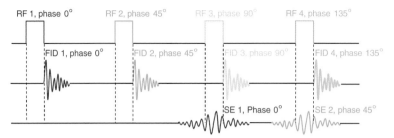

■ **FIGURE 12-38** Incoherent (spoiled) GRE acquisition: Persistent transverse magnetization is dephased by each RF pulse; the superposition of the FID from the current RF pulse with a stimulated-echo from the previous RF pulse is separable, because of differences in the phase of the generated signals. In an actual sequence with TR of 5 to 6 ms, several of stimulated echoes will contribute to the signal, along with the FID. Particular angles of phase increment (typically 117° or 123°) have been determined empirically to cause cancellation by destructive interference of the magnetization from the different coherence pathways to eliminate the signal, leaving only the signal from the FID. T1 contrast can be preferentially generated without contamination of the signals due to the T2 characteristics of the tissues.

phase locked, so that the receiver discriminates the phase of the GRE from the SE generated by the previous RF pulse, now out of phase, as shown in Figure 12-38. Mostly, T1-weighted contrast is obtained, with short TR, short TE, and moderate to large flip angle. This technique is widely used in high-resolution three-dimensional volume acquisitions because of the extremely short acquisition time allowed by the short TR of the GRE sequence and the good contrast rendition of the anatomy provided by T1 weighting (Fig. 12-39). The common acronyms of this technique include SPGR (*S*poiled *g*radient *r*ecalled) and FLASH (*F*ast *l*ow *a*ngle *sh*ot).

MR contrast agents (*e.g.*, gadolinium) produce greater contrast with T1-weighted SPGR than with a comparable T1-weighted SE sequence because of its fast acquisition speed and high resolution. The downsides of spoiled GRE techniques are the increased sensitivity to motion artifacts and non-uniform T1-weighting due to transmit RF field variations (note that small flip angles are more sensitive to RF field variations than larger flip angles like 90°).

Summary, Gradient Echo Contrast

For GRE acquisition in the realm of short TR, persistent transverse magnetization produces two signals: (1) the FID produced from the RF pulse just applied and (2)

■ **FIGURE 12-39** Incoherent (spoiled) GRE images. The ability to achieve T1 contrast weighting is extremely useful for rapid three-dimensional volume imaging. Bright blood (lower portion of each image) and magnetic susceptibility artifacts are characteristic of this sequence. TR = 8 ms, TE = 1.9 ms, flip angle = 20°.

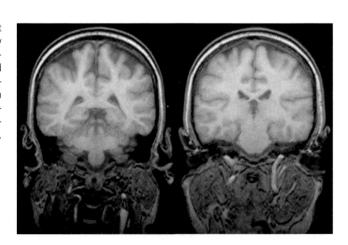

the stimulated echo from the residual transverse magnetization. From these two generated signals, coherent SSFP or spoiled GRE sequences are used in order to generate different contrast-weighting schemes. Coherent GRE uses the combined FID and SE signals and produces contrast mainly depending on the ratio of T2/T1 or T2*/T1; SSFP samples the SE signal only, thus producing signals that are more T2 weighted; and incoherent (or spoiled) GRE produces contrast mainly based on T1.

12.6.3 Tissue Suppression Techniques

One of the advantages of MRI is a capability of selectively suppressing unwanted signals (fat or CSF) in the anatomy that interfere with interpretation of images or cause image artifacts. This can be typically achieved by using two distinct characteristics: T1 relaxation or chemical shift.

Short Tau Inversion Recovery

Short Tau Inversion Recovery, or STIR, is a pulse sequence that uses a very short TI and magnitude image reconstruction, where M_z signal intensity is always positive (Fig. 12-40). In this situation, materials with short T1 have a lower signal intensity (the reverse of a standard T1-weighted image), and all tissues at some point during recovery have $M_z = 0$. This is known as the *bounce point* or tissue null. Selection of an appropriate TI can thus suppress tissue signals (*e.g.*, fats/lipids, CSF) depending on their T1 relaxation times. The signal null ($M_z = 0$) occurs at TI = ln(2) × T1, where ln is the natural log and ln(2) = 0.693. Since T1 for fat at 1.5 T is approximately 260 ms, TI is selected as 0.693 × 260 ms = 180 ms. A typical STIR sequence uses TI of 140 to 180 ms and TR of approximately 2,500 ms. Compared with a T1-weighted examination, STIR reduces distracting fat signals (Fig. 12-41) and chemical shift artifacts (explained in Chapter 13).

Fat Saturation RF Pulse

Besides the relatively short T1 of fat, another unique character of fat is chemical shift. Chemical shift refers to the resonance frequency variations resulting from intrinsic magnetic shielding of anatomic structures. Molecular structure and electron orbital characteristics produce fields that shield the main magnetic field and give rise to distinct peaks in the MR spectrum. The resonance frequency of fat is 3.5 ppm lower than that of water. Chemical shift artifact numerical calculation for field strength, with a

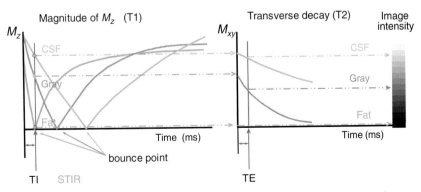

■ **FIGURE 12-40** IR longitudinal magnetization as a function of time, with magnitude signal processing. All tissues go through a null (the bounce point) at a time dependent on T1. The inversion time (TI) is adjusted to select a time to null a certain tissue type. Shown above is the STIR (Short Tau IR) used for suppressing the signal due to fat tissues, achieved with TI = approximately 150 ms (0.693 × 260 ms).

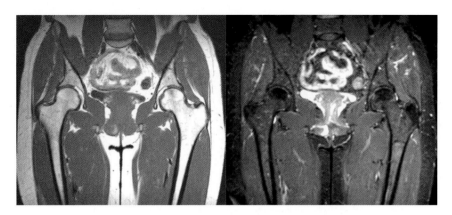

| T1 | STIR |

■ **FIGURE 12-41** SE T1-weighting versus STIR technique. Left: T1 W with TR = 750 ms, TE = 13 ms. Right: STIR with TR = 5,520 ms, TI = 150 ms, TE = 8 ms. The fat is uniformly suppressed in the STIR image, providing details of non-fat structures otherwise difficult to discern.

3.5-ppm (3.5×10^{-6}) variation in resonance frequency between fat and water, results in the following frequency differences:

$$1.5\,T : 63.8 \times 10^{6}\,Hz \times 3.5 \times 10^{-6} = 223\ Hz$$
$$3.0\,T : 127.7 \times 10^{6}\,Hz \times 3.5 \times 10^{-6} = 447\ Hz.$$

Figure 12-42 describes the spectra of fat and water and the pulse diagram of fat saturation RF pulse at 1.5 T. Firstly, a fat saturation RF pulse with the fat resonance frequency excites only fat signal. Its bandwidth (200 Hz) needs to be broad enough to excite the whole fat spectrum. The RF pulse width is at least 2/BW, which is 10 ms. Secondly, a spoiling gradient after the fat saturation RF pulse removes the transverse magnetization of fat. Lastly, a 90° on-resonance RF pulse excites only water signal. This fat saturation technique is mostly common at 1.0 T or higher because the pulse duration is short (in the same way, 5 ms at 3 T). Compared to the STIR technique, this technique maintains full water signal and, therefore, higher SNR can be achieved. However, it is sensitive to off-resonance fields and imperfect fat saturation is often observed on a large FOV. This technique is also referred to as Chem Sat (*Chemical saturation*) or CHESS (*Chemical shift selective*).

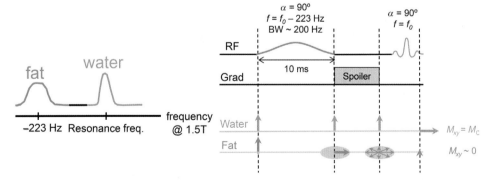

■ **FIGURE 12-42** Description of chemical saturation: Fat signal has a 223 Hz lower resonance frequency than water signal at 1.5 T because of chemical shift. A fat saturation RF pulse at the fat resonance frequency excites only fat signal and a spoiling gradient after the fat saturation RF pulse completely saturates the transverse magnetization of fat before a water excitation RF pulse.

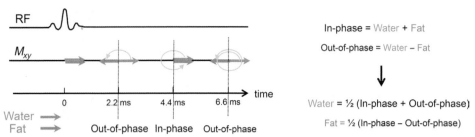

■ FIGURE 12-43 Description of a fat/water separation technique (Dixon method): Due to the chemical shift of fat, the fat and the water spins are out of phase at 2.2 ms, 6.6 ms, and so on while in phase at 0, 4.4 ms, and so on right after the excitation RF pulse is applied at 1.5 T. From the images collected while fat and water spins are in-phase and out-of-phase, the amount of fat and water can be estimated by the linear operation. The method produces four different images: in-phase, out-of-phase, water, and fat images.

Fat Separation

Previously described methods are to suppress fat signals in images, but there are needs to qualitatively or quantitatively visualize fat signal as well as water signal (*i.e.*, fat fraction in fatty liver or fat infiltration in muscles). In multi-echo GRE sequences, phase evolution of fat signal due to chemical shift distinguishes from water signal depending on the choice of echo times. Described previously, the chemical shift between fat and water yields the resonance frequency difference of 223 Hz at 1.5 T, which is interpreted as their being in-phase every 4.4 ms. As described in Figure 12-43, the fat and the water spins are out of phase at 2.2 ms, 6.6 ms, and so on, while in phase at 0, 4.4 ms, and so on, right after the excitation RF pulse is applied. From the images collected while fat and water spins are in-phase and out-of-phase, the amount of fat and water can be estimated as shown in Figure 12-44. This approach is called the 2-point Dixon method. The 2-point Dixon method is significantly sensitive to off-resonance fields because the estimation of fat or water contents is based on an assumption that water spins are on resonance. Another challenge in accurate fat quantification is that the intensities of two echoes are not identical due to T2* decays and even the T2* values of water and fat are different. In addition, iron deposition causing local field inhomogeneities in a certain organ makes accurate estimation even more difficult. To overcome these limitations, 3 or more echoes can be collected to additionally estimate T2* of fat and water and, ultimately, fat fraction.

Fluid Attenuated Inversion Recovery

The signal levels of CSF and other tissues with long T1 relaxation constants can be overwhelming in the magnitude IR image. Fluid attenuated IR, the *FLAIR* sequence, reduces CSF signal and other water-bound anatomy in the MR image by using a TI selected at or near the bounce point of CSF to permit better evaluation of the surrounding anatomy as shown in Figure 12-45. Reducing the CSF signal (T1 ≈ 2,500 ms at 1.5 T) requires TI = 0.693 × 2,500 ms, or ≈1,700 ms. A comparison of T1, T2, and FLAIR sequences demonstrates the contrast differences achievable by reducing signals of one tissue to be able to visualize another (see Fig. 12-46).

12.7 MR SIGNAL LOCALIZATION

Spatial localization is essential for creating MR images and determining the location of discrete sample volumes for MRS. This is achieved by superimposing linear magnetic field variations on the main (B_0) field to generate corresponding position-dependent

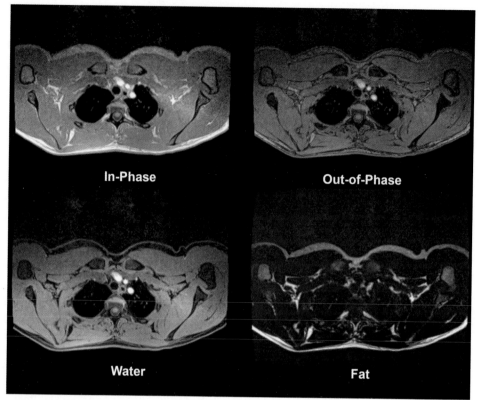

■ FIGURE 12-44 An example of 2-point Dixon method: In-phase and out-of-phase images were collected by a dual-echo GRE sequence with a TE of 2.6 ms and 1.4 ms, respectively, at 3 T.

variations in precessional frequency of the protons. Simultaneous application of an RF excitation (B_1 pulse) excites only those protons in resonance within the frequency bandwidth (BW) of the B_1 RF pulse by absorbing energy.

In the rotating frame of reference, incremental changes of frequency occur symmetrically about the null, and the positions of protons are encoded by frequency and phase. The frequency BW is the range of frequencies over the FOV, and the frequency BW per pixel is the BW divided by the number of discrete samples. Gradient amplitude can also be expressed in frequency per distance. For instance, a 10-mT/m

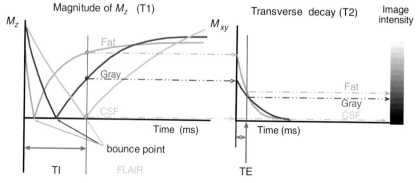

■ FIGURE 12-45 Shown above is the FLAIR acquisition, with the TI set to the null of CSF, which reduces the large CSF signals and allows the visualization of subtle details otherwise hidden. TE is short to not allow T2 "contamination" of the signals.

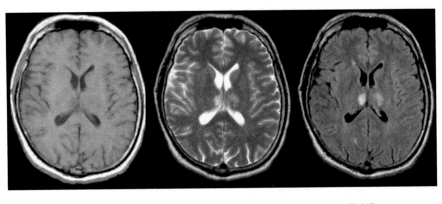

T1	T2	FLAIR

■ **FIGURE 12-46** Left: T1-weighted spin-echo axial brain image (TR = 549 ms, TE = 11 ms); Middle: T2 weighted spin-echo image (TR = 2,400 ms, TE = 90 ms); Right: FLAIR image (TR = 10,000 ms, TI = 2,400 ms, TE = 150 ms).

gradient can be expressed as 10 mT/m × 42.58 MHz/T × 1 T/1,000 mT = 0.4258 MHz/m, which is equivalent to 425.8 kHz/m or 425.8 Hz/mm (Table 12-5). The relationship of gradient strength and frequency BW across the FOV is independent of the main magnet field strength.

Localization of protons in the three-dimensional volume requires the application of three distinct gradients during the pulse sequence: slice selective, frequency encoding, and phase encoding. These gradients are sequenced in a specific order, depending on the pulse sequences employed. Often, the three gradients overlap partially or completely during the scan to achieve a desired spin state, or to leave protons in their original phase state after the application of the gradient(s).

12.7.1 Slice Selection

RF transmitters cannot spatially direct the RF energy to a specific region in the body; rather the RF pulse, when turned on during the application of the slice selective gradient (SSG), determines the slice location of protons in the tissues that absorb

TABLE 12-5 PRECESSIONAL FREQUENCY VARIATION AT 1.5 T ALONG AN APPLIED GRADIENT

Main magnetic field strength	1.5 T
Gradient field strength	10 mT/m = 425.8 Hz/mm
FOV	0.24 m = 240 mm
Linear gradient amplitude over FOV	2.4 mT; from −1.2 mT to +1.2 mT
Maximum magnetic field (frequency)	1.5012 T (63.921096 MHz)
Unchanged magnetic field at null	1.500000 T (63.8700000 MHz)
Minimum magnetic field	1.4988 T (63.818904 MHz)
Net frequency range across FOV[a]	0.102192 MHz = 102.192 kHz =102,192 Hz
Frequency range across FOV (1,278 Hz/cm)[b]	425.8 Hz/mm × 240 mm = 102,192 Hz
Frequency BW per pixel (256 samples)	102,192 Hz/256 = 399.2 Hz/pixel

[a]Calculated using the absolute precessional frequency range: 63.921096–63.18904 MHz.
[b]Calculated using the gradient strength expressed in Hz/mm.

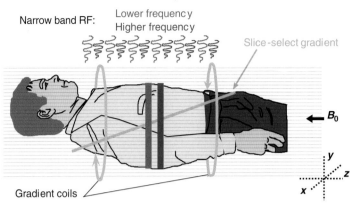

■ **FIGURE 12-47** The *SSG* disperses the precessional frequencies of the protons in a known way along the gradient. A narrow band RF pulse excites only a selected volume (slice) of tissues, determined by frequency, BW, and SSG strength. In the example above, two narrow-band RF pulses with different center frequencies irradiate the whole body during the application of the gradient, and only those protons at the same frequencies as the RF pulses will absorb energy. Note that the higher frequency slice is shifted towards the positive pole of the applied gradient.

energy. For axial MR images, the SSG is applied along the long (cranial-caudal) axis of the body. Under the influence of the gradient field, the proton precessional frequencies in the volume are incrementally increased or decreased dependent on their distance from the gradient isocenter. A selective, narrow band RF frequency pulse of a known duration and amplitude delivers energy to the total volume, but only those protons with precessional frequencies matching the RF BW frequencies will absorb energy within a defined slice of tissues as shown in Figure 12-47 (red vertical line indicates energy absorbed due to resonance). If the center frequency of the RF pulse is increased, then a different slab of protons absorbs energy (blue vertical line).

Slice thickness is chiefly determined by the frequency BW of the RF pulse and the gradient strength across the slice. For a fixed gradient strength, the RF pulse with a narrow BW excites protons within a thin slice, and a wide BW excites a thick slice (Fig. 12-48A). For a fixed RF BW, a high gradient strength produces a large range of frequencies across the FOV and decreases the slice thickness, whereas a low gradient strength produces a small range of frequencies and produces an increase in the slice thickness (Fig. 12-48B).

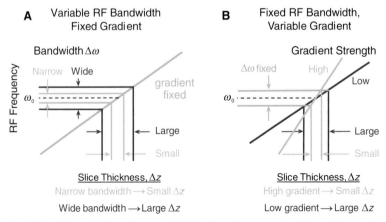

■ **FIGURE 12-48** Slice thickness is dependent on RF BW and gradient strength. **A.** For a fixed gradient strength, the RF BW determines the slice thickness. **B.** For a fixed RF BW, gradient strength determines the slice thickness.

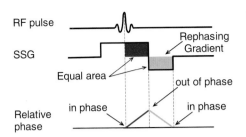

■ **FIGURE 12-49** SSG rephasing. At the peak of the RF pulse, all protons in the slice are in phase, but the SSG causes the spins to become dephased after the gradient is turned off. To reestablish phase coherence, a reverse polarity gradient is applied equal to one-half the area of the original SSG. At the next pulse, the relative phase will be identical.

A combination of a narrow BW and a low gradient strength or a wide BW and a high gradient strength can result in the same slice thickness. In general, a wide BW and a high gradient strength is preferred at a given slice thickness because RF pulse width is short and chemical shift artifacts through the slice direction are minimized.

After the SSG is turned off, the protons revert to the precessional frequency of the main magnetic field, but phase coherence across slice is lost. To reestablish the original phase of all stationary protons, a gradient of opposite polarity equal to one half of the area of the original SSG is applied (Fig. 12-49). For 180° refocusing RF excitations, the rephasing gradient is not necessary, as all protons maintain their phase relationships because of the symmetry of the RF pulse and spin inversion.

To summarize, the SSG is applied simultaneously with an RF pulse of a known BW to create proton excitation in a single plane with a known slice thickness, and to localize signals orthogonal to the gradient. It is the first of three gradients applied to the volume.

12.7.2 Frequency Encoding

The frequency encoding gradient (FEG), also known as the *readout gradient,* is applied in a direction perpendicular to the SSG, along the "logical" x-axis, during the evolution and decay of the induced echo. Net changes in precessional frequencies are distributed symmetrically from 0 at the gradient isocenter to $+f_{max}$ and $-f_{max}$ at the edges of the FOV (Fig. 12-50) under the applied FEG. The composite signal is amplified, digitized, and processed by the Fourier transform to convert frequency into spatial position (Fig. 12-51). A spatial "projection" is created by integrating the resultant Fourier transformed signal amplitudes perpendicular to the direction of the applied gradient at corresponding spatial positions. The frequency encoding can be described as an analogy of pressing multiple keys on a piano simultaneously. Each key on a piano has a unique pitch (*i.e.*, frequency) and pressure on a key is intensity at a certain frequency. When we apply Fourier transform of recorded sound, we have information of what keys were pressed and how hard each key was pressed.

Similar to SSG, the strength of FEG determines the bandwidth across FOV. Decisions depend chiefly on the SNR and the propensity for "chemical shift" artifacts. SNR is inversely proportional to the receiver BW: $SNR \propto \dfrac{1}{\sqrt{BW}}$; therefore, narrow BW and low gradient strength are preferred; however, artifacts due to *chemical shift* (see Chapter 13, Section 13.5, Chemical Shift Artifacts) is more pronounced and the allowable minimum TE, if desired, is longer. Consequently, trade-offs in image quality must be considered when determining the optimal RF BW and FEG field strength combinations (further described in Section 12.9.5).

The SSG in concert with an incremental rotation of the FEG direction about the object can produce data projections through the object as a function of angle, as shown in Figure 12-52. With a sufficient number of projections, filtered backprojection

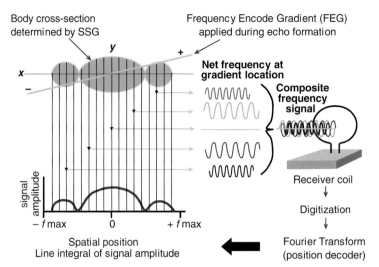

■ **FIGURE 12-50** The *FEG* is applied in an orthogonal direction to the SSG, and confers *a spatially dependent variation* in the precessional frequencies of the protons. Acting only on those protons in a slice determined by the SSG excitation, the composite signal is acquired, digitized, demodulated (Larmor frequency removed), and Fourier transformed into frequency and amplitude information. A one-dimensional array represents a *projection* of the slice of tissue (amplitude and position) at a specific angle. (Demodulation into net frequencies occurs *after* detection by the receiver coil; this is shown in the figure for clarity only.)

can be used for reconstructing a tomographic image (see Chapter 11 on CT Reconstruction). In fact, this is how some of the first MR images were reconstructed from individual projections, using a rotating FEG (variants of this scheme are described in Chapter 13). However, inefficient acquisition and complicated data handling

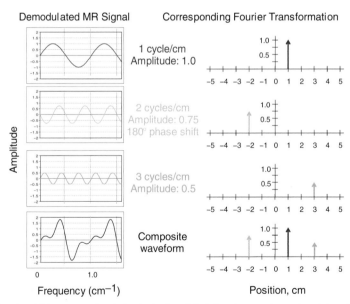

■ **FIGURE 12-51** Spatial frequency signals (cycles/cm) and their Fourier transforms (spatial position) are shown for three simple sinusoidal waveforms with a specific amplitude and phase. The Fourier transform decodes the frequency, phase, and amplitude variations in the spatial frequency domain into a corresponding position and amplitude in the spatial domain. A 180° phase shift (second from the top) is shifted in the negative direction from the origin. The composite waveform (a summation of all waveforms, lower left) is decoded by Fourier transformation into the corresponding positions and amplitudes (lower right).

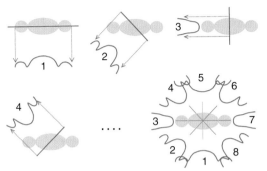

■ **FIGURE 12-52** A rotating FEG in the *x–y* plane allows the acquisition of individual projections as a function of angle, by repeating the SSG-FEG sequence with incremental change of the FEG direction. This example shows eight projections; to have sampling sufficient for high SNR and resolution would require hundreds of projections about the object.

due to unique artifacts have led to near-universal acquisition with phase encoding techniques.

12.7.3 Phase Encoding

Position of the protons in the third orthogonal dimension is determined with a phase encoding gradient (PEG), which is applied after the SSG but before the FEG, along the third orthogonal axis. Phase in this context represents a linear variation in the starting point of sinusoidal waves that precess at the same frequency. Phase changes are purposefully introduced by the application of a short duration PEG within each DAQ interval. Prior to the PEG, all protons have the same phase, and turning on the PEG introduces a linear variation in the precessional frequency of the protons according to their position along the gradient. After a brief interval, the PEG is turned off, all protons revert to the Larmor frequency, and linear phase shifts are manifested by a specific gradient strength and polarity. Incremental positive phase change is introduced for protons under the positive pole, negative phase change is introduced under the negative pole, and no phase change occurs for protons at the isocenter of the PEG. Throughout the acquisition sequence, the PEG strength and polarity is incrementally changed to introduce specific known phase changes as a function of position across the FOV for each acquisition interval (Fig. 12-53). Spatial encoding is determined by the amount of phase shift that has occurred. Protons located at the center of the FOV, the PEG isocenter, do not

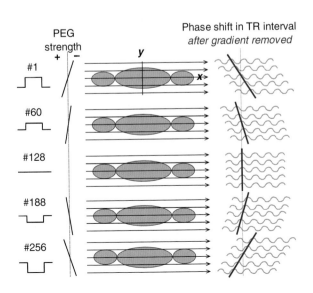

■ **FIGURE 12-53** The PEG is applied *before* the FEG and *after* the SSG. The PEG produces a spatially dependent variation in angular frequency of the excited spins for a brief duration, and generates a spatially dependent variation in phase when the spins return to the Larmor frequency. Incremental changes in the PEG strength for each TR interval spatially encodes the phase variations: protons at the isocenter of the PEG do not experience any phase change, while protons in the periphery experience a large phase change dependent on their distance from the null. The incremental variation of the PEG strength can be thought of as providing specific "views" of the volume because the SSG and FEG remain fixed throughout the acquisition.

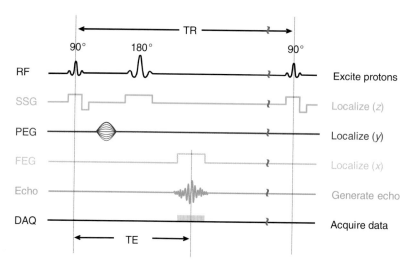

■ **FIGURE 12-54** A typical spin-echo pulse sequence diagram indicates the timing of the SSG, PEG, and FEG during the repetition time (TR) interval, synchronized with the RF pulses and the DAQ when the echo appears. Each TR interval is repeated with a different PEG strength (this appears as multiple lines in the illustration, but only one PEG strength is applied per TR as indicated by the bold line in this figure). *Note:* The amplitude of the FEG determines the bandwidth of the evolving echo and data acquisition.

exhibit a phase shift. Protons located at the edges of the FOV exhibit the largest positive to negative (or negative to positive) phase shifts. Protons located at intermediate distances from the isocenter experience intermediate phase shifts (positive or negative). Each location along the phase encode axis is spatially encoded by the amount of phase shifts experienced by the protons. For sequential acquisition sequences, each sample in the PEG direction is separated in time by the TR interval.

12.7.4 Gradient Sequencing

An acquisition of an *SE* pulse sequence is illustrated in Figure 12-54, showing the timing of the SSG in conjunction with the 90° RF excitation pulse, the application of a short duration PEG at a known strength, followed by a 180° refocusing RF pulse at TE/2, and the echo envelope with the peak amplitude occurring at TE. This sequence is repeated with slight incremental changes in the PEG strength to define the three dimensions in the image over the acquisition time.

12.8 "K-SPACE" DATA ACQUISITION AND IMAGE RECONSTRUCTION

MR data are initially stored in the *k*-space matrix, the "spatial frequency domain" repository (Fig. 12-55). *k*-Space describes a two-dimensional matrix of positive and negative spatial frequency values, encoded as complex numbers (e.g., $a + bi$, $i = \sqrt{-1}$). The matrix is divided into four quadrants, with the origin at the center representing frequency $= 0$. Frequency domain data are encoded in the k_x direction by the FEG, and in the k_y direction by the PEG in most image sequences. The lowest spatial frequency increment (the fundamental frequency) is the BW across each pixel (see Table 12-5). The maximum useful frequency (the Nyquist frequency) is equal to ½ frequency range across the k_x or k_y directions, as the frequencies are encoded from

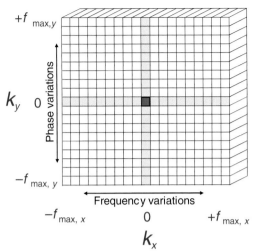

■ **FIGURE 12-55** The k-space matrix is the repository for spatial frequency signals acquired during the evolution and decay of the echo. The k_x axis (along the rows) and the k_y axis (along the columns) have units of cycles/unit distance. Each axis is symmetric about the center of k-space, ranging from $-f_{max}$ to $+f_{max}$ along the rows and the columns. The matrix is filled one row at a time in a conventional acquisition with the FEG-induced frequency variations mapped along the k_x axis and the PEG-induced phase variations mapped along the k_y axis.

$-f_{max}$ to $+f_{max}$. The periodic nature of the frequency domain has a built-in symmetry described by "symmetric" and "antisymmetric" functions (*e.g.*, cosine and sine waves). "Real," "imaginary," and "magnitude" describe specific phase and amplitude characteristics of the composite MR frequency waveforms. Partial acquisitions are possible (*e.g.*, one half of the k-space matrix plus one line) with complex conjugate symmetry filling the remainder (see Chapter 13, Section "Data Synthesis").

12.8.1 Two-Dimensional Data Acquisition

MR data are acquired as a complex, composite frequency waveform. With methodical variations of the PEG during each excitation, the k-space matrix is filled to produce the desired variations across the frequency and phase encoding directions as shown in Figure 12-56.

A summary description of the two-dimensional spin-echo image acquisition steps follows.

1. A narrow band RF excitation pulse simultaneously applied with the SSG causes a specific slab of tissues with protons at the same frequency to absorb energy. Transverse magnetization, M_{xy}, is produced with amplitude dependent on the saturation of the protons and the angle of excitation. A 90° flip angle produces the largest M_{xy}.
2. A PEG is applied for a brief duration, which introduces a phase difference among the protons along the phase encode direction to produce a specific "view" of the data along the k_y axis, corresponding to the strength of the PEG.
3. A refocusing 180° RF pulse is delivered at TE/2 to invert and reestablish the phase coherence of the transverse magnetization at time TE.
4. During the evolution and decay of the echo signal, the FEG is applied orthogonal to both the SSG and PEG directions, generating spatially dependent changes in the precessional frequencies of the protons.
5. Data sampling and acquisition of the complex signal occurs simultaneous to the FEG. A one-dimensional inverse Fourier transform converts the digital data into discrete frequency values and corresponding amplitudes to determine position along the k_x (readout) direction.
6. Data are deposited in the k-space matrix at a row location specifically determined by the strength of the PEG. For each TR, an incremental variation of the PEG strength sequentially fills each row. In some sequences, the phase encode

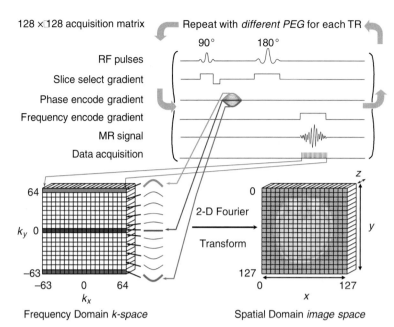

■ **FIGURE 12-56** MR data are acquired into *k*-space matrix, where each row in *k*-space represents spatially dependent frequency variations under a fixed FEG strength, and each column represents spatially dependent phase shift variations under an incrementally varied PEG strength. Data are placed in a specific row determined by the PEG strength for each TR interval. The grayscale image is constructed from the two-dimensional Fourier transformation of the *k*-space matrix by sequential application of one-dimensional transforms along each row, and then along each column of the intermediate transformed data. The output image matrix is arranged with the image coordinate pair, $x = 0$, $y = 0$ at the upper left of the image matrix.

data are acquired in non-sequential order to fill portions of *k*-space more pertinent to the requirements of the exam (*e.g.*, in the low-frequency, central area of *k*-space). Once filled, the *k*-space matrix columns contain positionally dependent variations in phase change along the k_y (phase encode) direction.

7. After all rows are filled, an inverse Fourier transform decodes the frequency domain variations in phase for each of the columns of *k*-space to produce the spatial domain representation.

8. The final image is scaled and adjusted to represent the proton density, T1, T2, and flow characteristics of the tissues using a grayscale range, where each pixel represents a voxel.

The bulk of image information representing the lower spatial frequencies is contained in the center of *k*-space, whereas the higher spatial frequencies are contained in the periphery, as shown in Figure 12-57, representing a grayscale rendition of *k*-space for a sagittal slice of a brain MR image acquisition. The innermost areas represent the bulk of the anatomy, while the outer areas of *k-space* represent the detail and resolution components of the anatomy, as shown by reconstructed images.

12.8.2 Two-Dimensional Multiplanar Acquisition

Direct axial, coronal, sagittal, or oblique planes can be obtained by energizing the appropriate gradient coils during the image acquisition, as shown in Figure 12-58. The SSG determines the orientation of the slices: axial uses *z*-axis coils; coronal uses *y*-axis coils; and sagittal uses *x*-axis coils for selection of the slice orientation. Oblique plane acquisition depends on a combination of the *x*-, *y*-, and *z*-axis coils energized simultaneously. SSG, PEG, and FEG applications are perpendicular to each other,

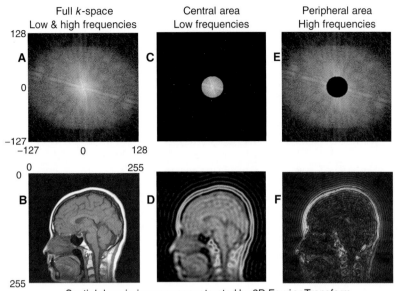

Full *k*-space
Low & high frequencies

Central area
Low frequencies

Peripheral area
High frequencies

Spatial domain images reconstructed by 2D Fourier Transform

■ **FIGURE 12-57 A.** Image representations of *k-space* segmentation show a concentration of information around the origin (the *k*-space images are logarithmically amplified for display of the lowest amplitude signals). **B.** Inverse two-dimensional Fourier transformation converts the data into a visible image. **C.** Segmenting a radius of 25 pixels out of 128 in the central area and zeroing out the periphery extracts a majority of the low-frequency information. **D.** The corresponding image demonstrates the majority of the image content is in the center of *k*-space. **E.** Zeroing out the central portion and leaving the peripheral areas isolates the higher spatial frequency signals. **F.** The resulting image is chiefly comprised of high frequency detail and resolution. Ringing that is visible in the image is due to the sharp masking transition from the image data to zero.

and acquisition of data into the *k*-space matrix remains the same, with the FEG along the k_x axis and the PEG along the k_y axis.

12.8.3 Three-Dimensional Image Acquisition

Three-dimensional image acquisition (volume imaging) requires the use of a broadband, non-selective, or "slab-selective" RF pulse to excite a large volume of protons simultaneously. Two phase gradients are discretely applied in the slice encode and phase encode directions, prior to the frequency encoding (readout) gradient (Fig. 12-59). A three-dimensional Fourier transform (three one-dimensional Fourier transforms) is applied for each column, row, and depth axis in the image matrix

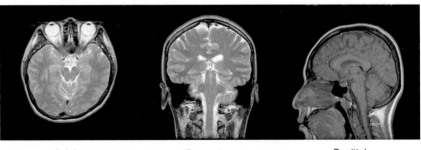

Axial   Coronal   Sagittal

■ **FIGURE 12-58** Direct acquisitions of axial, coronal, and sagittal tomographic images are possible by electronically energizing the magnetic field gradients in a different order without moving the patient. Oblique planes can also be obtained. PEG (k_y axis) and FEG (k_x axis) are perpendicular to the SSG.

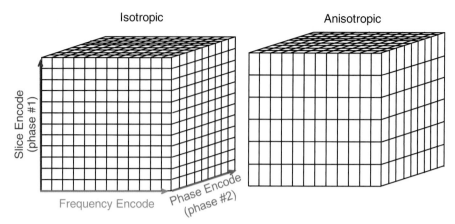

Isotropic   Anisotropic

Slice Encode (phase #1)

Frequency Encode   Phase Encode (phase #2)

■ **FIGURE 12-59** Three-dimensional image acquisition requires the application of a broadband RF pulse to excite all of the protons in the volume simultaneously, followed by a phase encode gradient along the slice encode direction, a phase encode gradient along the phase encode direction, and a frequency encode gradient in the readout direction. Spatial location is decoded sequentially by the Fourier transform along each encode path, storing intermediate results in the three-dimensional *k*-space matrix.

"cube." Volumes obtained can be either isotropic, the same size in all three directions, or anisotropic, where at least one dimension is different in size. The advantage of the former is equal resolution in all directions; reformations of images from the volume do not suffer from degradations of larger sample size from other directions. After the spatial domain data are obtained, individual two-dimensional slices in any arbitrary plane are extracted by interpolation of the cube data.

A major benefit to isotropic three-dimensional acquisition is the uniform resolution in all directions when extracting any two-dimensional image from the matrix cube. In addition, high SNR is achieved compared to a similar two-dimensional image, allowing reconstruction of very thin slices with good detail (less partial volume averaging) and high SNR. Downsides are the increased probability of motion artifacts and increased computer hardware requirements for data handling and storage.

12.9 MR IMAGE CHARACTERISTICS

12.9.1 Spatial Resolution and Contrast Sensitivity

Spatial resolution, contrast sensitivity, and SNR parameters form the basis for evaluating the MR image characteristics. The spatial resolution is dependent on the FOV, which determines pixel size; the gradient field strength, which determines the FOV; the receiver coil characteristics (head coil, body coil, and various surface coil designs); the sampling bandwidth; and the image matrix. Common image matrix sizes are 128 × 128, 256 × 128, 256 × 192, and 256 × 256, with 512 × 256, 512 × 512, and 1,024 × 512 becoming prevalent. In general, MR provides spatial resolution approximately equivalent to that of CT, with pixel dimensions on the order of 0.5 to 1.0 mm for a high-contrast object and a reasonably large FOV (greater than 250 mm). A 250 mm FOV and a 256 × 256 matrix will have a pixel size on the order of 1 mm. In small FOV acquisitions with high gradient strengths and with surface coil receivers, the effective pixel size can be smaller than 0.1 to 0.2 mm (of course, with a limited FOV of 25 to 50 mm). Slice thickness in MRI is usually 5 to 10 mm and represents the dimension that produces the most partial volume averaging.

Spatial resolution can be improved with higher field strength magnets due to a larger SNR, which allows thinner slice acquisition, and/or higher sampling rates (smaller pixels) for a given acquisition. However, with higher B_0, increased RF absorption, artifact production, and a lengthening of T1 relaxation occur. The latter decreases T1 contrast sensitivity because of increased saturation of the longitudinal magnetization.

Contrast sensitivity is the major attribute of MR. The spectacular contrast sensitivity of MR enables the exquisite discrimination of soft tissues and contrast due to blood flow. This sensitivity is achieved through differences in the T1, T2, proton density, and flow velocity characteristics. Contrast, which is dependent upon these parameters, is achieved through the proper application of pulse sequences, as discussed previously. MR contrast materials, usually susceptibility agents that disrupt the local magnetic field to enhance T2 decay or provide a relaxation mechanism for shorter T1 recovery time (*e.g.*, bound water in hydration layers), are becoming important enhancement agents for differentiation of normal and diseased tissues. The absolute contrast sensitivity of the MR image is ultimately limited by the SNR and presence of image artifacts.

12.9.2 Signal-to-Noise Ratio

There are numerous dependencies on the ultimate SNR achievable by the MR system. The intrinsic signal intensity based on T1, T2, and proton density parameters has been discussed; to summarize, the TR, TE, and flip angle will have an impact on the magnitude of the signal generated in the image. While there are many mitigating factors, a long TR increases the longitudinal magnetization recovery and increases the SNR; a long TE increases the transverse magnetization decay and reduces the SNR; a smaller flip angle (reduced from 90°) reduces the SNR. Therefore, SE pulse sequences with large flip angle, long TR, short TE, coarse matrix, large FOV, thick slices, and many averages will generate the best SNR; however, the resultant image may not be clinically relevant or desirable. While SNR is important, it's not everything.

For a given pulse sequence (TR, TE, flip angle), the SNR of the MR image is dependent on a number of variables, as shown in the equation below for a two-dimensional image acquisition:

$$\text{SNR} \propto I \times \text{voxel}_{x,y,z} \times \frac{\sqrt{\text{NEX}}}{\sqrt{\text{BW}}} \times f(\text{QF}) \times f(\boldsymbol{B}) \times f(\text{slice gap}) \times f(\text{reconstruction}),$$

where I is the intrinsic signal intensity based on pulse sequence; $\text{voxel}_{x,y,z}$ is the voxel volume, determined by FOV, image matrix, and slice thickness; NEX is the number of excitations, determined by the number (or fractional number) of repeated signal acquisitions into the same voxels; BW is the frequency bandwidth of the RF receiver; $f(\text{QF})$ is the function of the coil quality factor parameter (tuning the coil); $f(\boldsymbol{B})$ is the function of magnetic field strength, $\boldsymbol{B}$; $f(\text{slice gap})$ is the function of interslice gap effects; and $f(\text{reconstruction})$ is the function of the reconstruction algorithm.

The variables in the above equation are explained briefly below.

12.9.3 Voxel Volume

The voxel volume is equal to

$$\text{Volume} = \frac{\text{FOV}_x}{\text{No. of pixels}, \, x} \times \frac{\text{FOV}_y}{\text{No. of pixels}, \, y} \times \text{Slice thickness}, \, z.$$

SNR is linearly proportional to the voxel volume. Thus, by reducing the image matrix size from 256×256 to 256×128 over the same FOV, the effective voxel size increases by a factor of two, and therefore increases the SNR by a factor of two for the same image acquisition time (*e.g.*, 256 phase encodes with one average versus 128 phase encodes with two averages).

12.9.4 Signal Averages

Signal averaging (also known as number of excitations, NEX) is achieved by averaging sets of data acquired using an identical pulse sequence (same PEG strength). The SNR is proportional to the square root of the number of signal averages. A 2-NEX acquisition requires a doubling (100% increase) of the acquisition time for a 40% increase in the SNR($\sqrt{2} = 1.4$). Doubling the SNR requires 4 NEX. In some cases, less than 1 average (*e.g.*, ½ or ¾ NEX) can be selected. Here, the number of phase encode steps is reduced by ½ or ¼, and the missing data are synthesized in the *k*-space matrix. Imaging time is therefore reduced by a similar amount; however, a loss of SNR accompanies the shorter imaging times by the same square root factor.

12.9.5 RF Bandwidth

The receiver bandwidth defines the range of frequencies to which the detector is tuned during the application of the readout gradient. A narrow bandwidth (a narrow spread of frequencies around the center frequency) provides a higher SNR, proportional to $\dfrac{1}{\sqrt{BW}}$. A twofold reduction in RF bandwidth—from 8 to 4 kHz, for instance—increases the SNR by $1.4 \times$ (40% increase). This is mainly related to the fact that the white noise, which is relatively constant across the bandwidth, does not change, while the signal distribution changes with bandwidth. In the spatial domain, bandwidth is inversely proportional to the sample dwell time, ΔT to sample the signal: $BW = 1/\Delta T$. Therefore, a narrow bandwidth has a longer dwell time, which increases the signal height (Fig. 12-60), compared to the shorter dwell time for the broad bandwidth signal, thus spreading the signal over a larger range of frequencies. The SNR is reduced by the square root of the dwell time. However, any decrease in RF bandwidth must be coupled with a decrease in gradient strength to maintain the sampling across the FOV, which might be unacceptable if chemical shift artifacts are of concern (see Artifacts, Chapter 13). Narrower bandwidths also require a longer time for sampling, and therefore affect the minimum TE time that is possible for an imaging sequence. Clinical situations that can use narrow bandwidths are with T2-weighted images and long TEs that allow the echo to evolve over an extended period, particularly in situations where fat saturation pulses are used to reduce the effects of chemical shift in the acquired images. Use of broad bandwidth settings is necessary when very short TEs are required, such as in fast GRE imaging to reduce the sampling time.

12.9.6 RF Coil Quality Factor

The coil quality factor is an indication of RF coil sensitivity to induced currents in response to signals emanating from the patient. Coil losses that lead to lowered SNR are caused by patient "loading" effects and eddy currents, among other factors. Patient loading refers to the electric impedance characteristics of the body, which to a certain extent acts like an antenna. This effect causes a variation in the magnetic field that is different for each patient and must be measured and corrected for. Consequently, tuning the receiver coil to the resonance frequency is mandatory before

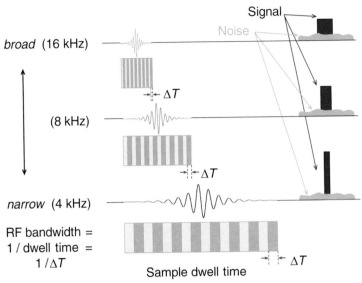

■ **FIGURE 12-60** RF Receiver Bandwidth is determined by the FEG strength, the FOV, and sampling rate. This figure illustrates the spatial domain view of SNR and corresponding sample dwell time. Evolution of the echo in the broad bandwidth situation occurs rapidly with minimal dwell time, which might be needed in situations where very short TE is required, even though the SNR is reduced. On the other hand, in T2 weighted images requiring a long TE, narrow bandwidth can improve SNR.

image acquisition. Eddy currents are signals that are opposite of the induced current produced by transverse magnetization in the RF coil and reduce the overall signal. Quadrature coils increase the SNR as two coils are used in the reception of the signal; phased array coils increase the SNR even more when the data from several coils are added together (see Parallel Imaging, Section 13.1). The proximity of the receiver coil to the volume of interest affects the coil quality factor, but there are trade-offs with image uniformity. Positioning of the coil with respect to the direction of the main magnetic field is also an issue that occurs with air core (horizontal B_0) to solid core (vertical B_0) magnets. Body receiver coils positioned in the bore of the magnet have a moderate quality factor, whereas surface coils have a high-quality factor. With the body coil, the signal is relatively uniform across the FOV; however, with surface coils, the signal falls off abruptly near the edges of the field, limiting the useful imaging depth and resulting in non-uniform brightness across the image.

12.9.7 Magnetic Field Strength

Magnetic field strength influences the SNR of the image by a factor of $B^{1.0}$ to $B^{1.5}$. Thus, one would expect a three- to fivefold improvement in SNR with a 1.5 T magnet over a 0.5 T magnet. Although the gains in the SNR are real, other considerations mitigate the SNR improvement in the clinical environment, including longer T1 relaxation times and greater RF absorption, as discussed previously.

12.9.8 Cross-Excitation

Cross-excitation occurs from the non-rectangular RF excitation profiles in the spatial domain and the resultant overlap of adjacent slices in multislice image acquisition sequences. This saturates the protons and reduces contrast and the contrast-to-noise ratio. To avoid cross-excitation, interslice gaps or interleaving procedures are necessary (see Artifacts section, Chapter 13).

12.9.9   Image Acquisition and Reconstruction Algorithms

Image acquisition and reconstruction algorithms have a profound effect on SNR. The various acquisition/reconstruction methods that have been used in the past and those used today are, in order of increasing SNR, point acquisition methods, line acquisition methods, two-dimensional Fourier transform acquisition methods, and three-dimensional Fourier transform volume acquisition methods. In each of these techniques, the volume of tissue that is excited is the major contributing factor to improving the SNR and image quality. Reconstruction filters and image processing algorithms will also affect the SNR. High-pass filtration methods that increase edge definition will generally decrease the SNR, while low-pass filtration methods that smooth the image data will generally increase the SNR at the cost of reduced resolution.

12.9.10   Summary, Image Quality

The best possible image quality is always desirable, but not always achievable because of the trade-off between SNR, scan speed, and spatial resolution. To increase one of these three components of image quality involves the consideration of reducing one or both of the other two. It is thus a balancing act that is chosen by the operator, the protocol, and the patient in order to acquire images with the best diagnostic yield. MR parameters that may be changed include TR, TE, TI, matrix size, slice thickness, FOV, BW, and NEX. Working with these parameters in the optimization of acquisition protocols to achieve high image quality is essential.

12.10   SUMMARY

The basics of magnetic resonance are covered in this chapter, including the simplest descriptions of magnetism, magnetic characteristics of the elements, and magnetization of tissue samples. Important is the description of the intrinsic decay constants T1, T2, T2*, and proton density in terms of tissue-specific structures and variation in the intrinsic and extrinsic local magnetic fields. Contrast between tissues is determined by pulse sequences including SE, IR, GRE, and their associated parameters TR, TE, TI, and flip angle. In addition to generating contrast, the ability to spatially localize the protons and create a two-dimensional image is as important, so that the differences can be appreciated in a grayscale rendition of the anatomy. The concepts of the frequency domain description of the signals and the k-space acquisition matrix are integral to the discussion, as well as the Fourier transform and the conversion of frequency to spatial domain representations of the data, necessary for visualization. In the next chapter, more details are given for image acquisition time, various pulse sequence designs, how image acquisition time is shortened, and characteristics of the image in terms of SNR, CNR, and artifacts. Unique capabilities for non-invasive "biopsy" of tissues, quality control, equipment, MR safety, and biological effects are also discussed.

SUGGESTED READING AND REFERENCES

Bottomley PA, Foster TH, Argersinger RE, Pfeifer LM. A review of normal tissue hydrogen NMR relaxation mechanisms from 1-100 MHz: dependence on tissue type, NMR frequency, temperature, species, excision, and age. *Med Phys.* 1984;11:425-448.

Chavhan GB, Babyn PS, Jankharia BG, Cheng HM, Shroff MM. Steady-state MR imaging sequences: physics, classification, and clinical applications. *Radiographics*. 2008;28:1147-1160.

Fullerton GD, Potter JL, Dornbluth NC. NMR relaxation of protons in tissues and other macromolecular water solutions. *Magn Reson Imaging*. 1982;1:209-228.

Hashemi RH, Lisanti CJ, Bradley W. *MRI: The Basics*. 4th ed. Philadelphia, PA: Wolters Kluwer; 2017.

NessAiver M. *All You Really Need to Know about MRI Physics*. Baltimore, MD: Simply Physics; 1997.

Pooley RA. AAPM/RSNA physics tutorial for residents: fundamental Physics of MR imaging. *Radiographics*. 2005;25:1087-1099.

Westbrook C, Kaut-Roth C, Talbot J. *MRI in Practice*. 3rd ed. Malden, MA: Blackwell Publishing; 2005.

12.10 Summary

Magnetic Resonance Imaging: Advanced Image Acquisition Methods, Artifacts, Spectroscopy, Quality Control, Siting, Bioeffects, and Safety

The essence of magnetic resonance imaging (MRI) in medicine is the acquisition, manipulation, display, and archive of datasets that have clinical relevance in the context of making a diagnosis or performing research for new applications and opportunities. There are many advantages and limitations of MRI and MR spectroscopy (MRS) as a solution to a clinical problem. Certainly, as described previously (note that this chapter assumes a working knowledge of Chapter 12 content), the great advantages of MR are the ability to generate images with outstanding tissue contrast and good resolution, without resorting to ionizing radiation. Capabilities of MR extend far beyond those basics, into fast acquisition sequences, perfusion and diffusion imaging, MR angiography (MRA), tractography, spectroscopy, and a host of other useful or potentially useful clinical applications. Major limitations of MR are also noteworthy, including extended acquisition times, MR artifacts, patient claustrophobia, tissue heating, and acoustic noise to name a few. MR safety, often ignored, is also of huge concern to the safety of the patient.

In this second of two MR chapters, advanced pulse sequences and fast image acquisition methods, methods for perfusion, diffusion, and angiography imaging, spectroscopy, image quality metrics, common artifacts, MR siting, as well as MR safety issues are described and discussed with respect to the underlying physics.

The concepts of image acquisition and timing issues for standard and advanced pulse sequences into k-space is discussed first, with several methods that can be used to reduce acquisition times and many of the trade-offs that must be considered.

13.1 IMAGE ACQUISITION TIME

A defining character of MRI is the tremendous range of acquisition time needed to image a patient volume. Times ranging from as low as 50 ms to tens of minutes are commonly required depending on the study, pulse sequence, number of images in the dataset, and desired image quality. When MR was initially considered to be a potential diagnostic imaging modality in the late 1970s, the prevailing conventional wisdom gave no chance for widespread applicability because of the extremely long times required to generate a single slice from a sequentially acquired dataset, which required several minutes or more per slice. Breakthroughs in technology, equipment design, RF coils, the unique attributes of the k-space matrix, and methods of acquiring data drastically shortened acquisition times (or effective acquisition times) quickly, and propelled the rapid adoption of MRI in the mid-1980s. By the early 1990s, MRI established its clinical value that continues to expand today.

13.1.1 Acquisition Time, Two-Dimensional Fourier Transform Spin Echo Imaging

The time to acquire an image is determined by the data needed to fill the fraction of k-space that allows the image to be reconstructed by Fourier transform methods. For a standard spin echo sequence, the relevant parameters are the TR, number of phase encoding steps, and number of excitations (NEX) (or averages) used for averaging identical repeat cycles, as

$$\text{Acquisition time} = \text{TR} \times \#\,\text{PEG Steps} \times \text{NEX}.$$

The matrix size that defines k-space is often not square (*e.g.*, 256 × 256, 128 × 128), but rectangular (*e.g.*, 256 × 192, 256 × 128) where the small matrix dimension is most frequently along the phase encode direction to minimize the number of incremental PEG strength applications during the acquisition. A 256 × 192 image matrix and two averages (NEX) per phase encode step with a TR = 600 ms (for T1 weighting) requires imaging time of 0.6 s × 192 × 2 = 230.4 s = 3.84 min for a single slice! For a proton density and T2-weighted double echo sequence with TR = 2,500 ms, this increases to 16 min, although two images are created in that time. Of course, a simple first-order method would be to eliminate the number of averages (NEX), which reduces the time by a factor of 2; however, the downsides are an increase in the statistical variability of the data, which decreases the image signal-to-noise ratio (SNR) and makes the image appear "noisy." Methods to reduce acquisition time and/or time per slice are crucial to making MR exam times reasonable, as described by various methods below.

13.1.2 Multislice Data Acquisition

The average acquisition time per reconstructed image slice in a single-slice spin echo sequence is clinically unacceptable. However, the average time per slice is significantly reduced using multislice acquisition methods, where several slices within the tissue volume are selectively excited in a sequential timing scheme during the TR interval to fully utilize the dead time waiting for longitudinal recovery in an adjacent slice, as shown in Figure 13-1. This requires cycling all of the gradients and tuning the RF excitation pulse many times during a single TR interval. The total number of slices that can be acquired simultaneously is a function of TR, TE, and machine limitations:

$$\text{Total Number of Slices} = \text{TR}/(\text{TE} + C),$$

where C is a constant dependent on the MR equipment capabilities (computer speed; gradient capabilities; sequence options; additional pulses, *e.g.*, spoiling pulses in standard SE; use of spatial saturation; and chemical shift, among others). Each slice and each echo, if multiecho, requires its own k-space repository to store data as they are acquired. Long TR acquisitions such as proton density and T2-weighted sequences can produce a greater number of slices over a given volume than T1-weighted sequences with a short TR. The chief trade-off is a loss of tissue contrast due to *cross-excitation* of adjacent slices due to non-square excitation profiles, causing undesired proton saturation as explained in Section 13.6 on artifacts.

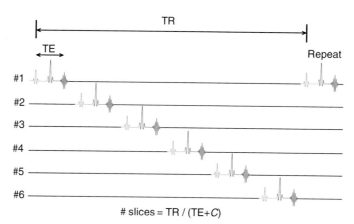

■ FIGURE 13-1 Multislice two-dimensional image acquisition is accomplished by discretely exciting different slabs of tissue during the TR period; appropriate changes of the RF excitation bandwidth, SSG, PEG, and FEG parameters are necessary. Because of diffuse excitation profiles, RF irradiation of adjacent slices leads to partial saturation and loss of contrast. The number of slices (volume) that can be obtained is a function of the TR, TE, and C, the latter representing the capabilities of the MR system and type of pulse sequence.

13.1.3 Acquisition Time, 3D Acquisition

The image acquisition time is equal to

$$\text{TR} \times \text{\# Phase Encode Steps}(z\text{-axis}) \times \text{\# Phase Encode Steps}(y\text{-axis}) \times \text{\# NEX}.$$

When using a standard TR of 600 ms with one average for a T1-weighted exam, a $128 \times 128 \times 128$ cube requires 163 min or about 2.7 h! Obviously, this is unacceptable for standard clinical imaging. GRE pulse sequences with TR of 50 ms acquire the same image volume in about 15 min. Another shortcut is with anisotropic voxels, where the phase encoding steps in one dimension are reduced, albeit with a loss of resolution.

13.2 FAST IMAGING TECHNIQUES

13.2.1 Fast Pulse Sequences

Fast Spin Echo (FSE) techniques use multiple PEG steps in conjunction with multiple 180° refocusing RF pulses to produce an echo train length (ETL) with corresponding digital data acquisitions per TR interval, as illustrated in Figure 13-2. Multiple k-space rows are filled during each TR equal to the ETL, which is also the reduction factor for acquisition time. "Effective echo time" is determined when the central views in k-space are acquired, which are usually the first echoes, and subsequent echoes are usually spaced apart via increased PEG strength with the same echo spacing time. *"Phase re-ordering"* optimizes SNR by acquiring the low-frequency information with the early echoes (lowest amount of T2 decay), and the high-frequency, peripheral information with late echoes, where the impact on overall image SNR is lower. The FSE technique has the advantage of spin echo image acquisition, namely immunity from external magnetic field inhomogeneities, with $4\times, 8\times,$ to $16\times$ faster acquisition time. However, each echo experiences different amounts of intrinsic T2 decay, which results in image contrast differences and image blurring in

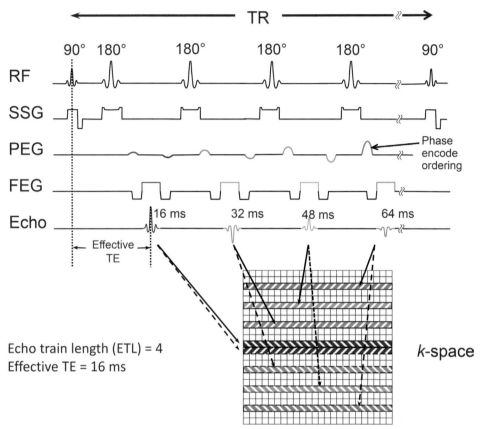

■ **FIGURE 13-2** Conventional FSE uses multiple 180° refocusing RF pulses per TR interval with incremental changes in the PEG to fill several views in *k*-space (the ETL). This example illustrates an ETL of four, with an "effective" TE equal to 16 ms. Total time of the acquisition is reduced by the ETL factor. The reversed polarity PEG steps reestablish coherent phase before the next gradient application. Slightly different PEG strengths are applied to fill the center of *k*-space first, and then the periphery with later echoes, continuing until all views are recorded. As shown, data can be mirrored using conjugate symmetry to reduce the overall time by another factor of two.

the phase encoding direction when compared with conventional spin echo images of similar TR and TE. Lower signal levels in the later echoes produce less SNR, and fewer images can be acquired in the image volume during the same acquisition. A T2-weighted spin echo image (TR = 2,000 ms, 256 phase encode steps, one average) requires approximately 8.5 min, while a corresponding FSE with an ETL of 4 (Fig. 13-2) requires about 2.1 min. Longer TR values allow for a greater ETL, which will offset the longer TR in terms of overall acquisition time, and will also allow more proton density weighting due to larger M_z recovery. Specific FSE sequences for T2 weighting and multiecho FSE are employed with variations in phase reordering and data acquisition. FSE is also known as "turbo spin echo" or "RARE" (rapid acquisition with refocused echoes).

Echo Planar Image (EPI) Acquisition is a technique that provides extremely fast imaging time. Spin Echo (SE-EPI) and Gradient Echo (GRE-EPI) are two methods used for acquiring data, and a third is a hybrid of the two, GRASE (Gradient and Spin Echo). Single-shot (all of the image information is acquired within 1 TR interval) or multishot EPI has been implemented with these methods. For single-shot SE-EPI (Fig. 13-3A), image acquisition typically begins with a standard 90° flip, then a PEG/FEG gradient application to initiate the acquisition of data in the periphery of the

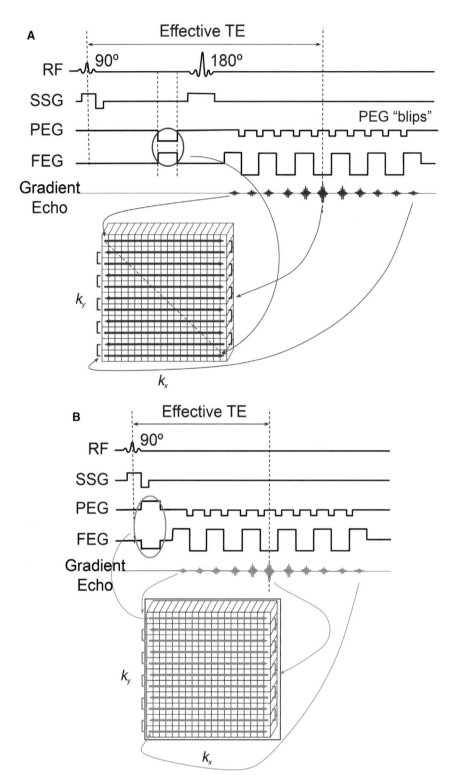

■ **FIGURE 13-3** Single shot Echo Planar Spin Echo image (SE-EPI) **(A)** and Single shot Echo Planar Gradient Recalled Echo image (GRE-EPI) **(B)** acquisition sequences. Data are deposited in *k*-space, initially positioned by a simultaneous PEG and FEG application to locate the initial row and column position (in this example, the upper left; for SE-EPI, the 180-degree pulse inverts starting location to upper left), followed by phase encode gradient "blips" simultaneous to FEG oscillations, to fill *k-space* line by line by introducing 1-row phase changes in a zigzag pattern. Image matrix sizes of 64 × 64 and 128 × 64 are common.

k-space, followed by a 180° echo-producing RF pulse. Immediately after, an oscillating readout gradient and phase encode gradient "blips" are continuously applied to form a gradient echo train and rapidly fill k-space in a stepped "zigzag" pattern. The "effective" echo time occurs at a time TE, when the maximum amplitude of the induced GREs occurs at the center of k-space. Acquisition of the data must proceed in a period less than T2* (around 50 ms), placing high demands on the sampling rate, the gradient coils (shielded coils are required, with low induced "eddy currents"), the RF transmitter/receiver, and RF energy deposition limitations. For GRE-EPI (Fig. 13-3B), a similar acquisition strategy is implemented but without a 180-degree refocusing RF pulse, allowing for faster acquisition time. SE-EPI is generally longer, but better image quality is achieved; on the other hand, larger RF energy deposition to the patient occurs. EPI acquisition can be preceded by any type of RF pulse, for instance FLAIR (EPI-FLAIR), which will produce images much faster than the corresponding conventional FLAIR sequence. EPI acquisitions typically have poor SNR, low resolution (matrices of 64 × 64 or 128 × 64 are typical), and many artifacts, particularly of chemical shift and magnetic susceptibility origin. Nevertheless, EPI offers real-time "snapshot" image capability with 50 ms total acquisition time. EPI is emerging as a clinical tool for studying time-dependent physiologic processes and functional imag-

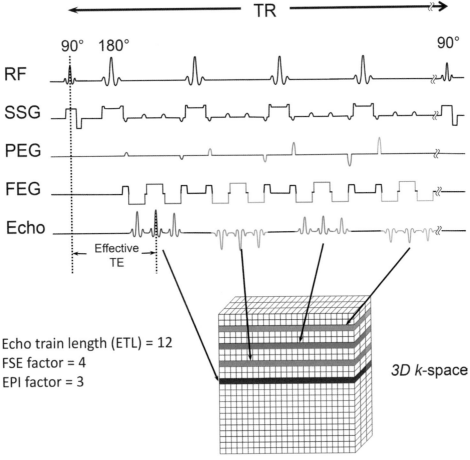

Echo train length (ETL) = 12
FSE factor = 4
EPI factor = 3

3D k-space

■ **FIGURE 13-4** A Gradient and Spin Echo (GRASE) sequence with three gradient echoes and four fast spin echoes. There are many strategies to efficiently collect 2D or 3D spaces and the example illustrates a case that gradient echoes fill the 3D matrix in the slice direction and spin echoes in the phase encoding direction. Effective TE can be determined by timing the collection of echoes at the center of k-space based on desired image contrast.

ing. Concerns of safety with EPI, chiefly related to the rapid switching of gradients and possible nerve stimulation of the patient, the associated acoustic noise, image artifacts, distortion, and chemical shift are components that limit use for many imaging procedures.

The **GRASE (Gradient and Spin Echo) sequence** combines the initial spin echo with a series of GREs, followed by an RF rephasing (180°) pulse, and the pattern is repeated until *k*-space is filled (Fig. 13-4). A GRASE sequence can be utilized for 2D multislice imaging or 3D imaging. The example in the figure describes a 3D imaging application. Although there are variations of terminologies across MRI vendors, general definitions are following: ETL is the number of total echoes acquired in a single TR, an FSE factor is the number of 180° inversion RF pulses inducing spin echoes, and an EPI factor is the number of gradient echoes in a single spin echo. This hybrid sequence achieves the benefits of both types of rephasing: the speed of the gradient and the ability of the RF pulse to compensate for T2* effects, providing significant improvements in image quality compared to the standard EPI methods. A trade-off is a longer acquisition time (*e.g.*, greater than 100 ms) and much greater energy deposition from the multiple 180° RF pulses.

13.2.2 *k*-Space Filling

Methods to fill *k*-space in a non-sequential way can increase signal, enhance contrast, and achieve rapid scan times as shown in Figure 13-5. **Centric k-space filling** has been discussed with FSE imaging (above), where the lower strength phase encode gradients are applied first, filling the center of *k*-space when the echoes have their highest amplitude. This type of filling is also important for fast GRE techniques, where the image contrast and the SNR fall quickly with time from the initial excitation pulse.

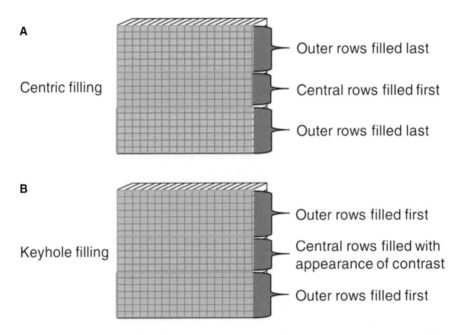

A

Centric filling

— Outer rows filled last

— Central rows filled first

— Outer rows filled last

B

Keyhole filling

— Outer rows filled first

— Central rows filled with appearance of contrast

— Outer rows filled first

■ **FIGURE 13-5** Alternate methods of filling *k*-space. **A.** Centric filling applies the lower strength PEGs first to maximize signal and contrast from the earliest echoes of a FSE or GRE sequence. **B.** Keyhole filling applies PEGs of higher strength first to fill the outer portions of *k*-space, and the central lines are filled only during a certain part of the sequence, such as with arrival of contrast signal.

Keyhole filling methods fill *k*-space similarly to centric filling, except the central lines are filled when important events occur during the sequence, in situations such as contrast-enhanced angiography. Outer areas of *k*-space are filled first, and when gadolinium appears in the imaging volume, the center areas are filled. At the end of the scan, the outer and central *k*-space regions are meshed to produce an image with both good contrast and resolution.

13.2.3   Non-Cartesian *k*-Space Acquisition

The conventional *k*-space acquisition collects the *k*-space data in a rectilinear pattern in a Cartesian grid. In some applications, particularly requiring rapid image acquisition, non-Cartesian *k*-space acquisition schemes have been widely used.

Radial Imaging

Radial imaging was the first method implemented to obtain MR images. However, radial imaging is more susceptible to off-resonance effect and system instabilities, such as field inhomogeneity, eddy-currents, gradient and data acquisition delays, and other effects. *k*-Space lines can be acquired in a rotating pattern in 2D space (Fig. 13-6A). 3D *k*-space can be filled with the radial sampling lines with slice encoding steps along *z*-axis (Fig. 13-6B). Field inhomogeneity, eddy-current, and gradient linearity have been improved in current MR systems. Due to the unique benefit of the tolerance of undersampling, interest in radial imaging has been expanded in volumetric imaging with high undersampling factors such as hybrid projection reconstruction (PR) and 3DPR.

In radial acquisition schemes, all radial spokes pass through the center of a circular *k*-space and the center has higher sampling density than the periphery. The non-uniform sampling density benefits applications of dynamic (or time-resolved) imaging that requires high temporal resolution, such as contrast-enhanced angiography and cardiac imaging. The redundant information near the center, containing the majority of image contrast, is selected based on the acquisition timing while the sparsely sampled periphery information is shared over different temporal frames, which is called *view-sharing*. Figure 13-7 describes an example of cardiac imaging using radial acquisitions.

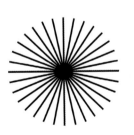
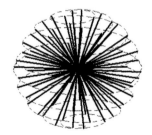
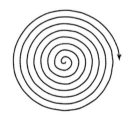

A. Radial   B. 3D Radial   C. Spiral

■ **FIGURE 13-6** Various non-Cartesian sampling methods: **(A)** 2D radial sampling with $G_x = G_0 \cos \phi$ and $G_y = G_0 \sin \phi$. where G_0 is the maximum gradient strength, ϕ is the azimuthal angle of radial line, and full radial lines are acquired with $0 < \phi < \pi$. **B.** 3D radial sampling with $G_x = G_0 \sin \theta \cos \phi$, $G_y = G_0 \sin \theta \sin \phi$, and $G_z = G_0 \cos \theta$ where θ and ϕ are the polar angle and the azimuthal angle of radial line, respectively. **C.** Spiral sampling with sinusoidal oscillation of the *x* and *y* gradients 90° out of phase with each other, with samples beginning in the center of *k*-space and spiraling out to the periphery.

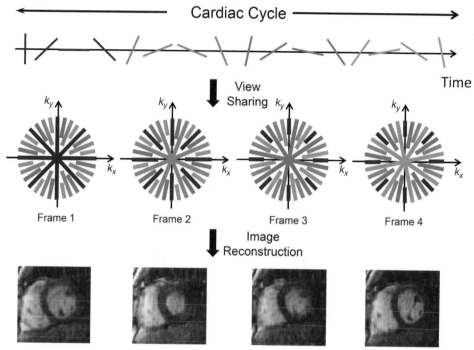

■ **FIGURE 13-7** Illustration of time-resolved cardiac imaging with 2D radial sampling. The radial lines are acquired in an interleaved fashion during one or multiple cardiac cycles. By view sharing, sharing high frequency (periphery of k-space) data with other time frames, the images do not suffer from undersampling artifacts while maintaining the contrast by utilizing full radial lines at a specific time frame.

Spiral Imaging

Spiral filling is an alternate method of filling k-space radially, which involves the simultaneous oscillation of equivalent encoding gradients to sample data points during echo formation in a spiral, starting at the origin (the center of the k-space) and spiraling outward to the periphery in the prescribed acquisition plane (Fig. 13-6C). The same contrast mechanisms are available in spiral sequences (*e.g.*, T1, T2, proton density weighting), and spin or gradient echoes can be obtained. After acquisition of the signals, an additional postprocessing step, re-gridding, is necessary to convert the spiral data into the rectilinear matrix for two-dimensional Fourier transform (2DFT). Spiral scanning is an efficient method for acquiring data and sampling information in the center of k-space, where the bulk of image information is contained.

Propeller

A variant of radial sampling with enhanced filling of the center of k-space is known generically as "blade" imaging, and commonly as **propeller**: Periodically Rotated Overlapping Parallel Lines with Enhanced Reconstruction, where a rectangular block of data is acquired and then rotated about the center of k-space. Redundant information concentrated in the center of k-space is used for improvement of SNR or for the identification of times during the scan in which the patient may have moved, so that those blocks of data can be processed with a phase-shifting algorithm to eliminate the movement effect on the data during the reconstruction process and to mitigate motion artifacts to a great extent. Filling of k-space for this method is shown in Figure 13-8.

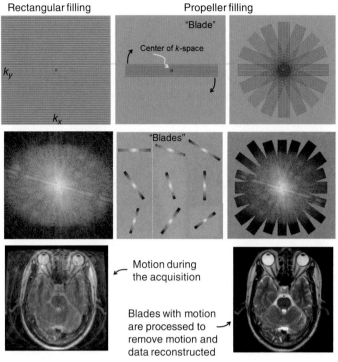

■ **FIGURE 13-8** The propeller data acquisition compared to a rectangular filling of k-space is shown above. Instead of acquiring single lines of information to fill k-space consecutively as shown in the upper left and middle left, a rectangular data acquisition at a specific angle (*e.g.*, 0°) is acquired encompassing several lines of k-space, which represents a "blade" of information. The partial acquisition is rotated about the center of k-space at angular increments, which provides a dense sampling of data at the center of k-space and less in the periphery as shown by the schematic (upper right illustration). If the patient moves during a portion of the examination (lower left image), the blades in which the motion occurred can be identified and reprocessed, and the image reconstructed without the motion artifacts (lower right image).

13.2.4 Data Synthesis

Data "synthesis" takes advantage of the symmetry and redundant characteristics of the frequency domain signals in k-space. The acquisition of as little as one half the data plus one row of k-space allows the mirroring of "complex conjugate" data to fill the remainder of the matrix (Fig. 13-9). In the phase encode direction, "half Fourier," "½ NEX," or "phase conjugate symmetry" (vendor-specific naming) techniques effectively reduce the number of required TR intervals by one half plus one line, and thus can reduce the acquisition time by nearly one half. In the frequency encoding direction, "fractional echo" or "read conjugate symmetry" refers to reading a fraction of the echo. While there is no scan time reduction when all the phase encode steps are acquired, there is a significant echo time reduction, which allows more slices to be covered in one TR or reduces motion-related artifacts, such as dephasing of blood. However, the penalty for either half Fourier or fractional echo techniques is a reduction in the SNR (caused by a reduced NEX or data sampling in the volume). If the approximations in the complex conjugation of the signals are not accurate mainly due to the factors causing phase incoherence of spins, artifacts may present and collecting k-space by more than a half (*i.e.*, 5/8 NEX) is desired. The factors yielding phase incoherence include inhomogeneities of the magnetic field, imperfect linear gradient fields, and the presence of magnetic susceptibility agents in the volume being imaged.

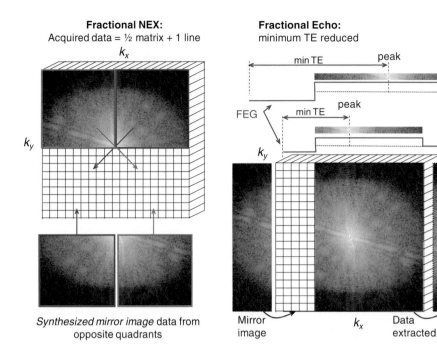

■ **FIGURE 13-9** Fractional NEX and fractional echo. Left: Data synthesis uses the redundant characteristics of the frequency domain. This is an example of phase conjugate symmetry, in which ½ of the PEG views +1 extra are acquired, and the complex conjugate of the data is reflected in the symmetric quadrants. Acquisition time is thus reduced by approximately $2\times$ (~50%) although image noise is increased by approximately $\sqrt{2}$ (40%). Right: Fractional echo acquisition is performed when only part of the echo is read during the application of the FEG. Usually, the peak of the echo is centered in the middle of the readout gradient, and the echo signals prior to the peak are identical mirror images after the peak. With fractional echo, the echo is no longer centered, and the sampling window is shifted such that only the peak echo and the dephasing part of the echo are sampled. As the peak of the echo is closer to the RF excitation pulse, TE can be reduced, which can improve T1 and proton density weighting contrast. A larger number of slices can also be obtained with a shorter TE in a multislice acquisition (see Fig. 13-2).

13.2.5 Parallel Imaging

Acquiring k-space information quickly is desired in many applications in order to reduce motion artifact as well as a scan time. Without compromise of image resolution, only a part of k-space can be acquired as shown in Figure 13-10A. However, because the field of view (FOV) dimension in the phase encode direction is inversely proportional to the spacing, the size of the effective FOV is reduced to $1/N$ its original size, and as a result, aliasing of signals outside of the FOV in the phase encode direction occurs.

Parallel imaging is a technique that overcomes the aliasing artifacts due to undersampling by using the response of multiple receive RF coils that are coupled together with independent channels, so that data can be acquired simultaneously. Specific hardware and software are necessary for the electronic orchestration of this capability. Typically, 2, 4, 8, 16, 24 (or more) coils are arranged around the area to be imaged; if a 4-coil configuration is used, then during each TR period, each coil acquires a view of the data as the acquisition sequence proceeds. Lines in k-space are defined only after the processing of linear combinations of the signals that are received by all of the coils. If 4 views of the data are acquired per TR interval, in the ideal situation, scan time can be decreased by a factor of 4 (known as the *reduction factor or acceleration factor*). One of the approaches, called SENSitivity Encoding (SENSE), uses the sensitivity profile of each coil to calculate where the signal is coming from relative to the coil based on its amplitude—the signal generated near the coil has a higher amplitude than the signal furthest away. Depending on the geometrical configuration of coils, an individual coil may have unique spatial information that other coils do not have. The unwrapped images can be expressed as a linear combination of acquired images from each coil times the coil sensitivity of each coil (Fig. 13-10B). With knowledge of the coil sensitivities, the unwrapped images can be generated by solving a linear equation per voxel. The coil sensitivity can be measured by a short separate calibration scan prior to the undersampling scan or by generating low resolution images from the image itself by acquiring additional lines near the center of k-space (referred to as self-calibration).

Parallel imaging can also be achieved by synthesizing the skipped k-space lines directly and generating unwrapped images from an individual coil. Coil sensitivity in image space corresponds to a convolution kernel in k-space (a multiplication in image space is equivalent to a convolution in frequency space). The convolution operation is essentially a linear operation of neighboring voxels, and the redundant information from multiple coil elements allows synthesizing the missing information as shown in Figure 13-10C. After the missing k-space lines are filled up, images from each coil are generated and combined to create the final images. Similar to coil sensitivity measurement, the convolution kernel of each coil can be estimated by acquiring additional

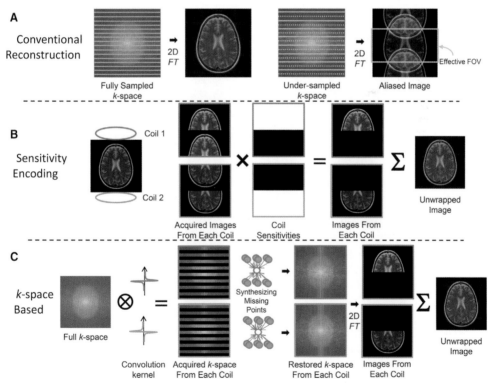

■ **FIGURE 13-10** Image reconstruction with undersampled k-space by acquiring a half of data (every odd line): **(A)** Conventional reconstruction showed imaging aliasing (wrap-around) because the size of the effective FOV is reduced to a half of its original size. **B.** Image based sensitivity encoding utilizes the sensitivity profile of each coil to calculate where the signal is coming from relative to the coil based on its amplitude. With *a priori* knowledge of the coil sensitivities, the unwrapped images can be generated by solving a linear equation per voxel. **C.** k-space based methods synthesize the skipped k-space lines directly and generate unwrapped images from an individual coil using coil specific convolution kernels estimated by auto-calibration.

lines near the center of k-space and a representative method is GeneRalized Autocalibrating Partially Parallel Acquisition (GRAPPA).

Parallel imaging can be used to either reduce scan time or improve resolution, in conjunction with most pulse sequences. In addition, it significantly reduces geometric distortion present in EPI. Downsides include image misalignment between a calibration scan and an actual scan due to patient motion and, more importantly, an SNR penalty. The SNR of parallel imaging is

$$SNR_{PI} = \frac{SNR_{Fully\ Sampled}}{\sqrt{R} \cdot g},$$

where $SNR_{Fully\ Sampled}$ is the SNR of fully sampled image, R is the scan time reduction factor, and g is the coil geometry factor. Although the example shown in Figure 13-10 has ideal coil sensitivities with sharp boundaries, the actual coil sensitivity is reduced as further apart from each coil location. Therefore, a part of image volume (usually the center) is detectable by multiple coil elements and the geometry factor, g-factor, is determined by the number of aliased replications on each voxel that varies by location across the image.

As the example shows, the acceleration is done in the phase encoding direction in 2D imaging; however, the acceleration can be done in either phase encoding or slice encoding directions in 3D imaging. Considering the direction of acceleration, the coil geometry should be reviewed. Choosing the acceleration direction into the direction that has the most coil elements guarantees the best performance in terms of SNR and residual aliasing artifacts. For example, if the parallel imaging direction is chosen in the A/P direction during a spine exam with a spine coil, parallel imaging will not be performed correctly and images will have severe aliasing artifacts.

13.2.6 Multiband Imaging

Multiband (MB) imaging (or simultaneous multislice [SMS]) is a technique to further accelerate image acquisition, primarily for 2D multislice imaging. Recent advances in parallel imaging enable unwrapping the aliased image in the slice direction when multiple slices are excited and acquired simultaneously. Figure 13-11 describes a simple example of MB imaging with an MB factor of 2, meaning two slices are excited together. In 2D axial acquisition, multiple slices can be excited by a single RF pulse that has two distinct resonance frequencies or two sequential RF pulses that each has a unique resonance frequency. When multiple slices are excited, the FOV of slices are shifted by a factor of FOV/MB in order to minimize the overlapped area and improve the g-factor in the reconstruction. For example, when two slices are excited, one of the slices that locates off the gradient isocenter is shifted by FOV/2 as shown in the figure. This is done by adding a small gradient in the z-direction. The acquired image with MB excitation shows multiple slices together, and the unwrapping is done by a parallel imaging technique applied in the slice encoding direction. Although the actual acquisition is done in 2D image space, the image reconstruction handles the data as 3D imaging. While parallel imaging has an SNR penalty because of reduced phase (or slice) encoding lines, MB imaging does not have this penalty and only the coil g-factor in the slice direction affects SNR. This SNR advantage allows high MB factors if a coil has very high number of channels, such as 32 or 64 channels. Thus, the MB imaging is often utilized in conjunction with parallel imaging for further acceleration. For example, an acceleration factor of 8 (MB factor of 4 × parallel imaging factor of 2) or higher is feasible without much SNR loss or artifacts.

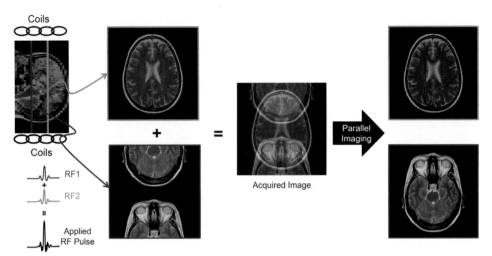

■ **FIGURE 13-11** Multiband imaging excites multiple slices simultaneously and unwraps the aliased image in the slice direction using a parallel imaging approach. There is no SNR penalty besides the coil geometry factor because a larger signal is received with multiple 2D slices. This enables a high acceleration factor along with parallel imaging.

13.3 SIGNAL FROM FLOW

The appearance of moving fluid (vascular and cerebrospinal fluid [CSF]) in MR images is complicated by many factors, including flow velocity, vessel orientation, laminar versus turbulent flow patterns, pulse sequences, and image acquisition modes. Flow-related mechanisms combine with image acquisition parameters to alter contrast. Signal due to flow covers the entire gray scale of MR signal intensities, from "black blood" to "bright blood" levels, and flow can be a source of artifacts. The signal from flow can also be exploited to produce MR angiographic images.

Low signal intensities (flow voids) are often a result of *high-velocity signal loss* (HVSL), in which protons in the flowing blood move out of the slice during echo reformation, causing a lower signal. *Flow turbulence* can also cause flow voids, by causing a dephasing of protons in the blood with a resulting loss of the tissue magnetization in the area of turbulence. With HVSL, the amount of signal loss depends on the velocity of the moving fluid. Pulse sequences to produce "black blood" in images can be very useful in cardiac and vascular imaging. A typical black blood pulse sequence uses a "double inversion recovery" method, whereby a non-selective 180° RF pulse is initially applied, inverting all protons in the active volume, and is followed by a selective 180° RF pulse that restores the magnetization in the selected slice. During the inversion time, blood with inverted protons outside of the excited slice flows into the slice, producing no signal; therefore, the blood appears dark.

13.3.1 Flow-Related Enhancement

Flow-related enhancement is a process that causes increased signal intensity due to flowing protons; it occurs during imaging of a volume of tissues. Flow enhancement in GRE images is pronounced for both venous and arterial structures, as well as CSF. The high intensity is caused by the wash-in (between subsequent RF excitations) of fully unsaturated protons into a volume of partially saturated protons due to the

■ **FIGURE 13-12** The repeated RF excitation within an imaging volume produces partial saturation of the tissue magnetization (top figure, gray area). Unsaturated protons flowing into the volume generate a large signal difference that is bright relative to the surrounding tissues. Bright blood effects can be reduced by applying presaturation RF pulses adjacent to the imaging volume, so that protons in inflowing blood will have a similar partial saturation (bottom figure; note no blood signal).

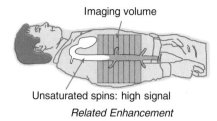

Imaging volume

Unsaturated spins: high signal

Related Enhancement

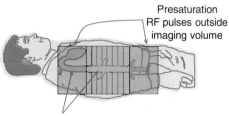

Presaturation RF pulses outside imaging volume

Presaturated spins: equal signal

Flow presaturation

short TR used with gradient imaging. During the next excitation, the signal amplitude resulting from the moving unsaturated protons is about 10 times greater than that of the non-moving saturated protons. With GRE techniques, the degree of enhancement depends on the velocity of the blood, the slice or volume thickness, and the TR. As blood velocity increases, unsaturated blood exhibits the greatest signal. Similarly, a thinner slice or decreased repetition time results in higher flow enhancement. In arterial imaging of high-velocity flow, it is possible to have bright blood throughout the imaging volume of a three-dimensional acquisition if unsaturated blood can penetrate into the volume prior to experiencing an RF pulse.

Signal from blood is dependent on the relative saturation of the surrounding tissues and the incoming blood flow in the vasculature. In a multislice volume, repeated excitation of the tissues and blood causes a partial saturation of the protons, dependent on the T1 characteristics and the TR of the pulse sequence. Blood outside of the imaged volume does not interact with the RF excitations, and therefore these unsaturated protons may enter the imaged volume and produce a large signal compared to the blood within the volume. This is known as flow-related enhancement. As the pulse sequence continues, the unsaturated blood becomes partially saturated and the protons of the blood produce a similar signal to the tissues in the inner slices of the volume (Fig. 13-12). In some situations, flow-related enhancement is undesirable and is eliminated with the use of "presaturation" pulses applied to volumes just above and below the imaging volume. These same saturation pulses are also helpful in reducing motion artifacts caused by adjacent tissues outside the imaging volume.

13.3.2 MR Angiography

Exploitation of blood flow enhancement is the basis for MRA. Two techniques to create images of vascular anatomy include time-of-flight and phase contrast angiography.

Time-of-Flight Angiography

The time-of-flight technique relies on the tagging of blood in one region of the body and detecting it in another. This differentiates moving blood from the surrounding stationary tissues. Tagging is accomplished by proton saturation, inversion, or

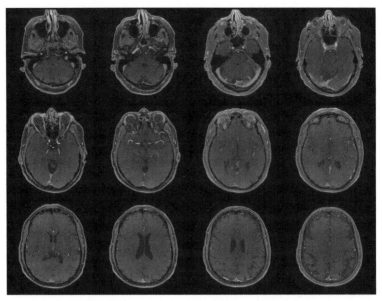

■ **FIGURE 13-13** The *time of flight* MRA acquisition collects each slice separately with a sequence to enhance blood flow. Exploitation of blood flow is achieved by detecting unsaturated protons moving into the volume, producing a bright signal. A coherent GRE image acquisition pulse sequence is shown, TR = 24 ms, TE = 3.1 ms, flip angle = 20°. Every 10th image in the stack is displayed above, from left to right and top to bottom.

relaxation to change the longitudinal magnetization of moving blood. The penetration of the tagged blood into a volume depends on the T1, velocity, and direction of the blood. Since the detectable range is limited by the eventual saturation of the tagged blood, long vessels are difficult to visualize simultaneously in a three-dimensional volume. For these reasons, a two-dimensional stack of slices is typically acquired, where even slowly moving blood can penetrate the region of RF excitation in thin slices (Fig. 13-13). Each slice is acquired separately, and blood moving in one direction (north or south, *e.g.*, arteries versus veins) can be selected by delivering a presaturation pulse on an adjacent slab superior or inferior to the slab of data acquisition. Thin slices are also helpful in preserving resolution of the flow pattern. Often used for the two-dimensional image acquisition is a "GRASS" or "FISP" GRE technique that produces relatively poor anatomic contrast yet provides a high-contrast "bright blood" signal. Magnetization transfer contrast sequences (see below) are also employed to increase the contrast of the signals due to blood by reducing the background anatomic contrast.

Two-dimensional TOF MRA images are obtained by projecting the content of the stack of slices at a specific angle through the volume. A maximum intensity projection (MIP) algorithm detects the largest signal along a given ray through the volume and places this value in the image (Fig. 13-14). The superimposition of residual stationary anatomy often requires further data manipulation to suppress undesirable signals. This is achieved in a variety of ways, the simplest of which is setting a window threshold. Another method is to acquire a dataset without contrast and subtract the non-contrast MIP from the contrast MIP to reduce background signals. Clinical MRA images show the three-dimensional characteristics of the vascular anatomy from several angles around the volume stack (Fig. 13-15) with some residual signals from the stationary anatomy. Time-of-flight angiography often produces variation in vessel intensity dependent on orientation with respect to the image plane, a situation that is less than optimal.

■ FIGURE 13-14 A simple illustration shows how the MIP algorithm extracts the highest (maximum) signals in the two-dimensional stack of images along a specific direction in the volume, and produces projection images with maximum intensity variations as a function of angle.

Projections are cast through the image stack (volume)
The *maximum* signal along each line is projected

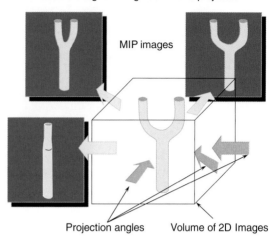

MIP images

Projection angles   Volume of 2D Images

Phase Contrast Angiography

Phase contrast imaging relies on the phase change that occurs in moving protons such as blood. One method of inducing a phase change is dependent on the application of a bipolar gradient in the direction of the bipolar gradients (one gradient with positive polarity followed by a second gradient with negative polarity, separated by a delay time ΔT). There are many factors other than flow that causes a phase offset, such as off-resonance fields, chemical shift, motion, and temperature. To remove this phase offset, another image is acquired with opposite gradients. In a second acquisition of the same view of the data (same PEG), the polarity of the bipolar gradients is reversed, and moving protons show phases in the opposite direction, while the

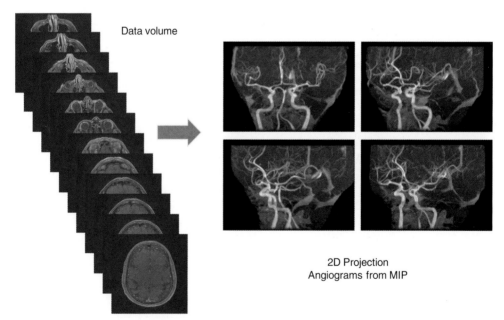

Data volume

2D Projection
Angiograms from MIP

■ FIGURE 13-15 A volume stack of bright blood images (left) is used with MIP processing to create a series of projection angiograms at regular intervals; the three-dimensional perspective is appreciated in a stack view, with virtual rotation of the vasculature.

bipolar velocity encoding gradients

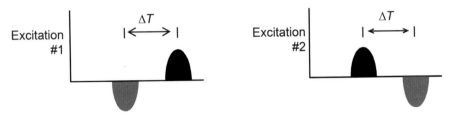

Excitation #1 phase — Excitation #2 phase ∝ velocity of spins

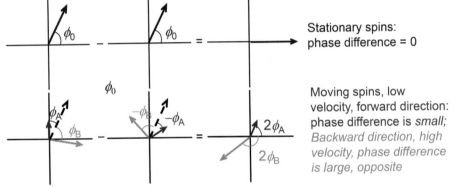

Stationary spins: phase difference = 0

Moving spins, low velocity, forward direction: phase difference is *small; Backward direction, high velocity, phase difference is large, opposite*

■ **FIGURE 13-16** Phase contrast angiography uses consecutive excitations that have a bipolar gradient encoding with the polarity reversed between the first and second excitation, as shown in the top row. Magnetization vectors (lower two rows) illustrate the effect of the bipolar gradients on stationary and moving spins for the first and second excitations. Subtracting the phases of two spins will cancel stationary tissue phase and enhance phase differences caused by the velocity of moving blood.

stationary protons exhibit no phase differences (Fig. 13-16). Subtracting the phase of the second excitation from the first cancels the phase of stationary protons but doubles the phase of moving protons. Alternating the bipolar gradient polarity for each subsequent excitation during the acquisition provides phase contrast image information. The degree of phase shift is directly related to the velocity encoding (VENC) time, ΔT, between the positive and negative lobes of the bipolar gradients, the area of velocity encoding gradients, and the velocity of the protons within the excited volume. Proper selection of the VENC time and gradient areas is necessary to avoid phase wrap error (exceeding 180° phase differences) and to ensure an optimal phase shift range for the velocities encountered. In the phase image, intensity variations are dependent on the amount of phase shift, where the brightest pixel values represent the largest forward (or backward) velocity, a mid-scale value represents 0 velocity, and the darkest pixel values represent the largest backward (or forward) velocity. Figure 13-17 shows a representative magnitude and phase contrast image of the cardiac vasculature. Unlike the time-of-flight methods, the phase contrast image is inherently quantitative and, when calibrated carefully, provides an estimate of the mean blood flow velocity and direction. Two- and three-dimensional phase contrast image acquisitions for MRA are possible.

13.3.3 Gradient Moment Nulling

In spin echo or gradient recalled echo imaging, the slice select and readout gradients are balanced, so that the uniform dephasing with the initial gradient application

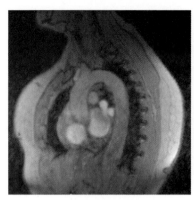 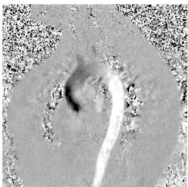

Magnitude Image   Phase Image

■ **FIGURE 13-17** Magnitude (left) and phase (right) images provide contrast of flowing blood. Magnitude images are sensitive to flow, but not to direction; phase images provide direction and velocity information. The blood flow from the heart shows forward flow in the ascending aorta (*dark* area) and forward flow in the descending aorta at this point in the heart cycle for the phase image. Some bright flow patterns in the ascending aorta represent backward flow to the coronary arteries. Grayscale amplitude is proportional to velocity, where intermediate grayscale is 0 velocity.

is rephased by an opposite polarity gradient of equal area. However, when moving protons are subjected to the gradients, the amount of phase dispersion is not compensated (Fig. 13-18). This phase dispersal can cause ghosting (faint, displaced copies of the anatomy) in images. It is possible, however, to rephase the protons by a gradient moment nulling technique. With constant velocity flow (first-order motion), all protons can be rephased using the application of a gradient triplet. In this technique, an initial positive gradient of unit area is followed by a negative gradient of twice the area, which creates phase changes that are compensated by a third positive gradient of unit area. The velocity compensated gradient (right graph in Fig. 13-18) depicts the evolution of the proton phase back to zero for both stationary and moving protons. Note that the overall applied gradient has a net area of zero—equal to the sum of the positive and negative areas. Higher order corrections such as second- or

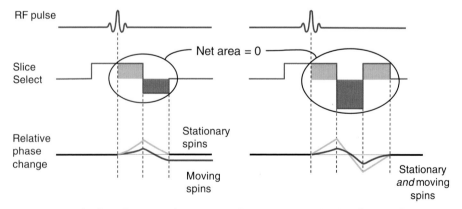

■ **FIGURE 13-18** Left: Phase dispersion of stationary and moving spins under the influence of an applied gradient (no flow compensation) as the gradient is inverted is shown. The stationary spins return to the original phase state, whereas the moving spins do not. Right: *Gradient moment nulling* of first order linear velocity (flow compensation) requires a doubling of the negative gradient amplitude followed by a positive gradient such that the total summed area is equal to zero. This will return both the stationary spins *and* the moving spins to their original phase state.

third-order moment nulling to correct for acceleration and other motions are possible, but these techniques require more complicated gradient switching. Gradient moment nulling can be applied to both the slice select and readout gradients to correct for problems such as motion ghosting as elicited by CSF pulsatile flow. This approach is also referred to as flow-compensation.

13.4 PERFUSION AND DIFFUSION CONTRAST IMAGING

Perfusion is the delivery of blood to a capillary bed in tissue and permits the delivery of oxygen and nutrients to the cells and removal of waste (*e.g.*, CO_2) from the cells. There are many perfusion parameters that are estimated using MRI. Blood flow is the rate at which blood is delivered to tissues. Blood volume is the fraction of blood volume in tissues. Mean transit time (MTT) is the average time during which a tracer resides within the system. Lastly, vessel permeability is the transfer of a tracer from intravascular space to extravascular-extracellular space. These parameters are related to the vascular physiology. Hyper or hypo metabolism or ischemia is reflected to the amount of blood flow. Abnormal vascularization such as angiogenesis of tumor or stenosis affects blood volume and MTT. In the brain, when the blood-brain barrier (BBB) is broken down, vessel permeability is also changed. Conventional perfusion measurements are based on the uptake and wash-out of radioactive tracers or other exogenous tracers that can be quantified from image sequences using well-characterized imaging equipment and calibration procedures. For MR perfusion images, exogenous and endogenous tracer methods are used. As an endogenous contrast, blood itself can be a contrast tracer because blood is freely diffusible into tissue including the interior of cells. Arterial spin labeling (ASL) technique uses the blood magnetization. Another approach uses Gadolinium (Gd) based contrast agent. Gd is a paramagnetic element that shortens T2/T2* and T1 of surrounding tissue. Most of the Gd based contrast agent is an extracellular tracer that passes through vessel walls, but not in the brain because of the blood-brain barrier. Dynamic susceptibility contrast (DSC) MRI and dynamic contrast enhanced (DCE) MRI are in this category.

13.4.1 Arterial Spin Labeling

ASL technique uses the blood magnetization and measures blood flow. There are two popular ASL techniques based on a blood tagging scheme (Fig. 13-19). One is pulsed ASL and the other is continuous ASL. In pulsed ASL, a 180° RF pulse inverts the blood signal in the neck, and a 90° saturation pulse is applied later to the same location in order to convert the spatial bolus into temporal bolus. After a 1–2 s waiting time for blood to be delivered to the tissue, images in the target region are obtained. Another set of images without blood inversion is acquired (called control) and subtracted from the images in which blood signals are inverted. The subtraction removes signals from static tissues. For continuous or pseudo-continuous ASL, a long RF pulse or a train of RF pulses is applied in the neck while the blood signal passing through the plane is inverted. After waiting time for blood to be delivered to the tissue (often called postlabeling delay), images in the target region are acquired. Same as pulsed ASL, another set of images is collected while blood signals are non-inverted and subtracted from the tagged images. The signals are derived from blood signals, which are a small fraction (1%–2%) of brain or tissue, so ASL imaging suffers from low SNR. 2D imaging needs multiple signal averages (20–60) to overcome the low SNR. 3D imaging, which provides higher SNR, is often preferred but is sensitive to motion. Background suppression is often applied with multiple inversion pulses in order to

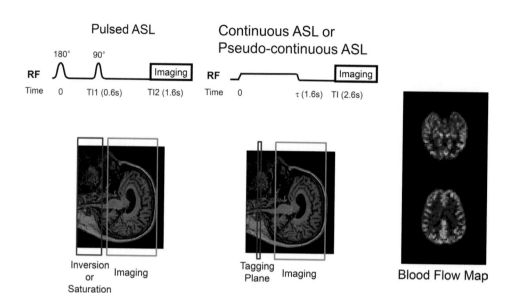

■ **FIGURE 13-19** Description of arterial spin labeling techniques: In-flowing blood spins are inverted by a single spatial inversion pulse (for pulsed ASL) or a long RF train at the tagging plane (for continuous ASL). Control and tag images are collected and perfusion-weighted images are generated by subtraction of two. Blood flow is estimated using a kinetic model with an assumption that the entire labeled signal is delivered to the tissues because the water in the blood is freely diffusible into the tissues.

reduce static signals, such as gray and white matter, and improve SNR of ASL images. The most important issue in ASL imaging is choice of the waiting time. If the images are acquired too early, the signals observed in image are only vascular signals, not true tissue perfusion. In case of a sufficiently long waiting time, only tissue perfusion signals are measured, but the SNR is decreased because of T1 decay of blood signals.

13.4.2 Dynamic Susceptibility Contrast

Figure 13-20 describes inflow of the Gd based contrast agent through a vessel including BBB leakage to extravascular space. The model in the figure shows the Gd concentration changes over time in artery and in tissue. The concentrations are measurable in the images. The response function is the "tissue residue function" and its magnitude represents the amount of flow. Blood flow can be estimated by deconvolution of this model. Cerebral blood volume (CBV) is the ratio of tissue concentration area and artery concentration area. Because the artery has 100% of blood, this represents the fraction of blood volume in tissue. Mean transit time (MTT) can be estimated by

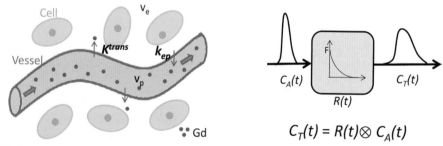

$$C_T(t) = R(t) \otimes C_A(t)$$

■ **FIGURE 13-20** Illustration of postcontrast model in tissues: Inflow of the contrast agent passes through a capillary with leakage to extravascular extracellular space. The tissue concentration measured from dynamic images is from convolution of the concentration in a large artery (arterial input function) and a response function.

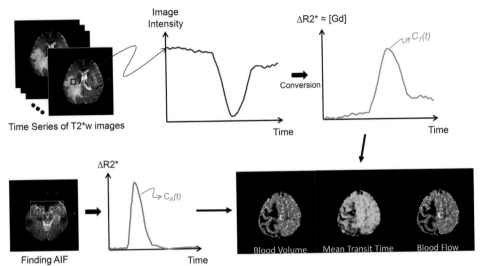

■ **FIGURE 13-21** Description of dynamic susceptibility contrast perfusion MRI: A series of dynamic T2*-weighted images is collected using 2D EPI. The signals are changed over time when the contrast passes through the area and the concentration changes of Gd are estimated from the T2* changes. After the arterial input function (AIF) is found, CBV, MTT, and CBF values are estimated using the concentration changes in the artery and in the tissues.

the ratio of CBV and cerebral blood flow (CBF) or an integral of the tissue residue function.

A series of dynamic T2 or T2* weighted images is collected using 2D multislice EPI with an echo time of 50–70 ms at 1.5 T and a TR of 1.5 seconds. The signal changes within a single voxel are heavily decreased while the contrast passes through the area (see Fig. 13-21). The dynamic T2 or T2* curve per voxel is analyzed to estimate perfusion parameters. The concentration of Gd is proportional to change of R2* (inverse of T2*). The signal intensity is converted into R2* signal change. The arterial input function is found by selecting an area manually or automatically and CBV, MTT, and CBF values are estimated using the concentration changes in the artery and in the tissues.

A concern in DSC is contrast agent leakage to the extravascular extracellular space. Because the conventional DSC model is based on no leakage, a leakage correction is often applied, or a small amount of contrast agent is preloaded prior to a DSC scan to fill up the possible leaky tissues.

13.4.3 Dynamic Contrast Enhanced

The purpose of DCE imaging is to measure the amount of leakage. As shown in Figure 13-20, K^{trans} is a transfer constant from intravascular space to extravascular space; V_e is the volume fraction of extravascular extracellular space; and k_{ep} is the rate constant for efflux back into plasma, which is K^{trans}/V_e. When CBV is assumed to be close to zero, the response function represents the K^{trans} and k_{ep}, which can be estimated by the "Tofts" model (Sourbron, 2011):

$$C_T(t) = R(t) \otimes C_A(t), \quad CBV \approx 0.$$

There is a model including plasma volume, v_p, called extended Tofts model:

$$C_T(t) = R(t) \otimes C_A(t) + v_p C_A(t).$$

In the Tofts and extended Tofts models, the response function, $R(t)$ is:

$$R(t) = K^{\text{trans}} e^{-k_{ep}t} = K^{\text{trans}} e^{\frac{-K^{\text{trans}}}{V_e}t}.$$

A dynamic T1-weighted pulse sequence such as SPGR is used for DCE, and Figure 13-22 describes an example of T1w signal change when Gd based contrast agent is injected. The Gd concentration is proportional to change of R1 (inverse of T1). In a T1-weighted sequence, such as SPGR, the signal is expressed in a complicated equation factoring flip angle, TR, and T1 of tissue. Tissue T1 is often measured with a separate scan or an assumed value of Tissue T1 is used to estimate R1 changes. After finding the arterial input function as DSC, K^{trans}, V_e, V_p, and k_{ep} are calculated based on the extended Tofts model. Please note that K^{trans} is not simply permeability but it is related to vessel surface area and blood flow as well.

Table 13-1 describes comparison of the perfusion MRI techniques. ASL does not use Gd based contrast agent, so it can be repeatable during a single scan session. And it is easy to quantify CBF value. However, ASL has transit delay effect and its spatial resolution is low because of low sensitivity of blood signal. For DSC, the scan time is short and the signal change is large, which brings robust quantification. However, its spatial resolution is also low and images suffer from susceptibility artifacts. Finally, DCE is good for evaluation of tumor, but its model is complicated.

13.4.4 Diffusion MRI

Molecular diffusion is the stochastic translational motion of molecules also known as Brownian motion. Interaction of the local cellular structure with the movement of water molecules produces anisotropic, directionally dependent diffusion (e.g., in the white matter of brain tissues). Diffusion sequences use strong MR gradients applied symmetrically about the refocusing pulse to produce signal

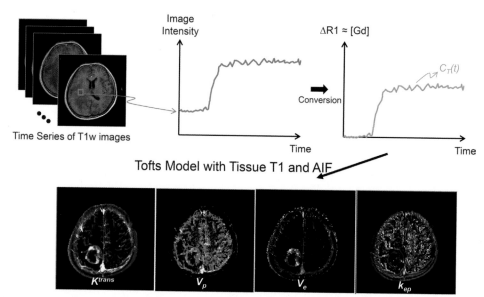

■ **FIGURE 13-22** Description of dynamic contrast enhanced perfusion MRI: DCE imaging is mainly to measure the amount of leakage. A series of dynamic T1-weighted images are used to estimate the Gd concentration in the tissue. Using Tofts model, the exchange parameters and volume fraction maps are generated.

TABLE 13-1 COMPARISON OF PERFUSION MRI TECHNIQUES

	ASL	DSC	DCE
GBCA	X	O	O
Contrast	Blood T1	T2/T2*	T1
Sequence	PASL or PCASL	T2w SE or T2*w GRE	T1w SPGR
Parameters	CBF	CBF, CBV, MTT	K^{trans}, k_{ep}, V_p, V_e
Pros	Repeatable Ease of quantification	Short scan time Large signal change	Evaluation of leakage
Cons	Transit delay effect Low spatial resolution	Low spatial resolution Susceptibility artifact	Complexity of model
Clinical use	Used to measure blood flow of brain, heart, kidney, muscle	Most widely used for brain (strokes/tumors) and heart (ischemia)	Most widely used for evaluating tumors/response to therapy in brain, breast, pelvis

ASL, arterial spin labeling; DSC, dynamic susceptibility contrast; DCE, dynamic contrast enhanced; GBCA, gadolinium based contrast agent; PASL, pulsed ASL; PCASL: pseudo-continuous ASL; CBF, cerebral blood flow; CBV, cerebral blood volume; MTT, mean transit time; K^{trans}, the rate constant from intravascular space to extravascular space; k_{ep}, the rate constant for efflux back into plasma; V_p, the volume fraction of plasma; V_e, the volume fraction of extravascular extracellular space.

differences based on the mobility and directionality of water diffusion, as shown in Figure 13-23. Tissues with more water mobility (normal) have a greater signal loss than those with lesser water mobility (injury) under the influence of the diffusion weighted imaging (DWI) gradients. With diffusion weighted gradients, the measurable transverse magnetization from this spin echo sequence can be expressed as:

$$M_{xy}(b,\text{TE}) = M_0 e^{-\text{TE}/T2} e^{-bD},$$

where the diffusion sensitivity factor is the b-value (s/mm²), and the diffusivity, D, of which free water molecules in water at 37°C, is 3×10^{-3} mm²/s.

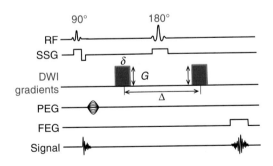

■ FIGURE 13-23 The basic elements of a DWI pulse sequence are shown. The diffusion weighting gradients are of amplitude G, duration of the gradients is δ, and time between gradients is Δ.

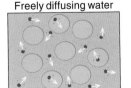

Normal Tissue

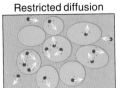

Ischemic Injury / Stroke

Various acquisition techniques are used to generate diffusion-weighted contrast. Standard spin echo and EPI pulse sequences with applied diffusion gradients of high strength are used. Challenges for DWI are the extreme sensitivity to motion of the head and brain, which is chiefly caused by the large pulsed gradients required for the diffusion preparation. Eddy currents are also an issue, which reduce the effectiveness of the gradient fields, so compensated gradient coils are necessary. Several strategies have been devised to overcome the motion sensitivity problem, including common electrocardiographic gating and motion compensation methods.

Diffusion Weighted Imaging

The in vivo structural integrity of certain tissues (healthy, diseased, or injured) can be measured using DWI, in which water diffusion characteristics are determined through the generation of apparent diffusion coefficient (ADC) maps. This requires two or more acquisitions with different DWI parameters: one is with a b-value close to zero and the others are with a high b-value (typically $b = 1,000$ in brain applications) in different diffusion directions. Trace weighted maps are generated by averaging all diffusion weighted images and include T2 weighted contrast as well. ADC maps are generated after applying diffusion gradients in three orthogonal directions, calculating a exponential decay due to a diffusivity in the specific direction and adding the diffusivities in three directions. A low ADC corresponds to high signal intensity on a DWI, which may represent reduced diffusion in infarcted region (Fig. 13-24). ADC maps of the brain and the spinal cord have shown promise in predicting and evaluating pathophysiology before it is visible on conventional T1- or T2-weighted images. DWI is also a sensitive indicator for early detection of ischemic injury. Areas of acute stroke show a drastic reduction in the diffusion coefficient compared with non-ischemic tissues.

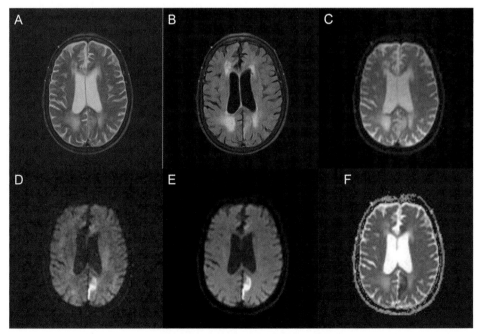

■ **FIGURE 13-24** Structural images of a brain infarction case: **(A)** T2 weighted image, **(B)** T2 FLAIR image, **(C)** $b = 0$ image, **(D)** DWI in a diffusion direction, **(E)** Trace weighted image, and **(F)** ADC map. The diffusion weighted images **(D, E, and F)** show clear distinctions between normal and infarcted regions.

Diffusion Tensor Imaging

The diffusivity of water molecules is often restricted by macromolecules and tissue structure surrounding them in biological tissues. This anisotropic mobility could provide the structure of surrounding tissues. For example, in a bundle of parallel fibers in brain white matter, molecular displacements to the perpendicular direction of fibers in intra-axonal and interstitial compartments are much more restricted than that to the parallel direction. The anisotropic directional diffusion coefficients can be expressed as a 3 × 3 symmetric diffusion tensor, **D**:

$$\mathbf{D} = \begin{bmatrix} D_{xx} & D_{xy} & D_{xz} \\ D_{xy} & D_{yy} & D_{yz} \\ D_{xz} & D_{yz} & D_{zz} \end{bmatrix}.$$

The diffusion tensor is diagonally symmetric (i.e., $D_{xy} = D_{yx}$) so a minimum of 6 diffusion encoding directions are required to generate the tensor but practically, 15 or 30 directions are played to improve SNR. Figure 13-25 describes a representation of white matter fibers to a diffusion ellipsoid measured from diffusion tensor

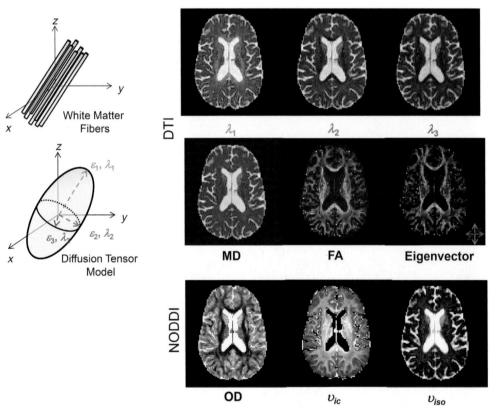

■ **FIGURE 13-25** Illustration of diffusion tensor model associated with white matter fibers represents eigenvalues and eigen vectors characterizing water diffusion and molecular structure within a voxel (left). From a DTI with a 1,000 b-value in 30 diffusion directions, three orthogonal eigenvalues are estimated and mean diffusivity (MD), fractional anisotropy (FA), and eigen vector color map showing the direction of the primary eigen vector (blue: S/I, red: R/L, and green: A/P directions) are calculated from the eigenvalues and eigen vectors (upper right). Neurite Orientation Dispersion and Density Images (NODDI) acquired with a b-value of 711 in 30 directions and a b-value of 2855 in 60 directions. The images shown represent neurite orientation dispersion (OD), intracellular volume fraction (v_{ic}), and isotropic volume fraction (v_{iso}) (lower right).

imaging (DTI). From a tensor matrix for each voxel, eigenvalues and eigen vectors of the voxel represent the water diffusion characteristics and the major direction of a fiber tract passing the specific voxel. DTI allows tractography, a 3D modeling technique visualizing white matter tracts (an example shown in Fig. 13-27).

Diffusion MRI measures mobilities of water molecules in tissues, which indirectly provides information of molecular structures. Diffusion MRI with a very high number of diffusion encoding directions can be acquired in a clinically relevant scan time because of recent advances in parallel imaging and MB imaging. Diffusion spectrum imaging (DSI) or high angular resolution diffusion imaging (HARDI) with more than 100 directions resolves intra-voxel heterogeneity caused by crossing fiber tracts. Multiple diffusion sensitivities, b-values (or diffusion shells), are used to estimate the tissue kurtosis, skewed distribution from Gaussian (diffusion kurtosis imaging), or neurite orientation dispersion and density (NODDI).

13.5 OTHER ADVANCED TECHNIQUES

13.5.1 Functional MRI

Functional MRI (fMRI) is based on the increase in blood flow to the local vasculature that accompanies neural activity in the specific areas of the brain, resulting in a local reduction of deoxyhemoglobin because the increase in blood flow occurs without an increase in oxygen extraction fraction although oxygen utilization is increased. As deoxyhemoglobin is a paramagnetic agent, it alters the T2*-weighted MRI image signal. Thus, this endogenous contrast enhancing agent serves as the signal for fMRI. Area voxels (represented by x-y coordinates and z slice thickness) of high metabolic activity resulting from a task-induced stimulus produce a correlated signal for blood oxygen level dependent (BOLD) acquisition techniques. A BOLD sequence produces multiple T2*-weighted images of the head before the application of the stimulus. The patient is repeatedly subjected to the stimulus and multiple BOLD images are acquired. Because the BOLD sequence produces images that are highly dependent on blood oxygen levels, areas of high metabolic activity will demonstrate a change in signal when the prestimulus image data set is subtracted, voxel by voxel, from poststimulus image data set. Voxel locations defined by significant signal changes indicate regions of the brain activated by a specific task. Stimuli in fMRI experiments can be physical (finger movement), sensory (light flashes or sounds), or cognitive (repetition of "good" or "bad" word sequences, complex problem solving), among others. To improve the SNR in the fMRI images, a stimulus is typically applied in a repetitive, periodic sequence, and BOLD images are acquired continuously, tagged with the timing of the stimulus. Regions in the brain that demonstrate time-dependent activity and correlate with the time-dependent application of the stimulus are statistically analyzed, and coded using a color scale, while voxels that do not show a significant intensity change are not colored. The resultant color map is overlaid onto a grayscale image of the brain for anatomic reference, as shown in Figure 13-26.

High-speed imaging and T2* weighting necessary for fMRI is typically achieved with GRE EPI acquisition techniques including 24 slices, slice thickness 4 mm, a 96 × 96 acquisition matrix, TR = 3 s, TE = 30 ms at 3 T, with 80 to 100 complete head acquisitions. Utilizing MB and parallel imaging, high spatial resolution (i.e., 2 mm isotropic resolution with a whole brain coverage) and fast temporal resolution (TR < 1 s) are achievable.

Bilateral finger tapping paradigm

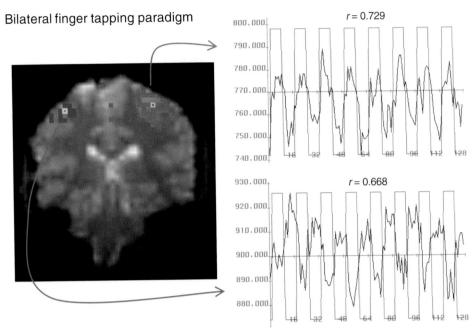

■ **FIGURE 13-26** Functional MR image bilateral finger tapping paradigm shows the areas of the brain activated by this repeated activity. The paradigm was a right finger tap alternated by a left finger tap (time sequence on the right side of the figure) and the correlated BOLD signals (black traces) derived from the echo planar image sequence. A voxel-by-voxel correlation of the periodic stimulus and MR signal is performed, and when exceeding a correlation threshold, a color overlay is added to the grayscale image. In this example, red indicates the right finger tap that excites the left motor cortex, which appears on the right side of the image, and blue the left finger tap. (Courtesy of the late M. H. Buonocore, MD, PhD, University of California Davis.)

Diffusion MRI and fMRI have been more often used clinically for presurgical planning. Figure 13-27 shows an example of how fMRI and DTI visualize function and structure surrounding the tumoral region prior to brain tumor resection.

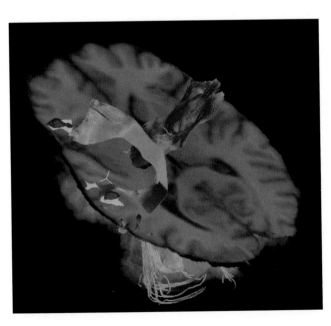

■ **FIGURE 13-27** Functional MRI (fMRI) and diffusion tensor imaging (DTI) tractography for presurgical evaluation of brain tumor resection. Significant fMRI activations were detected in both anterior (Broca's) and posterior (Wernicke's) areas of the language network in the left hemisphere when the patient was performing language tasks (blue: word generation, pink: category naming, yellow: sentence completion). Critical fiber bundles including corticospinal tract (motor) and arcuate fasciculus (language) were generated with fiber tracking of the DTI data. (Copyright held by, and used with permission of, The University of Texas MD Anderson Cancer Center.)

13.5.2   Susceptibility Weighted Imaging

Susceptibility weighted imaging (SWI), sensitive to local susceptibility differences from deoxyhemoglobin in venous blood, methemoglobin in blood hemorrhage, and iron deposition, is based on T2* weighted images obtained with a 3D GRE sequence. The technique utilizes small and local phase differences as well as magnitude change. Slowly changing phase variations due to field inhomogeneities are first removed using high pass phase filter. The filtered images are used to create phase masks ranging between 0 and 1, and SWI is generated by multiplying the magnitude images with the phase masks multiple times to emphasize the small phase deviations created by focal hemorrhage or iron deposit. For better visualization, minimum intensity projection (mIP) is created by selecting the minimum value through a projection plane, contrary to MIP. Figure 13-28 describes an example of SWI. Quantitative susceptibility mapping is also feasible with multiple gradient images more than 6 echoes.

13.5.3   MR Elastography

MR elastography (MRE) is a technique to evaluate the stiffness of tissues. GRE imaging with motion-encoding gradients (similar to phase-contrast MRA) is able to detect sub-micrometer motion in the direction of mechanical wave propagation. Typically 4–8 dynamic images are acquired while mechanical waves generated by a wave generator are transmitted through an organ, particularly liver. The displacement information at the applied mechanical frequency (~60 Hz) is extracted from the dynamic phase images while other frequency information is rejected. The spatial wavelength is inversely proportional to the wave speed, and the tissue stiffness is estimated from the wave speed (stiffer tissue shows faster wave speed). Figure 13-29 describes an example of MRE.

13.5.4   Magnetization Transfer Contrast

Magnetization transfer contrast is the result of selective observation of the interaction between protons in free water molecules and protons hydrated to the macromolecules of a protein. Magnetization exchange occurs between the two proton groups resulting from coupling or chemical exchange. Because the protons exist in slightly different magnetic environments, the selective saturation of the protons in the

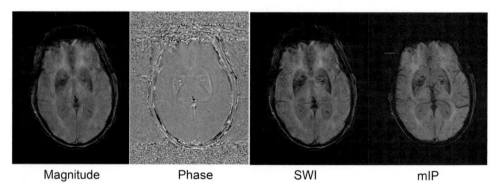

Magnitude   Phase   SWI   mIP

■ **FIGURE 13-28** Example of susceptibility weighted imaging: Magnitude and phase images are obtained with 3D T2* weighted images GRE sequence. In SWI, the small phase deviations hardly detectable in normal T2* weighted images are emphasized by multiplying the magnitude images with the phase masks multiple times. mIP is created by choosing the minimum value in multiple slices.

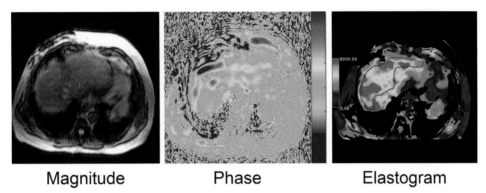

| Magnitude | Phase | Elastogram |

■ **FIGURE 13-29** Example of MR elastography: The phase of MRE shows the phase variation due to the mechanical vibration included by a wave generator. Elastogram shows tissue stiffness estimated based on the wave propagation.

hydration layer can be excited separately from the bulk water by using narrow-band RF pulses (because the Larmor frequencies are different). A transfer of the magnetization from the protons in the hydration layer partially saturates the protons in bulk water, even though these protons have not experienced an RF excitation pulse (Fig. 13-30). Reduced signal from the adjacent free water protons by the saturation "label" affects only those protons having a chemical exchange with the macromolecules and improves local image contrast in many situations by decreasing the otherwise large signal generated by the protons in the bulk water. This technique is used for anatomic MRI of the heart, the eye, multiple sclerosis, knee cartilage, and general MRA. Tissue characterization is also possible, because the image contrast in part is caused by the surface chemistry of the macromolecule and the tissue-specific factors that affect the magnetization transfer characteristics.

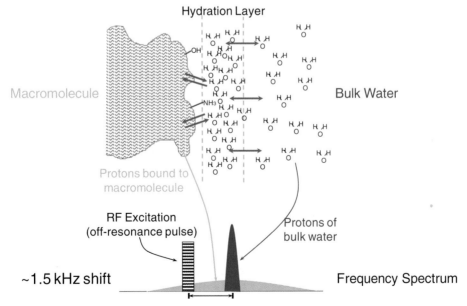

■ **FIGURE 13-30** Magnetization transfer contrast is implemented with an off-resonance RF pulse of about 1,500 Hz from the Larmor frequency. Excitation of hydrogen confined in the macromolecule hydration layer is transferred to adjacent "free-water" hydrogen atoms. A partial saturation of bulk water protons reduces the signals that would otherwise compete with signals from blood flow, making this useful for time-of-flight MRA.

Magnetization transfer contrast pulse sequences are often used in conjunction with MRA time-of-flight methods. Hydrogen atoms constitute a large fraction of macromolecules in proteins in a hydration layer, are tightly bound to these macromolecules, and have a very short T2 decay with a broad range of resonance frequencies compared to protons in free water. Selective excitation of these protons is achieved with an off-resonance RF pulse of approximately 1,500 Hz from the Larmor frequency, causing their saturation. The protons in the hydration layer bound to these molecules transfer their magnetization to the local unbound water protons, partially saturating and suppressing their signal as well, with an impact of reducing the contrast variation of the associated anatomy. As a result, the differential contrast of the flow-enhanced signals is increased, with overall better image quality angiographic sequence.

13.5.5 Magnetic Resonance Spectroscopy

MRS is a method to measure tissue chemistry (an "electronic" biopsy) by recording and evaluating signals from metabolites by identifying metabolic peaks caused by frequency shifts (in parts per million, ppm) relative to a frequency standard. In vivo MRS can be performed with ^{1}H (proton), ^{23}Na (sodium), and ^{31}P (phosphorus) nuclei, but proton spectroscopy provides a much higher SNR and can be included in a conventional MRI protocol with about 10 to 15 minutes of extra exam time. Uses of MRS include serial evaluation of biochemical changes in tumors; analyzing metabolic disorders, infections, and diseases; as well as evaluation of therapeutic oncology treatments for tumor recurrence versus radiation damage. Early applications were dedicated to brain disorders, but now breast, liver, and prostate MRS is also performed. Correlation of spectroscopy results and MR images are always advised before making a final diagnosis.

In MRS, signals are derived from the amplitude of proton metabolites in targeted tissues. In these metabolites, chemical shifts occur due to electron cloud shielding of the nuclei, causing slightly different resonance frequencies, which exist in a frequency range between water and fat. The very small signal amplitudes of the metabolites require suppression of the extremely large (~10,000 times higher) amplitudes due to bulk water and fat protons, as shown in Figure 13-31. This is achieved by using specific chemical saturation techniques, such as CHESS (Chemical Shift-Selective) or STIR (see Chapter 12). In many cases, the areas evaluated are away from fat

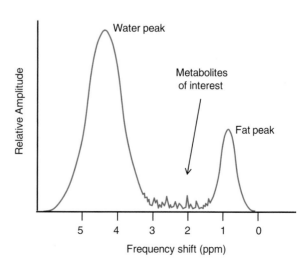

■ **FIGURE 13-31** MRS metabolites of interest in comparison to the water and fat peaks commonly used for imaging. In order to isolate the very small signals, chemical saturation of the water (and fat when present) signal is essential.

structures, and only bulk water signal suppression is necessary; however, in organs such as the liver and the breast, suppression of both fat and water is required. Once the water and fat signals are suppressed, localization of the targeted area volume is achieved by either a single voxel or multivoxel technique.

Single voxel MRS sampling areas, covering a volume of about 1 cm³, are delineated by a STEAM (STimulated Echo Acquisition Mode) or a PRESS (Point Resolved Spectroscopy) sequence. The STEAM method uses a 90° excitation pulse and 90° refocusing pulse to collect the signal in conjunction with gradients to define each dimension of the voxel. The PRESS sequence uses a 90° excitation and 180° refocusing pulse in each direction. STEAM achieves shorter echo times and superior voxel boundaries, but with lower SNR. After the voxel data are collected, a Fourier transform is applied to separate the composite signal into individual frequencies, which are plotted as a trace for a normal brain spectrum (Fig. 13-32). The resulting line widths are based on homogeneity of the main magnetic field as well as the magnetic field strength. Higher field strengths (e.g., 3.0 T) will improve resolution of the peaks and corresponding SNR.

Multivoxel MRS uses a CSI (Chemical Shift Imaging) technique to delineate multiple voxels of approximately 1 cm³ volume in 1, 2, or 3 planes over a rectangular block of several centimeters, achievable with more sophisticated equipment and longer scan times. This is followed by MRSI (Magnetic Resonance Spectroscopic Imaging) where the signal intensity of a single metabolite in each voxel is color encoded for each voxel according to concentration and the generated parameter maps superimposed on the anatomical MR image. In practice, the single voxel technique is used to make the initial diagnosis because the SNR is high and all metabolites are represented in the MRS trace. Then, a multivoxel acquisition to assess the distribution of a specific metabolite is performed.

Proton MRS can be performed with short (20 to 40 ms), intermediate (135 to 145 ms), or long (270 to 290 ms) echo times. For short TE, numerous resonances from metabolites of lesser importance (with shorter T2) can make the spectra more difficult to interpret, and with long echo times, SNR losses are too severe. Therefore, most MRS acquisitions use a TE of approximately 135 ms at 1.5 T. Metabolites of interest for brain spectroscopy are listed in Table 13-2.

Applications of MRS are achieved through the interpretation of the spectra that are obtained from the lesion, from its surroundings, and presumably healthy tissue

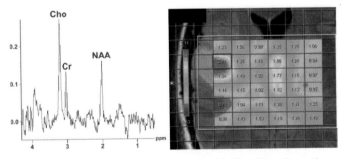

MR Spectrum from anaplastic oligoastrocytoma   Choline / Creatine ratio map

■ **FIGURE 13-32** Left: Intermediate echo (TE = 135 ms) single voxel spectrum is shown, positioned over an anaplastic oligoastrocytoma brain lesion. Note the elevated choline peak and lowered creatine and NAA peaks. Right: Multivoxel spectrum is color coded to the choline/creatine ratio, illustrating the regional variation of the metabolites corresponding to tumor. (Reprinted with permission from Al-Okaili RN, Krejza J, Wang S, Woo JH, Melhem ER. Advanced MR imaging techniques in the diagnosis of intraaxial brain tumors in adults. *Radiographics*. 2006;26:S173-S189. Copyright © Radiological Society of North America. doi: 10.1148/rg.26si065513.)

TABLE 13-2 METABOLITES IN MRS AT 1.5 T

ABBREVIATION	METABOLITE	SHIFT (PPM)	PROPERTIES/SIGNIFICANCE IN THE BRAIN
Cho	Phosphocholine	3.22	Membrane turnover, cell proliferation
Cr	Creatine	3.02 and 3.93	Temporary store for energy-rich phosphates
NAA	N-acetyl-L-aspartate	2.01	Presence of intact glioneural structures
Lactate		1.33 (inverted)	Anaerobic glycolysis
Lipids	Free fatty acids	1.2–1.4	Necrosis

in the same scan. Main criteria include the presence or absence of pathologic metabolites (lactate or lipids) and the relationships between the concentrations of choline, creatine, and NAA as ratios. Spectra are usually scaled to the highest peak, and y-axis values will usually differ between measurements, so caution must be observed to avoid potential misdiagnoses.

In a tumor, high cell turnover causes an increase in choline concentration along with a corresponding depression of the NAA peak caused by the loss of healthy glioneural structures. In addition, the creatine peak may also be reduced depending on the energy status of the tumor; it is often used to serve as an internal reference for calculating ratios of metabolites. When a lipid peak is observed, this is a sign of hypoxia and the likelihood of a high-grade malignancy. Table 13-3 lists qualitative findings for MRS spectroscopy in evaluating brain tumors for the ratios of NAA/Cr, NAA/Cho, and Cho/Cr. Examples of single voxel and multivoxel spectra are shown in Figure 13-32, illustrating the use of the spectral peaks for diagnostic interpretation of the ratios, and an MRSI color-encoded graphic display of the spatial distribution of findings. There is certainly much more than determining ratios, and differential diagnoses are often clouded by indistinct peaks, poor SNR, and tumor heterogeneity, among other causes. MRS at 3 T field strength enjoys much better SNR, improved spectral resolution, and faster scans. Because of the higher spectral resolution, familiar single target peaks at 1.5 T become a collection of peaks at 3 T.

13.6 MR ARTIFACTS

Artifacts manifest as positive or negative signal intensities that do not accurately represent the imaged anatomy. Although some artifacts are relatively insignificant and are easily identified, others can limit the diagnostic potential of the exam by obscuring or mimicking pathologic processes or anatomy. One must realize the impact of MR acquisition protocols and understand the etiology of artifact production to exploit the information they convey.

TABLE 13-3 RATIOS OF METABOLITE PEAKS IN MRS INDICATING "NORMAL" AND "ABNORMAL" STATUS

METABOLITE RATIO	NORMAL	ABNORMAL
NAA/Cr	2.0	<1.6
NAA/Cho	1.6	<1.2
Cho/Cr	1.2	>1.5

To minimize the impact of MR artifacts, a working knowledge of MR physics as well as image acquisition techniques is required. On the one hand, there are many variables and options available that complicate the decision-making process for MR image acquisition. On the other, the wealth of choices enhances the goal of achieving diagnostically accurate images. MR artifacts are classified into three broad areas—those based on the machine, on the patient, and on signal processing.

13.6.1 Magnetic Field Inhomogeneities

Magnetic field inhomogeneities are either global or focal field perturbations that lead to the mismapping of tissues within the image, and cause more rapid T2 relaxation. Distortion or misplacement of anatomy occurs when the magnetic field is not completely homogeneous. Proper site planning, self-shielded magnets, automatic shimming, and preventive maintenance procedures help to reduce inhomogeneities.

Focal field inhomogeneities arise from many causes. Ferromagnetic objects in or on the patient (*e.g.*, makeup, metallic implants, prostheses, surgical clips, dentures) produce field distortions and cause protons to precess at frequencies different from the Larmor frequency in the local area. Incorrect proton mapping, displacement, and appearance as a signal void with a peripherally enhanced rim of increased signal are common findings. Geometric distortion of surrounding tissue is also usually evident. Even non-ferromagnetic conducting materials (*e.g.*, aluminum) produce field distortions that disturb the local magnetic environment. Partial compensation by the spin echo (180° RF) pulse sequence reduces these artifacts; on the other hand, the gradient-refocused echo sequence accentuates distortions, since the protons always experience the same direction of the focal magnetic inhomogeneities within the patient.

13.6.2 Susceptibility Artifacts

Magnetic susceptibility is the ratio of the induced internal magnetization in a tissue to the external magnetic field. As long as the magnetic susceptibility of the tissues being imaged is relatively unchanged across the field of view, the magnetic field will remain uniform. Any drastic changes in the magnetic susceptibility will distort the magnetic field. The most common susceptibility changes occur at tissue-air interfaces (*e.g.*, lungs and sinuses), which cause a signal loss due to more rapid dephasing (T2*) at the tissue-air interface. Any metal (ferrous or not) may have a significant effect on the adjacent local tissues due to changes in susceptibility and the resultant magnetic field distortions (Fig. 13-33). Paramagnetic agents exhibit a weak magnetization and increase the local magnetic field causing an artifactual reduction in the surrounding T2* relaxation.

Magnetic susceptibility can be quite helpful in some diagnoses. Most notable is the ability to diagnose the age of a hemorrhage based on the signal characteristics of the blood degradation products, which are different in the acute, subacute, and chronic phases. Some of the iron-containing compounds (deoxyhemoglobin, methemoglobin, hemosiderin, and ferritin) can dramatically shorten T1 and T2 relaxation of nearby protons. The amount of associated free water, the type and structure of the iron-containing molecules, the distribution (intracellular versus extracellular), and the magnetic field strength all influence the degree of relaxation effect that may be seen. For example, in the acute stage, T2 shortening occurs due to the paramagnetic susceptibility of the organized deoxyhemoglobin in the local area, without any large effect on the T1 relaxation time. When red blood cells lyse during the subacute stage, the hemoglobin is altered into methemoglobin, and spin-lattice relaxation is

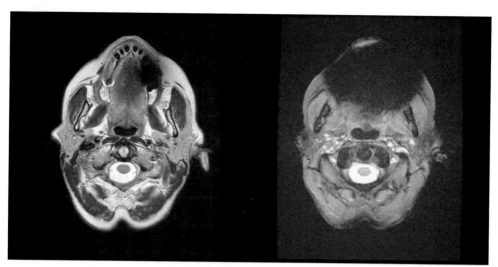

■ **FIGURE 13-33** Susceptibility artifacts due to dental fillings are shown in the same axial image slice. Left: Axial T2-weighted fast spin echo image illustrates significant suppression of susceptibility artifacts with 180° refocusing pulse. Right: Axial T2*-weighted gradient echo image illustrates significant image void exacerbated by the gradient echo, where external inhomogeneities are not canceled in the reformed echo.

enhanced with the formation of a hydration layer, which shortens T1 relaxation, leading to a much stronger signal on T1-weighted images. Increased signal intensity on T1-weighted images not found in the acute stage of hemorrhage identifies the subacute stage. In the chronic stage, hemosiderin, found in the phagocytic cells in sites of previous hemorrhage, disrupts the local magnetic homogeneity, causes loss of signal intensity, and leads to signal void, producing a characteristic dark rim around the hemorrhage site.

Gadolinium-based contrast agents (paramagnetic characteristics shorten T2 and hydration layer interactions shorten T1) are widely used in MRI. Tissues that uptake gadolinium contrast agents exhibit shortened T1 relaxation and demonstrate increased signal on T1-weighted images. Although focal inhomogeneities are generally considered problematic, there are certain physiologic and anatomic manifestations that can be identified and diagnostic information obtained.

13.6.3 Gradient Field Artifacts

Magnetic field gradients spatially encode the location of the signals emanating from excited protons within the volume being imaged. Accurate reconstruction requires linear, matched, and properly sequenced gradients. The slice select gradient defines the volume (slice). Phase and frequency encoding gradients provide the spatial information in the other two dimensions.

Since the reconstruction algorithm assumes ideal, linear gradients, any deviation or temporal instability will be represented as a distortion. Gradient strength has a tendency to fall off at the periphery of the FOV. Consequently, anatomic compression occurs, especially pronounced on coronal and sagittal images having a large FOV, typically greater than 35 cm (Fig. 13-34). Minimizing the spatial distortion entails reducing the FOV either by lowering the gradient field strength or by holding the gradient field strength and number of samples constant while decreasing the frequency bandwidth. Of course, gradient calibration is part of a continuous quality control (QC) checklist, and geometric accuracy must be periodically verified.

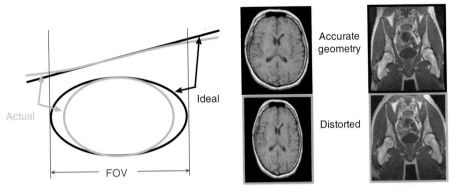

■ **FIGURE 13-34** Gradient non-linearity causes image distortions by mis-mapping anatomy. In the above examples, the strength of the gradient at the periphery is less than the ideal (orange line versus black line). This results in a compression of the imaged anatomy, with inaccurate geometry (images with orange border). For comparison, images acquired with linear corrections are shown above.

Anatomic proportions may simulate abnormalities, so verification of pixel dimensions in the PEG and FEG directions are necessary. If the strength of the FEG and the strength of the largest PEG are different, the height or width of the pixels can become distorted and produce inaccurate measurements. Ideally, the phase and frequency encoding gradients should be assigned to the smaller and larger dimensions of the object, respectively, to preserve spatial resolution while limiting the number of phase encoding steps. In practice, this is not always possible, because motion artifacts or high-intensity signals that need to be displaced away from important areas of interest after an initial scan might require swapping the frequency and phase encode gradient directions.

13.6.4 RF Coil Artifacts

RF surface coils produce variations in uniformity across the image caused by RF excitation variability, attenuation, mismatching, and sensitivity falloff with distance. Proximal to the surface coil, received signals are intense, whereas with distance, signal intensity is attenuated, resulting in grayscale shading and loss of brightness in the image. Non-uniform image intensities are the all-too-frequent result. Also, adjustment for the disturbance of the magnetic field by the patient is typically compensated by an automatic shimming calibration. When this is not performed, or performed inadequately, a significant negative impact on image quality occurs. Examples of variable response are shown in Figure 13-35.

Other common artifacts from RF coils occur with RF quadrature coils (coils that simultaneously measure the signal from orthogonal views) that have two separate amplifier and gain controls. If the amplifiers are imbalanced, a bright spot in the center of the image, known as a center point artifact, arises as a "0 frequency" direct current offset. Variations in gain between the quadrature coils can cause ghosting of objects diagonally in the image. The bottom line for all RF coils is the need for continuous measurement and consistent calibration of their response, so that artifacts are minimized.

13.6.5 RF Artifacts

RF pulses and precessional frequencies of MRI instruments occupy the same frequencies of common RF sources, such as TV and radio broadcasts, electric motors, fluorescent lights, and computers. Stray RF signals that propagate to the MRI antenna can

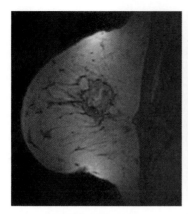 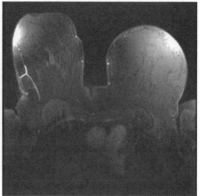

Coil close to skin   Inadequate shimming for fat saturation

■ **FIGURE 13-35** Signal intensity variations occur when surface RF receive coils are too close to the skin, as exemplified by the MR breast image on the left. With inadequate shimming calibration, saturation pulses for adipose tissue in the breast are uneven, causing a significant variation in the uniformity of the reconstructed image. (Left, reprinted by permission from Springer Nature. Hendrick RE. *Breast MRI: Fundamentals and Technical Aspects*. Copyright © 2008, Springer Science Business Media, LLC. Right, courtesy of R. Edward Hendrick, PhD.)

produce various artifacts in the image. Narrow-band noise creates noise patterns perpendicular to the frequency encoding direction. The exact position and spatial extent depend on the resonant frequency of the imager, applied gradient field strength, and bandwidth of the noise. A narrow band pattern of black/white alternating noise produces a "zipper" artifact. Broadband RF noise disrupts the image over a much larger area of the reconstructed image with diffuse, contrast-reducing "herringbone" artifacts. Appropriate site planning and the use of properly installed RF shielding materials (*e.g.*, a Faraday cage) reduce stray RF interference to an acceptably low level. An example RF zipper artifact is shown in Figure 13-48 in Section 13.7.

RF energy received by adjacent slices during a multislice acquisition excite and saturate protons in adjacent slices, chiefly due to RF pulses without sharp off/on/off transitions. This is known as cross-excitation. On T2-weighted images, the slice-to-slice interference degrades the SNR; on T1-weighted images, the extra partial saturation reduces image contrast by reducing longitudinal recovery during the TR interval. A typical truncated "sinc" RF profile and overlap areas in adjacent slices are shown in Figure 13-36. Interslice gaps reduce the overlap of the profile tails, and pseudo-rectangular RF pulse profiles reduce the spatial extent of the tails. Important anatomic findings could exist within the gaps, so *slice interleaving* is a technique to mitigate cross-excitation by reordering slices into two groups with gaps. During the first half of the TR, the first slices are acquired (slices 1 to 5), followed by the second group of slices that are positioned in the gap of the first group (slices 6 to 10). This method reduces cross-excitation by separating the adjacent slice excitations in time. The most effective method is to acquire two independent sets of gapped multislice images, but the image time is doubled. The most appropriate solution is to devise RF pulses that approximate a rectangular profile; however, the additional time necessary for producing such an RF pulse can be prohibitive.

13.6.6 *k*-Space Errors

Errors in *k*-space encoding affect all areas of the reconstructed image, and cause the artifactual superimposition of wave patterns across the FOV. Each individual pixel value in *k*-space contributes to all pixel values in image space as a frequency

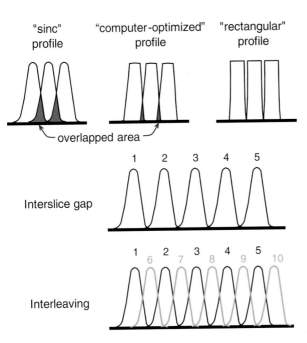

"sinc" profile   "computer-optimized" profile   "rectangular" profile

overlapped area

Interslice gap   1 2 3 4 5

Interleaving   1 6 2 7 3 8 4 9 5 10

FIGURE 13-36 Top: Poor pulse profiles are caused by truncated RF pulses, and resulting profile overlap causes unwanted partial saturation in adjacent slices, with a loss of SNR and CNR. Optimized pulses are produced by considering the trade-off of pulse duration versus excitation profile. Bottom: Reduction of cross-excitation is achieved with interslice gaps, but anatomy at the gap location might be missed. An interleaving technique acquires the first half of the images with an interslice gap, and the second half of the images are positioned in the gaps of the first images. The separation in time reduces the amount of contrast reducing saturation of the adjacent slices.

harmonic with a signal amplitude. One bad pixel introduces a significant artifact, rendering the image suboptimal, as shown in Figure 13-37.

13.6.7 Motion Artifacts

The most ubiquitous and noticeable artifacts in MRI arise with patient motion, including voluntary and involuntary movement, and flow (blood, CSF). Although motion artifacts are not unique to MRI, the long acquisition time of certain MRI sequences increases the probability of motion blurring and contrast resolution losses. Motion artifacts occur mostly along the phase encode direction, as adjacent phase encoding measurements in k-space are separated by a TR interval that can last 3,000 ms or longer. Even very slight motion can cause a change in the recorded phase variation across the FOV throughout the MR acquisition sequence. Examples of motion artifacts are shown in Figure 13-38. The frequency encode direction is less affected, especially by periodic motion, since the evolution of the echo signal, frequency encoding, and sampling occur simultaneously over several milliseconds. Ghost images, which are faint copies of the image displaced along the phase encode direction, are the visual result of patient motion.

Bad pixel in k-space   Resultant image

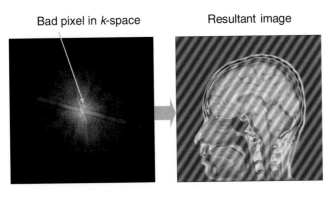

FIGURE 13-37 A single bad pixel in k-space causes a significant artifact in the reconstructed image. The bad pixel is located at $k_x = 2$, $k_y = 3$, which produces a superimposed sinusoidal wave on the spatial domain image as shown.

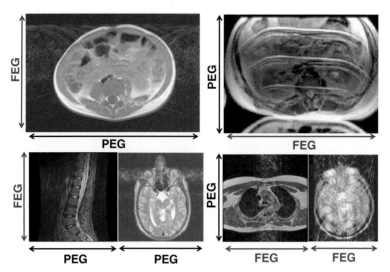

■ **FIGURE 13-38** Motion artifacts, particularly of flow patterns, are almost always displayed in the phase encode gradient direction. Slight changes in phase produce multiple ghost images of the anatomy, since the variation in phase caused by motion can be substantial between excitations.

Several techniques can compensate for motion-related artifacts. The simplest technique transposes the PEG and FEG to relocate the motion artifacts out of the region of diagnostic interest with the same pulse sequences. This does not reduce the magnitude of the artifacts, however, and often there is a mismatch when placing the PEG along the long axis of a rectangular FOV (*e.g.*, an exam of the thoracic spine) in terms of longer examination times or a significant loss of spatial resolution or of SNR.

There are other motion compensation methods:

1. Cardiac and respiratory gating—signal acquisition at a particular cyclic location synchronizes the phase changes applied across the anatomy (Fig. 13-39).

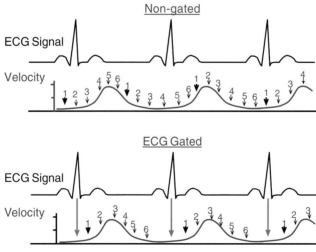

■ **FIGURE 13-39** Motion artifacts occur when data are acquired without consideration of physiologic periodicity. Top: The electrocardiogram measures the R-wave at each heartbeat, but data acquisition proceeds in a linear fashion without regard to reproducibility. The result is a set of images degraded with motion artifact, with diagnostic usefulness marginal, at best. Bottom: Acquisition of images proceeds with the detection of the R-wave signal and synchronization of the collection of image data in a stepwise fashion over the period between R-waves. A reduced number of images or extended acquisition time is required to collect the data.

2. Respiratory ordering of the phase encoding projections based on location within the respiratory cycle. Mechanical or video devices provide signals to monitor the cycle.

3. Signal averaging to reduce artifacts of random motion by making displaced signals less conspicuous relative to stationary anatomy.

4. Short TE spin echo sequences (limited to proton density, T1-weighted scans, fractional echo acquisition, Fig. 13-9). Note: Long TE scans (T2 weighting) are more susceptible to motion.

5. Gradient moment nulling (additional gradient pulses for flow compensation) to help rephase protons that are dephased due to motion. Most often, these techniques require a longer TE and are more useful for T2-weighted scans (Fig. 13-18).

6. Presaturation pulses applied outside the imaging region to reduce flow artifacts from inflowing protons, as well as other patient motions that occur in the periphery (Fig. 13-12).

7. Multiple redundant sampling in the center of k-space (*e.g.*, propeller) to identify and remove those sequences contributing to motion, without deleteriously affecting the image (Fig. 13-8).

13.6.8 Chemical Shift Artifacts of the First Kind

There are two types of chemical shift artifacts that affect the display of anatomy due to the precessional frequency differences of protons in fat versus protons in water. In the case of proton spectra, peaks correspond to water and fat, and in the case of breast imaging, silicone material is another material to consider. Lower frequencies of about 3.5 parts per million for protons in fat and 5.0 parts per million for protons in silicone occur, compared to the resonance frequency of protons in water (Fig. 13-40). Since resonance frequency increases linearly with field strength, the absolute difference between the fat and water resonance also increases, making high field strength magnets more susceptible to chemical shift artifact.

Data acquisition methods cannot directly discriminate a frequency shift due to the application of a frequency encode gradient or a chemical shift artifact. Water and fat differences therefore cannot be distinguished by the frequency difference induced by the gradient. The protons in fat resonate at a slightly lower frequency than the corresponding protons in water and cause a shift in the anatomy (misregistration of water and fat moieties) along the frequency encode gradient direction.

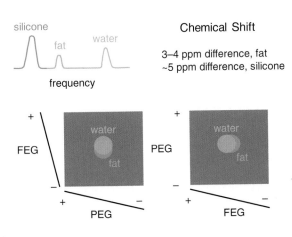

Chemical Shift

3–4 ppm difference, fat
~5 ppm difference, silicone

■ **FIGURE 13-40** Chemical shift refers to the slightly different precessional frequencies of protons in different materials or tissues. The shifts (in ppm) are referenced to water for fat and silicone. Fat chemical shift artifacts are represented by a shift of water and fat in the images of anatomical structure, mainly in the frequency encode gradient direction. Swapping the PEG and the FEG will cause a shift of the fat and water components of the tissues in the image.

A sample calculation in the example below demonstrates frequency variations in fat and water for two different magnetic field and gradient field strengths:

As described in Chapter 12, the resonance frequency between fat and water are

$$1.5\,T : 63.8 \times 10^6\,Hz \times 3.5 \times 10^{-6} = 223\,Hz$$

$$3.0\,T : 127.7 \times 10^6\,Hz \times 3.5 \times 10^{-6} = 447\,Hz.$$

Thus, the chemical shift is more severe for higher field strength magnets.

Chemical shift artifact numerical calculation for gradient strength results in the following numerical calculations for a 25-cm (0.25 m) FOV, 256 × 256 matrix:

Low gradient strength: 2.5 mT/m × 0.25 m = 0.000625 T variation, gives frequency range of 0.000625 T × 42.58 MHz/T = 26.6 kHz across FOV and 26.6 kHz/256 pixels = 104 Hz/pixel.

High gradient strength: 10 mT/m × 0.25 m = 0.0025 T variation, gives frequency range of 0.0025 T × 42.58 MHz/T = 106.5 kHz across FOV and 106.5 kHz/256 pixels = 416 Hz/pixel.

Thus, a chemical shift occurrence is more severe for lower gradient strengths, since displacement will occur over many pixels. With a higher gradient strength, water and fat are more closely contained within the broader pixel boundary bandwidths. Normal and low bandwidth images are illustrated in Figure 13-41.

RF bandwidth and gradient strength considerations can mitigate chemical shift artifacts. While higher gradient strength can confine the chemical shift of fat within the pixel bandwidth boundaries, a significant SNR penalty occurs with the broad RF bandwidth required to achieve a given slice thickness. A more widely used method is to use lower gradient strengths and narrow bandwidths in combination with off-resonance "chemical presaturation" RF pulses or use of STIR techniques described in Chapter 12.

13.6.9 Chemical Shift Artifacts of the Second Kind

Chemical shift artifacts of the second kind occur with GRE images, resulting from the rephasing and dephasing of the echo in the same direction relative to the main magnetic field. Signal appearance is dependent on the selection of TE. This happens because of constructive (in phase) or destructive (out of phase) transverse magnetization events that occur periodically due to the difference in precessional frequencies. At 1.5 T, the chemical shift is 220 Hz, and the periodicity of each peak (in phase)

■ FIGURE 13-41 MR images of the breast, containing glandular and adipose tissue, are acquired under a high bandwidth (32 kHz) and a low bandwidth (4 kHz), illustrating the more severe chemical shift with low readout gradient strength and bandwidth. (Courtesy of R. Edward Hendrick, PhD.)

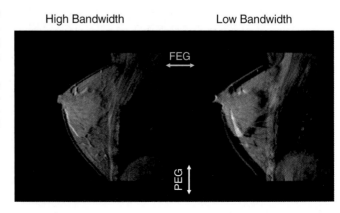

High Bandwidth   Low Bandwidth

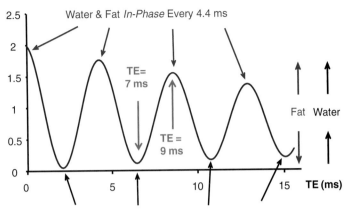

■ FIGURE 13-42 For GRE image sequences, signal intensity of a voxel containing both water and fat is dependent on the selection of TE, as shown above, because of 220 Hz lower precessional frequency of fat protons, where in-phase magnetization occurs every 4.4 ms (1/220 s^{-1}), and out-of-phase magnetization occurs every 4.4 ms shifted by ½ cycle (2.2 ms).

between water and fat occurs at 0, 4.5, 9.0, 13.5, ... ms, and each valley (out of phase) at 2.25, 6.75, 11.0, ... ms, as shown in Figure 13-42. Thus, selection of TE at 9 ms will lead to a constructive addition of water and fat, and TE at 7 ms will lead to a destructive addition of water and fat. The in-phase timing will lead to a conventional chemical shift image of the first kind, while the out-of-phase timing will lead to a chemical shift image of the second kind, manifesting a dark rim around heterogeneous water and fat anatomical structures, shown in Figure 13-43.

13.6.10 Ringing Artifacts

Ringing artifact (also known as Gibbs phenomenon) occurs near sharp boundaries and high-contrast transitions in the image, and appears as multiple, regularly spaced parallel bands of alternating bright and dark signal that slowly fades with

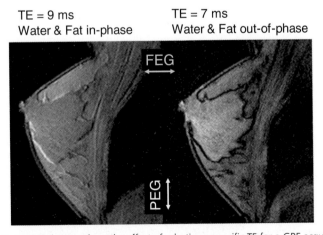

■ FIGURE 13-43 Breast MRI images show the effect of selecting a specific TE for a GRE acquisition. On the left, chemical shift of the "first kind" is shown with TE = 9 ms and water and fat in phase for transverse magnetization, shifted only due to the intrinsic chemical shift differences of fat and water. On the right, chemical shift of the second kind is additionally manifested with TE = 7 ms, due to fat and water being out of phase, creating a lower signal at all fat-water interfaces, and resulting in reduced intensity. (Adapted by permission from Springer Nature. Hendrick RE. *Breast MRI: Fundamentals and Technical Aspects.* Copyright © 2008, Springer Science Business Media, LLC.)

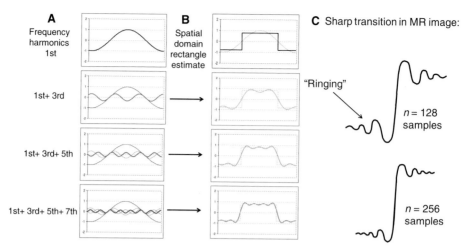

■ FIGURE 13-44 The synthesis of a spatial object occurs by the summation of frequency harmonics in the MR image. **A.** Left column: Frequency harmonics that estimate a rectangle function with progressively higher frequencies and lower amplitudes are shown. **B.** Middle column: As higher frequency harmonics are included, the summed result more faithfully represents the object shape, in this example a rectangle with two vertical edges. The number of frequencies encoded in the MR image is dependent on the matrix size. **C.** Right column: A sharp transition boundary in an MR image is represented with 256 samples better than with 128 samples (frequency harmonics in k-space). The amount of ringing caused by insufficient sampling is reduced with a larger number of samples.

distance. The cause is the insufficient sampling of high frequencies inherent at sharp discontinuities in the signal. Images of objects can be reconstructed from a summation of sinusoidal waveforms of specific amplitudes and frequencies, as shown in Figure 13-44 for a simple rectangular object. In the figure, the summation of frequency harmonics, each with a specific amplitude and phase, approximates the distribution of the object, but initially does very poorly, particularly at the sharp edges. As the number of higher frequency harmonics increases, a better estimate is achieved, although an infinite number of frequencies are theoretically necessary to reconstruct the sharp edge perfectly.

In the MR acquisition, the number of frequency samples is determined by the number of pixels (frequency, k_x, or phase, k_y, increments) across the k-space matrix. For 256 pixels, 128 discrete frequencies are depicted, and for 128 pixels, 64 discrete frequencies are specified (the k-space matrix is symmetric in quadrants and duplicated about its center). A lack of high-frequency signals causes the "ringing" at sharp transitions described as a diminishing hyper- and hypointense signal oscillation from the transition. Ringing artifacts are thus more likely for smaller digital matrix sizes (Fig. 13-45, 256 versus 128 matrix). Ringing artifact commonly occurs at skull/brain interfaces, where there is a large transition in signal amplitude.

13.6.11 Wraparound Artifacts

The wraparound artifact is a result of the mismapping of anatomy that lies outside of the FOV but within the slice volume. The anatomy is usually displaced to the opposite side of the image. It is caused by non-linear gradients or by undersampling of the frequencies contained within the returned signal envelope. For the latter, the sampling rate must be twice the maximal frequency that occurs in the object (the Nyquist sampling limit). Otherwise, the Fourier transform cannot

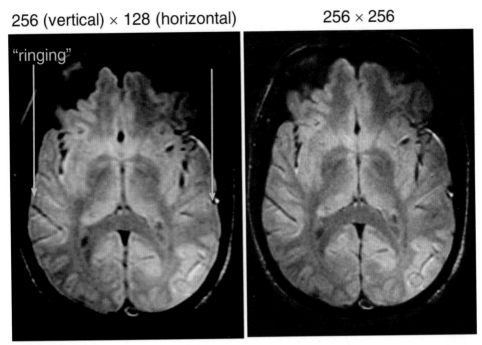

256 (vertical) × 128 (horizontal)   256 × 256

"ringing"

■ **FIGURE 13-45** Example of ringing artifacts caused by a sharp signal transition at the skull in a brain image for a 256 × 128 matrix (left) along the short (horizontal) axis, and the elimination of the artifact in a 256 × 256 matrix (right). The short axis defines the PEG direction.

distinguish frequencies that are present in the data above the Nyquist frequency limit, and instead assigns a lower frequency value to them (Fig. 13-46). Frequency signals will "wraparound" to the opposite side of the image, masquerading as low-frequency (aliased) signals.

In the frequency encode direction, a low-pass filter can be applied to the acquired time domain signal to eliminate frequencies beyond the Nyquist frequency.

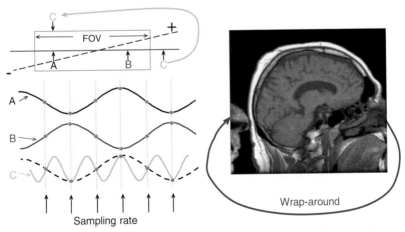

■ **FIGURE 13-46** Left: Wraparound artifacts are caused by aliasing. Shown is a fixed sampling rate and net precessional frequencies occurring at position *A* and position *B* within the FOV that have identical frequencies but different phases. If signal from position *C* is at *twice* the frequency of *B* and insufficiently sampled, the same frequency and phase will be assigned to *C* as that assigned to *A*, and therefore will appear at that location. Right: A wraparound artifact example displaces anatomy from one side of the image (or outside of the FOV) to the other side.

In the phase encode direction, aliasing artifacts can be reduced by increasing the number of phase encode steps (the trade-off is increased image time). Another approach is to move the region of anatomic interest to the center of the imaging volume to avoid the overlapping anatomy, which usually occurs at the periphery of the FOV. An "antialiasing" saturation pulse just outside of the FOV is yet another method of eliminating high-frequency signals that would otherwise be aliased into the lower frequency spectrum. This example of wrap-around artifact is easy to interpret. In some cases, the artifact is not as well delineated (*e.g.*, the top of the skull wrapping into the brain).

13.6.12 Partial Volume Artifacts

Partial volume artifacts arise from the finite size of the voxel over which the signal is averaged. This results in a loss of detail and spatial resolution. Reduction of partial volume artifacts is accomplished by using a smaller pixel size and/or a smaller slice thickness. With a smaller voxel, the SNR is reduced for a similar imaging time, resulting in a noisier signal with less low-contrast sensitivity. Of course, with a greater NEX (averages), the SNR can be maintained, at the cost of longer imaging time.

13.7 MAGNET SITING AND QUALITY CONTROL

13.7.1 Magnet Siting

Superconductive magnets produce extensive magnetic fringe fields and create potentially hazardous conditions in adjacent areas. In addition, extremely small signal amplitudes generated by the protons in the body during an imaging procedure have a frequency common to commercial FM broadcasts. Thus, two requirements must be considered for MR system siting: protect the local environment from the magnet system and protect the magnet system from the local environment.

Fringe fields from a high field strength magnet can extend quite far—roughly equal to αB_0, where α is a constant dependent on the magnet bore size and magnet configuration. Fringe fields can potentially cause a disruption of electronic signals and sensitive electronic devices. An unshielded 1.5-T magnet has a 1-mT fringe field at a distance of approximately 9.3 m, a 0.5-mT field at 11.5 m, and a 0.3-mT field at 14.1 m from the center of the magnet. Magnetic shielding is one way to reduce fringe field interactions in adjacent areas. Passive (*e.g.*, thick metal walls close to the magnet) and active (*e.g.*, electromagnet systems strategically placed in the magnet housing) magnetic shielding systems permit a significant reduction in the extent of the fringe fields for high field strength, air core magnets (Fig. 13-47). Patients with pacemakers or ferromagnetic aneurysm clips must avoid fringe fields above 0.5 mT. Magnetically sensitive equipment such as image intensifiers, gamma cameras, and color TVs are severely impacted by fringe fields of less than 0.3 mT, as electromagnetic focusing in these devices is disrupted.

Administrative control for magnetic fringe fields is 0.5 mT, requiring controlled access to areas that exceed this level. Magnetic fields below 0.5 mT are considered safe for the patient population. Disruption of the fringe fields can reduce the homogeneity of the active imaging volume. Any large metallic object (elevator, automobile, etc.) traveling through the fringe field can produce such an effect.

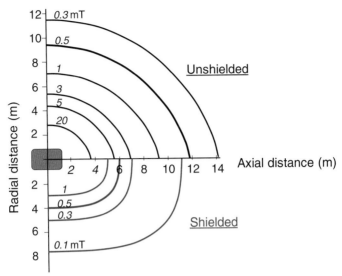

■ FIGURE 13-47 An unshielded (top half of diagram) and shielded (bottom half of diagram) 1.5 T magnet and the magnetic fringe field strengths plotted with radial distance (vertical axis) and axial distance (horizontal axis).

Environmental RF noise must be reduced to protect the extremely sensitive receiver within the magnet from interfering signals. The typical approach for stray RF signal protection is the construction of a Faraday cage, an internal enclosure consisting of RF attenuating copper sheet and/or copper wire mesh. The room containing the MRI system is typically lined with copper sheet (walls) and mesh (windows). This is a costly construction item but provides effective protection from stray RF noise (Fig. 13-48).

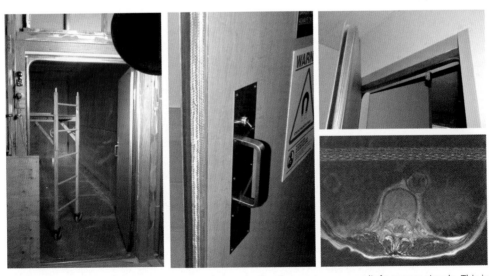

■ FIGURE 13-48 The MR scanner room requires protection from extraneous radiofrequency signals. This is achieved with the installation of a "Faraday cage" comprised of copper sheet that lines the inner walls of the room (left), copper mesh covering the operator viewing window (not shown), and a copper lined door and doorjamb with an inflatable bladder conductor (note switch above the door handle) to seal the door (middle and upper right). A leak in the Faraday cage will result in RF artifacts that will occur at specific frequencies as streaks across the image, perpendicular to the FEG direction, lower right. (FEG is vertical, PEG is horizontal.)

13.7.2   Field Uniformity

In addition to magnetic field strength, field uniformity is an important characteristic, expressed in parts per million (ppm) over a given volume, such as 40 cm^3. This is based upon the precessional frequency of the proton, which is determined from the proton gyromagnetic ratio. At 1.5 T, the precessional frequency is 1.5 T × 42.58 MHz/T = 63.8 MHz = 63.8 × 10^6 cycles/s, and a specification of 2 ppm homogeneity (2 × 10^{-6}) gives a frequency uniformity of about 128 cycles/s (Hz) over the volume. Typical homogeneities range from less than 1 ppm for a small FOV (*e.g.*, 150 mm) to greater than 10 ppm for a large FOV (*e.g.*, 400 mm). Field uniformity is achieved by manipulating the main field peripherally with passive and active "shim" coils, which exist in proximity to the main magnetic field. These coils interact with the fringe fields and adjust the variation of the central magnetic field.

13.7.3   Quality Control

Like any imaging system, the MRI scanner is only as good as the weakest link in the imaging chain. The components of the MR system that must be periodically checked include the magnetic field strength, magnetic field homogeneity, system field shimming, gradient linearity, system RF tuning, receiver coil optimization, environmental noise sources, power supplies, peripheral equipment, and control systems among others. A QC program should be designed to assess the basic day-to-day functionality of the scanner. A set of QC tests is listed in Table 13-4. Qualitative and quantitative measurements of system performance should be obtained on a periodic basis, with a test frequency dependent on the likelihood of detecting a change in the baseline values outside of normal operating limits.

The American College of Radiology has an MRI accreditation program that specifies requirements for system operation, QC, and the training requirements of technologists, radiologists, and physicists involved in scanner operation (ACR, 2020a). The accreditation process evaluates the qualifications of personnel, equipment performance, effectiveness of QC procedures, and quality of clinical images—factors that are consistent with the maintenance of a state-of-the-art facility.

TABLE 13-4 RECOMMENDED QC TESTS FOR MRI SYSTEMS
High-contrast spatial resolution
Slice thickness accuracy
Slice position accuracy
RF center frequency tuning
Geometric accuracy and spatial uniformity
Signal uniformity
Low-contrast detectability
Image artifact evaluation
Operational controls (*e.g.*, table movement control and alignment lighting checks)
Preventive maintenance logging and documentation
Review of system log book and operations

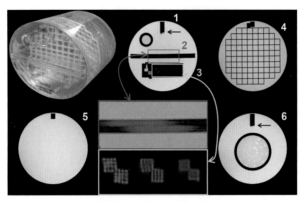

MRI Accreditation Phantom

■ FIGURE 13-49 The ACR MRI accreditation phantom (upper left) and selected MRI axial images from the phantom are shown. (1) First phantom slab containing slice position accuracy ramp (black arrow); (2) slice thickness ramp (magnified and enhanced image—red outline); (3) spatial resolution module (magnified image—yellow outline). Other phantom slabs include (4) geometric distortion module; (5) uniformity module; (6) low contrast resolution module and slice position accuracy ramp at other end of phantom. Not all images are shown; specific details are described in the large phantom MRI accreditation documentation—https://www.acraccreditation.org/media/Documents/; search for MRI large phantom guidance.

MRI phantoms are composed of materials that produce MR signals with carefully defined relaxation times. Some materials are aqueous paramagnetic solutions; pure gelatin, agar, silicone, or agarose; and organic doped gels, paramagnetic doped gels, and others. Water is most frequently used, but it is necessary to adjust the T1 and T2 relaxation times of (doped) water, so that images can be acquired using pulse sequence timing for patients (*e.g.*, this is achieved by adding nickel, aqueous oxygen, aqueous manganese, or gadolinium). For example, the ACR MR Accreditation phantom (Fig. 13-49) is a cylindrical phantom of 190 mm inside diameter and 148 mm inside length. It is filled with a 10 millimolar solution of nickel chloride and 75 millimolar sodium chloride. Inside the phantom are several structures that are used in a variety of tests for scanner performance. In this phantom, seven quantitative tests are made by scanning the phantom with specific instructions, and include geometric accuracy, high contrast spatial resolution, slice thickness accuracy, slice position accuracy, image intensity uniformity, percent signal ghosting, and low-contrast object detectability. Details on measurement analysis, recommended action criteria, and causes of failure/corrective action are included in the guidance (ACR, 2020a). Some phantoms have standards with known T1, T2, and proton density values to evaluate the quantitative accuracy of the scanner, and to determine the ability to achieve an expected contrast level for a given pulse sequence. A homogeneity phantom is imaged to determine the spatial uniformity of transmit and receive RF magnetic fields. Ideal performance is a spatially uniform excitation of the protons and a spatially uniform receiver sensitivity across the imaged object.

13.8   MR BIOEFFECTS AND SAFETY

Because ionizing radiation is not used with MRI and MRS, the perception of the general public is that MR is a very safe modality. Safety aspects are often an afterthought, particularly in terms of operational activities and training of personnel who work in the area and around the magnet. There are very many important bioeffects and safety issues to be considered for MR. These include the presence of strong magnetic fields, RF energy, time-varying magnetic gradient fields, cryogenic liquids, a confined imaging device (claustrophobia), and noisy operation (gradient coil activation and deactivation, creating acoustic noise). Patients with implants, prostheses, aneurysm clips, pacemakers, heart valves, etc., should be aware of considerable torque on the devices, which when placed in the magnetic field, could cause serious adverse effects. Non-metallic implant materials can also lead to significant heating under rapidly changing gradient fields. Consideration of the distortions and artifacts on the acquired images and possibility of misdiagnosis are also a concern. Ferromagnetic materials inadvertently brought into the imaging room (*e.g.*, an IV pole) are attracted to the magnetic field and can become a deadly projectile to the occupant within the bore of the magnet. Many unfortunate deaths have been attributed to carelessness and lack of a safety culture around an MR scanner. Signage exists in three categories to help identify MR-compatible materials. "MR safe" is a square green sign, and is put on materials and objects that are wholly non-metallic; "MR unsafe" is round red, and is placed on all ferromagnetic and many conducting metals; "MR conditional" signage is triangular yellow, placed on objects that may or may not be safe until further investigation is performed. Implanted devices (*e.g.*, pacemakers, neurostimulators) that have an MR *conditional* label allow patients to be scanned, but the safety of the exam is conditional on meeting the manufacturer's prerequisites such as reduced specific absorption rate, limitations on field strength, types of coils used, and setting the devices in "MR mode" when scanning, among other conditions. These signs are shown in Figure 13-50.

The magnet is *always* on. In extreme emergencies, the superconducting magnet can be turned off by a manually controlled "quench" procedure. Even under the best circumstances, the quench procedure subjects the magnet to a 260 K temperature difference in a short period of time. If performed too quickly, major physical damage to the magnet can occur. Because of risks to personnel, equipment, and physical facilities, manual quenches should only be initiated after careful considerations and preparation. Uncontrolled quenching is the result of a sudden loss of superconductivity in the main magnet coils, which can result in the explosive conversion of liquid helium to gas and jeopardize the safety of those in the room and adjacent areas. In the event of insufficient gas outflow, oxygen can be displaced and buildup of pressure in the room can prevent the entry door from being easily opened.

MRI is considered "safe" when used within the regulatory guidelines required of the manufacturers by the Food and Drug Administration (FDA; Table 13-5). Serious bioeffects are demonstrated with static and varying magnetic fields at strengths significantly higher (10 to 20 times greater) than those used for typical diagnostic imaging.

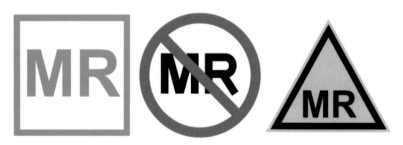

■ **FIGURE 13-50** MR labeling includes on the left, *MR safe* materials that have been found not to interact with the strong MR field or disrupt operation; in the middle, *MR unsafe* labels that contraindicate bringing materials with this designation past Zone 2 (see discussion later in this section); on the right, *MR conditional* labels indicate more consideration is required before bringing such labeled objects into the scan room.

TABLE 13-5 **MRI SAFETY GUIDELINES**

ISSUE	PARAMETER	VARIABLES	SPECIFIED VALUE
Static magnetic field	Magnetic field (B_0)	Maximum strength	3.0 T[a]
	Inadvertent exposure	Maximum	0.0005 T
Changing magnetic field (dB/dt)	Axial gradients	$\tau > 120$ μs	<20 T/s
		12 μs < τ < 120 μs	<2,400/τ (μs) T/s
		τ < 12 μs	<200 T/s
	Transverse gradients		<3× axial gradients
	System		
			<6 T/s
RF power deposition	Temperature	Core of body	<38°C
		Maximum head	<38°C
		Maximum trunk	<39°C
		Maximum extremities	<40°C
	Specific absorption rate (SAR)[b]	Whole body (average)	<4 W/kg
		Head (average)	<3.2 W/kg
		Head or torso per gram	<8 W/kg
		Extremities per gram	<12 W/kg
Acoustic noise levels		Peak pressure	200 pascals
		Average pressure	105 dBA

τ rise time of gradients.
[a]In some clinical applications, higher field strengths (e.g., 7.0 T) are allowed.
[b]"Normal" mode (suitable for all patients) is half the limit (2 W/kg); "First Level" mode (shown) is with medical supervision.

13.8.1 Static Magnetic Fields

The long-term biologic effects of high magnetic field strengths are not well known. At lower magnetic field strengths, there have not been any reports of deleterious or non-reversable biologic effects, either acute or chronic. With very high field strength magnets (e.g., 4 T or higher), there has been anecdotal mention of dizziness and disorientation of personnel and patients as they move through the field. With systems in excess of 20 T, enzyme kinetic changes have been documented, increased membrane permeability shown, and altered biopotentials have been measured. These effects have not been demonstrated in magnetic fields below 10 T. Effects on ECG traces have shown an increased amplitude of the T wave, presumably due to the magneto-hemodynamic effect, caused by conductive fluid such as blood moving across a magnetic field. When this occurs, sometimes the elevated T wave will be mistaken for the desired R wave, creating an insufficient gating situation. For this reason, it is recommended that ECG leads are not used for patient monitoring, but rather an alternative such as pulse oximetry be used.

13.8.2 Spatial Field Gradient

Although the static magnetic fields is stable over time, the distribution of the field is spatially varying (i.e., the magnetic field is stronger closer to the magnet). As an object or a patient slides into the magnet, the effective magnetic fields are changing. According to Lenz's law, the induced current in conductive material due to a change

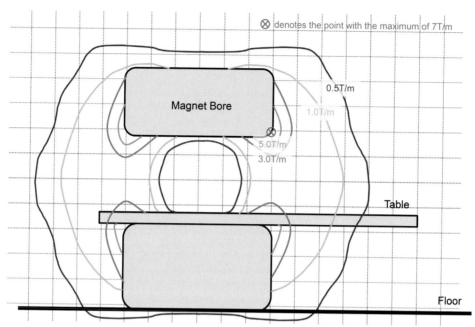

■ FIGURE 13-51 A spatial magnetic field gradient map specifies the magnetic field gradient distribution in the vertical cross section of an MRI scanner. The spatial field gradient along the passage of patient must be considered when a patient with an MR conditional implant or device is scanned.

in a magnetic field is directed to oppose the change in flux and to exert a mechanical force that opposes the motion. A conductive material (even though non-ferromagnetic) experiences mechanical force in the opposite direction when the surrounding magnetic field is changing. Therefore, MR conditional implants and devices have labeling that specifies a condition under the maximum spatial magnetic field gradient as well as the maximum static field (such as 1.5 T or 3 T). Figure 13-51 is an example of spatial field gradient map provided by an MRI scanner manufacturer. The location of the maximum spatial field gradient is also indicated on the map. As shown in the figure, the entry of the magnet shows the highest spatial field gradient, and extra care is needed when conditional implants or devices move over the area. Moving the table using a slow mode is one of the approaches to reduce the risk of mechanical force.

13.8.3 Varying Magnetic Field Effects

The time-varying magnetic fields encountered in the MRI system are due to the gradient switching used for localization of the protons. Magnetic fields that vary their strength with time are generally of greater concern than static fields because oscillating magnetic fields can induce electrical current flow in conductors. The maximum allowed changing gradient fields depend on the rise times of the gradients, as listed in Table 13-5. At extremely high levels of magnetic field variation, effects such as visual phosphenes (the sensation of flashes of light being seen) can result because of induced currents in the nerves or tissues. Other consequences such as bone healing and cardiac fibrillation have been suggested in the literature. The most common bioeffect of MR systems is tissue heating caused by RF energy deposition and/or by rapid switching of high strength gradients. RF coils and antennas can present burn hazards when electrical currents and conductive loops are present and must have proper insulation—both electrical and thermal. Patients can experience burns when they inadvertently create a conductive loop with parts of their body, such as touching their fingers directly on their torso, resulting in induced current that concentrates at the fingertips.

13.8.4 Specific Absorption Rate

Specific absorption rate (SAR) is a measure of the energy absorption rate when the human body is exposed to RF fields. For MR, the maximum allowed SAR values are listed in Table 13-5. Labeling of conditional devices and implants often specifies the maximum allowable SAR or B1+ rms (B1+ means the transmit RF fields and rms stands for root-mean-squared power). The type of coil, either a transmit and receive coil or a receive only coil, and pulse sequence parameters need to be modified to meet the conditions for the patient's safety.

13.8.5 RF Exposure, Acoustic Noise Limits

RF exposure causes heating of tissues. There are obvious effects of overheating, and therefore a power deposition limit is imposed by governmental regulations on the manufacturers for various aspects of MRI and MRS operation. RF coil safety requires regular inspection of the coil condition, including the conductive wires leading to the coils from the connectors. These wires have the capacity to transmit heat, which may burn the insulating material of the wires or burn the patient. It is important to ensure that the coils are not looped and do not touch the patient or the bore of the magnet. Damage to the insulation requires immediate repair, as this could result in extreme heating, fire, and potential harm to the patient.

The gradient coils are located inside the cylinder of the magnet and are responsible for the banging noise one hears during imaging. This noise is caused by the flexing and torque experienced by the gradient coil from the rapidly changing magnetic fields when energized. The acoustic noise levels and pressure amplitudes are determined from limits that are shown to have reversible (unaffected) outcomes for clinically approved sequences. Hearing protection should always be available to the patient. For research sequences and procedures that have not been approved by the FDA, patients or volunteers are to have hearing protection in place.

Table 13-5 lists some of the categories and the maximum values permitted for clinical use. The rationale for imposing limits on static and varying magnetic fields is based on the ability of the resting body to dissipate heat buildup caused by the deposition and absorption of thermal energy.

13.8.6 Pregnancy-Related Issues and Pediatric Patient Concerns

Pregnant healthcare staff and physicians are permitted to work in and around the MR environment throughout all stages of pregnancy and assist as needed in setting up the patient and the exam. However, they are not to remain in the magnet scanning room (Zone 4). Regarding the scanning of pregnant patients, current data have not yielded any deleterious effects on the developing fetus with common examinations, and no special considerations are warranted, as long as the benefit-risk ratio of doing the study is that for any other typical patient. Another consideration is the administration of contrast, which should not be routinely provided. A well-documented justification is required to administer contrast based on the overwhelming potential benefit to the patient or fetus relative to the risk of exposing them to gadolinium-based agents and potential deleterious effects of free gadolinium ions. There are studies documenting that gadolinium agents do pass the placental barrier and do enter the fetus.

For pediatric patients, the largest issues are sedation and monitoring. Special attention to sedation protocols, adherence to standards of care regarding sedation guidelines, and monitoring patients during the scan with MR-safe temperature monitoring and isolation transport units are crucial to maintaining patient safety.

13.8.7 MR Personnel and MR Safety Zones

The American College of Radiology has published a white paper in 2007 describing the recommendations for MR safety in general, and MR safety "zones" and MR personnel definitions (ACR, 2007). This has been updated in 2013 and 2019, with expanded commentary and precautions (ACR, 2013, 2020b). MR safety policies, procedures, and safe practices are suggested in the guidance. To maintain a buffer zone around the "always on" magnet, MR safety zones are categorized from Zone 1 to Zone 4. Zone 1 is the area freely accessible to the general public, everywhere outside of the MR magnet area and building. Zone 2 represents the interface between Zone 1 and Zone 3—typically the reception area, where patients are registered and MR screening questions take place. Zone 3 is a restricted area comprised of the MR control room and computer room that only specific personnel can access, namely, those specifically trained as MR personnel (described below) and appropriately screened patients and other individuals (nurses, support staff). Zone 4 represents the MR magnet room and is always located within the confines of Zone 3. Demarcation of these zones should be clearly marked and identified. Figure 13-52 illustrates the zoning concept.

Furthermore, there are personnel definitions describing criteria that must be achieved before access can be granted to Zone 3 and Zone 4 areas. *Non-MR personnel*

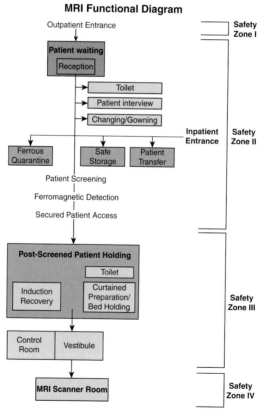

■ **FIGURE 13-52** Zoning concept for describing areas in an MR system environment include Zone 1, unrestricted access; Zone 2, interface between unrestricted and restricted areas; Zone 3, restricted area only allowed for MR personnel and screened individuals; Zone 4, the area of the scanner and high magnetic field strength. (Obtained from and modified with the permission of the Department of Veterans Affairs Office of Construction & Facilities Management, Strategic Management Office; reprinted from Kanal E, Barkovich AJ, Bell C, et al. ACR guidance document on MR safe practices: 2013. *J. Magn. Reson.* Imaging 2013;37:501-530. doi:10.1002/jmri.24011)

are patients, visitors, or staff who do not have the appropriate education or training that meet the criteria for Level 1 or Level 2 MR personnel. *Level 1 MR personnel* have passed minimal safety and education training on MR safety issues and have a basic understanding of the effects of MR magnets, dangers of projectiles, effects of strong magnetic fields, etc. These individuals can work in Zone 3 and Zone 4 areas without supervision or oversight; examples are MR office staff, patient aides, and custodial staff. *Level 2 MR personnel* are more extensively trained in the broader aspects of MR safety issues, for example, understanding the potential for thermal loading, burns, neuromuscular excitation, and induced currents from gradients. These individuals are the gatekeepers of access into Zone 4 and take the action and the leadership role in the event of a patient code, ensuring that only properly screened support staff are allowed access. Those responding to a code must be made aware of and comply with MR safety protocols. Examples of personnel designated as Level 2 include MR technologists, MR medical physicists, radiologists, and department nursing staff.

Designated personnel are required to continuously maintain their safety credentials, by acquiring continuous education credits throughout the year on MR safety aspects, and taking an annual test and achieving a minimum passing score.

13.8.8 Summary

Meeting the needs of the MR exam and using the equipment safely and effectively require the understanding of the basic physics underpinnings described in Chapter 12, and the details of advanced acquisition methods, image characteristics, artifacts/pitfalls, and MR safety/bioeffects covered in this chapter. The reader is encouraged to keep up with the rapid developments of MRI and MRS by referring to recent literature and websites dedicated to MRI education and technological advances.

SUGGESTED READING AND REFERENCES

ACR. American College of Radiology MRI Accreditation Program. Documentation for the MRI accreditation program, including MRI phantom test guidance. 2020a. https://www.acraccreditation.org/Modalities/MRI

ACR; ACR Committee on MR Safety, et al. ACR guidance document on MR safe practices: updates and critical information 2019. *J Magn Reson Imaging.* 2020b;51(2):331-338.

ACR; Expert Panel on MR Safety, et al. ACR guidance document on MR safe practices: 2013. *J Magn Reson Imaging.* 2013;37(3):501-530.

ACR; Kanal E, Barkovich AJ, Bell C, et al. ACR guidance document for safe MR practices. *AJR Am J Roentgenol.* 2007;188:1-27.

Alexander AL, Lee JE, Lazar M, Field AS. Diffusion tensor imaging of the brain. *Neurotherapeutics.* 2007;4(3):316-329.

Al-Okaili RN, Krejza J, Wang S, Woo JH, Melhem ER. Advanced MR imaging techniques in the diagnosis of intraaxial brain tumors in adults. *Radiographics.* 2006;26:S173-S189.

Hendrick RE. *Breast MRI: Fundamentals and Technical Aspects.* New York, NY: Springer; 2007.

NessAiver M. *All You Really Need to Know about MRI Physics.* Baltimore, MD: Simply Physics; 1997.

Sourbron SP, Buckley DL. On the scope and interpretation of the Tofts models for DCE MRI. *Magn Reson Med.* 2011;66:735-745.

Westbrook C, Kaut-Roth C, Talbot J. *MRI in Practice.* 3rd ed. Malden, MA: Blackwell Publishing; 2005.

CHAPTER 14

Ultrasound

In ultrasound imaging, a short burst of mechanical energy created by a transducer is introduced into the body through contact with the skin. The resulting ultrasound pulse travels at the speed of sound in the tissues interacting with the many boundaries between organs and parenchyma and creating echoes from changes in the acoustic properties that return to the transducer receiver. Collection and recording of the echo amplitudes over time provide depth information about the tissues and echogenicity along the path of travel, which are encoded as grayscale values. Repeating the process hundreds of times with a small incremental change in the direction of the pulse produces a tomographic image of the insonated region (Fig. 14-1). In addition to two-dimensional (2D) tomographic imaging, ultrasound allows for anatomical distance and volume measurements, motion studies, blood velocity measurements, tissue stiffness measurements, and 3D imaging.

Imaging systems using ultrasound have attained a large presence in medical care within and outside of radiology and across many clinical domains, particularly in the past 10 years. The success of ultrasound is attributed to several characteristics, including the non-ionizing nature of ultrasound waves, the ability to produce real-time images of tissue structures in the body to deliver timely patient care, and the high portability and relatively low cost of Point of Care (PoC) systems. While hands-on training and practice are essential for the ultrasound practitioner, an understanding of the basic physics of ultrasound is central to the effective and safe use of this technology for medical imaging. This chapter describes the characteristics, properties, and production of ultrasound; interaction with tissues; instrumentation and equipment; image acquisition, processing, and display; achievable measurements including tissue stiffness and blood velocity; common artifacts; bioeffects; and safety considerations.

14.1 CHARACTERISTICS OF SOUND

Sound is mechanical energy that propagates through a continuous medium by the compression (high pressure) and rarefaction (low pressure) of particles that comprise it. Tissues can be considered to be elastic, like a spring. A mechanical inward deformation by an external force, such as a piston that pushes inward, causes a local increase in pressure and compression of the spring. As the piston moves backward during its cycle, a negative force causes a local decrease in pressure, causing the spring to elongate, while the compressed part of the spring moves forward with time, transferring the imparted energy to adjacent components (particles) of the spring. With constant motion of the piston, the energy continues to travel cyclically, as shown in the top diagram of Figure 14-2.

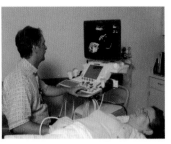
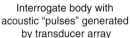
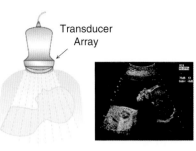

Interrogate body with acoustic "pulses" generated by transducer array

Acquire and record echoes arising from tissue interfaces

Construct "acoustic image" of tissues

■ **FIGURE 14-1** A major use of ultrasound is the acquisition and display of the acoustic properties of tissues. A transducer array (transmitter and receiver of ultrasound pulses) directs sound waves into the patient, receives the returning echoes, and converts the echo amplitudes into a 2D tomographic image using the ultrasound acquisition system. Exams requiring a high level of safety such as obstetrics are increasing the use of ultrasound in diagnostic radiology. (Photo credit: Emi Manning, UC Davis Health System.)

With ultrasound, the corresponding mechanical force is a transducer, made of an array of expanding and contracting crystal elements that form a surface area that is placed in contact with the tissues. During transducer surface expansion, an increase in the local pressure at the tissue surface occurs. Contraction follows, causing a decrease in pressure. The mechanical energy imparted at the surface is transferred to adjacent particles of the tissue, which travels at the speed of sound into the patient. Expansion and contraction of the transducer surface introduce energy into the medium as a series of compressions and rarefactions occurring every cycle, as shown in Figure 14-2 (middle diagram). A continuous tissue structure is necessary for mechanical energy transfer (*i.e.*, sound propagation) as the constituent "particles" of the tissue act to transfer the mechanical energy with very small back-and-forth displacements. Energy propagation occurs as a wavefront in the direction of travel, known as a longitudinal wave, as shown in the bottom diagram of Figure 14-2.

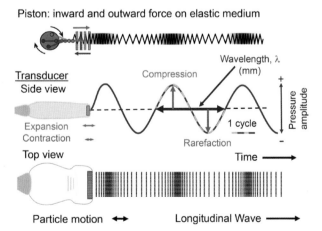

■ **FIGURE 14-2** Ultrasound energy is generated by mechanical displacement of an elastic medium, modeled as a compressible spring. An inward and outward force of a piston coupled to the medium creates increased pressure (compression) and decreased pressure (rarefaction) in a cyclical manner (top row). Constituents (particles) of the medium transfer energy to adjacent particles with minor back and forth displacement. The ultrasound transducer is the mechanical energy source that expands and contracts like the piston at very high frequency. This results in the introduction of ultrasound into the tissues, with propagation as a longitudinal wave. The wavelength is equal to the distance of one cycle.

14.1.1   Wavelength, Frequency, Speed

The *wavelength* (λ) is the distance between any two repeating points on the wave (a cycle) typically measured in millimeters (mm). The *frequency* (f) is the number of times the wave repeats per second (s), also defined in Hertz (Hz), where 1 Hz = 1 cycle/s. Frequency identifies the category of sound: less than 15 Hz is infrasound, 15 Hz to 20,000 Hz (20 kHz) is audible sound, and above 20 kHz, ultrasound. Medical ultrasound typically uses frequencies in the million (mega) cycles/s (MHz) range, from 1 to 20 MHz, with specialized ultrasound applications up to 50 MHz and beyond. The *period* is the time duration of one wave cycle and is equal to $1/f$. The *speed of sound*, c, is the distance traveled per unit time through a medium and is equal to the wavelength (distance) divided by the period (time). As the frequency is equal to 1/period, the product of wavelength and frequency is equal to the speed of sound:

$$c = \lambda f, \qquad\qquad [14\text{-}1]$$

where c is the speed of sound, typically expressed in units of m/s, and often in cm/s and mm/μs. The speed of sound varies substantially within different materials, based on compressibility, stiffness, and density characteristics of the medium. The wave speed is determined by the ratio of the bulk modulus, B (a measure of the stiffness of a medium and its resistance to being compressed), and the density of the medium:

$$c = \sqrt{\frac{B}{\rho}}.$$

SI units are kg/(ms^2), kg/m^3, and m/s for B, ρ, and c, respectively. Sound propagates through a highly compressible medium such as air slowly, while sound propagates more rapidly through a less compressible medium such as bone. Soft tissues have compressibility and density characteristics with speeds as listed in Table 14-1. To relate time with propagation distance traveled in the patient, medical ultrasound devices assume a speed of sound of 1,540 m/s, despite slight differences in actual speed for the various tissues encountered. The speed of sound in soft tissue can be expressed in different units to simplify conversion factors or estimating values. The most common are 154,000 cm/s and 1.54 mm/μs.

Wavelength is the parameter that affects spatial resolution in an ultrasound image, with shorter wavelengths providing better spatial resolution. In a homogeneous medium or tissue, ultrasound frequency and speed of sound are constant; thus, a higher ultrasound frequency results in a shorter wavelength. Examples of the wavelength change as a function of frequency and propagation medium are given below.

EXAMPLE: A 2-MHz beam has a wavelength in soft tissue of (from Eq. 14-1):

$$\lambda = \frac{c}{f} = \frac{1{,}540\,\text{m/s}}{2\times10^6\,/\text{s}} = 770\times10^{-6}\,\text{m} = 7.7\times10^{-4}\,\text{m}\times1{,}000\frac{\text{mm}}{\text{m}} = 0.77\,\text{mm}.$$

A 10-MHz ultrasound beam has a corresponding wavelength in soft tissue of

$$= \frac{1{,}540\,\text{m/s}}{10\times10^6\,/\text{s}} = 154\times10^{-6}\,\text{m} = 1.54\times10^{-4}\,\text{m}\times1{,}000\frac{\text{mm}}{\text{m}} \cong 0.15\,\text{mm}.$$

Higher frequency sound has shorter wavelength, as shown in Figure 14-3.

TABLE 14-1 DENSITY, SPEED OF SOUND, AND ACOUSTIC IMPEDANCE FOR TISSUES AND MATERIALS RELEVANT TO MEDICAL ULTRASOUND

MATERIAL	DENSITY (kg/m³)	c (m/s)	Z (rayls)[a]
Air	1.2	330	3.96×10^2
Lung	300	600	1.80×10^3
Fat	924	1,450	1.34×10^6
Water	1,000	1,480	1.48×10^6
"Soft Tissue"	1,050	1,540	1.62×10^6
Kidney	1,041	1,565	1.63×10^6
Blood	1,058	1,560	1.65×10^6
Liver	1,061	1,555	1.65×10^6
Muscle	1,068	1,600	1.71×10^6
Skull bone	1,912	4,080	7.8×10^6
PZT	7,500	4,000	3.0×10^7

[a]Acoustic impedance is the product of density and speed of sound. The named unit, rayl, has base units of kg/(m²s) for values listed in the column. Acoustic impedance directly relates to the propagation characteristics of ultrasound in each medium and is the basis for echo formation.

EXAMPLE: A 5-MHz beam travels from soft tissue into fat. Calculate the wavelength in each medium and determine the percent wavelength change.

In soft tissue,

$$\lambda = \frac{c}{f} = \frac{1,540 \text{ m/s}}{5 \times 10^6 /s} = 3.08 \times 10^{-6} \text{ m} \cong 0.31 \text{ mm.}$$

In fat,

$$= \frac{1,450 \text{ m/s}}{5 \times 10^6 /s} = 2.9 \times 10^{-6} \text{ m} \cong 0.29 \text{ mm.}$$

A *decrease* in wavelength of 5.8% occurs in going from soft tissue into fat, due to the differences in the speed of sound. This is depicted in Figure 14-3 for a 5-MHz ultrasound beam.

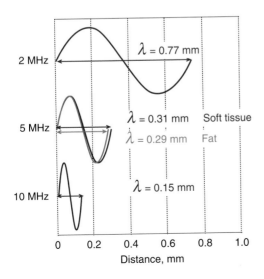

■ FIGURE 14-3 Ultrasound wavelength is determined by the frequency and the speed of sound in the propagation medium. Wavelengths in soft tissue are calculated for 2-, 5-, and 10-MHz ultrasound sources for soft tissue (*blue*). A comparison of wavelength in fat (*red*) to soft tissue at 5 MHz is also shown.

The wavelength in mm in soft tissue can be readily calculated by dividing the speed of sound in mm/μs (c = 1.54 mm/μs) by the frequency in MHz, as

$$\lambda \,(\text{mm, soft tissue}) = \frac{c}{f} = \frac{1.54\ \text{mm}}{f\,(\text{MHz})} = \frac{\dfrac{1.54\ \text{mm}}{10^{-6}\ \text{s}}}{f\left(\dfrac{10^{6}}{\text{s}}\right)} = \frac{1.54\ \text{mm}}{f\,(\text{MHz})}.$$

Thus, the wavelength of a 10-MHz beam is easily determined as 1.54/10 = 0.154 mm, and that of a 2-MHz beam is 1.54/2 = 0.77 mm by using this simple change in units.

The spatial resolution of the ultrasound image and the attenuation of the ultrasound beam energy depend on the wavelength and frequency, respectively. While higher frequencies provide better resolution, they are also more readily attenuated, and depth penetration can be inadequate for certain exams such as for the heart and abdomen.

14.1.2 Pressure and Intensity

Sound energy causes particle displacements and variations in local pressure amplitude, P, in the propagation medium. Pressure amplitude is defined as the peak maximum or peak minimum value from the average pressure on the medium in the absence of a sound wave. In the case of a symmetrical waveform, the positive and negative pressure amplitudes are equal (lower portion of Fig. 14-2); however, in most diagnostic ultrasound applications, the compressional amplitude significantly exceeds the rarefactional amplitude. The SI unit of pressure is the Pascal (Pa), defined as one Newton per square meter (N/m²). The average atmospheric pressure on earth at sea level is approximately equal to 100,000 Pa. Diagnostic ultrasound beams typically deliver peak pressure levels that exceed ten times the earth's atmospheric pressure, or about 1 MPa (mega Pascal). The pressure amplitude produced by a transducer element array during excitation producing the ultrasound pulse, and subsequently sensed by a transducer during echo reception (see Section 14.3) can exceed 6 orders of magnitude equal to a factor of one million.

Intensity, I, is a measure of average power (energy per unit time) per unit area and is proportional to the square of the pressure amplitude, $I \propto P^2$. Medical diagnostic ultrasound intensity levels are typically measured in units of milliwatts/cm². The absolute intensity level depends upon the method of ultrasound production (e.g., pulsed or continuous—a discussion of these parameters can be found in Section 14.11 of this chapter). Relative pressure and intensity levels are described as a unitless logarithmic ratio, the *decibel* (*dB*). The relative pressure and intensity in dB are expressed as

$$\text{Relative pressure (dB)} = 20 \log \frac{P_1}{P_2}, \qquad [14\text{-}2]$$

$$\text{Relative intensity (dB)} = 10 \log \frac{I_1}{I_2}, \qquad [14\text{-}3]$$

where P_1 and P_2 are pressure values (proportional to voltage values), I_1 and I_2 are intensity values that are compared as a *relative measure*, and "log" is the base 10 logarithm. In diagnostic ultrasound, the pressure and intensity ratios of the incident pulse to the returning echo can span a range of one million times or more. The logarithm function compresses the large ratios and expands the small ratios into a more

TABLE 14-2 INTENSITY RATIO AND CORRESPONDING DECIBEL VALUES

INTENSITY RATIO		DECIBELS (dB)
I_2/I_1	$log(I_2/I_1)$	$10 \times log(I_2/I_1)$
1	0	0
2	0.3	3
10	1	10
100	2	20
10,000	4	40
1,000,000	6	60
0.5	−0.3	−3
0.01	−2	−20
0.0001	−4	−40
0.000001	−6	−60

manageable number range. Pressure is proportional to voltage, and Equation 14-2 is important when comparing voltages that are induced by the reception of echoes by the transducer elements (see Section 14.4). Note: when considering pressure or voltage comparisons, the *dB* scale is a factor of 2 higher compared to intensity comparisons, so the *dB* scale must be used in context. Using Equation 14-3, an intensity ratio of 10^6 (*e.g.*, an incident intensity one million times greater than the returning echo intensity) is equal to 60 dB, whereas an intensity ratio of 10^2 is equal to 20 dB. A change of 10 in the relative intensity *dB* scale corresponds to an order of magnitude (10 times) change; a change of 20 corresponds to two orders of magnitude (100 times) change, and so forth. When the intensity ratio is greater than one (*e.g.*, the incident ultrasound intensity greater than the detected echo intensity), the *dB* values are positive; when less than one, the *dB* values are negative. A loss of 3 dB (−3 dB) represents a 50% loss of signal intensity. The tissue thickness that reduces the ultrasound intensity by 3 dB is considered the "half-value" thickness (*HVT*). In Table 14-2, intensity ratios, logarithms, and the corresponding intensity *dB* values are listed.

The amount of ultrasound energy imparted to the medium is dependent on the pressure amplitude variations generated by the degree of transducer expansion and contraction, controlled by the transmit gain applied to a transducer. Signals used for creating images are derived from ultrasound interactions and the returning intensity of echoes.

14.2 INTERACTIONS OF ULTRASOUND WITH TISSUES

Interactions of ultrasound are chiefly based on the acoustic impedance of tissues and result in reflection, refraction, scattering, and absorption of the ultrasound energy.

14.2.1 Acoustic Impedance

Acoustic impedance, Z, is a measure of tissue stiffness and flexibility, equal to the product of the density and speed of sound: $Z = \rho c$ where ρ is the density in kg/m³ and c is the speed of sound in m/s, with the combined units given the name rayl, where 1 rayl is equal to 1 kg/(m²s). Air, soft tissues, and bone represent the typical low, medium, and high ranges of acoustic impedance values encountered in the patient, as listed in Table 14-1, right column. The efficiency of sound energy transfer from one tissue to another is largely based upon the differences in acoustic impedance—if impedances are similar, a large fraction of the incident intensity at the boundary interface will be transmitted, and if the impedances are largely different, a large fraction will be reflected. In most soft tissues, these differences are typically small, allowing for ultrasound travel to large depths in the patient.

14.2.2 Reflection

When an ultrasound beam is traveling perpendicular (at normal incidence or 90°) to the boundary between two tissues that have a difference in acoustic impedance, *reflection* occurs as illustrated in Figure 14-4A. The fraction of incident intensity reflected back to the transducer is the *intensity reflection coefficient*, R_I, calculated as:

$$R_1 = \frac{I_r}{I_i} = \left(\frac{Z_2 - Z_1}{Z_2 + Z_1}\right)^2.$$ [14-4]

The subscripts 1 and 2 represent tissues that are proximal and distal to the ultrasound source, respectively.

The *intensity transmission coefficient, TI*, is defined as the fraction of the incident intensity that is transmitted across an interface, and is equal to $1 - R_I$. For a fat-muscle interface, the intensity reflection and transmission coefficients are calculated using Equation 14-4 as:

$$R_{1,(\text{fat}\to\text{muscle})} = \frac{I_r}{I_i} = \left(\frac{1.71 - 1.34}{1.71 + 1.34}\right)^2 = 0.015; \quad T_{1,(\text{fat}\to\text{muscle})} = 1 - R_{1,(\text{fat}\to\text{muscle})} = 0.985.$$

A high fraction of ultrasound is transmitted at tissue boundaries in which the tissues have similar acoustic impedance.

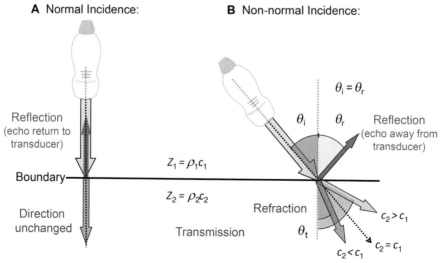

■ **FIGURE 14-4** Reflection and refraction of ultrasound occur at tissue boundaries with differences in acoustic impedance, Z. **A.** With perpendicular incidence (90°), a fraction of the beam is transmitted, and a fraction of the beam is reflected to the source at a tissue boundary. **B.** With non-perpendicular incidence ($\neq$90°), the reflected fraction of the beam is directed away from the transducer at an angle $\theta_r = \theta_i$. The transmitted fraction of the beam is refracted in the transmission medium at a transmitted refraction angle greater than the incident angle ($\theta_t > \theta_i$) when $c_2 > c_1$, and the refraction angle of the transmitted beam is less than that of the incident angle when $c_2 < c_1$.

TABLE 14-3 PRESSURE AND REFLECTION COEFFICIENTS FOR VARIOUS INTERFACES

TISSUE INTERFACE	PRESSURE REFLECTION[a]	INTENSITY REFLECTION
Liver-Kidney	−0.006	0.00003
Liver-Fat	−0.10	0.011
Fat-Muscle	0.12	0.015
Muscle-Bone	0.64	0.41
Muscle-Lung	−0.81	0.65
Muscle-Air	−0.99	0.99

[a]Note: the reflected pressure amplitude is calculated as the ratio of the difference divided by the sum of the acoustic impedances, so a change in sign to negative infers a phase change of the ultrasound reflection.

The ultrasound intensity reflected at a boundary is the product of the incident intensity and the reflection coefficient. For example, an intensity of 40 mW/cm² incident on a boundary with $R_I = 0.015$ reflects $40 \times 0.015 = 0.6$ mW/cm². Likewise, the transmitted intensity is $40 \times 0.985 = 39.4$ mW/cm². Examples of tissue interfaces and respective reflection coefficients are listed in Table 14-3. For a typical muscle-fat interface, approximately 1% of the ultrasound intensity is reflected, and thus almost 99% of the intensity is transmitted to greater depths in the tissues. At a muscle-air interface, nearly 100% of incident intensity is reflected, making anatomy unobservable beyond an air-filled cavity. Acoustic gel placed between the transducer and the patient's skin is a critical part of the standard ultrasound imaging procedure to ensure good transducer coupling to the skin and to eliminate air pockets that would reflect the ultrasound.

At non-normal angles (other than 90°) to a tissue boundary, the incident angle, θ_i of the ultrasound direction is measured with respect to normal incidence. The reflection of the ultrasound pulse occurs away from the transducer, at an angle, θ_r, which is equal to θ_i on the opposite side of the normal incidence trajectory, and is lost to detection.

14.2.3 Refraction

Refraction is a change in direction of the transmitted ultrasound pulse when the incident pulse is not perpendicular to the tissue boundary, *and* the speeds of sound in the two tissues are different. As frequency remains constant for stationary tissues and reflectors, the speed difference causes the wavelength to change, resulting in a redirection of the transmitted pulse at the boundary as shown in Figure 14-4B. The angle of refraction in the transmitted tissue, θ_t and its speed, c_2, is dependent on the change in wavelength, and is related to the incident angle, θ_i, and its speed, c_1 by Snell's law: $\dfrac{\sin\theta_t}{\sin\theta_i} = \dfrac{c_2}{c_1}$. For small angles, this can be approximated as $\dfrac{\theta_t}{\theta_i} \cong \dfrac{c_2}{c_1}$. Figure 14-4B illustrates the refraction angle when the speeds of sound in tissue 1 are greater than or less than tissue 2.

A situation called *total reflection* occurs when $c_2 \neq c_1$ and the angle of incidence of the sound beam with the boundary between two media exceeds an angle called the *critical angle*. In this case, the sound beam does not penetrate the second medium but travels along the boundary. The critical angle (θ_c) is calculated by setting $\theta_t = 90°$ in Snell's law (equation above), producing the equation $\sin\theta_c = c_1/c_2$.

14.2 Interactions of Ultrasound with Tissues

14.2.4 Scattering

Scattering arises from objects and interfaces within tissues that are about the size of the ultrasound wavelength or smaller. At low frequencies (1–5 MHz) wavelengths are relatively large, and tissue boundaries appear smooth or specular (mirror-like). A *specular reflector* represents a smooth boundary between two tissues. At higher frequencies (5–15 MHz), wavelengths are smaller, and on a smaller scale, the same boundaries manifest with irregular, non-normal interfaces causing echo reflection in many directions. This effect is enhanced with increased frequency. A *non-specular reflector* represents a boundary that presents many different angles to the ultrasound beam and of the returning echoes, only a fraction of the echo intensity will return to the transducer, resulting in a large signal attenuation (Fig. 14-5).

Many organs can be identified by a defined "signature" or "echo texture" caused by intrinsic structures that produce variations in the returning scatter intensity. Scatter amplitude differences from one tissue region to another result in corresponding brightness changes on the ultrasound display. In general, the echo signal amplitude from tissue or material depends on the number of scatterers per unit volume, the acoustic impedance differences at interfaces, the sizes of the scatterers, and the ultrasound frequency. Tissues generating higher scatter amplitude are called "hyperechoic" and tissues generating lower or no scatter amplitude tissues are called "hypoechoic" relative to the average background signal. Non-specular echo signals are more prevalent relative to specular echo signals when using higher ultrasound frequencies, making the images appear more echogenic and granular.

14.2.5 Absorption and Attenuation

Attenuation is the loss of intensity with distance traveled, caused by scattering and absorption of the incident beam. Scattering has a strong dependence with increasing ultrasound frequency. Absorption occurs by transferring energy to the tissues that result in heating or mechanical disruption of the tissue structure. The combined effects of scattering and absorption result in exponential attenuation of ultrasound intensity with distance traveled as a function of increasing frequency. When expressed in decibels (dB), a logarithmic measure of intensity, attenuation in dB/cm linearly increases with ultrasound frequency. An approximate rule of thumb for average ultrasound attenuation in soft tissue is 0.5 dB/cm times the frequency in MHz. Compared to a 1-MHz beam, a 2-MHz beam will have approximately twice the attenuation, a 5-MHz beam will have *five times* the attenuation, and a 10-MHz beam will have *ten times* the attenuation *per unit distance traveled*. Since the *dB* scale progresses

■ FIGURE 14-5 Specular and non-specular boundary characteristics are partially dependent on the wavelength of the incident ultrasound. For long wavelengths, tissue boundary interactions are smooth and mirror-like. As the wavelength reduces with higher frequency ultrasound, the boundary becomes "rough" with non-perpendicular surfaces that result in diffuse scattering from the surface.

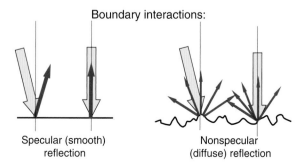

Boundary interactions:

Specular (smooth) reflection

Nonspecular (diffuse) reflection

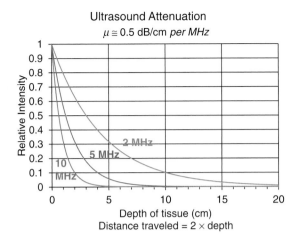

Ultrasound Attenuation
$\mu \cong 0.5$ dB/cm *per MHz*

Depth of tissue (cm)
Distance traveled = 2 × depth

■ **FIGURE 14-6** Ultrasound attenuation occurs exponentially with penetration depth and increases with increased frequency. The plots are estimates of a single frequency ultrasound wave with an attenuation coefficient of (0.5 dB/cm)/MHz of ultrasound intensity versus penetration depth. Note that the total distance traveled by the ultrasound pulse and echo is twice the penetration depth.

logarithmically to the base 10, the beam intensity is attenuated to the power of 10 with distance (See Fig. 14-6). Careful selection of the transducer frequency must be made in the context of the imaging depth needed for an exam. The loss of ultrasound intensity in decibels (dB) can be determined empirically for different tissues by measuring intensity as a function of distance traveled in centimeters (cm) and is the attenuation coefficient μ, expressed in dB/cm. For a given ultrasound frequency, tissues and fluids have widely varying attenuation coefficients chiefly resulting from structural and density differences, as indicated in Table 14-4 for a 1-MHz ultrasound beam.

Another attenuation measure is the ultrasound HVT, the thickness of tissue necessary to attenuate the incident intensity by 50%. This is determined by taking the ratio of 3 dB (a factor of 2 or 50% on the *dB* scale) by the attenuation coefficient (dB/cm) for a specified frequency. As the frequency increases, the HVT decreases and the depth of penetration decreases, as illustrated by the examples below.

TABLE 14-4 ATTENUATION COEFFICIENT μ(dB/cm-MHz) FOR TISSUES ENCOUNTERED IN ULTRASOUND

TISSUE	μ (1 MHz)[a]
Air	1.64
Blood	0.2
Bone	7–10
Brain	0.6
Cardiac	0.52
Connective tissue	1.57
Fat	0.48
Liver	0.5
Muscle	1.09
Tendon	4.7
Soft tissue (average)	**0.54**
Water	0.0022

[a]For higher frequency operation, multiply the transducer frequency in MHz by the attenuation coefficient.

EXAMPLE 1: Calculate the approximate intensity HVT in soft tissue for ultrasound beams of 2 and 10 MHz.

Answer: Information needed is (1) the attenuation coefficient approximation 0.5 (dB/cm)/MHz and (2) the HVT intensity expressed as a 3 dB loss. Given this information, the HVT in soft tissue for an ultrasound beam of frequency f (MHz) is

$$\text{HVT}_{f(\text{MHz})}(\text{cm}) = \frac{3\ \text{dB}}{\text{attenuation coefficient}\left(\dfrac{\text{dB}}{\text{cm}}\right)} = \frac{3\ \text{dB}}{\dfrac{0.5\left(\dfrac{\text{dB}}{\text{cm}}\right)}{\text{MHz}} \times f(\text{MHz})} = \frac{6}{f}\text{cm}$$

$$\text{HVT}_{2\,\text{MHz}}(\text{cm}) = \frac{6}{2} = 3\ \text{cm}$$

$$\text{HVT}_{10\,\text{MHz}}(\text{cm}) = \frac{6}{10} = 0.6\ \text{cm}.$$

EXAMPLE 2: Calculate the approximate intensity loss of a 5-MHz ultrasound wave traveling round-trip to a depth of 4 cm in the liver and reflected from an encapsulated air pocket (100% reflection at the boundary).

Answer: Using 0.5 dB/(cm-MHz) for a 5-MHz transducer, the attenuation coefficient is 2.5 dB/cm. The total distance traveled by the ultrasound pulse is 8 cm (4 cm to the depth of interest and 4 cm back to the transducer). Thus, the total attenuation is 2.5 dB/cm × 8 cm = 20 dB. The incident intensity relative to the returning intensity (100% reflection at the boundary) is

$$20\ \text{dB} = 10 \log\frac{I_{\text{Incident}}}{I_{\text{Echo}}}$$

$$2 = \log\frac{I_{\text{Incident}}}{I_{\text{Echo}}}$$

$$10^2 = \frac{I_{\text{Incident}}}{I_{\text{Echo}}}$$

Therefore, $I_{\text{Incident}} = 100 I_{\text{Echo}}$.

The echo intensity is one-hundredth of the incident intensity in this example or −20 dB. If the boundary reflected 1% of the incident intensity (a typical value), the returning echo intensity would be (100/0.01) or 10,000 times *less* than the incident intensity, or −40 dB. Considering the depth and travel distance of the ultrasound energy, the detector system must have a dynamic range of 60 to 70 dB relative intensity (120 to 140 dB relative pressure) to reliably detect acoustic echoes generated in the medium. When penetration to deeper structures is important, lower frequency ultrasound transducers must be used.

14.3   ULTRASOUND TRANSDUCERS

Ultrasound is transmitted and received with a *transducer array*, comprised of hundreds of small ceramic elements with electromechanical (piezoelectric) properties, connected to controlling electronics, aligned in a row, and contained in a handheld hardened plastic housing.

14.3.1   Piezoelectric Materials

Piezoelectric materials are materials that can generate an internal electrical charge from applied mechanical stress. The term piezo is a Greek derivation for "press." These same materials can exhibit the *inverse* piezoelectric effect with the internal generation of mechanical strain in response to an applied electrical field. Ultrasound transducers for medical imaging applications employ a synthetic piezoelectric ceramic, *lead-zirconate-titanate* (PZT), or a silicon-based capacitive micromachined ultrasound transducer (CMUT).

PZT is a manufactured compound with an internal molecular dipole (positive and negative charge) asymmetrical crystal lattice structure. When expanded or compressed under a mechanical force, the small displacements create polarization in proportion to the stress that produced it. Re-orientation of the internal dipole structure generates a positive and negative charge on each of the surfaces of the PZT crystal (Fig. 14-7A). To detect ultrasound, electrode wires are attached to each surface to measure the surface charge variations resulting from the compression and rarefaction of returning ultrasound echoes, generating a potential difference on the order of 10s to 100s of μV (μV = one-*millionth* of a volt). To generate ultrasound, the same electrode wires on the PZT crystal use the inverse piezoelectric effect by applying a voltage with a polarity to cause contraction or expansion of the transducer crystal thickness as illustrated in Figure 14-7B.

An alternate, relatively new electromechanical method of producing ultrasound is with silicon-based CMUT materials. The basic element of a CMUT is a capacitor cell with a fixed electrode (backplate) and a free electrode (membrane) that uses electrostatic transduction. An alternating voltage applied between the membrane and the backplate creates a modulating electrostatic force that results in membrane vibration with the generation of ultrasound. In the receive mode, the membrane is subject to an incident ultrasound wave that results in a capacitance change detected as a voltage signal. The main advantages of CMUT compared to PZT are better acoustic matching with the propagation medium, which allows wider bandwidth capabilities, improved resolution, and potentially lower costs with easier fabrication. While only beginning to emerge in diagnostic medical ultrasound, CMUT transducers show great promise for improvements in efficiency, speed, multi-bandwidth operation, and volumetric imaging.

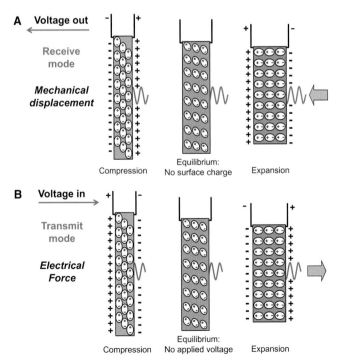

A Voltage out
Receive mode
Mechanical displacement
Compression   Equilibrium: No surface charge   Expansion

B Voltage in
Transmit mode
Electrical Force
Compression   Equilibrium: No applied voltage   Expansion

■ **FIGURE 14-7** The piezoelectric element is comprised of aligned molecular dipoles. **A.** Under the influence of mechanical pressure from an adjacent medium (*e.g.*, an ultrasound echo), the element thickness contracts (at the peak pressure amplitude), achieves equilibrium (with no pressure), or expands (at the peak rarefactional pressure) causing realignment of the electrical dipoles to produce positive and negative surface charge. Surface electrodes measure the amplitude of the charge in millivolt to microvolt output as a function of time in receive mode. **B.** An external voltage source (~100 V) applied to the element surfaces over several microseconds causes compression or expansion from equilibrium by realignment of the dipoles in response to the electrical attraction or repulsion force in transmit mode.

■ **FIGURE 14-8** A short-duration voltage spike causes the piezoelectric element to vibrate at its natural resonance frequency, f_0, which is determined by the thickness of the transducer equal to $\frac{1}{2}\lambda$. Low-frequency oscillation is produced with a thicker piezoelectric element.

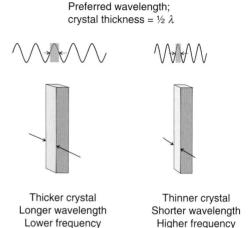

Preferred wavelength; crystal thickness = ½ λ

Thicker crystal
Longer wavelength
Lower frequency

Thinner crystal
Shorter wavelength
Higher frequency

14.3.2 Resonance Frequency, Damping, Absorbing and Matching Layers

Excitation of a PZT element is implemented with a voltage spike of 10–150 V over 1 to 2 μs with a polarity to re-orient dipoles and contract the crystal. Subsequent expansion and contraction result in vibration at a natural "resonance" frequency—dependent on crystal thickness. This is much like the way a "tuning" fork vibrates at a constant audible pitch (frequency) dependent on the distance between its tines. As shown in Figure 14-8, the PZT crystal thickness equal to one-half the wavelength of ultrasound is the preferred vibration frequency—thus, the manufactured thickness determines the center operating frequency. Crystal vibration will continue over an extended time at this natural frequency without any external contact, resulting in a long ultrasound pulse. In practice, many transducer elements are aligned in an array and individually controlled as shown in Figure 14-9. Each transducer element

■ **FIGURE 14-9 A.** A single-element crystal with surface electrodes, showing the thickness, width, and height dimensions. **B.** A section of a multielement transducer array at equilibrium (blue), thickness mode contraction (green), and expansion (red). With thickness mode variation there is also variation in the width and height of the array. The dashed double arrows represent the equilibrium dimensions.

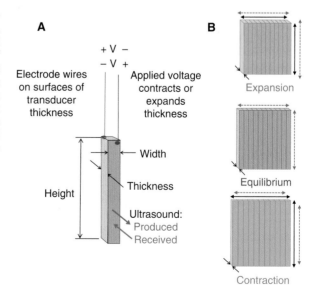

A

+ V −
− V +

Electrode wires on surfaces of transducer thickness

Applied voltage contracts or expands thickness

Height

Width

Thickness

Ultrasound:
Produced
Received

Single element PZT transducer

B

Expansion

Equilibrium

Contraction

Multi-element PZT transducers

functions in an excitation mode to transmit ultrasound energy, and in a reception mode to receive ultrasound energy. To be able to use the pulse-echo format, there is a need to shorten the pulse.

Other layers are necessary to control the spatial and transmission characteristics of the ultrasound pulse (Fig. 14-10). Layered on the backside of each element is a *damping block* to attenuate the transducer vibration duration in order to produce an ultrasound pulse with a short spatial pulse length (SPL). This preserves detail of organ boundaries and echogenic anatomy carried by the returning echoes. Dampening of the transducer crystal vibration (also known as "ring-down") introduces a range of frequencies above and below the center frequency and results in a broadband frequency spectrum. A term called the "*Q-Factor*" describes the ratio of the center frequency and the bandwidth of the pulse, as: $Q = \dfrac{f_0}{\text{bandwidth}}$, where f_0 is the center frequency and the bandwidth is the width of the frequency distribution. A high "*Q*" transducer operation has a narrow bandwidth and a long spatial pulse width, which is good for evaluating frequency shifts such as are used in pulsed Doppler studies for measuring blood velocities (Section 14.8). A low "*Q*" transducer has heavy damping and a rapid ring-down of the crystal vibration to achieve a short SPL for imaging studies.

Behind the damping block is an *absorbing* layer, which is present to reduce the backside-produced ultrasound energy and to attenuate stray ultrasound signals reflected from the transducer housing. On the front side of the transducer array is the *matching layer*, which provides the interface between the PZT element and the tissue. It consists of one or more layers of materials with acoustic properties intermediate to that of soft tissue and transducer element composition to minimize acoustic impedance differences and maximize the transmission of ultrasound into the tissues. The thickness of each layer is equal to ¼ wavelength, determined from the center operating frequency of the transducer and speed characteristics of the matching layer. For example, the wavelength of sound in a matching layer material with a speed of sound of 2,000 m/s for a 5-MHz ultrasound beam is 0.4 mm. The optimal matching layer thickness is equal to ¼λ = ¼ × 0.4 mm = 0.1 mm. In addition to the matching layer, acoustic coupling gel (with acoustic impedance similar to soft tissue) is used between the transducer and the skin of the patient to eliminate air pockets that could attenuate and reflect the ultrasound beam.

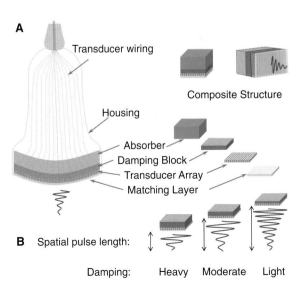

A

Transducer wiring

Composite Structure

Housing

Absorber

Damping Block

Transducer Array

Matching Layer

B Spatial pulse length:

Damping: Heavy   Moderate   Light

■ **FIGURE 14-10 A.** The transducer is comprised of a housing, electrical insulation, and a composite of active element layers, including the PZT crystal, damping block and absorbing material on the backside, and a matching layer on the front side of the multielement array. **B.** The ultrasound spatial pulse length is based upon the damping material causing a ring-down of the element vibration. For imaging, a pulse of 2 to 3 cycles is typical, with a wide frequency bandwidth, while for Doppler transducer elements, less damping provides a narrow frequency bandwidth.

14.3.3   Broad Bandwidth "Multifrequency" Transducer Operation

Unlike the simple resonance transducer design of pure PZT, the multifrequency piezoelectric crystal element is manufactured with many small rods and backfilled with an epoxy resin to create a smooth surface. The acoustic properties of these composite elements are closer to tissue than a pure PZT material and thus provide a greater transmission efficiency of the ultrasound beam without resorting to multiple matching layers. In terms of excitation, by varying the transmit voltage to the crystal electrodes in a specific way, the transducer crystal can be made to expand and contract over a selectable range of frequencies. Coupled with digital signal processing, "multifrequency" or "multihertz" transducer operation over a known frequency range is enabled, whereby the center frequency can be selected in the transmit mode. Broadband multifrequency transducers have bandwidths that exceed 80% of the center frequency (Fig. 14-11). For a given transducer, multifrequency operation allows the sonographer to interactively choose the appropriate frequency to emphasize spatial resolution or depth of penetration based upon the needs of the examination. Multihertz transducers are often identified with the frequency range of operation, for example, C4-10, where the letter indicates the transducer array type (*e.g.*, C = convex) and the numbers identify the operational frequency range.

Excitation of the multifrequency transducer elements is accomplished with a short square wave burst of approximately 150 V with one to three cycles, unlike the voltage spike used for resonance transducers. This allows the transmit frequency to be selected within the limits of the transducer bandwidth. Likewise, the broad bandwidth response permits the reception of echoes within a selected range of frequencies. For instance, ultrasound pulses can be transmitted at a low frequency and the echoes received at higher frequency as is accomplished with *harmonic imaging* (see Section 14.6).

14.3.4   Transducer Arrays

Most medical ultrasound systems employ transducers with linear, curvilinear (convex), or phased arrays, comprised of 10's to 1,000's of individual crystals. Transducer arrays operate over many selectable frequencies with multihertz broadband operation, have various physical dimensions and "footprints," and provide different image display formats.

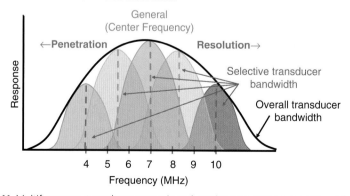

■ **FIGURE 14-11** Multifrequency transducer transmit and receive response to operational frequency bandwidths allows the operator to select an appropriate transmit and receive frequency depending on the type of exam, type of transducer, the transducer bandwidth range, and the need for penetration depth (selecting lower frequency) or spatial resolution (selecting higher frequency). The transducer response shown has a selectable frequency range of 4 to 10 MHz.

A   B

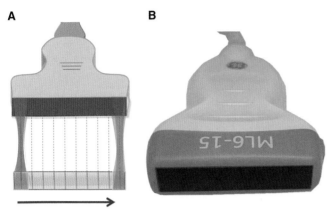

Linear   6–15 MHz transducer

■ **FIGURE 14-12 A.** The linear array transducer activates a subgroup of transducer elements to produce an ultrasound beam directed perpendicular to the array, repeating with incremental shifting of the subgroup element by element. A rectangular field of view is produced. **B.** A common linear array transducer with a 6 to 15 MHz range of operation is pictured.

Linear array transducers activate a subset of elements in a group, producing a single transmit beam at one location perpendicular to the aperture, and then listen for echoes in the receive mode. Within a fraction of a second when all echoes are received from the greatest depths, the next pulse is created by activating another element aperture group that is incrementally shifted along the transducer array, and the process repeats on the order of thousands of times per second to generate a rectangular image format with real-time frame rates and data acquisition (Fig. 14-12A). Linear arrays are comprised of hundreds to thousands of transducer elements, have small to large form factors, and generally operate at higher frequencies, from 5 to 20 MHz. These transducers are suited for imaging superficial structures such as the eyes, joints, muscles, and proximal blood vessels and for performing ultrasound-guided biopsy procedures. A 6–15 MHz linear array transducer is shown in Figure 14-12B. A small footprint "hockey stick" linear array is shown in Figure 14-31.

Curvilinear array transducers (often called convex arrays) have hundreds of elements in a convex geometry with a relatively larger housing and footprint than linear arrays. Like the linear array, a subset of piezoelectric elements defining an aperture are sequentially activated, producing a trapezoidal image format with an increased field of view at both proximal and distal depths as shown in Figure 14-13A. These transducers are ideal for imaging intraabdominal organs such as the liver, spleen, kidneys, and bladder that need large FOV coverage. Low to mid-range frequencies (1–10 MHz) are used. For depth penetration with larger patients, low-frequency operation limits spatial resolution, and at greater depths the ultrasound beam sampling becomes sparse. A 1–6 MHz curvilinear array is pictured in Figure 14-13B.

Phased array transducers (also known as sector scanners) are typically comprised of a tightly grouped array of ~60 to hundreds of transducer elements in a 3- to 5-cm-wide enclosure. All transducer elements are involved in producing the ultrasound beam and recording the returning echoes. The ultrasound beam is electronically steered by adjusting the delays applied to the individual transducer elements as illustrated in Figure 14-14A. This time delay sequence is varied from one transmit pulse to the next in order to incrementally change the sweep angle across the FOV in a sector scan format, as shown in Figure 14-14B. In receive mode, returning echoes are detected by all transducer elements in the array. Phased array transducers mostly operate at lower frequencies over a range of 1–5 MHz (although some operate at higher frequencies from 8 to 12 MHz). A narrow to wide sector field of view

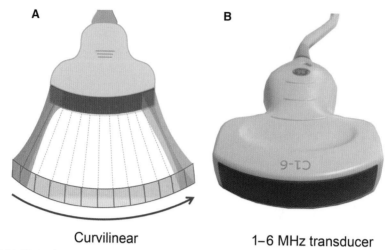

Curvilinear   1–6 MHz transducer

■ **FIGURE 14-13 A.** The curvilinear (also known as convex) array operates with subgroup transducer element excitation, like the linear array. A convex arrangement produces a trapezoidal field of view, with good coverage proximally and extended coverage distally. **B.** A common curvilinear array transducer with a 1 to 6 MHz range of operation is pictured.

can be interactively selected by the operator. The smaller physical dimension of the transducer array is useful for access to intercostal acoustic windows when performing heart and thoracic imaging exams. With a sector-scan format, the FOV dimension can be limited in regions proximal to the transducer array. A 1–5 MHz phased array transducer is shown in Figure 14-14C.

Other transducer arrays often found in a radiology ultrasound imaging suite include *intracavitary array* probes (Fig. 14-15A) for internal imaging, and *mechanically scanned* curved arrays in a larger protective housing (Fig. 14-15B) for volumetric imaging. Intracavitary probes are designed to operate inside a body cavity, have specialized shapes, and operate with a linear or phased array sequence based upon transducer array configurations. The proximity of the transducer to the tissue region allows a higher frequency range (5–8 MHz), with a wide field of view, and excellent image resolution. These transducers are used in trans-vaginal, trans-rectal, and

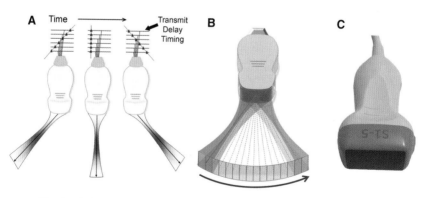

Electronic beam steering   Sector scan format   1–5 MHz transducer

■ **FIGURE 14-14 A.** A phased array transducer produces a beam from the near simultaneous excitation of all array elements. The beam can be electronically steered across the FOV using transmit delay excitation patterns—three are shown. **B.** A sector scan format is produced with incremental time delay patterns to control the direction and number of lines across the FOV. **C.** A common phased array transducer with a 1–5 MHz range of operation is pictured.

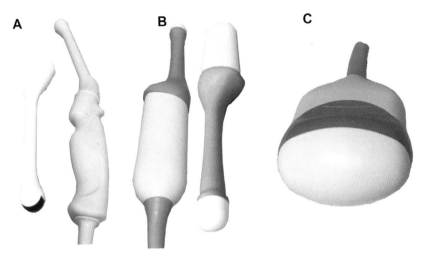

Intracavitary Arrays   3D mechanical scan curved array

■ **FIGURE 14-15** Intracavitary array probes exist in a variety of shapes and acquisition geometries to directly image internal organs with cavity access. **A.** Endovaginal curvilinear array with very wide 150° FOV and 5–9 MHz range of operation. **B.** Endovaginal probe using mechanically scanned curved array transducer for 3D imaging acquisitions, with 5–9 MHz range. **C.** Mechanically scanned curved array transducer assembly for the acquisition of 3D volumetric imaging of the fetus, with a 4–8 MHz operational range.

intraoral applications. The mechanically scanned curved array transducer is commonly used in obstetrical evaluations for 3D volume image acquisitions. Mechanical scanning of the curved array occurs simultaneously with 2D image acquisition and is synchronized to provide volumetric sampling over a ~90° by ~90° FOV range as a function of time. Shaded surface and volumetric rendering generate real-time 3D movies of the fetus, as discussed in Section 14.6.

There are many other transducer probes and types not discussed here, such as annular arrays, fully 2D electronic matrix arrays with thousands of transducer elements for real-time 3D and 4D imaging of the heart, and other specialized applications (Szabo and Lewin, 2013).

14.4 ULTRASOUND BEAM PROPERTIES

The ultrasound beam propagates as a longitudinal wave from the transducer surface into the propagation medium and exhibits two distinct beam patterns: a slightly converging beam out to a distance determined by the geometry and frequency of the transducer (the near field), and a diverging beam beyond that point (the far-field), as shown in Figure 14-16.

14.4.1 The Near Field

The near field, also known as the Fresnel zone, is adjacent to the transducer face and has a converging beam profile. Beam convergence occurs because of multiple constructive and destructive interference patterns of the ultrasound waves from the transducer surface. "Huygens' principle" describes a large transducer surface as an infinite number of point sources of sound energy where each point is characterized as a radial emitter (see Fig. 14-16, left middle diagram). As individual wave patterns interact, the peaks and troughs from adjacent sources constructively and destructively interfere causing the beam profile to be collimated. The ultrasound beam path is thus

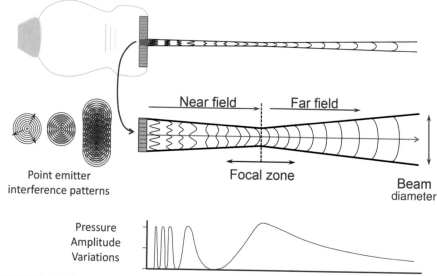

■ **FIGURE 14-16** A linear array transducer subgroup excitation (top) and the expanded beam profile (middle) shows the near-field and far-field characteristics of the ultrasound beam. The near field is characterized as a collimated beam, and the far field begins when the beam diverges. Point emitters (left middle) generate constructive and destructive interference patterns that cause beam collimation and large pressure amplitude variations in the near field (lower diagram). Beam divergence occurs in the far field, where pressure amplitude monotonically decreases with propagation distance.

largely confined to the dimensions of the active portion of the transducer surface, with the beam converging to approximately half the transducer area at the end of the near field. The near field length is dependent on the transducer area and inversely proportional to propagation wavelength, so higher transducer frequency results in an extended near field. Lateral resolution (the ability of the system to resolve objects in a direction perpendicular to the beam direction) depends on the lateral beam dimension and is best at the end of the near field for an unfocused transducer element aperture (*e.g.*, a subgroup of linear array transducer elements fired simultaneously).

Pressure amplitude changes caused by ultrasound propagation in the near field are very complex, produced by the individual transducer element excitations and the constructive and destructive interference wave pattern interactions of the ultrasound beam. Pressures vary rapidly from peak compression to peak rarefaction several times during transit through the near field. Peak ultrasound pressure occurs at the end of the near field, corresponding to the minimum beam area.

14.4.2 The Far Field

The far-field, also known as the Fraunhofer zone, begins at the distance from the transducer where the beam diverges, and lateral resolution degrades. The angle of divergence is directly proportional to the wavelength and inversely proportional to the transducer area. Less beam divergence occurs with higher-frequency and larger sub-element excitations in a linear array. Ultrasound intensity in the far-field decreases monotonically with distance (Fig. 14-16 bottom illustration).

14.4.3 Transducer Array Beam Focusing

Transducer elements in a linear array that are fired simultaneously produce an effective transducer width equal to the sum of the widths of the individual elements. Individual beams interact via "constructive" and "destructive" interference to produce a collimated beam that has properties like the properties of a single crystal area transducer of the same size. Thus, for a subgroup of simultaneously fired transducers in a linear array, the focal distance is a function of the transducer area (height/width) and the transducer frequency. With slight differences in excitation time for individual elements in the subgroup aperture (or full phased array), wave interactions and summations can focus the beam.

Transmit Focus

Array transducer electronics can apply specific timing delays between transducer elements in a subgroup for linear and curvilinear array transducers, and for all elements in a phased array transducer to cause the beam to converge at a specified closer distance. A shallow focal zone (close to the transducer surface) is produced by firing outer transducer elements before the inner elements in a symmetrical pattern, as shown in Figure 14-17A for a phased-array transducer (note that these principles also apply for the subgroup aperture elements in a linear or curvilinear array). Focal distances at greater depth are achieved by reducing the delay time differences amongst the transducer elements, resulting in more distal beam convergence.

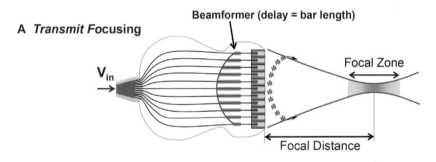

A *Transmit Focusing*

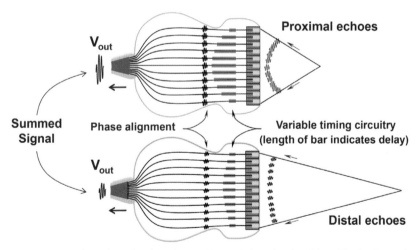

B *Dynamic Receive Focusing*

■ **FIGURE 14-17** Transmit and Receive focusing. **A.** Transmit focusing is achieved by implementing a programmable delay time (beamformer electronics) for the excitation of the individual transducer elements in a concave pattern with outer elements energized first. The individual ultrasound pulses converge to a minimum beam diameter (the focal distance) at a predictable depth in tissue. **B.** Dynamic receive focusing uses receive beamformer electronics to dynamically adjust delay times for processing the received echo signals. This compensates for differences in arrival time across the array as a function of time (depth of the echo) and results in phase alignment of the echo signals by all elements to achieve a good signal output as a function of time.

Receive Focus

The echoes received by the active transducer elements are summed together to create the ultrasound signal from a given depth as a function of time. Echoes received at the edge of the array travel a slightly longer distance than those received at the center, particularly at shallow depths, and are received later, causing phase misalignment during the summation of the individual transducer responses. *Dynamic receive focusing* is a method to align the phase by introducing electronic delays continuously as a function of depth (time). At shallow depths, delays between adjacent transducer element reception times are largest. With greater depth the returning beam is less concave, so the delays are less, as shown in Figure 14-17B. This is for both linear (subgroup) and phased array transducer operation.

Dynamic Aperture

The lateral spatial resolution of the linear array beam varies with depth, dependent on the linear dimension of the transducer width (aperture). A process termed *dynamic aperture* increases the number of active *receiving* elements in the linear array with reflector depth so that the lateral resolution does not degrade with the depth of propagation.

14.4.4 Side Lobes and Grating Lobes

Side lobes are unwanted emissions of ultrasound energy directed away from the main pulse, caused by the expansion and contraction of the transducer elements in the width and height dimensions during thickness contraction and expansion as explained earlier (see Fig. 14-9B). Side lobe emissions occur in a forward direction along the main beam (Fig. 14-18A). Individual transducer element widths that are less than ½ wavelength reduce the intensity of side lobe emissions. Side lobe emission intensity is also reduced with lower Q transducer operation (high damping) and when the amplitude of peripheral transducer element excitation voltages are less relative to the central element excitation voltages.

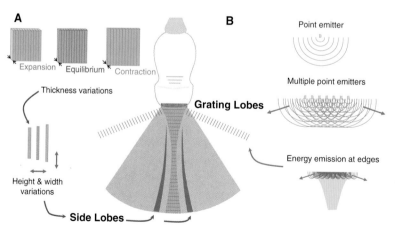

■ **FIGURE 14-18** Side lobes and grating lobes. **A.** Side lobes represent ultrasound energy produced outside of the main ultrasound beam along the same beam direction caused by height and width variations of the transducer elements. **B.** Grating lobes represent emission of energy at large angles relative to the direction of the beam caused by the discrete nature of the multielement transducer array. At the edges of the array, energy is emitted that does not undergo interference as shown by the inset diagram. The grating lobe intensity is low relative to the intensity of the main beam or side lobes.

Grating lobes result when ultrasound energy is emitted far off-axis by multielement arrays and are a consequence of the non-continuous, discrete element transducer surface. The grating lobe effect is equivalent to placing a grating in front of a continuous transducer element, producing coherent waves directed at a large angle away from the main beam (Fig. 14-18B). This misdirected energy of relatively low amplitude can reflect from off-axis tissue boundaries with high impedance mismatch and return to the transducer array.

In the receive mode of transducer operation, echoes generated from the side and grating lobes are unavoidably remapped as coming from the main beam, which can introduce artifacts in the image (see Section 14.9). For transducer operation with a narrow frequency bandwidth (high Q) the side lobe energy is a significant fraction of the total beam. In pulsed mode operation, the low Q, broadband ultrasound beam produces a spectrum of wavelengths that reduces the emission of side lobe energy.

14.4.5 Spatial Resolution

In ultrasound, the major factor that limits the spatial resolution and visibility of detail is the volume of the acoustic pulse. The axial, lateral, and elevational (slice-thickness) dimensions determine the minimal volume element (Fig. 14-19). Each dimension has an effect on the resolvability of objects in the image.

Axial Resolution

Axial resolution (also known as linear, range, longitudinal, or depth resolution) refers to the ability to discern two closely spaced objects in the direction of the beam. Achieving good axial resolution requires that the returning echoes from adjacent boundary reflectors be distinct without overlap. The ultrasound SPL, a product of the wavelength and the number of cycles emitted per pulse, determines axial resolution.

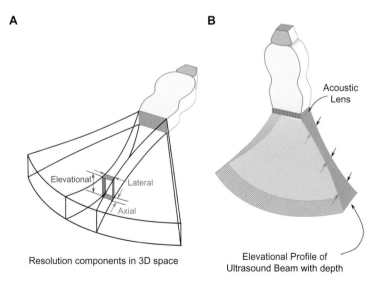

A

B

Acoustic Lens

Elevational Lateral

Axial

Resolution components in 3D space

Elevational Profile of Ultrasound Beam with depth

■ **FIGURE 14-19 A.** The axial, lateral, and elevational (slice-thickness) contributions in three dimensions are shown for a phased-array transducer ultrasound beam. Axial resolution, along the direction of the beam, is independent of depth; lateral resolution and elevational resolution are strongly depth dependent. Lateral resolution is determined by transmit and receive focus electronics; elevational resolution is determined by the height of the transducer elements. At the focal distance, axial is better than lateral, and lateral is better than elevational resolution. **B.** Elevational resolution profile with an acoustic lens across the transducer array produces a weak focal zone in the slice-thickness direction.

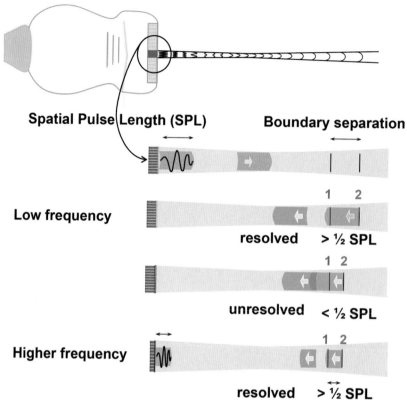

■ FIGURE 14-20 Axial resolution is equal to ½ SPL. Tissue boundaries that are separated by a distance greater than ½ SPL produce echoes from the first boundary that are completely distinct from echoes reflected from the second boundary, whereas boundaries with less than ½ SPL result in overlap of the returning echoes. Higher frequencies reduce the SPL and thus improve the axial resolution, as shown in the lower diagram.

Shorter pulses can be achieved with greater damping of the transducer element (to reduce the pulse duration and number of cycles) or with higher frequency (to reduce wavelength). The minimal required separation distance between two reflectors is one-half of the SPL to avoid the overlap of returning echoes, as the distance traveled between two reflectors is twice the separation distance. Objects spaced closer than ½ SPL will not be resolved (Fig. 14-20).

For imaging applications, the ultrasound pulse typically consists of three cycles. In tissue at 5 MHz (wavelength of 0.31 mm), the SPL is about $3 \times 0.31 = 0.93$ mm, which provides an axial resolution of ½ (0.93 mm) = 0.47 mm. At a given frequency, shorter pulse lengths require heavy damping and low Q, broad bandwidth operation. For a constant damping factor, higher frequencies (shorter wavelengths) give better axial resolution, but the imaging depth is reduced due to higher attenuation. The axial resolution remains constant with depth.

Lateral Resolution

Lateral resolution, also known as azimuthal resolution, refers to the ability to discern two closely spaced objects perpendicular to the beam direction as distinct. The beam width determines the lateral resolution (see Fig. 14-21). Since the beam width varies with distance from the transducer in the near and far-field, the lateral resolution is depth-dependent. The best lateral resolution occurs at the near field–far field interface. At this depth, the effective beam width is approximately equal to ½ the effective transducer width. In the far-field, the beam diverges and substantially reduces the lateral resolution.

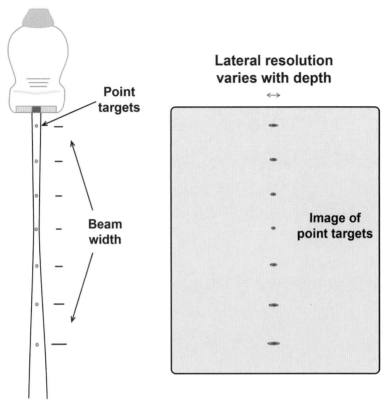

**Lateral resolution
varies with depth**

↔

Point
targets

Beam
width

Image of
point targets

■ **FIGURE 14-21** Lateral resolution is a measure of the ability to discern objects perpendicular to the direction of beam travel and is determined by the beam diameter. Point targets in the beam are averaged over the effective beam diameter in the ultrasound image as a function of depth. Best lateral resolution occurs at the focal distance; good resolution occurs over the focal zone.

As the beam width can be selectively varied as a function of depth with adjustable delay times for exciting the transducer elements (see Fig. 14-17A), lateral resolution can be improved. Moreover, multiple transmit/receive focal zones can be implemented to maintain lateral resolution as a function of depth for both linear and phased array transducer operation (Fig. 14-22). Each focal zone requires a separate pulse-echo sequence to acquire data. This is accomplished by acquiring data along one beam direction multiple times equal to the number of transmit focal zones, accepting only the echoes within each focal zone, and merging the data. Increasing the number of focal zones improves overall in-focus lateral resolution with depth, but the amount of time required to produce an image increases, with a consequent reduction in frame rate and/or number of scan lines per image.

Elevational Resolution

The elevational or slice-thickness dimension of the ultrasound beam is perpendicular to the image plane. Slice thickness plays a significant part in image resolution, particularly with respect to volume averaging of acoustic details in the regions close to the transducer and in the far-field beyond the focal zone. Elevational resolution is dependent on the transducer element height in much the same way that the lateral resolution is dependent on the transducer element width as shown in Figure 14-19B. The slice thickness dimension has the poorest

14.4 Ultrasound Beam Properties

■ **FIGURE 14-22** Linear and phased-array transducers have multiple user-selectable transmit and receive focal zones implemented by the beamformer electronics. In this example, a phased array transducer is illustrated. Each focal zone requires the transmit beamformer excitation of the active array for a given focal distance. Subsequent processing meshes the independently acquired data to enhance the lateral focal zone over a greater distance. Good lateral resolution over an extended depth can be achieved at the expense of reduced image frame rate.

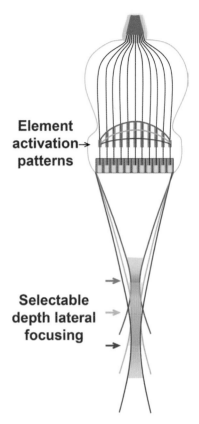

Element activation→ patterns

Selectable depth lateral focusing

resolvability for array transducers. The use of an acoustic lens across the entire array can provide improved elevational resolution at a fixed focal distance. Unfortunately, this compromises resolution before and after the elevational focal zone due to partial volume averaging.

Multiple linear array transducers with five to seven rows, known as *1.5D transducer arrays*, have the ability to steer and focus the beam in the elevational dimension. Elevational focusing is implemented with phased excitation of the outer to inner arrays to minimize the slice-thickness dimension at a given depth (Fig. 14-23). By using subsequent excitations with different focusing distances, multiple transmit

■ **FIGURE 14-23** Elevational resolution with multiple transmit focusing zones is achieved with "1.5D" transducer arrays to reduce the slice-thickness profile over an extended depth. Five to seven rows of discrete arrays replace the single array. Phase delay timing provides focusing in the elevational plane, like that used for lateral transmit and receive focusing.

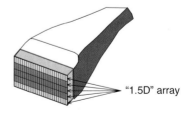

"1.5D" array

Multiple transmit focal zones: elevational plane

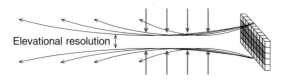

Elevational resolution ↕

focusing can produce smaller slice thickness over a range of tissue depths. A disadvantage of elevational focusing is a frame rate reduction penalty required for multiple excitations to build one image. The increased width of the transducer array also limits positioning flexibility. Extension to full 2D transducer arrays with enhancements in computational power allows 3D imaging with more uniform resolution throughout the image volume.

14.5 IMAGE DATA ACQUISITION AND PROCESSING

Images are acquired using a *pulse-echo* mode of ultrasound production and detection. Each pulse is directionally transmitted into the patient. Partial reflections from tissue boundaries at normal incidence create echoes that return to the transducer as a function of travel time and depth, along a corresponding line in the ultrasound image. The receiver detects the echoes, and the process is repeated incrementally across the field of view to sequentially construct the image line by line. Data acquisition and image formation using the pulse-echo approach requires several hardware components: the beamformer, pulser, receiver, amplifier, scan converter/image memory, and display system (Fig. 14-24A), complemented by the operating system and program software to orchestrate the acquisition, processing, display, and storage algorithms. These components are housed in the ultrasound system as pictured in Figure 14-24B, with the operator controls, various transducers, display monitor, and interfaces to information systems (PACS, RIS, EHR as discussed in Chapter 5). The detection and processing of the echo signals is the subject of this section.

14.5.1 Beamformer

The beamformer generates the electronic delays for individual transducer elements in an array to achieve transmit and receive focusing and beam steering. The digital beamformer logic controls the pulser, transmit/receive switch, timing logic for beam steering and focusing, the digital-to-analog (DAC) and analog-to-digital (ADC) converters, preamplification, and time-gain-compensation (TGC) circuitry. Each of these components is explained below.

14.5.2 Pulser

The pulser (also known as the transmitter) provides the electrical voltage for exciting the piezoelectric transducer elements and controls the output transmit power by adjustment of the applied voltage. A DAC determines the amplitude of the voltage. An increase in transmit amplitude creates higher intensity sound and improves echo detection from weaker reflectors. A direct consequence is a higher signal-to-noise ratio in the images but also higher power deposition to the patient. User controls of the output power are labeled "output," "power," "dB," or "transmit" by the manufacturer. In many systems, a low power setting for obstetric imaging reduces power deposition to protect the fetus from excessive thermal and mechanical energy. A method for indicating output power in terms of a thermal index (TI) and mechanical index (MI) is provided by ultrasound equipment manufacturers (see Section 14.11).

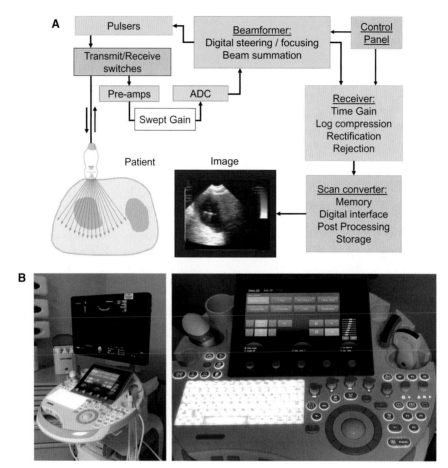

■ **FIGURE 14-24 A.** Components of the ultrasound imager. This schematic depicts the design of a **digital acquisition/digital beamformer system,** where **each** of the transducer elements in the array has a pulser, transmit-receive switch, preamplifier, swept gain, and analog to digital converter (ADC). Swept gain reduces the dynamic range of the signals prior to digitization. The beamformer provides focusing, steering, and summation of the beam; the receiver processes the data for optimal signal to noise ratio, and the scan converter produces the output image rendered on the monitor. **B.** A commercial ultrasound scanner system is comprised of a keyboard, various acquisition and processing controls including transmit gain and TGC, several transducer selections, an image display monitor, and other components/interfaces not shown.

14.5.3 Transmit/Receive Switch

The transmit/receive switch, synchronized with the pulser, isolates the high voltage associated with pulsing (~150 V) from the sensitive amplification stages during receive mode, with induced voltages ranging from approximately 1 V to 2 μV from the returning echoes. After the *ring-down* time, when the vibration of the piezoelectric material has stopped, the transducer electronics are switched to sensing surface charge variations of mechanical deflection caused by the returning echoes, over a period of up to about 1,000 μs (1 ms).

14.5.4 Pulse-Echo Operation

In the *pulse-echo* mode of transducer operation, the ultrasound beam is intermittently transmitted, with most of the time occupied by listening for echoes. The ultrasound pulse is created with a short voltage waveform provided by the *pulser* of the ultrasound system. This event is sometimes known as the *main bang*, generating a pulse of two to three cycles based on the damping characteristics of the transducer elements. The time, T (μs) between the transmitted pulse and the detection of an echo is directly related to the depth D (cm) of the reflector interface with the speed of sound in tissue expressed as 0.154 cm/μs, as

$$T(\mu s) = \frac{2D(cm)}{c\left(\dfrac{cm}{\mu s}\right)} = \frac{2D \; cm}{0.154\dfrac{cm}{\mu s}} = \frac{13 \; \mu s}{cm} \times D(cm),$$

$$D(cm) = \frac{0.154\dfrac{cm}{\mu s} \times T(\mu s)}{2} = 0.077 \times T(\mu s),$$

where the constant 2 in each equation accounts for two times the distance traveled by the ultrasound to the depth, D. One pulse-echo sequence produces one amplitude-modulated line (A-line) of image data. The timing of the data excitation and echo acquisition relates to the depth of the reflector (Fig. 14-25). Hundreds of repetitions of the pulse-echo sequence are necessary to construct an image from the individual A-lines.

Pulse Repetition Frequency and Pulse Repetition Period

The number of times the transducer is pulsed per second is known as the *pulse repetition frequency* (PRF). For imaging, the PRF typically ranges from 2,000 to 4,000 pulses per second (2 to 4 kHz). The time between pulses is the *pulse repetition period* (PRP), equal to the inverse of the PRF. An increase in PRF results in a decrease in echo listening time. The maximum PRF is determined by the time required for echoes from the most distant structures to reach the transducer. If a second pulse occurs before the detection of the most distant echoes, confusion of the late echoes from the first pulse with prompt echoes from the second pulse will result in "range ambiguity" artifacts. The *maximal range* in *cm* is the depth that all echoes will return to the transducer before the next pulse and is determined from the product of the speed of sound (cm/s)

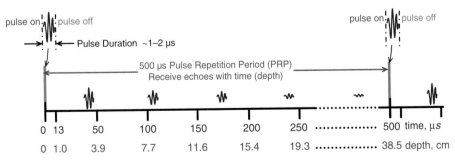

■ **FIGURE 14-25** In this example, the pulse-echo timing of data acquisition depicts the initial pulse occurring in a very short time span, the pulse duration, of 1 to 2 μs, and the time between pulses, the pulse repetition period (PRP), of 500 μs. The number of pulses per second, the pulse repetition frequency (PRF) is 2,000/s, or 2 kHz. The indicated depth is ½ of the total travel distance of the pulse/echo for the indicated time.

TABLE 14-5 TYPICAL PRF, PRP, AND DUTY CYCLE VALUES FOR ULTRASOUND OPERATION MODES

OPERATION MODE	PRF (Hz)	PRP (μs)	DUTY CYCLE (%)
M-mode	500	2,000	0.05
Real-time	2,000–4,000	500–250	0.2–0.4
Pulsed Doppler	4,000–12,000	250–83	0.4–1.2

Adapted with permission from Zagzebski J. *Essentials of Ultrasound Physics*. St. Louis, MO: Mosby-Year Book; 1996. Copyright Elsevier 1996.

and the PRP (s) divided by 2 (the factor of 2 accounts for travel to the depth and back to the transducer):

$$\text{Maximal range (cm)} = 154{,}000 \text{ cm/s} \times \text{PRP(s)}/2 = 77{,}000 \times \text{PRP} = 77{,}000/\text{PRF(s}^{-1}),$$

where PRP $= 1/\text{PRF}$. A 500 μs PRP corresponds to a PRF of 2 kHz (2,000 s^{-1}) and a maximal range of 38.5 cm. For a PRP of 250 μs (PRF of 4 kHz), the maximum depth is halved to 19.3 cm. Since higher ultrasound frequencies have limited penetration depth due to increased attenuation, larger PRFs can be used. Conversely, lower frequencies require a smaller PRF because echoes return from greater depths requiring a longer PRP.

Pulse Duration and Duty Cycle

Pulse duration is the ratio of the number of cycles in the pulse to the transducer frequency and is equal to the instantaneous "on" time. A pulse consisting of two cycles with a center frequency of 2 MHz has a duration of 1 μs. The *duty cycle*, the fraction of "on" time, is equal to the pulse duration divided by the PRP. For real-time imaging applications, the duty cycle is typically 0.2% to 0.4%, indicating that greater than 99.5% of the scan time is spent "listening" to echoes as opposed to producing acoustic energy. Intensity levels in medical ultrasonography are very low when averaged over time, as is the intensity when averaged over space due to the collimation of the beam. For clinical data acquisition, a typical range of PRF, PRP, and duty cycle values is listed in Table 14-5.

14.5.5 Preamplification and Analog-to-Digital Conversion

In multielement array transducers, preprocessing steps are performed in parallel. Each transducer element produces a voltage proportional to the pressure amplitude of the returning echoes that can span a range of 120 dB (a factor of a million in terms of voltage, see Eq. 14.2) during the PRP. An initial preamplification to increase the detected voltages to useful signal levels is combined with swept gain, to compensate for the exponential attenuation of the echo amplitudes. This reduces the overall voltage range to about 60 dB or about a factor of 1,000 for digitization.

For high-end ultrasound transducers, each piezoelectric element has its own preamplifier, swept gain, and ADC electronics as shown in Figure 14-26. A typical sampling rate of 20 to 40 MHz with 12 bits (1 out of 4096 or ~0.02%) precision is used.

14.5.6 Beam Steering, Dynamic Focusing, and Signal Summation

Echo reception includes electronic delays to adjust for beam direction and dynamic receive focusing to align the phase of detected echoes from the individual elements in the array as a function of echo depth. Following phase alignment, the preprocessed

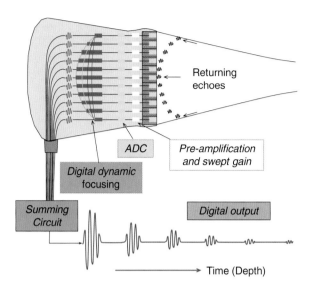

■ FIGURE 14-26 A phased-array transducer (also applicable to linear array operation) produces a pulsed beam that is focused at a programmable depth and receives echoes during the PRP. This figure shows a digital beam former system, with front-end digital electronics (swept gain and ADC) converting the signals prior to beamformer receive focusing. Electronic delays are adjusted as a function of receive time and position to align the phase of the echoes received by each transducer element. The output is summed to form the ultrasound echo train along a specific beam direction.

digital signals from all active transducer elements are summed (Fig. 14-26). The output signal represents the acoustic information gathered during the PRP along a single beam direction. This information is sent to the receiver for further processing before rendering it into a 2D image.

14.5.7 Receiver

The receiver accepts data from the beamformer during the PRP, which represents echo reception as a function of time (depth). Subsequent signal processing occurs in the following sequence (Fig. 14-27):

1. **Time Gain Compensation adjustments and dynamic frequency tuning.** *Time Gain Compensation (TGC)*, also known as *Time Varied Gain and Depth Compensation*, is a user-adjustable amplification of the returning echo signals as a function of time, to further compensate for beam attenuation to meet the needs of a specific imaging application. The ideal TGC curve makes all equally reflective boundaries equal in signal amplitude, regardless of the depth of the boundary (Fig. 14-28), so that acoustic impedance differences between tissue boundaries are properly depicted. User adjustment is typically achieved by multiple slider potentiometers, where each slider represents a given depth in the image, or by a 3-knob TGC control, which controls the initial gain, slope, and far gain of the echo signals. When set properly, TGC effectively reduces the maximum to minimum range of the echo voltages as a function of time.

   Dynamic frequency tuning is a feature of some broadband receivers that changes the sensitivity of the tuner bandwidth with time, so echoes from shallow depths are tuned to a higher frequency range, while echoes from deeper structures are tuned to lower frequencies. This accommodates for increased attenuation of higher frequencies in a broad bandwidth pulse as a function of depth. Dynamic frequency tuning allows the receiver to make the most efficient use of the ultrasound frequencies incident on the transducer as a function of time.

2. **Dynamic range and logarithmic compression.** *Dynamic range* defines the effective operational range of an electronic device from the threshold signal level to the saturation level. The ultrasound imaging chain component most

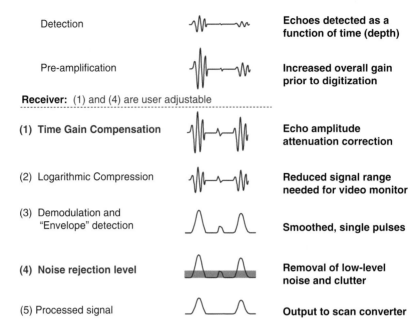

| Detection | Echoes detected as a function of time (depth) |
| Pre-amplification | Increased overall gain prior to digitization |

Receiver: (1) and (4) are user adjustable

(1) Time Gain Compensation	Echo amplitude attenuation correction
(2) Logarithmic Compression	Reduced signal range needed for video monitor
(3) Demodulation and "Envelope" detection	Smoothed, single pulses
(4) Noise rejection level	Removal of low-level noise and clutter
(5) Processed signal	Output to scan converter

■ **FIGURE 14-27** A snapshot of data streaming from the beamformer is described. Left column is the processing step, middle is the illustration of the signal, and right is the described output. The user can adjust the time gain compensation (TGC) levels and the noise rejection level.

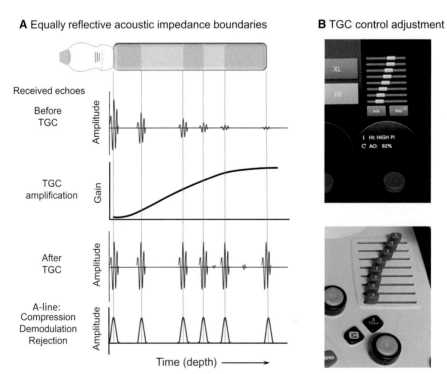

A Equally reflective acoustic impedance boundaries

B TGC control adjustment

Received echoes

Before TGC

Amplitude

TGC amplification

Gain

After TGC

Amplitude

A-line: Compression Demodulation Rejection

Amplitude

Time (depth) ⟶

■ **FIGURE 14-28** TGC amplifies the acquired signals with respect to time after the initial pulse by operator adjustments. **A.** Equally reflective boundaries are expected to produce equal echo amplitudes. Appropriate TGC amplification settings provide the correct adjustments. **B.** On the operator console, the sonographer interactively adjusts TGC with a set of electronic calipers or slide potentiometers that represent a range of image depths to optimize the gain.

affected by wide dynamic range signals is the display monitor. For viewing at a fixed brightness accommodation level, display monitors have a useful dynamic range of about 100:1 to 150:1 and therefore require a reduced range of input signal amplitudes to accurately render the visual display output. Thus, after TGC, the range of incoming signals is further compressed by using *logarithmic compression* to increase the smallest echo amplitudes and to decrease the largest amplitudes to avoid signal thresholding or saturation.

3. **Rectification, demodulation, and envelope detection.** *Rectification* inverts the negative amplitude signals to positive values. *Demodulation and envelope detection* convert the rectified amplitudes of the echo into a smoothed pulse.

4. **Noise Rejection** adjustment sets the lower threshold signal level allowed to pass to the scan converter. This removes a significant amount of undesirable low-level noise and clutter generated from scattered sound or by the electronics.

5. Processed signals are optimized for gray-scale range and passed to the scan converter to render the information into a 2D image matrix for display.

Of the steps listed above, the operator can control the TGC and noise/clutter rejection level.

The amount of amplification (overall gain) necessary is dependent on the initial power (transmit gain) settings of the ultrasound system. Higher intensities are achieved by exciting the transducer elements with larger voltages. This increases the amplitude of the returning echoes and reduces the need for electronic amplification gain but also deposits more energy into the patient, where heating or mechanical interactions can be significant. Conversely, lower ultrasound power settings, such as those used in obstetrical ultrasound, require a greater overall electronic gain to amplify weaker echo signals. TGC allows the operator to manipulate depth-dependent gain to improve image uniformity and compensate for unusual imaging situations. Inappropriate adjustment of TGC can lead to artifactual enhancement of tissue boundaries and tissue texture, as well as non-uniform response versus depth (see example in Section 14.9—equipment settings). The noise rejection level sets a threshold to clean up low-level signals in the electronic signal. It is usually adjusted in conjunction with the transmit power level setting of the ultrasound instrument.

14.5.8 Echo Signal Modes

A-mode

A-mode (A for amplitude) is the *processed* echo amplitude versus time generated as output by the receiver. As echoes return from tissue boundaries and scatterers, digital signals proportional to echo amplitudes produce one "A-line" of data per PRP for conventional line by line acquisition. Since the speed of sound equates to depth, the tissue interfaces along the ultrasound beam path are localized by distance from the transducer. A-mode acquisition and analysis was the earliest application of ultrasound in medicine for determining the midline position of the brain for revealing possible mass effect of brain tumors. *Direct* use of A-mode and A-line information is limited to accurate measurements such as ophthalmology applications to determine precise distance measurements of the eye.

B-mode

B-mode (B for brightness) is the electronic conversion of the A-mode amplitude information into brightness-modulated signals along the A-line trajectory. Brightness is encoded as a grayscale value proportional to the echo signal amplitude. B-mode is intrinsic to M-mode and 2D gray-scale imaging.

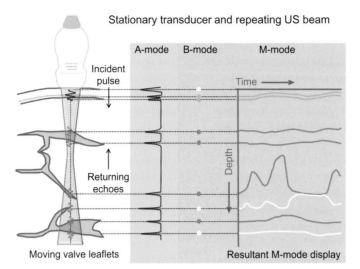

Stationary transducer and repeating US beam

■ **FIGURE 14-29** M (motion)-mode acquisition. Data are acquired with a stationary ultrasound beam positioned over moving anatomy such as heart valves. The A-mode data (vertical amplitude-modulated trace) represent echo amplitudes during one pulse-echo period. The amplitudes are encoded to brightness (B-mode) as a series of variable intensity dots. The A-mode line and corresponding B-mode dots vertically change position as the valve leaflets positionally move within the stationary beam. By deflecting the dots horizontally in time, the traces create motion graphs (M-mode) that depict the periodic (or lack of periodic) motion.

M-mode

M-mode (M for motion) also known as T-M (time-motion) mode, is a technique that uses B-mode information from a *stationary ultrasound beam* to track echoes generated from moving reflectors, such as the valve leaflets in the vasculature (Fig. 14-29). Echo data generated by moving anatomy in the beam are acquired and displayed as a function of time, represented by reflector depth on the vertical axis (beam path direction) and time on the horizontal axis. M-mode can provide excellent temporal resolution of periodic (or aperiodic) motion patterns, allowing functional evaluation of heart valves and cardiac and vascular anatomy. Only one dimension of anatomy is represented by the M-mode technique, and with advances in real-time 2D echocardiography, Doppler, and color flow imaging, this display mode is less important than in the past.

14.5.9 Scan Converter

The *scan converter* generates 2D ultrasound images from B-mode data streaming from the receiver. Scan conversion is necessary because the image acquisition frame of reference and display formats are different. During image acquisition, the B-mode digital signals are inserted into the digital image matrix at memory addresses that correspond as closely as possible to the relative reflector positions in the body, determined by beam orientation, direction, and echo reception time. Misalignment between the digital image matrix and the beam trajectory, particularly for sector-scan and curvilinear formats at larger depths, requires data interpolation to fill in empty or partially filled pixels. Each pixel has a memory address that uniquely defines its location within the matrix. The dimensions of the digital image matrix are a function of the transducer being used, the acquisition settings, and the manufacturer of the ultrasound device. With digital scan converter technology, data manipulation, image processing, and storage are handled directly.

14.6 IMAGE ACQUISITION

A 2D ultrasound image is acquired by sweeping a pulsed ultrasound beam sequentially in a plane over the volume of interest. Most acquisitions involve real-time data acquisition "video clips," with subsequent selection of relevant static images extracted from each of the acquired clips for review and diagnosis. The matrix size and frame rate are dependent on several factors including ultrasound frequency, PRF, the field of view, depth of penetration, number of lines per frame, and line density. Many different matrix dimensions are used to format the data into grayscale and color representations.

Improvements in image acquisition rate are achievable with advanced techniques such as multi-line acquisition (MLA), multi-line transmission (MLT), plane, and diverging wave imaging. These advances provide frame rates that go well beyond conventional line by line acquisitions and create high temporal resolution imaging of several hundred to thousands of frames per second.

14.6.1 Real-Time Imaging: Frame Rate, FOV, Depth, Sampling Trade-Offs

The 2D image (a single *frame*) is created from a number N of A-lines (typically 100 to 1,000+), acquired across the FOV. A larger N will produce a higher quality image as there will be a greater line density (LD) across the FOV; however, the finite time for pulse-echo propagation places an upper limit on N that also impacts temporal resolution. For *line by line* pulse-echo acquisition, the time required for each line, T_{line}, to a maximum penetration depth, D_{max}, is equal to 13 µs/cm × D_{max} (cm), where a depth of 1 cm requires a travel distance of 2 cm (Fig. 14-25). Thus, the time necessary per frame, T_{frame}, is given by.

$$T_{frame} = N \times T_{line} = N \times 13 \, \mu s/cm \times D_{max} (cm).$$

The *frame rate per second* is the reciprocal of the time required per frame:

$$Frame \ rate \ (s^{-1}) = \frac{1}{T_{frame}} = \frac{1}{N \times 13 \, \mu s/cm \times D_{max} (cm)} = \frac{0.077 \, cm/\mu s}{N \times D_{max} (cm)} = \frac{77,000 \, cm/s}{N \times D_{max} (cm)}.$$

This equation describes the maximum frame rate possible in terms of N and D_{max}. If either N or D_{max} increases without a corresponding decrease of the other variable, then the maximum frame rate will decrease.

The line density (LD—number of lines per unit distance in the lateral direction) is determined by N and the FOV. The lateral spatial sampling of the ultrasound beam remains constant with depth for the rectangular format (linear array) and decreases with depth for sector and trapezoidal scan formats. Insufficient LD can cause the image to appear pixelated from the interpolation of several pixels in the matrix to fill unscanned volumes and can cause the loss of lateral resolution, particularly at greater depths. This might happen when one chooses high temporal resolution (high frame rates) at the expense of LD. For a given procedure, the sonographer must consider the compromises among frame rate, D_{max}, PRF, FOV, and LD. As the PRF is ultimately limited by D_{max}, higher frame rates can be achieved by reducing D_{max} (and increasing PRF) or reducing the FOV or LD as illustrated in Figure 14-30.

Another factor that affects frame rate is transmit focusing, whereby the ultrasound beam (each A-line) can be focused at multiple depths for improved lateral resolution (see Fig. 14-22). The frame rate is decreased by a factor approximately equal to the

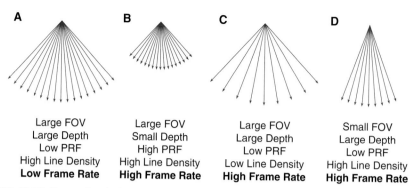

A	**B**	**C**	**D**
Large FOV	Large FOV	Large FOV	Small FOV
Large Depth	Small Depth	Large Depth	Large Depth
Low PRF	High PRF	Low PRF	Low PRF
High Line Density	High Line Density	Low Line Density	High Line Density
Low Frame Rate	**High Frame Rate**	**High Frame Rate**	**High Frame Rate**

■ **FIGURE 14-30** Conventional ultrasound acquisitions are acquired as video clips with frame rates that depend on the field of view (FOV), depth of penetration (*D*), pulse repetition frequency (PRF), and line density (*LD*—the number of lines over the FOV). **A.** Low frame rate: the baseline situation requires a low PRF because of large *D*; large FOV for anatomic coverage; and high *LD* for image quality. Ways to achieve high frame rate are **B.** Increased PRF with lower *D* (e.g., with higher frequency transducer). **C.** Lower *LD* to maintain FOV. **D.** Small FOV to maintain *LD*.

number of transmit focal zones placed on the image since the beamformer electronics must transmit an independent set of pulses for each focal zone.

14.6.2 Multi-Line Acquisition

Overcoming the frame rate limitation of pulse-echo ultrasound is achievable with several methods. Described here is *Multi-line Acquisition* (MLA). With this technique, the beam does not need to be the same in the transmit and receive phases as in *line by line* pulse-echo acquisitions. The approach uses a wide transmit beam, produced by excitation of a small element aperture to insonate the volume. In receive mode, a larger group of adjacent elements are used with receive beamforming logic to form several A-lines along different directions for each transmission event. Multiple lines formed in parallel, as shown in Figure 14-31A, can be used to increase the frame rate and improve temporal resolution. The receive phase is defined by how the different signals received by the array elements are combined to form a line in the image, by using different phase masks and sophisticated frequency processing, also known as parallel receive beamforming. Compared to conventional transmit-receive acquisition, axial spatial resolution is comparable, but the lateral resolution is diminished with MLA

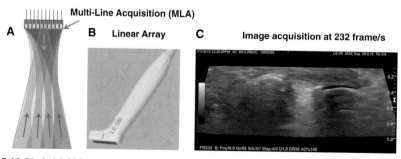

Multi-Line Acquisition (MLA)

A   **B**   **Linear Array**   **C**   **Image acquisition at 232 frame/s**

■ **FIGURE 14-31 A.** Multi-line acquisition (MLA) scheme shows a wide transmit beam profile (orange) generated by a small aperture excitation of a linear array transducer. The receive beams shown in shades of blue are generated in parallel from the single pulse; in this case, 4 lines are acquired. **B.** A "hockey stick" linear array 8–18 MHz transducer has MLA capabilities. **C.** An ultrasound image depicting gas from a knuckle-cracking experiment using the transducer operated at 18 MHz, maximum depth of 1 cm, lateral FOV of 2.5 cm, matrix size of 960 × 649, and 4:1 MLA for a frame rate of 232/s (4.3 ms/frame). Gas emission timing by knuckle-cracking was possible within a 5 ms error. (Courtesy of Robert Downey Boutin, MD, Stanford University.)

because the transmission pressure is lower with the diverging transmit beam and focusing is applied only during the receive phase.

MLA can be applied to improve the frame rate but can also be applied to improve the signal to noise ratio of the images by averaging consecutive images acquired at higher temporal resolution. Also, a larger FOV can be imaged, where the gain in frame rate can be used to widen the area covered. A linear array transducer operating at 18 MHz, 1 cm depth, high PRF, 4:1 MLA, at 232 frames/s, and a single frame from the video sequence are shown in Figure 14-31B and C, respectively.

Other methods that are used to improve ultrasound real-time acquisition rates include *Multi-Line Transmission* beamforming, *Plane and Diverging Wave* beamforming, and *Synthetic Aperture* beamforming (Demi, 2018). These techniques rely upon parallel fast processing using graphic processing units, sub-band transducer bandwidth capabilities, frequency division multiplexing, and a host of additional high-level processing algorithms. In general, the gains achieved in temporal resolution result in a loss in performance with respect to other image features such as resolution, SNR, and generation of ghost artifacts. Nevertheless, there are many applications in which plane wave imaging is being used, most notably in ultrasound elastography (covered later in this section) where images can be acquired at rates higher than 1,000 frames per second.

14.6.3 Spatial Compounding

Spatial compounding is a method in which ultrasound information is obtained from several angles of insonation and averaged to produce a single image. In linear and phased array transducer systems, electronic beam steering allows the redirection of the ultrasound beam from multiple angles (typically from 3 to 5 or more) as shown in Figure 14-32. By averaging the data, the resultant compound image improves image quality in a variety of applications including imaging of the breast, thyroid, atherosclerotic plaque, and musculoskeletal anatomy. Since each compound image is produced from multiple beam angles, the probability that one of these angles is perpendicular

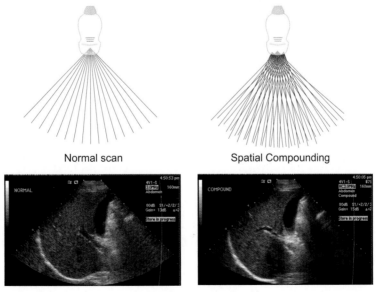

Normal scan   Spatial Compounding

■ **FIGURE 14-32** A phased array transducer (upper left) in the normal acquisition mode yields a sector image (lower left). Compound scanning (upper right) uses ultrasound beams produced at several angles achieved by electronic steering (three are shown) to acquire multi-directional acoustic image data with oversampling and a frame rate reduced by the number of angles. The compound image (lower right) demonstrates lower noise, better boundary delineation, and some motion blurring.

to a specular reflector is increased, and in turn, higher echo amplitudes are generated for better definition. Also, curved surfaces appear more continuous. Speckle noise, a random source of image variation, is reduced by the averaging process of forming the compound image, with a corresponding increase in signal-to-noise ratio. Downsides to spatial compounding are the persistence effect of frame averaging, the loss of temporal resolution, and the increase in spatial blurring of moving objects, so it is not particularly useful in situations with voluntary and involuntary patient motion.

14.6.4 Contrast-Enhanced Ultrasound

The basis for contrast-enhanced ultrasound is the large difference in acoustic impedance between gas and tissues that generate echoes with 100% reflection. Contrast agents are comprised of encapsulated microbubbles of 3 to 5 μm diameter containing gaseous compounds such as sulfur hexafluoride, perfluorobutane, and other perfluorocarbons. Encapsulation materials made of phospholipids provide stability for a reasonable time in the vasculature after injection to allow contrast agent propagation to specific anatomical vascular areas that are targeted for imaging. Because of the small size of the encapsulated bubbles, perfusion of tissues is possible, but the bubbles must remain extremely stable during the time required for tissue uptake.

Ultrasound contrast agents for cardiovascular and lesion imaging are important from the clinical perspective to make a differential diagnosis based upon the temporal evaluation of pre- and post-contrast signals in ultrasound scans. The microbubbles are small compared with the wavelength of the ultrasound beam and thus become a point source of sound, producing strong reflections in all directions. In addition, the compressibility of microbubbles compared to the incompressible tissues that are displaced produces shifts in the returning frequency of the echoes and introduction of harmonics in the returning echoes as integer multiples of the original ultrasound frequencies (see next section on harmonics). To fully use the properties of contrast agents, imaging techniques apart from standard B-mode scans are necessary and are based upon the non-linear compressibility of the gas bubbles and the frequency harmonics that are generated. An example of a contrast-enhanced ultrasound study is shown in Figure 14-33,

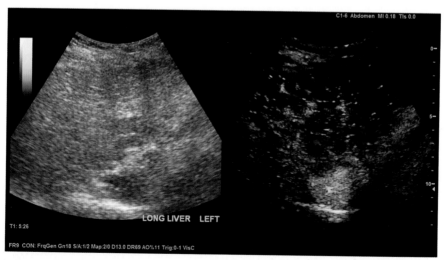

■ **FIGURE 14-33** Contrast-enhanced ultrasound exam of the left upper lobe of the liver. Left image is the grayscale B-mode image and the right is the corresponding contrast-processed image from a real-time video clip sequence. The hypo-echoic mass on the grayscale image correlates with contrast uptake on the enhancement image. In the real-time video sequence, there was rapid contrast enhancement followed by washout of the mass, consistent with hepatocellular carcinoma.

illustrating contrast uptake in a liver lesion. Destruction of the microbubbles occurs with the incident ultrasound pulse and therefore requires temporal delays between video clip acquisitions to allow circulating contrast agent to appear.

14.6.5 Harmonic Imaging

Harmonic imaging is a method to use higher frequencies generated by non-linear propagation of ultrasound in tissues that introduce harmonics, which are integer multiples (*e.g.*, 2×, 3×) of the incident frequency, f_0. A distortion of the wave occurs, as the high-pressure compression part of the wave travels faster than the low-pressure rarefaction, introducing higher-order frequency harmonics that increase with depth and localize in the central area of the low-frequency beam as shown in Figure 14-34A. The returning harmonic echoes

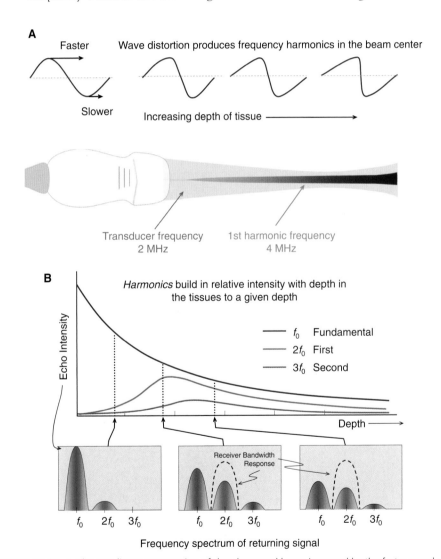

■ **FIGURE 14-34 A.** The non-linear propagation of the ultrasound beam is caused by the faster speed of the compression relative to the rarefaction, resulting in wave distortion that introduces harmonic frequencies that form in the center area of the beam. A 2-MHz beam introduces a 4-MHz harmonic. **B.** The fundamental frequency amplitude drops as ultrasound harmonic frequencies build and continuously change with depth (upper illustration). The frequency spectrum of the returning echoes is illustrated in the lower figure with first and second order harmonic spectra ($2f_0$, $3f_0$) at three points in time.

travel only slightly greater than one-half the distance to the transducer and, despite the higher attenuation, have less but substantial amplitude compared to the fundamental frequency (Fig. 14-34B). Reflected echoes of the harmonic frequencies (typically the 1st harmonic—$2 \times f_0$) are detected by the use of a multifrequency transducer set to the higher frequency. For instance, a transmit frequency of 2 MHz has the receive frequency tuned to 4 MHz as shown in Figure 14-35A. Low-frequency echo clutter occurring in the shallow regions of the image is reduced because the receive bandwidth is set to the 1st harmonic frequency after the pulse. Since the harmonic frequencies concentrate in the central area of the beam, lateral resolution is improved by the smaller effective beamwidth. Reduced side lobe artifacts and removal of multiple reverberation artifacts caused by anatomy adjacent to the transducer are other advantages. Comparison of conventional and harmonic right kidney images demonstrates better image quality (Fig. 14-35B), typical of many examinations. While not always advantageous, native tissue harmonic imaging is best applied in exams requiring a lower transmit transducer frequency for depth penetration, allowing for the harmonics to build and return as a higher frequency harmonic echo, without too much attenuation returning to the transducer. With the receiver frequency switched to a higher frequency harmonic, the outcome is improved spatial resolution and substantially less clutter from proximal low-frequency echoes.

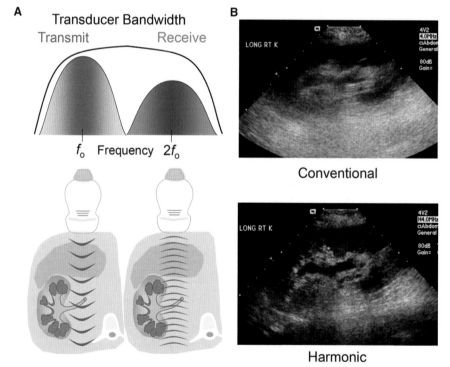

■ **FIGURE 14-35 A.** Native tissue harmonic imaging uses a lower transmit bandwidth (2 MHz center frequency) and receives echoes from the higher harmonics (4 MHz spectrum). **B.** Conventional (top) and harmonic image (bottom) of the kidney. The harmonic image shows better image quality resulting from reduced echo clutter, increased contrast, and superior resolution. (Courtesy of Kiran Jain, MD, University of California Davis Health.)

14.6.6 Ultrasound Elastography

Ultrasound elastography is an extension of ultrasound imaging that can enable qualitative and quantitative assessment of tissue stiffness. Identification of the elasticity of soft tissues resulting from pathological or physiological processes has important ramifications in differential diagnoses and identifying targets for biopsy procedures. For instance, fibrosis associated with chronic liver diseases causes less compliance than normal tissues, and many solid tumors exhibit greater stiffness than either benign or normal tissues. Thus, ultrasound elastography can be used to differentiate affected from normal tissues.

The underlying physics of elastography is based on the tendency of tissue to resist deformation with an applied force, or to regain the original shape after the force is removed. There are three types of elastic moduli defined for tissues by the method of deformation: Young's modulus (E), shear modulus (G), and bulk modulus (B). These are measurable quantities generated from an applied stress (σ), equal to force per unit area (N/m^2) quantified in kilopascals (kPa), and the resultant strain (ε), which manifests as expansion or compression per unit length of the tissue object (a dimensionless ratio). Of importance for ultrasound elastography is Young's modulus, relating an applied normal (perpendicular) stress to a normal strain as $E = \sigma_n/\varepsilon_n$. If the strain response ε_n is small, E will be large, indicating a stiffer tissue. The shear modulus relates a shear (tangential) stress to a shear strain as $G = \sigma_s/\varepsilon_s$. Shear waves are generated with the tangential force and have a speed much slower than the speed of sound. The shear wave speed can be directly related to Young's modulus in assessing tissue stiffness as explained later in this section. Thus, tissue stiffness can be estimated with ultrasound using strain or shear wave methods, the former using speckle tracking to identify particle displacement, ΔI, and the latter measuring the shear wave speed. While details are beyond the scope of this chapter, for more information and expanded explanations of the underlying physics, consult the recommended reading list (Sigrist et al., 2017). A brief explanation of each method follows.

Strain elastography measures the displacement of tissues under an applied force, either static or dynamic. Static compression methods use an acquisition of an ultrasound reference image, then a manual compression of the tissues with the transducer and acquisition of a second image. The applied normal stress (σ_n) induces deformation and strain (ε_n) on the tissues subjected to the force. A difference image is generated and 2D correlation processing identifies the local tissue displacement (or lack thereof). Relative stiffness of the tissues in the reference image is identified as a range of colors designated as "hard" (little or no displacement) to "soft" (substantial displacement) mapped as a 2D overlay on the reference grayscale image (Fig. 14-36). Dynamic strain imaging uses an Acoustic Radiation Force Impulse (ARFI) excitation to create tissue displacement within a designated volume, followed by high-speed acquisitions to measure the resultant tissue displacement by speckle tracking using correlated processing similar to the static method. Static compression methods are limited to the assessment of superficial tissues. Lack of control on the amount of applied force can affect reproducibility, and assessment of tissue stiffness for strain elastography is relative and qualitative over a range of "soft" to "hard" tissues.

Shear wave elastography is dependent upon the generation of shear waves from an applied stress and the measurement of the resultant shear wave speeds within the volume to correlate with tissue stiffness. Shear waves have a speed of 1–10 m/s, a

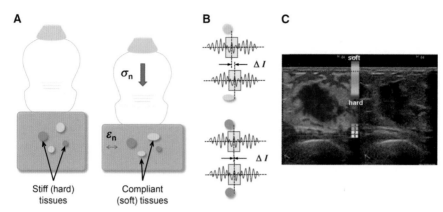

A

σ_n ↓

ε_n ↔

Stiff (hard)
tissues

Compliant
(soft) tissues

B

Δ*I*

Δ*I*

C

soft

hard

■ **FIGURE 14-36** Static compression ultrasound elastography. **A.** A conventional "reference" image is acquired and followed by a manual applied stress σ_n, by compressing the tissue volume with the transducer and acquiring a second image. The resultant strain (ε_n) causes compliant (soft) tissues to change shape in the perpendicular direction while stiffer (hard) tissues do not. **B.** Changes in object shape are detected with echo correlation and define the amount of tissue displacement Δ*I*, to *identify* the hard (stiff) or soft (elastic) tissue properties. **C.** Tissue stiffness properties are mapped using a relative color scale representing the degree of soft (red color) versus hard (blue color) tissues superimposed on the reference image.

factor of more than 1,000 to 100 times slower than the speed of ultrasound in soft tissue. The shear wave speed is a function of the shear modulus: $c_s = \sqrt{\dfrac{G}{\rho}}$, where c_s is the shear wave speed and ρ is the density of the tissue. For hard tissues, the shear wave speed is faster than for soft tissues. It can be shown that the shear modulus and Young's modulus are related (Sigrist et al., 2017) resulting in $c_s = \sqrt{\dfrac{E}{3\rho}}$. Thus, E can be determined by measurement of the shear wave speed, given by $E = 3\rho c_s^2$. With a known shear stress, the ability to measure the shear wave speed with ultrasound allows the quantitative assessment of tissue stiffness in terms of shear wave speed (m/s) and Young's modulus (kPa).

Transient elastography uses a low-frequency vibrator source (10 to 500 Hz) attached to an ultrasound transducer that produces spherical compression waves as well as spherical shear waves generated axially along the axis of vibration. The displacement as a function of depth and time is estimated by correlation of echoes recorded using a 1D ultrasound pulse at ~2.5 to ~5 MHz (depending on large to small patient size) operating in M-mode with an acquisition rate higher than 1,000 pulses/s. By measuring the phase of the returning A-line for each depth, the phase speed of the shear wave at the central frequency can be determined, leading to the estimation of E when assuming the tissues are homogeneous and non-viscous. Multiple locations are measured to identify a volume of tissue. While not an imaging method (although crude images can be produced from the M-mode data), the technique can assist in quantifying hepatic fibrosis from 20 to 60 mm depth and has become a reference standard in the evaluation of chronic liver disease.

Two-dimensional shear wave elastography (2D-SWE) uses transducer-generated ARFI excitations focused at multiple depths. Multiple focal zones are generated in rapid succession in a time period much faster than the shear wave speed. This creates a cylindrical shear wave cone emanating in the perpendicular direction to the applied force as shown in Figure 14-37. Real-time monitoring with high-speed plane wave imaging (greater than 1,000 frames/s) measures particle displacement as a function of time using speckle tracking over the volume of interest to determine the local

14.6 Image Acquisition

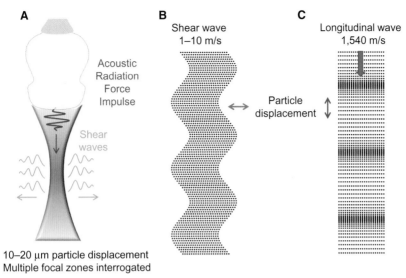

■ **FIGURE 14-37** Generation of shear waves. **A.** A high intensity Acoustic Radiation Force Impulse (ARFI) delivered to a focal depth causes particle displacement perpendicular to the force, generating shear waves in the same direction. Multiple ARFI pulses delivered to various depths create 2D shear wave volumes. **B.** Shear waves travel at 1–10 m/s in tissues. **C.** Right: Longitudinal ultrasound waves travel at 1,540 m/s with particle displacement occurring in the direction of ultrasound propagation. High speed ultrasound waves can measure slower speed shear wave particle displacement.

shear wave speed c_s. Tissue stiffness is mapped as shear wave speed in m/s or E in kPa from the relationship $E = 3\rho c_s^2$ using color-encoded quantitative elastograms superimposed on the grayscale ultrasound image (Fig. 14-38). The operator can guide the transducer to locations of anatomical tissue stiffness interactively based on real-time

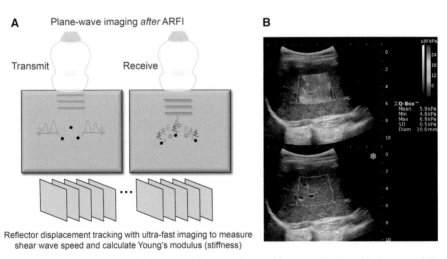

■ **FIGURE 14-38** Two-dimensional shear wave elastography. **A.** After several ARFI excitations are delivered, high frame rate imaging follows and uses plane-wave transmit and receive to acquire thousands of frames/s. Displacement of particles is mapped by speckle tracking, and corresponds to the local shear shear wave speed over the tissue volume. This allows the calculation of Young's modulus, a measure of tissue stiffness, in kPa, as a quantitative measure at the same tissue locations (see text). **B.** Example of a 2D-shear wave elastography evaluation of liver stiffness. (**B,** reprinted with permission from Barr RG, Ferraioli G, Palmeri ML et.al. Elastography Assessment of Liver Fibrosis: Society of Radiologists in Ultrasound Consensus Conference Statement. *Radiology* 2015;276: 845-861. Copyright © Radiological Society of North America. doi: 10.1148/radiol.2015150619)

feedback and, likewise, avoid structures such as blood vessels. This is currently the latest ultrasound elastography method.

Limitations of strain and shear wave elastography are related to the assumptions made about the tissues being examined in order to simplify the analysis and interpretation of the measurements. Core assumptions include linear behavior (the resulting strain increases as a function of incremental stress); elasticity (tissue deformation is not dependent on stress rate, with a return to the original, non-deformed state after the force is removed); isotropic response (tissues are symmetrical and homogeneous, and respond to stress from all directions in the same manner); and incompressibility (overall volume of tissues remains the same under the stress applied). In principle, these assumptions violate the conventional models that describe soft tissue mechanical properties as complex, comprised of heterogeneous materials with both a viscous and an elastic mechanical response when probed. There is an ultrasound frequency dependence on quantitative measurements that further complicates matters. Comparison of shear wave speed measurements amongst different vendors indicates a great need for standardization and improvement of methods. Nevertheless, ultrasound elastography in its current state is an important adjunct in the evaluation of liver, breast, thyroid, kidney, prostate, and lymph node disease.

14.6.7 Ultrasound Biopsy Guidance

Ultrasound is extremely useful for the guidance of biopsy procedures of suspicious solid masses or signs of abnormal tissue change with ultrasound imaging. Fine needle or core needle biopsy is used in many areas of the body, such as the breast, prostate, thyroid, and abdominopelvic organs. This is made possible by the excellent needle visibility due to the reflection and scattering of ultrasound under real-time image acquisition and guidance.

14.6.8 Intravascular Ultrasound

Intravascular ultrasound (IVUS) devices are catheter-mounted, typically with a rotating single transducer or phased-array transducer (up to 64 acoustic elements) design, and commonly used in interventional radiology and cardiology procedures. Transducer operating frequencies from 10 MHz up to 60 MHz are typical. Selection of PRFs from 15 to 80 kHz create high-resolution (80 to 100 μm detail) acoustic images inside the vessel. The high attenuation and minimal range of the ultrasound allow high PRF sampling. To render the vessel volume, a stack of cylindrical images can be created as the catheter is pulled back through the vasculature of interest. Intravascular transducers are used to assess vessel wall morphology, to differentiate plaque types (fibrous, fibrofatty, necrotic core, dense calcium), to estimate stenosis, and to determine the efficacy of vascular intervention. Figure 14-39 shows IVUS transducer types, depiction of the ultrasound beam, and cylindrical images demonstrating a normal and a diseased vessel lumen.

14.6.9 Three-Dimensional Imaging

3D ultrasound imaging acquires 2D tomographic image data in a series of individual B-scans of a volume of tissue. Forming the 3D dataset requires the location of each individual 2D image using known acquisition geometries. Volume sampling can be achieved in several ways with a transducer array: (1) linear translation, (2) freeform motion with external localizers to a reference position, (3) rocking motion either

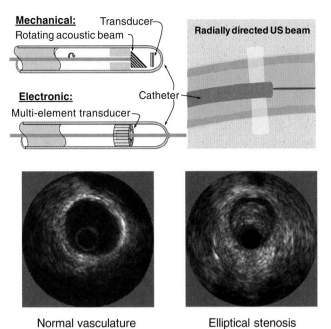

Mechanical: Transducer
Rotating acoustic beam

Catheter

Electronic:
Multi-element transducer

Radially directed US beam

■ **FIGURE 14-39** Intravascular ultrasound: devices and images. Catheter-mounted transducer arrays provide an acoustic analysis of the vessel lumen and wall from the inside out. Mechanical (rotating shaft and acoustic mirror with a single transducer) and electronic phased-array transducer assemblies are used. Images show a normal vessel lumen (lower left) and reduced luminal stenosis and plaque buildup (lower right).

Normal vasculature   Elliptical stenosis

mechanical or electronic and (4) rotation of the scan (Fig. 14-40A). Three-dimensional image acquisition as a function of time (4D) allows visualization of motion during the scan and rendering of the 3D data using real-time mechanical or electronic scanning transducer arrays. With the volume dataset acquisition geometry known, generating a surface display (Fig. 14-40B) by maximum intensity projection processing or volume surface rendering is achieved with data reordering. Applications of various 3D imaging protocols are being actively pursued, particularly in obstetric

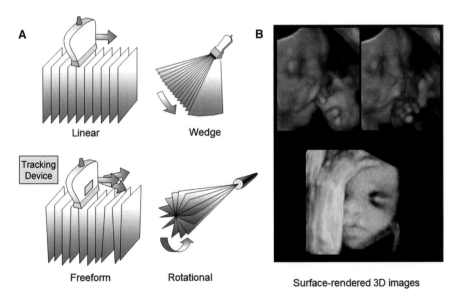

A

Linear   Wedge

Tracking Device

Freeform   Rotational

B

Surface-rendered 3D images

■ **FIGURE 14-40 A.** 3D ultrasound acquisitions can be accomplished in several ways as depicted, and include linear, wedge, freeform, and circular formats. **B.** Reconstruction of the dataset provides 3D surface-shaded and/or wire mesh renditions of the anatomy. The top images on the right are from a 4D acquisition of a fetus at two different points in time. The bottom image shows the 3D surface evaluation of a fetus with a cleft lip.

imaging. Features such as organ boundaries are identified in each image, and the computer calculates the 3D surface, complete with shading effects or false color for the delineation of anatomy.

14.7 IMAGE QUALITY, STORAGE, AND MEASUREMENTS

14.7.1 Image Quality

Image quality is dependent on the ultrasound equipment, transducers, frequency, modes of imaging selected, positioning skills of the operator, and acquisition protocols, which should be set with examination-specific needs in mind. The operator has control over equipment parameters such as the selection of transducer frequency, ultrasound intensity through the transmit gain settings, TGC curves, lateral focal zone placement(s), and noise threshold settings, among others. Measures of image quality include spatial resolution, contrast resolution, temporal resolution, image uniformity, and noise characteristics. Additionally, image artifacts can enhance or degrade the diagnostic value of the ultrasound image, as covered in the section on ultrasound artifacts.

As previously described, ultrasound spatial resolution, includes axial, lateral, and elevational. Axial and lateral resolutions are in the plane of the image. Elevational (slice-thickness) resolution, perpendicular to the plane of the image, is not directly discernable. It varies as a function of depth like lateral resolution but is typically fixed and not adjustable. Contrast resolution is the ability to discern differences in acoustic impedance that are assigned certain grayscale values as rendered on the display monitor. Degradations can limit contrast, including insufficient signal strength with transmit gain set too low, very large patients, inappropriate TGC adjustments, anatomical clutter, excessive electronic noise, transducer element malfunction, image artifacts, display monitor quality/calibration and room viewing conditions, many of which the operator has no control over. Harmonic imaging improves image contrast by reducing proximal low-frequency clutter and improving spatial resolution by receiving only the 1st order harmonic frequency signals ($2f_0$) in the returning echoes.

Image noise is chiefly generated by electronic amplification of weaker signals with depth, so deeper anatomical regions have less contrast to noise ratio values. Image processing that specifically reduces noise, such as temporal or spatial averaging, can increase the contrast-to-noise ratio; however, trade-offs include reduced temporal resolution and/or poorer spatial resolution. For instance, spatial compounding better depicts tissue boundaries with multiple angle incidence of the ultrasound beam and reduces stochastic speckle and electronic noise through averaging. While these and other tools and acquisition modes can assist in delivering the best image quality possible, it is also very important to recognize the limitations that can only be partially mitigated.

Image Modifications

Grayscale ultrasound images can be modified by window width and window level adjustments at the control panel to non-destructively modify the brightness and contrast of the displayed image, implemented with look-up-table (LUT) transformations. The pixel density can limit the quality and resolution of the displayed image. A "zoom" feature on many ultrasound instruments can enhance the image to delineate details within the image that are otherwise blurred. Two methods, "read" zoom and "write" zoom, are usually available. "Read" zoom enlarges a user-defined region of

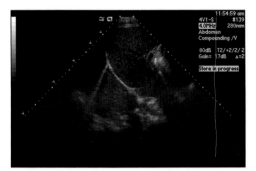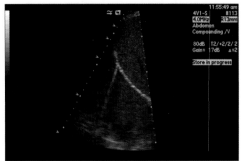

■ **FIGURE 14-41** Large FOV sector scan image (left) and corresponding reduced FOV write zoom image with improved sampling and fidelity (right).

the stored image and expands the information over a larger number of pixels in the displayed image with replication and interpolation. Even though the displayed region becomes larger, the resolution of the image itself does not change. Using "write" zoom requires the operator to rescan the area of the patient that corresponds to the user-selectable area. When enabled, the transducer scans the selected area, echo data within the limited region are acquired, and line density is increased to improve image data sampling, spatial resolution, and contrast (Fig. 14-41).

Besides the B-mode data used for the 2D image, other information from M-mode and Doppler signal processing (to be discussed) can also be displayed. During the operation of the ultrasound scanner, information in the memory is continuously updated in real-time and stored as video clips. When ultrasound scanning is stopped, the last image acquired is displayed on the screen until ultrasound scanning resumes.

14.7.2 Image Storage

Ultrasound images are commonly acquired in real-time video clip sequences of 10s of seconds long for each series with matrix sizes that depend on the manufacturer, type of transducer used (linear, curvilinear, sector), the field of view, frame rate, and type of study (B-mode grayscale, M-mode, elastography, Doppler, color flow) among many parameters. Often, relevant images out of each video sequence are extracted as single image frames for review and diagnosis in lieu of saving any or all video files. Typical matrix sizes include 600 × 800, 649 × 850, 748 × 982, 768 × 1,024, 899 × 1,442, among many variations, stored with 8 bits per pixel (256 gray levels). For color encoding using red-green-blue (RGB) enhanced images, three bytes (24 bits) per pixel are required.

It is common to use lossy compression algorithms on multi-frame video clip sequences to keep the ultrasound study storage size reasonable and comparable to other imaging modalities for a patient study. The DICOM-compliant Joint Photographic Experts Group (JPEG) standard for image compression is used by ultrasound vendors for single and multi-frame studies at a lossy compression level that is considered clinically equivalent in image quality to lossless image compression, yet reduces the file sizes considerably. Compression ratios from 5:1 to 25:1 are typical for multi-frame video ultrasound sequences. For a study with 25 lossy compressed video clips, a few hundred megabytes of storage are needed. Without compression, complete organ studies would easily require gigabytes of storage.

Ultrasound images that use RGB color encoding such as Doppler, color flow, and elastography, are compressed into 8 bits with an alternate color-coding scheme called YBR (also known as YCbCr) that represents the colors as brightness and difference signals from two colors. This scheme is more robust for compression. The Y is the brightness (luma), Cb is blue minus luma (B-Y) and Cr is red minus luma (R-Y), the values of which combine to create the output color on the monitor. In the image pixel array, flags are used to recognize YBR encoding to distinguish color pixels from 8-bit grayscale pixels when combined as a color/grayscale image.

14.7.3 Distance, Area, and Volume Measurements and Structured Reporting

Measurements of distance, area, and volume are performed routinely in diagnostic ultrasound examinations. This is possible because the speed of sound in soft tissue is known to within about =1% accuracy (1,540 ± 15 m/s), and calibration of the instrument can be easily performed based on round-trip time of the pulse and the echo. A notable example of common distance evaluations is for fetal age determination by measuring anatomical dimensions of the fetus (Fig. 14-42A). Measurement accuracy is achieved by careful selection of reference positions, such as the leading edge to the leading edge of the reflector echo signals along the axis of the beam, as these points are less affected by variations in echo signal amplitude. Measurements between points along the direction of the ultrasound beam are usually more reliable because axial spatial resolution provides the best detail. Points measured laterally tend to be smeared out over a larger area due to the poorer lateral resolution of the system. Thus, horizontal and oblique measurements in the image will likely be less accurate.

■ **FIGURE 14-42 A.** Ultrasound provides accurate distance measurements. Fetal age is often determined from measurements of biparietal diameter, circumference measurements (top), and femur length, abdominal circumference (bottom). Based upon known correlation methods, the gestational age can be calculated for each of the measurements. **B.** The structured report captures and summarizes the data in a tabular format as part of the reporting mechanism.

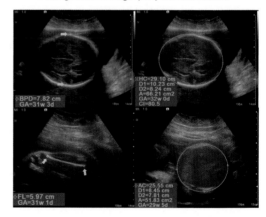

A   Fetal gestational age (GA) measurements

BPD: Biparietal diameter   HC: Head circumference
FL: Femur Length   AC: Abdominal circumference

B   Structured report with composite data

The circumference of a circular object can easily be calculated from the measured diameter (d) or radius (r), using the relationship: circumference $= 2\pi r = \pi d$. Distance measurements extend to two dimensions (area) straightforwardly by assuming a specific geometric shape. Similarly, area measurements in each image plane extend to 3D volumes by estimating the slice thickness (elevational resolution).

Measurements of features in images in ultrasound (and in fact of all radiology exams) are a standard requirement for many diagnoses (Fig. 14-42B). Translation of measurements from the modality to the PACS and/or to the interpretive report with manual human effort is very prone to error. DICOM structured reports with automatic capture of generated data from the images provide a solution to ensure accurate reporting of information that is automatically transferred.

14.8 DOPPLER ULTRASOUND

Doppler ultrasound assesses the velocity of moving reflectors, typically blood cells in the vasculature, based upon frequency shifts occurring with the incident pulse and returning echo as illustrated in Figure 14-43. A familiar analogy is an observer encounter with a train and its whistle that has a high pitch as the train moves toward

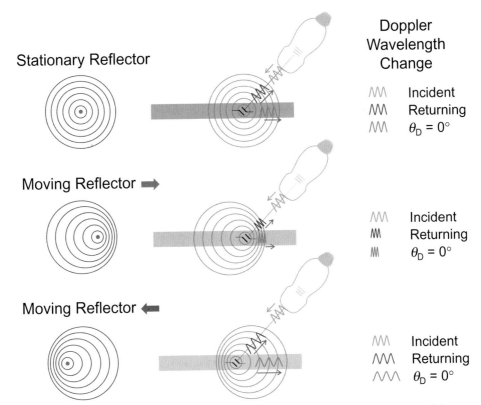

FIGURE 14-43 A moving reflector such as a blood cell in a vessel changes the wavelength of the returning echo, and thus the frequency, the degree to which is proportional to the velocity of motion and angle of the echo trajectory. For the reflector moving toward the transducer, the wavelength is shortened, and the frequency is increased (middle illustration), while the opposite occurs for the reflector moving away from the transducer (bottom illustration). When at an angle to the reflector direction, the measured wavelength (frequency) is not equal to that along the direction of the reflector, except in the case of a stationary reflector, where there is no change in wavelength or frequency (top illustration). θ_D is the Doppler angle (see Fig. 14-44).

the person and changes to a low pitch as the train passes and moves away. The approaching sound waves are compressed with motion, resulting in decreased distance between the source and observer causing a shorter wavelength and higher frequency. The opposite, longer wavelength and lower frequency occur as the sound waves recede from the observer. The magnitude of the frequency shift is dependent on the velocity of the train relative to the observer, and the angle with respect to the direction of motion.

By comparing the incident ultrasound frequency with the reflected ultrasound frequency from the blood cells, it is possible to discern the velocity and direction of blood flow. In the example shown in Figure 14-43, for moving blood cells of equal velocity, the *net* frequency shift will be equal, but for cells moving towards the transducer the shift will be positive, and away from the transducer negative. Not only can blood velocity (and indirectly blood flow) be measured, but the information provided by Doppler techniques can also be used to create color blood flow maps of the vasculature. The interpretation of Doppler signals in clinical practice, however, requires the extraction of information about the blood flow from the potential confounding aspects related to the technique itself. Therefore, an understanding of the physical principles of Doppler ultrasound is an important prerequisite for the accurate interpretation of the acquired information.

14.8.1 Doppler Frequency Shift

When an ultrasound wave of known frequency reflects from blood cells in a vessel moving towards the transducer, the echoes have a higher frequency, and if moving away from the transducer will have a lower frequency. The generated frequency shift is a fraction of the initial ultrasound (transducer) frequency, proportional to the ratio of the velocity of the blood cells relative to the velocity of the speed of sound plus the reflector speed. The *Doppler shift*, f_D, is the difference between the incident frequency f_i and reflected frequency f_r from the blood cells for *parallel incidence* of the blood cells with the ultrasound beam, as

$$f_D = f_i - f_r = 2 \times f_i \frac{\text{reflector speed}}{\text{reflector speed} + \text{speed of sound}} = 2 f_0 \frac{v}{c},$$

where v is the velocity of the blood cells (reflector), c is the velocity of ultrasound, and f_0 is the center frequency of the transducer, renamed from the incident frequency, f_i, to be consistent with previous nomenclature. The factor of 2 arises as the Doppler effect is twice as great for reflection of the ultrasound back to the source, and the final equality is simplified in the denominator by considering the speed of sound (154,000 cm/s) is much greater than the velocity range of blood cells (~100 cm/s). Thus, the Doppler shift is proportional to the velocity of the blood cells.

When the sound waves and blood cells are not moving in parallel directions, the equation must be modified to account for a deviation in the measured Doppler shift to the Doppler shift parallel to the direction of motion (see Fig. 14-43). The angle between the direction of blood flow and the direction of the sound source is called the Doppler angle, θ_D (Fig. 14-44), formed from the adjacent side (vector component of the blood velocity in the direction of the sound) and hypotenuse (vector component of blood velocity along the vessel) of a right triangle. By trigonometry rules, the hypotenuse multiplied by the *cosine* of the angle is equal to the adjacent side. The generalized Doppler shift equation is adjusted to include the Doppler angle.

$$f_D = 2 f_0 \frac{v}{c} \cos(\theta_D). \qquad \text{[14-5]}$$

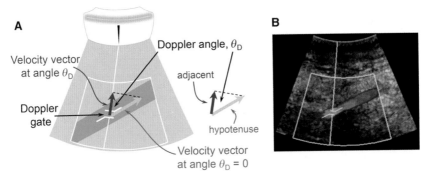

■ **FIGURE 14-44 A.** Doppler evaluation of frequency shift associated with blood velocity, illustrating the Doppler gate, the Doppler angle, and the calculated velocity vectors in the direction of blood flow and in the direction of the transducer. The right triangle geometry and vector relationships are shown to the right. **B.** Image acquired with duplex acquisition and color flow active area (trapezoidal white boundary, see section on color flow imaging for explanation) shows the vessel location that aids in placing the Doppler gate.

Solving for velocity:

$$v = \frac{f_D}{\cos(\theta_D)} \times \frac{c}{2f_0}.$$ [14-6]

Thus, the *measured* Doppler shift at Doppler angle θ_D is adjusted by $1/\cos(\theta_D)$ to estimate the actual velocity. As the Doppler angle increases from 0° to 90°, the cosine of the angle non-linearly decreases from 1 to 0 (cos 0° = 1, cos 30° = 0.87, cos 45° = 0.707, cos 60° = 0.5, cos 90° = 0). At a Doppler angle of 60°, the measured Doppler frequency is ½ the actual Doppler frequency; at 90°, the Doppler frequency can't be measured. The *preferred* Doppler angle ranges from 30° to 60°. At too large an angle (greater than 60°), the measured Doppler shift becomes diminishingly small, and minor errors in angle accuracy can result in very large errors in the corrected velocity (Table 14-6). On the other hand, at too small an angle (*e.g.*, less than 20°), refraction and critical angle interactions can cause problems, as can aliasing of the signal in pulsed Doppler studies (covered in the next section).

The Doppler frequency shifts for moving blood occur in the audible range. It is both customary and convenient to convert these frequency shifts into an audible signal through a loudspeaker that can be heard by the sonographer to aid in positioning and to assist in diagnosis.

TABLE 14-6 DOPPLER ANGLE AND ERROR ESTIMATES OF BLOOD VELOCITY FOR A +3° ANGLE ACCURACY ERROR

ACTUAL ANGLE (°)	SET ANGLE (°)	ACTUAL VELOCITY (cm/s)	ESTIMATED VELOCITY (cm/s)	PERCENT ERROR (%)
0	3	100	100.1	0.14
25	28	100	102.6	2.65
45	48	100	105.7	5.68
60	63	100	110.1	10.1
80	83	100	142.5	42.5

EXAMPLE: Given: f_0 = 5 MHz, v = 35 cm/s, and θ_D = 45°, calculate the Doppler shift frequency. Using Equation 14-5,

$$f_D = 2 \times 5 \times 10^6 \, s^{-1} \times \frac{35 \, cm/s}{154,000 \, cm/s} \times \cos(45°) = 1.6 \times 10^3 \, s^{-1} = 1.6 \, kHz.$$

The frequency shift of 1.6 kHz is in the audible range (15 Hz to 20 kHz). With an increased Doppler angle, the *measured* Doppler shift is *decreased* according to $\cos(\theta_D)$ since the projection of the velocity vector toward the transducer decreases.

14.8.2 Continuous Doppler Operation

The continuous wave Doppler system is the simplest and least expensive device for measuring blood velocity. Two transducers are required, with one transmitting the incident ultrasound and the other detecting the resultant continuous echoes (Fig. 14-45). An oscillator produces a resonant frequency to drive the transmit transducer and provides the same frequency signal to the demodulator, which compares the returning frequency to the incident frequency. The receiver amplifies the returning signal and extracts the residual information containing the Doppler shift frequency by using a "low-pass" filter, which removes the superimposed high-frequency oscillations. The Doppler signal from vessel walls and other specular reflector motion contain very low-frequency signals that are removed by an adjustable *wall filter* to clean up unwanted signal clutter. An audio amplifier increases the audible sound level of the Doppler signal, and a recorder tracks spectrum changes as a function of time for analysis of transient pulsatile flow.

Continuous-wave Doppler suffers from depth selectivity with accuracy affected by object motion within the beam path. Multiple overlying vessels will result in

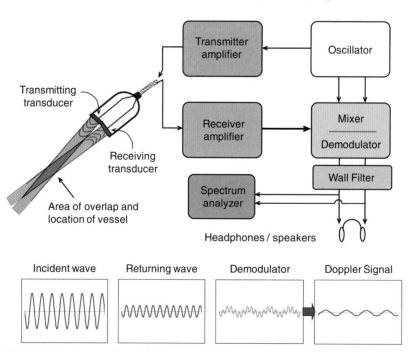

■ **FIGURE 14-45** Block diagram of a continuous wave Doppler system. Two transducers are required: one as a transmitter and the other as a receiver. The area of overlap determines the position of blood velocity measurement. Signals from the receiver are mixed with the original frequency to extract the Doppler signal. A low-pass filter removes the highest frequencies in the demodulated signals, and a high-pass filter (Wall filter) removes the lowest frequencies due to tissue and transducer motion to extract the desired Doppler shift.

superimposition, making it difficult to distinguish a specific Doppler signal. Spectral broadening of the frequencies occurs with a large sample area across the vessel profile (composed of high velocity in the center and slower velocities at the edge of the vessels). Advantages of continuous mode include high accuracy of the Doppler shift measurement because a narrow frequency bandwidth is used, and no aliasing occurs when high velocities are measured, as occurs with pulsed Doppler operation.

14.8.3   Quadrature Detection

The demodulation technique measures the magnitude of the Doppler shift but does not reveal the direction of the Doppler shift—that is, whether the flow is toward or away from the transducers. A method of signal processing called quadrature detection is phase-sensitive and can indicate the direction of flow either toward or away from the transducers.

14.8.4   Pulsed Doppler Operation

Pulsed Doppler ultrasound combines the velocity determination of continuous-wave Doppler systems and the range discrimination of pulse-echo imaging. A "duplex" mode of operation (see next section) allows the user to simultaneously perform gray-scale B-mode imaging and pulsed Doppler evaluation, the latter with a separate transducer element group within the transducer array. The SPL for Doppler transducer elements is longer (a minimum of 5 cycles per pulse up to 25 cycles per pulse) to provide a higher Q factor and improve the measurement accuracy of the frequency shift (axial resolution is not as important for pulsed Doppler). Depth selection is achieved with an electronic time gate circuit to reject all echo signals except those falling within the gate window, as determined by the operator. In some systems, multiple gates

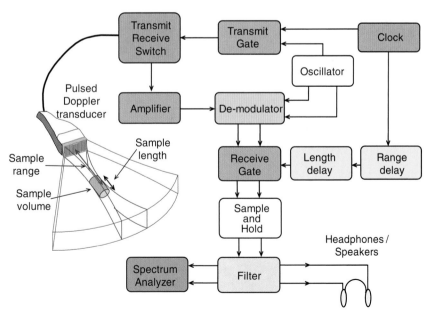

■ **FIGURE 14-46** Block diagram of a pulsed Doppler system. Isolation of a selected area is achieved by gating the time of echo return and analyzing only those echoes that fall within the time window of the gate. In the pulsed mode, the Doppler signal is discretely sampled in time to estimate the frequency shifts occurring in the Doppler gate. Because axial resolution isn't as important as narrow bandwidths to better estimate the Doppler shift, a long spatial pulse width (high Q factor) is employed.

provide profile patterns of velocity values across a vessel. Figure 14-46 illustrates a simple block diagram of the pulsed Doppler system and the system subcomponents necessary for data processing.

A single Doppler pulse does not contain enough information to completely determine the Doppler shift, but only a sample of the shifted frequencies measured as a phase change. A stationary object within the sample volume does not generate a phase change in the returning echo when compared to the oscillator phase, but a moving object does. Repeated echoes from the active gate are analyzed in the sample/hold circuit, and a Doppler signal is gradually built up (Fig. 14-47A). The discrete measurements acquired at the Doppler pulse repetition frequency, PRF_D, produce the synthesized Doppler signal. According to the Nyquist sampling theory (see Chapter 4 for an in-depth explanation), a signal can be reconstructed unambiguously if the frequency (e.g., the Doppler shift) is equal to or less than half the sampling rate. Thus, the *maximum* Doppler shift, $f_{D\,max} = \frac{1}{2}PRF_D$, and therefore the PRF_D must be at least twice the maximal Doppler frequency shift encountered in the measurement.

The maximum Doppler shift $f_{D\,max}$ correlates with the maximum pulsatile velocity of the blood, v_{max}, for pulsed Doppler operation from Equation 14-5 as:

$$f_{Dmax} = \frac{PRF_D}{2} = 2f_0 \frac{v_{max}}{c} \cos(\theta_D).$$

Rearranging per Equation 14-6 in terms of PRF_D and solving for v_{max}:

$$v_{max} = \frac{c}{4} \times \frac{PRF_D}{f_0 \cos(\theta_D)},$$

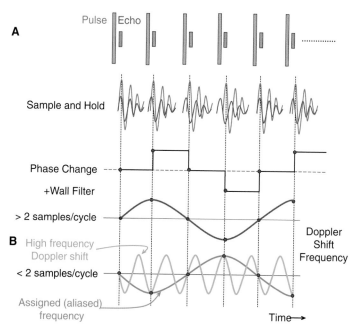

■ FIGURE 14-47 A. The returning ultrasound pulses from the Doppler gate are sampled over several pulse-echo cycles (in this example, six times to estimate Doppler shifts). A sample and hold circuit measures signal with time (the echo [**purple line**] and the pulse [**blue line**] vary in phase, analyzed by Fourier transform methods to determine the Doppler shift). The wall filter removes the low-frequency degradations caused by transducer and patient motion. **B.** Aliasing occurs when the Doppler shift frequencies are greater than ½ the PRF (sampling frequency). In this example, a signal of twice the frequency is analyzed as if it were the lower frequency with reverse phase, and thus mimics (aliases) the higher frequency with slower, reverse flow.

illustrates the acquisition parameter adjustments available to increase the maximum velocity that can accurately be measured—namely, an increase in PRF_D, an increase in the Doppler angle towards 90°, or a decrease in the center operating frequency of the Doppler transducer. Of these, the most interactive is adjustment of the Doppler angle by the operator.

For Doppler shift frequencies exceeding one-half PRF_D, aliasing will occur, causing a potentially significant error in the velocity estimation of the blood (Fig. 14-47B). A 1.6-kHz Doppler shift requires a minimum PRF_D of 2×1.6 kHz = 3.2 kHz. One cannot simply increase PRF to arbitrarily high values, because of insufficient echo transit time and possible echo ambiguity. Use of a larger angle between the ultrasound beam direction and the blood flow direction up to about 60° reduces the measured Doppler shift. At larger angles (*e.g.*, 60° to 90°), however, small errors in angle estimation cause significant errors in the estimation of blood velocity (see Table 14-6).

A 180° phase shift in the Doppler frequency represents blood that is moving away from the transducer. Beyond the Nyquist sampling frequency, higher frequency Doppler shifts will be interpreted as lower frequency signals with a 180° phase shift, such that the highest blood velocities in the center of a vessel are measured as having reverse flow, as shown in Figure 14-47B. This is a manifestation of aliasing.

14.8.5 Duplex Scanning

Duplex scanning refers to the combination of 2D B-mode imaging and pulsed Doppler data acquisition. Without visual guidance to the vessel of interest, pulsed Doppler systems would be of little use. A duplex scanner operates in the imaging mode and creates a real-time image. The Doppler gate is positioned over the vessel of interest with size (length and width) appropriate for evaluation of blood velocity, and oriented at the Doppler angle (see Fig. 14-44). When switched to Doppler mode with activation of the pulsed Doppler transducer elements, the scanner electronics extract data only from within the user-defined gate.

The duplex system allows estimation of the blood velocity directly from the Doppler shift frequency, since the velocity of sound and the transducer frequency are known, while the Doppler angle is determined from the B-mode image and input into the scanner computer for calculation. Once the velocity is known, flow (in units of cm^3/s) is estimated as the product of the vessel's cross-sectional area (cm^2) times the velocity (cm/s).

Errors in the flow volume may occur. The vessel axis might not lie totally within the scanned plane, the vessel might be curved, or flow might be altered from the perceived direction. The beam-vessel angle (Doppler angle) could be in error, which is much more problematic for very large angles, particularly those greater than 60°, as explained previously. The Doppler gate (sample area) could be mispositioned or of inappropriate size, such that the velocities are an overestimate (gate area too small in the center of the vessel) or underestimate (gate area too large including the edges of the vessel) of the average velocity. Non-circular cross sections will cause errors in the area estimate if a circular area is assumed, and therefore errors in the flow volume.

Multi-gate pulsed Doppler systems operate with several parallel channels closely spaced across the lumen of a single large vessel. The outputs from all of the gates can be combined to estimate the *velocity profile* across the vessel, which represents the variation of flow velocity within the vessel lumen. Velocities mapped with a color scale visually separate the flow information from the gray-scale image, and a real-time color flow Doppler ultrasound overlay indicates the direction of flow through color coding. However, time is insufficient to complete the computations necessary for determining the Doppler shifts from too many gates to get real-time image update rates over the whole image, particularly for those located at depth. This is solved with 2D color flow imaging by using correlation techniques described in the color flow subsection (Section 14.8.7).

14.8.6 Doppler Spectrum and Spectral Doppler Waveform

The Doppler signal is typically represented by a spectrum of frequencies resulting from a range of velocities contained within the sampling gate at a specific point in time. Blood flow can exhibit blunt, laminar, vortex, or turbulent flow patterns, depending upon the vessel wall characteristics, the size and shape of the vessel, and the flow rate. Fast, laminar flow exists in the center of large, smooth wall vessels, while slower blood flow occurs near the vessel walls, due to frictional forces. Vortex flow represents localized swirling or stagnant blood flow that has separated from the central streamline within the vessel, and frequently occurs at vascular bifurcations, and areas distal to stenoses. Turbulent flow is the disruption of laminar characteristics, with non-linear and chaotic flow patterns, occurring at vessel wall narrowing caused by plaque buildup and stenosis. A large Doppler gate that is positioned to encompass the entire lumen of the vessel will contain a large range of blood velocities, while a smaller gate positioned in the center of the vessel will have a smaller, faster range of velocities. A Doppler gate positioned near a stenosis in the turbulent flow pattern will measure the largest range of velocities.

With the pulsatile nature of blood flow, the spectral characteristics vary with time. Interpretation of the frequency shifts and direction of blood flow is accomplished with the fast Fourier transform, which mathematically analyzes the detected signals and generates an amplitude versus frequency distribution profile known as the *Doppler spectrum*, measured over a dwell time Δt as shown in Figure 14-48A for two instances in time. In a clinical instrument, the Doppler spectrum is continuously updated in a real-time *spectral Doppler waveform* (Fig. 14-48B). This information is displayed on the monitor, typically below the 2D B-mode image, as a moving trace,

■ **FIGURE 14-48 A.** The Doppler spectrum represents a distribution of frequencies (x-axis) and corresponding amplitudes (y-axis) measured within the Doppler gate over a dwell time Δt. A broad spectrum represents turbulent flow, while a narrow spectrum represents laminar flow. Two spectra are shown, acquired at different times Δt_1 and Δt_2. **B.** The spectral Doppler display is a plot of the Doppler shift frequency spectrum displayed vertically, versus time, displayed horizontally. The amplitude of the shift frequency is encoded as grayscale or color intensity variations.

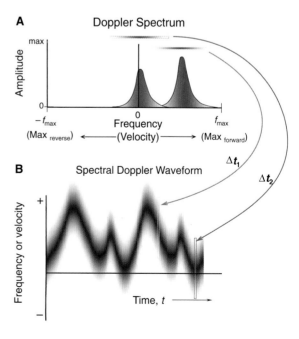

with the blood velocity (proportional to Doppler frequency) plotted on the vertical axis (from $-V_{max}$ to $+V_{max}$) and time plotted on the horizontal axis. Blood flow moving toward the transducer has a positive velocity (frequency) and moving away has a negative velocity (phase shift of the frequency). As new data arrive, the information is updated and scrolled from left to right. Pulsatile blood takes on the appearance of a choppy sinusoidal wave through the periodic cycle of the heartbeat. The waveform characteristics depend on the vessel (arterial or venous), the location of the vessel being evaluated, and the size and position of the Doppler gate. The range of frequencies in the Doppler spectrum are strongly affected by the range of velocities by type of blood flow measured within the gate: blunt (narrow), laminar (less narrow), turbulent (wide), vortex (wide with reverse flow). A corresponding appearance of the spectral waveform envelope identified by the maximum frequency shift of the distribution as a function of time will be a line, broad line, filled-in trace, and filled-in trace with negative values, respectively.

Spectral Doppler Waveform Interpretation

Interpretation of the spectral Doppler waveform can determine the presence, direction, and characteristics of velocity, pulsatility, and turbulence associated with flow. More difficult is the determination of a lack of flow, since it is also necessary to ensure that the lack of signal is not due to other acoustical or electrical system parameters or problems. The direction of flow (positive or negative Doppler shift) is best determined with a smaller Doppler angle (about 30°). Normal flow is typically characterized by a specific spectral Doppler display waveform, which is a consequence of the hemodynamic features of vessels. Disturbed and turbulent flow produce Doppler spectra that are correlated with disease processes. In these latter situations, the spectral curve could be filled in with a wide distribution of frequencies representing a wide range of velocities, as might occur with a vascular stenosis.

Vascular pulsatile velocity changes that are concurrent with the circulation and heart cycle can be tracked by spectral Doppler waveform analysis. The peak value represents the peak systolic frequency shift "S" and the minimum value represents the end diastolic frequency shift "D." The time averaged value of the maximum frequency shift envelope over one cardiac cycle is "A" (Fig. 14-49A). Pertinent quantitative measures are resistive index: $RI = (S - D)/S$, pulsatility index: $PI = (S - D)/A$, and S/D

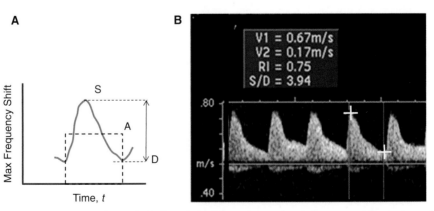

■ **FIGURE 14-49 A.** Spectral Doppler indices derived from the maximum frequency shift envelope of one cardiac cycle. *S:* the peak systolic frequency shift; *D:* the peak diastolic frequency shift; *A:* temporal average frequency shift over one cycle. **B.** Spectral Doppler waveform is evaluated with cursors to extract values: $S = 0.67$ m/s, $D = 0.17$ m/s. From these values, a resistive index RI = 0.75 and *S/D* ratio = 3.75 are determined. See text for details.

ratio. These indices are determined from a spectral waveform analysis (Fig. 14-49B). and are used to assess the hemodynamic information of the vascular system (Maulik, 2005).

Spectral Doppler Waveform Velocity Aliasing

Aliasing, as described earlier, is an error caused by an insufficient sampling rate (PRF) relative to the high-frequency Doppler signals generated by high velocity blood. Doppler frequencies just above the Nyquist frequency experience a 180° phase shift and reflect into the spectrum as maximum negative velocities. Even higher Doppler frequencies are mapped to lower negative velocities as shown in Figure 14-50A. Upon inspection of the spectral Doppler waveform, a significant fraction of the blood flow for this measurement is towards the transducer, so a straightforward method to reduce or eliminate the aliasing error is to allocate a larger frequency sampling range for reflectors moving toward the transducer by readjusting the baseline (Fig. 14-50B).

Other methods that can eliminate aliasing include increasing the PRF_D, which has the effect of increasing the velocity scale values, but the details of the waveform are suppressed. (See the example in the artifacts section, Fig. 14-62). Increasing the Doppler angle will allow higher velocities to be measured without aliasing, but errors in the Doppler angle measurement can lead to large errors in the actual velocity determination.

14.8.7 Color Flow Imaging

Color flow imaging provides a 2D real-time visual display of moving blood in the vasculature, superimposed upon the conventional gray-scale image as shown in Figure 14-51. Point by point evaluation of Doppler shifts over the full image area is not possible, simply due to a lack of processing time and parallel channels that would be required. Instead, a subregion of the image is indicated by the sonographer for evaluation of flow, and within the region, coarse evaluation samples are spread throughout to determine velocity and direction. Analysis of each sample is performed, not by Fourier analysis of the full Doppler spectrum, but by phase-shift autocorrelation or time domain correlation techniques. Velocities and directions are determined for all samples within the image subarea and then color encoded (*e.g.*, shades of red for blood moving toward the transducer, and shades of blue for blood moving away from the transducer).

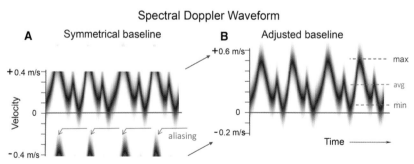

Spectral Doppler Waveform

■ **FIGURE 14-50 A.** Aliasing is present in the spectral Doppler waveform due to insufficient sampling, where the highest velocity signals are mapped to reverse flow. **B.** Adjustment of the spectral Doppler waveform baseline from −0.4 m/s/+0.4 m/s to −0.2 m/s/+0.6 m/s allocates more sampling in the faster flow direction to eliminate aliasing. The maximum, average, and minimum values of the waveform are important indices for assessing hemodynamic conditions.

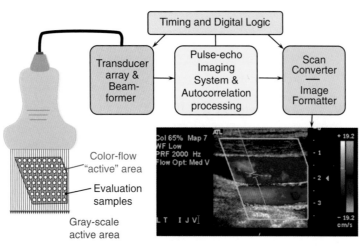

■ **FIGURE 14-51** Color flow acquisition produces dynamic gray-scale B-mode images with color-encoded velocity map data in a user-defined active area of multiple evaluation samples. Each sample is analyzed by an autocorrelation processor to identify motion and estimate its velocity and direction. The scan converter and image formatter create a color map by interpolation of adjacent samples. Color assignments depict the direction of blood flow where red represents flow toward the transducer and blue away from the transducer. A color scale (positioned on the right edge of the image) indicates the velocity range. Also note the Doppler gate (in the blue region), which allows the acquisition of a spectral Doppler waveform.

Phase-shift autocorrelation is a technique to measure the similarity of one scan line measurement to another when the maximum correlation (overlap) occurs. The autocorrelation processor compares the entire echo pulse of one A-line with that of a previous echo pulse separated by a time equal to the PRP. This "self-scanning" algorithm detects changes in phase between two A-lines of data due to any motion over the time Δt. The output correlation varies proportionately with the phase change, which in turn varies proportionately with the velocity at the point along the echo pulse trace. In addition, the direction of the moving object (toward or away from the transducer) is preserved through phase detection of the echo amplitudes. Generally, four to eight traces are used to determine the presence of motion along one A-line of the scanned region. Therefore, the beam must remain stationary for short periods of time before evaluating another region in the imaging volume. Additionally, because a gray-scale B-mode image must be acquired at the same time, the flow information must be interleaved with the image information. The motion data are mapped with a color scale and superimposed on the gray-scale image. FOV determines the processing time necessary to evaluate the color flow data. A smaller FOV delivers a faster frame rate but, of course, sacrifices the area evaluated for flow.

Time domain correlation is another method for color flow image processing, based upon the measurement that a reflector has moved over a time Δt between consecutive pulse-echo acquisitions (Fig. 14-52). Correlation mathematically determines the degree of similarity between two quantities. From echo train one, a series of templates are formed, which are mathematically manipulated over echo train two to determine the time shifts that result in the best correlation. Stationary reflectors need no time shift for high correlation; moving reflectors require a time Δt (either positive or negative) to produce the maximal correlation. The displacement of the reflector (Δx) is determined by the range equation as $\Delta x = (c\Delta t)/2$, where c is the speed of sound. Measured velocity (v_m) is the displacement divided by the time between pulses (PRP): $v_m = \Delta x/\text{PRP}$. Finally, correction for the angle (θ_D) between the beam axis and the direction of motion (like the standard Doppler correction) is $v = v_m/\cos(\theta_D)$.

■ **FIGURE 14-52** Time domain correlation uses a short SPL and an echo "template" to determine positional change of moving reflectors from subsequent echoes. The template scans the echo train to find maximum correlation in each A-line; the displacement between the maximum correlations of each A-line divided by the PRP is the measured velocity.

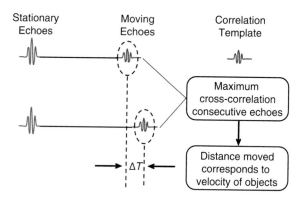

Stationary Echoes   Moving Echoes   Correlation Template

Maximum cross-correlation consecutive echoes

ΔT

Distance moved corresponds to velocity of objects

The sign of the displacement determines red (towards) or blue (away) color, velocity determines brightness of color, and the images appear similar to Doppler-processed images. Multiple pulse-echo sequences are typically acquired to provide a good estimate of reflector displacements, and frame rates are reduced corresponding to the number of repeated measurements per line. With time domain correlation methods, short transmit pulses can be used, unlike the longer transmit pulses required for Doppler acquisitions where longer pulses are necessary to achieve narrow bandwidth pulses. Axial resolution is thus improved. Aliasing effects are reduced compared to Doppler methods because greater time shifts can be tolerated in the returning echo signals from one pulse to the next, which means that higher velocities can be measured.

There are several limitations with color flow imaging. Noise and clutter of slowly moving, solid structures can overwhelm smaller echoes returning from moving blood cells in the color flow image. The spatial resolution of the color display is much poorer than the gray-scale image, and variations in velocity are not well resolved in a large vessel. Since the color flow map does not fully describe the Doppler frequency spectrum, many color 2D units also provide a duplex scanning capability to provide a spectral analysis of specific questionable areas indicated by the color flow examination. Aliasing artifacts due to insufficient sampling of the phase shifts are also a problem that affects the color flow image, causing apparent reversed flow in areas of high velocity (*e.g.*, stenosis).

14.8.8 Power Doppler

Doppler analysis places a constraint on the sensitivity to motion, because the signals generated by motion must be extracted to determine *velocity and direction* from the Doppler and phase shifts in the returning echoes within each gated region. In color flow imaging, the frequency shift encodes the pixel value and assigns a color, which is further divided into positive and negative directions. *Power Doppler* is a signal processing method that relies on the total strength of the Doppler signal (amplitude) and ignores directional (phase or displacement direction) information. The power mode of signal acquisition is dependent on the amplitude of all Doppler signals, regardless of their frequency shift. This dramatically improves the sensitivity to motion (*e.g.*, slow blood flow) at the expense of directional and quantitative flow information.

Compared to conventional color flow imaging, power Doppler produces images that have more sensitivity to motion and are not affected as much by the Doppler angle (largely non-directional). Aliasing is not a problem as only the power of the frequency shifted signals are analyzed, and not the phase. Greater sensitivity allows detection and interpretation of very subtle and slow blood flow. On the other hand,

Color Flow   Power

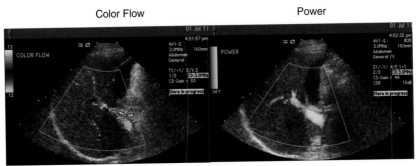

■ **FIGURE 14-53** A comparison of color Doppler (left) and power Doppler (right) studies shows the enhanced sensitivity of the power Doppler acquisition, particularly in areas perpendicular to the beam direction, where the signal is lost in the color Doppler image. Flow directionality, however, is not available in the power Doppler image.

frame rates tend to be slower for the power Doppler imaging mode, and a significant amount of "flash artifacts" occur, which are related to color signals arising from moving tissues, patient motion, or transducer motion. The name "power Doppler" is sometimes mistakenly understood as implying the use of increased transmit power to the patient, but, in fact, the power levels are typically the same as in a standard color flow procedure. The difference is in the processing of the returning signals, where sensitivity is achieved at the expense of direction and quantitation. Images acquired with color flow and power Doppler are illustrated in Figure 14-53.

14.9   ULTRASOUND ARTIFACTS

Ultrasound artifacts represent false portrayal of image anatomy or image degradations related to assumptions regarding the propagation and interaction of ultrasound with tissues, as well as malfunctioning or maladjusted equipment. Understanding how artifacts are generated and how they can be recognized is crucial, which places high demands on the knowledge of the sonographer and the interpreting physician. Most artifacts arise from violations of assumptions in the creation of the ultrasound image, including but not limited to the following:

1. *Ultrasound travels at a constant speed in all tissues (1,540 m/s).* The reality is that sound travels at different speeds in different media based upon compressibility and density characteristics. The ultrasound system uses the average speed in soft tissue of 1,540 m/s to map echo amplitude depths as a function of time in the image matrix. Most notably, fat with a speed of 1,450 m/s (about a 6% difference) causes echoes along the trajectory including fat structures to be displaced further in depth from the actual location.

2. *Ultrasound travels in a straight path.* Even minor differences in ultrasound speed between tissues alter the transmitted beam direction from a straight-line trajectory when the incident ultrasound beam is non-perpendicular to the boundary, causing a change in wavelength (ultrasound frequency remains constant in stationary tissues). The transmitted beam is redirected at an angle of transmission different from the angle of incidence (known as refraction), potentially causing mis-mapped anatomical locations.

3. *Ultrasound echoes are produced from one interaction at perpendicular incidence for each boundary.* Multiple reflections of ultrasound occur from all directions within the complex environment of the human body, complicating the mapping of anatomical boundaries in the ultrasound image.

4. *Attenuation of transmitted ultrasound and reflected echoes is uniform.* Ultrasound attenuation in typical tissues and structures varies from high to low, with resultant artifactual shadowing or enhancement of tissues at greater depths in the image.

5. *The ultrasound main beam contains all of the energy emitted by the transducer array.* Transducer crystal expansion and contraction in the thickness mode produces the main ultrasound beam, but at the same time height and width contraction and expansion also occurs. This results in ultrasound energy emitted outside of the main beam producing echoes that can appear in the beam, creating false information in the image.

6. *The operator has properly adjusted ultrasound acquisition settings, including transmit and receive gain.* Improper use of user-adjusted overall receive gain or TGC results in images that may not be representative of the acoustic properties at a given depth in the image. PRF settings must ensure adequate time for listening for echoes before the next pulse. Additionally, proper transducer frequencies must be selected to achieve the desired depth of penetration in the image.

7. *All imaging system components are operating optimally.* The ultrasound system is dependent on all components of the imaging chain to be functioning normally, from the transducer array, gain and filter settings, and image display. When there are component failures or miscalibrations, the ultrasound images may not be accurately portrayed.

Fortunately, most ultrasound artifacts can be identified by the experienced sonographer because of obvious effects on the image or transient nature of mis-mapped anatomy that appears and disappears during the scan. Some artifacts can be used to advantage as a diagnostic aid in characterization of tissue structures and composition. The following descriptions represent some typical artifacts encountered in diagnostic ultrasound.

14.9.1 Refraction

Refraction represents a change in the transmitted ultrasound pulse direction at a boundary with non-perpendicular incidence, when the two adjacent tissues support a different speed of sound. Misplaced anatomy can occur in the image from the beam redirection as the echoes propagate back to the transducer over a similar return path (Fig. 14-54A). The sonographer must be aware of objects appearing and disappearing with slight differences in orientation of the transducer array. At the edges of smooth-rounded organs, refraction of the beam at non-normal incidence can redirect the beam away from the edge, creating a shadow of reduced intensity beyond the edge, resulting in an edge artifact (Fig. 14-54B). In many situations, the cause of the refraction artifact can be traced back to anatomical structures.

14.9.2 Shadowing and Enhancement

Acoustic shadowing is the result of several physical mechanisms. Objects with high attenuation, such as kidney stones and gallstones, can assist in diagnosis by producing shadowing or streaks (Fig. 14-55), but also can be a hindrance if a large size attenuator such as a rib produces shadows that precludes optimal imaging of distal anatomy. Shadowing is also the result of reflection and refraction, as shown in Figure 14-54 of edge shadowing artifact. Acoustic enhancement occurs distal to low-attenuation fluid-filled structures such as cysts and bladder where increased transmission of sound occurs, resulting in distal hyperintense signals. "Through transmission" is commonly described for this occurrence.

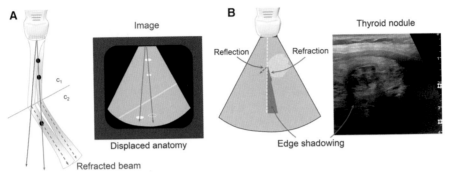

■ **FIGURE 14-54 A.** Refraction artifacts arise from a change of direction of the ultrasound beam at a tissue boundary with non-perpendicular incidence caused by a speed of sound difference and a change in wavelength. The illustration on the left demonstrates how anatomy can be displaced as the ultrasound beam sweeps over the field of view, where the actual co-linear structures are incorrectly mapped. **B.** Edge shadowing occurs at the edges of rounded tissue structures caused by reflection away from the beam at the boundary edge and refraction of the beam within the structure. These interactions result in an edge shadow, an example of which is shown for a thyroid nodule on the right image. (Reprinted from Seibert JA, Fananapazir G. Ultrasound artifacts, chapter 2. In: McGahan JP, Schick MA, Mills LD, eds. *Fundamentals of Emergency Ultrasound.* 27-40. Copyright 2020, with permission from Elsevier.)

14.9.3 Reverberation, Comet Tail, and Ring-Down

Reverberation artifacts arise from multiple echoes generated between highly reflective and parallel structures that interact at a perpendicular angle to the ultrasound beam. These artifacts are often caused by reflections between a reflective interface and the transducer or between reflective interfaces such as metallic objects (*e.g.*, bullet fragments), calcified tissues, or air pocket/partial liquid areas of the anatomy, and are

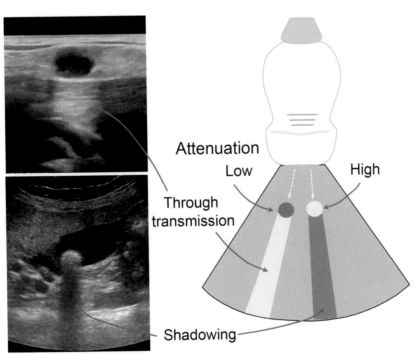

■ **FIGURE 14-55** Image enhancement and shadowing are created by anatomy with low attenuation, such as fluid-filled cysts, and high attenuation, such as calcifications. Anatomical examples illustrate through transmission (enhancement) distal to a cyst and shadowing distal to a gallstone. (Reprinted from Seibert JA, Fananapazir G. Ultrasound artifacts, chapter 2. In: McGahan JP, Schick MA, Mills LD, eds. *Fundamentals of Emergency Ultrasound.* 27-40. Copyright 2020, with permission from Elsevier.)

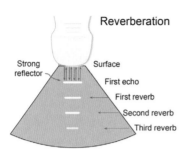

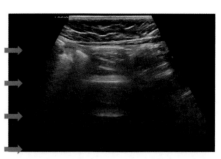

Reverberation

Strong reflector
Surface
First echo
First reverb
Second reverb
Third reverb

■ **FIGURE 14-56** Left: Reverberation artifacts arise from a highly reflective boundary close to the transducer surface. The echo returns to the transducer (itself a highly reflective surface) and back to the boundary several times, creating many equally spaced structures that diminish in intensity with depth. Right: Ultrasound image of a pediatric abdomen and reverberation of the transducer and the first very strong reflector, with distal repetitions of the boundary.

typically manifested as multiple, equally spaced parallel lines at progressive depth with decreasing amplitude (Fig. 14-56). Comet tail artifact is a form of reverberation between two closely spaced reflectors and appears as bright lines along the direction of ultrasound propagation. It is manifested as a tapering shape and decreasing width with depth of travel (Fig. 14-57A). Reverberation artifacts are useful in assessing the characteristic structures of tissues but can also hinder visualization of deeper anatomy. Effects of reverberation can be reduced by adjusting the transducer angle of incidence or by decreasing the distance between the reflective structure and the transducer. Harmonic imaging reduces these artifacts by receiving the first harmonic frequency and filtering out the fundamental frequency.

Ring-down artifacts arise from resonant vibrations within fluid trapped between a tetrahedron of air bubbles, which creates a continuous sound wave that is transmitted back to the transducer and displayed as a series of parallel bands extending posterior to a collection of gas (Fig. 14-57B).

14.9.4 Speed Displacement

The speed displacement artifact results from the substantial variability of sound speed in fat (1,450 m/s) relative to soft tissues (1,540 m/s)—about a 6% slower propagation speed. Anatomical borders are displaced distally when ultrasound interacts with structures containing fat compared to the non-displaced borders through the soft tissues (Fig. 14-58A). In the situation of a soft tissue structure surrounded by a fatty liver, the border is proximally displaced behind the soft tissue structure (Fig. 14-58B).

A Comet tail **B Ringdown**

■ **FIGURE 14-57 A.** Comet tail artifacts are generated from closely spaced, highly reflective interfaces such as may be seen in calcified objects, creating a repeated and closely spaced emission of reflected echoes distal to the object. **B.** Ring-down artifacts are generated by resonant vibrations in air bubbles contained in abscesses, emphysematous infections, and other processes that contain air pockets. (Reprinted from Seibert JA, Fananapazir G. Ultrasound artifacts, chapter 2. In: McGahan JP, Schick MA, Mills LD, eds. *Fundamentals of Emergency Ultrasound.* 27-40. Copyright 2020, with permission from Elsevier.)

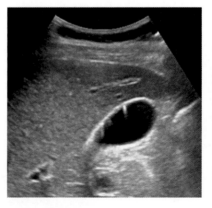

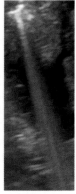

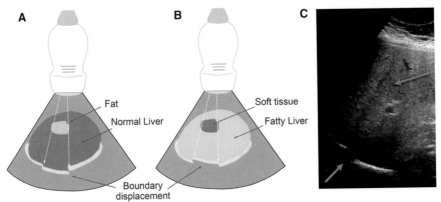

■ **FIGURE 14-58** Boundary displacement is caused by the speed of sound differences in soft tissues (1,540 m/s) to fat (1,450 m/s). Artifactual separation of boundaries and errors in distance measurements along the direction of ultrasound beam travel are the result. **A.** A fat mass in a normal liver, demonstrating distal boundary displacement. **B.** Fatty replaced liver with a soft tissue structure, causing a proximal displacement of the boundary. **C.** Ultrasound of the liver with irregular fatty deposits (upper red arrow) and resultant distal displacement of the diaphragm due to the slower speed of sound in fat (lower red arrow). (Reprinted from Seibert JA, Fananapazir G. Ultrasound artifacts, chapter 2. In: McGahan JP, Schick MA, Mills LD, eds. *Fundamentals of Emergency Ultrasound*. 27-40. Copyright 2020, with permission from Elsevier.)

An image of a liver with a fatty region demonstrates a displacement and disruption of the distal border (Fig. 14-58C). The differences in speed also impact the accuracy of distance measurements along the direction of ultrasound travel when fat is present in the beam.

14.9.5   Mirror Image and Multipath Reflection

Mirror image artifacts occur when the ultrasound beam encounters a highly reflective non-perpendicular or curved boundary such as the diaphragm. The redirected beam encounters a specular reflector, producing a series of echoes that are reflected along the same path back to the transducer. As the field of view is scanned, the beam interacts with the same specular reflector to record its true position. Later echoes of the specular reflector from the redirected beam arrive and are mapped as distal objects on the opposite side of the strong reflector, appearing as a mirror image because of the double reflection. A common mirror image artifact occurs at the interface of the liver and the diaphragm in abdominal imaging. In one direction, the ultrasound beam correctly positions the echoes emanating from a lesion in the liver. As the ultrasound beam moves through the liver, echoes are strongly reflected from the curved diaphragm away from the main beam to interact with the lesion, generating echoes that travel back to the diaphragm and ultimately back to the transducer. The back and forth travel distance of these echoes creates artifactual anatomy that resembles a mirror image of the mass, placed beyond the diaphragm that would otherwise not have anatomy present in the image (Fig. 14-59). Other strong reflectors that generate mirror image artifacts include pericardium and bowel, which might be more difficult to detect due to the presence of other anatomical structures in the same area.

14.9.6   Side Lobes and Grating Lobes

Ultrasound energy produced outside of the main longitudinal wave arises from the height and width expansion and contraction of the piezoelectric element that occurs when the crystal thickness mode undergoes contraction and expansion. The

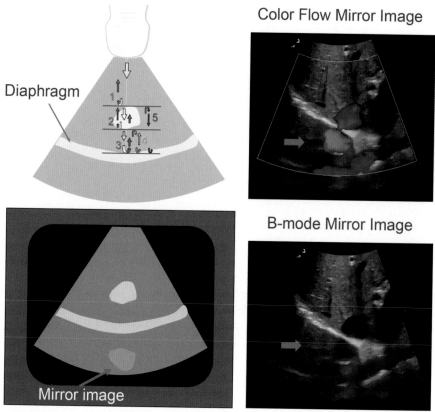

■ **FIGURE 14-59** Mirror image artifact. Top left: White arrows depict the ultrasound pulse traveling along the dashed path creating echoes when interacting at tissue boundaries (1st and 2nd echoes) generating the acoustic image of the anatomy in the normal mode. At the diaphragm, a large fraction of ultrasound is reflected indicated as a red arrow (3rd echo). The returning energy generates echoes from the distal (4th echo) and proximal (5th echo) boundaries of the anatomy. These echoes return to the diaphragm, are reflected, and arrive at the transducer later in time with proximal and distal boundaries reversed. The events are repeated along each ultrasound A-line during the scan. Bottom left: A mirror image of the anatomy is generated distal to the diaphragm where no ultrasound signals should be detected. Top right: Mirror image artifact of color flow image shows reversal of blood flow direction (blue to red) on opposite sides of the diaphragm. Bottom right: B-mode grayscale image of the mirror image artifact.

resultant ultrasound energy is slightly off-axis from the main beam and creates side lobe emissions (see Fig. 14-18). Tissues along the trajectory of the side lobes can create echoes that are positioned in the image as if they occurred along the main beam, generating artifactual signals. This is quite noticeable when side lobes redirect diffuse echoes from adjacent soft tissues into an organ that is normally hypo- or anechoic. For instance, in imaging of the gallbladder, the side lobes can produce artifactual "pseudo-sludge" in an otherwise echo-free organ (Fig. 14-60). Side lobe artifacts are reduced with lower transmit gain (at the loss of penetration depth), with a process called apodization (excitations from the center of the transducer array are modified to reduce the amplitude of the side lobes), or with the use of harmonic imaging (higher order frequency harmonics are generated in the center of the main ultrasound beam). Most often, if artifacts from side lobes are suspected, the sonographer should scan the anatomy from a different direction to determine if the signals persist.

Grating lobes are caused by the division of the multielement transducer surface into small discrete emitters, each creating a diverging radial wave pattern. The individual waves interact with constructive and destructive interference (in-phase and

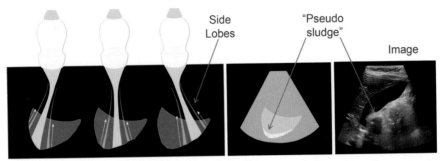

■ **FIGURE 14-60** Common side lobe artifacts are manifested when imaging curved hypo-echoic structures such as the gallbladder, where the side lobe energy echoes adjacent to the beam are integrated within the beam. The example in the illustration demonstrates artifactual "pseudo-sludge" in the gallbladder that can be ameliorated by scanning at a different angle.

out-of-phase frequencies) to produce the forward directed main beam; however, a small fraction of the emitted energy escapes at large angles relative to the main beam direction, resulting in the presence of grating lobe energy (Fig. 14-18). While weak in intensity, grating lobes generate signals in the main beam from off-axis highly reflective objects that can be recognized in hypo-echoic structures. Design of transducer arrays with elements less than one-half wavelength spacing can somewhat mitigate grating lobe energy emission. These artifacts are more likely present when using phased array transducers, as the leakage occurs most at the edges of the array.

14.9.7 Ambiguity

Range ambiguity artifacts are caused by a high PRF acquisition that decreases the time allocated to listening for echoes during the PRP. Returning echoes arriving from depth at a time longer than the PRP will be detected after the next pulse excitation and mis-mapped to shallow positions in the image. These artifacts are most easily identified in regions of low attenuation and echogenicity, such as a fluid-filled cyst in the proximal field of the transducer. Ambiguity artifacts can be eliminated by decreasing the PRF, but lower acquisition frame rate and/or reduced image quality will occur as a trade-off. When possible, selecting a higher operational transducer frequency will reduce penetration depth so that echoes from depth are insignificant in amplitude.

14.9.8 Twinkling Artifact

Two-dimensional color-flow imaging detects blood flow in a selected sub-region in the image and displays moving blood as red or blue (or selectable color) on the monitor, depending on direction and velocity. In the presence of a small, strong reflector such as a calculus, a rapidly changing mixture of colors often appears, and can be mistaken for an aneurysm. This artifactual appearance is caused by echoes undergoing frequency changes of narrow band "ringing" from the small reflectors. Twinkling artifact may be used to identify small renal stones (Fig. 14-61) and differentiate echogenic foci from calcifications within kidney, gallbladder, and liver. Turning off color-flow acquisition allows the differentiation of calcific from other anatomic structures.

14.9.9 Doppler Spectrum and Color Flow Artifacts

Artifacts caused by insufficient sampling of the Doppler shift frequencies (refer to Section 14.7 for details on the Nyquist sampling requirements) cause signal aliasing.

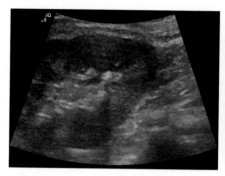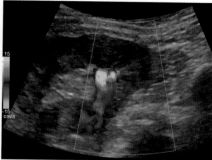

■ **FIGURE 14-61** Left: B-mode longitudinal image of the left kidney with a high-attenuation object and distal shadowing. Right: Color flow image with an obvious multi-color "twinkle" related to the object, due to ultrasound beam interactions with the calcified structure and associated narrow-band ringing. (Reprinted from Seibert JA, Fananapazir G. Ultrasound artifacts, chapter 2. In: McGahan JP, Schick MA, Mills LD, eds. *Fundamentals of Emergency Ultrasound.* 27-40. Copyright 2020, with permission from Elsevier.)

In measurements containing frequencies beyond the minimum sampling rate of two times the maximum frequency results in wrap-around to lower frequencies. In the Doppler spectrum (Fig. 14-62), the highest frequency Doppler signals are cut off and appear as negative velocity (moving away from the transducer). By increasing the PRF (sampling rate) from 1.6 to 2.6 kHz, the velocity range is extended, and the full Doppler spectrum is properly measured. Color flow images are similarly affected, as shown in Figure 14-63 where high velocity blood in the center of the vessel (red arrow) is color encoded as blood with high velocity in the opposite direction. In some situations, aliasing may be a useful indicator of high velocity flow caused by the presence of a stenosis. A straightforward adjustment to reduce or eliminate the aliasing error is to increase the PRF to enable a wider velocity scale range for the Doppler spectrum. If the maximum PRF is reached, then the spectral baseline can be readjusted to allocate a greater frequency sampling in the direction with the highest frequency shift. The sonographer can adjust the transducer for a larger Doppler angle, which lowers the measured Doppler shift and enables use of a lower PRF to meet the Nyquist criterion. Subsequent correction by $1/\cos(\theta_D)$ determines the actual blood velocity. At angles larger than 60°, however, small errors in angle measurement can cause large errors in estimates of blood velocity.

Pseudoflow artifacts are generated by color flow imaging in a fluid medium other than flowing blood, caused by the motion of particles in the fluid. The frequency

A 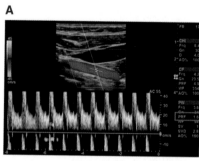   **B**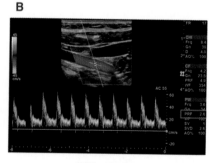

PRF = 1.6 kHz   **PRF = 2.6 kHz**

■ **FIGURE 14-62 A.** Aliasing in the Doppler spectral display is demonstrated by wrap-around of the high velocity signals (lower traces in the image). The Doppler pulse repetition frequency of 1.6 kHz was insufficient to provide an adequate sampling. **B.** A Doppler pulse repetition frequency of 2.6 kHz extends the velocity range to measure the peak velocity accurately without aliasing. (Adapted from Seibert JA, Fananapazir G. Ultrasound artifacts, chapter 2. In: McGahan JP, Schick MA, Mills LD, eds. *Fundamentals of Emergency Ultrasound.* 27-40. Copyright 2020, with permission from Elsevier.)

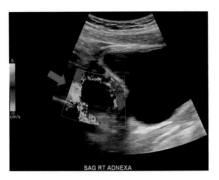

SAG RT ADNEXA

■ **FIGURE 14-63** Color flow image shows artifactual reverse blood flow in the center of a blood vessel of high velocity (turquoise—see velocity color scale on the left) resulting from insufficient sampling by correlation methods and signal wrap-around from yellow to turquoise to blue. (Adapted from Seibert JA, Fananapazir G. Ultrasound artifacts, chapter 2. In: McGahan JP, Schick MA, Mills LD, eds. *Fundamentals of Emergency Ultrasound*. 27-40. Copyright 2020, with permission from Elsevier.)

change will be detected and transformed into a velocity, with color assigned to the flow, which can occur with ascites, urinary bladder imaging with ureteral jets, and moving sludge in the gallbladder, among other causes. This finding will also be manifested in power Doppler imaging. One way to distinguish the pseudoflow artifact is with the use of spectral Doppler and analysis of generated waveforms to differentiate pseudoflow from the periodic flow exhibited by vascular hemodynamics.

Blooming artifact occurs in color flow imaging with the color gain setting set too high, causing the rendered color to bleed over the vessel wall (such as might happen with a non-occlusive thrombus) and demonstrate a fully patent vessel when in fact the thrombus does exist. In this situation, the operator can lower the color gain or use power Doppler, which doesn't amplify the received signal.

Edge artifact is generated at the surface of a strong echogenic reflector such as a calculus (see twinkling artifact above), bone, diaphragm, or other static structures. On the color flow display, the edge artifact appears as a continuous rim of color along the edge of the structure. This artifact can be recognized by the absence of a vessel on the grayscale image, or with spectral Doppler analysis illustrating an absence of a waveform. This artifact can be eliminated with a higher wall filter setting or with an increase in the PRF of the color flow acquisition.

Power Doppler is a way to improve motion sensitivity to slow blood flow by eliminating directionality and quantitation capabilities of color Doppler. Aliasing is not a problem as only the strength of the frequency shifted signals are analyzed, and not the phase, but the greater sensitivity leads to significant *flash artifacts* related to moving tissues, patient motion, or transducer motion.

14.9.10 Beam Width and Slice Thickness

Beam width artifact results from the variable width of the in-plane ultrasound beam as a function of depth, resulting in poor lateral resolution proximal and even poorer lateral resolution distal to the focal zone. The artifact refers to the lateral blurring of objects as a function of beam width. Objects at proximal and deeper depths beyond the focal zone appear to be horizontally stretched (Fig. 14-64). In addition, if two adjacent small objects are separated by less than the beam width, they will not be resolved. A solution to the beam width artifact is to implement a lateral focal zone at the depth of interest; multiple depths can be selected, but at the cost of temporal resolution. Use of higher frequency transducer operation results in a narrower beam width, which can improve lateral resolution, as can the use of harmonic imaging with the generation of harmonic frequencies in the center of the beam, as discussed in Section 14.6.

The slice thickness profile, perpendicular to the displayed ultrasound image, varies with depth similar to the in-plane lateral beam width. Proximal to the transducer array, the slice thickness is broad, becomes narrower at the mid-depth zone, and widens with greater depth. Consequences are loss of signal from objects smaller than

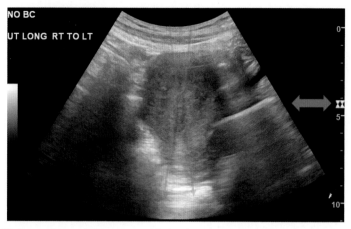

■ **FIGURE 14-64** Beam width variations occur with depth in the ultrasound image, causing horizontal lateral spread of anatomy and loss of lateral resolution proximal and distal (red arrows) to the focal zone depth (red arrow). (Reprinted from Seibert JA, Fananapazir G. Ultrasound artifacts, chapter 2. In: McGahan JP, Schick MA, Mills LD, eds. *Fundamentals of Emergency Ultrasound*. 27-40. Copyright 2020, with permission from Elsevier.)

the slice thickness due to partial volume averaging, and inclusion of signals from highly reflective objects adjacent to the imaging plane. Usually there is no specific solution to slice-thickness artifacts, although 1.5D and 2D array transducers can aid in creating a narrower slice thickness over selected depths.

14.9.11 Equipment Settings and Equipment Failures

Artifacts can be caused by inappropriate equipment settings and protocols. Variations in image echogenicity and uniformity are affected by TGC settings inappropriately adjusted by the user as shown in Figure 14-65. Inappropriate wall filter settings can significantly affect the Doppler spectrum by overcompensating the low frequency cut-off, which can have significant repercussions on the determination of quantitative values such as resistive index (Fig. 14-66).

Loss of transducer element function in a multielement array can be difficult to detect, as adjacent transducers and image processing can compensate for malfunctions. Specialized electronic equipment is often needed to evaluate and detect functionality of individual transducer elements. When two or more adjacent elements are malfunctioning, a uniformity phantom can assist in indicating the location and

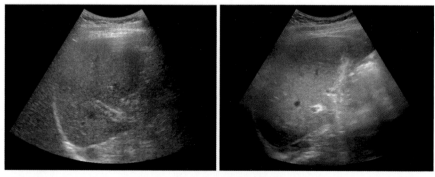

■ **FIGURE 14-65** Time Gain Compensation can be improperly adjusted, resulting in under- or overemphasis of anatomical features in terms of grayscale and echogenicity, potentially leading to misdiagnosis or other untoward outcomes. Left: Liver image with proper TGC. Right: Liver image with too much gain in the mid depths and insufficient gain in the proximal and distal areas of the image. (Reprinted from Seibert JA, Fananapazir G. Ultrasound artifacts, chapter 2. In: McGahan JP, Schick MA, Mills LD, eds. *Fundamentals of Emergency Ultrasound*. 27-40. Copyright 2020, with permission from Elsevier.)

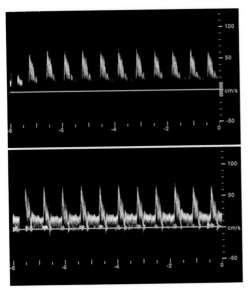

■ **FIGURE 14-66** Improper wall filter settings can result in loss of information in the spectral Doppler waveform when the wall filter settings to eliminate low frequency motion are set too high (top) compared to a proper wall filter setting (bottom). (Adapted from Seibert JA, Fananapazir G. Ultrasound artifacts, chapter 2. In: McGahan JP, Schick MA, Mills LD, eds. *Fundamentals of Emergency Ultrasound*. 27–40. Copyright 2020, with permission from Elsevier.)

effects on the image, as vertical dark streaks (Fig. 14-67). Horizontal banding in the ultrasound image is attributed to miscalibration of the beamformer logic to set a focal zone at a given depth, or with the use of multiple focal zones and improper combination of the individual focal zone acquisitions from timing errors when creating the composite image. The banding artifact occurs at depths coincident with the location of the focal zones (Fig. 14-68). Service calibration adjustment is necessary to correct this artifact.

14.9.12 Summary, Artifacts

Artifacts, resulting from violations of the underlying assumptions used for acquiring and creating an ultrasound image or from improper equipment settings or malfunctioning equipment, are common and widespread, so understanding the physical principles and underlying causes are important in recognizing and diminishing those that interfere with image interpretation. At the same time, some artifacts can reveal important information regarding tissue structure and composition that can assist in diagnosis. Periodic quality control is an important and useful activity to identify component failure effects on the ultrasound images and to direct repair and replacement by service engineers to maintain optimal image quality.

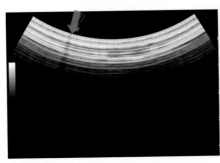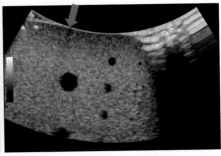

■ **FIGURE 14-67** Transducer element dropout. Left: In-air operation of curvilinear transducer array shows several elements malfunctioning. Right: Same transducer array showing effect on an ultrasound quality control phantom. The effect on the image is less noticeable, particularly with compound scanning activated. (Reprinted from Seibert JA, Fananapazir G. Ultrasound artifacts, chapter 2. In: McGahan JP, Schick MA, Mills LD, eds. *Fundamentals of Emergency Ultrasound*. 27–40. Copyright 2020, with permission from Elsevier.)

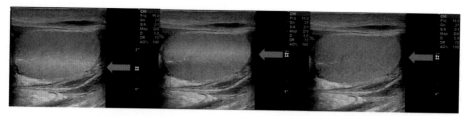

Focal zone banding   After calibration

■ **FIGURE 14-68** Lateral focal zones are user-defined depths within the image to increase lateral resolution. Focal zone (horizontal) banding occurs at the location of a user-placed lateral focal zone shown for two depths (left and middle). After calibration, the image is uniform (right). (Reprinted from Seibert JA, Fananapazir G. Ultrasound artifacts, chapter 2. In: McGahan JP, Schick MA, Mills LD, eds. *Fundamentals of Emergency Ultrasound.* 27-40. Copyright 2020, with permission from Elsevier.)

14.10 ULTRASOUND SYSTEM PERFORMANCE AND QUALITY ASSURANCE

The American College of Radiology (ACR) has a technical standard that specifies medical physics performance monitoring for ultrasound equipment throughout its lifetime (ACR, 2016). Documentation of program goals, policies, and responsible personnel are the important first steps for a quality assurance program. Included are testing procedures and equipment, the frequency of tests, and their passing criteria. Results of the performance measures and actions taken to address problems are key outcomes. Initial acceptance includes evaluation of image uniformity, geometric accuracy, system sensitivity, spatial resolution, contrast resolution, and fidelity of displays. All transducers and transducer ports should be individually tested. Since each ultrasound system may also have other capabilities such as harmonic imaging, elastography, Doppler, and color flow, these must also be evaluated and documented to meet published specifications and tolerances. To ensure the performance, accuracy, and safety of ultrasound equipment, periodic QC measurements and documentation are essential. The periodic QC testing frequency of ultrasound components should be adjusted to the probability of finding instabilities or maladjustment. This can be assessed by initially performing tests frequently, reviewing logbooks over an extended period, and, with documented stability, reducing the testing rate as appropriate.

14.10.1 Ultrasound Quality Control

Equipment QC is essentially performed every day during routine scanning by the sonographer, who should and can recognize major problems with the images and the equipment. Ensuring ultrasound image quality, however, requires implementation of a QC program with periodic measurement of system performance to identify problems before serious malfunctions occur. Required are tissue-mimicking phantoms with acoustic targets of various sizes and echogenic features embedded in a medium of uniform attenuation and speed of sound characteristic of soft tissues. Various multipurpose phantoms are available to evaluate the clinical capabilities of the ultrasound system.

A generic phantom comprised of three modules is illustrated in Figure 14-69A–C. The phantom gel filler has tissue-like attenuation of 0.5 to 0.7 dB/cm-MHz (higher attenuation provides a more challenging test) and low-contrast targets within a matrix of small scatterers to mimic tissue background. Small, high-contrast reflectors are positioned at known depths for measuring the axial and lateral spatial resolution, for assessing the accuracy of horizontal and vertical distance measurements, and for measuring the depth of the dead zone (the non-imaged area immediately adjacent to the transducer). Another module contains low-contrast, small-diameter spheres (or cylinders) of 2 and 4 mm diameter uniformly spaced with depth, to measure elevational resolution (slice-thickness) variation with depth. The third module is composed of a uniformly distributed scattering material for testing image uniformity and penetration depth.

Spatial resolution, contrast resolution, and distance accuracy are evaluated with one module (Fig. 14-69A). Axial resolution is evaluated by the ability to resolve high-contrast targets separated by 2, 1, 0.5, and 0.25 mm at three different depths. In an optimally functioning system, the axial resolution should be consistent with depth and improve with higher operational frequency. Lateral resolution is evaluated by measuring the lateral spread of the high-contrast targets as a function of depth and transmit focus. Contrast resolution is evaluated with "gray-scale" objects of lower and higher attenuation than the tissue-mimicking gel; more sophisticated phantoms have contrast resolution targets of varying contrast and size. Contrast resolution should improve with increased transmit power. Dead zone depth is determined with the first high-contrast target (positioned at several depths from 0 to ~1 cm) visible in the image. Horizontal and vertical distance measurement accuracy uses the small high-contrast targets. Vertical targets (along the axial beam direction) should have higher precision and accuracy than the corresponding horizontal targets (lateral resolution), and all measurements should be within 5% of the known distance.

Elevational resolution and partial volume effects are evaluated with the "sphere" module (Fig. 14-69B). The ultrasound image of the spherical targets illustrates the effects of slice-thickness variation with depth and the dependence of resolvability on object size. With 1.5D and 2D transducer arrays as well as 3D imaging capabilities, multiple transmit focal zones to reduce slice thickness at various depths are becoming important, as is the need to verify elevational resolution performance.

Uniformity and penetration depth are measured with the uniformity module (Fig. 14-69C). With a properly adjusted and operating ultrasound system, a uniform response is expected up to the penetration depth capabilities of the transducer array. Higher operational frequencies will display a lower penetration depth. Evidence of vertical-directed shadowing for linear arrays or angular-directed shadowing for phased arrays is an indication of malfunction of a transducer element or its associated circuitry. Horizontal variations indicate inadequate handling of transitions between focal zones when in the multifocal mode.

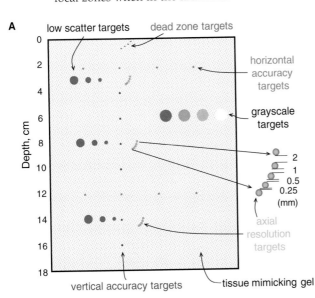

■ **FIGURE 14-69 A.** General-purpose ultrasound quality assurance phantoms are comprised of several scanning modules. System resolution targets (axial and lateral), dead zone depth, vertical and horizontal distance accuracy targets, contrast resolution (grayscale targets), and low scatter targets positioned at several depths (to determine penetration depths) are placed in a tissue mimicking (acoustic scattering) gel.

B

Elevational resolution phantom

Image of phantom

2 mm spheres   4 mm spheres

0.5 cm ↕

0.75 cm ↕

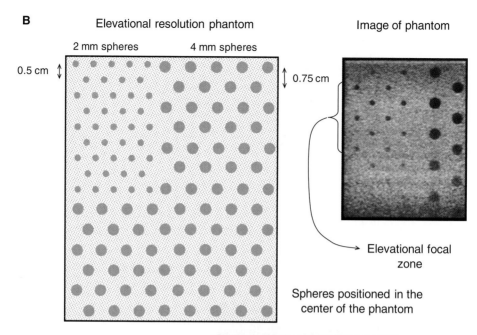

→ Elevational focal zone

Spheres positioned in the center of the phantom

■ **FIGURE 14-69** (*Continued*) **B.** Elevational resolution is determined with spheres equally distributed along a plane in tissue mimicking gel. An image of the phantom shows the effects of partial volume averaging and variations in elevational resolution with depth. **C.** The system uniformity module elucidates possible problems with image uniformity. Shown in this figure is a multi-focal zone banding problem indicated by the horizontal bands. A transducer element dropout is indicated by the vertical band at the surface of the phantom, and the maximum penetration depth is identified with a drop-off of image intensity.

C

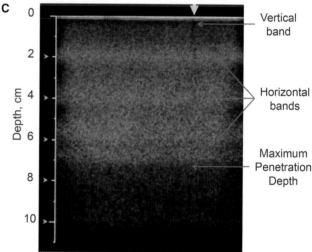

Vertical band

Horizontal bands

Maximum Penetration Depth

During acceptance testing of a new unit, all transducers should be evaluated, and baseline performance should be measured against manufacturer specifications. The maximum depth of visualization is determined by identifying the deepest low contrast scatterers in a uniformity phantom that can be perceived in the image. This depth is dependent on the type of transducer and its operating frequency and should be measured to verify that the transducer and instrument components are operating at their designed sensitivity levels. In a 0.7-dB/cm-MHz attenuation medium, a depth of 18 cm for abdominal and 8 cm for small-parts transducers is the goal for visualization when a single-transmit focal zone is placed as deeply as possible with maximum transmit power level and optimal TGC adjustments. For a multifrequency transducer, the mid frequency setting should be used. With the same settings, the uniformity section of the phantom without targets assesses gray level and image uniformity. Power and gain settings of the machine can have a significant effect on the apparent size of point-like targets (*e.g.*, high receive gain reveals only large-size tar-

TABLE 14-7 RECOMMENDED ROUTINE QC TESTS FOR AN ULTRASOUND PROGRAM

TEST (GRAYSCALE IMAGING MODE) FOR EACH SCANNER	FREQUENCY
System sensitivity and/or depth penetration capability	Semiannually
Image uniformity and artifact survey	Semiannually
Low contrast detectability (optional)	Semiannually
Assurance of electrical and mechanical safety	Semiannually
Geometric accuracy (mechanically scanned transducers in the mechanically scanned direction)	Semiannually
Horizontal and vertical distance accuracy	At acceptance
Transducer ports/transducers (of different scan format)	Ongoing basis
Ultrasound scanner electronic image display performance	Semiannually

gets and has poorer resolution). One method to improve test reproducibility is to set the instrument to the threshold detectability of the targets and to rescan with an increased transmit gain of 20 dB.

Recommended QC procedures are listed in Table 14-7. Routine QC testing must occur regularly and is typically performed by appropriately trained sonographers or equipment service engineers. The same tests must be performed during each testing period, so that changes can be monitored over time and effective corrective action can be taken. Testing results, corrective action, and the effects of corrective action must be documented and maintained on site. Other equipment-related issues involve cleaning air filters, checking for loose or frayed cables, and checking handles, wheels, and wheel locks as part of the QC tests.

The most frequently reported source of performance instability of an ultrasound system is related to the display on maladjusted video monitors. Drift of the ultrasound instrument settings and/or poor viewing conditions (for instance, portable ultrasound performed in a very bright patient room, potentially causing inappropriately gain-adjusted images) can lead to suboptimal images on the softcopy monitor. The contrast and brightness settings for the monitor should be properly established during installation; monitor calibration should be performed according to the DICOM Grayscale Standard Display Function at least semiannually (see Chapter 5) and verified with image test patterns (*e.g.*, the SMPTE pattern).

14.10.2 Doppler Performance Measurements

Doppler techniques are becoming more common in the day-to-day use of medical ultrasound equipment. Reliance on flow measurements to make diagnoses requires demonstration of accurate data acquisition and processing. QC phantoms to assess velocity and flow contain one or more tubes in tissue-mimicking materials at various depths. A blood-mimicking fluid is pushed through the tubes with carefully calibrated pumps to provide a known velocity for assessing the accuracy of the Doppler velocity measurement. Several tests can be performed, including maximum penetration depth at which flow waveforms can be detected, alignment of the sample volume with the duplex B-mode image, accuracy of velocity measurements, and volume flow. For color-flow systems, sensitivity and alignment of the color flow image with the B-scan gray-scale images are assessed.

14.11 ACOUSTIC POWER AND BIOEFFECTS

Power is the rate of energy production, absorption, or flow. The SI unit of power is the watt (W), defined as one joule of energy per second. Acoustic intensity is the rate at which sound energy flows through a unit area and is usually expressed in units of watts per square centimeter (W/cm^2) or milliwatts per square centimeter (mW/cm^2).

Ultrasound acoustic power levels are strongly dependent on the operational characteristics of the system, including the transmit power, PRF, transducer frequency, and operation mode. Biological effects (bioeffects) are predominately related to the heating of tissues caused by high intensity levels of ultrasound used to enhance image quality and functionality. For diagnostic imaging, the intensity levels are kept below the threshold for documented bioeffects.

14.11.1 Intensity Measures of Pulsed Ultrasound

Measurement of ultrasound pressure amplitude within a beam is performed with a hydrophone, a device containing a small (*e.g.*, 0.5-mm-diameter) piezoelectric element coupled to external conductors and mounted in a protective housing. When placed in an ultrasound beam, the hydrophone produces a voltage that is proportional to the variations in pressure amplitude at that point in the beam as a function of time, permitting determination of peak compression and rarefaction amplitude as well as pulse duration and PRP (Fig. 14-70A). Calibrated hydrophones provide absolute measures of pressure, from which the acoustic intensity can be calculated if the acoustic impedance of the medium is accurately known.

In the pulsed mode of ultrasound operation, the instantaneous intensity varies greatly with time and position. At a particular location in tissue, the instantaneous intensity is quite large while the ultrasound pulse passes through the tissue, but the pulse duration is only about a microsecond or less, and for the remainder of the PRP, the intensity is nearly zero.

The temporal peak, I_{TP}, is the highest instantaneous intensity in the beam, the temporal average, I_{TA}, is the time-averaged intensity over the PRP, and the pulse average, I_{PA}, is the average intensity of the pulse (Fig. 14-70B). The spatial peak, I_{SP}, is the highest intensity spatially in the beam, and the spatial average, I_{SA}, is the average intensity over the beam area, usually taken to be the area of the transducer (Fig. 14-70C).

The acoustic power contained in the ultrasound beam (watts), averaged over at least one PRP and divided by the beam area (usually the area of the transducer face), is the spatial average–temporal average intensity I_{SATA}. Other meaningful measures for pulsed ultrasound intensity are determined from I_{SATA}, including

1. The spatial average–pulse average intensity, $I_{SAPA} = I_{SATA}/$duty cycle, where $I_{PA} = I_{TA}/$duty cycle
2. The spatial peak–temporal average intensity, $I_{SPTA} = I_{SATA} \times [I_{SP}/I_{SA}]$, which is a good indicator of thermal ultrasound effects
3. The spatial peak–pulse average intensity, $I_{SPPA} = I_{SATA} \times [I_{SP}/I_{SA}]/$duty cycle, an indicator of potential mechanical bioeffects and cavitation

For acoustic ultrasound intensity levels, $I_{SPPA} > I_{SPTA} > I_{SAPA} > I_{SATA}$. Typical acoustical power outputs are listed in Table 14-8. The two most relevant measures are the I_{SPPA} and the I_{SPTA}. Both measurements are required by the US Food and Drug Administration (FDA) for certification of instrumentation. Values of I_{SPTA} for diagnostic imaging are usually below 100 mW/cm^2 for imaging, but for certain Doppler applications, I_{SPTA} can exceed 1,000 mW/cm^2. I_{SPPA} can be several orders of magnitude greater than I_{SPTA}, as shown in Table 14-8. For real-time scanners, the combined

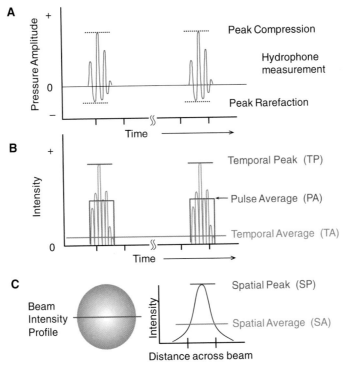

■ **FIGURE 14-70 A.** Pressure amplitude variations are measured with a hydrophone and include peak compression and peak rarefaction variations with time. **B.** Temporal intensity variations of pulsed ultrasound vary widely, from the temporal peak and temporal average values; pulse average intensity represents the average intensity measured over the pulse duration. **C.** Spatial intensity variations of pulsed ultrasound are described by the spatial peak value and the spatial average value, measured over the beam profile.

intensity descriptors must be modified to consider dwell time (the time the ultrasound beam is directed at a particular region) and the acquisition geometry and spatial sampling. These variations help explain the measured differences between the I_{SPTA} and I_{SPPA} values indicated, which are much less than the duty cycle values that are predicted by the equations above.

Thermal and mechanical indices of ultrasound operation are now the accepted method of determining power levels for real-time instruments that provide the operator with quantitative estimates of power deposition in the patient. These indices are selected for their relevance to risks from biological effects and are displayed on the monitor during real-time scanning. The sonographer can use these indices to minimize power deposition to the patient (and fetus) consistent with obtaining useful clinical images in the spirit of the ALARA (As Low As Reasonably Achievable) concept.

TABLE 14-8 TYPICAL INTENSITY MEASURES FOR ULTRASOUND DATA COLLECTION MODES

MODE	PRESSURE AMPLITUDE (MPa)	I_{SPTA} (mW/cm²)	I_{SPPA} (W/cm²)	POWER (mW)
B-scan	1.68	19	174	18
M-mode	1.68	73	174	4
Pulsed Doppler	2.48	1,140	288	31
Color flow	2.59	234	325	81

Adapted with permission from Zagzebski J. *Essentials of Ultrasound Physics.* St. Louis, MO: Mosby-Year Book; 1996. Copyright Elsevier 1996. Note the difference in units for I_{SPTA} (mW/cm²) versus I_{SPPA} (W/cm²).

Thermal Index

The *thermal index*, *TI*, is the ratio of the acoustical power produced by the transducer to the power required to raise tissue in the beam area by 1°C. This is estimated by the ultrasound system using algorithms that consider the ultrasonic frequency, the beam area, and the acoustic output power of the transducer. Assumptions are made for attenuation and thermal properties of the tissues with long, steady exposure times. An indicated *TI* value of 2 signifies a possible 2°C increase in the temperature of the tissues when the transducer is stationary. *TI* values are associated with the I_{SPTA} measure of intensity.

On some scanners, other thermal indices that might be encountered are *TIS* (*S* for soft tissue), *TIB* (*B* for bone), and *TIC* (*C* for cranial bone). These quantities are useful because of the increased heat buildup that can occur at a bone–soft tissue interface when present in the beam, particularly for obstetric scanning of late-term pregnancies, and with the use of Doppler ultrasound (where power levels can be substantially higher).

Mechanical Index

Cavitation is a consequence of the negative pressures (rarefaction of the mechanical wave) that induce bubble formation from the extraction of dissolved gases in the medium. The *mechanical index*, *MI*, is a value that estimates the likelihood of cavitation by the ultrasound beam. The *MI* is directly proportional to the peak rarefactional (negative) pressure and inversely proportional to the square root of the ultrasound frequency (in MHz). An attenuation of 0.3 dB/cm-MHz is assumed for the algorithm that estimates the *MI*. As the ultrasound output power (transmit pulse amplitude) is increased, the *MI* increases linearly, while an increase in the transducer frequency (say from 2 to 8 MHz) decreases the *MI* by the square root of 4 or by a factor of two. *MI* values are associated with the I_{SPPA} measure of intensity.

14.11.2 Biological Mechanisms and Effects

Diagnostic ultrasound has established a remarkable safety record. Significant deleterious bioeffects on either patients or operators of diagnostic ultrasound imaging procedures have not been reported in the literature. Despite the lack of evidence that any harm can be caused by diagnostic intensities of ultrasound, it is prudent and indeed an obligation of the physician to consider issues of benefit versus risk when performing an ultrasound exam and to take all precautions to ensure maximal benefit with minimal risk. The American Institute of Ultrasound in Medicine recommends adherence to the ALARA principles. US FDA requirements for new ultrasound equipment include the display of acoustic output indices (*MI* and *TI*) to give the user feedback regarding the power deposition to the patient.

At high intensities, ultrasound can cause biological effects by thermal and mechanical mechanisms. Biological tissues absorb ultrasound energy, which is converted into heat; thus, heat will be generated at all parts of the ultrasonic field in the tissue. Thermal effects are dependent not only on the rate of heat deposition in a volume of the body but also on how fast the heat is removed by blood flow and other means of heat conduction. The best indicator of heat deposition is the I_{SPTA} measure of intensity and the calculated *TI* value. Heat deposition is determined by the average ultrasound intensity in the focal zone and the absorption coefficient of the tissue. Absorption increases with the frequency of the ultrasound and varies with tissue type. Bone has a much higher attenuation (absorption) coefficient than soft tissue, which can cause significant heat deposition at a tissue-bone interface. In diagnostic ultrasound applications, the heating effect is typically well below a temperature rise (*e.g.*, 1°C to 2°C) that would be considered potentially damaging, although some Doppler instruments can approach these levels with high pulse repetition frequencies and longer pulse duration.

Non-thermal mechanisms include mechanical movement of the particles of the medium due to radiation pressure (that can cause force or torque on tissue structures) and acoustic streaming, which can give rise to a steady circulatory flow. With higher energy deposition over a short period, *cavitation* can occur, broadly defined as sonically generated activity of highly compressible bodies composed of gas and/or vapor. Cavitation can be subtle or readily observable and is typically unpredictable and sometimes violent. *Stable cavitation* generally refers to the pulsation (expansion and contraction) of persistent bubbles in the tissue that occur at low and intermediate ultrasound intensities (as used clinically). Chiefly related to the peak rarefactional pressure, the *MI* is an estimate for producing cavitation. At higher ultrasound intensity levels, *transient cavitation* can occur, whereby the bubbles respond non-linearly to the driving force, causing a collapse approaching the speed of sound. At this point, the bubbles might dissolve, disintegrate, or rebound. In the minimum volume state, conditions exist that can dissociate the water vapor into free radicals such as H• and OH•, which can cause chemical damage to biologically important molecules such as DNA. Short, high amplitude pulses such as those used in imaging are good candidates for transient cavitation; however, the intensities used in diagnostic imaging are far below the transient cavitation threshold (*e.g.*, 1 kW/cm^2 peak pulse power is necessary for transient cavitation to be evoked).

Although biological effects have been demonstrated at much higher ultrasound power levels and longer durations, the levels and durations for typical imaging and Doppler studies are below the threshold for known undesirable effects. At higher output power, outcomes include macroscopic damage (*e.g.*, rupturing of blood vessels, breaking up cells—indeed, the whole point of shock wave lithotripsy—the breakup of kidney stones) and microscopic damage (*e.g.*, breaking of chromosomes, changes in cell mitotic index). No bioeffects have been shown below I_{SPTA} of 100 mW/cm^2 (Fig. 14-71). Even though ultrasound is considered safe when used properly, prudence dictates that ultrasound exposure be limited to only those patients for whom a definite benefit will be obtained.

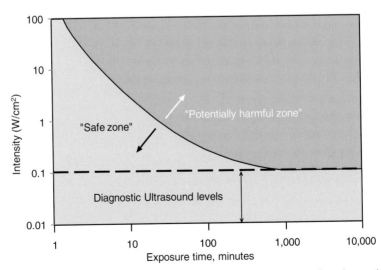

■ **FIGURE 14-71** A diagram of potential bioeffects from ultrasound delineates **safe** and potentially **harmful** regions according to ultrasound intensity levels and exposure time. The dashed line shows the upper limit of intensities typically encountered in diagnostic imaging applications.

Summary

Ultrasound uses mechanical energy to generate acoustic maps of the body, providing valuable diagnostic information in a very safe and efficient manner. However, quality of the exam is extremely operator-dependent. Of all medical imaging modalities, performing ultrasound examinations is an art that requires extensive knowledge and understanding of the underlying basic physics for the operator to be considered a true "artist." This is also true of the interpreting radiologist who must use the knowledge of ultrasound interactions, image generation, limitations, potential artifacts, and possible pitfalls that are present to make confident diagnoses. Despite the purported safety of ultrasound, precautions must be taken to ensure the appropriateness of the examination and the potential misdiagnoses and deleterious bioeffects that can occur with misuse.

SUGGESTED READING AND REFERENCES

ACR-AAPM. *Technical Standard for Diagnostic Medical Physics Performance Monitoring of Real Time Ultrasound Equipment.* 2016. https://www.acr.org/-/media/ACR/Files/Practice-Parameters/US-Equip.pdf. Accessed July 18, 2020.

AIUM. *Official Statements and Reports.* American Institute of Ultrasound in Medicine; 2020. Available at the AIUM web site: http://www.aium.org. Accessed April 30, 2020.

Barr RG, Ferraioli G, Palmeri ML, et al. Elastography assessment of liver fibrosis: Society of Radiologists in Ultrasound Consensus Conference Statement. *Radiology.* 2015;276:845-861.

Demi L. Practical guide to ultrasound beam forming: beam pattern and image reconstruction analysis. *Appl Sci.* 2018;8:1544. Open Access.

Feldman MK. US artifacts. *Radiographics.* 2009;29:1179-1189.

Maulik D. Spectral Doppler sonography: waveform analysis and hemodynamic interpretation. Chapter 4. In: Maulik D, ed. *Doppler Ultrasound in Obstetrics and Gynecology.* New York, NY: Springer Publishing; 2005.

Nelson TR, Fowlkes JB, Abramowicz JS, Church CC. Ultrasound biosafety considerations for the practicing sonographer and sonologist. *J Ultrasound Med.* 2009;28:139-150.

Sigrist RMS, Liau J, El Kaffas A, Chammas MC, Willmann JK. Ultrasound elastography: review of techniques and clinical applications. *Theranostics.* 2017;7(5):1303-1329. Open Access.

Szabo TL, Lewin PA. Ultrasound transducer selection in clinical imaging practice. *J Ultrasound Med.* 2013;32(4):573-582. Open Access.

Wood MM, Romine LE, Lee YK, et al. Spectral doppler signature waveforms in ultrasonography: a review of normal and abnormal waveforms. *Ultrasound Q.* 2010;26(2):83-99.

Zagzebski, J. *Essentials of Ultrasound Physics.* St. Louis, MO: Mosby-Year Book; 1996.

Nuclear Medicine

CHAPTER 15

Radioactivity and Nuclear Transformation

Roentgen had discovered x-rays in early November 1895. Even in the absence of the virtually instantaneous worldwide communication networks known today, this discovery spread very quickly and ignited the imagination of scientists and the general public alike. One of those scientists was Henri Becquerel who was studying the phenomenon of phosphorescence following the absorption of light by different minerals. Becquerel was intrigued by Roentgen's discovery and wondered if any of the minerals in his collection might emit a similar type of ray that could penetrate visually opaque objects when exposed to strong sunlight. The experiment he planned was simple. He wrapped an unexposed photographic plate in black paper, placed the mineral to be tested on the top of the paper, and left it out in strong sunlight to see if this would "activate" the mineral to produce x-rays and produce a darkening of the photographic plate when it was developed. The experiment with the mineral uranium was set up but delayed due to cloudy skies and placed in a desk drawer. Later, and by accident, one of Becquerel's assistants developed the plate. To their surprise, the uranium sulfate had left a faint impression of its granules on the plate. Becquerel soon discovered that the properties of this mineral (uranium) were quite unique and that the type of radiation was being emitted spontaneously without the uranium salts having to be illuminated by the sun. He also showed that the "rays" emitted, which for many years were named after their discoverer, differed from x-rays in that they could be deflected by electric or magnetic fields. In 1975 the General Conference on Weights and Measures decided to honor Henri Becquerel by accepting a proposal from the International Commission for Radiation Units and Measurements (ICRU) to adopt the special name of becquerel (Bq) as the official SI derived unit of activity (the quantity of radioactive material). Prior to 1975, the unit of activity was the Curie (Ci) named in honor of Marie Curie, one of the most accomplished women in the history of science.

Becquerel's discovery inspired Marie and her husband Pierre Curie to further investigate this phenomenon. They examined many substances and minerals for signs of radioactivity. They found that the mineral pitchblende was more radioactive than uranium and concluded that it must contain other radioactive substances. From it, they managed to extract two previously unknown elements, polonium (Po) and radium (Ra). Marie Curie named polonium in honor of her homeland, Poland, and radium (a rare, brilliant white, luminescent, and highly radioactive metallic element) whose name is derived from the Latin word radius, meaning "ray." Noting that the number of radiated emissions per unit time per unit mass from both Ra and Po was much more frequent than with uranium Marie Curie coined the term "radioactivity."

Marie Curie was a woman of many "firsts" and her research paved the way for numerous remarkable applications of radiation in science, technology, and medicine. In 1903, she was the first woman in the world to earn a Doctor of Science degree. That same year she was the first woman to be awarded a Nobel Prize in Physics and in 1911 she was the only women to be awarded a second Nobel Prize, this time in Chemistry. She was also the first woman Professor and Chair of physical sciences at the Sorbonne. In 1935, the Curies' daughter, Irene Joliot-Curie and her husband

629

Frederic Joliot won the Nobel Prize for Chemistry, making them the only mother and daughter to share this honor.

Marie Curie's relentless resolve and insatiable curiosity made her an icon in the world of modern science. She championed the use of radiation in medicine and fundamentally changed our understanding of radioactivity. Today many people fear anything to do with the word radiation or radioactivity. In the following pages, we will discuss the types of radioactive transformations common to the radionuclides used in medical imaging. It would be prudent to remember the words of Dr. Curie at this juncture who said:

"Nothing in life is to be feared, it is only to be understood. Now is the time to understand more, so that we may fear less"

15.1 RADIONUCLIDE DECAY TERMS AND RELATIONSHIPS

15.1.1 Activity

The quantity of radioactive material, expressed as the number of radioactive atoms undergoing nuclear transformation per unit time (t), is called *activity* (A). Described mathematically, activity is equal to the change (dN) in the total number of radioactive atoms (N) in a given period of time (dt), or

$$A = -dN/dt. \qquad [15\text{-}1]$$

The minus sign indicates that the number of radioactive atoms decreases with time. Activity has traditionally been expressed in units of curies (Ci). One Ci is defined as 3.70×10^{10} disintegrations per second (dps), which is roughly equal to the rate of disintegrations from 1 g of radium-226 (Ra-226). A curie is a large amount of radioactivity. In nuclear medicine, activities from 0.1 to 30 mCi of a variety of radionuclides are typically used for imaging studies, and up to 300 mCi of iodine-131 is used for therapy. Although the curie is still the most common unit of radioactivity in the United States, the majority of the world's scientific literature uses the SI unit for radioactivity, the becquerel, defined as 1 dps. One millicurie (mCi) is equal to 37 megabecquerels (1 mCi = 37 MBq). Table 15-1 lists the units and prefixes describing various amounts of radioactivity.

TABLE 15-1 UNITS AND PREFIXES ASSOCIATED WITH VARIOUS QUANTITIES OF RADIOACTIVITY

QUANTITY	SYMBOL	DPS	DPM
Gigabecquerel	GBq	1×10^9	6×10^{10}
Megabecquerel	MBq	1×10^6	6×10^7
Kilobecquerel	kBq	1×10^3	6×10^4
Curie	Ci	3.7×10^{10}	2.22×10^{12}
Millicurie	mCi (10^{-3} Ci)	3.7×10^7	2.22×10^9
Microcurie	µCi (10^{-6} Ci)	3.7×10^4	2.22×10^6
Nanocurie	nCi (10^{-9} Ci)	3.7×10^1	2.22×10^3
Picocurie	pCi (10^{-12} Ci)	3.7×10^{-2}	2.22

Multiply mCi by 37 to obtain MBq or divide MBq by 37 to obtain mCi (*e.g.*, 1 mCi = 37 MBq).

15.1.2 Decay Constant

Radioactive decay is a random process. From moment to moment, it is not possible to predict which radioactive atoms in a sample will decay. However, observation of a larger number of radioactive atoms over a period of time allows the average rate of nuclear transformation (decay) to be established. The number of atoms decaying per unit time (dN/dt) is proportional to the number of unstable atoms (N) that are present at any given time:

$$dN/dt \propto N. \qquad [15\text{-}2]$$

A proportionality can be transformed into an equality by introducing a constant. This constant is called the *decay constant* (λ).

$$-dN/dt = \lambda N \qquad [15\text{-}3]$$

The minus sign indicates that the number of radioactive atoms decaying per unit time (the decay rate or activity of the sample) decreases with time. The decay constant is equal to the fraction of the number of radioactive atoms remaining in a sample that decay per unit time. The relationship between activity A and the decay constant λ can be seen by considering Equation 15-1 and substituting A for $-dN/dt$ in Equation 15-3:

$$A = \lambda N. \qquad [15\text{-}4]$$

The decay constant is characteristic of each radionuclide. For example, the decay constants for technetium-99m (Tc-99m) and molybdenum-99 (Mo-99) are 0.1151 h^{-1} and 0.252 day^{-1}, respectively.

15.1.3 Physical Half-Life

A useful parameter related to the decay constant is the physical half-life ($T\frac{1}{2}$ or $T_p\frac{1}{2}$). The half-life is defined as the time required for the number of radioactive atoms in a sample to decrease by one half. The number of radioactive atoms remaining in a sample and the number of elapsed half-lives are related by the following equation:

$$N = N_0/2^n, \qquad [15\text{-}5]$$

where N is the number of radioactive atoms remaining, N_0 is the initial number of radioactive atoms, and n is the number of half-lives that have elapsed. The relationship between time and the number of radioactive atoms remaining in a sample is demonstrated with Tc-99m ($T_p\frac{1}{2} \approx 6$ h) in Table 15-2.

After 10 half-lives, the number of radioactive atoms in a sample is reduced by approximately a factor of a thousand. After 20 half-lives, the number of radioactive atoms is reduced to approximately one millionth of the initial number.

The decay constant and the physical half-life are related as follows:

$$\lambda = \ln 2/T_p\frac{1}{2} = 0.693/T_p\frac{1}{2}, \qquad [15\text{-}6]$$

where ln 2 denotes the natural logarithm of 2. Note that the derivation of this relationship is identical to that between the half-value layer (HVL) and the linear attenuation coefficient (μ) in Chapter 3 (Eq. 3-9).

The physical half-life and the decay constant are physical quantities that are inversely related and unique for each radionuclide. Half-lives of radioactive materials range from billions of years to a fraction of a second. Radionuclides used in nuclear medicine typically have half-lives on the order of hours or days. Examples of $T_p\frac{1}{2}$ and λ for radionuclides commonly used in nuclear medicine are listed in Table 15-3.

TABLE 15-2 RADIOACTIVE DECAY FOR Tc-99m[a]

TIME (DAY)	NO. OF PHYSICAL HALF-LIVES	EXPRESSION	N	$(N/N_0) \times 100 = \%$ REMAINING
0	0	$N_0/2^0$	10^6	100%
0.25	1	$N_0/2^1$	5×10^5	50%
0.5	2	$N_0/2^2$	2.5×10^5	25%
0.75	3	$N_0/2^3$	1.25×10^5	12.5%
1	4	$N_0/2^4$	6.25×10^4	6.25%
2.5	10	$N_0/2^{10}$	$\approx 10^3$	$\approx 0.1\%\ (1/1{,}000)N_0$
5	20	$N_0/2^{20}$	≈ 1	$\approx 0.000001\%\ (1/1{,}000{,}000)N_0$

[a]The influence of radioactive decay on the number of radioactive atoms in a sample is illustrated with technetium-99m, which has a physical half-life of 6 h (0.25 day). The sample initially contains one million (10^6) radioactive atoms (N).

15.1.4 Fundamental Decay Equation

By applying the integral calculus to Equation 15-3, a useful relationship is established between the number of radioactive atoms remaining in a sample and time—the fundamental decay equation:

$$N_t = N_0 e^{-\lambda t} \quad \text{or} \quad A_t = A_0 e^{-\lambda t}, \qquad [15\text{-}7]$$

where N_t is the number of radioactive atoms at time t, A_t is the activity at time t, N_0 is the initial number of radioactive atoms, A_0 is the initial activity, e is the base of natural logarithm = 2.718 ..., λ is the decay constant = $\ln 2/T_p\frac{1}{2} = 0.693/T_p\frac{1}{2}$, and t is the elapsed time.

TABLE 15-3 PHYSICAL HALF-LIFE ($T_p\frac{1}{2}$) AND DECAY CONSTANT (λ) FOR RADIONUCLIDES COMMONLY USED IN NUCLEAR MEDICINE

RADIONUCLIDE	$T_p\frac{1}{2}$	λ
Rubidium-82 (^{82}Rb)	75 s	0.0092 s^{-1}
Fluorine-18 (^{18}F)	110 min	0.0063 min^{-1}
Technetium-99m (^{99m}Tc)	6.02 h	0.1151 h^{-1}
Iodine-123 (^{123}I)	13.27 h	0.0522 h^{-1}
Samarium-153 (^{153}Sm)	1.93 d	0.3591 d^{-1}
Yttrium-90 (^{90}Y)	2.69 d	0.2575 d^{-1}
Molybdenum-99 (^{99}Mo)	2.75 d	0.2522 d^{-1}
Indium-111 (^{111}In)	2.81 d	0.2466 d^{-1}
Thallium-201 (^{201}Tl)	3.04 d	0.2281 d^{-1}
Gallium-67 (^{67}Ga)	3.26 d	0.2126 d^{-1}
Xenon-133 (^{133}Xe)	5.24 d	0.1323 d^{-1}
Lutetium-177 (^{177}Lu)	6.7 d	0.1034 d^{-1}
Iodine-131 (^{131}I)	8.02 d	0.0864 d^{-1}
Ra-223 (^{223}Ra)	11.4 d	0.0608 d^{-1}
Strontium-82 (^{82}Sr)	25.60 d	0.0271 d^{-1}
Cobalt-57 (^{57}Co)	271.79 d	0.0117 d^{-1}

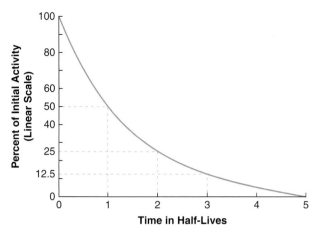

■ **FIGURE 15-1** Percentage of initial activity as a function of time (linear scale).

Problem: A nuclear medicine technologist injects a patient with 400 µCi of indium-111–labeled autologous leukocytes ($T_p\frac{1}{2} = 2.81$ days). Twenty-four hours later, the patient is imaged. Assuming that none of the activity was excreted, how much activity remains at the time of imaging?

Solution:

$A = A_0 e^{-\lambda t}$

Given:

$A_0 = 400 \, \mu Ci$

$\lambda = 0.693/2.81 \, \text{days} = 0.247 \, \text{day}^{-1}$

$t = 1 \, \text{day}$

Note: t and $T_p\frac{1}{2}$ must be in the same units of time.

$A_t = 400 \, \mu Ci \, e^{-(0.247 \, \text{day}^{-1})(1 \, \text{day})}$

$A_t = 400 \, \mu Ci \, e^{-0.247}$

$A_t = (400 \, \mu Ci)(0.781)$

$A_t = 312 \, \mu Ci$

A plot of activity as a function of time on a linear scale results in a curvilinear exponential relationship in which the total activity asymptotically approaches zero (Fig. 15-1). If the logarithm of the activity is plotted versus time (semilog plot), this exponential relationship appears as a straight line (Fig. 15-2).

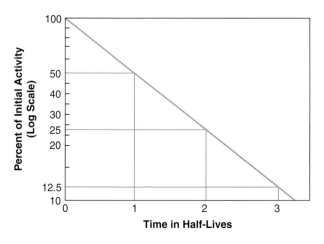

■ **FIGURE 15-2** Percentage of initial activity as a function of time (semilog plot).

15.2 NUCLEAR TRANSFORMATION

As mentioned previously, when an unstable (*i.e.*, radioactive) atomic nucleus undergoes the spontaneous transformation, called *radioactive decay*, radiation is emitted. If the decay product nucleus is stable, this spontaneous transformation ends. If the decay product is also unstable, the process continues until a stable nuclide is reached. Most radionuclides decay in one or more of the following ways: (1) alpha decay, (2) beta-minus emission, (3) beta-plus (positron) emission, (4) electron capture, or (5) isomeric transition.

15.2.1 Alpha Decay

Alpha (α) decay is the spontaneous emission of an alpha particle (identical to a helium nucleus consisting of two protons and two neutrons) from the nucleus (Fig. 15-3). Alpha decay typically occurs with heavy nuclides ($A > 150$) and is often followed by γ and characteristic x-ray emissions. These photon emissions are often accompanied by the competing processes of internal conversion and Auger electron emission. Alpha particles are the heaviest and least penetrating form of radiation considered in this chapter. They are emitted from the atomic nucleus with discrete energies in the range of 2 to 10 MeV. An alpha particle is approximately four times heavier than a proton or neutron and carries an electronic charge twice that of the proton. Alpha decay can be described by the following equation:

$$\underset{Z}{\overset{A}{}}X \rightarrow \underset{Z-2}{\overset{A-4}{}}Y + \underset{2}{\overset{4}{}}\underset{\substack{\text{alpha} \\ \text{particle}}}{He^{2+}} + \text{transition energy.} \qquad [15\text{-}8]$$

EXAMPLE:

$$\underset{86}{\overset{220}{}}Rn \rightarrow \underset{84}{\overset{216}{}}Po + \underset{2}{\overset{4}{}}He^{2+} + 6.4 \text{ MeV transition energy.}$$

Alpha decay results in a large energy transition and a slight increase in the ratio of neutrons to protons (*N/Z* ratio):

$$\underset{86}{\overset{220}{}}Rn \xrightarrow{\;\;\alpha+2\;\;} \underset{84}{\overset{216}{}}Po$$

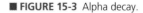

$$N/Z = 134/86 = 1.56 \qquad\qquad N/Z = 132/84 = 1.57.$$

Alpha particles are not used in medical imaging because their ranges are limited to approximately 1 cm/MeV in air and typically less than 100 μm in tissue. Even the most energetic alpha particles cannot penetrate the dead layer of the skin. However, the intense ionization tracks produced by this high linear energy transfer (LET) radiation (*e.g.*, mean LET of alpha particles is ~100 keV/μm compared to ~3 keV/μm for

■ **FIGURE 15-3** Alpha decay.

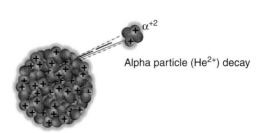

Alpha particle (He²⁺) decay

energetic electrons set in motion by the interaction of diagnostic x-rays in tissue as discussed in Chapter 3) make them a potentially serious health hazard should alpha-emitting radionuclides enter the body via ingestion, inhalation, or a wound. Research continues to assess the potential therapeutic effectiveness of alpha-emitting radionuclides such as astatine-212, bismuth-212, and bismuth-213 (At-211, Bi-212, and Bi-213) chelated to monoclonal antibodies to produce stable radioimmunoconjugates directed against various tumors as radioimmunotherapeutic agents.

15.2.2 Beta-Minus (Negatron) Decay

Beta-minus (β^-) decay, or negatron decay, characteristically occurs with radionuclides that have an excess number of neutrons compared with the number of protons (*i.e.*, a high N/Z ratio). Beta-minus decay can be described by the following equation:

$$\underset{Z}{\overset{A}{X}} \rightarrow \underset{Z+1}{\overset{A}{Y}} + \underset{\text{(negatron)}}{\beta^-} + \underset{\text{(antineutrino)}}{\overline{v}} + \text{energy.} \qquad [15\text{-}9]$$

This mode of decay results in the conversion of a neutron into a proton with the simultaneous ejection of a negatively charged beta particle (β^-) and an antineutrino ($\overline{v}$), (Fig. 15-4). With the exception of their origin (the nucleus), beta particles are identical to ordinary electrons. The antineutrino is an electrically neutral subatomic particle whose mass is much smaller than that of an electron. The absence of charge and the infinitesimal mass of antineutrinos make them very difficult to detect because they rarely interact with matter. Beta-decay increases the number of protons by 1 and thus transforms the atom into a different element with an atomic number $Z + 1$. However, the concomitant decrease in the neutron number means that the mass number remains unchanged. Decay modes in which the mass number remains constant are called *isobaric transitions*. Radionuclides produced by nuclear fission are "neutron-rich," and therefore most decay by β^- emission. Beta-minus decay decreases the N/Z ratio, bringing the decay product closer to the line of stability (see Chapter 2):

EXAMPLE:

$$\underset{15}{\overset{32}{P}} \xrightarrow{\quad \beta^- \quad} \underset{16}{\overset{32}{S}}$$

$$N/Z = 17/15 = 1.13 \qquad N/Z = 16/16 = 1.00.$$

Although the β^- particles emitted by a specific radionuclide has a discrete maximal energy (E_{max}), almost all are emitted with energies lower than the maximum. The average energy of the β^- particles is approximately 1/3 E_{max}. The balance of the energy

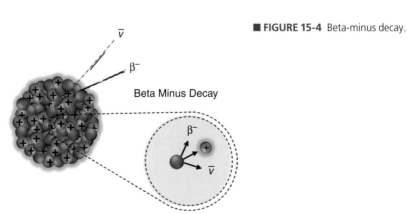

■ **FIGURE 15-4** Beta-minus decay.

Beta Minus Decay

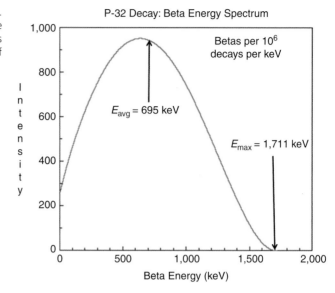

■ **FIGURE 15-5** P-32 example. Distribution of beta-minus particle kinetic energy. Number of beta-minus particles emitted per 10^6 decays of P-32 as a function of energy.

is given to the antineutrino (*i.e.*, $E_{max} = E_{\beta^-} + E_{\bar{\nu}}$). Thus, beta-minus decay results in a polyenergetic spectrum of β^- energies ranging from zero to E_{max} (Fig. 15-5). Any excess energy in the nucleus after beta decay is emitted as γ-rays, internal conversion electrons, and other associated radiations.

15.2.3 Beta-Plus Decay (Positron Emission)

Just as beta-minus decay is driven by the nuclear instability caused by excess neutrons, "neutron-poor" radionuclides (*i.e.*, those with a low N/Z ratio) are also unstable. Many of these radionuclides decay by beta-plus (positron) emission, which increases the neutron number by one. Beta-plus decay can be described by the following equation:

$$^A_Z X \rightarrow ^A_{Z-1} + \underset{(\text{positron})}{\beta^+} + \underset{(\text{neutrino})}{\nu} + \text{energy}.$$

[15-10]

The net result is the conversion of a proton into a neutron with the simultaneous ejection of the positron (β^+) and a neutrino (ν). Positron decay decreases the number of protons (atomic number) by 1 and thereby transforms the atom into a different element with an atomic number of $Z - 1$ (Fig. 15-6). The decay product atom, with one less proton in the nucleus, initially has one too many orbital electrons and thus

■ **FIGURE 15-6** Beta-plus decay.

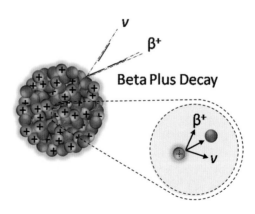

Beta Plus Decay

is a negative ion. However, the decay product quickly releases the extra orbital electron to the surrounding medium and becomes a neutral atom. Positron decay can only occur if the mass of the parent atom exceeds that of the decay product atom by at least the masses of the two electrons (positron and orbital electron). According to Einstein's mass-energy equivalence formula, $E = mc^2$, 511 keV is the energy equivalent of the rest mass of an electron (positively or negatively charged). Therefore, there is an inherent threshold for positron decay equal to the sum of the rest mass energy equivalent of two electrons (*i.e.*, 2×511 keV, or 1.02 MeV).

The number of neutrons is increased by 1; therefore, the transformation is isobaric because the total number of nucleons is unchanged. Accelerator-produced radionuclides, which are typically neutron deficient, often decay by positron emission. Positron decay increases the N/Z ratio, resulting in a nuclide closer to the line of stability.

EXAMPLE:

$$^{18}_{9}\text{F} \xrightarrow{\;\beta^+\;} {}^{18}_{8}\text{O}$$
$$N/Z = 9/9 = 1 \qquad N/Z = 10/8 = 1.25.$$

The energy distribution between the positron and the neutrino is similar to that between the negatron and the antineutrino in beta-minus decay; thus positrons are polyenergetic with average energy equal to approximately $1/3 \; E_{max}$. As with β^- decay, excess energy following positron decay is released as γ-rays and other associated radiation.

Although β^+ decay has similarities to β^- decay, there are also important differences. The neutrino and antineutrino are *antiparticles*, as are the positron and negatron. The prefix *anti-* before the name of an elementary particle denotes another particle with certain symmetry characteristics. In the case of charged particles such as the positron, the antiparticle (*i.e.*, the negatron) has a charge equal but opposite to that of the positron and a magnetic moment that is oppositely directed with respect to spin. In the case of neutral particles such as the neutrino and antineutrino, there is no charge; therefore, differentiation between the particles is made solely on the basis of differences in magnetic moment. Other important differences between the particle and antiparticle are their lifetimes and their eventual fates. As mentioned earlier, negatrons are physically identical to ordinary electrons and as such lose their kinetic energy as they traverse matter via excitation and ionization. When they lose all (or almost all) of their kinetic energy, they may be captured by an atom or absorbed into the free electron pool. Positrons undergo a similar process of energy deposition via excitation and ionization; however, when they come to rest, they react violently with their antiparticles (electrons). This process results in the entire rest mass of both particles being instantaneously converted to energy and emitted as two oppositely directed (*i.e.*, ~180° apart) 511-keV *annihilation photons* (Fig. 15-7). Medical imaging of annihilation radiation from positron-emitting radiopharmaceuticals, called positron emission tomography (PET), is discussed in Chapter 19.

15.2.4 Electron Capture Decay

Electron capture (ε) is an alternative to positron decay for neutron-deficient radionuclides. In this decay mode, the nucleus captures an orbital (usually a K- or L-shell) electron, with the conversion of a proton into a neutron and the simultaneous

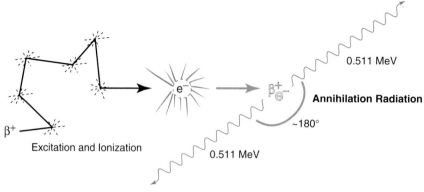

■ **FIGURE 15-7** Annihilation radiation.

ejection of a neutrino (Fig. 15-8). Electron capture can be described by the following equation:

$$_{Z}^{A}X + e^{-} \rightarrow _{Z-1}^{A}Y + \underset{(neutrino)}{\nu} + energy. \qquad [15\text{-}11]$$

The net effect of electron capture is the same as positron emission: the atomic number is decreased by 1, creating a different element, and the mass number remains unchanged. Therefore, electron capture is isobaric and results in an increase in the N/Z ratio.

EXAMPLE:

$$\underset{N/Z = 120/81 = 1.48}{_{81}^{201}Tl} \quad \xrightarrow{\quad \varepsilon \quad} \quad \underset{N/Z = 121/80 = 1.51}{_{80}^{201}Hg} \quad + \quad energy$$

The capture of an orbital electron creates a vacancy in the electron shell, which is filled by an electron from a higher energy shell. As discussed in Chapter 2, this electron transition results in the emission of characteristic x-rays and/or Auger electrons. For example, thallium-201, (Tl-201) decays to mercury-201 (Hg-201) by electron capture, resulting in the emission of characteristic x-rays. It is these x-rays that are primarily used to create the images in Tl-201 myocardial perfusion studies. As with other modes of decay, if the nucleus is left in an excited state following electron capture, the excess energy will be emitted as γ-rays and other radiations.

As previously mentioned, positron emission requires a mass energy difference between the parent and decay product (daughter) atoms of at least 1.02 MeV.

■ **FIGURE 15-8** Electron capture decay.

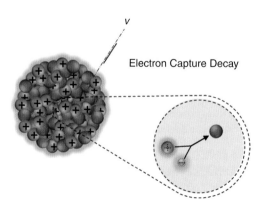

Neutron-poor radionuclides below this threshold energy decay exclusively by electron capture. Nuclides for which the energy difference between the parent and progeny exceed 1.02 MeV may decay by electron capture or positron emission, or both. Heavier proton-rich nuclides are more likely to decay by electron capture, whereas lighter proton-rich nuclides are more likely to decay by positron emission. This is a result of the closer proximity of the *K*- or *L*-shell electrons to the nucleus and the greater magnitude of the coulombic attraction from the positive charges. Although the capture of a *K*- or *L*-shell electron is the most probable, electron capture can occur with higher energy shell electrons.

The quantum mechanical description of the atom is essential for understanding electron capture. The Bohr model describes electrons in fixed orbits at discrete distances from the nucleus. This model does not permit electrons to be close enough to the nucleus to be captured. However, the quantum mechanical model describes orbital electron locations as probability density functions in which there is a finite probability that an electron will pass close to or even through the nucleus.

Electron capture radionuclides used in medical imaging decay to atoms in excited states that subsequently emit externally detectable x-rays, γ-rays, or both.

15.2.5 Isomeric Transition

Often during radioactive decay, a decay product is formed in an "excited state", (*i.e.*, an intermediate nuclear energy state between that of the parent and that of final decay product). γ-rays are emitted as the nucleus undergoes an internal transition from its excited state to a lower energy state. Once created, most excited states transition almost instantaneously (on the order of 10^{-12} s) to lower energy states with the emission of γ-radiation. However, some excited states persist for longer periods, with half-lives ranging from nanoseconds (10^{-9} s) to more than 30 years. These excited states are called metastable or isomeric states and those with half-lives exceeding a millisecond (10^{-3} s) are denoted by the letter "*m*" after the mass number (*e.g.*, Tc-99m). Isomeric transition is a decay process that yields γ-radiation without the emission or capture of a particle by the nucleus. There is no change in atomic number, mass number, or neutron number. Thus, this decay mode is isobaric and isotonic, and it occurs between two nuclear energy states with no change in the *N/Z* ratio.

Isomeric transition can be described by the following equation:

$$^{Am}_{Z}X \rightarrow {}^{A}_{Z}X + (\text{energy}).\qquad [15\text{-}12]$$

The energy is released in the form of γ-rays, internal conversion electrons, or both.

15.2.6 Decay Schemes

Each radionuclide's decay process is a unique characteristic of that radionuclide. The majority of the pertinent information about the decay process and its associated radiation can be summarized in a line diagram called a *decay scheme* (Fig. 15-9). Decay schemes identify the parent, decay product (i.e. progeny or daughter), mode of decay, energy levels including those of excited and metastable states, radiation emissions, and sometimes physical half-life and other characteristics of the decay sequence. The top horizontal line represents the parent, and the bottom horizontal line represents the decay product. Horizontal lines between those two represent intermediate excited or metastable states. By convention, a diagonal arrow to the right indicates an increase in Z, which occurs with beta-minus decay. A diagonal arrow to the left indicates a

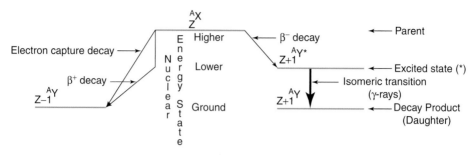

■ **FIGURE 15-9** Elements of the generalized decay scheme.

decrease in Z such as decay by electron capture. A vertical line followed by a diagonal arrow to the left is used to indicate alpha decay and in some cases to indicate positron emission when a radionuclide decays by both electron capture and positron emission (*e.g.*, F-18). Vertical down-pointing arrows indicate γ-ray emission, including those emitted during isomeric transition. These diagrams are often accompanied by decay data tables, which provide information on all the significant ionizing radiations emitted from the atom as a result of the nuclear transformation. Examples of these decay schemes and data tables are presented in this section.

Figure 15-10 shows the alpha decay scheme of radon-220 (Rn-220). Rn-220 has a physical half-life of 55 s and decays by one of two possible alpha transitions. Alpha 1 (α_1) at 5.747 MeV occurs 0.07% of the time and is followed immediately by a 0.55-MeV γ-ray (γ_1) to the ground state. The emission of alpha 2 (α_2) with an energy of 6.287 MeV occurs 99.9% of the time and leads directly to the ground state. The decay data table lists these radiations together with the decay product atom, which has a -2 charge and a small amount of kinetic energy as a result of recoil from the alpha particle emission.

Phosphorus-32 (P-32) is still used in some nuclear medicine departments as a therapeutic agent in the treatment of diseases such as polycythemia vera, and serous effusions. P-32 has a half-life of 14.3 days and decays directly to its ground state by

■ **FIGURE 15-10** Principal decay scheme of radon-220.

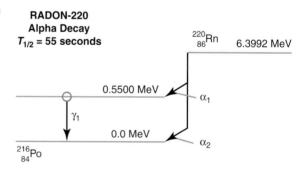

RADON-220
Alpha Decay
$T_{1/2}$ = 55 seconds

Decay Data Table

Radiation		Mean Number per Disintegration	Mean Energy per Particle (MeV)
Alpha	1	0.0007	5.7470
Recoil Atom		0.0007	0.1064
Alpha	2	0.9993	6.2870
Recoil Atom		0.9993	0.1164
Gamma	1	0.0006	0.5500

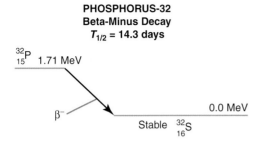

PHOSPHORUS-32
Beta-Minus Decay
$T_{1/2}$ = **14.3 days**

■ **FIGURE 15-11** Principal decay scheme of phosphorus-32.

Decay Data Table

Radiation	Mean Number per Disintegration	Mean Energy per Particle (MeV)
Beta Minus	1.000	0.6948

emitting a beta-minus particle with an E_{max} of 1.71 MeV (Fig. 15-11). The average (mean) energy of the beta-minus particle is approximately 1/3 E_{max} (0.6948 MeV), with the antineutrino carrying off the balance of the transition energy. There are no excited energy states or other radiation emitted during this decay; therefore, P-32 is referred to as a "*pure beta emitter.*"

A somewhat more complicated decay scheme is associated with the beta-minus decay of Mo-99 to Tc-99 (Fig. 15-12). Eight of the ten possible beta-minus decay transitions are shown with probabilities ranging from 0.822 for beta-minus 8 (*i.e.*, 82.2% of all decays of Mo-99 are by β_8^- transition) to 0.0004 (0.04%) for β_6^-. The sum of all transition probabilities (β_1^- to β_{10}^-) is equal to 1. The average energy of beta particles from the transition is 0.4519 MeV. The β_8^- transition leads directly to a metastable state of technetium 99, Tc-99m, which is 0.1427 MeV above the ground state and decays with a half-life of 6.02 h. Tc-99m is the most widely used radionuclide in nuclear medicine.

After beta decay, there are a number of excited states created that transition to lower energy levels via the emission of γ-rays and/or internal conversion electrons. As previously described, the ejection of an electron by internal conversion of the γ-ray results in the emission of characteristic x-rays, Auger electrons, or both. All of these radiations, their mean energies, and associated probabilities are included in the decay data table.

The process of γ-ray emission by isomeric transition is of primary importance to nuclear medicine because most procedures performed depend on the emission and detection of γ-radiation. Figure 15-13 shows the decay scheme for Tc-99m. There are three γ-ray transitions as Tc-99m decays to Tc-99. The gamma 1 transition (γ_1) occurs very infrequently because 99.2% of the time this energy is internally converted resulting in the emission of either an M-shell internal conversion electron (86.2%) with a mean energy of 1.8 keV or an N-shell internal conversion electron (13.0%) with a mean energy of 2.2 keV. After internal conversion, the nucleus is left in an excited state, which is followed almost instantaneously by gamma 2 (γ_2) transition at 140.5 keV to ground state. The γ_2 transition occurs 89.1% of the time with the balance of the transitions from 140.5 keV to ground state occurring primarily via internal conversion. Gamma 2 is the principal photon imaged in nuclear medicine. Like gamma 1, the gamma 3 transition at 142.7 keV occurs very infrequently relative to the probability of internal conversion electron emission. Here again, the vacancies

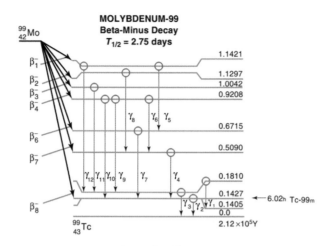

Decay Data Table

Radiation		Mean Number per Disintegration	Mean Energy per Particle (MeV)	Radiation		Mean Number per Disintegration	Mean Energy per Particle (MeV)
Beta Minus	1	0.0010	0.0658	Gamma	4	0.0119	0.3664
Beta Minus	3	0.0014	0.1112	Gamma	5	0.0001	0.4706
Beta Minus	4	0.1640	0.1331	Gamma	6	0.0002	0.4115
Beta Minus	6	0.0004	0.2541	Gamma	7	0.0006	0.5288
Beta Minus	7	0.0114	0.2897	Gamma	8	0.0002	0.6207
Beta Minus	8	0.8220	0.4428	Gamma	9	0.1367	0.7397
Gamma	1	0.0105	0.0406	K Int Con Elect		0.0002	0.7186
K Int Con Elect		0.0428	0.0195	Gamma	10	0.0426	0.7779
L Int Con Elect		0.0053	0.0377	K Int Con Elect		0.0000	0.7571
M Int Con Elect		0.0017	0.0401	Gamma	11	0.0013	0.8230
Gamma	2	0.0452	0.1405	Gamma	12	0.0010	0.9608
K Int Con Elect		0.0058	0.1194	K Alpha-1 X-Ray		0.0253	0.0183
L Int Con Elect		0.0007	0.1377	K Alpha-2 X-Ray		0.0127	0.0182
Gamma	3	0.0600	0.1811	K Beta-1 X-Ray		0.0060	0.0206
K Int Con Elect		0.0085	0.1600	KLL Auger Elect		0.0087	0.0154
L Int Con Elect		0.0012	0.1782	KLX Auger Elect		0.0032	0.0178
M Int Con Elect		0.0004	0.1806	LMM Auger Elect		0.0615	0.0019
				MXY Auger Elect		0.1403	0.0004

■ **FIGURE 15-12** Principal decay scheme of molybdenum-99. Auger electron nomenclature: KXY Auger Elect is an Auger electron emitted from the "Y" shell as a result of a transition of an electron of the "X" shell to a vacancy in the K shell. "X" and "Y" are shells higher than the K shell. For example, KLL Auger Elect is an Auger electron emitted from the L shell as a result of a transition of another L shell electron to a vacancy in the K shell.

created in orbital electron shells following internal conversion result in the production of characteristic x-rays and Auger electrons.

As discussed previously, positron emission and electron capture are competing decay processes for neutron-deficient radionuclides. As shown in Figure 15-14, fluorine-18 (F-18) decays by both modes. F-18 decays by positron emission (represented by a solid vertical line followed by a diagonal arrow to the left) 97% of the time. The length of the vertical part of the line in the diagram represents the sum of the rest mass energy equivalent of the positron and electron (i.e., 1.02 MeV). Electron capture (represented by a diagonal arrow to the left) occurs 3% of the time. The dual mode of decay results in an "effective" decay constant (λ_e) that is the sum of the positron (λ_1) and electron capture (λ_2) decay constants: $\lambda_e = \lambda_1 + \lambda_2$. The decay data table shows that positrons are emitted 97% of the time with an average energy of 0.2496 MeV ($\sim$1/3 of 0.635 MeV, which is E_{max}). Furthermore, the interaction of the positron with an electron results in the production of two 511-keV annihilation radiation photons. Because two photons are produced for each positron, their abundance is 2 × 97% or 194%. ^{18}F is the most widely used radionuclide for PET imaging.

A summary of the characteristics of radionuclide decay modes previously discussed is provided in Table 15-4.

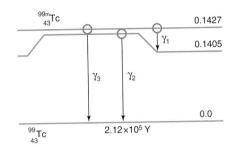

TECHNETIUM 99m
Isomeric Transition
$T_{1/2}$ = 6.02 hrs.

Decay Data Table

Radiation		Mean Number per Disintegration	Mean Energy per Particle (MeV)
Gamma	1	0.0000	0.0021
M Int Con Elect		0.8620	0.0018
N Int Con Elect		0.1300	0.0022
Gamma	2	0.8910	0.1405
K Int Con Elect		0.0892	0.1194
L Int Con Elect		0.0109	0.1375
M Int Con Elect		0.0020	0.1377
Gamma	3	0.0003	0.1426
K Int Con Elect		0.0088	0.1215
L Int Con Elect		0.0035	0.1398
M Int Con Elect		0.0011	0.1422
K Alpha-1 x-ray		0.0441	0.0183
K Alpha-2 x-ray		0.0221	0.0182
K Beta-1 x-ray		0.0105	0.0206
KLL Auger Elect		0.0152	0.0154
KLX Auger Elect		0.0055	0.0178
LMM Auger Elect		0.1093	0.0019
MXY Auger Elect		1.2359	0.0004

■ **FIGURE 15-13** Principal decay scheme of technetium-99m. Auger electron nomenclature: KXY Auger Elect is an Auger electron emitted from the "Y" shell as a result of a transition of an electron of the "X" shell to a vacancy in the K shell. "X" and "Y" are shells higher than the K shell. For example, KLL Auger Elect is an Auger electron emitted from the L shell as a result of a transition of another L shell electron to a vacancy in the K shell.

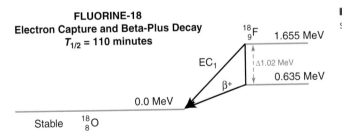

FLUORINE-18
Electron Capture and Beta-Plus Decay
$T_{1/2}$ = 110 minutes

■ **FIGURE 15-14** Principal decay scheme of fluorine-18.

Decay Data Table

Radiation	Mean Number per Disintegration	Mean Energy Particle (MeV)
Beta Plus	0.9700	0.2496
Annih. Radiation	1.9400	0.5110

TABLE 15-4 **SUMMARY OF RADIONUCLIDE DECAY**

TYPE OF DECAY	PRIMARY RADIATION EMITTED	OTHER RADIATION EMITTED	NUCLEAR TRANSFORMATION	CHANGE IN		NUCLEAR CONDITION PRIOR TO TRANSFORMATION
				Z	A	
Alpha	$_2^4 He^{+2}(\pm)$	γ-rays C x-rays AE, ICE	$_Z^A X \rightarrow _Z^A X \rightarrow^{-2} + _2^4 He^{2+} + energy$	-2	-4	$Z > 83$
Beta minus	β^{-1}	γ-rays C x-rays AE, ICE, $\bar{v}$	$_Z^A X \rightarrow _{Z+1}^A Y + \beta^- + \bar{v} + energy$	$+1$	0	N/Z too large
Beta plus	β^{+1}	γ-rays C x-rays AE, ICE, v	$_Z^A X \rightarrow _{Z-1}^A Y + \beta^+ + v + energy$	-1	0	N/Z too small
Electron capture	C x-rays	γ-rays AE, ICE, v	$_Z^A X + e^- \rightarrow _{Z-1}^A Y + v + energy$	-1	0	N/Z too small
Isomeric transition	γ-rays	C x-rays AE, ICE	$_Z^{Am} X \rightarrow _Z^A X + energy$	0	0	Excited or metastable nucleus

ICE, internal conversion e^{-1}; AE, Auger e^{-1}; C x-rays, characteristic x-rays; γ-rays, gamma rays; $\bar{v}$, antineutrino; v, neutrino.

SUGGESTED READING AND REFERENCES

Centers for Disease Control and Prevention. What is radiation? Properties of radioactive isotopes. https://www.cdc.gov/nceh/radiation/isotopes.html

Cherry SR, et al. *Physics in Nuclear Medicine.* 4th ed. Philadelphia, PA: Saunders; 2012.

International Atomic Energy Agency. *Nuclear Medicine Physics.* Vienna: IAEA; 2015. https://www-pub.iaea.org/MTCD/Publications/PDF/Pub1617web-1294055.pdf

International Atomic Energy Agency. Nuclear Data Services. https://www.iaea.org/resources/databases/nuclear-data-services

Mould RF. *A Century of X-Rays and Radioactivity in Medicine: With Emphasis on Photographic Records of the Early Years.* UK: CRC Press; 2018.

CHAPTER 16

Radionuclide Production, Radiopharmaceuticals, and Internal Dosimetry

16.1 RADIONUCLIDE PRODUCTION

Although many naturally occurring radioactive nuclides exist, all of those commonly administered to patients in nuclear medicine are artificially produced. Artificial radioactivity was discovered in 1934 by Irene Curie (daughter of Marie and Pierre Curie) and Frederic Joliot, who induced radioactivity in boron and aluminum targets by bombarding them with alpha (α) particles from polonium. Positrons continued to be emitted from the targets after the alpha source was removed. Today, more than 2,500 artificial radionuclides have been produced by a variety of methods. Most radionuclides used in nuclear medicine are produced by particle accelerators (e.g., cyclotrons), nuclear reactors, or radionuclide generators.

16.1.1 Cyclotron-Produced Radionuclides

Cyclotrons and other charged-particle accelerators produce radionuclides by bombarding stable nuclei with high-energy charged particles. Positively charged ions such as protons (H^+), deuterons ($^2H^+$), and alpha particles ($^4He^{2+}$) as well as negatively charged hydrogen ions (H^-) are commonly used to produce radionuclides used in medicine. Charged particles must be accelerated to high kinetic energies to overcome and penetrate the repulsive coulombic barrier of the target atoms' nuclei.

In 1930, Cockcroft and Walton applied a clever scheme of cascading a series of transformers, each capable of stepping up the voltage by several hundred thousand volts. The large potentials generated were used to produce artificial radioactivity by accelerating particles to high energies and using them to bombard stable nuclei.

In Berkeley, California, in 1931, E.O. Lawrence capitalized on this development but added a unique dimension in his design of the cyclotron (Fig. 16-1). A cyclotron has a vacuum chamber between the poles of an electromagnet. Inside the vacuum chamber is a pair of hollow, semicircular electrodes, each shaped like the letter D and thus referred to as "dees." The two dees are separated by a small gap. An alternating high voltage is applied between the two dees. When positive ions are injected into the center of the cyclotron, they are attracted to and accelerated toward the negatively charged dee. The static magnetic field constrains the ions to travel in a circular path, whereby the radius of the circle increases as the ions gain kinetic energy (Fig. 16-2). Halfway around the circle, the ions approach the gap between the dees; at this time, the polarity of the electrical field between the two dees is reversed, causing the ions to be accelerated toward the negative dee. This cycle is repeated again and again, with the particles accelerated each time they cross the gap, acquiring additional kinetic energy and sweeping out larger and larger circles. As the length of the path between successive accelerations increases, the speed of the particle also increases; hence,

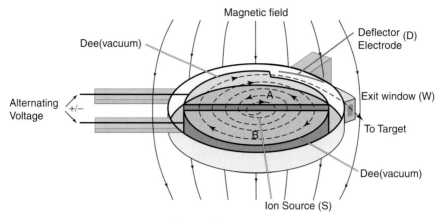

Top and bottom magnet removed

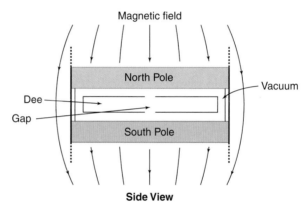

Side View

■ **FIGURE 16-1** Schematic view of a cyclotron. Two "dees" **(A and B)** are separated by a small gap.

the time interval between accelerations remains constant. The cyclic nature of these events led to the name "cyclotron." The final kinetic energy achieved by the accelerated particles depends on the type of particle (*e.g.*, protons or deuterons), the diameter of the dees, and the strength of the static magnetic field. Finally, as the ions reach the periphery of the dees, they are removed from their circular path by a negatively

■ **FIGURE 16-2** A constant magnetic field imposes a force (**F**) on a moving charged particle that is perpendicular to the direction of the particle's velocity (**v**). This causes an ion in a cyclotron to move in a circular path. The diameter of the circular path is proportional to the speed of the ion.

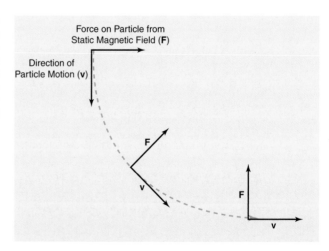

charged deflector plate (if positive ions are accelerated) or electron stripping foil (if H^- ions are accelerated), emerge through the window, and strike the target. Depending on the design of the cyclotron, particle energies can range from a few million electron volts (MeV) to several hundred MeV.

The accelerated ions collide with the target nuclei, causing nuclear reactions. An incident particle may leave the target nucleus after interacting, transferring some of its energy to it, or it may be completely absorbed. The specific reaction depends on the type and energy of the bombarding particle as well as the composition of the target. In either case, target nuclei are left in an excited state, and this excitation energy is disposed of through the emission of particulate (protons and neutrons) and electromagnetic (γ-rays) radiations. Gallium-67 (Ga-67) is an example of a cyclotron-produced radionuclide. The production reaction is written as follows:

$$^{68}Zn\,(p, 2n)\,^{67}Ga, \qquad [16\text{-}1]$$

where the target material is zinc-68 (Zn-68), the bombarding particle is a proton (p) accelerated to approximately 20 MeV, two neutrons (2n) are emitted, and Ga-67 is the product radionuclide. In some cases, the nuclear reaction produces a radionuclide that decays to the clinically useful radionuclide (see iodine-123 and thallium-201 production below). Most cyclotron-produced radionuclides are neutron poor and therefore decay by positron emission or electron capture. The production methods of several cyclotron-produced radionuclides important to nuclear medicine are shown below (EC = electron capture, $T_{1/2}$ = physical half-life).

Iodine-123 production:

$$^{127}I\,(p, 5n)\,^{123}Xe \xrightarrow[T_{1/2}2h]{EC} {}^{123}I \quad \text{or}$$

$$^{124}Xe\,(p, 2n)\,^{123}Cs \xrightarrow[T_{1/2}1s]{EC\ or\ \beta^+} {}^{123}Xe \xrightarrow[T_{1/2}2h]{EC} {}^{123}I. \qquad [16\text{-}2]$$

Indium-111 production:

$$^{109}Ag\,(\alpha, 2n)\,^{111}In \quad \text{or} \quad ^{111}Cd\,(p, n)\,^{111}In \quad \text{or} \quad ^{112}Cd\,(p, 2n)\,^{111}In.$$

Cobalt-57 production:

$$^{56}Fe\,(d, n)\,^{57}Co.$$

Thallium-201 production:

$$^{203}Tl\,(p, 3n)\,^{201}Pb \xrightarrow[T_{1/2}9.4h]{EC\ or\ \beta^+} {}^{201}Tl.$$

Industrial cyclotron facilities that produce large activities of clinically useful radionuclides are very expensive and require substantial cyclotron and radiochemistry support staff and facilities. Cyclotron-produced radionuclides are usually more expensive than those produced by other technologies.

Much smaller, specialized cyclotrons, installed in commercial radiopharmacies serving metropolitan areas or in hospitals, have been developed to produce positron-emitting radionuclides for positron emission tomography (PET) (Fig. 16-3). These cyclotrons operate at lower energies (10 to 30 MeV) than industrial cyclotrons and commonly accelerate H^- ions, which is a proton with two orbital electrons. In such a cyclotron, the beam is extracted by passing it through a carbon stripping foil, which removes the electrons thus creating an H^+ ion (proton) beam.

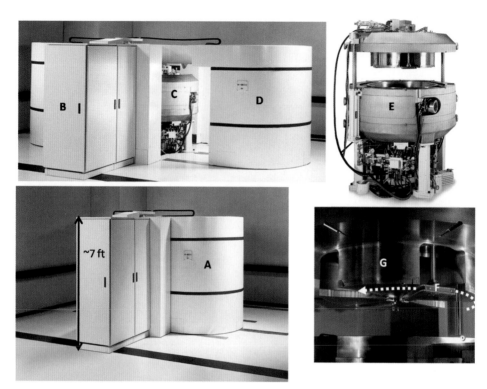

■ FIGURE 16-3 Commercial self-shielded cyclotron for radionuclide production capable of producing a 60 μA beam of protons accelerated to −11 MeV is shown with the radiation shields closed **(A)**. The unit is designed with a small footprint to fit into a relatively small room (24′ × 23′ × 14′ height). **(B)** Power supply and control cabinet. **(C)** Cyclotron assembly approximately 10,000 kg (22,000 lb). **(D)** Retractable radiation shielding (open) approximately 14,500 kg (32,000 lb) of borated concrete and polyethylene. Neutrons and γ radiation are an unavoidable by-product of the nuclear reactions that are used to produce the desired radioactive isotopes. Boron and polyethylene are added to the radiation shield to absorb neutrons. The shielding is designed so that radiation exposure rates are reduced to the point where technologists and other radiation workers can occupy the room while the accelerator is in operation (less than 20 μSv/h at 24 ft from the center of the cyclotron). **(E)** Cyclotron assembly open. Hydrogen gas line at the top of the cyclotron assembly provides the source of hydrogen ions to be accelerated. **(F)** One of four cyclotron dees. The acceleration potential is supplied by high frequency voltage. In this system, four dees provide eight accelerations per orbit, thus reducing acceleration path length and beam loss. **(G)** Beam shaping magnets act as powerful lenses to confine ions to the midplane. The *dotted white arrow* shows the beam path through one of the dees. The radiochemicals produced (in gas or liquid) are sent through tubing in a shielded channel running under the floor to the automated radiochemistry unit located in a shielded enclosure in a room next to the cyclotron. A typical production run from a cyclotron in a commercial radiopharmacy serving a metropolitan area will produce approximately 131 GBq (3.5 Ci) of F-18 during a 2 h irradiation. The radiopharmacy may have three to four production runs a day depending on the clinical demand in the area. (© Siemens Healthineers 2019. Used with permission.)

Because of the change in the polarity of the charge on each particle, the direction of the forces on the moving particles from the magnetic field is reversed and the beam is diverted out of the cyclotron and onto a target. These commercially available specialized medical cyclotrons have a number of advantages, including automated cyclotron operation and radiochemistry modules, allowing a technologist with proper training to operate the unit. Radiation shielding of cyclotrons is always an important consideration; however, the use of negative ions avoids the creation of unwanted radioactivity in the cyclotron housing and thus reduces the amount of radiation shielding necessary. These features substantially reduce the size and weight of the cyclotron facility allowing it to be placed within the hospital close to the PET imaging facilities. Production methods of clinically useful positron-emitting radionuclides are listed below.

$$
\begin{aligned}
&\text{Fluorine-18 production}: {}^{18}\text{O}\,(\text{p, n})\,{}^{18}\text{F} && (T_{1/2} = 110\text{ min})\\
&\text{Nitrogen-13 production}: {}^{16}\text{O}\,(\text{p}, \alpha)\,{}^{13}\text{N} && (T_{1/2} = 10\text{ min})\\
&\text{Oxygen-15 production}: {}^{14}\text{N}\,(\text{d, n})\,{}^{15}\text{O}\text{ or }{}^{15}\text{N}\,(\text{p, n})\,{}^{15}\text{O} && (T_{1/2} = 2.0\text{ min})\\
&\text{Carbon-11 production}: {}^{14}\text{N}\,(\text{p}, \alpha)\,{}^{11}\text{C} && (T_{1/2} = 20.4\text{ min})
\end{aligned}
\qquad [16\text{-}3]
$$

In the interests of design simplicity and cost, some medical cyclotrons accelerate only protons. These advantages may be offset for particular productions such as ^{15}O when an expensive rare isotope ^{15}N that requires proton bombardment must be used in place of the cheap and abundant ^{14}N isotope that requires deuteron bombardment. The medical cyclotrons are usually located near the PET imaging system because of the short half-lives of the radionuclides produced. Fluorine-18 (F-18) is an exception to this generalization owing to its longer half-life (110 min). Regional production and distribution of ^{18}F is thus an option for this commonly used PET radionuclide.

16.1.2 Nuclear Reactor–Produced Radionuclides

Nuclear reactors are another major source of clinically used radionuclides. Neutrons, being uncharged, have an advantage in that they can penetrate the nucleus without being accelerated to high energies. There are two principal methods by which radionuclides are produced in a reactor: nuclear fission and neutron activation.

Nuclear Fission

Fission is the splitting of an atomic nucleus into two smaller nuclei. Whereas some unstable nuclei fission spontaneously, others require the input of energy to overcome the nuclear binding forces. This energy is often provided by the absorption of neutrons. Neutrons can induce fission only in certain very heavy nuclei. Whereas high-energy neutrons can induce fission in several such nuclei, there are only three nuclei of reasonably long half-life that are fissionable by neutrons of all energies; these are called fissile nuclides.

The most widely used fissile nuclide is uranium-235 (U-235). Elemental uranium exists in nature primarily as U-238 (99.3%) with a small fraction of U-235 (0.7%). U-235 has a high fission cross section (*i.e.*, high fission probability); therefore, its concentration is usually enriched (typically to 3% to 5%) to make the fuel used in nuclear reactors.

When a U-235 nucleus absorbs a neutron, the resulting nucleus (U-236) is in an extremely unstable excited energy state that usually promptly fissions into two smaller nuclei called *fission fragments*. The fission fragments separate with very high kinetic energies, with the simultaneous emission of γ radiation and the ejection of two to five neutrons per fission (Eq. 16-4).

$$
{}^{235}_{92}\text{U} + {}^{1}_{0}\text{n}_{\text{thermal}} \rightarrow \left[{}^{235}_{92}\text{U}\right] \nearrow {}^{134}_{50}\text{Sn} \atop \searrow {}^{99}_{42}\text{Mo} \qquad +3{}^{1}_{0}\text{n}_{\text{fast}} + \gamma +{\sim}200\text{ MeV} \qquad [16\text{-}4]
$$

The fission of uranium creates fission fragment nuclei having a wide range of mass numbers. More than 200 radionuclides with mass numbers between 70 and 160 are

■ **FIGURE 16-4** Fission yield as a percentage of total fission products from uranium 235.

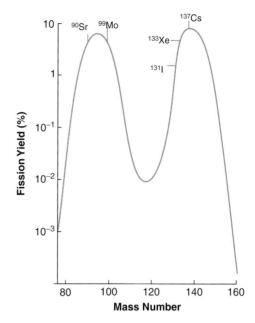

produced by the fission process (Fig. 16-4). These fission products are neutron-rich and therefore almost all of them decay by beta-minus (β^-) particle emission.

Nuclear Reactors and Chain Reactors

The energy released by the nuclear fission of a uranium atom is more than 200 MeV. Under the right conditions, this reaction can be perpetuated if the fission neutrons interact with other U-235 atoms, causing additional fissions and leading to a self-sustaining nuclear chain reaction (Fig. 16-5). The probability of fission with U-235 is greatly enhanced as neutrons slow down or *thermalize*. The neutrons emitted from fission are very energetic (called *fast neutrons*) and are slowed (*moderated*) to thermal energies (~0.025 eV) as they scatter in water in the reactor core. Good moderators are low-Z materials that slow the neutrons without absorbing a significant fraction of them. Water is the most commonly used moderator, although other materials, such as graphite (used in the reactors at the Chernobyl plant in Ukraine) and heavy water (^2H_2O), are also used.

Some neutrons are absorbed by non-fissionable material in the reactor, while others are moderated and absorbed by U-235 atoms and induce additional fissions. The ratio of the number of fissions in one generation to the number in the previous generation is called the *multiplication factor*. When the number of fissions per generation is constant, the multiplication factor is 1 and the reactor is said to be *critical*. When the multiplication factor is greater than 1, the rate of the chain reaction increases, at which time the reactor is said to be *supercritical*. If the multiplication factor is less than 1 (*i.e.*, more neutrons being absorbed than produced), the reactor is said to be *subcritical* and the chain reaction will eventually cease.

This chain reaction process is analogous to a room whose floor is filled with mousetraps, each one having a ping-pong ball placed on the trap. Without any form of control, a self-sustaining chain reaction will be initiated when a single ping-pong ball is tossed into the room and springs one of the traps. The nuclear chain reaction is maintained at the desired level by limiting the number of available neutrons through the use of neutron-absorbing *control rods* (containing boron, cadmium, indium, or a mixture of these elements), which are placed in the reactor core between the fuel elements. Inserting the control rods deeper into the core absorbs more neutrons,

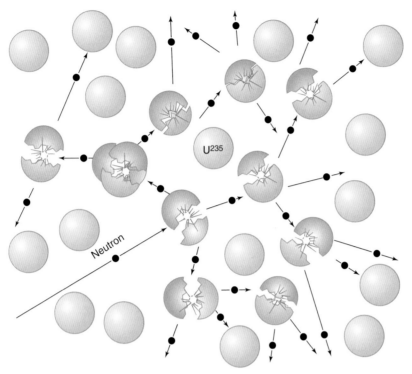

■ **FIGURE 16-5** Schematic of a nuclear chain reaction. The neutrons (shown as small blackened circles) are not drawn to scale with respect to the uranium atoms.

reducing the reactivity (*i.e.*, causing the neutron fluence rate and power output to decrease with time). Removing the control rods has the opposite effect. If a nuclear reactor accident results in loss of the coolant, the fuel can overheat and melt (so-called *meltdown*). However, because of the design characteristics of the reactor and its fuel, an atomic explosion, like those from nuclear weapons, is impossible.

Figure 16-6 is a diagram of a typical radionuclide production reactor. The fuel is processed into rods of uranium-aluminum alloy approximately 6 cm in diameter and 2.5 m long. These *fuel rods* are encased in zirconium or aluminum, which have favorable neutron and heat transport properties. There may be as many as 1,000 fuel rods in the reactor, depending on the design and the neutron fluence rate requirements. Water circulates between the encased fuel rods in a closed loop, whereby the heat generated from the fission process is transferred to cooler water in the heat exchanger. The water in the reactor and heat exchanger are in separate closed loops that do not come into direct physical contact with the fuel. The heat transferred to the cooling water is released to the environment through cooling towers, evaporation ponds, or heat exchangers that transfer the heat to a large body of water. The cooled water is pumped back toward the fuel rods, where it is reheated and the process is repeated.

In commercial nuclear power electric generation stations, the heat generated from the fission process produces high-pressure steam that is directed through a steam turbine, which powers an electrical generator. The steam is then condensed to water by the condenser.

Nuclear reactor safety design principles dictate numerous barriers between the radioactivity in the core and the environment. For example, in commercial power reactors, the fuel is encased in metal fuel rods that are surrounded by water and enclosed in a sealed, pressurized, approximately 30-cm-thick steel

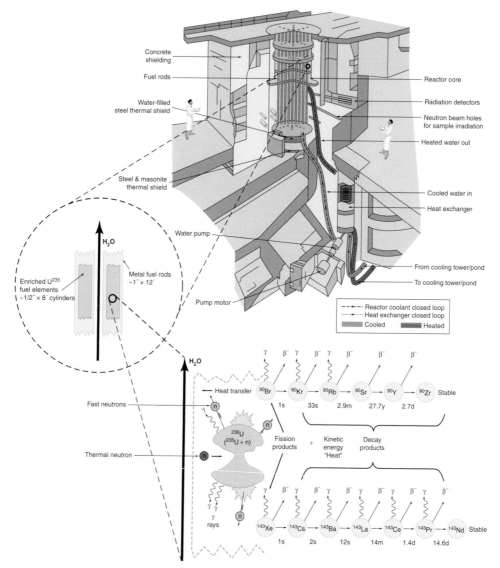

FIGURE 16-6 NRU Radionuclide research/production reactor. (Adapted from diagram provided courtesy of Atomic Energy of Canada and Chalk River Laboratories, Chalk River, Ontario.) Fuel rod assemblies and the fission process are illustrated to show some of the detail and the relationships associated with fission-produced radionuclides.

reactor vessel. These components, together with other highly radioactive reactor systems, are enclosed in a large steel-reinforced concrete shell (~1 to 2 m thick), called the *containment structure*. In addition to serving as a moderator and coolant, the water in the reactor acts as a radiation shield, reducing the radiation levels adjacent to the reactor vessel. Specialized nuclear reactors are used to produce clinically useful radionuclides from fission products or neutron activation of stable target material.

Fission-Produced Radionuclides

The fission products most often used in nuclear medicine are molybdenum-99 (Mo-99), iodine-131 (I-131), and xenon-133 (Xe-133). These products can be chemically separated from other fission products with essentially no stable isotopes (*carrier*) of the radionuclide present. Thus, the concentration or specific activity (measured in MBq or Ci per gram) of these "carrier-free" fission-produced radionuclides is very high. High-specific-activity, carrier-free nuclides are preferred in radiopharmaceutical preparations to increase the labeling efficiency of the preparations and minimize the mass and volume of the injected material.

Neutron Activation–Produced Radionuclides

Neutrons produced by the fission of uranium in a nuclear reactor can be used to create radionuclides by bombarding stable target material placed in the reactor. Ports exist in the reactor core between the fuel elements where samples to be irradiated are inserted. This process, called *neutron activation*, involves the capture of neutrons by stable nuclei, which results in the production of radioactive nuclei. The most common neutron capture reaction for thermal (slow) neutrons is the (n,γ) reaction, in which the capture of the neutron by a nucleus is immediately followed by the emission of a γ-ray. Other thermal neutron capture reactions include the (n,p) and (n,α) reactions, in which the neutron capture is followed by the emission of a proton or an alpha particle, respectively. However, because thermal neutrons can induce these reactions only in a few, low-atomic-mass target nuclides, most neutron activation uses the (n,γ) reaction. Almost all radionuclides produced by neutron activation decay by beta-minus particle emission. Examples of radionuclides produced by neutron activation useful to nuclear medicine are listed below.

$$\text{Phosphorus-32 production}: {}^{31}\text{P}\,(n,\gamma)\,{}^{32}\text{P} \quad (T_{1/2}=14.3\,\text{days})$$
$$\text{Chromium-51 production}: {}^{50}\text{Cr}\,(n,\gamma)\,{}^{51}\text{Cr} \quad (T_{1/2}=27.8\,\text{days})$$

[16-5]

A radionuclide produced by an (n,γ) reaction is an isotope of the target element. As such, its chemistry is identical to that of the target material, making chemical separation techniques useless. Furthermore, no matter how long the target material is irradiated by neutrons, only a small fraction of the target atoms will undergo neutron capture and become activated. Therefore, the material removed from the reactor will not be carrier-free because it will always contain stable isotopes of the radionuclide. In addition, impurities in the target material will cause the production of other radionuclides. The presence of carrier in the mixture limits the ability to concentrate the radionuclide of interest and therefore lowers the specific activity. For this reason, many of the clinically used radionuclides that could be produced by neutron activation (*e.g.*, ${}^{131}\text{I}$, ${}^{99}\text{Mo}$) are instead produced by nuclear fission to maximize specific activity. An exception to the limitations of neutron activation is the production of ${}^{125}\text{I}$, in which neutron activation of the target material, ${}^{124}\text{Xe}$, produces a radioisotope, ${}^{125}\text{Xe}$, that decays to form the desired radioisotope (Eq. 16-6). In this case, the product radioisotope can be chemically or physically separated from the target material. Various characteristics of radionuclide production are compared in Table 16-1.

$$ {}^{14}\text{Xe}\,(n,\gamma)\,{}^{125}\text{Xe} \xrightarrow[T_{1/2}17\,h]{EC\ or\ \beta^{+}} {}^{125}\text{I} $$

[16-6]

16.1.3 Radionuclide Generators

Since the mid-1960s, technetium-99m (Tc-99m) has been the most important radionuclide used in nuclear medicine for a wide variety of radiopharmaceutical applications. However, its relatively short half-life (6 h) makes it impractical to store even

TABLE 16-1 COMPARISON OF RADIONUCLIDE PRODUCTION METHODS

CHARACTERISTIC	PRODUCTION METHOD			
	Linear Accelerator/ Cyclotron	*Nuclear Reactor (Fission)*	*Nuclear Reactor (Neutron Activation)*	*Radionuclide Generator*
Bombarding particle	Proton, alpha	Neutron	Neutron	Production by decay of parent
Product	Neutron poor	Neutron excess	Neutron excess	Neutron poor or excess
Typical decay pathway	Positron emission, electron capture	Beta-minus	Beta-minus	Several modes
Typically carrier free	Yes	Yes	No	Yes
High specific activity	Yes	Yes	No	Yes
Relative cost	High	Low	Low	Low (^{99m}TC) High (^{82}Rb)
Radionuclides for nuclear medicine applications	^{11}C, ^{13}N, ^{15}O, ^{18}F, ^{57}Co, ^{67}Ga, ^{68}Ge, ^{111}In, ^{123}I, ^{201}Tl	^{99}Mo, ^{131}I, ^{133}Xe	^{32}P, ^{51}Cr, ^{89}Sr, ^{125}I, ^{153}Sm	^{68}Ga, ^{81m}Kr, ^{82}Rb, ^{90}Y, ^{99m}Tc

a weekly supply. This supply problem is overcome by obtaining the parent Mo-99, which has a longer half-life (67 h) and continually produces Tc-99m. The Tc-99m is collected periodically in sufficient quantities for clinical operations. A system for holding the parent in such a way that the daughter can be easily separated for clinical use is called a *radionuclide generator*.

Molybdenum-99/Technetium-99m Radionuclide Generator

In a molybdenum-99/technetium-99m radionuclide generator, Mo-99 (produced by nuclear fission of U-235 to yield a high-specific-activity, carrier-free parent) is loaded, in the form of ammonium molybdenate ($NH4^+$)(MoO_4^-), onto a porous column containing 5 to 10 g of an alumina (Al_2O_3) resin. The ammonium molybdenite becomes attached to the surface of the alumina molecules (a process called *adsorption*). The porous nature of the alumina provides a large surface area for the adsorption of the parent.

As with all radionuclide generators, the chemical properties of the parent and daughter are different. In the Mo-99/Tc-99m or "moly" generator, the Tc-99m is much less tightly bound than the Mo-99. The daughter is removed (*eluted*) by the flow of isotonic (normal, 0.9%) saline (the "eluant") through the column. When the saline solution is passed through the column, the chloride ions easily exchange with the TcO_4^- (but not the MoO_4^-) ions, producing sodium pertechnetate, $Na^+(^{99m}TcO_4^-)$. Technetium-99m pertechnetate ($^{99m}TcO_4^-$) is produced in a sterile, pyrogen-free form with high specific activity and a pH (~5.5) that is ideally suited for radiopharmaceutical preparations.

Commercially moly generators have a large reservoir of oxygenated saline (the eluant) connected by tubing to one end of the column and a vacuum extraction vial to the other. On insertion of the vacuum collection vial (contained in a shielded elution tool), saline is drawn through the column and the eluate is collected during elution, which takes about 1 to 2 min. Figure 16-7 is a picture and cross-sectional diagram of a moly generator together with an insert that shows details of the generator column. Sterility is achieved by a Millipore filter connected to the end of the column, by the

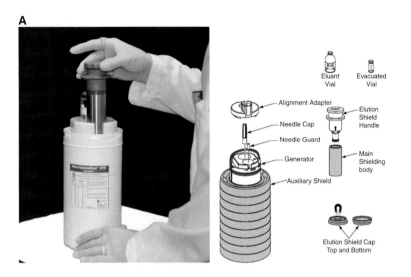

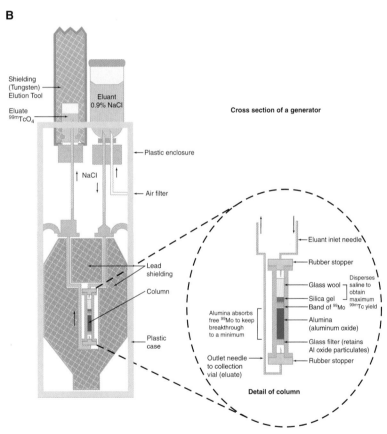

■ **FIGURE 16-7 A.** Picture of a "wet" molybdenum 99/technetium 99m generator in the process of being eluted (left). A spent generator that is no longer radioactive was used in order to minimize dose. For picture clarity, the shielding normally surrounding the generator is not shown [as illustrated in the accompanying diagram (right)]. However, correct radiation safety principles (discussed further in Chapter 21) are shown including the use of disposable gloves, finger ring and body dosimeters, and disposable plastic backed absorbent paper on the bench top to minimize the spread of any contamination. An explosion diagram depicting the generator components, and auxiliary radiation shielding is shown on the right. **B.** A cross-sectional diagram of the generator interior and column detail. Consult the text for additional information on the elution process. (Adapted from photo and diagrams provided courtesy of Curium US LLC, St. Louis, MO.)

use of a bacteriostatic agent in the eluant, or by autoclave sterilization of the loaded column by the manufacturer.

Moly generators are typically delivered with approximately 37 to 740 GBq (1 to 20 Ci) of Mo-99, depending on the workload of the department. The larger activity generators are typically used by commercial radiopharmacies supplying radiopharmaceuticals to multiple nuclear medicine departments. The generators are shielded by the manufacture with lead, tungsten, or, in the case of higher activity generators, depleted uranium. Additional shielding is typically placed around the generator to reduce the exposure of staff during elution. The activity of the daughter at the time of elution depends on the following:

1. The activity of the parent
2. The rate of formation of the daughter, which is equal to the rate of decay of the parent (*i.e.*, $A_0 e^{-\lambda_p t}$)
3. The decay rate of the daughter
4. The time since the last elution
5. The elution efficiency (typically 80% to 90%)

Transient Equilibrium

Between elutions, the daughter (Tc-99m) builds up or "grows in" as the parent (Mo-99) continues to decay. After approximately 23 h, the Tc-99m activity reaches a maximum, at which time the production rate and the decay rate are equal and the parent and daughter are said to be in *transient equilibrium*. Once transient equilibrium has been achieved, the daughter activity decreases, with an apparent half-life equal to the half-life of the parent. Transient equilibrium occurs when the half-life of the parent is greater than that of the daughter by a factor of approximately 10. In the general case of transient equilibrium, the daughter activity will exceed the parent at equilibrium. If all of the (Mo-99) decayed to Tc-99m, the Tc-99m activity would slightly exceed (~10% higher) that of the parent at equilibrium. However, approximately 12% of Mo-99 decays directly to Tc-99 without first producing Tc-99m, Figure 16-8.

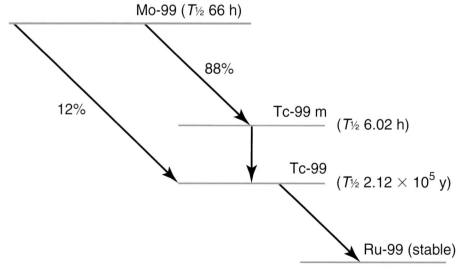

■ **FIGURE 16-8** Simplified decay scheme of Mo-99. Mo-99 decays to Tc-99m approximately 88% of the time. Thus is due to the β_8 transition directly to Tc-99m (~82.2%) along with several other beta transitions to excited states that emit γ-rays (principally the β_4 γ_{10} and β_7 γ_4) to yield Tc-99m. The balance (12%) of Mo-99 decays occurs by other beta transitions to excited states that ultimately yield Tc-99 bypassing the metastable form of Tc (Tc-99m).

Therefore, at equilibrium, the Tc-99m activity will be only approximately 97% (1.1 × 0.88) that of the parent (Mo-99) activity.

Moly generators (sometimes called "cows") are usually delivered weekly and eluted (a process referred to as "milking the cow") each morning, allowing maximal yield of the daughter. The elution process is approximately 90% efficient. This fact, together with the limitations on Tc-99m yield in the Mo-99 decay scheme, results in a maximum elution yield of approximately 85% of the Mo-99 activity at the time of elution. Therefore, a typical elution on Monday morning from a moly generator with 55.5 GBq (1.5 Ci) of Mo-99 yields approximately 47.2 GBq (1.28 Ci) of Tc-99m in 10 mL of normal saline (a common elution volume). By Friday morning of that same week, the same generator would be capable of delivering only about 17.2 GBq (0.47 Ci). The moly generator can be eluted more frequently than every 23 h; however, the Tc-99m yield will be less. Approximately half of the maximal yield will be available 6 h after the last elution. Figure 16-9 shows a typical time-activity curve for a moly generator.

Secular Equilibrium

Although the moly generator is by far the most widely used in nuclear medicine, other generator systems produce clinically useful radionuclides. When the half-life of the parent is much longer than that of the daughter (*i.e.*, more than about 100 times longer), *secular equilibrium* occurs after approximately five to six half-lives of the daughter. In secular equilibrium, the activity of the parent and the daughter are the same if all of the parent atoms decay directly to the daughter. Once secular equilibrium is achieved, the daughter will have an apparent half-life equal to that of

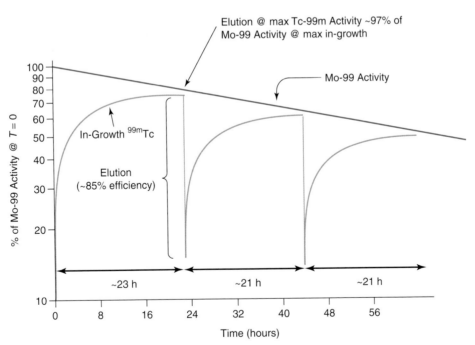

■ **FIGURE 16-9** Time-activity curve of a molybdenum 99/technetium 99m radionuclide generator system demonstrating the ingrowth of Tc-99m and subsequent elution. The time to maximum Tc-99m activity, approximately 23 h, assumes there is no residual Tc-99m from a previous elution of the column. Typical elution efficiency is approximately 85% (~15% residual Tc-99m), thus time to maximum Tc-99m activity following the first elution is approximately 21 h. Approximately 50% of the maximum Tc-99m activity is obtained in 6 h. The maximum Tc-99m activity in the eluate is typically 80% to 90% of Mo-99 activity.

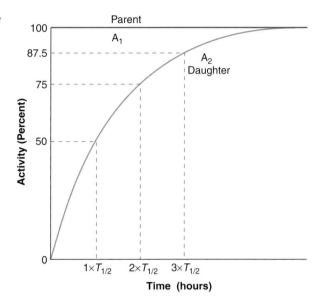

■ **FIGURE 16-10** Time-activity curve demonstrating secular equilibrium.

the parent. The strontium-82/rubidium-82 (Sr-82/Rb-82) generator, with parent and daughter half-lives of 25.5 d and 75 s, respectively, reach secular equilibrium within approximately 7.5 min after elution. Figure 16-10 shows a time-activity curve demonstrating secular equilibrium. The characteristics of radionuclide generator systems are compared in Table 16-2.

Quality Control

The users of moly generators are required to perform molybdenum and alumina breakthrough tests. Mo-99 contamination in the Tc-99m eluate is called *molybdenum breakthrough*. Mo-99 is an undesirable contaminant because its long half-life and highly energetic betas increase the radiation dose to the patient without providing any clinical information. The high-energy γ-rays (~740 and 780 keV) are very penetrating and cannot be efficiently detected by scintillation cameras. The *U.S. Pharmacopeia* (USP) and the U.S. Nuclear Regulatory Commission (NRC) limit the Mo-99 contamination to 0.15 μCi of Mo-99 per mCi of Tc-99m or (0.15 kBq/MBq) at the time of administration. Contaminant limits are specified in 10CFR35.204 and include

TABLE 16-2 CLINICALLY USED RADIONUCLIDE GENERATOR SYSTEMS IN NUCLEAR MEDICINE

PARENT	DECAY MODE AND (HALF-LIFE)	DAUGHTER	TIME OF MAXIMAL INGROWTH (EQUILIBRIUM)	DECAY MODE AND (HALF-LIFE)	DECAY PRODUCT
^{68}Ge	EC (271 d)	^{68}Ga	~6.5 h (S)	β$^+$ EC (68 min)	^{68}Zn (stable)
^{90}Sr	β$^-$ (28.8 y)	^{90}Y	~1 mo (S)	β$^-$ (2.67 d)	^{90}Zr (stable)
^{81}Rb	β$^+$ EC (4.6 h)	^{81m}Kr	~80 s (S)	IT (13.5 s)	^{81}Kr[a]
^{82}Sr	EC (25.5 d)	^{82}Rb	~7.5 min (S)	β$^+$ (75 s)	^{82}Kr (stable)
^{99}Mo	β$^-$ (67 h)	^{99m}Tc	~24 h (T)	IT (6 h)	^{99}Tc[a]

Note: Decay modes: EC, electron capture; β$^+$, positron emission; β$^-$, beta-minus; IT, isometric transition (*i.e.*, γ-ray emission). Radionuclide equilibrium: T, transients; S, secular.
[a]These nuclides have half-lives greater than 10^5 years and for medical applications can be considered to be essentially stable.

those for the Rb-82 generators: 0.02 µCi of Sr-85 per mCi of Rb-82 or (0.02 kBq/MBq). The Mo-99 contamination is evaluated by placing the Tc-99m eluate in a thick (~6 mm) lead container (provided by the dose calibrator manufacturer), which is placed in the dose calibrator. The high-energy photons of Mo-99 can be detected, whereas virtually all of the Tc-99m 140-keV photons are attenuated by the lead container. Eluates from moly generators rarely exceed permissible Mo-99 contamination limits. The quality control procedures to evaluate breakthrough of radionuclidic contaminates in the eluates from Mo-99/Tc-99m and Sr-82/Rb-82 generators are discussed further in Chapter 17 in the context of dose calibrator operations and quality control. It is also possible (although rare) for some of the alumina from the column to contaminate the Tc-99m eluate. Alumina interferes with the preparation of some radiopharmaceuticals (especially sulfur colloid and Tc-99m-labeled red blood cell preparations). The USP limits the amount of alumina to no more than 10 mg alumina per mL of Tc-99m eluate. Commercially available paper test strips and test standards are used to assay for alumina concentrations.

16.2 RADIOPHARMACEUTICALS

16.2.1 Characteristics, Applications, Quality Control, and Regulatory Issues in Medical Imaging

The vast majority of radiopharmaceuticals in nuclear medicine today use Tc-99m as the radionuclide. Most Tc-99m radiopharmaceuticals are easily prepared by aseptically injecting a known quantity of Tc-99m pertechnetate into a sterile vial containing the lyophilized (freeze-dried) pharmaceutical. The radiopharmaceutical complex is, in most cases, formed instantaneously and can be used for multiple doses over a period of several hours. Radiopharmaceuticals can be prepared in this fashion (called "kits") as needed in the nuclear medicine department, or they may be delivered to the department by a centralized commercial radiopharmacy that serves several hospitals in the area. Although most Tc-99m radiopharmaceuticals can be prepared rapidly and easily at room temperature, several products (e.g., Tc-99m sulfur colloid), require multiple steps such as boiling the Tc-99m reagent complex for several minutes. In almost all cases, however, the procedures are simple and the labeling efficiencies are very high (typically greater than 95%).

Other radionuclides common to diagnostic nuclear medicine imaging include ^{123}I, ^{67}Ga, ^{111}In, ^{133}Xe, and ^{201}Tl. Positron-emitting radionuclides are used for PET. F-18, as fluorodeoxyglucose (FDG), is used in approximately 85% of all clinical PET applications. Rubidium-82 (^{82}Rb) is used to assess myocardial perfusion using PET/CT imaging systems, in place of Tl-201 and Tc-99m based myocardial perfusion agents that are imaged using scintillation cameras. A wide variety of other positron-emitting radionuclides are currently being evaluated for their clinical utility, including carbon-11 (^{11}C), nitrogen-13 (^{13}N), oxygen-15 (^{15}O), and gallium-68 (^{68}Ga). The physical characteristics, most common modes of production, decay characteristics, and primary imaging photons (where applicable) of the radionuclides used in nuclear medicine are summarized in Table 16-3.

16.2.2 Ideal Diagnostic Radiopharmaceuticals

Although there are no truly "ideal" diagnostic radiopharmaceuticals, it is helpful to think of currently used agents in light of a set of ideal characteristics for radiopharmaceuticals applied to medical imaging of disease or evaluating the progress of prescribed therapy.

TABLE 16-3 PHYSICAL CHARACTERISTICS OF CLINICALLY USED RADIONUCLIDES

RADIONUCLIDE	METHOD OF PRODUCTION	MODE OF DECAY (%)	PRINCIPAL PHOTONS keV (% ABUNDANCE)	PHYSICAL HALF-LIFE	COMMENTS
Radionuclides Used in Diagnostic Nuclear Medicine Imaging (Planar Imaging and SPECT)					
Chromium-51 (^{51}Cr)	Neutron activation	EC (100)	320 (9)	27.8 d	Used for in vivo red cell mass determinations (not used for imaging; samples counted in a NaI(Tl) well counter).
Cobalt-57 (^{57}Co)	Cyclotron produced	EC (100)	122 (86) 136 (11)	271 d	Principally used as a uniform flood field source for scintillation camera quality control.
Gallium-67 (^{67}Ga)	Cyclotron produced	EC (100)	93 (40) 184 (20) 300 (17) 393 (4)	78 h	Typically use the 93, 184, and 300 keV photons for imaging.
Indium-111 (^{111}In)	Cyclotron produced	EC (100)	171 (90) 245 (94)	2.8 d	Typically used when the kinetics require imaging more than 24 h after injection. Both photons are used in imaging.
Iodine-123 (^{123}I)	Cyclotron produced	EC (100)	159 (83)	13.2 h	Has replaced ^{131}I for diagnostic imaging to reduce patient radiation dose.
Iodine 125 (^{125}I)	Neutron activation	EC (100)	35 (6) 27 (39) XR 28 (76) XR 31 (20) XR	60.2 d	Typically used as ^{125}I albumin for in vivo blood/plasma volume determinations (not used for imaging; samples counted in a NaI(Tl) well counter).
Krypton-81m (^{81m}Kr)	Generator product	IT (100)	190 (67) 181 (6) 740 (12)	13 s	This ultrashort-lived generator-produced radionuclide is a gas and is used to perform serial lung ventilation studies with very little radiation exposure to patient or staff. The expense and short $T_{1/2}$ of the parent (^{81}Rb, 4.6 h) limits its use.
Molybdenum-99 (^{99}Mo)	Nuclear fission (^{235}U)	β⁻ (100)	740 (12) 780 (4)	67 h	Parent material for Mo/Tc generator. Not used directly as a radiopharmaceutical; 740- and 780-keV photons used to identify "moly breakthrough."
Technetium-99m (^{99m}Tc)	Generator product	IT (100)	140 (88)	6.02 h	This radionuclide is used in radiopharmaceuticals that account for >70% of all nuclear medicine imaging studies.
Xenon-133 (^{133}Xe)	Nuclear fission (^{235}U)	β⁻ (100)	81 (37)	5.3 d	^{133}Xe is a heavier-than-air gas. Low abundance and low energy of photon reduces image resolution.

Radionuclide	Production	Half-life	Decay Mode (%)	Principal Photons keV (%)	Comments
Thallium-201 (^{201}Tl)	Cyclotron produced	73.1 h	EC (100)	69–80 (94) XR	The majority of clinically used photons are low-energy x-rays (69–80 keV) from mercury 201 (^{201}Hg), the daughter of ^{201}Tl. Although these photons are in high abundance (94%), their low energy results in significant patient attenuation. This issue is of particular concern in female patients in whom breast artifacts may appear in myocardial imaging.
Radionuclides Used in Diagnostic Nuclear Medicine Imaging (PET)					
Carbon-11 (^{11}C)	Cyclotron produced	20.4 min	β^+ (99.8)	511 AR (200)	Carbon-11 production: 14N (p,α) ^{11}C Short half-life requires on-site cyclotron for imaging. Primarily clinical research applications.
Fluorine-18 (^{18}F)	Cyclotron produced	110 min	β^+ (97) EC (3)	511 AR (193)	This radionuclides accounts for more than 70%–80% of all clinical PET studies; typically formulated as FDG Cyclotron produced via ^{18}O (p,n)^{18}F reaction.
Nitrogen-13 (^{13}N)	Cyclotron produced	10 min	β^+ (99.8)	511 AR (200)	Cyclotron produced via ^{16}O (p,α)^{13}N reaction. Short half-life requires on-site cyclotron for imaging. Primarily clinical research applications.
Oxygen-15 (^{15}O)	Cyclotron produced	122 s	β^+ (99.9)	511 AR (200)	Cyclotron produced via ^{14}N(d,n)^{15}O or ^{15}N(p,n)^{15}O. Short half-life requires on-site cyclotron for imaging. Primarily clinical research applications.
Gallium-68 (^{68}Ga)	Generator product	68 min	β^+ (89) EC (11)	511 AR (184)	Ga-68 is a generator decay product of Ge-68, which is linear accelerator produced via a ^{69}Ga(p,2n)^{68}Ge reaction.
Rubidium-82 (^{82}Rb)	Generator product	78 s	β^+ (95) EC (15)	511 AR (190) 776 (13)	Rb-82 is a generator decay product of Sr-82, which in turn is cyclotron produced via the 85Rb(p,4n)82Sr reaction. The half-life of Sr-82 is 25 d (or 600 h). Sr-82 is thus in secular equilibrium with Rb-82 within ~8 min after elution.
Radionuclides Used in Radiopharmaceutical Therapy (Alpha-Emitters)					
Astatine-211 (^{211}At)	Cyclotron produced	7.2 h	α (42) EC (5)	^{211}Po x-rays ^{211}Po γ-rays	^{211}Po (α), ^{207}Bi (β^-), and ^{207}Pb (stable)
Lead-212 (^{212}Pb)	Generator product	10.6 h	β^- (100)	239 (43)	^{212}Pb is the parent of ^{212}Bi (see below)
Bismuth-212 (^{212}Bi)	Generator product or decay of ^{232}Th	1.0 h	α (36) β^- (64)	67–91 220–257	^{208}Tl (β^-), ^{212}Po (α), ^{208}Pb (stable)

(Continued)

TABLE 16-3 PHYSICAL CHARACTERISTICS OF CLINICALLY USED RADIONUCLIDES (Continued)

RADIONUCLIDE	METHOD OF PRODUCTION	MODE OF DECAY (%)	PRINCIPAL PHOTONS keV (% ABUNDANCE)	PHYSICAL HALF-LIFE	COMMENTS
Bismuth-213 (^{213}Bi)	Generator product	α (2) β⁻ (98)	440 (26)	45.6 m	^{209}Tl (β⁻), ^{213}Po (α), ^{209}Pb (β⁻), ^{209}Bi (stable)
Radium-223 (^{223}Ra)	Neutron activation	α (100)	154, 270, 351, 405 (progeny)	11.4 d	^{219}Rn (α), ^{214}Po (α), ^{211}Pb (β⁻), ^{211}Bi (α/β⁻), ^{207}Tl (β⁻), ^{211}Po(α), ^{207}Pb (stable)
Actinium-225 (^{225}Ac)	Cyclotron produced or decay of ^{233}U	α (100)	440 (26) of ^{213}Bi	10.0 d	^{211}Fr (α), ^{217}At (α), and followed by ^{213}Bi (see above)
Thorium-227 (^{227}Th)	Neutron activation of decay of ^{235}U	α (100)	12.3, 15.2, 236	18.7 d	^{227}Th is the parent of ^{223}Ra (see above)
Radionuclides Used in Radiopharmaceutical Therapy (Beta-Emitters)					
Phosphorus-32 (^{32}P)	Neutron activation	β⁻ (100)	None	14.3 d	Prepared as either sodium phosphate for treatment of myeloproliferative disorders such as polycythemia vera and thrombocytosis or colloidal chromic phosphate for intracavitary therapy of malignant ascites, malignant pleural effusions, malignant pericardial effusions, and malignant brain cysts.
Strontium-89 (^{89}Sr)	Neutron activation	β⁻ (100)	Bremsstrahlung x-rays	50.5 d	As strontium chloride for pain relief from metastatic bone lesions.
Yttrium-90 (^{90}Y)	Generator product daughter of ^{90}Sr	β⁻ (100)	Bremsstrahlung x-rays (0.0032) AR	2.7 d	The radionuclide is bound to microspheres (glass or resin) for intrahepatic arterial delivery of the Y-90 microspheres for the treatment of unresectable metastatic liver tumors ^{90}Y-DOTATOC and ^{90}Y-DOTATATE are therapy radiopharmaceutical for treatment of neuroendocrine tumors that express somatostatin receptors. ^{90}Y-ibritumomab is used for therapy of CD20+ relapsed or refractory, low-grade or follicular B-cell non-Hodgkin's lymphoma.

Radionuclide	Production Method	Decay Mode (%)	Photon Energies keV (%)	Half-Life	Comments
Iodine-124 (^{124}I)	Cyclotron produced		511 (46) AR	4.2 d	I-124 is an alternative to 131 for treatment of differentiated thyroid cancer, which further allows PET imaging of its biodistribution.
Iodine-131 (^{131}I)	Neutron activation or nuclear fission (^{235}U)	β^- (100)	80 (2.6) 284 (6) 364 (82) 637 (7) 732 (1.8)	8.0 d	Used for treatment of hyperthyroidism and thyroid cancer: 364-keV photon used for imaging. Resolution and detection efficiency are poor due to high energy of photons. High patient dose, mostly from β-particles. Used as the therapy radionuclide for ^{131}I-MIBG (metaiodobenzylguanidine) for the treatment of neuroblastoma in children and young adults. Prior to 2014, ^{131}I-tositumomab was used for therapy of CD20+ relapsed or refractory, low-grade or follicular B-cell non-Hodgkin's lymphoma.
Samarium-153 (^{153}Sm)	Neutron activation	β^- (100)	69 (4.8) 103 (30) 635 (32)	46.3 h	As ^{153}Sm ethylene diamine tetra methylene phosphonic acid (EDTMP) used for pain relief from metastatic bone lesions. Advantage compared to ^{89}Sr is that the ^{153}Sm distribution can be imaged.
Lutetium-177 (^{177}Lu)	Neutron activation	β^- (100)	133 (6) 208 (11)	6.7 d	^{177}Lu-DOTATATE is a therapy radiopharmaceutical for treatment of neuroendocrine tumors that express somatostatin receptors.
Rhenium-186 (^{186}Re)	Neutron activation	β^- (92.5) EC (7.5)	137 (9)	3.7 d	^{186}Re-HEDP has been used as an alternative to ^{153}Sm-EDTMP for pain relief from metastatic bone lesions. The radionuclide has also be used in radiopharmaceuticals for prostate, breast, colon, lung, and skin cancer therapy.
Rhenium-188 (^{188}Re)	Neutron activation	β^- (100)	155 (15) 478 (1) 633 (1)	17 h	^{188}Re-HEDP has been used as an alternative to ^{153}Sm-EDTMP for pain relief from metastatic bone lesions. The radionuclide has also be used in radiopharmaceuticals for prostate, breast, colon, lung, and skin cancer therapy.
Radionuclides Used in Radiopharmaceutical Therapy (Auger Electron-Emitters)					
Palladium-103 (^{103}Pd)	Neutron activation	EC (100)	20–27 (7) XR	17.0 d	Pd-103 is been traditionally used as a therapy radionuclide for brachytherapy seeds in the treatment of prostate and cervical cancer. The radionuclide is also a potential therapy agent as labeled to albumin microspheres (AMS).

(Continued)

TABLE 16-3 PHYSICAL CHARACTERISTICS OF CLINICALLY USED RADIONUCLIDES (Continued)

RADIONUCLIDE	METHOD OF PRODUCTION	MODE OF DECAY (%)	PRINCIPAL PHOTONS keV (% ABUNDANCE)	PHYSICAL HALF-LIFE	COMMENTS
Indium-111 (^{111}In)	Cyclotron produced	EC (100)	171 (90) 245 (94)	2.8 d	High-administered activity ^{111}In-octreotide therapy has been used for patients with disseminated neuroendocrine tumors (NET) with high somatostatin receptor (SSR)
Tin-117m (^{117}Sn)	Neutron activation	IT (100)	156 (2) 159 (86)	13.6 d	Sn-117m diethylenetriaminepentaacetic acid (^{117m}Sn DTPA) is a radiopharmaceutical agent for the palliation of pain from bony metastases.
Iodine-123 (^{123}I)	Cyclotron produced	EC (100)	159 (83)	13.2 h	I-123 is used in pretherapy scans of patients with thyroid cancer to provide information on the amount of thyroid remnant, sometimes indicating the need for two-step I-131 ablation. It may also detect unsuspected local lymph node involvement or distant metastases, indicating the requirement for a higher I-131 dose after thyroidectomy.
Iodine-125 (^{125}I)	Neutron activation	EC (100)	35 (6) 27 (39) XR 28 (76) XR 31 (20) XR	60.2 d	Use as ^{125}I Iotrex liquid brachytherapy source in Proxima GliaSite radiation therapy system for treatment of recurrent gliomas and metastatic brain tumors.
Platinum-193m (^{193m}Pt)	Cyclotron produced	IT (100)	135 (0.11) 65–79 (14)	4.3 d	Potential radionuclide for chemoradiotherapy in which the chemotherapy drug cisplatin forms DNA-platinum adducts that are targeted to cancer cells. Cisplatin and Auger-electron radiation has demonstrated synergism in their cell killing effects.
Platinum-195m (^{195m}Pt)	Neutron activation	IT (100)	31 (2) 99 (11) 130 (3)	4.2 d	Potential radionuclide for chemoradiotherapy in which the chemotherapy drug cisplatin forms DNA-platinum adducts that are targeted to cancer cells. Cisplatin and Auger-electron radiation has demonstrated synergism in their cell killing effects.

Note: α, alpha decay; β−, beta-minus decay; β+, beta-plus (positron) decay; AR, annihilation radiation; EC, electron capture; IT, isomeric transition (*i.e.*, γ-ray emission), XR, x-ray.

Low Radiation Dose

It is important to minimize radiation exposure to patients while preserving the diagnostic quality of the image. Radionuclides can be selected that have few particulate emissions and a high abundance of clinically useful photons. Most modern scintillation cameras are optimized for photon energies close to 140 keV, which is a compromise among patient attenuation, spatial resolution, and detection efficiency. Photons whose energies are too low are largely attenuated by the body, increasing the patient dose without contributing to image formation. High-energy photons are more likely to escape the body but have poor detection efficiency and easily penetrate collimator septa of scintillation cameras (see Chapter 18). A radiopharmaceutical should have an effective half-life long enough to complete the study with an adequate concentration in the tissues of interest, but short enough to minimize the patient dose.

High Target-to-Non-Target Activity

The ability to detect and evaluate lesions depends largely on the concentration of the radiopharmaceutical in the organ, tissue or, lesion of interest or on a clinically useful uptake and clearance pattern. Maximizing the concentration of the radiopharmaceutical in the target tissues of interest while minimizing the uptake in surrounding (non-target) tissues and organs improves contrast and the ability to detect subtle abnormalities in the radiopharmaceutical's biodistribution. Maximizing this target/non-target ratio is characteristic of all clinically useful radiopharmaceuticals and is improved by observing the recommended interval between injection and imaging for the specific agent. This interval is a compromise between the uptake of the activity in the target tissue, washout of the activity in the background (non-target) tissues, and practical considerations of clinic operations. With some radiopharmaceuticals such as the bone scanning agent, Tc-99m labeled methylene-diphosphonate (99m Tc-MDP), instructions to the patient, needed both to improve image quality and to reduce radiation dose to patient and technologist, might include the request to be well hydrated and to void the urinary bladder just prior to imaging. Abnormalities can be identified as localized areas of increased radiopharmaceutical concentration, called "hot spots" (*e.g.*, a stress fracture in a bone scan), or as "cold spots" or "photopenic regions" in which the radiopharmaceutical's normal localization in tissue is altered by a disease process (*e.g.*, perfusion defect in a lung scan with ^{99m}Tc-MAA). Disassociation of the radionuclide from the radiopharmaceutical alters the desired biodistribution, thus degrading image quality. Good quality control over radiopharmaceutical preparation helps to ensure that the radionuclide continues to be chemically bound to the pharmaceutical throughout the imaging session.

Safety, Convenience, and Cost Effectiveness

Low chemical toxicity is enhanced by the use of high-specific-activity, carrier-free radionuclides that also facilitate radiopharmaceutical preparation and minimize the required amount of the isotope. For example, 3.7 GBq (100 mCi) of I-131 contains only 0.833 µg of iodine. Radionuclides should also have a chemical form, pH, concentration, and other characteristics that facilitate rapid complexing with the pharmaceutical under normal laboratory conditions. The compounded radiopharmaceutical should be stable, with a shelf life compatible with clinical use, and should be readily available from several manufacturers to minimize cost.

16.2.3 Therapeutic Radiopharmaceuticals

Radiopharmaceuticals are also used for the treatment of a number of diseases. The goal of radiopharmaceutical therapy is to deliver a sufficiently large dose to the target organ, tissue, or cell type while limiting the dose to non-targeted tissues to minimize deterministic effects such as bone marrow suppression and to minimize the risk of cancer. Prior to 2013, all approved therapeutic radiopharmaceuticals were based radionuclides that decayed either through beta-particle emission (^{32}P, ^{89}Sr, ^{90}Y, ^{124}I, ^{131}I, ^{153}Sm, ^{177}Lu, ^{186}Re, and ^{188}Re) or Auger electron emission (^{103}Pd, ^{111}In, ^{117m}Sn, ^{123}I, ^{125}I, ^{193m}Pt, or ^{195m}Pt). In May of 2013, the U.S. FDA approved the first therapy radiopharmaceutical using an alpha-particle emitter: Xofigo (radium Ra 223 dichloride) for the treatment of patients with castration-resistant prostate cancer (CRPC), symptomatic bone metastases, and no known visceral metastatic disease. Since that milestone, there has been significant research activities and ongoing clinical trials in the development of other alpha-emitter therapy radiopharmaceuticals across a variety of cancer types such as breast, prostate, neuroendocrine tumors, and leukemia. Alpha-emitters of current interest in radiopharmaceutical therapy include ^{211}At, ^{212}Pb, ^{212}Bi, ^{213}Bi, ^{223}Ra, ^{225}Ac, and ^{227}Th. Further details for therapeutic radionuclides – alpha, beta, and Auger emitters – are given in Table 16-3.

16.2.4 Radiopharmaceutical Mechanism of Localization

Radiopharmaceutical concentration in tissue is driven by one or more of the following mechanisms: (1) compartmental localization and leakage, (2) cell sequestration, (3) phagocytosis, (4) passive diffusion, (5) active transport, (6) capillary blockade, (7) perfusion, (8) chemotaxis, (9) antibody-antigen complexation, (10) receptor binding, and (11) physiochemical adsorption. Each of these mechanisms is reviewed briefly below.

Compartmental Localization and Leakage

Compartmental localization refers to the introduction of the radiopharmaceutical into a well-defined anatomic compartment. Examples include Xe-133 gas inhalation into the lung, intraperitoneal instillation of P-32 chromic phosphate, and Tc-99m labeled RBCs injected into the circulatory system. Compartmental leakage is used to identify an abnormal opening in an otherwise closed compartment, as when labeled RBCs are used to detect gastrointestinal bleeding.

Cell Sequestration

To evaluate splenic morphology and function, RBCs are withdrawn from the patient, labeled with Tc-99m, and slightly damaged by in vitro heating in a boiling water bath for approximately 30 min. After they have been reinjected, the spleen's ability to recognize and remove (i.e., sequester) the damaged RBCs is evaluated.

Phagocytosis

The cells of the reticuloendothelial system are distributed in the liver (~85%), spleen (~10%), and bone marrow (~5%). These cells recognize small foreign substances in the blood and remove them by phagocytosis. In a liver scan, for example, Tc-99m-labeled sulfur colloid particles (~100 nm) are recognized, being substantially smaller than circulating cellular elements, and are rapidly removed from circulation.

Passive Diffusion

Passive diffusion is simply the free movement of a substance from a region of high concentration to one of lower concentration. Anatomic and physiologic mechanisms exist in the brain tissue and surrounding vasculature that allow essential nutrients, metabolites, and lipid-soluble compounds to pass freely between the plasma and brain tissue while many water-soluble substances (including most radiopharmaceuticals) are prevented from entering healthy brain tissue. This system, called the blood-brain barrier, protects and regulates access to the brain. Disruptions of the blood-brain barrier can be produced by trauma, neoplasms, and inflammation. The disruption permits radiopharmaceuticals such as Tc-99m diethylenetriaminepentaacetic acid (DTPA), which is normally excluded by the blood-brain barrier, to follow the concentration gradient and enter the affected brain tissue.

Active Transport

Active transport involves cellular metabolic processes that expend energy to concentrate the radiopharmaceutical into a tissue against a concentration gradient and above plasma levels. The classic example in nuclear medicine is the trapping and organification of radioactive iodide. Trapping of iodide in the thyroid gland occurs by transport against a concentration gradient into follicular cells, where it is oxidized to a highly reactive iodine by a peroxidase enzyme system. Organification follows, resulting in the production of radiolabeled triiodothyronine (T3) and thyroxine (T4). Another example is the localization of thallium (a potassium analog) in muscle tissue. The concentration of Tl-201 is mediated by the energy-dependent Na^+/K^+ ionic pump. Non-uniform distribution of Tl-201 in the myocardium indicates a myocardial perfusion deficit. F-18 FDG is a glucose analog that concentrates in cells that rely upon glucose as an energy source, or in cells whose dependence on glucose increases under pathophysiological conditions. F-18 FDG is actively transported into the cell where it is phosphorylated and trapped for several hours as FDG-6-phosphate. The retention and clearance of FDG reflect glucose metabolism in a given tissue. F-18 FDG is used to assist in the evaluation of malignancy in patients with known or suspected diagnoses of cancer. In addition, F-18 FDG is used to assess regional cardiac glucose metabolism for the evaluation of hibernating myocardium (*i.e.*, the reversible loss of systolic function) in patients with coronary artery disease.

Capillary Blockade

When particles slightly larger than RBCs are injected intravenously, they become trapped in the capillary beds. A common example in nuclear medicine is in the assessment of pulmonary perfusion by the injection of Tc-99m-MAA, which is trapped in the pulmonary capillary bed. Imaging the distribution of Tc-99m-MAA provides a representative assessment of pulmonary perfusion. The "microemboli" created by this radiopharmaceutical do not pose a significant clinical risk because only a very small percentage of the pulmonary capillaries are blocked and the MAA is eventually removed by biodegradation.

Perfusion

Relative perfusion of a tissue or organ system is an important diagnostic element in many nuclear medicine procedures. For example, the perfusion phase of a three-phase bone scan helps to distinguish between an acute process (*e.g.*, osteomyelitis) and remote fracture. Perfusion is also an important diagnostic element in examinations such as renograms, cerebral and hepatic blood flow studies, and myocardial perfusion studies.

Chemotaxis

Chemotaxis describes the movement of a cell such as a leukocyte in response to a chemical stimulus. [111]In- and ^{99m}Tc-labeled leukocytes respond to products formed in immunologic reactions by migrating and accumulating at the site of the reaction as part of an overall inflammatory response.

Antibody-Antigen Complexation

An antigen is a biomolecule (typically a protein) that is capable of inducing the production of, and binding to, an antibody in the body. The antibody has a strong and specific affinity for the antigen. An in vitro test called radioimmunoassay (RIA) makes use of the competition between a radiolabeled antigen and the same antigen in the patient's serum for antibody binding sites. RIA, developed by Berson and Yalow in the late 1950s (Yalow and Berson, 1960a, 1960b), led to a Nobel Prize in Medicine for Yalow in 1977, five years after the untimely death of Berson. RIA techniques have been employed to measure minute quantities of various enzymes, antigens, drugs, and hormones; however, many of these tests have been replaced by immunoassays using non-radioactive labels. At equilibrium, the more unlabeled serum antigen that is present, the less radiolabeled antigen (free antigen) will become bound to the antibody (bound antigen). The serum level is measured by comparing the ratio between bound and free antigen in the sample to a known standard for that particular assay.

Antigen-antibody complexation is also used in diagnostic imaging with such agents as In-111-labeled monoclonal antibodies for the detection of colorectal carcinoma. This class of immunospecific radiopharmaceuticals promises to provide an exciting new approach to diagnostic imaging. In addition, a variety of radiolabeled (typically with I-131 or Y-90) monoclonal antibodies directed toward tumors are being used in an attempt to deliver tumoricidal radiation doses. This procedure, called radioimmunotherapy, has proven effective in the treatment of some non-Hodgkin's lymphomas and is under clinical investigation for other malignancies.

Receptor Binding

This class of radiopharmaceuticals is characterized by their high affinity to bind to specific receptor sites. For example, the uptake of In-111-octreotide, used for the localization of neuroendocrine and other tumors, is based on the binding of a somatostatin analog to receptor sites in tumors.

Physiochemical Adsorption

The localization of methylene diphosphonate (MDP) occurs primarily by adsorption in the mineral phase of the bone. MDP concentrations are significantly higher in amorphous calcium than in mature hydroxyapatite crystalline structures, which helps to explain its concentration in areas of increased osteogenic activity. A summary of the characteristics and clinical utility of commonly used radiopharmaceuticals is provided in Appendix F-1.

16.2.5 Radiopharmaceutical Quality Control

Aside from the radionuclidic purity quality control performed on the 99mTc-pertechnetate generator eluate, the most common radiopharmaceutical quality control procedure is the test for radiochemical purity. The radiochemical purity assay identifies the fraction of the total radioactivity that is in the desired chemical form. Radiochemical impurity can occur as the result of temperature changes, presence of unwanted oxidizing or reducing agents, pH changes, or radiation damage to the radiopharmaceutical (called autoradiolysis). The presence of radiochemical impurities compromises the diagnostic utility of the radiopharmaceutical by reducing uptake in the organ of interest and increasing background activity, thereby degrading image quality. In addition to lowering the diagnostic quality of the examination, radiochemical impurities unnecessarily increase patient dose.

The most common method to determine the amount of radiochemical impurity in a radiopharmaceutical preparation is thin-layer chromatography. This test is performed by placing a small aliquot (~1 drop) of the radiopharmaceutical preparation approximately 1 cm from one end of a small rectangular paper (*e.g.*, Whatman filter paper) or a silica-coated plastic strip. This strip is called the "stationary phase." The end of the strip with the spot of radiopharmaceutical is then lowered into a glass vial containing an appropriate solvent (*e.g.*, saline, acetone, or 85% methanol), such that the solvent front begins just below the spot. The depth of the solvent in the vial must be low enough so that the spot of radiopharmaceutical on the strip is above the solvent. The solvent will slowly move up the strip and the various radiochemicals will partition themselves at specific locations identified by their reference values (R_f), which ranges from 0 to 1 along the strip, according to their relative solubilities. The reference value number is the fraction of the total distance on the strip, (from the origin, where the spot of the radiopharmaceutical is placed to a predetermined line near the top of the strip where the solvent front ends), traveled by a particular radiochemical. Once the solvent front has reached the top, the strip is removed and dried. The strip is cut into sections, and the percentage of the total radioactivity on each section of the strip is assayed and recorded. The movements of radiopharmaceuticals and their contaminants have been characterized for several solvents. Comparison of the results with these reference values allows the identities and percentages of the radiochemical impurities to be determined.

The two principal radiochemical impurities in technetium-labeled radiopharmaceuticals are free (*i.e.*, unbound) Tc-99m-pertechnetate and hydrolyzed Tc-99m. The Tc-99m radiopharmaceutical complex and its associated impurities will, depending upon the solvent, either remain at the origin ($R_f = 0$) or move with the solvent front to a location near the end of the strip. For example, with Whatman 31 ET chromatography paper as the stationary phase in an acetone solvent, Tc-99m-MAA remains at the origin and any free pertechnetate or hydrolyzed Tc-99m migrates close to the solvent front ($R_f = 0.9$). On the other hand, I-131 (as bound NaI) moves with the solvent front ($R_f = 1$) in an 85% methanol solvent, while the impurity (unbound iodide) moves approximately 20% of the distance from the origin ($R_f = 0.2$). These assays are easy to perform and should be used as part of a routine radiopharmacy quality control program, and whenever there is a question about the radiochemical integrity of a radiopharmaceutical preparation.

16.3 INTERNAL DOSIMETRY

Radiation doses to patients from diagnostic imaging procedures are an important issue and, in the absence of a medical physicist at an institution (*e.g.*, private practice radiology), radiologists and nuclear medicine physicians are often consulted as the local experts. Radiation dosimetry is primarily of interest because radiation dose quantities serve as indices of the risk from diagnostic imaging procedures using ionizing radiation. Dosimetry also plays an important role in radiopharmaceutical therapy where estimates of activity necessary to produce tumoricidal doses must be weighed against potential radiotoxicity to healthy tissue. In nuclear medicine procedures, the chemical form of the radiopharmaceutical, its route of administration (*e.g.*, intravenous injection, ingestion, inhalation), the administered activity, the radionuclide, and patient-specific disease states and pharmacokinetics determine the patient dose.

16.3.1   MIRD and ICRP Schema

The radiation absorbed dose to internal organs of a patient following the administration of a radiopharmaceutical for either diagnostic or therapeutic purposes is not a directly measurable quantity, and thus it must be computed using an internal dosimetry formalism based upon typically a combination of pre-computed quantities and data obtained by measurement on the individual patient. The original mathematical methods, models, equations, nuclear decay data, and biokinetic parameters needed for computing radiation absorbed dose to internal organs were developed by the Medical Internal Radiation Dose (or MIRD) Committee of the Society of Nuclear Medicine and Molecular Imaging (SNMMI) in the late 1950s to early 1960s. The most recent revision of the MIRD schema for internal organ dosimetry was published in 2009 as MIRD Pamphlet No. 21 in the Journal of Nuclear Medicine. In the 1970s, the International Commission on Radiological Protection (ICRP) developed its own set of expression, quantities, and terminology for the same purpose – estimating dose to internal organs following intake of both radionuclides and radiopharmaceuticals. With the issue of ICRP Publication 130 (in 2015) and ICRP Publication 133 (in 2016), however, a harmonization of the dosimetry schema for internal organ dosimetry was made, thus providing a consistent terminology and approach to the field of internal dosimetry.

Radiation dose assessment requires information regarding the amount of radionuclide or radioactivity present over a defined time period, the spatial distribution of the radiopharmaceutical, the geometric boundaries relative to defined regions of dosimetric interest, and the tissue mass density in which radiations traverse, interact, and deposit energy. For convenience in dose assessment, we define both source regions and target regions. A source region (r_S) is an organ or tissue containing the radiopharmaceutical and thus it defines the tissue region in which radiation decay products (photons or charged particles) are emitted within the patient. A target region (r_T) is an organ or tissue region for which the radiation absorbed dose is calculated (see Fig. 16-11). Due to the limited ranges of many low-energy charged particles and photons, each source region is generally also a target region within the MIRD schema. Other non-source target regions include those organs or tissues that are within the spatial range of the radiation particles emitted from the source regions that are also of dosimetric interest due to their physiological importance and radiosensitivity. Obtaining the necessary information regarding the radiopharmaceutical activity in

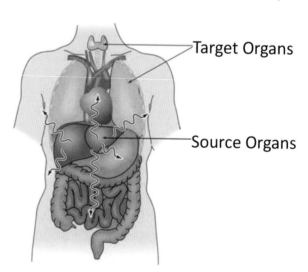

■ **FIGURE 16-11** Illustration of source and target organ concept for calculation of the dose to the lungs and thyroid gland (target organs) from a radiopharmaceutical (*e.g.*, technetium-99m sulfur colloid) primarily located in the liver (source organ). Note that the relative geometry and mass of the source and target organs together with the physical decay characteristic of the radionuclide and its associated radiopharmaceutical kinetics all play a part in determining the dose to any particular organ.

the source region requires the ability to assess radionuclide uptake, retention, distribution, and clearance by redistribution, excretion, and radioactive decay. In many cases, multiple source regions may contribute energy to a given target region. The absorbed dose to a target region is simply the total energy imparted by all source regions divided by the target mass. Multicellular dosimetry represents an extreme example of this where radiations from thousands to millions of source cells may contribute to the energy imparted to a given target cell. Details regarding the computation of the absorbed dose are given below.

Mean Absorbed Dose Rate

The mean absorbed dose $D(r_T)$ is defined as the mean energy imparted to target tissue (or region) r_T per unit tissue mass. The rate at which the absorbed dose is delivered $\dot{D}(r_T,t)$ to target tissue r_T within a patient from a radiopharmaceutical distributed uniformly within source tissue r_S at time t following radiopharmaceutical administration is given as:

$$\dot{D}(r_T,t) = \sum_{r_S} A(r_S,t)\, S(r_T \leftarrow r_S,t), \qquad [16\text{-}7]$$

where $A(r_S,t)$ is the time-dependent activity of the radiopharmaceutical in source tissue r_S and $S(r_T \leftarrow r_S,t)$ is a quantity called the radionuclide S value (or S coefficient). We first note that this expression involves a summation over all possible source regions r_S that might contribute absorbed dose to the target region r_T. For short-range radiations emitted by the radionuclide, the relevant source tissue may only be the target tissue itself (i.e., $r_T = r_S$). For source tissues that emit photons (γ-rays or x-rays), the relevant source tissues may be adjacent to or even at a distance from the target tissue (i.e., $r_T \neq r_S$) and may also include the target tissue itself (i.e., $r_T = r_S$). The time-dependent activity $A(r_S,t)$ represents the rate of nuclear decays in the source tissue r_S at time t, while the S value represents the absorbed dose rate to the target tissue r_T per radionuclide activity in the source region r_S also at time t.

The S value is characteristic of the radionuclide and the anatomic model chosen to represent the internal body anatomy of the patient. In many cases, "reference" anatomic models are used to compute the S value. These may be anatomic models of either the averaged sized male or female patients at fixed ages – newborn, 1-year-old, 5-year-old, 10-year-old, 15-year-old, and the adult (see Fig. 16-12). This choice of a "reference"

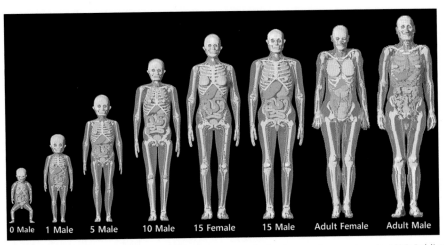

0 Male   1 Male   5 Male   10 Male   15 Female   15 Male   Adult Female   Adult Male

■ **FIGURE 16-12** Frontal views of the ICRP reference voxel phantom series as given in ICRP Publication 110 (adults) and ICRP Publication 143 (pediatric series).

patient is perfectly adequate for patient organ dosimetry under the MIRD schema for diagnostic nuclear medicine. In radionuclide therapy, however, it may be desirable to compute S values that are truly unique to the individual organ anatomy of the patient based upon CT or MR images. In general, however, the source and target regions r_S and r_T, respectively, are those defined within the anatomic model, and may represent the full range of configurations including whole organs, sub-organ tissue regions, voxels from SPECT or PET images, tumors and cell clusters, individual cells, or cell components. If an absorbed dose distribution is desired as related to voxels defined in a SPECT or PET image, then the MIRD schema is applied at the voxel level (Bolch et al., 1999).

Mean Absorbed Dose: Time-Independent Formulation

In Equation 16-7, the absorbed dose rate to the target tissue r_T is shown to be given as the sum of the product of two terms—the activity of the radiopharmaceutical activity in the source tissue $A(r_S, t)$ and the radionuclide S value for the source/target organ pair of interest $S(r_T \leftarrow r_S, t)$. While the first term is clearly a function of time since administration, the second term—the S value—may typically be considered not to vary with time during the period when the absorbed dose is delivered. Thus, the corresponding expression for the mean absorbed dose $D(r_T, \tau)$ to target tissue r_T may be written as:

$$D(r_T, \tau) = \int_0^\tau \dot{D}(r_T, t) dt = \sum_{r_S} \tilde{A}(r_S, \tau) S(r_T \leftarrow r_S) \qquad [16\text{-}8]$$

with

$$\tilde{A}(r_S, \tau) = \int_0^\tau A(r_S, t) dt, \qquad [16\text{-}9]$$

where $\tilde{A}(r_S, \tau)$ is the time-integrated activity (TIA) in source tissue r_S over the dose-integration period τ. The time-integrated activity represents the total number of decays within the source organ.

The magnitude of the organ dose $D(r_T, \tau)$ is directly proportional to the activity of the radiopharmaceutical administered to the patient, A_0. Thus, doubling or tripling A_0 will then double or triple the organ doses resulting from that nuclear medicine study. It is then convenient to normalize organ dose by the value of A_0, thus reporting the organ dose per activity administered (mGy per MBq). If the ratio of $A(r_S, t)$ to the administrated activity A_0 is denoted as $a(r_S, t)$, then we can define the absorbed dose coefficient $d(r_T, \tau)$ in the target tissue r_T as:

$$d(r_T, \tau) = \sum_{r_S} \tilde{a}(r_S, \tau) S(r_T \leftarrow r_S) \qquad [16\text{-}10]$$

with

$$\tilde{a}(r_S, \tau) = \int_0^\tau \frac{A(r_S, t)}{A_0} dt = \int_0^\tau a(r_S, t) dt, \qquad [16\text{-}11]$$

where $a(r_S, t)$ is the fraction of administered activity in the source tissue r_S at time t after administration, and the quantity $\tilde{a}(r_S, \tau)$ is the time-integrated activity coefficient (TIAC). The time-dependent activity in source tissues of the patient may be obtained directly via quantitative imaging, including 2D planar imaging, 3D SPECT, or 3D PET, or by tissue sampling (e.g., blood or urine collection). In the case of preclinical animal studies, this may also be determined by the radioactivity counting of individual organs or tissues of the experimental animals. Alternatively, in the absence of direct measurement, the time-dependent activity in the source tissue may be obtained by a numeric solution of a set of first-order coupled differential equations defined by compartment models for all organs and sub-organ tissues of interest.

The second term in Equations 16-8 and 16-10 is the S value, a quantity in the MIRD schema that is specific to the radionuclide and to the computational anatomic model defining the spatial relationship and tissue compositions of r_S and r_T, as well as their intervening tissues. In equation form, the S value is defined as:

$$S(r_T \leftarrow r_S) = \frac{1}{m(r_T)} \sum_i E_i\, Y_i\, \phi(r_T \leftarrow r_S, E_i) = \frac{1}{m(r_T)} \sum_i \Delta_i\, \phi(r_T \leftarrow r_S, E_i), \qquad [16\text{-}12]$$

where E_i is the mean (or individual) energy per particle of the ith radiation emitted; Y_i is the number of ith radiation emitted per nuclear decay; Δ_i is their product (mean energy of the ith radiation emitted per nuclear decay); $\phi(r_T \leftarrow r_S, E_i)$ is the absorbed fraction (fraction of E_i emitted within r_S that is absorbed in the target tissue r_T); and $m(r_T)$ is the mass of the target tissue r_T in the model.

The specific absorbed fraction $\Phi(r_T \leftarrow r_S, E_i)$ is further defined as the ratio of the absorbed fraction and the target mass:

$$\Phi(r_T \leftarrow r_S, E_i) = \frac{\phi(r_T \leftarrow r_S, E_i)}{m(r_T)} \qquad [16\text{-}13]$$

such that

$$S(r_T \leftarrow r_S) = \sum_i \Delta_i\, \Phi(r_T \leftarrow r_S, E_i). \qquad [16\text{-}14]$$

Mean Absorbed Dose: Time-Dependent Formulation

In the vast majority of the applications of the MIRD schema for radiopharmaceutical dosimetry, the dose integration period τ is taken to be infinity, as radionuclides of general use in nuclear medicine have relatively short physical half-lives. However, there may be instances in radiobiological modeling where a non-infinite time-integration period would be adopted, one dictated by time scales of DNA repair and cell re-population, or alternatively, limited to a time point beyond which the radiobiological effect (cell kill) of the dose rate is low compared to cell re-population. Furthermore, there may be situations, such as in radiopharmaceutical therapy, where the target tissue mass $m(r_T)$ and/or the source tissue mass $m(r_S)$ changes during the dose integration period. In such cases, the radionuclide S value itself might be a function of time during the period of dose assessment. We can thus update the MIRD schema equations above to include a time dependence of both the target mass and radionuclide S value:

$$D(r_T, \tau) = \int_0^\tau \dot{D}(r_T, t)\,dt = \sum_{r_S} \int_0^\tau A(r_S, t)\, S(r_T \leftarrow r_S, t)\,dt \qquad [16\text{-}15]$$

$$d(r_T, \tau) = \frac{D(r_T, \tau)}{A_0} = \sum_{r_S} \int_0^\tau a(r_S, t)\, S(r_T \leftarrow r_S, t)\,dt \qquad [16\text{-}16]$$

with

$$S(r_T \leftarrow r_S, t) = \frac{1}{m(r_T, t)} \sum_i E_i\, Y_i\, \phi(r_T \leftarrow r_S, E_i, t)$$

$$= \frac{1}{m(r_T, t)} \sum_i \Delta_i\, \phi(r_T \leftarrow r_S, E_i, t). \qquad [16\text{-}17]$$

16.3.2 Models of Time-Dependent Activity in Source Regions

There are two general approaches to modeling time-dependent activity in the body following radiopharmaceutical administration. The first is based upon image-based quantification of source organ/region activity as described in Chapters 18 and 19, followed by mathematical fits to these data as sums of exponential terms. The second is the construction of new or the use of existing compartmental models of systemic activity flow within the body. Both approaches are summarized below.

Time-Dependent Activity as Sums of Exponential Expressions

Radiopharmaceuticals may be introduced into the body via a variety of routes including intravenous, intra-arterial, or intrathecal injection, or oral or inhaled administration. The tissue regions that incorporate the radioactivity become source regions, and radiation emitted by the radioactivity in the source regions is absorbed in target regions. Once introduced into the body, the radiopharmaceutical undergoes biological uptake and clearance in various source organs and tissues of the body. The kinetics of biological uptake (bu) and biological clearance (bc) are often of an exponential form with half-times denoted as T_{bu} and T_{bc}, respectively. Similarly, the rate constants for biological uptake and biological clearance are denoted as λ_{bu} and λ_{bc}, respectively, with $\lambda = \ln 2/T$. Biological uptake and biological clearance, coupled with physical radionuclide decay, results in values of effective uptake and effective clearance rate constants (λ_{eu} and λ_{ec}) and effective uptake and effective clearance half-times (T_{eu} and T_{ec}) as given by the following expressions:

$$\lambda_{eu} = \lambda_{bu} + \lambda_p \quad \text{and} \quad T_{eu} = \frac{T_{bu}T_p}{T_{bu} + T_p}, \quad \text{[16-18]}$$

$$\lambda_{ec} = \lambda_{bc} + \lambda_p \quad \text{and} \quad T_{ec} = \frac{T_{bc}T_p}{T_{bc} + T_p}. \quad \text{[16-19]}$$

The time-dependent activity in source region $A(r_S, t)$ can thus be given as the product of the administered activity A_0, the fraction f_s of the total administered activity taken up by a single identified source region r_S, and the difference of time-dependent exponential terms for radiopharmaceutical clearance and radiopharmaceutical uptake, respectively:

$$A(r_S, t) = A_0 f_s \left[e^{-\lambda_{ec}t} - e^{-\lambda_{eu}t} \right]. \quad \text{[16-20]}$$

While radiopharmaceutical clearance from tissue source regions is, in general, adequately expressed by a single exponential term, there are frequently situations in which two or more exponential terms are required to sufficiently model radiopharmaceutical clearance from the source region. As an example, Equation 16-20 would be modified to the following if radiopharmaceutical clearance were better expressed using two exponential terms:

$$A(r_S, t) = A_0 \left[f_{s_1} e^{-\lambda_{ec_1}t} + f_{s_2} e^{-\lambda_{ec_2}t} - (f_{s_1} + f_{s_2}) e^{-\lambda_{eu}t} \right], \quad \text{[16-21]}$$

where λ_{ec_1} and λ_{ec_2} are the effective clearance rate constants for the first and second compartment for radiopharmaceutical clearance, respectively, and f_{s_1} and f_{s_2} are the fractions of the administered activity that localize within these same two compartments of source tissue region r_S. The time-integrated activity within the source region, assuming the two-exponential model of Equation 16-21, is then given as:

$$\bar{A}(r_s,\tau) = \int_0^\tau A(r_s,t)dt$$

$$= \frac{A_0\, f_{s_1}}{\lambda_{ec_1}}\Big[1-e^{-\lambda_{ec_1}\tau}\Big] + \frac{A_0\, f_{s_2}}{\lambda_{ec_2}}\Big[1-e^{-\lambda_{ec_2}\tau}\Big] - \frac{A_0\,(f_{s_1}+f_{s_2})}{\lambda_{eu}}\Big[1-e^{-\lambda_{eu}\tau}\Big]. \quad [16\text{-}22]$$

Time-Dependent Activity from Compartmental Models of Systemic Biodistribution

An alternative approach to assessing time-integrated activities of the radiopharmaceutical in various source regions of the body is to utilize compartmental models of systemic biodistribution. Compartments in these models may be identifiable organs or tissue sub-organ regions, or they may be mathematical constructs needed to trace observable time-dependent changes in radioactivity within a given source tissue similar to the two-term exponential clearance terms of Equation 16-21. The compartmental model defines a system of first-order differential equations of activity flow from donor to receiving compartments and in-situ physical decay of the radionuclide. In the case of some alpha-emitter therapeutic radionuclides, one must additionally consider the ingrowth of radioactive progeny following the administration of the radiopharmaceutical (labeled with the parent radionuclide) (see Table 16-3 for alpha-emitter progeny).

The system of differential equations must be solved using suitable numerical methods. The system is generally solved for the initial conditions that at time $t = 0$, all compartments have zero activity except the compartment of intake (e.g., blood in the case in an intravenous administration). To compute values of time-dependent activity $A(r_s, t)$, it is necessary to associate each biokinetic compartment with anatomical regions of the patient's body – source regions indexed as r_s. The source regions may or may not be living tissue, as in the example of the contents of the stomach or urinary bladder. The solutions of the system of differential equations yield values of $A(r_s, t)$, which then may be time-integrated to give values of time-integrated activity (i.e., the total number of nuclear transformations) $\bar{A}(r_s, \tau)$.

As an example, Figure 16-13 gives the compartmental structure of the biokinetic model for systemic iodine used by the ICRP for both radiological protection and nuclear medicine dose assessments. The model is applicable to all radioisotopes of iodine and is based on the work of Leggett (2010). The model describes the biokinetics of systemic iodine in terms of three subsystems: (1) circulating (extra-thyroidal) inorganic iodine, (2) thyroidal iodine (trapping and organ binding of iodide, and synthesis, storage, and secretion of thyroid hormones), and (3) extra-thyroidal organic iodine. The structure of the model includes connections with the alimentary tract. Baseline transfer coefficients (defined as the fraction of activity in the donor compartment that is transferred to the receiving compartment per unit time) for normal adult males and females are listed in Table 16-4. These values may be adjusted to represent individual patient iodine metabolism, including those with hyperthyroidism or thyroid cancer, by iterative adjustment of selected transfer coefficients so as to statistically approach measured time-activity data in various tissues compartments. For further information on the systemic biokinetic model used by the ICRP, the reader is referred to Chapter 5 of ICRP Publication 137.

Example Dose Calculation

The simplest example of an internal organ dose calculation would be a situation in which the radiopharmaceutical did the following:

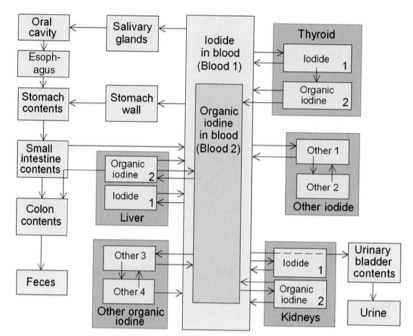

■ **Figure 16-13** Structure of the biokinetic model for systemic iodine used in ICRP Publication 137.

1. The radiopharmaceutical localized in a single organ (*e.g.*, liver) such that $f_s = 1$ in Equation 16-20.
2. The radiopharmaceutical remains in this single source organ with no biological clearance (such that $T_{bc} \to \infty$ and thus $\lambda_{bc} = 0$ and $\lambda_{ec} = \lambda_{bc} + \lambda_p = \lambda_p$). In this way, activity in the organ decreases over time due only to in-situ physical radioactive decay.
3. The radiopharmaceutical exhibits no uptake phase (such that $T_{bu} \to 0$ and $\lambda_{eu} = \lambda_{bu} + \lambda_p \to \infty$ and $e^{-\lambda_{eu}t} \to 0$). At the time of radiopharmaceutical injection ($t = 0$), the administered activity A_0 is fully present within this single source organ. Under these conditions, we can rewrite Equation 16-20 as follows:

$$A(r_S,t) = A_0 \left[e^{-\lambda_p t} \right].$$
[16-22]

EXAMPLE: A patient is injected with 100 MBq of Tc-99m sulfur colloid. Estimate the absorbed dose to the (1) liver, (2) testes, and (3) active (red) bone marrow.
Assumptions:

1. All of the injected activity uniformly distributes throughout the liver.
2. The uptake of Tc-99m sulfur colloid in the liver from the blood is instantaneous.
3. There is no biologic removal of Tc-99m sulfur colloid from the liver.

In this case, the testes and red bone marrow are target organs, whereas the liver is both a source organ and a target organ. The mean absorbed dose to any target organ can be estimated by applying the MIRD schema from Equation 16-8, where the time integration is carried out to infinity (all physical decay has occurred) and the source organ summation is not needed, as there is only one source organ:

$$D(r_T) = \int_0^\infty \dot{D}(r_T,t)dt = \tilde{A}(\text{liver}) \, S(r_T \leftarrow \text{liver}).$$
[16-23]

STEP 1. Calculate the time-integrated activity (number of radioactive decays) in the source organ (*i.e.*, liver) using Equations 16-9 and 16-22.

$$\tilde{A}(\text{liver}) = \int_0^\infty A(\text{liver},t)dt = \int_0^\infty A_0 \left[e^{-\lambda_p t} \right] dt = \frac{A_0}{\lambda_p} = \frac{T_p A_0}{\ln 2} = 1.443 T_p A_0$$
[16-24]

TABLE 16-4 BASELINE PARAMETER VALUES FOR THE ICRP PUBLICATION 137 BIOKINETIC MODEL FOR SYSTEMIC IODINE IN THE NORMAL ADULT MALE OR FEMALE

PATHWAY	TRANSFER COEFFICIENT (d^{-1})	NOTES
Blood 1 to Thyroid 1	7.26	A
Blood 1 to Urinary Bladder Content	11.86	
Blood 1 to Salivary Glands	5.16	
Blood 1 to Stomach Wall	8.6	
Blood 1 to Other 1	600	B
Blood 1 to Kidneys 1	25	
Blood 1 to Liver 1	15	
Salivary Gland to Oral Cavity	50	
Stomach Wall to Stomach Contents	50	
Thyroid 1 to Thyroid 2	95	
Thyroid 1 to Blood 1	36	
Thyroid 2 to Blood 2	0.0077	C
Thyroid 2 to Blood 1	0	D
Other 1 to Blood 1	330	B
Other 1 to Other 2	35	B
Other 2 to Other 1	56	B
Kidneys 1 to Blood 1	100	
Liver 1 to Blood 1	100	
Blood 2 to Other 3	15	B
Other 3 to Blood 2	21	B
Other 3 to Other 4	1.2	B
Other 4 to Other 3	0.62	B
Other 4 to Blood 1	0.14	B
Blood 2 to Kidneys 2	3.6	
Kidneys 2 to Blood 2	21	
Kidneys 2 to Blood 1	0.14	
Blood 2 to Liver 2	21	
Liver 2 to Blood 2	21	
Liver 2 to Blood 1	0.14	
Liver 2 to Right Colon Contents	0.08	

Notes:
A – Depends on the Y/S ratio where Y (μg/d) is the dietary intake of stable iodine and S (μg/d) is the rate of secretion of hormonal stable iodine by the thyroid.
B – For dosimetric purposes, each of the compartments Other 1, Other 2, Other 3, and Other 4 are assumed to be uniformly distributed in all remaining (not explicitly identified) tissues.
C – For high intake of stable iodine, the outflow form Thyroid 2 is split between Blood 2 and Blood 1 as described in Leggett (2010).
D – Non-zero only for high intake of stable iodine (see Leggett (2010)).

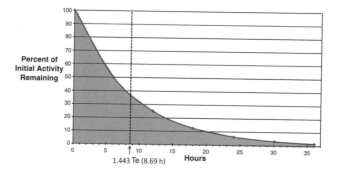

■ **FIGURE 16-14** Time-activity curve for a hypothetical Tc-99m labeled radiopharmaceutical that has a very long biological half-life (Tb) compared to the 6.02 h physical half-life (Tp) of Tc-99m; thus Te = Tp. The cumulated activity is equal to the area under the curve, which is numerically equal to A_0 (1.443 Tp) representing the total number of nuclear transformations (nt) in the specified source organ.

With a physical half-life of 6.02 h for Tc-99m and an administered activity of 100 MBq (where 1 Bq = 1 nuclear transformation or nt), the time-integrated activity within the liver source organ is

$$\bar{A}(\text{liver}) = 1.443\,(6.02\,\text{h})\left(\frac{3{,}600\,\text{s}}{\text{h}}\right)(100\,\text{MBq}) = 3.13 \times 10^6\,\text{MBq-s}$$

$$\text{or} \quad 3.13 \times 10^{12}\,\text{nt}.$$

[16-25]

The time-activity curve for this example problem is shown in Figure 16-14, where the y-axis is a relative scale showing the percentage of the administered activity in the liver present as a function of time post-administration. Recall that in this example, we assume no biological uptake of the radiopharmaceutical (thus all activity appears in the liver at $t = 0$), and all the administered activity A_0 is taken up by the liver. In more a realistic case, the 100% value of liver activity at $t = 0$ would be some fraction f_{liver} of the administered activity A_0.

STEP 2. Find the appropriate radionuclide S values for each source/target organ pair for the radionuclide of interest (*i.e.*, Tc-99m) from Table 16-5. The appropriate S values are found at the intersection of the source organ's column (in this case, the liver) and the individual target organ's row (in this case the liver, testes, and red bone marrow).

TARGET (r_T)	SOURCE (r_s)	S VALUE (mGy/MBq-s)
Liver	Liver	3.16×10^{-6}
Red bone marrow	Liver	8.32×10^{-8}
Testes	Liver	1.57×10^{-9}

STEP 3. Organize the assembled information in a table of organ absorbed doses:

TARGET ORGAN (r_T)	Ã(LIVER) (MBq-s)	S VALUES (mGy/MBq-s)	ORGAN DOSE D_{LIVER} (mGy)
Liver	3.13×10^6	3.16×10^{-6}	9.9
Red bone marrow	3.13×10^6	8.32×10^{-8}	0.26
Testes	3.13×10^6	1.57×10^{-9}	0.0049

It is notable that the self-dose to the liver (as $r_s = r_T$) is 38 times that of the red marrow dose and over 2,000 times that of the testes dose. This is attributed to the fact these two target organs receive their radiation dose only from the more penetrating photon emissions (γ-rays and x-rays) emitted from Tc-99m decay from within the liver. These photons must escape the liver and traverse body tissues situated between the liver and two target tissues before they can deposit a fraction of their residual energy (such as in photoelectric absorptions or Compton scattering events). The self-dose to the liver is much higher as all radiation emissions from the decay of Tc-99m (to include beta particles, γ-rays, x-rays, conversion electrons, and Auger and Coster-Kronig electrons) may contribute all or up to a non-negligible fraction of their emission energy to the absorbed dose to the liver.

TABLE 16-5 Tc-99m RADIONUCLIDE S-VALUES (mGy/MBq-s) FOR SOME SOURCE/TARGET ORGAN COMBINATIONS[a]

	SOURCE ORGANS										
TARGET ORGANS	Adrenals	Brain	LLI Contents	SI Content	Stomach Contents	ULI Contents	Heart Contents	Heart Wall	Kidneys	Liver	Lungs
Adrenals	1.80E−04	4.18E−10	2.25E−08	7.46E−08	2.73E−07	9.58E−08	2.53E−07	2.85E−07	7.24E−07	4.35E−07	2.33E−07
Brain	4.18E−10	4.23E−06	1.57E−11	3.91E−11	4.27E−10	4.68E−11	3.14E−09	2.54E−09	1.58E−10	8.16E−10	7.63E−09
Breasts	5.05E−08	3.17E−09	2.28E−09	7.35E−09	5.73E−08	8.00E−09	2.41E−07	2.61E−07	1.99E−08	6.82E−08	2.33E−07
Gallbladder wall	3.57E−07	1.54E−10	6.49E−08	4.38E−07	3.05E−07	7.53E−07	1.03E−07	1.22E−07	4.09E−07	8.70E−07	7.46E−08
LLI wall	1.98E−08	1.32E−11	1.23E−05	5.92E−07	9.10E−08	2.14E−07	4.06E−09	4.90E−09	5.50E−08	1.44E−08	3.29E−09
Small intestine	7.46E−08	3.91E−11	7.16E−07	4.22E−06	2.08E−07	1.25E−06	1.57E−08	2.06E−08	2.13E−07	1.16E−07	1.35E−08
Stomach wall	2.85E−07	2.52E−10	1.24E−07	2.13E−07	8.53E−06	2.86E−07	1.66E−07	2.65E−07	2.53E−07	1.48E−07	1.19E−07
ULI Wall	9.41E−08	4.76E−11	3.10E−07	1.36E−06	2.65E−07	8.37E−06	2.12E−08	2.65E−08	2.12E−07	1.88E−07	1.81E−08
Heart wall	2.85E−07	2.54E−09	5.42E−09	2.06E−08	2.33E−07	2.97E−08	5.48E−06	1.19E−05	8.22E−08	2.33E−07	4.40E−07
Kidneys	7.24E−07	1.58E−10	7.10E−08	2.13E−07	2.73E−07	2.12E−07	6.45E−08	8.22E−08	1.32E−05	2.93E−07	6.66E−08
Liver	4.35E−07	8.16E−10	1.80E−08	1.16E−07	1.47E−07	1.87E−07	2.13E−07	2.33E−07	2.93E−07	*3.16E−06*	1.97E−07
Lungs	2.33E−07	7.63E−09	4.50E−09	1.35E−08	1.10E−07	1.77E−08	4.59E−07	4.40E−07	6.66E−08	2.09E−07	3.57E−06
Muscle	1.12E−07	2.21E−08	1.23E−07	1.12E−07	9.96E−08	1.07E−07	8.83E−08	9.20E−08	9.79E−08	7.52E−08	9.34E−08
Ovaries	3.14E−08	1.52E−11	1.26E−06	9.23E−07	5.85E−08	7.71E−08	4.55E−09	6.15E−09	7.02E−08	3.81E−08	5.39E−09
Pancreas	1.09E−06	4.15E−10	5.21E−08	1.42E−07	1.23E−06	1.62E−07	2.65E−07	3.57E−07	4.97E−07	3.86E−07	1.74E−07
Red marrow	2.53E−07	1.01E−07	2.01E−07	1.79E−07	7.50E−08	1.43E−07	1.11E−07	1.11E−07	1.71E−07	*8.32E−08*	1.11E−07
Osteogenic cells	2.67E−07	2.99E−07	1.82E−07	1.49E−07	1.03E−07	1.27E−07	1.60E−07	1.60E−07	1.62E−07	1.24E−07	1.66E−07
Skin	3.41E−08	3.97E−08	3.62E−08	3.01E−08	3.41E−08	3.09E−08	3.41E−08	3.70E−08	3.79E−08	3.62E−08	4.02E−08

(Continued)

TABLE 16-5 Tc-99m RADIONUCLIDE S-VALUES (mGy/MBq-s) FOR SOME SOURCE/TARGET ORGAN COMBINATIONS[a] (Continued)

TARGET ORGANS	SOURCE ORGANS										
	Adrenals	Brain	LLI Contents	SI Content	Stomach Contents	ULI Contents	Heart Contents	Heart Wall	Kidneys	Liver	Lungs
Spleen	4.58E−07	5.19E−10	6.53E−08	1.01E−07	7.83E−07	1.05E−07	1.24E−07	1.67E−07	6.63E−07	7.22E−08	1.64E−07
Tests	1.54E−09	1.46E−12	1.40E−07	2.61E−08	2.90E−09	1.92E−08	5.16E−10	6.16E−10	3.10E−09	*1.57E−09*	3.67E−10
Thymus	5.66E−08	6.88E−09	2.04E−09	4.66E−09	3.65E−08	5.43E−09	8.87E−07	7.35E−07	1.73E−08	5.93E−08	2.85E−07
Thyroid	8.11E−09	1.35E−07	2.48E−10	4.87E−10	2.62E−09	7.69E−10	5.17E−08	4.33E−08	2.95E−09	8.64E−09	8.82E−08
Urinary bladder wall	7.55E−09	6.02E−12	4.98E−07	2.12E−07	1.73E−08	1.61E−07	2.22E−09	2.17E−09	1.87E−08	1.16E−08	1.33E−09
Uterus	1.89E−08	1.31E−11	5.17E−07	8.37E−07	5.05E−08	3.97E−07	4.87E−09	5.47E−09	6.42E−08	3.29E−08	4.10E−09
Total body	1.72E−07	1.25E−07	1.49E−07	1.59E−07	1.17E−07	1.41−07	1.17E−07	1.65E−07	1.58E−07	1.59E−07	1.44E−07

Note: Bold italicized correspond to values in MIRD example problem.

[a]OLINDA/EXM v1.0.

GI, gastrointestinal; SI, small intestine; ULI, upper large intestine; LLI, lower large intestine; E, exponential (e.g., 4.6E−05 = 4.6 × 10^{-5}).

16.3.3 Role of Internal Dosimetry in Diagnostic Nuclear Medicine

Clinical applications of diagnostic nuclear medicine allow functional imaging of normal and diseased tissue. Although they may cover almost all clinical specialties, the localization of malignant tissue and its potential metastatic spread, as well as assessment of myocardial perfusion, are amongst the most common procedures. In these applications, the amount of administered activity is such that the absorbed dose to both imaged and non-imaged tissues is typically very low and thus stochastic risks such as cancer induction are greatly outweighed by the diagnostic benefit of the imaging procedure. Nevertheless, these tissue doses and their stochastic risks should be quantified, and placed in context of both their cumulative values received over multiple imaging sessions, and of doses and risks received by other diagnostic imaging procedures they may have (fluoroscopy and computed tomography, for example). The role of internal dosimetry in diagnostic nuclear medicine is thus to provide the basis for stochastic risk quantification. Once this risk is quantified, it may be used to optimize the amount of administered activity in order to maximize image quality while minimizing patient risk. This optimization process is of particular importance for pediatric patients owing to their enhanced organ radiosensitivities and years over which any stochastic effects may become manifest. This optimization should consider, as much as possible, patient age, sex, and body morphometry, and pharmacokinetics, along with all available image acquisition and processing techniques.

Two options exist for quantification of $\tilde{A}$ in diagnostic nuclear medicine. The most patient-specific method entails serial imaging of the patient (2D planar, 3D SPECT, or 3D PET), data processing of these images to yield time-activity curves, and then integration of these time-activity curves. In the development of new diagnostic imaging agents, this approach is required for regulatory approval and should be conducted under standardized protocols to yield the greatest amount of information on agent pharmacokinetics and patient dosimetry. For existing diagnostic imaging agents, one may rely on reference biokinetic models, which when coupled to phantom-based radionuclide S values via the MIRD schema, yield organ dose coefficients—organ dose per unit administered activity. These reference models, however, should be based upon extensive human data sets and should include, where possible, variations accounting for patient disease states, as well as age and sex dependencies.

16.3.4 Role of Internal Dosimetry in Therapy Nuclear Medicine

In many forms of radiation cancer therapy, including external beam radiotherapy and brachytherapy, radiation dosimetry is an integral component to treatment planning, where the objective is to maximize the tumor absorbed dose while avoiding or minimizing normal tissue toxicities. In therapeutic nuclear medicine, tumor dosimetry may be problematic owing to (1) lack of imaging data to define the tumor, especially for disseminated and diffuse disease, (2) the dynamic nature of radiopharmaceutical uptake, retention, and washout, (3) non-uniformities in the spatial distribution of the agent at the cellular level, and (4) time-dependent dose rates. Consequently, there is a paucity of data on tumor dose-response relationships, upon which values of prescribed tumor dose may be assessed. Exceptions do occur, such as in the treatment of solid tumors and malignant and benign thyroid disease, but even here, there are no standardized clinically accepted protocols for radionuclide treatment planning based upon delivery of a dose prescription to the tumor.

Resultantly, current dosimetry practice in therapeutic nuclear medicine is to assess the absorbed dose to radiosensitive tissues, and based upon a general understanding of toxicity thresholds (taken primarily from previous experience in external beam radiotherapy), adjust administered activities to the cancer patient to maximize uptake and dose to the tumor while avoiding normal organ toxicities. The dose to the tumor is neither quantified nor prescribed.

In contrast to diagnostic nuclear medicine dosimetry, more sophisticated methods of dosimetry are generally required in therapeutic nuclear medicine in order to provide predictive indices of tissue toxicities. In the context of therapy, patient variability in terms of both agent pharmacokinetics and body morphometry must be explicitly considered on an individual patient basis to assure optimized treatment. Factors that have been shown to be relevant, if not essential, to predicting biological response include (1) the spatial distribution of the radiopharmaceutical at a resolution commensurate with the scale of the radiosensitive structures, (2) dose rate, (3) radiation quality, and (4) prior treatment history. These considerations require the application of radiobiological concepts to translate absorbed dose distributions to biological effects. This is an area of ongoing research involving pre-clinical and in-vitro studies.

In current clinical practice in nuclear medicine therapy, treatment is delivered based upon an administered activity prescription. This prescribed activity is typically established in a Phase I clinical trial from the toxicity response of only three to six patients and is then applied to all subsequent patients. The failure to account for patient variability will lead, in the majority of cases, to patient undertreatment. The relevant quantity for assuring therapeutic efficacy and avoiding organ toxicities is the radiation absorbed dose, and thus patient-specific dosimetry is essential for optimal efficacy and patient safety. Recent studies using patient-specific dosimetry have demonstrated the ability to establish dose-response relationships for toxicity avoidance. It is thus now clear that the application of patient-specific dosimetry is an essential element in optimizing radiopharmaceutical therapy.

16.4 REGULATORY ISSUES

16.4.1 Investigational Radiopharmaceuticals

All pharmaceuticals for human use, whether radioactive or not, are regulated by the U.S. Food and Drug Administration (FDA). A request to evaluate a new radiopharmaceutical for human use is submitted to the FDA in an application called a "Notice of Claimed Investigational Exemption for a New Drug" (IND). The IND can be sponsored by either an individual physician or a radiopharmaceutical manufacturer, who will work with a group of clinical investigators to collect the necessary safety and efficacy data. The IND application includes the names and credentials of the investigators, the clinical protocol, details of the research project, details of the manufacturing of the drug, and animal toxicology data. The clinical investigation of the new radiopharmaceutical occurs in three stages. Phase I focuses on a limited number of patients and is designed to provide information on the pharmacologic distribution, metabolism, dosimetry, toxicity, optimal dose schedule, and adverse reactions. For therapeutic pharmaceuticals, a maximum permissible dose (MPD) or recommended Phase-II dose (RP2D) for use in subsequent clinical studies is determined. Phase II studies include a limited number of patients with specific diseases to begin the assessment of the drug's efficacy, refine the dosing schedule, and collect more information on safety and efficacy. Phase III clinical trials involve a much larger number of patients (and are typically conducted by several institutions) to provide more extensive (*i.e.*, statistically significant) information on efficacy, safety, and dose administration, often in a randomized, blinded fashion. To obtain approval to market a new radiopharmaceutical, a "New Drug Application" (NDA) must be submitted to and approved by the FDA. Approval of a new radiopharmaceutical typically requires 5 to 10 years from laboratory work to NDA. The package insert of an approved radiopharmaceutical describes the intended purpose of the radiopharmaceutical, the suggested dose, dosimetry, adverse reactions, clinical pharmacology, and contraindications.

Any research involving human subjects conducted, supported, or otherwise regulated by a federal department or agency must be conducted in accordance with the Federal Policy for the Protection of Human Subjects (Federal Register, 2017); this policy is codified in the regulations of 15 federal departments and agencies. This policy requires that all research involving human subjects be reviewed and approved by an institutional review board (IRB) and that informed consent be obtained from each research subject. Most academic medical institutions have IRBs. An IRB comprises clinical, scientific, legal, and other experts as well as a patient advocate and must include at least one member who is not otherwise affiliated with the institution. Informed consent must be sought in a manner that minimizes the possibility of coercion and provides the subject sufficient opportunity to decide whether or not to participate. The information presented must be in language understandable to the subject. It must include a statement that the study involves research, the purposes of the research, a description of the procedures, and identification of any procedures that are experimental; a description of any reasonably foreseeable risks or discomforts; a description of any likely benefits to the subject or to others; a disclosure of alternative treatments; and a statement that participation is voluntary, that refusal will involve no penalty or loss of benefits, and that the subject may discontinue participation at any time.

An additional mechanism for limited investigational use of radiopharmaceuticals is a Radioactive Drug Research Committee (RDRC) protocol. An institution can form its own RDRC or request another institution's RDRC to review a protocol. RDRC approval places a number of limitations on the types of human investigational studies that are allowed. The intent is to allow the collection of data for basic research studies regarding the agent (*e.g.*, to obtain an understanding of the metabolism, pharmacokinetics, and dosimetry of the agent). The following limitations apply: (1) No more than 30 patients are allowed to be initially enrolled in a specific RDRC approved protocol; (2) RDRC protocols are not intended for immediate management of patients; (3) these studies are not intended to determine the safety and effectiveness of a radiopharmaceutical; and (4) they must comply with radiation dose limits outlined in 21CFR361.1. These dose limits are as follows:

1. Whole-body, active (red) bone marrow, eye lens, and gonads (testes or ovaries): 30 mSv for a single administration and 50 mSv annually for multiple administrations.
2. All other organs and tissues: 50 mSv for a single administration and 150 mSv annual for multiple administrations.

NCRP Report No. 185, Evaluating and Communicating Radiation Risks for Studies Involving Human Subjects: Guidance for Researchers and Institutional Review Boards, is a unique, comprehensive document providing guidance to researchers in preparing protocols that include ionizing radiation exposure to human subjects as well as recommendations for IRBs reviewing such protocols (NCRP, 2020). The document includes guidance on the estimation of risk, the optimization of radiation dose, and the formulation of informed consent statements that are based on consistent, comprehensive, and accurate language.

16.4.2 By-Product Material, Authorized Users, Written Directives, and Medical Events

Medical Use of By-Product Material

Although the production of radiopharmaceuticals is regulated by the FDA, the medical use of radioactive material is regulated under the terms of a license issued to a specific legal entity (such as a clinic or hospital that is the *licensee*) by the U.S. Nuclear Regulatory Commission (NRC) or, a comparable state agency (*i.e.*, an agreement state, which is discussed further in Chapter 21). NRC regulations do not, however, specify permissible administered activities or patient radiation doses, as any such regulations would be considered as excessively intrusive on the practice of medicine. The NRC's regulations apply to the use of *by-product material*. Until recently, the regulatory definition of by-product material included radionuclides that were the by-products of nuclear fission or nuclear activation but excluded others such as accelerator-produced radionuclides. The current NRC's definition of by-product material, however, has been broadened to include virtually all radioactive material used in medicine. The regulations regarding the medical use of radioactive material are contained in Title 10, Part 35, of the *Code of Federal Regulations* (10 CFR 35).

Authorized User

An *authorized user* (AU), in the context of the practice of nuclear medicine, is a physician who is responsible for the medical use of radioactive material and is designated by name on a license for the medical use of radioactive material or is approved by the radiation safety committee of a medical institution whose license authorizes such actions. Such a physician may be certified by a medical specialty board, such as the American Board of Radiology, whose certification process includes all of the requirements identified in Part 35 for the medical use of unsealed sources of radioactive materials for diagnosis and therapy. Alternatively, a physician can apply to the NRC or comparable state agency for AU status by providing documentation of the specific education, training, and experience requirements contained in 10 CFR 35.

Written Directive

The NRC requires that, before the administration of a dosage of I-131 sodium iodide greater than 1.11 MBq (30 μCi) or any therapeutic dosage of unsealed by-product material, a *written directive* must be signed and dated by an AU. The written directive must contain the patient or human research subject's name and must describe the radioactive drug, the activity, and (for radionuclides other than I-131) the route of administration. In addition, the NRC requires the implementation of written procedures to provide, for each administration requiring a written directive, high confidence that the patient or human research subject's identity is verified before the administration and that each administration is performed in accordance with the written directive.

Medical Events

The NRC defines certain errors in the administration of radiopharmaceuticals as *medical events* and requires specific actions to be taken within specified time periods following the recognition of the error. The initial report to the NRC (or, in an agreement state, the comparable state agency) must be made by telephone no later than the next calendar day after the discovery of the event and must be followed by a written report within 15 days. This report must include specific information such as a description of the incident, the cause of the medical event, the effect (if any) on the individual or individuals involved, and proposed corrective actions. The referring physician must be notified of the medical event, and the patient must also be notified, unless the referring physician states that he or she will inform the patient or that, based on medical judgment, notification of the patient would be harmful. Additional details regarding these reporting requirements can be found in 10 CFR 35.

The NRC defines a medical event as:

A. The administration of NRC-licensed radioactive materials that results in one of the following conditions (1, 2, or 3 below) unless its occurrence was as the direct result of patient intervention (*e.g.*, an I-131 therapy patient takes only one half of the prescribed treatment and then refuses to take the balance of the prescribed dosage):

1. A dose that differs from the prescribed dose or dose that would have resulted from the prescribed *dosage* (*i.e.*, administered activity) by more than 0.05 Sv (5 rem) effective dose equivalent, 0.5 Sv (50 rem) to an organ or tissue, or 0.5 Sv (50 rem) shallow dose equivalent to the skin; and one of the following conditions (i or ii) has also occurred.

   (i) The total dose delivered differs from the prescribed dose by 20% or more;

   (ii) The total dosage delivered differs from the prescribed dosage by 20% or more or falls outside the prescribed dosage range. Falling outside the prescribed dosage range means the administration of activity that is greater or less than a predetermined range of activity for a given procedure that has been established by the licensee.

2. A dose that exceeds 0.05 Sv (5 rem) effective dose equivalent, 0.5 Sv (50 rem) to an organ or tissue, or 0.5 Sv (50 rem) shallow dose equivalent to the skin from any of the following:

   (i) An administration of a wrong radioactive drug containing by-product material;

   (ii) An administration of a radioactive drug containing by-product material through the wrong route of administration;

   (iii) An administration of a dose or dosage to the wrong individual or human research subject.

3. A dose to the skin or an organ or tissue other than the treatment site that exceeds by 0.5 Sv (50 rem) and 50% or more of the dose expected from the administration defined in the written directive.

B. Any event resulting from intervention of a patient or human research subject in which the administration of by-product material or radiation from by-product material results or will result in unintended permanent functional damage to an organ or a physiological system, as determined by a physician.

This definition of a medical event was summarized from NRC regulations. It applies only to the use of unsealed by-product material and omits the definition of a medical event involving the use of sealed sources of by-product material to treat patients (*e.g.*, conventional brachytherapy treatment of prostate cancer with I-125 seeds by radiation oncologists). The complete regulations regarding written directives, AUs, and medical events can be found in 10 CFR 35. State regulatory requirements should be consulted as well, because they may differ from federal regulations.

SUGGESTED READING AND REFERENCES

Bolch WE, Eckerman KF, Sgouros G, Thomas SR. MIRD Pamphlet No. 21: a generalized schema for radiopharmaceutical dosimetry—standardization of nomenclature. *J Nucl Med.* 2009;50:477-484.

Bolch WE, Bouchet LG, Robertson JS, et al. MIRD Pamphlet No. 17: the dosimetry of nonuniform activity distributions—radionuclide S values at the voxel level. *J Nucl Med.* 1999;40:11S-36S.

Calabria F, Schillaci O. (Eds.) *Radiopharmaceuticals a Guide to PET/CT and PET/MRI*. 2nd ed. Switzerland: Springer International Publishing; 2020.

Dash A, Knapp FF. *Radiopharmaceuticals for Therapy*. India: Springer India; 2016.

Federal Register 2017: Federal Register. *Federal Policy for the Protection of Human Subjects*. January 19, 2017:7149-7274.

ICRP 2015: ICRP Publication 128. Radiation dose to patients from radiopharmaceuticals – a compendium of current information related to frequently used substances. *Ann ICRP*. 2015;44:1-321.

ICRP 2016: ICRP Publication 133. The ICRP computational framework for internal dose assessment for reference adults: specific absorbed fractions. *Ann ICRP*. 2016;45:1-74.

ICRP 2019: ICRP Publication 140. Radiological protection in therapy with radiopharmaceuticals. *Ann ICRP*. 2019;48:1-106.

International Atomic Energy Agency. *Quality Control in the Production of Radiopharmaceuticals*. IAEA-TEC-DOC-1856. Vienna: IAEA; 2018.

Leggett RW. A physiological systems model for iodine for use in radiation protection *Radiat Res*. 2010;174:496-516.

Michae M, Lim D, Gnerre J, Gerard P. Mechanisms of uptake of common radiopharmaceuticals Radio-Graphics fundamentals. Published Online: September 12, 2018. https://pubs.rsna.org/do/10.1148/rg.2018180072.pres/full/. Accessed June 4, 2020.

Mettler FA, Guiberteau MJ. *Essentials of Nuclear Medicine and Molecular Imaging*. Philadelphia, PA: Elsevier Health Sciences; 2018.

NCRP Report. *Evaluating and Communicating Radiation Risks for Studies Involving Human Subjects: Guidance for Researchers and Institutional Review Boards*. NCRP Report No. 185. Bethesda, MD: National Council on Radiation Protection and Measurements; 2020.

Saha GB. *Fundamentals of Nuclear Pharmacy*. 7th ed. New York, NY: Springer-Verlag; 2018.

Sgouros G, Allen BJ, Back T, et al. *MIRD Radiobiology and Dosimetry for Radiopharmaceutical Therapy with Alpha-Particle Emitters*. Reston, VA: Society of Nuclear Medicine and Molecular Imaging; 2015.

Sgouros G. Dosimetry, radiobiology, and synthetic lethality: radiopharmaceutical therapy (RPT) with alpha-particle-emitters. *Semin Nucl Med*. 2020;50:124-132.

Stabin MG. Uncertainties in internal dose calculations for radiopharmaceuticals. *J Nucl Med*. 2008;49: 853-860.

Yalow RS, Berson SA. Immunoassay of endogenous plasma insulin in man. *J Clin invest*. 1960a;39:1157-1175.

Yalow RS, Berson SA. Plasma insulin concentrations in nondiabetic and early diabetic subjects. Determinations by a new sensitive immuno-assay technic. *Diabetes*. 1960b;9:254-260.

16.4 Regulatory Issues

CHAPTER 17

Radiation Detection and Measurement

The detection and measurement of ionizing radiation are the basis for the majority of diagnostic imaging. In this chapter, the basic concepts of radiation detection and measurement are introduced, followed by a discussion of the characteristics of specific types of detectors. The electronic systems used for pulse height spectroscopy and the use of sodium iodide (NaI) scintillators to perform γ-ray spectroscopy are described, followed by a discussion of detector applications. The use of radiation detectors in imaging devices is covered in other chapters.

All detectors of ionizing radiation require the interaction of the radiation with matter. Ionizing radiation deposits energy in matter by ionization and excitation. *Ionization* is the removal of electrons from atoms or molecules. (An atom or molecule stripped of an electron has a net positive charge and is called a *cation*. In many gases, the free electrons become attached to uncharged atoms or molecules, forming negatively charged *anions*. An ion pair consists of a cation and its associated free electron or anion.) *Excitation* is the elevation of electrons to excited states in atoms, molecules, or a crystal. Excitation and ionization may produce chemical changes or the emission of visible light or ultraviolet (UV) radiation. Most energy deposited by ionizing radiation is ultimately converted into thermal energy.

The amount of energy deposited in matter by a single interaction is very small. For example, a 140-keV γ ray deposits 2.24×10^{-14} J if completely absorbed. To raise the temperature of 1 g of water by 1°C (*i.e.*, 1 calorie) would require the complete absorption of 187 trillion (187×10^{12}) of these photons. For this reason, most radiation detectors provide signal amplification. In detectors that produce an electrical signal, the amplification is electronic. In photographic film, the amplification is achieved chemically.

17.1 TYPES OF DETECTORS AND BASIC PRINCIPLES

Radiation detectors may be classified by their detection method. A *gas-filled detector* consists of a volume of gas between two electrodes. Ions produced in the gas by the radiation are collected by the electrodes, resulting in an electrical signal.

The interaction of ionizing radiation with certain materials produces UV radiation and/or visible light. These materials are called *scintillators*. They are commonly attached to or incorporated in devices that convert the UV radiation and light into an electrical signal. For other applications, photographic film is used to record the light emitted by the scintillators. Many years ago, in physics research and medical fluoroscopy, the light from scintillators was viewed directly with dark-adapted eyes.

Semiconductor detectors are especially pure crystals of silicon, germanium, or other semiconductor materials to which trace amounts of impurity atoms have been added so that they act as diodes. A diode is an electronic device with two terminals that permits a large electrical current to flow when a voltage is applied in one direction, but very little current when the voltage is applied in the opposite direction. When used to detect radiation, a voltage is applied in the direction in which little current flows. When an interaction occurs in the crystal, electrons are raised to an excited state, allowing a momentary pulse of electrical current to flow through the device.

Detectors may also be classified by the type of information produced. Detectors, such as Geiger-Mueller (GM) detectors, that indicate the number of interactions occurring in the detector are called *counters*. Detectors that yield information about the energy distribution of the incident radiation, such as NaI scintillation detectors, are called *spectrometers*. Detectors that indicate the net amount of energy deposited in the detector by multiple interactions are called *dosimeters*.

17.1.1 Pulse and Current Modes of Operation

Many radiation detectors produce an electrical signal after each interaction of a particle or photon. The signal generated by the detector passes through a series of electronic circuits, each of which performs a function such as signal amplification, signal processing, or data storage. A detector and its associated electronic circuitry form a *detection system*. There are two fundamental ways that the circuitry may process the signal—pulse mode and current mode. In *pulse mode*, the signal from each interaction is processed individually. In *current mode*, the electrical signals from individual interactions are averaged together, forming a net current signal.

There are advantages and disadvantages to each method of handling the signal. GM detectors are operated in pulse mode, whereas most ionization chambers, including ion chamber survey meters and the dose calibrators used in nuclear medicine, are operated in current mode. Scintillation detectors are operated in pulse mode in nuclear medicine applications, but in current mode in direct digital radiography, fluoroscopy, and x-ray computed tomography (CT).

In this chapter, the term *interaction* typically refers to the interaction of a single photon or charged particle, such as the interaction of a γ-ray by the photoelectric effect or Compton scattering. The term *event* may refer to a single interaction, or it may refer to something more complex, such as two nearly simultaneous interactions in a detector. In instruments that process the signals from individual interactions or events in pulse mode, an interaction or event that is registered is referred to as a *count*.

Effect of Interaction Rate on Detectors Operated in Pulse Mode

The main problem with using a radiation detector or detection system in pulse mode is that two interactions must be separated by a finite amount of time if they are to produce distinct signals. This interval is called the *dead time* of the system. If a second interaction occurs during this time interval, its signal will be lost; furthermore, if it is close enough in time to the first interaction, it may even distort the signal from the first interaction. The fraction of counts lost from dead-time effects is smallest at low interaction rates and increases with increasing interaction rate.

The dead time of a detection system is largely determined by the component in the series with the longest dead time. For example, the detector usually has the longest dead time in GM counter systems, whereas in multichannel analyzer (MCA) systems (see later discussion), the analog-to-digital converter (ADC) generally has the longest dead time.

The dead times of different types of systems vary widely. GM counters have dead times ranging from tens to hundreds of microseconds, whereas most other systems have dead times of less than a few microseconds. It is important to know the count-rate behavior of a detection system; if a detection system is operated at too high an interaction rate, an artificially low count rate will be obtained.

There are two mathematical models describing the behavior of detector systems operated in pulse mode—paralyzable and non-paralyzable. Although these models are simplifications of the behavior of real detection systems, real systems may behave like one or the other model. In a *paralyzable* system, an interaction that occurs during the dead time after a previous interaction extends the dead time; in a *non-paralyzable* system, it does not. Figure 17-1 shows the count rates of paralyzable and non-paralyzable detector systems as a function of the rate of interactions in the detector. At very high interaction rates, a paralyzable system will be unable to detect any interactions after the first, because subsequent interactions will extend the dead time, causing the system to indicate a count rate of zero!

Current Mode Operation

When a detector is operated in current mode, all information regarding individual interactions is lost. For example, neither the interaction rate nor the energies deposited by individual interactions can be determined. However, if the amount of electrical charge collected from each interaction is proportional to the energy deposited by that interaction, then the net electrical current is proportional to the dose rate in the detector material. Detectors subject to very high interaction rates are often operated in current mode to avoid dead-time information losses. Image-intensifier tubes and flat panel image receptors in fluoroscopy, detectors in x-ray CT machines, direct digital radiographic image receptors, ion chambers used in phototimed radiography, and most nuclear medicine dose calibrators are operated in current mode.

17.1.2 Spectroscopy

The term *spectroscopy*, literally the viewing of a spectrum, is commonly used to refer to measurements of the energy distributions of radiation fields, and a *spectrometer* is a detection system that yields information about the energy distribution of the incident radiation. Most spectrometers are operated in pulse mode, and the amplitude of each pulse is proportional to the energy deposited in the detector by the interaction causing that pulse. *The energy deposited by an interaction, however, is not always*

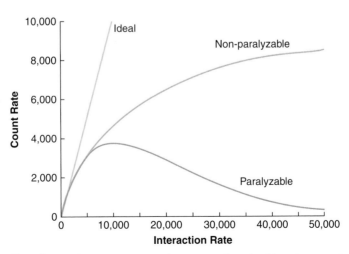

■ **FIGURE 17-1** Effect of interaction rate on measured count rate of paralyzable and non-paralyzable detectors. The "ideal" line represents the response of a hypothetical detector that does not suffer from dead-time count losses (*i.e.*, the count rate is equal to the interaction rate). Note that the *y*-axis scale is expanded with respect to that of the *x*-axis; the "ideal" line would be at a 45° angle if the scales were equal.

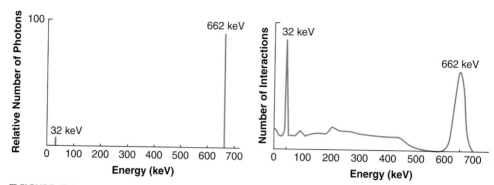

■ **FIGURE 17-2** Energy spectrum of cesium-137 (left) and resultant pulse height spectrum from a detector (right).

the total energy of the incident particle or photon. For example, a γ-ray may interact with the detector by Compton scattering, with the scattered photon escaping the detector. In this case, the deposited energy is the difference between the energies of the incident and scattered photons. A *pulse height spectrum* is usually depicted as a graph of the number of interactions depositing a particular amount of energy in the spectrometer as a function of energy (Fig. 17-2). Because the energy deposited by an interaction may be less than the total energy of the incident particle or photon and also because of random variations in the detection process, *the pulse height spectrum produced by a spectrometer is not identical to the actual energy spectrum of the incident radiation.* The energy resolution of a spectrometer is a measure of its ability to differentiate between particles or photons of different energies. Pulse height spectroscopy is discussed later in this chapter.

17.1.3 Detection Efficiency

The *efficiency (sensitivity)* of a detector is a measure of its ability to detect radiation. The efficiency of a detection system operated in pulse mode is defined as the probability that a particle or photon emitted by a source will be detected. It is measured by placing a source of radiation in the vicinity of the detector and dividing the number of particles or photons detected by the number emitted:

$$\text{Efficiency} = \frac{\text{Number detected}}{\text{Number emitted}}. \qquad [17\text{-}1]$$

This equation can be written as follows:

$$\text{Efficiency} = \frac{\text{Number reaching detector}}{\text{Number emitted}} \times \frac{\text{Number detected}}{\text{Number reaching detector}}.$$

Therefore, the detection efficiency is the product of two terms, the geometric efficiency and the intrinsic efficiency:

$$\text{Efficiency} = \text{Geometric efficiency} \times \text{Intrinsic efficiency}, \qquad [17\text{-}2]$$

where the *geometric efficiency* of a detector is the fraction of emitted particles or photons that reach the detector and the *intrinsic efficiency* is the fraction of those particles or photons reaching the detector that are detected. Because the total, geometric, and intrinsic efficiencies are all probabilities, each ranges from 0 to 1.

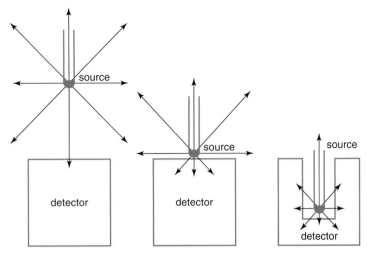

■ **FIGURE 17-3** Geometric efficiency. With a source far from the detector (left), the geometric efficiency is less than 50%. With a source against the detector (center), the geometric efficiency is approximately 50%. With a source in a well detector (right), the geometric efficiency is greater than 50%.

The geometric efficiency is determined by the geometric relationship between the source and the detector (Fig. 17-3). It increases as the source is moved toward the detector and approaches 0.5 when a point source is placed against a flat surface of the detector, because in that position one half of the photons or particles are emitted into the detector. For a source inside a well-type detector, the geometric efficiency approaches 1, because most of the particles or photons are intercepted by the detector. (A well-type detector is a detector containing a cavity for the insertion of samples.)

The intrinsic efficiency of a detector in detecting photons, also called the *quantum detection efficiency* (QDE), is determined by the energy of the photons and the atomic number, density, and thickness of the detector. If a parallel beam of monoenergetic photons is incident upon a detector of uniform thickness, the intrinsic efficiency of the detector is given by the following equation:

$$\text{Intrinsic efficiency} = 1 - e^{-\mu x} = 1 - e^{-(\mu/\rho)\rho x}, \qquad [17\text{-}3]$$

where μ is the linear attenuation coefficient of the detector material, ρ is the density of the material, μ/ρ is the mass attenuation coefficient of the material, and x is the thickness of the detector. This equation shows that the intrinsic efficiency for detecting x-rays and γ-rays increases with the thickness of the detector and the density and the mass attenuation coefficient of the detector material. The mass attenuation coefficient increases with the atomic number of the material and, within the range of photon energies used in diagnostic imaging, decreases with increasing photon energy, with the exception of absorption edges (Chapter 3).

17.2 GAS-FILLED DETECTORS

17.2.1 Basic Principles

A gas-filled detector (Fig. 17-4) consists of a volume of gas between two electrodes, with an electric potential difference (voltage) applied between the electrodes. Ionizing radiation forms ion pairs in the gas. The positive ions (cations)

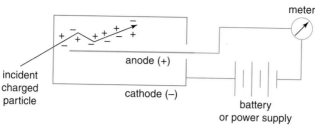

■ **FIGURE 17-4** Gas-filled detector. A charged particle, such as a beta particle, is shown entering the detector from outside and creating ion pairs in the gas inside the detector. This can occur only if the detector has a sufficiently thin wall. When a thick-wall gas-filled detector is used to detect x-rays and γ-rays, the charged particles causing the ionization are mostly electrons generated by Compton and photoelectric interactions of the incident x-rays or γ-rays in the detector wall or in the gas in the detector.

are attracted to the negative electrode (cathode), and the electrons or anions are attracted to the positive electrode (anode). In most detectors, the cathode is the wall of the container that holds the gas or a conductive coating on the inside of the wall, and the anode is a wire inside the container. After reaching the anode, the electrons travel through the circuit to the cathode, where they recombine with the cations. This electrical current can be measured with a sensitive ammeter or other electrical circuitry.

There are three types of gas-filled detectors in common use—ionization chambers, proportional counters, and GM counters. The type of detector is determined primarily by the voltage applied between the two electrodes. In an ionization chamber, the two electrodes can have almost any configuration: they may be two parallel plates, two concentric cylinders, or a wire within a cylinder. In proportional counters and GM counters, the anode must be a thin wire. Figure 17-5 shows the amount of electrical charge collected after a single interaction as a function of the electrical potential difference (voltage) applied between the two electrodes.

Ionizing radiation produces ion pairs in the gas of the detector. If no voltage is applied between the electrodes, no current flows through the circuit because there is no electric field to attract the charged particles to the electrodes; the ion pairs merely recombine in the gas. When a small voltage is applied, some of the cations are attracted to the cathode and some of the electrons or anions are attracted to the anode before they can recombine. As the voltage is increased, more ions are collected and fewer recombine. This region, in which the current increases as the voltage is raised, is called the *recombination region* of the curve.

As the voltage is increased further, a plateau is reached in the curve. In this region, called the *ionization chamber region*, the applied electric field is sufficiently strong to collect almost all ion pairs; additional increases in the applied voltage do not significantly increase the current. Ionization chambers are operated in this region.

Beyond the ionization region, the collected current again increases as the applied voltage is raised. In this region, called the *proportional region*, electrons approaching the anode are accelerated to such high kinetic energies that they cause additional ionization. This phenomenon, called *gas multiplication*, amplifies the collected current; the amount of amplification increases as the applied voltage is raised.

At any voltage through the ionization chamber region and the proportional region, the amount of electrical charge collected from each interaction is *proportional* to the amount of energy deposited in the gas of the detector by the interaction. For example, the amount of charge collected after an interaction depositing 100 keV is one tenth of that collected from an interaction depositing 1 MeV.

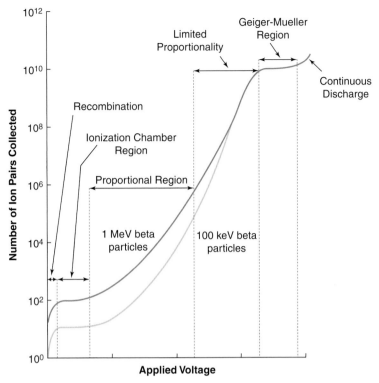

■ **FIGURE 17-5** Amount of electrical charge collected after a single interaction as a function of the electrical potential difference (voltage) applied between the two electrodes of a gas-filled detector. The lower curve shows the charge collected when a 100-keV electron interacts, and the upper curve shows the result from a 1-MeV electron.

Beyond the proportional region is a region in which the amount of charge collected from each event is the same, regardless of the amount of energy deposited by the interaction. In this region, called the *Geiger-Mueller region* (GM region), the gas multiplication spreads the entire length of the anode. The size of a pulse in the GM region tells us nothing about the energy deposited in the detector by the interaction causing the pulse. Gas-filled detectors cannot be operated at voltages beyond the GM region because they continuously discharge.

17.2.2 Ionization Chambers (Ion Chambers)

Because gas multiplication does not occur at the relatively low voltages applied to ionization chambers, the amount of electrical charge collected from a single interaction is very small and would require huge amplification to be detected. For this reason, ionization chambers are seldom used in pulse mode. The advantage to operating them in current mode is the almost complete freedom from dead-time effects, even in very intense radiation fields. In addition, as shown in Figure 17-5, the voltage applied to an ion chamber can vary significantly without appreciably changing the amount of charge collected.

Almost any gas can be used to fill the chamber. If the gas is air and the walls of the chamber are of a material whose effective atomic number is similar to air, the amount of current produced is proportional to the *exposure rate* (exposure is the amount of electrical charge produced per mass of air). Air-filled ion chambers are used in portable survey meters and can accurately indicate exposure rates from less than 1 mR/h to tens or hundreds of roentgens per hour (Fig. 17-6). Air-filled ion chambers are also used for performing quality-assurance testing of diagnostic and therapeutic x-ray machines, and they are the detectors in most x-ray machine phototimers. Measurements using an air-filled ion chamber that is open to the atmosphere are affected by the density of the air in the chamber, which is determined by ambient air pressure and temperature. Measurements using such chambers that require great accuracy must be corrected for these factors.

In very intense radiation fields, there can be signal loss due to recombination of ions before they are collected at the electrodes, causing the current from an ion chamber to deviate from proportionality to the intensity of the radiation. An ion chamber intended for use in such fields may have a small gas volume, a low gas density, and/or a high applied voltage to reduce this effect.

Gas-filled detectors tend to have low intrinsic efficiencies for detecting x-rays and γ-rays because of the low densities of gases and the low atomic numbers of most common gases. The sensitivity of ion chambers to x-rays and γ-rays can be enhanced

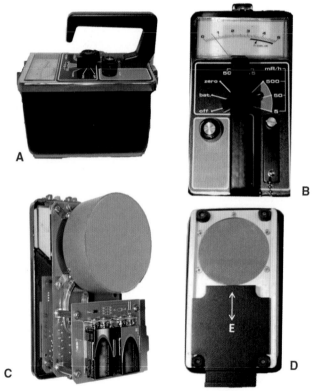

■ **FIGURE 17-6** Portable air-filled ionization chamber survey meter **(A)**. This particular instrument measures exposure rates ranging from about 0.1 mR/h to 50 R/h. The exposure rate is indicated by the position of the red needle on the scale. The scale is selected using the range knob located below the scale **(B)**. In this case, the needle is pointing to a value of 0.6 on the scale, and the range selector is set at 50 mR/h. Thus, the exposure rate being shown is 6 mR/h. The interior of the instrument is shown **(C)** and the ion chamber, covered with a thin Mylar membrane, is easily seen. On the bottom of the meter case **(D)** is a slide **(E)** that can cover or expose the thin Mylar window of the ion chamber. This slide should be opened when measuring low-energy x-ray and γ-ray radiation. The slide can also be used to determine if there is a significant beta radiation component in the radiation being measured. If there is no substantial change in the measured exposure rate with the slide open (where beta radiation can penetrate the thin membrane and enter the ion chamber) or closed (where the ion chamber is shielded from beta radiation), the radiation can be considered to be comprised primarily of x-rays or γ-rays.

by filling them with a gas that has a high atomic number, such as argon ($Z = 18$) or xenon ($Z = 54$), and pressurizing the gas to increase its density. Well-type ion chambers called dose calibrators are used in nuclear medicine to assay the activities of dosages of radiopharmaceuticals to be administered to patients; many are filled with pressurized argon. Xenon-filled pressurized ion chambers were formerly used as detectors in some CT machines.

Air-filled ion chambers are commonly used to measure the related quantities air kerma and exposure rate. These quantities were defined in Chapter 3. Air kerma is the initial kinetic energy transferred to charged particles, in this case electrons liberated in air by the radiation, per mass air and exposure is the amount of electrical charge created in air by ionization caused by these electrons, per mass air. There is a problem measuring the ionization in the small volume of air in an ionization chamber of reasonable size. The energetic electrons released by interactions in the air have long ranges in air, and many of them would escape the air in the chamber and cause much of their ionization elsewhere. This problem can be partially solved by building the ion chamber with thick walls of a material whose effective atomic number is similar to that of air. In this case, the number of electrons escaping the volume of air is approximately matched by a similar number of electrons released in the chamber wall entering the air in the ion chamber. This situation, if achieved, is called *electronic equilibrium*. For this reason, most ion chambers for measuring exposure or air kerma have thick air-equivalent walls, or are equipped with removable air-equivalent buildup caps to establish electronic equilibrium. The thickness of material needed to establish electronic equilibrium increases with the energy of the x- or γ-rays. However, thick walls or buildup caps may significantly attenuate low energy x- and γ-rays. Many ion chamber survey meters have windows that may be opened in the thick material around the ion chamber to permit more accurate measurement of low energy x- and γ-rays. Electronic equilibrium, also called charged particle equilibrium, is discussed in detail in more advanced texts (Attix, 1986; Knoll, 2010).

17.2.3 Proportional Counters

Unlike ion chambers, which can function with almost any gas, including air, a proportional counter must contain a gas with low electron affinity, so that few free electrons become attached to gas molecules. Because gas multiplication can produce a charge-per-interaction that is hundreds or thousands of times larger than that produced by an ion chamber, proportional counters can be operated in pulse mode as counters or spectrometers. They are commonly used in standards laboratories, in health physics laboratories, and for physics research. They are seldom used in medical centers.

Multiwire proportional counters, which indicate the position of an interaction in the detector, have been studied for use in nuclear medicine imaging devices. They have not achieved acceptance because of their low efficiencies for detecting x-rays and γ-rays from the radionuclides commonly used in nuclear medicine.

17.2.4 Geiger-Mueller Counters

GM counters must also contain gases with specific properties, discussed in more advanced texts. Because gas multiplication produces billions of ion pairs after an interaction, the signal from a GM detector requires little additional amplification. For this reason, GM detectors are often used for inexpensive survey meters.

GM detectors have high efficiencies for detecting charged particles that penetrate the walls of the detectors; almost every such particle reaching the interior of a detector is counted. Many GM detectors are equipped with thin windows to allow beta particles and conversion electrons to reach the gas and be detected. Very weak charged particles, such as the beta particles emitted by tritium (^{3}H, $E_{max} = 18$ keV), which is extensively used in biomedical research, cannot penetrate the windows; therefore, contamination by ^{3}H cannot be detected with a GM survey meter. Flat, thin-window GM detectors, called "pancake"-type detectors, are very useful for finding radioactive contamination (Fig. 17-7).

In general, GM survey meters are very inefficient detectors of x-rays and γ-rays, which tend to pass through the gas without interaction. Most of those that are detected have interacted with the walls of the detectors, with the resultant electrons scattered into the gas inside the detectors.

The size of the voltage pulse from a GM tube is independent of the energy deposited in the detector by the interaction causing the pulse: an interaction that deposits 1 keV causes a voltage pulse of the same size as one caused by an interaction that deposits 1 MeV. Therefore, GM detectors cannot be used as spectrometers or precise dose-rate meters. Many portable GM survey meters display measurements in units of

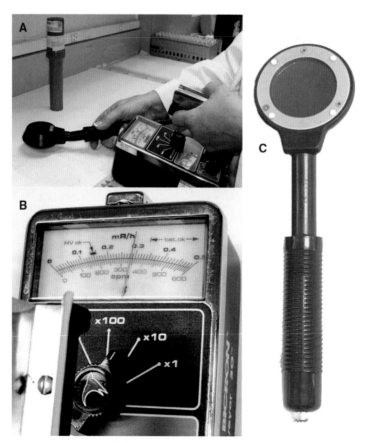

■ **FIGURE 17-7** Portable GM survey meter with a thin-window "pancake" probe. In the upper left **(A)**, a survey for radioactive contamination is being performed. In the lower left **(B)**, the range knob below the display is set to ×10 and so the red needle on the meter indicates a count rate of about 3,500 counts per minute (cpm). The thin window of the GM probe **(C)** is designed to permit beta particles and conversion electrons whose energies exceed about 45 keV to reach the sensitive volume inside the tube, and the large surface area of the detector reduces the time needed to survey a surface.

milliroentgens per hour. However, the GM counter cannot truly measure exposure rates, and so its reading must be considered only an approximation. If a GM survey meter is calibrated to indicate exposure rate for 662-keV γ-rays from ^{137}Cs (commonly used for calibrations), it may overrespond by as much as a factor of 5 for photons of lower energies, such as 80 keV. If an accurate measurement of exposure rate is required, an air-filled ionization chamber survey meter should be used.

This overresponse of a GM tube to low-energy x-rays and γ-rays can be partially corrected by placing a thin layer of a material with a moderately high atomic number (*e.g.*, tin) around the detector. The increasing attenuation coefficient of the material (due to the photoelectric effect) with decreasing photon energy significantly flattens the energy response of the detector. Such GM tubes are called *energy-compensated detectors*. The disadvantage of an energy-compensated detector is that its sensitivity to lower energy photons is substantially reduced and its energy threshold, below which photons cannot be detected at all, is increased. Energy-compensated GM detectors commonly have windows that can be opened to expose the thin tube walls so that high-energy beta particles and low-energy photons can be detected.

GM detectors suffer from extremely long dead times, ranging from tens to hundreds of microseconds. For this reason, GM counters are seldom used when accurate measurements are required of count rates greater than a few hundred counts per second. A portable GM survey meter may become paralyzed in a very high radiation field and yield a reading of zero. Ionization chamber instruments should always be used to measure high intensity x-ray and γ-ray fields.

17.3 SCINTILLATION DETECTORS

17.3.1 Basic Principles

Scintillators are materials that emit visible light or UV radiation after the interaction of ionizing radiation with the material. Scintillators are the oldest type of radiation detectors; Roentgen discovered x-radiation and the fact that x-rays induce scintillation in barium platinocyanide in the same fortuitous experiment. Scintillators are used in conventional film-screen radiography, many direct digital radiographic image receptors, fluoroscopy, scintillation cameras, CT scanners, and positron emission tomography (PET) scanners.

Although the light emitted from a single interaction can be seen if the viewer's eyes are dark adapted, most scintillation detectors incorporate a means of signal amplification. In conventional film-screen radiography, photographic film is used to amplify and record the signal. In other applications, electronic devices such as photomultiplier tubes (PMTs), photodiodes, or image-intensifier tubes convert the light into electrical signals. PMTs and image-intensifier tubes amplify the signal as well. However, most photodiodes do not provide amplification; if amplification of the signal is required, it must be provided by an electronic amplifier. A *scintillation detector* consists of a scintillator and a device, such as a PMT, that converts the light into an electrical signal.

When ionizing radiation interacts with a scintillator, electrons are raised to an excited energy level. Ultimately, these electrons fall back to a lower energy state, with the emission of visible light or UV radiation. Most scintillators have more than one mode for the emission of visible light or UV radiation, and each mode has its characteristic decay constant. *Luminescence* is the emission of light after excitation. *Fluorescence* is the prompt emission of light, whereas *phosphorescence* (also called *afterglow*) is the delayed emission of light. When scintillation detectors are operated in current mode, the prompt signal from an interaction cannot be separated from the phosphorescence caused by previous interactions. When a scintillation detector is operated in pulse mode, afterglow is less important because electronic circuits can separate the rapidly rising and falling components of the prompt signal from the slowly decaying delayed signal resulting from previous interactions.

It is useful, before discussing actual scintillation materials, to consider properties that are desirable in a scintillator.

1. The *conversion efficiency*, the fraction of deposited energy that is converted into light or UV radiation, should be high. (Conversion efficiency should not be confused with detection efficiency.)
2. For many applications, the decay times of excited states should be short. (Light or UV radiation is emitted promptly after an interaction.)
3. The material should be transparent to its own emissions. (Most emitted light or UV radiation escapes reabsorption.)
4. The frequency spectrum (color) of emitted light or UV radiation should match the spectral sensitivity of the light receptor (PMT, photodiode, or film).
5. If used for x-ray and γ-ray detection, the attenuation coefficient (μ) should be large, so that detectors made of the scintillator have high detection efficiencies. Materials with large atomic numbers and high densities have large attenuation coefficients.
6. The material should be rugged, unaffected by moisture, and inexpensive to manufacture.

In all scintillators, the amount of light emitted after an interaction increases with the energy deposited by the interaction. Therefore, scintillators may be operated in pulse mode as spectrometers. When a scintillator is used for spectroscopy, its energy resolution (ability to distinguish between interactions depositing different energies) is primarily determined by its conversion efficiency. A high conversion efficiency is required for superior energy resolution.

There are several categories of materials that scintillate. Many organic compounds exhibit scintillation. In these materials, the scintillation is a property of the molecular structure. Solid organic scintillators are used for timing experiments in particle physics because of their extremely prompt light emission. Organic scintillators include the liquid scintillation fluids that are used extensively in biomedical research. Samples containing radioactive tracers such as ^{3}H, ^{14}C, and ^{32}P are mixed in vials with liquid scintillators, and the light flashes are detected and counted by PMTs and associated electronic circuits. Organic scintillators are not used for medical imaging because the low atomic numbers of their constituent elements and their low densities make them poor x-ray and γ-ray detectors. When photons in the diagnostic energy range do interact with organic scintillators, it is primarily by Compton scattering.

There are also many inorganic crystalline materials that exhibit scintillation. In these materials, the scintillation is a property of the crystalline structure: if the crystal is dissolved, the scintillation ceases. Many of these materials have much larger average atomic numbers and higher densities than organic scintillators and therefore are excellent photon detectors. They are widely used for radiation measurements and imaging in radiology.

Most inorganic scintillation crystals are deliberately grown with trace amounts of impurity elements called *activators*. The atoms of these activators form preferred sites in the crystals for the excited electrons to return to the ground state. The activators modify the frequency (color) of the emitted light, the promptness of the light emission, and the proportion of the emitted light that escapes reabsorption in the crystal.

17.3.2 ## Inorganic Crystalline Scintillators in Radiology

No one scintillation material is best for all applications in radiology. Sodium iodide activated with thallium [NaI(Tl)] is used for most nuclear medicine applications. It is coupled to PMTs and operated in pulse mode in scintillation cameras, thyroid probes, and γ-well counters. Its high content of iodine ($Z = 53$) and high density provide a high photoelectric absorption probability for x-rays and γ-rays emitted by common nuclear medicine radiopharmaceuticals (70 to 365 keV). It has a very high conversion efficiency; approximately 13% of deposited energy is converted into light. Because a light photon has an energy of about 3 eV, approximately one light photon is emitted for every 23 eV absorbed by the crystal. This high conversion efficiency gives it a very good energy resolution. It emits light very promptly (decay constant, 250 ns), permitting it to be used in pulse mode at interaction rates greater than 100,000/s. Very large crystals can be manufactured; for example, the rectangular crystals of one modern scintillation camera are 59 cm (23 inches) long, 44.5 cm (17.5 inches) wide, and 0.95 cm thick. Unfortunately, NaI(Tl) crystals are fragile; they crack easily if struck or subjected to rapid temperature change. Also, they are hygroscopic (*i.e.*, they absorb water from the atmosphere) and therefore must be hermetically sealed.

PET, discussed in Chapter 19, requires high detection efficiency for 511-keV annihilation photons and a prompt signal from each interaction because the signals must be processed in pulse mode at high interaction rates. PET detectors are thick crystals of high-density, high atomic number scintillators optically coupled to PMTs. For many years, bismuth germanate ($Bi_4Ge_3O_{12}$, often abbreviated as "BGO") was the preferred scintillator. The high atomic number of bismuth ($Z = 83$) and the high density of the crystal yield a high intrinsic efficiency for the 511-keV positron annihilation photons. The primary component of the light emission is sufficiently prompt (decay constant, 300 ns) for PET. NaI(Tl) was used in early and some less-expensive PET scanners. Today, lutetium oxyorthosilicate (Lu_2SiO_4O, abbreviated LSO), lutetium yttrium oxyorthosilicate (Lu_xYSiO_4O, abbreviated LYSO), and gadolinium oxyorthosilicate (Gd_2SiO_4O, abbreviated GSO), all activated with cerium, are used in newer PET scanners. Their densities and effective atomic numbers are similar to those of BGO, but their conversion efficiencies are much larger and they emit light much more promptly.

Calcium tungstate ($CaWO_4$) was used for many years in intensifying screens in film-screen radiography. It was largely replaced by rare-earth phosphors, such as gadolinium oxysulfide activated with terbium. The intensifying screen is an application of scintillators that does not require very prompt light emission, because the film usually remains in contact with the screen for at least several seconds after exposure. Cesium iodide activated with thallium is used as the phosphor layer of many indirect-detection thin-film transistor radiographic and fluoroscopic image receptors, described in Chapters 7 and 9. Cesium iodide activated with sodium is used as the input phosphor and zinc cadmium sulfide activated with silver is used as the output phosphor of image-intensifier tubes in fluoroscopes.

Scintillators coupled to photodiodes are used as the detectors in CT scanners, as described in Chapter 10. The extremely high x-ray flux experienced by the detectors necessitates current mode operation to avoid dead-time effects. With the rotational speed of CT scanners as high as three rotations per second, the scintillators used in CT must have very little afterglow. Cadmium tungstate and gadolinium ceramics are scintillators used in CT. Table 17-1 lists the properties of several inorganic crystalline scintillators of importance in radiology and nuclear medicine.

TABLE 17-1 INORGANIC SCINTILLATORS USED IN MEDICAL IMAGING

MATERIAL	ATOMIC NUMBERS	DENSITY (g/cm³)	WAVELENGTH OF MAXIMAL EMISSION (nm)	CONVERSION EFFICIENCY[a] (%)	DECAY CONSTANT (μS)	AFTER GLOW (%)	USES
NaI(Tl)	11, 53	3.67	415	100	0.25	0.3–5 at 6 ms	Scintillation cameras
$Bi_4Ge_3O_{12}$	83, 32, 8	7.13	480	12–14	0.3	0.005 at 3 ms	PET scanners
$Lu_2SiO_4O(Ce)$	71, 14, 8	7.4	420	75	40	—	PET scanners
CsI(Na)	55, 53	4.51	420	85	0.63	—	Input phosphor of image-intensifier tubes
CsI(Tl)	55, 53	4.51	550	45[b]	1.0	0.5–5 at 6 ms	Thin-film transistor radiographic and fluoroscopic image receptors
ZnCdS(Ag)	30, 48, 16	—	—	—	—	—	Output phosphor of image-intensifier tubes
$CdWO_4$	48, 74, 8	7.90	475	40	14	0.1 at 3 ms	Computed tomographic (CT) scanners
$CaWO_4$	20, 74, 8	6.12	—	14–18	0.9–20	—	Radiographic screens
$Gd_2O_2S(Tb)$	64, 8, 16	7.34	—	—	560	—	Radiographic screens

[a]Relative to NaI(Tl), using a PMT to measure light.
[b]The light emitted by CsI(Tl) does not match the spectral sensitivity of PMTs very well; its conversion efficiency is much larger if measured with a photodiode.
Data on NaI(Tl), BGO, CsI(Na), CsI(Tl), and CdWO₄ courtesy of Saint-Gobain Crystals, Hiram, OH. Data on LSO from Ficke DC, Hood JT, Ter-Pogossian MM. A spheroid positron emission tomograph for brain imaging: a feasibility study. *J Nucl Med*. 1996;37:1222.

17.3.3 Conversion of Light into an Electrical Signal

Photomultiplier Tubes

PMTs perform two functions—conversion of UV and visible light photons into an electrical signal and signal amplification, on the order of millions to billions. As shown in Figure 17-8, a PMT consists of an evacuated glass tube containing a *photocathode*, typically 10 to 12 electrodes called *dynodes*, and an *anode*. The photocathode is a very thin electrode, located just inside the glass entrance window of the PMT, which emits electrons when struck by visible light. Photocathodes are inefficient; approximately one electron is emitted from the photocathode for every five UV or light photons incident upon it. A high-voltage power supply provides a voltage of approximately 1,000 V, and a series of resistors divides the voltage into equal increments. The first dynode is given a voltage of about +100 V with respect to the photocathode; successive dynodes have voltages that increase by approximately 100 V per dynode. The electrons emitted by the photocathode are attracted to the first dynode and are accelerated to kinetic energies equal to the potential difference between the photocathode and the first dynode. (If the potential difference is 100 V, the kinetic energy of each electron is 100 eV.) When these electrons strike the first dynode, about five electrons are ejected from the dynode for each electron hitting it. These electrons are then attracted to the second dynode, reaching kinetic energies equal to the potential difference between the first and second dynodes, and causing about five electrons to be ejected from the second dynode for each electron hitting it. This process continues down the chain of dynodes, with the number of electrons being multiplied by a factor of 5 at each stage. The total amplification of the PMT is the product of the individual multiplications at each dynode. If a PMT has ten dynodes and the amplification at each stage is 5, the total amplification will be

$$5 \times 5 \times 5 \times 5 \times 5 \times 5 \times 5 \times 5 \times 5 \times 5 = 5^{10} \approx 10,000,000.$$

The amplification can be adjusted by changing the voltage applied to the PMT.

When a scintillator is coupled to a PMT, an optical coupling material is placed between the two components to minimize reflection losses. The scintillator is usually surrounded on all other sides by a highly reflective material, often magnesium oxide powder.

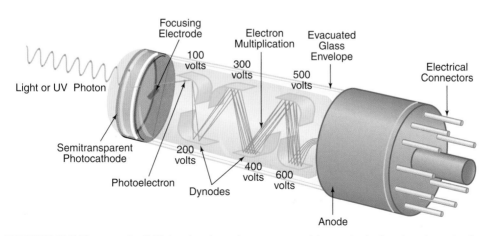

■ **FIGURE 17-8** Diagram of a PMT showing the main components (photocathode, focusing electrode, dynodes, and anode) and illustrating the process of electron multiplication. Actual PMTs typically have 10 to 12 dynodes.

Photodiodes

Photodiodes are semiconductor diodes that convert light into electrical signals. (The principles of operation of semiconductor diodes are discussed later in this chapter.) In use, photodiodes are reverse biased. *Reverse bias* means that the voltage is applied with the polarity such that essentially no electrical current flows. When the photodiode is exposed to light, an electrical current is generated that is proportional to the intensity of the light. Photodiodes are sometimes used with scintillators instead of PMTs. Photodiodes produce more electrical noise than PMTs do, but they are smaller and less expensive. Most photodiodes, unlike PMTs, do not amplify the signal. However, a type of photodiode called an avalanche photodiode does provide signal amplification, although not as much as a PMT. Photodiodes coupled to $CdWO_4$ or other scintillators are used in current mode in CT scanners. Photodiodes are also essential components of indirect-detection thin-film transistor radiographic and fluoroscopic image receptors, which use scintillators to convert x-ray energy into light.

Multi-Pixel Photon Counters, "Silicon Photomultipliers" (SiPMs)

Another solid-state electronic device that can detect and measure visible light and/or UV radiation from a scintillator is a rectangular array of tiny (typically 10-100 μm) avalanche photodiodes operated in Geiger mode, with the outputs summed (Fig. 17-9). Such diode arrays have been given several names, including multi-pixel photon counters, but perhaps are most commonly referred to as silicon photomultipliers (SiPMs).

As mentioned previously, an avalanche photodiode is a photodiode operated at a sufficiently high voltage that a hole-electron pair caused by the absorption of a single photon can, in turn, create a number of additional hole-electron pairs. If the applied voltage is kept below a value called the breakdown voltage, the number of hole-electron pairs is approximately proportional to the light or UV energy absorbed, whether from one or multiple photons. However, if the voltage applied to an avalanche photodiode is above the breakdown voltage, a single light photon can trigger a much larger avalanche in the photodiode that produces an electrical charge that is

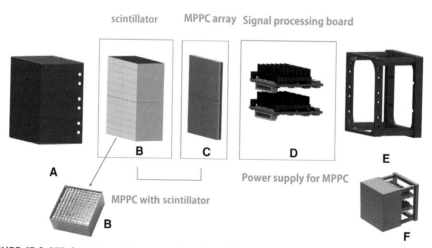

■ **FIGURE 17-9** PET detector module, consisting of multiple subcomponents within an outside shroud **(A)** including a square array of scintillation crystals **(B)**, optically coupled to an MPPC (SiPM) array **(C)**. The MPPC array converts the light from the scintillation crystals to electrical signals. The signal processing electronics **(D)** produce position, timing, and energy signals for each interaction of an annihilation photon. An MPPC array might be a 12 × 12 array of 144 independent 4 mm × 4 mm channels, with each channel being a square array of 75 μm avalanche photodiodes. These components are mounted to a metal frame **(E)** and the assembled unit is shown in **(F)**. (Modified with permission from Hamamatsu Photonics.)

several orders of magnitude larger than that produced by an avalanche photodiode operated below the breakdown voltage. This is known as Geiger mode operation and is analogous to the operation of a Geiger-Muller tube.

A Geiger mode avalanche is self-sustaining in the diode and, in practical applications, must be terminated ("quenched"). This is commonly done by placing a resistor in series with each avalanche photodiode. When an avalanche occurs, the electrical current through the resistor causes a voltage across the resistor. This, in turn, reduces the voltage across the photodiode to below the breakdown voltage, quenching the avalanche.

After an avalanche occurs in a photodiode, a recovery time (deadtime) elapses before the voltage across the diode again exceeds the breakdown voltage and another avalanche can occur. The diode is insensitive during this period.

The electrical charge released by a Geiger mode avalanche in a single diode is independent of the number of photons triggering the avalanche and so the resultant signal tells nothing about the number of photons absorbed or the energy they deposited. However, the net electrical charge from the entire SiPM after a burst of light, such as that from a γ-ray or annihilation photon interacting with a scintillator, is proportional to the number of photodiodes in which avalanches occurred and, provided that the number of incident photons is not much, much greater than the number of photodiodes in the SiPM, provides information regarding the number of photons incident on the SiPM. If the number of incident photons is sufficiently small such that most photodiodes receive only one or no photons, the signal from the SiPM will be nearly proportional to the number of incident photons, which is approximately proportional to the energy deposited in the scintillator. The range of light pulse intensities over which an SiPM produces a proportional (linear) response increases as the cross-sectional active areas of the individual photodiodes is reduced.

An SiPM provides a very large electrical charge amplification, nearly equivalent to that of a PMT.

SiPMs produce dark currents larger than those of PMTs, due to thermally generated hole-electron pairs. The dark current can be reduced by cooling the SiPM. However, thermally generated avalanches in individual photodiodes produce output pulses from the SiPM that are much smaller than those produced by pulses of light from a scintillator and so do not have much of an adverse impact in nuclear medicine imaging applications.

Although the QDE of photodiodes in general considerably exceeds that of PMTs across the UV and visible light spectra, the QDE of SiPMs may be similar to or barely exceed that of PMTs. A main reason for this is the insensitive dead space separating the individual photodiodes in an SiPM.

An important advantage of SiPMs over PMTs is that, like photodiodes in general, SiPMs are not significantly affected by magnetic fields. SiPMs are also much more compact than PMTs. SiPMs are commonly packaged in square arrays, of 4×4 or 8×8 separate SiPMs. SiPMs are used instead of PMTs in some new PET scanners.

17.3.4   Scintillators with Trapping of Excited Electrons

In most applications of scintillators, the prompt emission of light after an interaction is desirable. However, there are inorganic scintillators in which electrons become trapped in excited states after interactions with ionizing radiation. These trapped electrons can be released by heating or exposure to light; the electrons then fall to their ground state with the emission of light, which can be detected by a PMT or other sensor. These trapped electrons, in effect, store information about the radiation exposure. Such scintillators can be used for dosimetry or for radiographic imaging.

Thermoluminescent Dosimeters and Optically Stimulated Luminescent Dosimeters

As mentioned above, scintillators with electron trapping can be used for dosimetry. In the case of *thermoluminescent dosimeters* (TLDs), to read the signal after exposure to ionizing radiation, a sample of TLD material is heated, the light is detected and converted into an electrical signal by a PMT, and the resultant signal is integrated and displayed. The amount of light emitted by the TLD increases with the amount of energy absorbed by the TLD, but may deviate from proportionality, particularly at higher doses. After the TLD has been read, it may be baked in an oven to release the remaining trapped electrons and reused.

Lithium fluoride (LiF) is one of the most useful TLD materials. It is commercially available in forms with different trace impurities (Mg and Ti or Mg, Cu, and P), giving differences in properties such as sensitivity and linearity of response with dose. LiF has trapping centers that exhibit almost negligible release of trapped electrons at room temperature, so there is little loss of information with time from exposure to the reading of the TLD. The effective atomic number of LiF is close to that of tissue, so the amount of light emission is almost proportional to the tissue dose over a wide range of x-ray and γ-ray energies. It is commonly used instead of photographic film for personnel dosimetry.

In optically stimulated luminescense (OSL), the trapped excited electrons are released by exposure to light, commonly produced by a laser, of a frequency optimal for releasing the trapped electrons. The most commonly used OSL material is aluminum oxide (Al_2O_3) activated with a small amount of carbon. The effective atomic number of aluminum oxide is significantly higher than that of soft tissue, and so dose to this material is not proportional to dose to soft tissue over the full range of energies used in medical imaging. Methods for compensating for this effect are discussed in Chapter 21.

Photostimulable Phosphors

Photostimulable phosphors (PSPs), like TLDs, are scintillators in which a fraction of the excited electrons become trapped. PSP plates are used in radiography as image receptors, instead of film-screen cassettes. Although the trapped electrons could be released by heating, a laser is used to scan the plate and release them. The electrons then fall to the ground state, with the emission of light. Barium fluorohalide activated with europium is commonly used for PSP imaging plates. In this material, the wavelength that is most efficient in stimulating luminescence is in the red portion of the spectrum, whereas the stimulated luminescence itself is in the blue-violet portion of the spectrum. The stimulated emissions are converted into an electrical signal by PMTs. After the plate is read by the laser, it may be exposed to light to release the remaining trapped electrons that can be reused. The use of PSPs in radiography has been discussed further in Chapter 7.

17.4 SEMICONDUCTOR DETECTORS

Semiconductors are crystalline materials whose electrical conductivities are less than those of metals but more than those of crystalline insulators. Silicon and germanium are common semiconductor materials.

In crystalline materials, electrons exist in energy bands, separated by forbidden gaps. In metals (*e.g.*, copper), the least tightly bound electrons exist in a partially occupied band, called the conduction band. The conduction-band electrons are mobile, providing high electrical conductivity. In an insulator or a semiconductor, the valence electrons exist in a filled valence band. In semiconductors, these valence-band electrons participate in covalent bonds and so are immobile. The next higher energy band, the conduction band, is empty of electrons. However, if an electron is placed in the conduction band, it is mobile, as are the upper band electrons in metals. The difference between insulators and semiconductors is the magnitude of the energy gap between the valence and conduction bands. In insulators, the band gap is greater than 5 eV, whereas in semiconductors, it is about 1 eV or less (Fig. 17-10). In semiconductors, valence-band electrons can be raised to the conduction band by ionizing radiation, visible light or UV radiation, or thermal energy.

When a valence-band electron is raised to the conduction band, it leaves behind a vacancy in the valence band. This vacancy is called a *hole*. Because a hole is the absence of an electron, it is considered to have a net positive charge, equal but opposite to that of an electron. When another valence-band electron fills the hole, a hole is created at that electron's former location. Thus, holes behave as mobile positive charges in the valence band even though positively charged particles do not physically move in the material. The hole-electron pairs formed in a semiconductor material by ionizing radiation are analogous to the ion pairs formed in a gas by ionizing radiation.

A crystal of a semiconductor material can be used as a radiation detector. A voltage is placed between two terminals on opposite sides of the crystal. When ionizing radiation interacts with the detector, electrons in the crystal are raised to an excited state, permitting an electrical current to flow, similar to a gas-filled ionization chamber. Unfortunately, the radiation-induced current, unless it is very large, is masked by a larger current induced by the applied voltage.

To reduce the magnitude of the voltage-induced current so that the signal from radiation interactions can be detected, the semiconductor crystal is "doped" with a trace amount of impurities so that it acts as a diode (see earlier discussion of types of detectors). The impurity atoms fill sites in the crystal lattice that would otherwise be occupied by atoms of the semiconductor material. If atoms of the impurity material have more valence electrons than those of the semiconductor material, the impurity atoms provide mobile electrons in the conduction band. A semiconductor material containing an electron-donor impurity is called an *n-type material* (Fig. 17-11). N-type material has mobile electrons in the conduction band. On the other hand, an impurity with fewer valence electrons than the semiconductor material provides sites in the valence band that can accept electrons. When a valence-band electron fills one

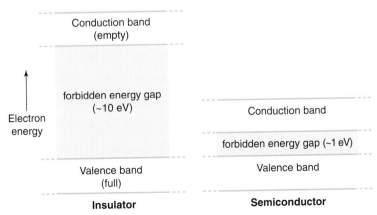

■ **FIGURE 17-10** Energy band structure of a crystalline insulator and a semiconductor material.

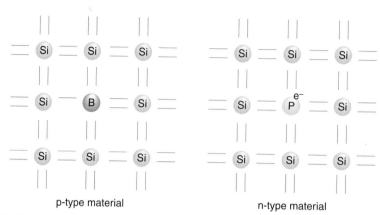

p-type material   n-type material

■ **FIGURE 17-11** P-type and n-type impurities in a crystal of a semiconductor material, silicon in this example. N-type impurities provide mobile electrons in the conduction band, whereas p-type impurities provide acceptor sites in the valence band. When filled by electrons, these acceptor sites create holes that act as mobile positive charges. Si, silicon; B, boron; P, phosphorus.

of these sites, it creates a hole at its former location. Semiconductor material doped with a hole-forming impurity is called *p-type material*. P-type material has mobile holes in the valence band.

A semiconductor diode consists of a crystal of semiconductor material with a region of n-type material that forms a junction with a region of p-type material (Fig. 17-12). If an external voltage is applied with the positive polarity on the p-type side of the diode and the negative polarity on the n-type side, the holes in the p-type material and the mobile conduction-band electrons of the n-type material are drawn to the junction. There, the mobile electrons fall into the valence band to fill holes. Applying an external voltage in this manner is referred to as *forward bias*. Forward bias permits a current to flow with little resistance.

On the other hand, if an external voltage is applied with the opposite polarity— that is, with the negative polarity on the p-type side of the diode and the positive polarity on the n-type side—the holes in the p-type material and the mobile conduction-band electrons of the n-type material are drawn away from the junction.

■ **FIGURE 17-12** Semiconductor diode. When no bias is applied, a few holes migrate into the n-type material and a few conduction-band electrons migrate into the p-type material. With forward bias, the external voltage is applied with the positive polarity on the p-side of the junction and negative polarity on the n-side, causing the charge carriers to be swept into the junction and a large current to flow. With negative bias, the charge carriers are drawn away from the junction, creating a region depleted of charge carriers that acts as a solid-state ion chamber.

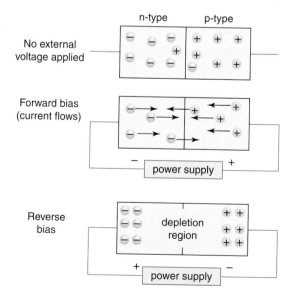

Applying the external voltage in this polarity is referred to as *reverse bias*. Reverse bias draws the charge carriers away from the n-p junction, forming a region depleted of current carriers. Very little electrical current flows when a diode is reverse biased.

A reverse-biased semiconductor diode can be used to detect visible light and UV radiation or ionizing radiation. The photons of light or ionization and excitation produced by ionizing radiation can excite lower energy electrons in the depletion region of the diode to higher energy bands, producing hole-electron pairs. The electrical field in the depletion region sweeps the holes toward the p-type side and the conduction-band electrons toward the n-type side, causing a momentary pulse of current to flow after the interaction.

Photodiodes are semiconductor diodes that convert light into an electrical current. As mentioned previously, they are used in conjunction with scintillators as detectors in CT scanners. Scintillation-based thin-film transistor radiographic and fluoroscopic image receptors incorporate a photodiode in each detector element.

Semiconductor detectors are semiconductor diodes designed for the detection of ionizing radiation. The amount of charge generated by an interaction is proportional to the energy deposited in the detector by the interaction; therefore, semiconductor detectors are spectrometers. Because thermal energy can also raise electrons to the conduction band, many types of semiconductor detectors used for x-ray and γ-ray spectroscopy must be cooled with liquid nitrogen.

The energy resolution of germanium semiconductor detectors is greatly superior to that of NaI(Tl) scintillation detectors. Liquid nitrogen–cooled germanium detectors are widely used for the identification of individual γ-ray–emitting radionuclides in mixed radionuclide samples because of their superb energy resolution.

Semiconductor detectors are seldom used for medical imaging devices because of high expense, because of low quantum detection efficiencies in comparison to scintillators such as NaI(Tl) (Z of iodine = 53, Z of germanium = 32, Z of silicon = 14), because they can be manufactured only in limited sizes, and because many such devices require cooling.

Efforts are being made to develop semiconductor detectors of higher atomic number than germanium that can be operated at room temperature. A leading candidate to date is cadmium zinc telluride (CZT). A small-field-of-view nuclear medicine camera using CZT detectors has been developed.

A layer of a semiconductor material, amorphous selenium (Z = 34), is used in some radiographic image receptors, including those in some mammography systems. The selenium is commonly referred to as a "photoconductor." In these image receptors, the selenium layer is electrically coupled to a rectangular array of thin film transistor detector elements that collect and store the mobile electrical charges produced in the selenium by x-ray interactions during image acquisition. These image receptors are discussed in Chapters 7 and 8.

17.5 PULSE HEIGHT SPECTROSCOPY

Many radiation detectors, such as scintillation detectors, semiconductor detectors, and proportional counters, produce electrical pulses whose amplitudes are proportional to the energies deposited in the detectors by individual interactions. *Pulse height analyzers* (PHAs) are electronic systems that may be used with these detectors to perform pulse height spectroscopy and energy-selective counting. In energy-selective counting, only interactions that deposit energies within a certain energy range are counted. Energy-selective counting can be used to reduce the effects of background radiation, to reduce the effects of scatter, or to separate events caused by different radionuclides in a sample containing multiple radionuclides. Two types of PHAs are *single-channel analyzers* (SCAs) and *multichannel analyzers* (MCAs). MCAs determine spectra much more efficiently than do SCA systems, but they are more expensive. Pulse height discrimination circuits are incorporated in scintillation cameras and other nuclear medicine imaging devices to reduce the effects of scatter on the images.

17.5.1 Single-Channel Analyzer Systems

Function of a Single-Channel Analyzer System

Figure 17-13 depicts an SCA system. Although the system is shown with an NaI(Tl) crystal and PMT, it could be used with any pulse-mode spectrometer. The high-voltage power supply typically provides 800 to 1,200 V to the PMT. The series of resistors divides the total voltage into increments that are applied to the dynodes and anode of the PMT. Raising the voltage increases the magnitude of the voltage pulses from the PMT.

The detector is often located some distance from the majority of the electronic components. The pulses from the PMT are usually routed to a preamplifier (pre-amp), which is connected to the PMT by as short a cable as possible. The function of the preamp is to amplify the voltage pulses further, so as to minimize distortion and attenuation of the signal during transmission to the remainder of the system. The pulses from the preamp are routed to the amplifier, which further amplifies the pulses and modifies their shapes. The gains of most amplifiers are adjustable.

The pulses from the amplifier then proceed to the SCA. The user is allowed to set two voltage levels, a lower level and an upper level. If a voltage pulse whose amplitude is less than the lower level or greater than the upper level is received from the amplifier, the SCA does nothing. If a voltage pulse whose amplitude is greater than the lower level but less than the upper level is received from the amplifier, the SCA produces a single logic pulse. A logic pulse is a voltage pulse of fixed amplitude and duration. Figure 17-14 illustrates the operation of an SCA. The counter counts the logic pulses from the SCA for a time interval set by the timer.

Many SCAs permit the user to select the mode by which the two knobs set the lower and upper levels. In one mode, usually called *LL/UL mode*, one knob directly sets the lower level and the other sets the upper level. In another mode, called *window*

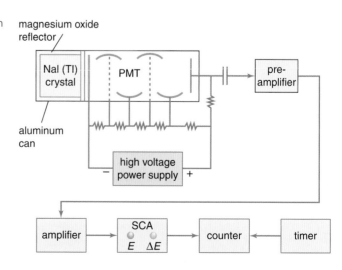

■ **FIGURE 17-13** SCA system with NaI(Tl) detector and PMT.

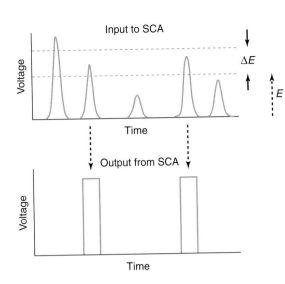

■ **FIGURE 17-14** Illustration of the function of an SCA. Energy discrimination occurs by rejection of pulses above or below the energy window set by the operator.

mode, one knob (often labeled E or energy) sets the midpoint of the range of acceptable pulse heights and the other knob (often labeled ΔE or window) sets the range of voltages around this value. In this mode, the lower level voltage is $E - \Delta E/2$ and the upper level voltage is $E + \Delta E/2$. (In some SCAs, the range of acceptable pulse heights is from E to $E + \Delta E$.) Window mode is convenient for plotting a spectrum.

Plotting a Spectrum Using a Single-Channel Analyzer

To obtain the pulse height spectrum of a sample of radioactive material using an SCA system, the SCA is placed in window mode, the E setting is set to zero, and a small window (ΔE) setting is selected. A series of counts is taken for a fixed length of time per count, with the E setting increased before each count but without changing the window setting. Each count is plotted on graph paper as a function of baseline (E) setting.

Energy Calibration of a Single-Channel Analyzer System

On most SCAs, each of the two knobs permits values from 0 to 1,000 to be selected. By adjusting the amplification of the pulses reaching the SCA—either by changing the voltage produced by the high-voltage power supply or by changing the amplifier gain—the system can be calibrated so that these knob settings directly indicate keV.

A ^{137}Cs source, which emits 662-keV γ-rays, is usually used. A narrow window is set, centered about a setting of 662. For example, the SCA may be placed into LL/UL mode with lower level value of 655 and an upper level value of 669 selected. Then the voltage produced by the high-voltage power supply is increased in steps, with a count taken after each step. The counts first increase and then decrease. When the voltage that produces the largest count is selected, the two knobs on the SCA directly indicate keV. This procedure is called *peaking* the SCA system.

17.5.2 Multichannel Analyzer Systems

An MCA system permits an energy spectrum to be automatically acquired much more quickly and easily than does an SCA system. Figure 17-15 is a diagram of a counting system using an MCA. The detector, high-voltage power supply, preamp, and amplifier are the same as were those described for SCA systems. The MCA consists of an ADC, a memory containing many storage locations called *channels,* control circuitry, and a timer. The memory of an MCA typically ranges from 256 to

■ **FIGURE 17-15** Diagram of an MCA system with NaI(Tl) detector.

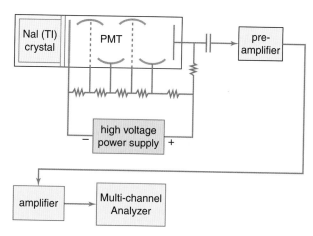

8,192 channels, each of which can store a single integer. When the acquisition of a spectrum begins, all of the channels are set to zero. When each voltage pulse from the amplifier is received, it is converted into a binary digital signal, the value of which is proportional to the amplitude of the analog voltage pulse. This digital signal designates a particular channel in the MCA's memory. The number stored in that channel is then incremented by 1. As many pulses are processed, a spectrum is generated in the memory of the MCA. Figure 17-16 illustrates the operation of an MCA. Today, most MCAs are interfaced to digital computers that store, process, and display the resultant spectra.

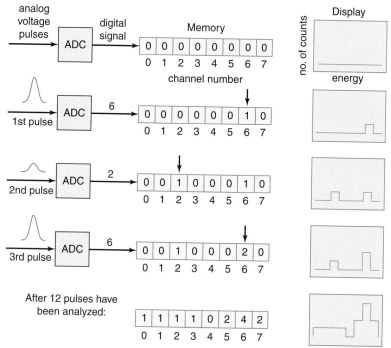

■ **FIGURE 17-16** Acquisition of a spectrum by an MCA. The digital signal produced by the ADC is a binary signal. After the analog pulses are digitized by the ADC, they are sorted into bins (channels) by height, forming an energy spectrum. Although this figure depicts an MCA with 8 channels, actual MCAs have as many as 8,192 channels.

17.5.3 X-ray and γ-ray Spectroscopy with Sodium Iodide Detectors

X-ray and γ-ray spectroscopy is best performed with semiconductor detectors because of their superior energy resolution. However, high detection efficiency is more important than ultrahigh energy resolution for most nuclear medicine applications, so most spectroscopy systems in nuclear medicine use NaI(Tl) crystals coupled to PMTs.

17.5.4 Interactions of Photons with a Spectrometer

There are a number of mechanisms by which an x-ray or γ-ray can deposit energy in the detector, several of which deposit only a fraction of the incident photon energy. As illustrated in Figure 17-17, an incident photon can deposit its full energy by a photoelectric interaction (A) or by one or more Compton scatters followed by a photoelectric interaction (B). However, a photon will deposit only a fraction of its energy if it interacts by Compton scattering and the scattered photon escapes the detector (C). In that case, the energy deposited depends on the scattering angle, with larger angle scatters depositing larger energies. Even if the incident photon interacts by the photoelectric effect, less than its total energy will be deposited if the inner-shell electron vacancy created by the interaction results in the emission of a characteristic x-ray that escapes the detector (D).

Most detectors are shielded to reduce the effects of natural background radiation and nearby radiation sources. Figure 17-17 shows two ways by which an x-ray or γ-ray interaction in the shield of the detector can deposit energy in the detector. The photon may Compton scatter in the shield, with the scattered photon striking the detector (E), or a characteristic x-ray from the shield may interact with the detector (F).

Most interactions of x-rays and γ-rays with an NaI(Tl) detector are with iodine atoms, because iodine has a much larger atomic number than sodium does. Although thallium has an even larger atomic number, it is only a trace impurity.

17.5.5 Spectrum of Cesium-137

The spectrum of ^{137}Cs is often used to introduce pulse height spectroscopy because of the simple decay scheme of this radionuclide. As shown at the top of Figure 17-18,

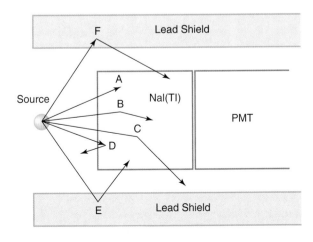

■ **FIGURE 17-17** Interactions of x-rays and γ-rays with an NaI(Tl) detector. See text for description.

^{137}Cs decays by beta particle emission to ^{137m}Ba, whose nucleus is in an excited state. The ^{137m}Ba nucleus attains its ground state by the emission of a 662-keV γ-ray 90% of the time. In 10% of the decays, a conversion electron is emitted instead of a γ-ray. The conversion electron is usually followed by the emission of an approximately 32-keV K-shell characteristic x-ray as an outer-shell electron fills the inner-shell vacancy.

In the left in Figure 17-18 is the actual energy spectrum of ^{137}Cs, and on the right is its pulse height spectrum obtained with the use of an NaI(Tl) detector. There are two reasons for the differences between the spectra. First, there are a number of mechanisms by which an x-ray or γ-ray can deposit energy in the detector, several of which deposit only a fraction of the incident photon energy. Second, there are random variations in the processes by which the energy deposited in the detector is converted into an electrical signal. In the case of an NaI(Tl) crystal coupled to a PMT, there are random variations in the fraction of deposited energy converted into light, the fraction of the light that reaches the photocathode of the PMT, and the number of electrons ejected from the back of the photocathode per unit energy deposited by the light. These factors cause random variations in the size of the voltage pulses produced by the detector, even when the incident x-rays or γ-rays deposit exactly the same energy. The energy resolution of a spectrometer is a measure of the effect of these random variations on the resultant spectrum.

In the pulse height spectrum of ^{137}Cs, on the right in Figure 17-18, the photopeak (A) is caused by interactions in which the energy of an incident 662-keV photon is entirely absorbed in the crystal. This may occur by a single photoelectric interaction or by one or more Compton scattering interactions followed by a photoelectric interaction. The Compton continuum (B) is caused by 662-keV photons that scatter in the

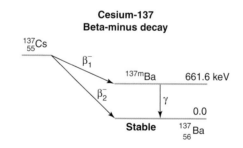

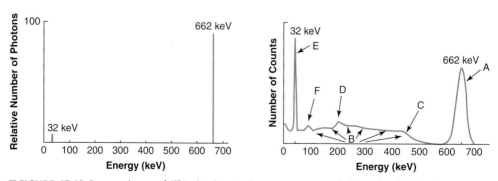

■ **FIGURE 17-18** Decay scheme of ^{137}Cs (top), actual energy spectrum (left), and pulse height spectrum obtained using an NaI(Tl) scintillation detector (right). See text for description of pulse height spectrum. (*A*) photopeak, due to complete absorption of 662-keV γ-rays in the crystal; (*B*) Compton continuum; (*C*) Compton edge; (*D*) backscatter peak; (*E*) barium x-ray photopeak; and (*F*) photopeak caused by absorption of lead K-shell x-rays (72 to 88 keV) from the shield.

crystal, with the scattered photons escaping the crystal. Each portion of the continuum corresponds to a particular scattering angle. The Compton edge (C) is the upper limit of the Compton continuum. The backscatter peak (D) is caused by 662-keV photons that scatter from the shielding around the detector into the detector. The barium x-ray photopeak (E) is a second photopeak caused by the absorption of barium K-shell x-rays (31 to 37 keV), which are emitted after the emission of conversion electrons. Another photopeak (F) is caused by lead K-shell x-rays (72 to 88 keV) from the shield.

17.5.6   Spectrum of Technetium-99m

The decay scheme of ^{99m}Tc is shown at the top in Figure 17-19. ^{99m}Tc is an isomer of ^{99}Tc that decays by isomeric transition to its ground state, with the emission of a 140.5-keV γ-ray. In 11% of the transitions, a conversion electron is emitted instead of a γ-ray.

   The pulse height spectrum of ^{99m}Tc is shown at the bottom of Figure 17-19. The photopeak (A) is caused by the total absorption of the 140-keV γ-rays. The escape peak (B) is caused by 140-keV γ-rays that interact with the crystal by the photoelectric effect but with the resultant iodine K-shell x-rays (28 to 33 keV) escaping the crystal. There is also a photopeak (C) caused by the absorption of lead K-shell x-rays from the shield. The Compton continuum is quite small, unlike the continuum in the spectrum of ^{137}Cs, because the photoelectric effect predominates in iodine at 140 keV.

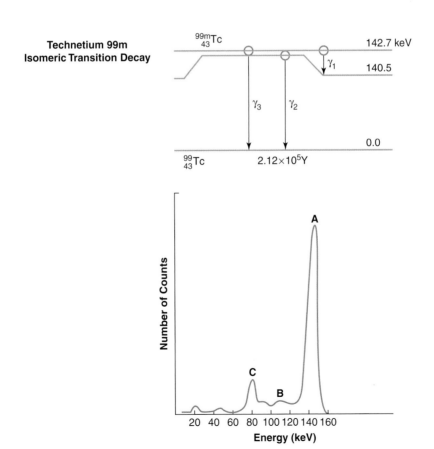

■ **FIGURE 17-19** Decay scheme of ^{99m}Tc (top) and its pulse height spectrum on an NaI(Tl) scintillation detector (bottom). See text for details.

17.5.7 Spectrum of Iodine-125

[125]I decays by electron capture followed by the emission of a 35.5-keV γ-ray (6.7% of decays) or a conversion electron. The electron capture usually leaves the daughter nucleus with a vacancy in the K-shell. The emission of a conversion electron usually also results in a K-shell vacancy. Each transformation of an ^{125}I atom therefore results in the emission, on the average, of 1.47 x-rays or γ-rays with energies between 27 and 36 keV.

Figure 17-20 shows two pulse height spectra from [125]I. The spectrum on the left was acquired with the source located 7.5 cm from an NaI(Tl) detector, and the one on the right was collected with the source in an NaI(Tl) well detector. The spectrum on the left shows a large photopeak at about 30 keV, whereas the spectrum on the right shows a peak at about 30 keV and a smaller peak at about 60 keV. The 60-keV peak in the spectrum from the well detector is a *sum peak* caused by two photons simultaneously striking the detector. The sum peak is not apparent in the spectrum with the source 7.5 cm from the detector because the much lower detection efficiency renders unlikely the simultaneous interaction of two photons with the detector.

17.5.8 Performance Characteristics

Energy Resolution

The energy resolution of a spectrometer is a measure of its ability to differentiate between particles or photons of different energies. It can be determined by irradiating the detector with monoenergetic particles or photons and measuring the width of the resultant peak in the pulse height spectrum. Statistical effects in the detection

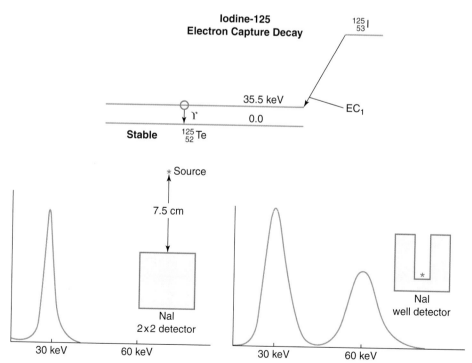

■ **FIGURE 17-20** Decay scheme and spectrum of ^{125}I source located 7.5 cm from solid NaI(Tl) crystal (left) and in NaI(Tl) well counter (right).

process cause the amplitudes of the pulses from the detector to randomly vary about the mean pulse height, giving the peak a gaussian shape. (These statistical effects are one reason why the pulse height spectrum produced by a spectrometer is not identical to the actual energy spectrum of the radiation.) A wider peak implies a poorer energy resolution.

The width is usually measured at half the maximal height of the peak, as illustrated in Figure 17-21. This is called the full width at half maximum (FWHM). The FWHM is then divided by the pulse amplitude corresponding to the maximum of the peak:

$$\text{Energy resolution} = \frac{\text{FWHM}}{\text{Pulse amplitude at center of peak}} \times 100\%. \qquad [17\text{-}4]$$

For example, the energy resolution of a 5-cm-diameter and 5-cm-thick cylindrical NaI(Tl) crystal, coupled to a PMT and exposed to the 662-keV γ-rays of ^{137}Cs, is typically about 7% to 8%.

Count-Rate Effects in Spectrometers

In pulse height spectroscopy, count-rate effects are best understood as pulse pileup. Figure 17-22 depicts the signal from a detector in which two interactions occur, separated by a very short time interval. The detector produces a single pulse, which is the sum of the individual signals from the two interactions, having a higher amplitude than the signal from either individual interaction. Because of this effect, operating a pulse height spectrometer at a high count rate causes loss of counts and misplacement of counts in the spectrum.

17.6 NON-IMAGING DETECTOR APPLICATIONS

17.6.1 Sodium Iodide Thyroid Probe and Well Counter

Thyroid Probe

A nuclear medicine department typically has a thyroid probe for measuring the uptake of ^{123}I or ^{131}I by the thyroid glands of patients and for monitoring the activities of ^{131}I in the thyroid glands of staff members who handle large activities of ^{131}I.

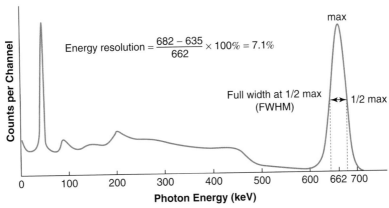

■ **FIGURE 17-21** Energy resolution of a pulse height spectrometer. The spectrum shown is that of ^{137}Cs, obtained by an NaI(Tl) scintillator coupled to a PMT.

■ **FIGURE 17-22** Pulse pileup. The dashed lines represent the signals produced by two individual interactions in the detector that occur at almost the same time. The solid line depicts the actual pulse produced by the detector. This single pulse is the sum of the signals from the two interactions.

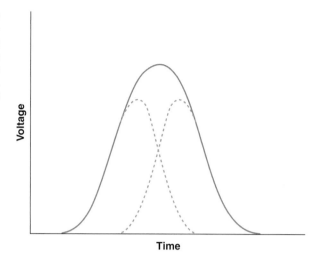

A thyroid probe, as shown in Figures 17-23 and 17-24, usually consists of a 5.1-cm (2-inch)-diameter and 5.1-cm-thick cylindrical NaI(Tl) crystal coupled to a PMT, which in turn is connected to a preamplifier. The probe is shielded on the sides and back with lead and is equipped with a collimator so that it detects photons only from a limited portion of the patient. The thyroid probe is connected to a high-voltage power supply and either an SCA or an MCA system.

Thyroid Uptake Measurements

Thyroid uptake measurements may be performed using one or two capsules of ^{123}I or ^{131}I sodium iodide. A neck phantom, consisting of a Lucite cylinder of diameter

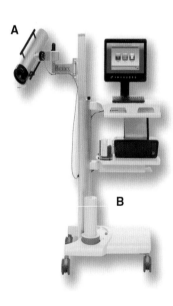

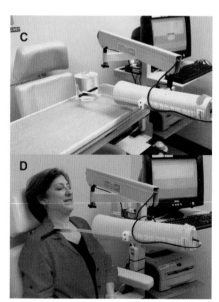

■ **FIGURE 17-23** Thyroid probe system **(A)**. The personal computer has added circuitry and software so that it functions as an MCA. An NaI(Tl) well detector **(B)**, discussed later in this chapter, for counting samples for radioactivity is part of this system. (**A** and **B**, photo courtesy of Biodex Medical Systems, Inc.) For thyroid uptake tests, the radioiodine capsules are placed in a Lucite neck phantom before patient administration and counted individually **(C)**. At 4 to 6 h and again at about 24 h after administration, the radioactivity in the patient's neck is counted at the same distance from the probe as was the neck phantom **(D)**.

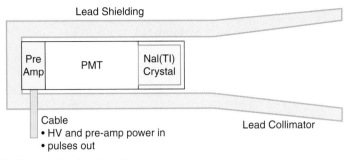

FIGURE 17-24 Diagram of a thyroid probe.

similar to the neck and containing a hole parallel to its axis for a radioiodine capsule, is required. In the two-capsule method, the capsules should have almost identical activities. Each capsule is placed in the neck phantom and counted separately. Then, one capsule is swallowed by the patient. The other capsule is called the "standard." Next, the emissions from the patient's neck are counted, typically at 4 to 6 h after administration, and again at 24 h after administration. Each time that the patient's thyroid is counted, the patient's distal thigh is also counted for the same length of time, to approximate non-thyroidal activity in the neck, and a background count is obtained. All counts are performed with the NaI crystal at the same distance, typically 20 to 30 cm, from the thyroid phantom or the patient's neck or thigh. (This distance reduces the effects of small differences in distance between the detector and the objects being counted.) Furthermore, each time that the patient's thyroid is counted, the remaining capsule is placed in the neck phantom and counted. Finally, the uptake is calculated for each neck measurement:

$$\text{Uptake} = \frac{\left(\text{Thyroid count} - \text{Thigh count}\right)}{\left(\text{Count of standard in phantom} - \text{Background count}\right)} \times \frac{\text{Initial count of standard in phantom}}{\text{Initial count of patient capsule in phantom}}.$$

Some nuclear medicine laboratories instead use a method that requires only one capsule. In this method, a single capsule is obtained, counted in the neck phantom, and swallowed by the patient. As in the previous method, the patient's neck and distal thigh are counted, typically at 4 to 6 h and again at 24 h after administration. The times of the capsule administration and the neck counts are recorded. Finally, the uptake is calculated for each neck measurement:

$$\frac{\left(\text{Thyroid count} - \text{Thigh count}\right)}{\left(\text{Count of capsule in phantom} - \text{Background count}\right)} \times e^{0.693_t / T_{1/2}},$$

where $T_{1/2}$ is the physical half-life of the radionuclide and t is the time elapsed between the count of the capsule in the phantom and the thyroid count. The single-capsule method avoids the cost of the second capsule and requires fewer measurements, but it is more susceptible to instability of the equipment, technologist error, and dead-time effects.

Sodium Iodide Well Counter

A nuclear medicine department also usually has an NaI(Tl) well counter, shown in Figures 17-23B and 17-25. The NaI(Tl) well counter may be used for clinical tests

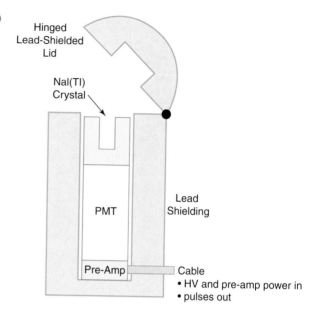

■ **FIGURE 17-25** Diagram of an NaI(Tl) well counter.

such as Schilling tests (a test of vitamin B_{12} absorption), plasma or red blood cell volume determinations, and radioimmunoassays, although radioimmunoassays have been largely replaced by immunoassays that do not use radioactivity. The well counter is also commonly used to assay wipe test samples to detect radioactive contamination. The well counter usually consists of a cylindrical NaI(Tl) crystal, either 5.1 cm (2 inches) in diameter and 5.1 cm thick or 7.6 cm (3 inches) in diameter and 7.6 cm thick, with a hole in the crystal for the insertion of samples. This configuration gives the counter an extremely high efficiency, permitting it to assay samples containing activities of less than 1 nCi (10^{-3} µCi). The crystal is coupled to a PMT, which in turn is connected to a preamplifier. A well counter in a nuclear medicine department should have a thick lead shield, because it is used to count samples containing nanocurie activities in the vicinity of millicurie activities of high-energy γ-ray emitters such as ^{67}Ga, ^{111}In, and ^{131}I. The well counter is connected to a high-voltage power supply and either an SCA or an MCA system. Departments that perform large numbers of radioimmunoassays often use automatic well counters, such as the one shown in Figure 17-26, to count large numbers of samples.

Sample Volume and Dead-Time Effects in Sodium Iodide Well Counters

The position of a sample in a sodium iodide well counter has a dramatic effect on the detection efficiency. When liquid samples in vials of a particular shape and size are counted, the detection efficiency falls as the volume increases. Most nuclear medicine in vitro tests require the comparison of a liquid sample from the patient with a reference sample. It is crucial that both samples be in identical containers and have identical volumes.

In addition, the high efficiency of the NaI well counter can cause unacceptable dead-time count losses, even with sample activities in the microcurie range. It is important to ensure that the activity placed in the well counter is sufficiently small so that dead-time effects do not cause a falsely low count. In general, well counters should not be used at apparent count rates exceeding about 5,000 cps, which limits samples of ^{125}I and ^{57}Co to activities less than about 0.2 µCi. However, larger activities of some radionuclides may be counted without significant losses; for example,

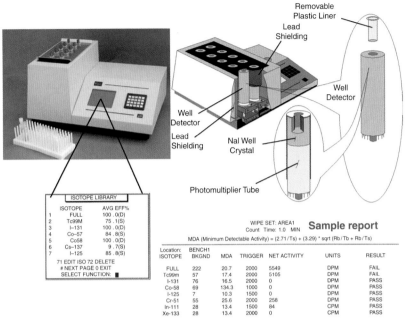

Removable
Plastic Liner
Lead
Shielding

Well
Detector

NaI Well
Crystal

Photomultiplier Tube

Lead
Shielding

Well
Detector

ISOTOPE LIBRARY	
ISOTOPE	AVG EFF%
1 FULL	100 . 0(D)
2 Tc99M	75 . 1(S)
3 I–131	100 . 0(D)
4 Co–57	84 . 8(S)
5 Co58	100 . 0(D)
6 Cs–137	9 . 7(S)
7 I–125	85 . 8(S)

71 EDIT ISO 72 DELETE
NEXT PAGE 0 EXIT
SELECT FUNCTION: ▮

WIPE SET: AREA1   **Sample report**
Count Time: 1.0 MIN

MDA (Minimum Detectable Activity) = (2.71 / Ts) + (3.29) * sqrt (Rb / Tb + Rb / Ts)

Location:	BENCH1					
ISOTOPE	BKGND	MDA	TRIGGER	NET ACTIVITY	UNITS	RESULT
FULL	222	20.7	2000	5549	DPM	FAIL
Tc99m	57	17.4	2000	5105	DPM	FAIL
I-131	76	16.5	2000	0	DPM	PASS
Co-58	69	134.3	1000	0	DPM	PASS
I-125	7	10.3	1500	0	DPM	PASS
Cr-51	55	25.6	2000	258	DPM	PASS
In-111	28	13.4	1500	84	CPM	PASS
Xe-133	28	13.4	2000	0	CPM	PASS

■ **FIGURE 17-26** Automatic γ well counter. (Courtesy of Laboratory Technologies, Inc.)

activities of ^{51}Cr as large as 5 μCi may be counted, because only about one out of every ten decays yields a γ-ray.

Quality Assurance for the Sodium Iodide Thyroid Probe and Well Counter

Both of these instruments should have energy calibrations (as discussed earlier for an SCA system) performed daily, with the results recorded. A background count and a constancy test, using a source with a long half-life such as ^{137}Cs, also should be performed daily for both the well counter and the thyroid probe to test for radioactive contamination or instrument malfunction. On the day the constancy test is begun, a counting window is set to tightly encompass the photopeak, and a count is taken and corrected for background. Limits called "action levels" are established, which, if exceeded, cause the person performing the test to notify the chief technologist, physicist, or physician. On each subsequent day, a count is taken using the same source, window setting, and counting time; corrected for background; recorded; and compared with the action levels. If each day's count were mistakenly compared with the previous day's count instead of the first day's count, slow changes in the instrument would not be discovered. Periodically, a new first day count and action levels should be established, accounting for decay of the radioactive source. This will prevent the constancy test count from exceeding an action level because of decreasing source activity. Also, spectra should be plotted annually for commonly measured radionuclides, usually ^{123}I and ^{131}I for the thyroid probe and perhaps ^{57}Co (Schilling tests), ^{125}I (radioimmunoassays), and ^{51}Cr (red cell volumes and survival studies) for the well counter, to verify that the SCA windows fit the photopeaks. This testing is greatly simplified if the department has an MCA.

17.6.2 Dose Calibrator

A dose calibrator, shown in Figure 17-27, is used to measure the activities of dosages of radiopharmaceuticals to be administered to patients. The U.S. Nuclear Regulatory

■ **FIGURE 17-27** Dose calibrator. The detector is a well-geometry ion chamber filled with pressurized argon. The syringe and vial holder **(A)** is used to place radioactive material, in this case in a syringe, into the detector. This reduces exposure to the hands and permits the activity to be measured in a reproducible geometry. The removable plastic insert **(B)** prevents contamination of the well.

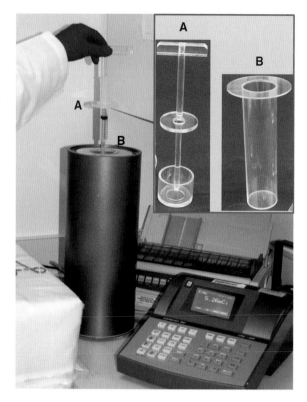

Commission (NRC) and state regulatory agencies require that dosages of x-ray– and γ-ray–emitting radiopharmaceuticals be determined before administration to patients. NRC allows administration of a "unit dosage" (an individual patient dosage prepared by a commercial radiopharmacy, without any further manipulation of its activity by the nuclear medicine department that administers it) without measurement. It also permits determination of activities of non-unit dosages by volumetric measurements and mathematical calculations. Most dose calibrators are well-type ionization chambers that are filled with argon ($Z = 18$) and pressurized to maximize sensitivity. Most dose calibrators have shielding around their chambers to protect users from the radioactive material being assayed and to prevent nearby sources of radiation from affecting the measurements.

A dose calibrator cannot directly measure activity. Instead, it measures the intensity of the radiation emitted by a dosage of a radiopharmaceutical. The manufacturer of a dose calibrator determines calibration factors relating the magnitude of the signal from the detector to activity for specific radionuclides commonly used in nuclear medicine. The user pushes a button or turns a dial on the dose calibrator to designate the radionuclide being measured, thereby specifying a calibration factor, and the dose calibrator displays the measured activity.

Operating Characteristics

Dose calibrators using ionization chambers are operated in current mode, thereby avoiding dead-time effects. They can accurately assay activities as large as 2 Ci. For the same reasons, they are relatively insensitive and cannot accurately assay activities less than about 1 μCi. In general, the identification and measurement of activities of radionuclides in samples containing multiple radionuclides is not possible. The measurement accuracy is affected by the position in the well of the dosages being measured, so it is important that all measurements be made with the dosages at the same position. Most dose calibrators have large wells, which reduce the effect of position on the measurements.

Dose calibrators using large well-type ionization chambers are in general not significantly affected by changes in the sample volume or container for most radionuclides. However, the measured activities of certain radionuclides, especially those such as ^{111}I, ^{123}I, ^{125}I, and ^{133}Xe that emit weak x-rays or γ-rays, are highly dependent on factors such as whether the containers (*e.g.*, syringe or vial) are glass or plastic and the thicknesses of the containers' walls. There is currently no generally accepted solution to this problem. Some radiopharmaceutical manufacturers provide correction factors for these radionuclides; these correction factors are specific to the radionuclide, the container, and the model of dose calibrator.

There are even greater problems with attenuation effects when assaying the dosages of pure beta-emitting radionuclides, such as ^{32}P and ^{89}Sr. For this reason, the NRC does not require unit dosages of these radionuclides to be assayed in a dose calibrator before administration. However, most nuclear medicine departments assay these, but only to verify that the activities as assayed by the vendor are not in error by a large amount.

Dose Calibrator Quality Assurance

Because the assay of activity using the dose calibrator is often the only assurance that the patient is receiving the prescribed activity, quality assurance testing of the dose calibrator is required by the NRC and state regulatory agencies. The NRC requires the testing to be in accordance with nationally recognized standards or the manufacturer's instructions. The following set of tests is commonly performed to satisfy this requirement.

The device should be tested for *accuracy* upon installation and annually thereafter. Two or more sealed radioactive sources (often ^{57}Co and ^{137}Cs) whose activities are known within 5% are assayed. The measured activities must be within 10% of the actual activities.

The device should also be tested for *linearity* (a measure of the effect that the amount of activity has on the accuracy) upon installation and quarterly thereafter. The most common method requires a vial of ^{99m}Tc containing the maximal activity that would be administered to a patient. The vial is measured two or three times daily until it decays to less than 30 μQ; the measured activities and times of the measurements are recorded. One measurement is assumed to be correct and, from this measurement, activities are calculated for the times of the other measurements. No measurement may differ from the corresponding calculated activity by more than 10%. An alternative to the decay method for testing linearity is the use of commercially available lead cylindrical sleeves of different thickness that simulate radioactive decay via attenuation (Fig. 17-28). These devices must be calibrated prior to first use by comparing their simulated decay with the decay method described above.

The device should be tested for *constancy* before its first use each day. At least one sealed source (usually ^{57}Co) is assayed, and its measured activity, corrected for decay, must not differ from its measured activity on the date of the last accuracy test by more than 10%. (Most laboratories perform a daily accuracy test, which is more rigorous, in lieu of a daily constancy test.)

Finally, the dose calibrator should be tested for geometry dependence on installation. This is usually done by placing a small volume of a radiochemical, often ^{99m}Tc pertechnetate, in a vial or syringe and assaying its activity after each of several dilutions. If volume effects are found to affect measurements by more than 10%,

■ **FIGURE 17-28** Set of cylindrical lead sleeves used to test dose calibrator linearity. These color-coded sleeves of different thicknesses use attenuation to simulate radioactive decay over periods of 6, 12, 20, 30, 40, and 50 h for ^{99m}Tc. Additional sleeves are available that can extend the simulated decay interval up to 350 h. (This research was originally published in JNM. Zanzonico, P. Routine quality control of clinical nuclear medicine instrumentation: a brief review. *J Nucl Med*. 2008;49:1114-1131. Figure 1. © SNMMI.)

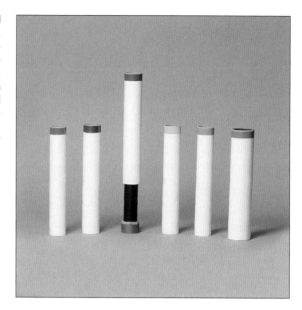

correction factors must be determined. The geometry test must be performed for syringe and vial sizes commonly used. Dose calibrators should also be appropriately tested after repair or adjustment.

The calibration factors of individual radionuclide settings should be verified for radionuclides assayed for clinical purposes. This can be performed by placing a source of any radionuclide in the dose calibrator, recording the indicated activity using a clinical radionuclide setting (*e.g.*, ^{131}I), recording the indicated activity using the setting of a radionuclide used for accuracy determination (*e.g.*, ^{57}Co or ^{137}Cs), and verifying that the ratio of the two indicated activities is that specified by the manufacturer of the dose calibrator.

17.6.3 Molybdenum-99 Concentration Testing

When a ^{99}Mo/^{99m}Tc generator is eluted, it is possible to obtain an abnormally large amount of ^{99}Mo in the eluate. (Radionuclide generators are discussed in Chapter 16.) If a radiopharmaceutical contaminated with ^{99}Mo is administered to a patient, the patient will receive an increased radiation dose (^{99}Mo emits high-energy beta particles and has a 66-h half-life) and the quality of the resultant images may be degraded by the high-energy ^{99}Mo γ-rays. The NRC requires that any ^{99m}Tc to be administered to a human must not contain more than 0.15 kBq of ^{99}Mo per MBq of ^{99m}Tc (0.15 μCi of ^{99}Mo per mCi of ^{99m}Tc) at the time of administration and that the first elution of a generator must be assayed for ^{99}Mo concentration.

The concentration of ^{99}Mo is most commonly measured with a dose calibrator and a special lead container that is supplied by the manufacturer. The walls of the lead container are sufficiently thick to stop almost all of the γ-rays from ^{99m}Tc (140 keV) but thin enough to be penetrated by many of the higher energy γ-rays from ^{99}Mo (740 and 778 keV). To perform the measurement, the empty lead container is first assayed in the dose calibrator. Next, the vial of ^{99m}Tc is placed in the lead container and assayed. Finally, the vial of ^{99m}Tc alone is assayed. The ^{99}Mo concentration is then obtained using the following equation:

$$\text{Concentration} = K \cdot \frac{A_{\text{vial-in-container}} - A_{\text{empty-container}}}{A_{\text{vial}}}, \qquad [17\text{-}5]$$

where K is a correction factor supplied by the manufacturer of the dose calibrator that accounts for the attenuation of the ^{99}Mo γ-rays by the lead container.

17.6.4 ^{82}Sr and ^{85}Sr Concentration Testing

Myocardial perfusion can by assessed by PET using the radiopharmaceutical ^{82}Rb chloride. In clinical practice, ^{82}Rb chloride is obtained from an ^{82}Sr/^{82}Rb generator. (These generators are discussed in Chapter 16.) When an ^{82}Sr/^{82}Rb generator is eluted, it is possible to obtain an abnormally large amount of ^{82}Sr or ^{85}Sr, a radioactive contaminant in the production of ^{82}Sr, in the eluate. The NRC requires that any ^{82}Rb chloride to be administered to a human not contain more than 0.02 kBq of ^{82}Sr or 0.2 kBq of ^{85}Sr per MBq of ^{82}Rb at the time of administration and that the concentrations of these radionuclides be measured before the first patient use each day. A dose calibrator is generally used to assay the concentration of the unwanted contaminants ^{82}Sr and ^{85}Sr in the eluate. The measurement procedures are contained in the package insert provided by the manufacturer of the generators. The eluate is allowed to decay for an hour so that only ^{82}Sr and ^{85}Sr remain. The sample is then assayed in the dose calibrator, and the amounts of ^{82}Sr and ^{85}Sr are estimated from an assumed ratio.

17.7   COUNTING STATISTICS

17.7.1   Introduction

Sources of Error

There are three types of errors in measurements. The first is *systematic error*. Systematic error occurs when measurements differ from the correct values in a systematic fashion. For example, systematic error occurs in radiation measurements if a detector is used in pulse mode at too high an interaction rate; dead-time count losses cause the measured count rate to be lower than the actual interaction rate. The second type of error is *random error*. Random error is caused by random fluctuations in whatever is being measured or in the measurement process itself. The third type of error is the *blunder* (*e.g.*, setting the SCA window incorrectly for a single measurement).

Random Error in Radiation Detection

The processes by which radiation is emitted and interacts with matter are random in nature. Whether a particular radioactive nucleus decays within a specified time interval, the direction of an x-ray emitted by an electron striking the target of an x-ray tube, whether a particular x ray passes through a patient to reach the film cassette of an x-ray machine, and whether a γ-ray incident upon a scintillation camera crystal is detected are all random phenomena. Therefore, all radiation measurements, including medical imaging, are subject to random error. Counting statistics enable judgments of the validity of measurements that are subject to random error.

17.7.2   Characterization of Data

Accuracy and Precision

If a measurement is close to the correct value, it is said to be *accurate*. If measurements are reproducible, they are said to be *precise*. Precision does not imply accuracy; a set of measurements may be very close together (precise) but not close to the correct value (*i.e.*, inaccurate). If a set of measurements differs from the correct value in a systematic fashion (systematic error), the data are said to be *biased*.

Measures of Central Tendency—Mean and Median

Two measures of central tendency of a set of measurements are the *mean* (average) and the median. The mean (*x*) of a set of measurements is defined as follows:

$$\bar{x} = \frac{x_1 + x_2 + \cdots + x_N}{N},$$ [17-6]

where N is the number of measurements.

To obtain the *median* of a set of measurements, they must first be put in order by size. The median is the middle measurement if the number of measurements is odd, and it is the average of the two midmost measurements if the number of measurements is even. For example, to obtain the median of the five measurements 8, 14, 5, 9, and 12, they are first sorted by size: 5, 8, 9, 12, and 14. The median is 9. The advantage of the median over the mean is that the median is less affected by outliers. An outlier is a measurement that is much greater or much less than the others.

Measures of Variability—Variance and Standard Deviation

The variance and standard deviation are measures of the variability (spread) of a set of measurements. The variance (σ^2) is determined from a set of measurements by subtracting the mean from each measurement, squaring the differences, summing the squares, and dividing by one less than the number of measurements:

$$\sigma^2 = \frac{\left(x_1 - \bar{x}\right)^2 + \left(x_2 - \bar{x}\right)^2 + \cdots + \left(x_N - \bar{x}\right)^2}{N-1},$$ [17-7]

where N is the total number of measurements and $\bar{x}$ is the sample mean.

The *standard deviation* (σ) is the square root of the variance:

$$\sigma = \sqrt{\sigma^2}.$$ [17-8]

The *fractional standard deviation* (also referred to as the *fractional error* or *coefficient of variation*) is the standard deviation divided by the mean:

$$\text{Fractional standard deviation} = \sigma/\bar{x}.$$ [17-9]

17.7.3 Probability Distribution Functions for Binary Processes

Binary Processes

A *trial* is an event that may have more than one outcome. A *binary process* is a process in which a trial can only have two outcomes, one of which is arbitrarily called a *success*. A toss of a coin is a binary process. The toss of a die can be considered a binary process if, for example, a "two" is selected as a success and any other outcome is considered to be a failure. Whether a particular radioactive nucleus decays during a specified time interval is a binary process. Whether a particular x-ray or γ-ray is detected by a radiation detector is a binary process. Table 17-2 lists examples of binary processes.

TABLE 17-2 BINARY PROCESSES

TRIAL	DEFINITION OF A SUCCESS	PROBABILITY OF A SUCCESS
Toss of a coin	"Heads"	1/2
Toss of a die	"A four"	1/6
Observation of a radioactive nucleus for a time "t"	It decays	$1 - e^{-\lambda t}$
Observation of a detector of efficiency E placed near a radioactive nucleus for a time "t"	A count	$E(1 - e^{-\lambda t})$

Adapted from Knoll GF. *Radiation Detection and Measurement.* 4th ed. Copyright © 2010, John Wiley and Sons.

A measurement consists of counting the number of successes from a specified number of trials. Tossing ten coins and counting the number of "heads" is a measurement. Placing a radioactive sample on a detector and recording the number of events detected is a measurement.

Probability Distribution Functions—Binomial, Poisson, and Gaussian

A probability distribution function (pdf) describes the probability of obtaining each outcome from a measurement—for example, the probability of obtaining six "heads" in a throw of ten coins. There are three probability distribution functions relevant to binary processes—the binomial, the Poisson, and the gaussian (normal). The binomial distribution exactly describes the probability of each outcome from a measurement of a binary process:

$$P(x) = \frac{N!}{x!(N-x)!} p^x (1-p)^{N-x}, \qquad [17\text{-}10]$$

where N is the total number of trials in a measurement, p is the probability of success in a single trial, and x is the number of successes. The mathematical notation $N!$, called *factorial notation,* is simply shorthand for the product

$$N! = N \cdot (N-1) \cdot (N-2) \cdots 3 \cdot 2 \cdot 1. \qquad [17\text{-}11]$$

For example, $5! = 5 \cdot 4 \cdot 3 \cdot 2 \cdot 1 = 120$. If we wish to know the probability of obtaining two heads in a toss of four coins, $x = 2$, $N = 4$, and $p = 0.5$. The probability of obtaining two heads is

$$P(\text{two-heads}) = \frac{4!}{2!(4-2)!}(0.5)^2 (1-0.5)^{4-2} = 0.375.$$

Figure 17-29 is a graph of the binomial distribution. It can be shown that the sum of the probabilities of all outcomes for the binomial distribution is 1.0 and that the mean (x) and standard deviation (σ) of the binomial distribution are as follows:

$$\bar{x} = pN \text{ and } \sigma = \sqrt{pN(1-p)}. \qquad [17\text{-}12]$$

If the probability of a success in a trial is much less than 1 (not true for a toss of a coin, but true for most radiation measurements), the standard deviation is approximated by the following:

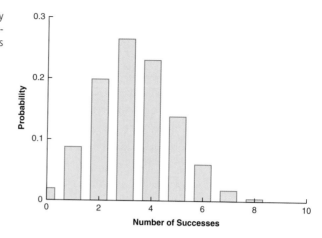

FIGURE 17-29 Binomial probability distribution function when the probability of a success in a single trial (p) is 1/3 and the number of trials (N) is 10.

$$\sigma = \sqrt{pN(1-p)} \approx \sqrt{pN} = \sqrt{x}. \qquad [17\text{-}13]$$

Because of the factorials in Equation 17-10, it is difficult to use if either x or N is large. The Poisson and gaussian distributions are approximations to the binomial pdf that are often used when x or N is large. Figure 17-30 shows a gaussian distribution.

17.7.4 Estimating the Uncertainty of a Single Measurement

Estimated Standard Deviation

The standard deviation can be estimated, as previously described, by making several measurements and applying Equations 17-7 and 17-8. Nevertheless, if the process being measured is a binary process, the standard deviation can be estimated from a single measurement. The single measurement is probably close to the mean. Because the standard deviation is approximately the square root of the mean, it is also approximately the square root of the single measurement:

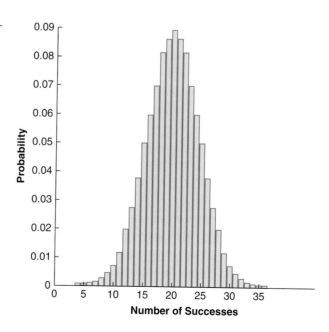

FIGURE 17-30 Gaussian probability distribution function for $pN = 20$.

$$\sigma \approx \sqrt{x}, \qquad\qquad\qquad [17\text{-}14]$$

where x is the single measurement. The fractional standard deviation of a single measurement may also be estimated as:

$$\text{Fractional error} = \frac{\sigma}{x} \approx \frac{\sqrt{x}}{x} = \frac{1}{\sqrt{x}}. \qquad\qquad [17\text{-}15]$$

For example, a single measurement of a radioactive source yields 1,256 counts. The estimated standard deviation is

$$\sigma \approx \sqrt{1,256 \text{ cts}} = 35.4 \text{ cts.}$$

The fractional standard deviation is estimated as

$$\text{Fractional error} = 35.4 \text{ cts} / 1,256 \text{ cts} = 0.028 = 2.8\%.$$

Table 17-3 lists the estimated fractional errors for various numbers of counts. The fractional error decreases with the number of counts.

Confidence Intervals

Table 17-4 lists intervals about a measurement, called *confidence intervals*, for which the probability of containing the true mean is specified. There is a 68.3% probability that the true mean is within one standard deviation (1σ) of a measurement, a 95% probability that it is within 2σ of a measurement, and a 99.7% probability that it is within 3σ of a measurement, assuming that the measurements follow a gaussian distribution.

For example, a count of 853 is obtained. Determine the interval about this count in which there is a 95% probability of finding the true mean.

First, the standard deviation is estimated as

$$\sigma \approx \sqrt{853 \text{ cts}} = 29.2 \text{ cts.}$$

From Table 17-4, the 95% confidence interval is determined as follows:

$$853 \text{ cts} \pm 1.96\sigma = 853 \text{ cts} \pm 1.96 \left(29.2 \text{ cts}\right) = 853 \text{ cts} \pm 57.2 \text{ cts.}$$

So, the 95% confidence interval ranges from 796 to 910 counts.

17.7.5 Propagation of Error

In nuclear medicine, calculations are frequently performed using numbers that incorporate random error. It is often necessary to estimate the uncertainty in the results of

TABLE 17-3 FRACTIONAL ERRORS (PERCENT STANDARD DEVIATIONS) FOR SEVERAL NUMBERS OF COUNTS

COUNT	FRACTIONAL ERROR (%)
100	10.0
1,000	3.2
10,000	1.0
100,000	0.32

TABLE 17-4 CONFIDENCE INTERVALS

INTERVAL ABOUT MEASUREMENT	PROBABILITY THAT MEAN IS WITHIN INTERVAL (%)
$\pm 0.674\sigma$	50.0
$\pm 1\sigma$	68.3
$\pm 1.64\sigma$	90.0
$\pm 1.96\sigma$	95.0
$\pm 2.58\sigma$	99.0
$\pm 3\sigma$	99.7

Adapted from Knoll GF. *Radiation Detection and Measurement*. 4th ed. Copyright © 2010, John Wiley and Sons.

these calculations. Although the standard deviation of a count may be estimated by simply taking its square root, it is incorrect to calculate the standard deviation of the result of a calculation by taking its square root. Instead, the standard deviations of the actual counts must first be calculated and entered into propagation of error equations to obtain the standard deviation of the result.

Multiplication or Division of a Number with Error by a Number without Error

It is often necessary to multiply or divide a number containing random error by a number that does not contain random error. For example, to calculate a count rate, a count (which incorporates random error) is divided by a counting time (which does not involve significant random error). If a number x has a standard deviation σ and is multiplied by a number c without random error, the standard deviation of the product cx is $c\sigma$. If a number x has a standard deviation σ and is divided by a number c without random error, the standard deviation of the quotient x/c is σ/c.

For example, a 5-min count of a radioactive sample yields 952 counts. The count rate is 952 cts/5 min = 190 cts/min. The standard deviation and percent standard deviation of the count are

$$\sigma \approx \sqrt{952 \text{ cts}} = 30.8 \text{ cts}$$

$$\text{Fractional error} = 30.8 \text{ cts}/952 \text{ cts} = 0.032 = 3.2\%.$$

The standard deviation of the count rate is

$$\sigma = 30.8 \text{ cts}/5\,\text{min} = 6.16 \text{ cts}/\text{min}$$

$$\text{Fractional error} = 6.16 \text{ cts}/190 \text{ cts} = 3.2\%.$$

Notice that the percent standard deviation is not affected when a number is multiplied or divided by a number without random error.

Addition or Subtraction of Numbers with Error

It is often necessary to add or subtract numbers with random error. For example, a background count may be subtracted from a count of a radioactive sample. Whether two numbers are added or subtracted, the same equation is used to calculate the standard deviation of the result, as shown in Table 17-5.

For example, a count of a radioactive sample yields 1,952 counts, and a background count with the sample removed from the detector yields 1,451 counts.

TABLE 17-5 PROPAGATION OF ERROR EQUATIONS

DESCRIPTION	OPERATION	STANDARD DEVIATION
Multiplication of a number with random error by a number without random error	cx	$c\sigma$
Division of a number with random error by a number without random error	x/c	σ/c
Addition of two numbers containing random errors	$x_1 + x_2$	$\sqrt{\sigma_1^2 + \sigma_2^2}$
Subtraction of two numbers containing random errors	$x_1 - x_2$	$\sqrt{\sigma_1^2 + \sigma_2^2}$

Note: c is a number without random error, σ is the standard deviation of x, σ_1 is the standard deviation of x_1, and σ_2 is the standard deviation of x_2.

The count of the sample, corrected for background, is

$$1,952 \text{ cts} - 1,451 \text{ cts} = 501 \text{ cts}.$$

The standard deviation and percent standard deviation of the original sample count are

$$\sigma_{s+b} \approx \sqrt{1,952 \text{ cts}} = 44.2 \text{ cts}$$

Fractional error $= 44.2 \text{ cts}/1,952 \text{ cts} = 2.3\%.$

The standard deviation and percent standard deviation of the background count are

$$\sigma_b \approx \sqrt{1,451 \text{ cts}} = 38.1 \text{ cts}$$

Fractional error $= 38.1 \text{ cts}/1,451 \text{ cts} = 2.6\%.$

The standard deviation and percent standard deviation of the sample count corrected for background are

$$\sigma_s \approx \sqrt{(44.4 \text{ cts})^2 + (38.3 \text{ cts})^2} = 58.3 \text{ cts}$$

Fractional error $= 58.1 \text{ cts}/501 \text{ cts} = 11.6\%.$

Note that the fractional error of the difference is much larger than the fractional error of either count. The fractional error of the difference of two numbers of similar magnitude can be much larger than the fractional errors of the two numbers.

Combination Problems

It is sometimes necessary to perform mathematical operations in series, for example, to subtract two numbers and then to divide the difference by another number. The standard deviation is calculated for each intermediate result in the series by entering the standard deviations from the previous step into the appropriate propagation of error equation in Table 17-5.

For example, a 5-min count of a radioactive sample yields 1,290 counts and a 5-min background count yields 451 counts. What is the count rate due to the sample alone and its standard deviation?

First, the count is corrected for background:

$$\text{Count} = 1{,}290 \text{ cts} - 451 \text{ cts} = 839 \text{ cts}.$$

The estimated standard deviation of each count and the difference are calculated:

$$\sigma_{s+b} \approx \sqrt{1{,}290 \text{ cts}} = 35.9 \text{ cts and } \sigma_b \approx \sqrt{451 \text{ cts}} = 21.2 \text{ cts}$$

$$\sigma_2 \approx \sqrt{(35.9 \text{ cts})^2 + (21.2 \text{ cts})^2} = 41.7 \text{ cts}.$$

Finally, the count rate due to the source alone and its standard deviation are calculated:

$$\text{Count rate} = 839 \text{ cts}/5 \text{ min} = 168 \text{ cts}/\text{min}$$

$$\sigma_2/c = 41.7 \text{ cts}/5 \text{ min} = 8.3 \text{ cts}/\text{min}.$$

SUGGESTED READING AND REFERENCES

Attix FH. *Introduction to Radiological Physics and Radiation Dosimetry*. New York, NY: John Wiley; 1986.

Knoll GF. *Radiation Detection and Measurement*. 4th ed. New York, NY: John Wiley; 2010.

Patton JA, Harris CC. Gamma well counter. In: Sandler MP, et al., eds. *Diagnostic Nuclear Medicine*. 3rd ed. Baltimore, MD: Williams & Wilkins; 1996:59-65.

Ranger NT. The AAPM/RSNA physics tutorial for residents: radiation detectors in nuclear medicine. *Radiographics*. 1999;19:481-502.

Roncali E, Cherry S. Application of silicon photomultipliers to positron emission tomography. *Ann Biomed Eng*. 2011;39(4):1358-1377.

Rzeszotarski MS. The AAPM/RSNA physics tutorial for residents: counting statistics. *Radiographics*. 1999;19:765-782.

Simon CR, et al. *Physics in Nuclear Medicine*. 4th ed. Philadelphia, PA: Saunders; 2011.

CHAPTER 18

Nuclear Imaging—The Gamma Camera

Nuclear imaging produces images of the distributions of radionuclides in patients. Because charged particles from radioactivity in a patient are almost entirely absorbed within the patient, nuclear imaging uses γ-rays, characteristic x-rays (usually from radionuclides that decay by electron capture), or annihilation photons (from positron-emitting radionuclides) to form images.

To form a projection image, an imaging system must determine not only the photon flux density (number of x- or γ-rays per unit area) at each point in the image plane but also the directions of the detected photons. In x-ray transmission imaging, the primary photons travel known paths diverging radially from a point (the focal spot of the x-ray tube). In contrast, the x- or γ-rays from the radionuclide in each volume element of a patient are emitted isotropically (equally in all directions). Nuclear medicine instruments designed to image x- and γ-ray–emitting radionuclides (gamma cameras) use *collimators* that permit photons following certain trajectories to reach the detector but absorb most of the rest. A heavy price is paid for using collimation—the vast majority (typically well over 99.95%) of emitted photons is wasted. Thus, collimation, although necessary for the formation of projection images, severely limits the performance of these devices. Instruments for imaging positron (β^+)-emitting radionuclides can avoid collimation by exploiting the unique properties of annihilation radiation to determine the directions of the photons. Positron-emission nuclear imaging devices are discussed in Chapter 19.

The earliest widely successful nuclear medicine imaging device, the rectilinear scanner, which dominated nuclear imaging from the early 1950s through the late 1960s, used a moving radiation detector to sample the photon fluence at a small region of the image plane at a time.[1] This was improved upon by the use of a large-area position-sensitive detector (a detector indicating the location of each interaction) to sample simultaneously the photon fluence over the entire image plane. The Anger scintillation gamma camera, which currently dominates single-photon x- and γ-ray nuclear imaging, is an example of the latter method. The scanning detector system is less expensive, but the position-sensitive detector system permits more rapid image acquisition and has replaced single scanning detector systems.

Gamma cameras using gas-filled detectors (such as multiwire proportional counters) have been developed in the past. Unfortunately, the low densities of gases, even when pressurized, yield low detection efficiencies for the x- and γ-ray energies commonly used in single-photon nuclear imaging. To obtain a sufficient number of interactions to form statistically valid images without imparting an excessive radiation dose to the patient, nearly all gamma cameras in routine clinical use utilize solid inorganic scintillators as detectors because of their superior detection efficiency. However, gamma cameras using semiconductor detectors have been developed. These devices utilize high atomic number, high-density semiconductor material of sufficient

---

[1]Cassen B, Curtis L, Reed A, Libby RL. Instrumentation for I-131 use in medical studies. *Nucleonics.* 1951;9:46-49.

thickness for absorbing the x- and γ-rays commonly used in nuclear imaging, and that can be operated at room temperature. The leading detector material in use to date is cadmium zinc telluride (CZT). Both small and large field of view (FOV) cameras using CZT semiconductor detectors are now commercially available.

The attenuation of x-rays in the patient is useful in radiography, fluoroscopy, and x-ray computed tomography and, in fact, is necessary for image formation. However, in nuclear imaging, attenuation is usually a hindrance; it causes a loss of information and, especially when it is very non-uniform, it is a source of artifacts.

The quality of a nuclear medicine image is determined not only by the performance of the nuclear imaging device but also by the properties of the radiopharmaceutical used. For example, the degree to which a radiopharmaceutical preferentially accumulates in a lesion of interest largely determines the smallest such lesion that can be detected. Furthermore, the dosimetric properties of a radiopharmaceutical determine the maximal activity that can be administered to a patient, which in turn affects the amount of statistical noise (quantum mottle) in the image. For example, in the 1950s and 1960s, radiopharmaceuticals labeled with I-131 and Hg-203 were commonly used. The long half-lives of these radionuclides and their beta particle emissions limited administered activities to approximately 150 microcuries (μCi). These low administered activities and the high-energy γ-rays of these radionuclides resulted in high statistical noise images and required the use of collimators providing poor spatial resolution. Many modern radiopharmaceuticals are labeled with technetium-99m (Tc-99m), whose short half-life (6.01 h) and isomeric transition decay (~88% of the energy is emitted as 140-keV γ-rays; only ~12% is given to conversion electrons and other emissions unlikely to escape the patient) permit activities of up to about 35 millicuries (mCi) to be administered. The high γ-ray flux from such an activity permits the use of high-resolution (low-efficiency) collimators. Radiopharmaceuticals are discussed in Chapter 16.

18.1 PLANAR NUCLEAR IMAGING: THE ANGER SCINTILLATION CAMERA

The Anger scintillation gamma camera, developed by Hal O. Anger at the Donner Laboratory in Berkeley, California, in the 1950s, is by far the most common nuclear medicine imaging device.[2] However, it did not begin to replace the rectilinear scanner significantly until the late 1960s, when its spatial resolution became comparable to that of the rectilinear scanner and Tc-99m-labeled radiopharmaceuticals, for which it is ideally suited, became commonly used in nuclear medicine. Most of the advantages of the scintillation camera over the rectilinear scanner stem from its ability simultaneously to collect data over a large area of the patient, rather than one small area at a time. This permits the more rapid acquisition of images and enables dynamic studies that depict the redistribution of radionuclides to be performed. Because the scintillation camera wastes fewer x- or γ-rays than earlier imaging devices, its images have less quantum mottle (statistical noise) and it can be used with higher resolution collimators, thereby producing images of better spatial resolution. The scintillation camera is also more flexible in its positioning, permitting images to be obtained from almost any angle. Although it can produce satisfactory images using x- or γ-rays ranging in energy from about 70 keV (Tl-201) to 364 keV (I-131) or perhaps even 511 keV (F-18), the scintillation camera is best suited for imaging photons with energies in the range of 100 to 200 keV. Figure 18-1 shows a modern scintillation camera.

---

[2]Anger HA. Scintillation camera. *Rev Sci Instr.* 1958;29:27-33.

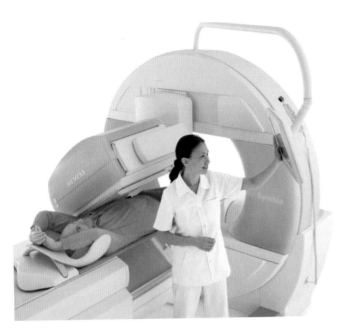

■ **FIGURE 18-1** Modern dual rectangular head scintillation camera. The two heads are in a 90° orientation for cardiac SPECT imaging (discussed in Chapter 19). (© Siemens Healthineers 2019. Used with permission.)

Gamma cameras of other designs have been devised (briefly described later in this chapter) and have recently achieved commercial success. However, the overall superior cost-effectiveness, versatility and performance of the Anger camera across the entire spectrum of clinical (including tomographic) applications have caused it to remain dominant in nuclear imaging. The term *scintillation camera* will refer exclusively to the Anger scintillation camera throughout this chapter.

18.1.1 Design and Principles of Operation

Detector and Electronic Circuits

A scintillation camera head (Fig. 18-2) contains a disk-shaped (mostly on older cameras) or rectangular thallium-activated sodium iodide [NaI(Tl)] crystal, typically 0.95 cm (⅜ inch) thick, optically coupled to a large number (typically 37 to 91) of 5.1- to 7.6-cm (2- to 3-inch) diameter photomultiplier tubes (PMTs). PMTs and NaI(Tl) scintillation crystals were described in Chapter 17. The NaI(Tl) crystals of modern cameras have large areas; the rectangular crystals of one manufacturer are 59 × 44.5 cm (23 × 17.4 inches), with an FOV of about 53 by 39 cm. Some camera designs incorporate a Lucite light pipe between the glass cover of the crystal and PMTs; in others, the PMTs are directly coupled to the glass cover. In most cameras, a preamplifier is connected to the output of each PMT. Between the patient and the crystal is a collimator, usually made of lead, that only allows x- or γ-rays approaching from certain directions to reach the crystal. The collimator is essential; a scintillation camera without a collimator does not generate meaningful images. Figure 18-2 shows a parallel-hole collimator.

The lead walls, called *septa*, between the holes in the collimator absorb most photons approaching the collimator from directions that are not aligned with the holes. Most photons approaching the collimator from a nearly perpendicular direction pass through the holes; many of these are absorbed in the sodium iodide crystal, causing the emission of visible light and ultraviolet (UV) radiation. The light and UV photons are converted into electrical signals and amplified by the PMTs. These signals are

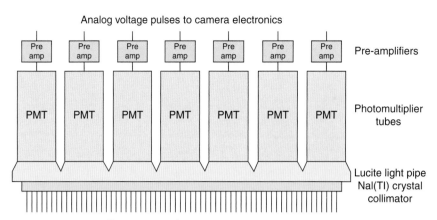

■ FIGURE 18-2 Scintillation camera detector.

further amplified by the preamplifiers (preamps). The amplitude of the electrical pulse produced by each PMT is proportional to the amount of light it received following an x- or γ-ray interaction in the crystal.

Because the collimator septa intercept most photons approaching the camera along paths not aligned with the collimator holes, the pattern of photon interactions in the crystal forms a two-dimensional projection of the three-dimensional activity distribution in the patient. The PMTs closest to each photon interaction in the crystal receive more light than those that are more distant, causing them to produce larger voltage pulses. The relative amplitudes of the pulses from the PMTs following each interaction contain sufficient information to determine the location of the interaction in the plane of the crystal within a few mm.

Early scintillation cameras formed images on photographic film using only analog electronic circuitry. In the late 1970s, digital circuitry began to be used for some functions. Modern scintillation cameras have an analog-to-digital converter (ADC) for the signal from the preamp following each PMT (Fig. 18-3). ADCs are described in Chapter 5. The remaining circuits used for signal processing and image formation are digital. The

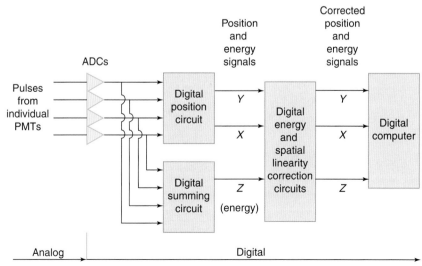

■ FIGURE 18-3 Electronic circuits of a modern digital scintillation camera. An actual scintillation camera has many more than four PMTs and ADCs.

digitized signals from the preamps are sent to two circuits. The position circuit receives the signals from the individual preamps after each x- or γ-ray interaction in the crystal and, by determining the centroid of these signals, produces an X-position signal and a Y-position signal that together specify the position of the interaction in the plane of the crystal. (This method of determining the position of an interaction is sometimes referred to as "Anger logic.") The summing circuit adds the signals from the individual preamps to produce an energy (Z) signal proportional in amplitude to the total energy deposited in the crystal by the interaction. These digital signals are then sent to correction circuits, described later in this chapter, to correct position-dependent systematic errors in event position assignment and energy determination (see Spatial Linearity and Uniformity, below). These correction circuits greatly improve the spatial linearity and uniformity of the images. The corrected energy (Z) signal is sent to an energy discrimination circuit. An interaction in the camera's crystal is recorded as a count in the image only if the energy (Z) signal is within a preset energy window. Scintillation cameras permit as many as four energy windows to be set for imaging radionuclides, such as Ga-67 and In-111, which emit useful photons of more than one energy. Following energy discrimination, the X- and Y-position signals are sent to a digital computer, where they are formed into a digital projection image, as described in Section 18.2 below, that can be displayed on a monitor.

Collimators

The collimator of a scintillation camera forms the projection image by permitting x- or γ-ray photons approaching the camera from certain directions to reach the crystal while absorbing most of the other photons. Collimators are made of high atomic number, high-density materials, usually lead. The most commonly used collimator is the *parallel-hole collimator*, which contains thousands of parallel holes (Fig. 18-4). The holes may be round, square, or triangular; however, most

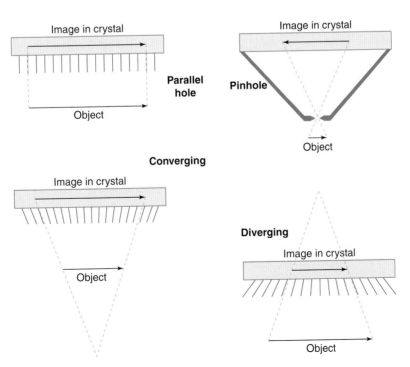

■ **FIGURE 18-4** Collimators.

state-of-the-art collimators have hexagonal holes and are usually made from lead foil, although some are cast. The partitions between the holes are called *septa*. The septa must be thick enough to absorb most of the photons incident upon them. For this reason, collimators designed for use with radionuclides that emit higher energy photons have thicker septa. There is an inherent compromise between the spatial resolution and efficiency (sensitivity) of collimators. Modifying a collimator to improve its spatial resolution (*e.g.*, by reducing the size of the holes or lengthening the collimator) reduces its efficiency. Most scintillation cameras are provided with a selection of parallel-hole collimators. These may include "low-energy, high-sensitivity"; "low-energy, all-purpose" (LEAP); "low-energy, high-resolution"; "medium-energy" (suitable for Ga-67 and In-111); "high-energy" (for I-131); and "ultra–high-energy" (for F-18) collimators. The size of the image produced by a parallel-hole collimator is not affected by the distance of the object from the collimator. However, its spatial resolution degrades rapidly with increasing collimator-to-object distance. The FOV of a parallel-hole collimator does not change with distance from the collimator.

A *pinhole collimator* (Fig. 18-4) is commonly used to produce magnified views of small objects, such as the thyroid gland or a hip joint. It consists of a small (typically 3- to 5-mm diameter) hole in a piece of lead or tungsten mounted at the apex of a leaded cone. Its function is identical to the pinhole in a pinhole photographic camera. As shown in the figure, the pinhole collimator produces a magnified image whose orientation is reversed. The magnification of the pinhole collimator decreases as an object is moved away from the pinhole. If an object is as far from the pinhole as the pinhole is from the crystal of the camera, the object is not magnified and, if the object is moved yet farther from the pinhole, it is minified. (Clinical imaging is not performed at these distances.) There are pitfalls in the use of pinhole collimators due to the decreasing magnification with distance. For example, a thyroid nodule deep in the mediastinum can appear to be in the thyroid itself. Pinhole collimators are used extensively in pediatric nuclear medicine. On some pinhole collimators, the part containing the hole can be removed and replaced with a part with a hole of another diameter; this allows the hole size to be varied for different clinical applications.

A *converging collimator* (Fig. 18-4) has many holes, all aimed at a focal point in front of the camera. As shown in the figure, the converging collimator magnifies the image. The magnification increases as the object is moved away from the collimator. A disadvantage of a converging collimator is that its FOV decreases with distance from the collimator. A *diverging collimator* (Fig. 18-4) has many holes aimed at a focal point behind the camera. It produces a minified image in which the amount of minification increases as the object is moved away from the camera. A diverging collimator may be used to image a part of a patient using a camera whose FOV, if a parallel-hole collimator were used, would be smaller than the body part to be imaged. For example, a diverging collimator could enable a mobile scintillation camera with a 25- or 30-cm-diameter crystal to perform a lung study of a patient in the intensive care unit. If a diverging collimator is reversed on a camera, it becomes a converging collimator. The diverging collimator is seldom used today, because it has inferior imaging characteristics to the parallel-hole collimator and the large rectangular crystals of most modern cameras render it unnecessary. The converging collimator is also seldom used; its imaging characteristics are superior, in theory, to the parallel-hole collimator, but its decreasing FOV with distance and varying magnification with distance have discouraged its use. However, a hybrid of the parallel-hole and converging collimator, called a *fan-beam collimator,* may be used in single photon emission computed tomography (SPECT) to take advantage of the favorable imaging properties of the converging collimator (see Chapter 19).

Many special-purpose collimators, such as the seven-pinhole collimator, have been developed. However, most of them have not enjoyed wide acceptance. The performance characteristics of parallel-hole, pinhole, and fan-beam collimators are discussed below (see Performance).

Principles of Image Formation

In nuclear imaging, which can also be called emission imaging, the photons from each point in the patient are emitted isotropically. Figure 18-5 shows the fates of the x- and γ-rays emitted in a patient being imaged. Some photons escape the patient without interaction, some scatter within the patient before escaping, and some are absorbed within the patient. Many of the photons escaping the patient are not detected because they are emitted in directions away from the image receptor. The collimator absorbs the vast majority of those photons that reach it. As a result, only a tiny fraction of the emitted photons (about 1 to 2 in 10,000 for typical low-energy parallel-hole collimators) has trajectories permitting passage through the collimator holes; thus, well over 99.9% of the photons reaching the gamma camera during imaging are wasted. Some photons penetrate the septa of the collimator without interaction. Of those reaching the crystal, some are absorbed in the crystal, some scatter from the crystal, and some pass through the crystal without interaction. The relative probabilities of these events depend on the energies of the photons and the thickness of the crystal. Of those photons absorbed in the crystal, some are absorbed by a single photoelectric absorption, whereas others undergo one or more Compton scatters before a photoelectric absorption. It is also possible for two photons to interact simultaneously with an Anger γ crystal; if the energy (Z) signal from the coincident

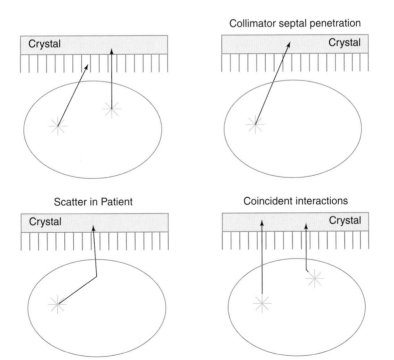

■ **FIGURE 18-5** Ways that x- and γ-rays interact with a scintillation camera. All of these, other than the ones depicted in the upper left, cause a loss of contrast and spatial resolution and add statistical noise. However, interactions by photons that have scattered though large angles and many coincident interactions are rejected by pulse height discrimination circuits.

interactions is within the energy window of the energy discrimination circuit, the result will be a single count mispositioned in the image. The fraction of simultaneous interactions increases with the interaction rate of the camera.

Interactions in the crystal of photons that have been scattered in the patient, photons that have penetrated the collimator septa, photons that undergo one or more scatters in the crystal, and coincident interactions in an Anger camera crystal reduce the spatial resolution and image contrast and increase random noise. The function of the camera's energy discrimination circuits (also known as pulse height analyzers) is to reduce this loss of resolution and contrast by rejecting photons that scatter in the patient or result in coincident interactions. Unfortunately, the limited energy resolution of the camera causes a wide photopeak, and low-energy photons can scatter through large angles with only a small energy loss. For example, a 140-keV photon scattering 45° will only lose 7.4% of its energy. An energy window that encompasses most of the photopeak will unfortunately still accept a significant fraction of the scattered photons and coincident interactions.

It is instructive to compare single photon emission imaging with x-ray transmission imaging (Table 18-1). In x-ray transmission imaging, including radiography and fluoroscopy, an image is projected on the image receptor because the x-rays originate from a very small source that approximates a point. In comparison, the photons in nuclear imaging are emitted isotropically throughout the patient and therefore collimation is necessary to form a projection image. Furthermore, in x-ray transmission imaging, x-rays that have scattered in the patient can be distinguished from primary x-rays by their directions and thus can be largely removed by grids. In emission imaging, primary photons cannot be distinguished from scattered photons by their directions. The collimator removes about the same fraction of scattered photons as it does primary photons and, unlike the grid in x-ray transmission imaging, does not reduce the fraction of counts in the resultant image due to scatter. Scattered photons in nuclear imaging can only be differentiated from primary photons by energy, because scattering reduces photon energy. In emission imaging, energy discrimination is used to reduce the fraction of counts in the image caused by scattered radiation. Finally, nuclear imaging devices must use pulse mode (the signal from each interaction is processed separately) for event localization and so that interaction-by-interaction energy discrimination can be employed; x-ray transmission imaging systems typically produce much larger photon fluxes and so most such systems do not detect, discriminate, and record on a photon-by-photon basis.

18.1.2 Alternative Camera Design—The Multielement Camera

An alternative to the Anger scintillation camera for nuclear medicine imaging is the multi-detector element (also known as pixelated) camera. An image receptor of such

TABLE 18-1 COMPARISON OF SINGLE-PHOTON NUCLEAR IMAGING WITH X-RAY TRANSMISSION IMAGING

	PRINCIPLE OF IMAGE FORMATION	SCATTER REJECTION	PULSE OR CURRENT MODE
X-ray transmission imaging	Point source	Grid or air gap	Current
Scintillation camera	Collimation	Pulse height discrimination	Pulse

a camera is a two-dimensional array of many small independent detector elements. Such cameras are used with collimators for image formation, as are Anger scintillation cameras.

The first such camera to achieve clinical acceptance (albeit limited) in the 1970s and early 1980s consisted of 294 NaI(Tl) scintillation crystals arranged in an array of 14 rows and 21 columns. A clever arrangement of light pipes was used to route the light from the crystals to 35 PMTs, with all crystals in a row connected to one PMT and all crystals in a column being connected to another PMT. Light signals being simultaneously received by the PMT for a column and another PMT for a row identified the crystal in which a x- or γ-ray interaction occurred. Since that time, other multielement cameras have been developed and become commercially available. One scintillator-based design (indirect conversion to an electrical signal, as is the case for an Anger camera), consists of a 64 × 48 array of 2.96 mm × 2.96 mm × 6 mm thick NaI(Tl) crystals, each 8 × 8 sub-array of which is coupled to an independent position-sensitive PMT, thus not requiring Anger logic for event positioning. Each detector element of another such scintillator-based multielement camera is a 3.3 mm × 3.3 mm × 6 mm thick thallium-activated cesium iodide (CsI[Tl]) crystal optically coupled to a silicon photodiode, in a 120 × 96 array of crystals (Fig. 18-6 right). In a second, so-called direct-conversion design, each detector element is a CZT semiconductor-based crystal, whereby the interaction of a x- or γ-ray in the crystal produces a current of electrons and holes directly, the total charge of which is proportional to the energy imparted. One such CZT camera is a breast-specific γ imager containing ninety-six 5 mm thick CZT crystals, each pixelated electronically into a 16 × 16 array of 1.6 mm × 1.6 mm detector elements. Two other such cameras from one manufacturer are a dedicated breast imaging (Fig. 18-6) and a large FOV camera, respectively, with 2.46 mm × 2.46 mm × 5 mm thick (750b, 96 × 64 array) or 7.25 mm thick (870, 208 × 160 array) detector elements, manufactured as 39.36 mm × 39.36 mm CZT crystals that are pixelated electronically.

The intrinsic spatial resolution of a multielement detector camera is determined by the physical dimensions of the independent detector elements. One advantage to the multielement camera design is that very high interaction rates can be tolerated with only limited dead-time losses because of the independent detectors in the image

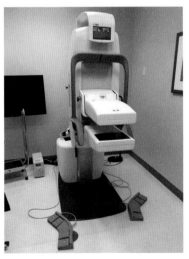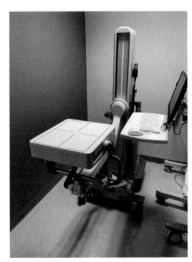

■ **FIGURE 18-6** Modern multielement gamma cameras. GE NM 750b molecular breast imager (left) and Digirad Ergo portable (right).

receptor. A second advantage is improved energy resolution afforded by the alternative detector material and method of processing events. A disadvantage is the complexity of the electronics needed to process the signals from such a large number of independent detectors. A limitation of current semiconductor multielement cameras is a maximum imaging x- or γ-ray energy of about 200 keV, due to a restriction on crystal thickness.

18.1.3 Performance

Measures of Performance

Measures of the performance of a gamma camera with the collimator attached are called *system* or *extrinsic* measurements. Measures of camera performance with the collimator removed are called *intrinsic* measurements. System measurements give the best indication of clinical performance, but intrinsic measurements are often more useful for comparing the performance of different cameras, because they isolate camera performance from collimator performance.

Uniformity is a measure of a camera's response to uniform irradiation of the detector surface. The ideal response is a perfectly uniform image. Intrinsic uniformity is usually measured by placing a point radionuclide source (typically 1 mCi of Tc-99m) in front of the uncollimated camera. The source should be placed at least four times the largest dimension of the detector away to ensure uniform irradiation of the camera surface and at least five times that distance away, if the uniformity image is to be analyzed quantitatively using a computer. System uniformity, which reveals collimator as well as camera defects, is assessed by placing a uniform planar radionuclide source in front of the collimated camera. Solid planar sealed sources of Co-57 (typically 5 to 10 mCi when new) and planar sources that may be filled with a Tc-99m solution are commercially available. A planar source should be large enough to cover the entire detector of the camera. The uniformity of the resultant images may be analyzed by a computer or evaluated visually.

Spatial resolution is a measure of a camera's ability to accurately portray spatial variations in activity concentration and to distinguish as separate radioactive objects in close proximity. The *system spatial resolution* is evaluated by acquiring an image of a line source, such as a capillary tube filled with Tc-99m, using a computer interfaced to the collimated camera and determining the line spread function (LSF). (System resolution for a multielement gamma camera should be measured at a distance, typically 100 mm, as resolution is essentially the detector element width and height at the collimator face.) The LSF, described in Chapter 4, is a cross-sectional profile of the image of a line source. The full-width-at-half-maximum (FWHM), the full-width-at-tenth-maximum, and the modulation transfer function (described in Chapter 4) may all be derived from the LSF.

The system spatial resolution, if measured in air so that scatter is not present, is determined by the collimator resolution and the intrinsic resolution of the camera. The *collimator resolution* is defined as the FWHM of the radiation transmitted through the collimator from a line source (Fig. 18-7). It is not directly measured, but calculated from the system and intrinsic resolutions. The *intrinsic resolution* of an Anger camera is determined quantitatively by acquiring an image, with a sheet of lead containing one or more thin slits placed against the uncollimated camera, using a point source. (The evaluation of multielement camera intrinsic resolution is not applicable, as it is simply the detector element width and length.) The point source should be positioned at least five times the largest dimension of the camera's detector away.

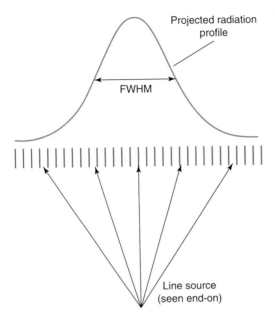

Projected radiation profile

FWHM

Line source (seen end-on)

■ **FIGURE 18-7** Collimator resolution.

The system (R_S), collimator (R_C), and intrinsic (R_I) resolutions, as indicated by the FWHMs of the LSFs, are related by the following equation:

$$R_S = \sqrt{R_C^2 + R_I^2}.$$ [18-1]

Some types of collimators magnify (converging, pinhole) or minify (diverging) the image. For these collimators, the system and collimator resolutions should be corrected for the collimator magnification, so that they refer to distances in the object rather than distances in the camera detector:

$$R_S' = \sqrt{R_C'^2 + (R_I/m)^2},$$ [18-2]

where $R_S' = R_S/m$ is the system resolution corrected for magnification, $R_C' = R_C/m$ is the collimator resolution corrected for magnification, and m is the collimator magnification (image size in detector/object size). The collimator magnification is determined as follows:

$m = 1.0$ for parallel-hole collimators

$m = $ (pinhole-to-crystal distance)/(object-to-pinhole distance) for pinhole collimators

$m = f/(f - x)$ for converging collimators

$m = f/(f + x)$ for diverging collimators,

where f is the distance from the crystal to the focal point of the collimator and x is the distance of the object from the crystal. It will be seen later in this section that the collimator and system resolutions degrade (FWHM of the LSF, corrected for collimator magnification, increases) with increasing distance between the line source and collimator.

As can be seen from Equation 18-2, collimator magnification reduces the deleterious effect of intrinsic spatial resolution on the overall system resolution. Geometric magnification in x-ray transmission imaging reduces the effect of image receptor blur for the same reason.

In routine practice, the spatial resolution is semiquantitatively evaluated by imaging a parallel line or a four-quadrant bar phantom (Fig. 18-8) in contact with the camera face, using a planar radionuclide source if the camera is collimated (system resolution) or a distant point source if the collimator is removed (intrinsic resolution), and visually noting the smallest bars that are resolved. (Bar phantom resolution evaluation is not applicable to multielement cameras, as both intrinsic and system resolutions are fixed, and the images may contain aliasing or moire artifacts due to the pixelated nature of the detector and/or collimator hole-detector element mismatch.) By convention, the widths of the bars are the same as the widths of the spaces between the bars. The size of the smallest bars that are resolved is approximately related to the FWHM of the LSF:

$$(\text{FWHM of the LSF}) \approx 1.7 \times (\text{Size of smallest bars resolved}). \qquad [18\text{-}3]$$

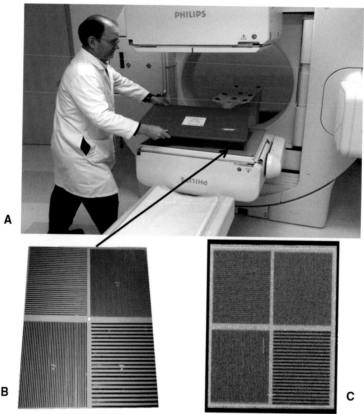

■ **FIGURE 18-8** Use of a bar phantom for evaluating spatial resolution. A plastic rectangular flood source containing up to 10 mCi (370 MBq) of uniformly distributed Co-57 **(A)** is placed on top of the bar phantom **(B)**, which is resting on top of the camera head collimator. The bar phantom has four quadrants, each consisting of parallel lead bars with a specific width and spacing between the bars. An image **(C)** is acquired with approximately 10 million counts and the lines are visually inspected for linearity and determination of closest spacing between the bars that can be seen resolved as separate lines. A typical four-quadrant bar phantom for a modern scintillation camera might have 2.0-, 2.5-, 3.0-, and 3.5-mm wide lead bars, with the widths of the spaces equal to the widths of the bars. This extrinsic resolution test (performed with the collimator attached to the camera) evaluates the system resolution. An intrinsic resolution test is performed with the collimator removed from the camera head. In this case, the bar phantom is placed against the crystal of the uncollimated camera head and irradiated by a point source containing 100 to 200 μCi (3.7 to 7.4 MBq) of Tc-99m in a syringe placed at least four camera crystal diameters away.

Spatial linearity (lack of spatial distortion) is a measure of the camera's ability to portray the shapes of objects accurately. It is determined from the images of a bar phantom, line source, or other phantom by assessing the straightness of the lines in the image. Spatial non-linearities can significantly degrade the uniformity, as will be discussed later in this chapter.

Multienergy spatial registration, commonly called *multiple window spatial registration*, is a measure of the camera's ability to maintain the same image magnification, regardless of the energies deposited in the crystal by the incident x- or γ-rays. (It is not applicable to multielement cameras.) (Image magnification is defined as the distance between two points in the image divided by the actual distance between the two points in the object being imaged.) Higher energy x- and γ-ray photons produce larger signals from the individual PMTs than do lower energy photons. The position circuit of the scintillation camera normalizes the *X*- and *Y*-position signals by the energy signal, so that the position signals are independent of the deposited energy. If a radionuclide emitting useful photons of several energies, such as Ga-67 (93-, 185-, and 300-keV γ-rays), is imaged and the normalization is not properly performed, the resultant image will be a superposition of images of different magnifications (Fig. 18-9). The multienergy spatial registration can be tested by imaging several point sources of Ga-67, offset from the center of the camera, using only one major γ-ray at a time. The centroid of the count distribution of each source should be at the same position in the image for all three γ-ray energies.

The *system efficiency* (sensitivity) of a gamma camera is the fraction of x- or γ-rays emitted by a source that produces counts in the image. The system efficiency is important because it, in conjunction with imaging time, determines the amount of quantum mottle (graininess) in the images. The system efficiency (E_s) is the product of three factors: the collimator efficiency (E_c), the intrinsic efficiency of the crystal (E_i), and the fraction (f) of interacting photons accepted by the energy discrimination circuits:

$$E_s = E_c \times E_i \times f. \tag{18-4}$$

The *collimator efficiency* is the fraction of photons emitted by a source that penetrate the collimator holes. In general, it is a function of the distance between the source and the collimator and the design of the collimator. The *intrinsic efficiency*, the fraction of

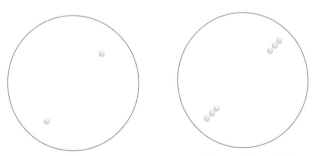

■ **FIGURE 18-9** Multienergy spatial registration. Left: A simulated image of two point sources of a radionuclide emitting γ-rays of three different energies, illustrating proper normalization of the *X*- and *Y*-position signals for deposited energy. Right: A simulated image of the same two point sources, showing improper adjustment of the energy normalization circuit. The maladjustment causes higher energy photons to produce larger *X* and *Y* values than lower energy photons interacting at the same position in the camera's crystal, resulting in multiple images of each point source. A less severe maladjustment would cause each point source to appear as an ellipse, rather than three discrete dots.

photons penetrating the collimator that interact with the crystal, is determined by the thickness of the crystal and the energy of the photons:

$$E_i = 1 - e^{-\mu x},$$ [18-5]

where μ is the linear attenuation coefficient of the crystal and x is the thickness of the crystal. The last two factors in Equation 18-4 can be combined to form the *photopeak efficiency*, defined as the fraction of photons reaching the crystal that produce counts in the photopeak of the energy spectrum:

$$E_p = E_i \times f.$$ [18-6]

This equation assumes that the window of the energy discrimination circuit has been adjusted to encompass the photopeak exactly. In theory, the system efficiency and each of its components range from zero to one. In reality, low-energy all-purpose parallel-hole collimators have efficiencies of about 2×10^{-4} and low-energy high-resolution parallel-hole collimators have efficiencies of about 1×10^{-4}.

The *energy resolution* of a gamma camera is a measure of its ability to distinguish between interactions depositing different energies in its crystal. A camera with superior energy resolution is able to reject a larger fraction of photons that have scattered in the patient or have undergone coincident interactions, thereby producing images of better contrast and less relative random noise. The energy resolution is measured by exposing the camera to a point source of a radionuclide, usually Tc-99m, emitting monoenergetic photons and acquiring a spectrum of the energy (Z) pulses, using either the nuclear medicine computer interfaced to the camera, if it has the capability, or a multichannel analyzer. The energy resolution is calculated from the FWHM of the photopeak (see Pulse Height Spectroscopy in Chapter 17). The FWHM is divided by the energy of the photon (140 keV for Tc-99m) and is expressed as a percentage. A wider FWHM implies poorer energy resolution.

Gamma cameras are operated in pulse mode (see Design and Principles of Operation, above) and therefore suffer from dead-time count losses at high interaction rates. Anger scintillation cameras behave as paralyzable systems (see Chapter 17); the indicated count rate initially increases as the imaged activity increases, but ultimately reaches a maximum and decreases thereafter. (Multielement cameras are much less susceptible to such count losses, due to their detector elements operating independently and their different method of processing events.) The count-rate performance of a camera is usually specified by (1) the observed count rate at 20% count loss and (2) the maximal count rate. These count rates may be measured with or without scatter. Both are reduced when measured with scatter. Table 18-2 lists typical values for modern cameras. These high count rates are usually achieved by implementing a high count-rate mode that degrades the spatial and energy resolutions.

Some scintillation cameras can correctly process the PMT signals when two or more interactions occur simultaneously in the crystal, provided that the interactions are separated by sufficient distance. This significantly increases the number of interactions that are correctly registered at high interaction rates.

18.1.4 Design Factors Determining Performance

Intrinsic Spatial Resolution and Intrinsic Efficiency

The intrinsic spatial resolution of a scintillation camera is determined by the types of interactions by which the x- or γ-rays deposit energy in the camera's crystal and the statistics of the detection of the visible light and UV photons emitted following

TABLE 18-2 TYPICAL INTRINSIC PERFORMANCE CHARACTERISTICS OF A MODERN SCINTILLATION CAMERA, MEASURED BY NEMA PROTOCOL

Intrinsic spatial resolution (FWHM of LSF for 140 keV)[a]	2.7–4.2 mm
Energy resolution (FWHM of photopeak for 140 keV photons)	9.2%–11%
Integral uniformity (max. pixel − min. pixel)/(max. pixel + min. pixel)	2%–5%
Absolute spatial linearity	<1.5 mm
Observed count rate at 20% count loss (measured without scatter)	110,000–260,000 counts/s
Observed maximal count rate (measured without scatter)	170,000–500,000 counts/s

[a]Intrinsic spatial resolution is for a 0.95-cm (3/8-inch) thick crystal; thicker crystals cause slightly worse spatial resolution.
FWHM, full width at half maximum; LSF, line spread function; NEMA, National Electrical Manufacturers Association.

these interactions. The most important of these is the random error associated with the collection of UV and visible light photons and subsequent production of electrical signals by the PMTs. Approximately one UV or visible light photon is emitted in the NaI(Tl) crystal for every 25 eV deposited by an x- or γ-ray. For example, when a 140-keV γ-ray is absorbed by the crystal, approximately 140,000/25 = 5,600 UV or visible light photons are produced. About two thirds of these, approximately 3,700 photons, reach the photocathodes of the PMTs. Only about one out of every five of these causes an electron to escape a photocathode, giving rise to about 750 electrons. These electrons are divided among the PMTs, with the most being produced in the PMTs closest to the interaction. Thus, only a small number of photoelectrons is generated in any one PMT after an interaction. Because the processes by which the absorption of a γ-ray causes the release of electrons from a photocathode are random, the pulses from the PMTs after an interaction contain significant random errors that, in turn, cause errors in the X and Y signals produced by the position circuit of the camera and the energy (Z) signal. These random errors limit both the intrinsic spatial resolution and the energy resolution of the camera. The energy of the incident x- or γ-rays determines the amount of random error in the event localization process; higher energy photons provide lower relative random errors and therefore superior intrinsic spatial resolution. For example, the γ-rays from Tc-99m (140 keV) produce better spatial resolution than do the x-rays from Tl-201 (69 to 80 keV), because each Tc-99m γ-ray produces about twice as many light photons when absorbed. There is relatively little improvement in intrinsic spatial resolution for γ-ray energies above 250 keV, because the improvement in spatial resolution due to more visible light photons is largely offset by the increased likelihood of scattering in the crystal before photoelectric absorption (discussed below).

The quantum detection efficiency of the PMTs in detecting the UV and visible light photons produced in the crystal is the most significant factor limiting the intrinsic spatial resolution (typically only 20% to 25% of the UV and visible light photons incident on a photocathode contribute to the signal from the PMT). The size of the PMTs also affects the spatial resolution slightly; using PMTs of smaller diameter improves the spatial resolution by providing better sampling of the light emitted following each interaction in the crystal.

A thinner NaI(Tl) crystal provides better intrinsic spatial resolution than a thicker crystal. A thinner crystal permits less spreading of the light before it reaches the PMTs. Furthermore, a thinner crystal reduces the likelihood of an incident x- or γ-ray undergoing one or more Compton scatters in the crystal followed by photoelectric absorption. Compton scattering in the crystal can cause the centroid of the energy

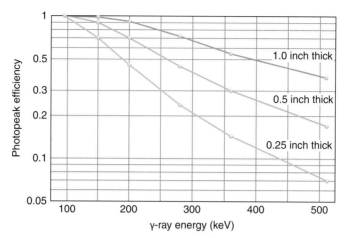

■ **FIGURE 18-10** Calculated photopeak efficiency as a function of x- or γ-ray energy for NaI(Tl) crystals. (Data from Anger HO, Davis DH. Gamma-ray detection efficiency and image resolution in sodium iodide. *Rev Sci Instr.* 1964;35(6):693-697.)

deposition to be significantly offset from the site of the initial interaction in the crystal. The likelihood of one or more scatters in the crystal preceding the photoelectric absorption increases with the energy of the x- or γ-ray.

The intrinsic efficiency of a gamma camera is determined by the thickness of the crystal and the energy of the incident x- or γ-rays. Figure 18-10 is a graph of photopeak efficiency (fraction of incident x- or γ-rays producing counts in the photopeak) as a function of photon energy for NaI(Tl) crystals 0.635 cm (¼ inch), 1.27 cm (½ inch), and 2.54 cm (1 inch) thick. Most modern scintillation cameras have 0.95-cm (⅜ inch) thick crystals. The photopeak efficiency of these crystals is greater than 80% for the 140-keV γ-rays from Tc-99m, but less than 30% for the 364-keV γ-rays from I-131. Some cameras, designed primarily for imaging radionuclides such as Tl-201 and Tc-99m, which emit low-energy photons, have 0.635-cm (¼ inch) thick crystals. Other cameras, designed to provide greater intrinsic efficiency for imaging radionuclides such as I-131, which emit high-energy γ-rays, have 1.27- to 2.5-cm (½ to 1 inch) thick crystals.

There is a design compromise between the intrinsic efficiency of the scintillation camera, which increases with crystal thickness, and intrinsic spatial resolution, which degrades with crystal thickness. This design compromise is similar to the design compromise between the spatial resolution of scintillator-based image receptors used in radiography and fluoroscopy, which deteriorates with increasing phosphor layer thickness, and detection efficiency, which improves with increasing thickness.

Collimator Resolution and Collimator Efficiency

The collimator spatial resolution, as defined above, of multihole collimators (parallel-hole, converging, and diverging) is determined by the geometry of the holes. The spatial resolution improves (narrower FWHM of the LSF) as the diameters of the holes are reduced and the lengths of the holes (thickness of the collimator) are increased. Unfortunately, changing the hole geometry to improve the spatial resolution in general reduces the collimator's efficiency. *The resultant compromise between collimator efficiency and collimator resolution is the single most significant limitation on gamma camera performance.*

The spatial resolution of a parallel-hole collimator decreases (*i.e.*, FWHM of the LSF increases) linearly as the collimator-to-object distance increases. This degradation of collimator spatial resolution with increasing collimator-to-object distance is also one of the most important factors limiting gamma camera performance. However, the efficiency of a parallel-hole collimator is nearly constant over the collimator-to-object distances used for clinical imaging. Although the number of photons passing through a particular collimator hole decreases as the square of the distance, the number of holes through which photons can pass increases as the square of the distance. The efficiency of a parallel-hole collimator, neglecting septal penetration, is approximately

$$E_c \approx \frac{A}{4\pi l^2} g,$$ [18-7]

where A is the cross-sectional area of a single collimator hole, l is the length of a hole (i.e., the thickness of the collimator), and g is the fraction of the frontal area of the collimator that is not blocked by the collimator septa (g = total area of holes in collimator face/area of collimator face).

Figure 18-11 depicts the LSF of a parallel-hole collimator as a function of source-to-collimator distance. The width of the LSF increases with distance. Nevertheless, the area under the LSF (total number of counts) does not significantly decrease with distance.

The spatial resolution of a pinhole collimator, along its central axis, corrected for collimator magnification, is approximately equal to

$$R'_c \approx d\frac{f + x}{f},$$ [18-8]

where d is the diameter of the pinhole, f is the distance from the crystal to the pinhole, and x is the distance from the pinhole to the object. The efficiency of a pinhole collimator, along its central axis, neglecting penetration around the pinhole, is

$$E_c = d^2/16x^2.$$ [18-9]

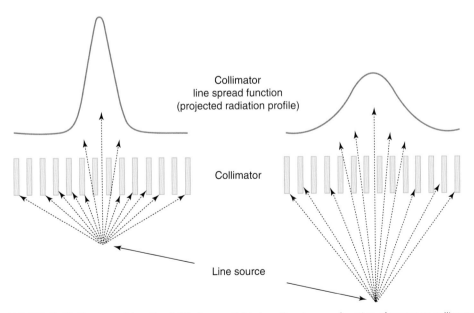

Collimator
line spread function
(projected radiation profile)

Collimator

Line source

■ **FIGURE 18-11** Line spread function (LSF) of a parallel-hole collimator as a function of source-to-collimator distance. The full-width-at-half-maximum (FWHM) of the LSF increases linearly with distance from the source to the collimator; however, the total area under the LSF (photon fluence through the collimator) decreases very little with source to collimator distance. (In both figures, the line source is seen "end-on.")

TABLE 18-3 THE EFFECT OF INCREASING COLLIMATOR-TO-OBJECT DISTANCE ON COLLIMATOR PERFORMANCE PARAMETERS

COLLIMATOR	SPATIAL RESOLUTION[a]	EFFICIENCY	FIELD SIZE	MAGNIFICATION
Parallel hole	Decreases	Approximately constant	Constant	Constant ($m = 1.0$)
Converging	Decreases	Increases	Decreases	Increases ($m > 1$ at collimator surface)
Diverging	Decreases	Decreases	Increases	Decreases ($m < 1$ at collimator surface)
Pinhole	Decreases	Decreases	Increases	Decreases (m largest near pinhole)

[a]Spatial resolution corrected for magnification.

Thus, the spatial resolution of the collimator improves (*i.e.*, R'_C decreases) as the diameter of the pinhole is reduced, but the collimator efficiency decreases, as it is proportional to the square of the pinhole diameter. Both the collimator spatial resolution and the efficiency are best for objects close to the pinhole (small x). The efficiency decreases rapidly with increasing pinhole-to-object distance.

The spatial resolution of all collimators decreases with increasing x- or γ-ray energy because of increasing collimator septal penetration or, in the case of pinhole collimators, penetration around the pinhole. Table 18-3 compares the characteristics of different types of collimators.

System Spatial Resolution and Efficiency

The system spatial resolution and efficiency are determined by the intrinsic and collimator resolutions and efficiencies, as described by Equations 18-2 and 18-4. Figure 18-12 (top) shows the effect of object-to-collimator distance on system spatial resolution. The system resolutions shown in this figure are corrected for magnification. *The system spatial resolution, when corrected for magnification, is degraded (i.e., FWHM of the LSF increases) as the collimator-to-object distance increases for all types of collimators.* This degradation of resolution with increasing patient-to-collimator distance is among the most important factors in image acquisition. Technologists should make every effort to minimize this distance during clinical imaging.

Figure 18-12 (bottom) shows the effect of object-to-collimator distance on system efficiency. The system efficiency with a parallel-hole collimator is nearly constant with distance over the range of distances used for clinical imaging. The system efficiency with a pinhole collimator decreases significantly with distance. The system efficiency of a fan-beam collimator (described in the following chapter) increases with collimator-to-object distance.

Modern scintillation cameras with 0.95-cm (⅜ inch) thick crystals typically have intrinsic spatial resolutions slightly less than 4.0 mm FWHM for the 140-keV γ-rays of Tc-99m. (Modern multielement camera intrinsic resolution, defined by detector element dimensions, is typically less than 3.5 mm.) One manufacturer's low-energy high-resolution parallel-hole collimator has a resolution of 1.5 mm FWHM at the face of the collimator and 6.4 mm at 10 cm from the collimator. The system resolutions, calculated from Equation 18-1, are as follows:

$$R_S = \sqrt{(1.5 \text{ mm})^2 + (4.0 \text{ mm})^2} = 4.3 \text{ mm at 0 cm,} \qquad \text{[18-10a]}$$

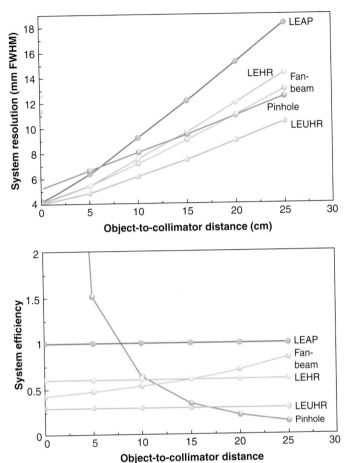

■ **FIGURE 18-12** System spatial resolution (top) and efficiency (bottom) as a function of object-to-collimator distance (in cm). System resolutions for pinhole and fan-beam collimators are corrected for magnification. System efficiencies are relative to a low-energy, all-purpose (LEAP) parallel-hole collimator (system efficiency 340 cpm/μCi Tc-99m for a 0.95-cm-thick crystal). LEHR, low-energy, high-resolution parallel-hole collimator; LEUHR, low-energy, ultra-high-resolution parallel-hole collimator. (Data courtesy of the late William Guth of Siemens Healthineers, Nuclear Medicine Group.)

and

$$R_S = \sqrt{(6.4 \text{ mm})^2 + (4.0 \text{ mm})^2} = 7.5 \text{ mm at } 10 \text{ cm}. \qquad \text{[18-10b]}$$

Thus, the system resolution is only slightly worse than the intrinsic resolution at the collimator face, but is largely determined by the collimator resolution at typical imaging distances for internal organs.

Spatial Linearity and Uniformity

Fully analog scintillation cameras, now obsolete, suffered from significant spatial non-linearity and non-uniformity. These distortions were caused by systematic (non-random) effects, which vary with position on the face of the camera, in the detection and collection of signals from individual x- or γ-rays. Because these position-dependent effects are not random, corrections for them can be made. Modern digital cameras use tables of position-specific correction factors for this function.

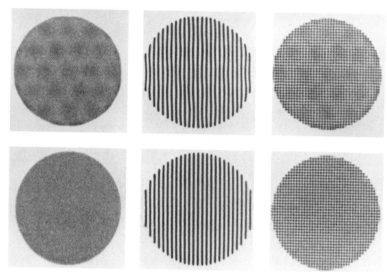

■ **FIGURE 18-13** Pairs of uniformity images, lead slit-mask (lead sheet with thin slits) images, and orthogonal hole phantom (lead sheet with a rectangular array of holes) images, with scintillation camera's digital correction circuitry disabled (top) to demonstrate non-uniformities and spatial non-linearities inherent to a scintillation camera and with correction circuitry functioning (bottom), demonstrating effectiveness of linearity and energy (Z) signal correction circuitry. (© Siemens Healthineers 2019. Used with permission.)

Spatial non-linearity (Fig. 18-13 top center and top right) is caused by the non-random (*i.e.*, systematic) mispositioning of events. It is mainly due to the calculated locations of the interactions being shifted in the resultant image toward the center of the nearest PMT by the position circuit of the camera. Modern cameras have digital circuits that use tables of correction factors to correct each pair of X- and Y-position signals for spatial non-linearities (Fig. 18-14). One lookup table contains an X-position correction for each portion of the crystal, and another table contains corrections for the Y direction. Each pair of digital position signals is used to "look up" a pair of X and Y corrections in the tables. The corrections are added to the uncorrected X and Y values. The corrected X and Y values (X' and Y' in Fig. 18-14) are sent to a computer or other device that accepts them in digital form for image formation. (Multielement cameras do not suffer from spatial non-linearity, as it is a phenomenon unique to Anger cameras.)

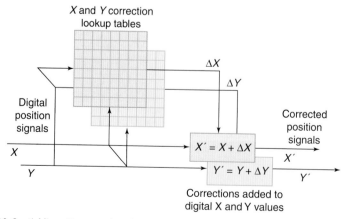

■ **FIGURE 18-14** Spatial linearity correction circuitry of a scintillation camera.

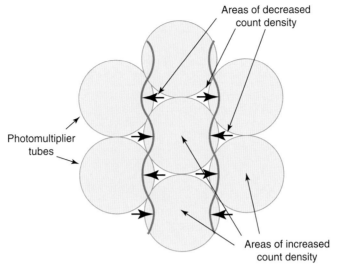

Areas of decreased
count density

Photomultiplier
tubes

Areas of increased
count density

■ **FIGURE 18-15** Spatial non-linearities cause non-uniformities. The two vertical wavy lines represent straight lines in the object that have been distorted. The scintillation camera's position circuit causes the locations of individual counts to be shifted toward the center of the nearest photomultiplier tube (PMT), causing an enhanced count density toward the center of the PMT and a decreased count density between the PMTs, as seen in the *top left image* in Figure 18-13.

There are three major causes of non-uniformity. The first is spatial non-linearities. As shown in Figure 18-15, the systematic mispositioning of events imposes local variations in the count density. Spatial non-linearities that are almost imperceptible can cause significant non-uniformities. The linearity correction circuitry previously described effectively corrects this source of non-uniformity.

The second major cause of non-uniformity is that the position of the interaction in the crystal affects the magnitude of the energy (Z) signal. In an Anger camera, it may be caused by local variations in the crystal in the light generation and light transmission to the PMTs and by variations in the light detection and gains of the PMTs. In a multielement camera, it may be due to local variations in light output from detector elements and/or signal output from the position-sensitive PMTs or photodiodes (scintillator-based); or variation in the electrical signal amplitude among detector elements (semiconductor-based). If these regional variations in energy signal are not corrected, the fraction of interactions rejected by the energy discrimination circuits will vary with position in the detector. These positional variations in the magnitude of the energy signal are corrected by digital electronic circuitry in modern cameras (Fig. 18-16). Multielement cameras also typically contain a number of detector elements that produce either no, extremely high, or unstable signals, due to either manufacturing defects or failure during use. A map of these so-called *bad* detector elements is created, and the corresponding pixel values in the resultant images are computed by averaging the pixel values corresponding to neighboring functional detector elements post-acquisition.

The third major cause of non-uniformity is local variations in the efficiency of the camera in absorbing x- or γ-rays, such as manufacturing defects or damage to the collimator. These may be corrected by acquiring an image of an extremely uniform planar source using a computer interfaced to the camera. A correction factor is determined for each pixel in the image by dividing the average pixel count by that pixel count. Each pixel in a clinical image is multiplied by its correction factor to compensate for this cause of non-uniformity.

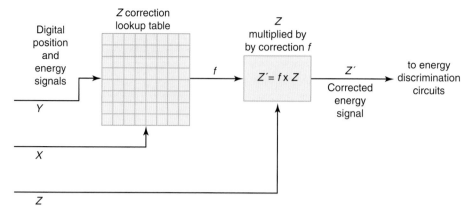

■ **FIGURE 18-16** Energy (*Z*) signal correction circuitry of a scintillation camera. The digital *X*- and *Y*-position signals are used to "look up" a position-dependent correction factor. The uncorrected *Z* value is multiplied by the correction factor. Finally, the corrected *Z* value is transmitted to the energy discrimination circuits.

The digital spatial linearity and energy correction circuits of a modern Anger or multielement camera do not directly affect its intrinsic spatial resolution. However, the obsolete fully analog Anger cameras, which lacked these corrections, used means such as thick light pipes and light absorbers between the crystal and PMTs to improve spatial linearity and uniformity. These reduced the amount of light reaching the PMTs. As mentioned previously, Anger camera intrinsic spatial resolution and energy resolution are largely determined by the statistics of the detection of light photons from the crystal. The loss of signal from light photons in fully analog cameras significantly limited their intrinsic spatial and energy resolutions. The use of digital linearity and energy correction permits camera designs that maximize light collection, thereby providing much better intrinsic spatial resolution and energy resolution than fully analog cameras.

NEMA Specifications for Performance Measurements of Gamma Camera

The National Electrical Manufacturers Association (NEMA) publishes a document that specifies standard methods for measuring camera performance.[3] All manufacturers of scintillation and multielement cameras publish NEMA performance measurements of their cameras, which are used by prospective purchasers in comparing cameras and for writing purchase specifications. Before the advent of NEMA standards, manufacturers measured the performance of scintillation gamma cameras in a variety of ways, making it difficult to compare the manufacturers' specifications for different cameras objectively. The measurement methods specified by NEMA require specialized equipment and are not intended to be performed by the nuclear medicine department. However, it is possible to perform simplified versions of the NEMA tests to determine whether a newly purchased camera meets the published specifications. Unfortunately, the NEMA protocols omit testing of a number of important camera performance parameters.

18.1.5 Effects of Scatter, Collimator Spatial Resolution, and Attenuation on Projection Images

Ideally, a nuclear medicine projection image would be a two-dimensional projection of the three-dimensional activity distribution in the patient. If this were the case,

---

[3]Performance Measures of Gamma Cameras, NEMA NU 1-2018.

the number of counts in each point in the image would be proportional to the average activity concentration along a straight line through the corresponding anatomy of the patient. There are three main reasons why nuclear medicine images are not ideal projection images—attenuation of photons in the patient, inclusion of Compton scattered photons in the image, and the degradation of spatial resolution with distance from the collimator. Furthermore, because most nuclear medicine images are acquired over periods of many seconds or even minutes, patient motion, particularly respiratory motion, is a source of image blurring.

Attenuation in the patient by Compton scattering and the photoelectric effect prevents some photons that would otherwise pass through the collimator holes from contributing to the image. The amount of attenuation is mainly determined by the path length through tissue and the densities of the tissues between a location in the patient and the corresponding point on the camera face. Thus, photons from structures deeper in the patient are much more heavily attenuated than photons from structures closer to the camera face. Attenuation is more severe for lower energy photons, such as the 69- to 80-keV characteristic x-rays emitted by Tl-201 ($\mu \approx 0.19$ cm^{-1} for soft tissue), than for higher energy photons, such as the 140-keV γ-rays from Tc-99m ($\mu = 0.15$ cm^{-1}) Non-uniform attenuation, especially in thoracic and cardiac nuclear imaging, presents a particular problem in image interpretation.

The vast majority of the interactions with soft tissue by x- and γ-rays of the energies used for nuclear medicine imaging are by Compton scattering. Some photons that have scattered in the patient pass through the collimator holes and are detected. As in x-ray transmission imaging such as radiography and CT, the relative number of scattered photons is greater when imaging thicker parts of the patient, such as the abdomen, and the main effects of counts in the image from scattered photons are a loss of contrast and an increase in random noise. As was mentioned earlier in this chapter, the number of scattered photons contributing to the image is reduced by pulse height discrimination. However, setting an energy window of sufficient width to encompass most of the photopeak permits a considerable amount of the scatter to contribute to image formation. (As mentioned earlier, one advantage of a CZT multielement camera is improved energy resolution, which allows a narrower energy window, which in turn reduces the amount of scatter in the photopeak image.)

18.1.6 Operation and Routine Quality Control

Peaking a gamma camera means to adjust its energy discrimination windows to center them on the photopeak or photopeaks of the desired radionuclide. Modern cameras display the spectrum as a histogram of the number of interactions as a function of pulse height (Fig. 18-17), like the display produced by a multichannel analyzer (see Chapter 17). On this display, the energy window limits are shown as vertical lines. A narrower energy window provides better scatter rejection, but also reduces the number of unscattered photons recorded in the image.

Peaking may be performed manually by adjusting the energy window settings while viewing the spectrum or automatically by the camera. Older scintillation cameras with mostly analog electronics required adjustment of the energy windows before the first use each day and again before imaging another radionuclide. In modern gamma cameras, the energy calibration and energy window settings are very stable. For such cameras, peaking is typically adjusted and assessed only at the beginning of each day of use with a single radionuclide, commonly using the Tc-99m or Co-57 source that is used for uniformity assessment. If other radionuclides are imaged during the day, preset energy windows for these radionuclides are used

■**FIGURE 18-17** Displays of a pulse-height spectrum used for "peaking" the scintillation camera (centering the pulse height analyzer window on the photopeak). The radionuclide is Tc-99m. The energy window is shown by the two vertical lines around the photopeak. **A.** A properly adjusted 20% window. **B.** An improperly adjusted 20% window. **C.** A properly adjusted 15% window.

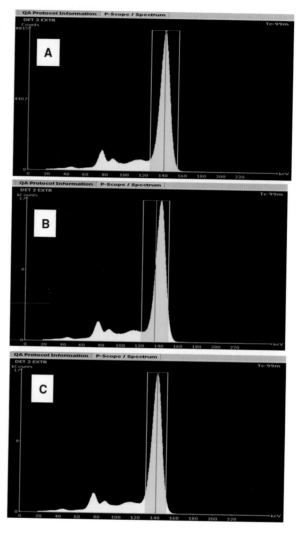

without adjusting them for the actual energy spectra. Adjustment of the energy discrimination windows for the photopeaks of other radionuclides (e.g., In-111, I-123, I-131, Xe-133, and Tl-201) that might be imaged is performed infrequently, such as after major calibrations of the camera. A nearly scatter-free source should be used to assess or adjust the energy windows; using the radiation emitted by a patient to assess or adjust the energy windows would constitute poor practice because of its large scatter component.

The uniformity of the camera should be assessed daily and after each repair. The assessment may be made intrinsically by using a Tc-99m point source, or the system uniformity may be evaluated by using a Co-57 planar source or a fillable flood source. Uniformity images must contain sufficient counts so that quantum mottle does not mask clinically significant uniformity defects. The number of counts needed increases with the useful area of the camera. As many as 5 to 15 million counts should be obtained for the daily test of a modern large area, rectangular head camera. Uniformity images can be evaluated visually or can be analyzed by a computer program, avoiding the subjectivity of visual evaluation. The uniformity test will reveal most malfunctions of a gamma camera. Figure 18-18 shows uniformity images from a modern scintillation camera. Multi-hole collimators are easily damaged by careless

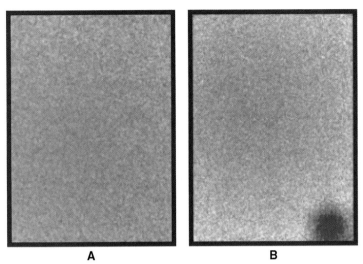

A   **B**

■ **FIGURE 18-18** Uniformity images. **A.** Image from a modern high-performance camera with digital spatial linearity and energy signal correction circuitry. **B.** The other head of the same camera, with an optically decoupled photomultiplier tube. (Courtesy Carol Moll, CNMT.)

handling, such as by striking them with an imaging table or dropping heavy objects on them. Technologists should inspect the collimators on each camera daily and whenever changing collimators. Old damage should be marked. The uniformity of each collimator should be evaluated periodically, by using a Co-57 planar source or a fillable flood source and whenever damage is suspected. The frequency of this testing depends on the care taken by the technologists to avoid damaging the collimators and their reliability in visually inspecting the collimators and reporting new damage.

The spatial resolution and spatial linearity of an Anger camera are typically assessed at least weekly. (As stated earlier, this assessment is not applicable to a multielement camera.) If a four-quadrant bar phantom (Fig. 18-8) is used, it should be imaged four times with a 90° rotation between images to ensure all quadrants of the camera are evaluated. If a parallel-line phantom is used, it should be imaged twice with a 90° rotation between images.

The efficiency of each camera head should be measured periodically. It can be monitored during uniformity tests by always performing the test with the source at the same distance, determining the activity of the source, recording the number of counts and counting time, and calculating the count rate per unit activity.

Each camera should also have a complete evaluation at least annually, which includes not only the items listed above but also multienergy spatial registration (Anger cameras only), energy resolution, and count-rate performance. Table 19-1 in Chapter 19 contains a recommended schedule for quality control testing of gamma cameras. Relevant tests should also be performed after each repair or adjustment of a camera.

New cameras should receive acceptance testing by an experienced medical physicist to determine if the camera's performance meets the purchase specifications and to establish baseline values for routine quality control testing.

18.1.7 Computers, Whole Body Scanning, and SPECT

All gamma cameras are now connected to digital computers. The computer is used for the acquisition, processing, and display of digital images and for control of the movement of the camera heads. Computers used with gamma cameras are discussed later in this chapter.

Many large-FOV gamma cameras can perform whole-body scanning. Some older systems move the camera past a stationary patient, but most now move the patient table past a stationary camera. Moving camera systems require less floor space. In either case, the system must sense the position of the camera relative to the patient table and must add values that specify the position of the camera relative to the table to the X- and Y-position signals. Older systems with round or hexagonal crystals usually had to make two passes over each side of the patient. Modern large-area rectangular head cameras can scan each side of all but extremely obese patients with a single pass, saving considerable time and producing superior image statistics.

Many modern computer-equipped gamma cameras have heads that can rotate automatically around the patient and acquire images from different views. The computer mathematically manipulates these images to produce cross-sectional images of the activity distribution in the patient. This is called SPECT and is discussed in detail in Chapter 19.

18.1.8 Obtaining High-Quality Images

Attention must be paid to many technical factors to obtain high-quality images. Imaging procedures should be optimized for each type of study. Sufficient counts must be acquired so that quantum mottle in the image does not mask lesions. Imaging times must be as long as possible consistent with patient throughput and lack of patient motion. The camera or table scan speed should be sufficiently slow during whole-body scans to obtain adequate image statistics. The use of a higher resolution collimator may improve spatial resolution, and the use of a narrower energy window to reduce scatter may improve image contrast.

Because the spatial resolution of a gamma camera is degraded significantly as the collimator-to-patient distance is increased, the camera heads should always be as close to the patient as possible. In particular, thick pillows and mattresses on imaging tables should be discouraged when images are acquired with the camera head below the table.

Significant non-uniformities can be caused by careless treatment of the collimators. Collimators are easily damaged by collisions with imaging tables or by placing them on top of other objects when they are removed from the camera.

Patient motion and metal objects worn by patients or in the patients' clothing are common sources of artifacts. Efforts should be made to identify metal objects and to remove them from the patient or from the FOV. The technologist should remain in the room during imaging to minimize patient motion. Furthermore, for safety, a patient should never be left unattended under a moving camera, either in whole-body or in SPECT mode.

18.2 COMPUTERS IN NUCLEAR IMAGING

Most nuclear medicine computer systems consist of commercially available computers with additional components to enable them to acquire, process, and display images from a gamma camera. A manufacturer may incorporate a computer for image acquisition and camera control in the camera itself and provide a separate computer for image processing and display, or provide a single computer for both purposes.

Modern gamma cameras create the pairs of *X*- and *Y*-position signals using digital circuitry and transfer them to the computer in digital form. The formation of a digital image is described in the following section.

18.2.1 Digital Image Formats in Gamma Camera Imaging

As discussed in Chapter 5, a digital image consists of a rectangular array of numbers, and an element of the image represented by a single number is called a pixel. In nuclear medicine, each pixel represents the number of counts detected from activity in a specific location within the patient. Common image formats are 64^2 and 128^2 pixels, reflecting the low spatial resolution of scintillation cameras. Whole-body images are stored in larger formats, such as 256 by 1,024 pixels. If one byte (8 bits) is used for each pixel, the image is said to be in *byte mode*; if two bytes are used for each pixel, the image is said to be in *word mode*. A single pixel can store as many as 255 counts in byte mode and 65,535 counts in word mode. Modern nuclear medicine computers may allow only word-mode images.

18.2.2 Image Acquisition

Frame-Mode Acquisition

Image data in nuclear medicine are acquired in either frame or list mode. Figure 18-19 illustrates frame-mode acquisition. Before acquisition begins, a portion of the computer's memory is designated to contain the image. All pixels within this image are

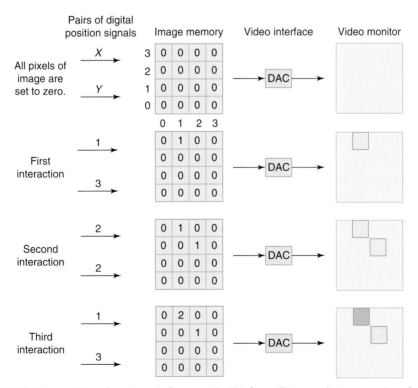

■ **FIGURE 18-19** Acquisition of an image in frame mode. This figure illustrates the incorporation of position data from the first three interactions into an image. This example shows a 4 by 4 pixel image for the purpose of illustration. Actual nuclear medicine projection images are typically acquired in formats of 64 × 64 or 128 × 128 pixels.

set to zero. After acquisition begins, pairs of X- and Y-position signals are received from the camera, each pair corresponding to the detection of a single x- or γ-ray. Each pair of numbers designates a single pixel in the image. One count is added to the counts in that pixel. As many pairs of position signals are received, the image is formed.

There are three types of frame-mode acquisition: *static*, *dynamic*, and *gated*. In a static acquisition, a single image is acquired for either a preset time interval or until the total number of counts in the image reaches a preset number. In a dynamic acquisition, a series of images is acquired one after another, for a preset time per image. Dynamic image acquisition is used to study dynamic processes, such as the first transit of a bolus of a radiopharmaceutical through the heart or the extraction and excretion of a radiopharmaceutical by the kidneys.

Some dynamic processes occur too rapidly for them to be effectively portrayed by dynamic image acquisition; each image in the sequence would have too few counts to be statistically valid. However, if the dynamic process is repetitive, such as the cardiac cycle, gated image acquisition may permit the acquisition of an image sequence that accurately depicts the dynamic process. Gated acquisition is most commonly used for evaluating cardiac mechanical performance in cardiac blood pool studies and, sometimes, in myocardial perfusion studies. Gated acquisition requires a physiologic monitor that provides a trigger pulse to the computer at the beginning of each cycle of the process being studied. In gated cardiac studies, an electrocardiogram (ECG) monitor provides a trigger pulse to the computer whenever the monitor detects a QRS complex.

Figure 18-20 depicts the acquisition of a gated cardiac image sequence. First, space for the desired number of images (usually 16 to 24 for gated cardiac blood pool imaging) is reserved in the computer's memory. Next, several cardiac cycles are timed and the average time per cycle is determined. The time per cycle is divided by the number of images in the sequence to obtain the time T per image. Then the acquisition begins. When the first trigger pulse is received, the acquisition interface sends the data to the first image in the sequence for a time T. Then it is stored in the second image in the sequence for a time T, after which it is stored in the third image for a time T. This process proceeds until the next trigger pulse is received. Then the process begins anew, with the data being added to that in the first image for a time T, then the second image for a time T, etc. This process is continued until a preset time

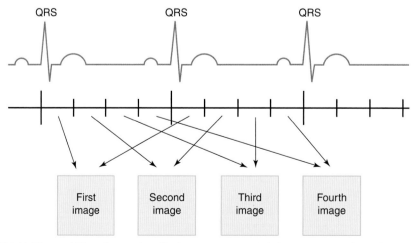

■ **FIGURE 18-20** Acquisition of a gated cardiac image sequence. Only four images are shown here. Sixteen to twenty-four images are typically acquired.

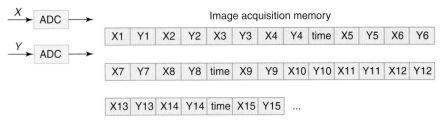

■ **FIGURE 18-21** Acquisition of image data in list mode. The digital *X*- and *Y*-position signals are stored as a list. Periodically, a timing signal is also stored. The image or images cannot be viewed until the list-mode data are formed into an image matrix or matrices.

interval, typically 10 min, has elapsed, enabling sufficient counts to be collected for the image sequence to form a statistically valid depiction of an average cardiac cycle.

List-Mode Acquisition

In *list-mode acquisition*, the pairs of *X*- and *Y*-position values are stored in a list (Fig. 18-21), instead of being immediately formed into an image. Periodic timing marks are included in the list. If a physiologic monitor is being used, as in gated cardiac imaging, trigger marks are also included in the list. After acquisition is complete, the list-mode data are reformatted into conventional images for display. The advantage of list-mode acquisition is that it allows great flexibility in how the *X* and *Y* values are combined to form images. The disadvantages of list-mode acquisition are that it generates large amounts of data, requiring more memory to acquire and disk space to store than frame-mode images, and that the data must be subsequently processed into standard images for viewing.

18.2.3 Image Processing in Nuclear Medicine

A major reason for the use of computers in nuclear medicine is that they provide the ability to present the data in the unprocessed images in ways that are of greater use to the clinician. Although it is not within the scope of this section to provide a comprehensive survey of image processing in nuclear medicine, the following are common examples.

Image Subtraction

When one image is subtracted from another, each pixel count in one image is subtracted from the corresponding pixel count in the other. Negative numbers resulting from these subtractions are set to zero. The resultant image depicts the change in activity that occurs in the patient during the time interval between the acquisitions of the two images.

Regions of Interest and Time-Activity Curves

A *region of interest* (ROI) is a closed boundary that is superimposed on an image. It may be drawn manually or it may be drawn automatically by the computer. The sum of the counts in all pixels in the ROI is an indication of the activity in the corresponding portion of the patient.

To create a *time-activity curve* (TAC) for a dynamic study, a ROI must first be drawn on one image of the dynamic image sequence. The same ROI is then superimposed on each image in the sequence by the computer and the total number of counts within the ROI is determined for each image. Finally, the counts within the ROI are plotted as a function of image number. The resultant curve is an indication of the activity in the corresponding portion of the patient as a function of time. Figure 18-22

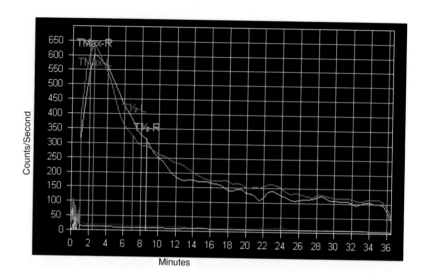

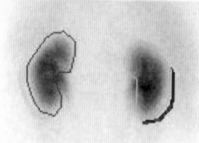

■ **FIGURE 18-22** Renal Tc-99m MAG-3 regions of interest (bottom) and time-activity curves (top).

shows ROIs over both kidneys of a patient and TACs describing the uptake and excretion of the radiopharmaceutical Tc-99m MAG-3 by the kidneys.

Spatial Filtering

Nuclear medicine images have a grainy appearance because of the statistical nature of the acquisition process. This quantum mottle can be reduced by a type of spatial filtering called *smoothing*. Unfortunately, smoothing also reduces the spatial resolution of the image. Images should not be smoothed to the extent that clinically significant detail is lost. Smoothing is a type of convolution filtering, which is described in detail in Chapter 4 and Appendix G.

Left Ventricular Ejection Fraction

The left ventricular ejection fraction (LVEF) is a measure of the mechanical performance of the left ventricle (LV) of the heart. It is defined as the fraction of the end-diastolic volume ejected during a cardiac cycle:

$$LVEF = (V_{ED} - V_{ES})/V_{ED},$$ [18-11]

where V_{ED} is the end-diastolic (ED) volume and V_{ES} is the end-systolic (ES) volume of the ventricle. In nuclear medicine, it can be determined from an equilibrium-gated blood pool image sequence, using Tc-99m–labeled red blood cells. The image sequence is acquired from a left anterior oblique (LAO) projection, with the camera positioned at the angle demonstrating the best separation of the two ventricles, after sufficient time has elapsed for the administered activity to reach a uniform concentration in the blood.

The calculation of the LVEF is based on the assumption that the counts from left ventricular activity are approximately proportional to the ventricular volume throughout the cardiac cycle. An ROI is first drawn around the left ventricular cavity, and a TAC is obtained by superimposing this ROI over all images in the sequence. The first image in the sequence depicts end diastole, and the image containing the least counts in the ROI depicts end systole. The total left ventricular counts in the ED and ES images are determined. Some programs use the same ROI around the LV for both images, whereas, in other programs, the ROI is drawn separately in the ED and ES images or in each individual image to better fit the varying shape and size of the ventricle. (If ED and ES ROIs only are drawn, the final TAC is an interpolation of the two ROIs' ED-to-ES and then ES-to-ED TACs.) Unfortunately, each of these counts is due not only to activity in the left ventricular cavity but also to activity in surrounding tissues, chambers, and great vessels (including in front of and in back of the projection of the LV). To compensate for this "crosstalk" (commonly called "background activity"), another ROI is drawn just beyond the wall of the LV (typically at ES), avoiding active structures such as the spleen, cardiac chambers, and great vessels. The number of counts in the left ventricular ROI due to crosstalk is estimated as follows:

$$\text{Counts crosstalk} = \frac{(\text{Counts in crosstalk ROI})(\text{Pixels in LV ROI})}{(\text{Pixels in crosstalk ROI})}. \qquad [18\text{-}12]$$

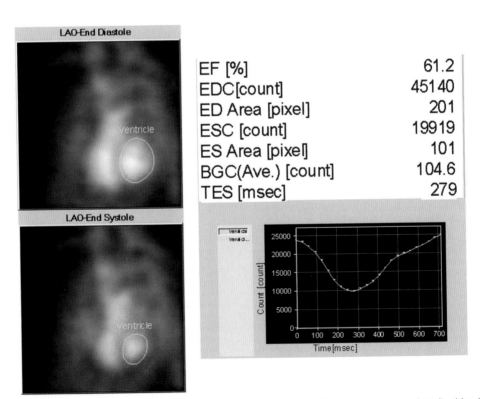

■ **FIGURE 18-23** End-diastolic (top left) and end-systolic (ES bottom left) images from a gated cardiac blood-pool study, showing ROIs used to determine the left ventricular ejection fraction (LVEF). The small red ROI below and to the right of the LV ROI in the ES image is used to determine and correct for the extracardiac ("background") counts. Calculated LVEF and volume curve are shown on the right.

Figure 18-23 shows ED and ES images of the heart from the LAO projection and the ROIs used to determine the LVEF. The LVEF is then calculated using the following equation:

$$LVEF = \frac{(Counts\ ED - Counts\ crosstalk\ ED) - (Counts\ ES - Counts\ crosstalk\ ES)}{(Counts\ ED - Counts\ crosstalk\ ED)}. \quad [18\text{-}13]$$

Other Quantitative Nuclear Medicine Imaging Studies

There exist a number of other quantitative planar nuclear medicine imaging studies that require computer post-processing. Examples are: (1) regional lung ventilation (Xe-133, Tc-99m DTPA aerosol or Tc-99m pertechnetate superheated gas)/Tc-99m MAA perfusion (V/Q) mismatch; (2) radioiodine or Tc-99m pertechnetate thyroid uptake; (3) gastric emptying (Tc-99m sulfur colloid solid, Tc-99m or In-111 DTPA liquid), including simultaneous dual-energy Tc-99m solid/In-111 liquid imaging; and (4) Tc-99m HIDA with CCK stimulation gallbladder ejection fraction.

18.3 SUMMARY

This chapter described the principles of operation of the gamma camera, which forms images depicting the distribution of x- and γ-ray–emitting radionuclides in patients, using either a planar crystal of the scintillator NaI(Tl) optically coupled to a two-dimensional array of PMTs (Anger scintillation camera) or a multielement (pixelated) camera, which uses either scintillation (NaI(Tl) or CsI(Tl)) or solid-state semiconductor (CZT) detector elements. The collimator, necessary for formation of projection images, imposes a compromise between spatial resolution and sensitivity in detecting x- and γ-rays. Because of the collimator, the spatial resolution of the images degrades with distance from the face of the camera. In Chapter 19, the use of the scintillation camera to perform computed tomography, called *SPECT*, is described.

SUGGESTED READINGS AND REFERENCES

Anger HO. Radioisotope cameras. In: Hine GJ, ed. *Instrumentation in Nuclear Medicine*, vol. 1. New York, NY: Academic Press; 1967:485-552.

Gelfand MJ, Thomas SR. *Effective Use of Computers in Nuclear Medicine.* New York, NY: McGraw-Hill; 1988.

Graham LS, Levin CS, Muehllehner G. Anger scintillation camera. In: Sandler MP, et al., eds. *Diagnostic Nuclear Medicine.* 4th ed. Baltimore, MD: Lippincott Williams & Wilkins; 2003:31-42.

Groch MW. Cardiac function: gated cardiac blood pool and first pass imaging. In: Henkin RE, et al., eds. *Nuclear Medicine*, vol. 1. St. Louis, MO: Mosby; 1996:626-643.

Simmons GH, ed. *The Scintillation Camera.* New York, NY: Society of Nuclear Medicine; 1988.

Yester MV, Graham LS, eds. *Advances in Nuclear Medicine: The Medical Physicist's Perspective.* Proceedings of the 1998 Nuclear Medicine Mini Summer School, American Association of Physicists in Medicine, June 21–23, 1998, Madison, WI.

CHAPTER 19

Nuclear Tomographic Imaging— Single Photon and Positron Emission Tomography (SPECT and PET)

The formation of projection images in nuclear medicine was discussed in the previous chapter. A nuclear medicine projection image depicts a two-dimensional projection of the three-dimensional activity distribution in the patient. The disadvantage of a projection image is that the contributions to the image from structures at different depths overlap, hindering the ability to discern the image of a structure at a particular depth. Tomographic imaging is fundamentally different—it attempts to depict the activity distribution in a single cross section of the patient.

There are two fundamentally different types of tomography: conventional tomography, also called geometric or focal plane tomography, and computed tomography. In conventional tomography, structures out of a focal plane are not removed from the resultant focal plane image; instead, they are blurred by an amount proportional to their distances from the focal plane. Those close to the focal plane suffer little blurring and remain apparent in the image. Even those farther away, although significantly blurred, contribute to the image, thereby reducing contrast and adding noise. In distinction, computed tomography uses mathematical methods to remove overlying structures completely. Computed tomography requires the acquisition of a set of projection images from at least a 180° arc about the patient. The projection image information is then mathematically processed by a computer to form images depicting cross sections of the patient. Just as in x-ray transmission imaging, both conventional and computed tomography are possible in nuclear medicine imaging. Both single photon emission computed tomography (SPECT) and positron emission tomography (PET) are forms of computed tomography.

19.1 FOCAL PLANE TOMOGRAPHY IN NUCLEAR MEDICINE

Focal plane tomography once had a significant role in nuclear medicine, but is seldom used today. The rectilinear scanner, when used with focused collimators, is an example of conventional tomography. A number of other devices have been developed to exploit conventional tomography in nuclear medicine. The Anger tomoscanner used two small scintillation cameras with converging collimators, one above and one below the patient table, to scan the patient in a raster pattern; a single scan produced multiple whole-body images, each showing structures at a different depth in the patient in focus. The seven-pinhole collimator was used with a conventional scintillation camera and computer to produce short-axis images of the heart, each showing structures at a different depth in focus. The rectilinear scanner and the Anger tomoscanner are no longer produced. The seven-pinhole collimator, which never enjoyed wide acceptance, has been almost entirely displaced by SPECT.

The gamma camera itself, when used for planar imaging with a parallel-hole collimator, produces a weak tomographic effect. The system's spatial resolution decreases with distance, causing structures farther from the camera to be more blurred than closer structures. Furthermore, attenuation of photons increases with depth in the patient, also enhancing the visibility of structures closer to the camera. This effect is perhaps most clearly evident in planar skeletal imaging of the body. In the anterior images, for example, the sternum and anterior portions of the ribs are clearly shown, whereas the spine and posterior ribs are barely evident.

19.2 SINGLE PHOTON EMISSION COMPUTED TOMOGRAPHY

19.2.1 Design and Principles of Operation

SPECT generates transverse images depicting the distribution of x- or γ-ray–emitting nuclides in patients. Standard planar projection images are acquired from an arc of 180° (most cardiac SPECT) or 360° (most non-cardiac SPECT) about the patient. Although these images could be obtained by any collimated imaging device, the vast majority of SPECT systems use one or more camera heads that revolve around the patient. The SPECT system's digital computer then reconstructs the transverse images using either filtered backprojection or an iterative reconstruction method, which are described later in this chapter, as does the computer in an x-ray CT system. Figure 19-1 shows a variety of SPECT systems.

SPECT was invented by David Kuhl and others in the early 1960s, about 10 years before the invention of x-ray CT by Hounsfield (Kuhl and Edwards, 1963). However, in contrast to x-ray CT, most features of interest in SPECT images were also visible in planar nuclear medicine images and SPECT did not come into routine clinical use until the late 1980s.

Image Acquisition

The camera head or heads of a SPECT system revolve around the patient, acquiring projection images. The head or heads may acquire the images while moving

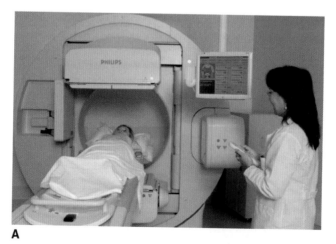

A

■ **FIGURE 19-1 A.** SPECT/CT system with two scintillation camera heads in a fixed 180° orientation and a non-diagnostic x-ray CT system for attenuation correction and anatomic correlation. The x-ray source is on the right side of the gantry and a flat-panel x-ray image receptor is on the left. (Photo credit: Emi Manning, UC Davis Health System.)

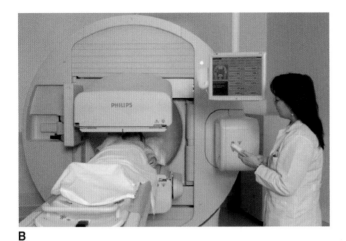

B

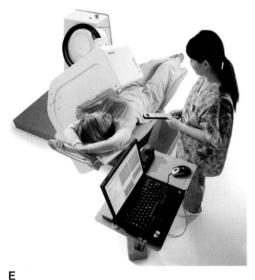

C

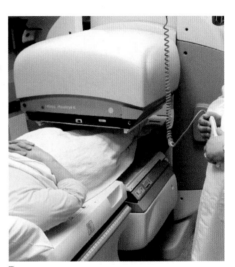

D

E

F

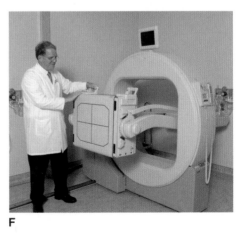

■ **FIGURE 19-1** *(Continued)* **B.** Technologist moving the upper camera head closer to the patient for SPECT imaging. (Photo credit: Emi Manning, UC Davis Health System.) Dual head, variable angle SPECT/CT camera with heads in the 90° orientation **(C)** for cardiac SPECT and in the 180° orientation **(D)** for other SPECT or whole-body planar imaging. **E.** Dual head, fixed 90° SPECT camera for cardiac imaging. (© Siemens Healthineers 2019. Used with permission.) **F.** Single head SPECT camera, with head in a position for planar imaging. (Courtesy Emi Manning, UC Davis Health System.)

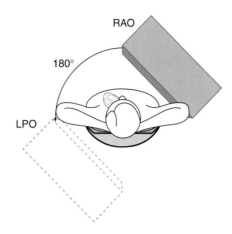

■ **FIGURE 19-2** 180° cardiac orbit.

(continuous acquisition) or may stop at predefined evenly spaced angles to acquire the images ("step and shoot" acquisition). If the camera heads of a SPECT system produced ideal projection images (*i.e.*, no attenuation by the patient and no degradation of spatial resolution with distance from the camera), projection images from opposite sides of the patient would be mirror images, and projection images over a 180° arc would be sufficient for transverse image reconstruction. However, in SPECT, attenuation greatly reduces the number of photons from activity in the half of the patient opposite the camera head, and this information is greatly blurred by the distance from the collimator. Therefore, for most non-cardiac studies, such as bone SPECT, the projection images are acquired over a complete revolution (360°) about the patient. However, most nuclear medicine laboratories acquire cardiac SPECT studies, such as myocardial perfusion studies, over a 180° arc symmetric about the heart, typically from the 45° right anterior oblique view to the 45° left posterior oblique view (Fig. 19-2). The 180° acquisition produces reconstructed images of superior contrast and resolution because the projection images of the heart from the opposite 180° have poor spatial resolution and contrast due to greater distance and attenuation. Although studies have shown that the 180° acquisition can introduce artifacts (Liu et al., 2002), the 180° acquisition is more commonly used than the 360° acquisition for cardiac studies.

SPECT projection images are usually acquired in either a 64^2 or a 128^2 pixel format. Using too small a pixel format reduces the spatial resolution of the projection images and of the resultant reconstructed transverse images, due to too large physical pixel dimensions. (A zoom factor of ~1.5 is often employed for 64^2 cardiac SPECT, to reduce the pixel dimensions, thereby improving spatial resolution.) When the 64^2 format is used, typically 60 or 64 projection images are acquired and, when a 128^2 format is chosen, 120 or 128 projection images are acquired. Using too few projections creates radial streak artifacts in the reconstructed transverse images.

The camera heads on older SPECT systems followed circular orbits around the patient while acquiring images. Circular orbits are satisfactory for SPECT imaging of the brain, but cause a loss of spatial resolution in body imaging because the circular orbit causes the camera head to be many centimeters away from the surface of the body during the anterior and perhaps the posterior portions of its orbit (Fig. 19-3). Modern SPECT systems provide non-circular orbits (also called "body contouring") that keep the camera heads in close proximity to the surface of the body throughout the orbit. For some systems, the technologist specifies the non-circular orbit by placing the camera head as close as possible to the patient at several angles, from which the camera's computer determines the orbit. Other systems perform automatic body

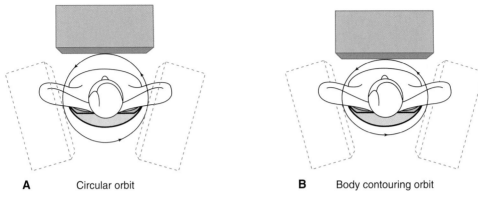

A   Circular orbit   **B**   Body contouring orbit

■ **FIGURE 19-3** Circular **(A)** and body-contouring **(B)** orbits.

contouring, using sensors on the camera heads to determine their proximity to the patient at each angle.

In brain SPECT, it is usually possible for the camera head to orbit with a much smaller radius than in body SPECT, thereby producing images of much higher spatial resolution. In many older cameras, a large distance from the physical edge of the camera head to the useful portion of the detector often made it impossible to orbit at a radius within the patient's shoulders while including the base of the brain in the images. These older systems were therefore forced to image the brain with an orbit outside the patient's shoulders, causing a significant loss of resolution. Most modern SPECT systems permit brain imaging with orbits within the patient's shoulders, although a patient's head holder extending beyond the patient table is generally necessary.

Transverse Image Reconstruction

After the projection images are acquired, they are corrected for non-uniformities and for center-of-rotation (COR) misalignments. (These corrections are discussed below, "Quality Control in SPECT.") Following these corrections, transverse image reconstruction is performed using either filtered backprojection or iterative methods.

As described in Chapter 10, filtered backprojection consists of two steps. First, the projection images are mathematically filtered. Then, to form a particular transverse image (also known as a slice), simple backprojection is performed of the row of each projection image corresponding to that transverse image. For example, the fifth row of each projection image is backprojected to form the fifth transverse image. A SPECT study produces transverse images covering the entire field of view (FOV) of the camera in the axial direction from each revolution of the camera head or heads.

Mathematical theory specifies that the ideal filter kernel, when displayed in the spatial frequency domain, is the ramp filter (Fig. 19-4). (The spatial frequency domain is discussed in Appendix G, Convolution and Fourier Transforms.) However, the actual projection images contain considerable statistical noise, from the random nature of radioactive decay and photon interactions, due to the relatively small number of counts in each pixel. If the images were filtered using a ramp filter kernel and then backprojected, the resultant transverse images would contain an unacceptable amount of statistical noise.

In the spatial frequency domain, statistical noise predominates in the high-frequency portion. Furthermore, the spatial resolution characteristics of the gamma camera cause a reduction of higher spatial frequency information that increases with the distance of the structure being imaged from the camera. To smooth the projection images before backprojection, the ramp filter kernel is modified to "roll-off" at

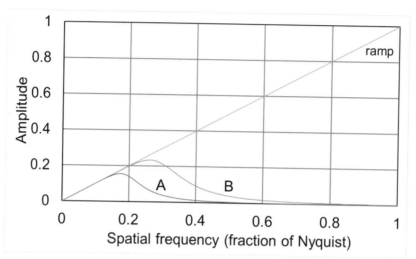

■ **FIGURE 19-4** Typical filter kernels used for filtered backprojection. The kernels are shown in frequency space. Filter Kernel A is a Butterworth filter of fifth order with a critical frequency of 0.20 Nyquist and Filter Kernel B is a Butterworth filter of fifth order with a critical frequency of 0.30 Nyquist. Filter Kernel A provides more smoothing than Filter Kernel B. A ramp filter, which provides no smoothing, is also shown.

higher spatial frequencies. Unfortunately, this reduces the spatial resolution of the projection images and thus of the reconstructed transverse images. A compromise must therefore be made between spatial resolution and the statistical noise of the transverse images.

Typically, a different filter kernel is selected for each type of SPECT study; for example, a different kernel would be used for Tc-99m HMPAO brain SPECT than would be used for Tc-99m sestamibi myocardial perfusion SPECT. The choice of filter kernel for a particular type of study is determined by the amount of statistical noise in the projection images (mainly determined by the injected activity, collimator, and acquisition time per image) and their spatial resolution (determined by the collimator and distances of the camera head(s) from the organ being imaged). The preference of the interpreting physician regarding the appearance of the images also plays a role. Projection images of better spatial resolution and less quantum mottle require a filter with a higher spatial frequency cutoff to avoid unnecessary loss of spatial resolution in the reconstructed transverse images, whereas projection images of poorer spatial resolution and greater quantum mottle require a filter with a lower spatial frequency cutoff to avoid excessive quantum mottle in the reconstructed transverse images. Although the SPECT camera's manufacturer may suggest filters for specific imaging procedures, the filters are usually empirically optimized in each nuclear medicine laboratory. Figure 19-5 shows a SPECT image created using three different filter kernels, illustrating too much smoothing, proper smoothing, and no smoothing.

Filtered backprojection is computationally efficient. However, it is based upon the assumption that the projection images are perfect projections of a three-dimensional object. As discussed in the previous chapter, this is far from true in gamma camera imaging, mainly because of attenuation of photons in the patient, the inclusion of Compton scattered photons in the image, and the degradation of spatial resolution with distance from the collimator.

In SPECT, iterative reconstruction methods are increasingly being used instead of filtered backprojection. In iterative methods, an initial activity (typically uniform) distribution in the patient is assumed. (Alternatively, an activity distribution created by simple backprojection could be used.) Then, projection images are calculated

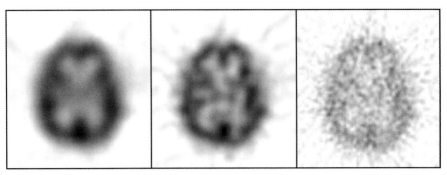

■ **FIGURE 19-5** SPECT images created by filtered backprojection. The projection images were filtered using the filter kernels shown in Figure 19-4. The image on the left, produced using Filter Kernel A, exhibits a significant loss of spatial resolution. The image in the center was produced using Filter Kernel B, which provides a proper amount of smoothing. The image on the right, produced using the ramp filter, shows good spatial resolution, but excessive statistical noise.

from the initial assumed activity distribution, using a model of the imaging characteristics of the gamma camera and the patient. The calculated projection images are compared with the actual projection images and, based upon this comparison, the assumed activity distribution is adjusted. This process is repeated several times, with successive adjustments to the assumed activity distribution, until the calculated projection images approximate the actual projection images (Fig. 19-6).

As was stated above, in each iteration, projection images are calculated from the assumed activity distribution. The calculation of projection images can incorporate the system resolution point spread function (PSF) of the gamma camera, which takes into account the decreasing spatial resolution with distance from the camera face. If a map of the attenuation characteristics of the patient is available, the calculation of the projection images can include the effects of attenuation. Furthermore, the PSF can be modified to incorporate the effect of photon scattering in the patient. Alternatively,

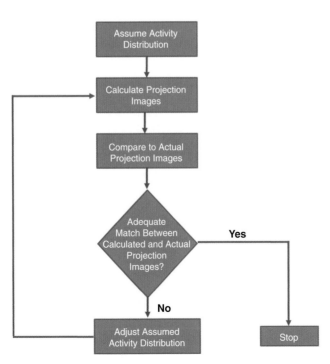

■ **FIGURE 19-6** Flowchart for iterative reconstruction. In some implementations, iterative reconstruction is performed for a specified number of iterations, instead of being terminated when a sufficiently good approximation is achieved.

modeling scatter within the photopeak based on either secondary energy window images (dual- or triple-energy-window method) or projection using the photopeak transverse images and attenuation and material density maps (effective scatter source estimation) is now more commonly applied. If all this is done, iterative methods will partially compensate for the effects of decreasing spatial resolution with distance, as well as attenuation and photon scattering in the patient. Iterative reconstruction can be used to produce higher quality tomographic images than filtered backprojection, or it can be used to produce images of similar quality to those produced by filtered backprojection, but with less administered activity or shorter acquisition times.

Iterative methods are computationally less efficient than filtered backprojection. However, the increasing speed of computers, the small image matrix sizes used in nuclear imaging, and the development of computationally efficient algorithms, such as the ordered-subset expectation maximization method (Hudson and Larkin, 1994), have made iterative reconstruction feasible for SPECT. Since iteratively reconstructed SPECT transverse images will contain substantial noise due to relatively poor counting statistics, three-dimensional spatial filtering is commonly applied after reconstruction for noise reduction.

Attenuation Correction in SPECT

Radioactivity whose x- or γ-rays must traverse long paths through the patient produces fewer counts, due to attenuation, than does activity closer to the surface of the patient adjacent to the camera. For this reason, transverse slices of a phantom with a uniform activity distribution, such as a cylinder filled with a well-mixed solution of radionuclide, will show a gradual decrease in activity toward the center (Fig. 19-7, on the left). Attenuation effects are more severe in body SPECT than in brain SPECT.

Approximate methods are available for attenuation correction. One of the most common, the Chang method, presumes a constant attenuation coefficient throughout the patient (Chang, 1978). Approximate attenuation corrections can overcompensate or undercompensate for attenuation. If such a method is to be used, its proper functioning should be verified using phantoms before its use in clinical studies.

These methods are only appropriate for filtered backprojection reconstruction. Furthermore, attenuation is not uniform in the patient, particularly in the thorax, and these approximate methods cannot compensate for non-uniform attenuation.

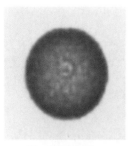 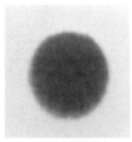 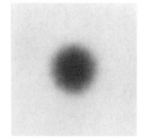

No Attenuation Correction	Attenuation Coefficient 0.12 cm⁻¹	Attenuation Coefficient 1 cm⁻¹

■ FIGURE 19-7 Attenuation correction. On the left is a reconstructed transverse image slice of a cylindrical phantom containing a well-mixed radionuclide solution. This image shows a decrease in activity toward the center due to attenuation. (A small ring artifact, unrelated to the attenuation, is also visible in the center of the image.) In the center is the same image corrected by the Chang method, using a linear attenuation coefficient of 0.12 cm^{-1}, demonstrating proper attenuation correction. On the right is the same image, corrected by the Chang method using an excessively large attenuation coefficient.

In the 1990s, several manufacturers provided SPECT cameras with sealed radioactive sources (commonly containing Gd-153, which emits 97 and 103-keV γ-rays) to measure the attenuation through the patient. The sources were used to acquire transmission data from projections around the patient. After acquisition, the transmission projection data were reconstructed to provide maps of tissue attenuation characteristics across transverse sections of the patient, similar to x-ray CT images. Finally, these attenuation maps were used during an iterative SPECT image reconstruction process to provide attenuation-corrected SPECT images.

The transmission sources were available in several configurations. These included scanning collimated line sources that were used with parallel-hole collimators, arrays of fixed line sources used with parallel-hole collimators, and a fixed line source located at the focal point of a fan-beam collimator.

The transmission data were usually acquired simultaneously with the acquisition of the emission projection data because performing the two separately can pose significant problems in the spatial alignment of the two data sets and greatly increases the total imaging time. The radionuclide used for the transmission measurements was chosen to have primary γ-ray emissions that differed significantly and were lower in energy from those of the radiopharmaceutical. Separate energy windows were used to differentiate the photons emitted by the transmission source from those emitted by the radiopharmaceutical. However, scattering of the higher energy emission photons in the patient and in the detector caused some cross-talk in the lower energy window.

Major manufacturers of nuclear medicine imaging systems now provide systems combining two camera heads capable of planar imaging and SPECT and an x-ray CT scanner, with a single patient bed. These systems have supplanted systems with radioactive transmission sources, and are referred to as SPECT/CT systems. In SPECT/CT systems, the x-ray CT attenuation image data can be used to correct the radionuclide emission data for attenuation by the patient. This is discussed in more detail later in this chapter.

Attenuation correction using radioactive transmission sources and x-ray CT-derived attenuation maps has been extensively studied in myocardial perfusion SPECT, where attenuation artifacts can mimic perfusion defects. These studies have shown that attenuation correction reduces attenuation artifacts and produces modest improvement in diagnostic performance when the studies are read by experienced clinicians (Hendel et al., 2002; Masood et al., 2005). However, other studies have shown that attenuation correction can cause artifacts, particularly when there is spatial misalignment of the emission data with respect to the attenuation maps determined from the transmission information. Furthermore, a period of transition is required, for even experienced clinicians to retrain themselves to interpret attenuation-corrected images. Therefore, it remains common for SPECT myocardial perfusion imaging to be performed without attenuation correction, although that may change with the increasing implementation of cardiac SPECT/CT.

Generation of Coronal, Sagittal, and Oblique Images

The pixels from the transverse slices may be reordered to produce coronal and sagittal slices. For cardiac imaging, it is desirable to produce oblique images oriented either parallel (vertical and horizontal long-axis images) or perpendicular (short-axis images) to the long axis of the left ventricle. Because there is considerable anatomic variation among patients regarding the orientation of the long axis of the left ventricle, the long axis of the heart must be determined before the computer can create the oblique images. This task is commonly performed manually by a technologist, although the software on most systems is now capable of correct automatic reorientation of myocardial perfusion images, with operator verification and override.

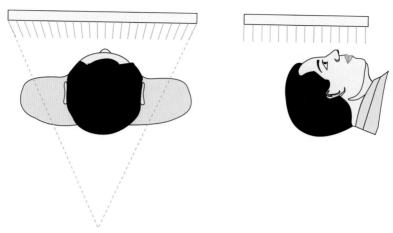

■ FIGURE 19-8 Fan-beam collimator.

Collimators for SPECT

Most SPECT is performed using parallel-hole collimators. However, specialized collimators have been developed for SPECT. The fan-beam collimator, shown in Figure 19-8, is a hybrid of the converging and parallel-hole collimator. Because it is a parallel-hole collimator in the y-direction, each row of pixels in a projection image corresponds to a single transaxial slice of the subject. In the x-direction, it is a converging collimator, with spatial resolution and efficiency characteristics superior to those of a parallel-hole collimator (see Fig. 18-12). Because a fan-beam collimator is a converging collimator in the cross-axial direction, its FOV decreases with distance from the collimator. For this reason, the fan-beam collimator is mainly used for brain SPECT; if the collimator is used for body SPECT, portions of the body are excluded from the FOV, which can cause artifacts, called "truncation artifacts," in the reconstructed images. One manufacturer offers a variable-focal-length converging collimator for cardiac imaging, where the focal length increases from the center outward, ending up as a parallel-hole collimator at the edge (to eliminate truncation artifacts), in both the transaxial and axial directions. Along with a heart-centric camera head orbit, an approximate factor of four improvement in sensitivity in the region of the heart is achieved (Fig. 19-9).

Multihead SPECT Cameras

To reduce the limitations imposed on SPECT by collimation and limited time per view, camera manufacturers provide SPECT systems with two camera heads that revolve around the patient (Fig. 19-1) and, in the past, SPECT systems with three heads were commercially available from at least two manufacturers. The use of multiple camera heads permits the use of higher resolution collimators, for a given level of quantum mottle in the tomographic images, than would a single head system. However, the use of multiple camera heads poses considerable technical challenges for the manufacturer. It places severe requirements upon the electrical and mechanical stability of the camera heads. In particular, the X and Y offsets and X and Y magnification factors of all the heads must be precisely matched throughout the rotation about the patient. Today's multihead systems are very stable and provide high-quality tomographic images for a variety of clinical applications.

Multihead gamma cameras are available in several configurations. Double-head cameras with opposed heads (180° head configuration) are good for head and body SPECT and whole-body planar scans (Fig. 19-1A and B). Triple-head, fixed-angle cameras are good for head and body SPECT, but less suitable for whole-body planar scans because

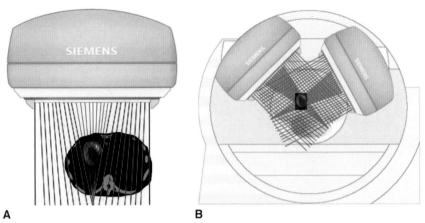

A   **B**

■ **FIGURE 19-9 A.** Illustration of Siemens Healthineers' IQ•SPECT SMARTZOOM collimator. The focal length increases from the center outward in both the radial and axial directions. **B.** Illustration of IQ•SPECT cardiocentric orbit acquisition. (Adapted with permission from Siemens Healthineers.)

of the limited width of the crystals. Double-head, variable-angle cameras are highly versatile, capable of head and body SPECT and whole-body planar scans with the heads in the 180° configuration and cardiac SPECT in the 90° configuration (Fig. 19-1C and D). (The useful portion of the crystal does not extend all the way to the edge of a camera head. If the two camera heads are placed at an angle of exactly 90° to each other, both heads cannot be close to the patient without parts of the patient being outside of the FOVs. For this reason, one manufacturer provides the option of SPECT acquisitions with the heads at a 76° angle to each other, as well as zoom from the corner where the two heads meet instead of in the center of the two detectors' FOVs.)

Multielement Detector SPECT Cameras

SPECT systems that employ a multitude of small or curved detectors and alternative scanning techniques, as opposed to conventional rotating gantry SPECT scanners with two or three large FOV detectors, are now commercially available. Spectrum Dynamics Medical's Veriton is a general-purpose (energy range 40–220 keV) scanner that has twelve detectors equally spaced over 360° around the patient. Each detector consists of a 6-mm-thick rectangular CZT crystal with 16 (transaxial dimension) × 128 (axial dimension), 2.46 mm × 2.46 mm detector elements, and an integrated parallel-hole tungsten collimator. Scanning of each (31.5 cm axial) SPECT FOV is achieved by a combination of detector swivel, rotation, and auto-contouring, with an increase in volume sensitivity on the order of 3 times compared to a conventional large FOV, dual-detector rotating gantry SPECT with LEHR collimation (Fig. 19-10). A scanner dedicated to cardiac SPECT, the NM530c from GE Healthcare, contains nine 8 cm × 8 cm and 5-mm-thick CZT crystals with 2.46 mm × 2.46 mm elements, equally spaced along a stationary L-shaped gantry. Strategic orientation of each detector and pinhole collimation allows all views to be acquired simultaneously without detector motion, resulting in an approximate fivefold increase in counting efficiency compared to conventional NaI(Tl)-LEHR (Fig. 19-11A and B). Spectrum Dynamics Medical also developed a dedicated cardiac CZT SPECT scanner (D-SPECT) Cardio, with nine 4 cm × 16 cm and 6 mm thick crystals, with 2.46 mm × 2.46 mm elements and parallel-hole tungsten collimation, in an L-shaped gantry, where scanning of the heart is achieved by translation and swivel of each detector, resulting in an approximate eightfold increase in sensitivity (Fig. 19-11C and D). A

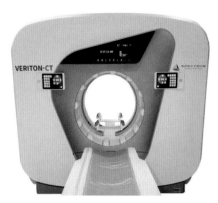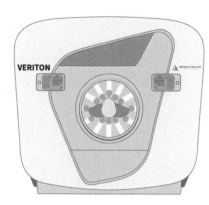

■ **FIGURE 19-10** Veriton-CT multiple detector SPECT/CT system. View into the gantry from the SPECT side, showing the twelve CZT detector modules equally spaced over 360° retracted (left). Illustration of body contoured acquisition (right). (With permission from Spectrum Dynamics Medical.)

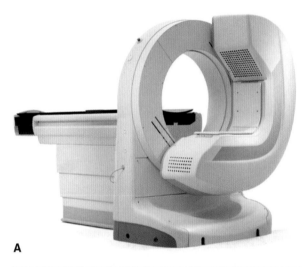

A

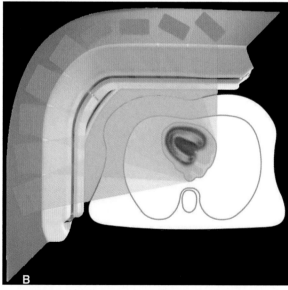

B

■ **FIGURE 19-11** Dedicated multiple CZT detector cardiac SPECT scanners. **A.** Discovery NM530c. **B.** Illustration of Discovery NM530c myocardial perfusion imaging (MPI) SPECT acquisition. (**A** and **B**, used with permission of GE Healthcare.) **C.** D-SPECT Cardio. **D.** Illustration of D-SPECT Cardio MPI SPECT acquisition (**C** and **D**, with permission from Spectrum Dynamics Medical.)

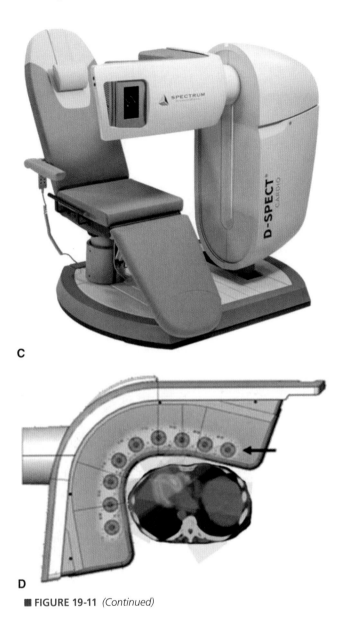

C

D

■ **FIGURE 19-11** *(Continued)*

third, NaI(Tl)-based dedicated cardiac SPECT scanner is CardiArc Inc.'s CardiArc, which employs three adjacent curved crystals and an array of PMTs. "Slit-hole" scanning is performed, whereby one series of lead sheets with horizontal gaps remains stationary while a curved lead sheet with six vertical slits rotates back and forth in electronic synchrony with six corresponding regions of the crystals, resulting in a sensitivity gain of about four.

19.2.2 Performance

Spatial Resolution

The spatial resolution of a SPECT system can be measured by acquiring a SPECT study of a line source, such as a capillary tube filled with a solution of Tc-99m, placed parallel to the axis of rotation (AOR). The National Electrical Manufacturers

Association (NEMA) has a protocol for measuring spatial resolution in SPECT. This protocol specifies a cylindrical plastic water-filled phantom, 22 cm in diameter, containing three line sources (Fig. 19-12, on the left) for measuring spatial resolution. The full widths at half maximum (FWHMs) of the line sources are measured from the reconstructed transverse images, as shown on the right in Figure 19-12. A ramp filter is used in the filtered backprojection so that the filtering does not reduce the spatial resolution. The NEMA spatial resolution measurements are primarily determined by the collimator used. The tangential resolution for the peripheral sources (typically 7 to 8 mm FWHM for low-energy high-resolution parallel-hole collimators) is superior to both the central resolution (typically 9.5 to 12 mm) and the radial resolution for the peripheral sources (typically 9.4 to 12 mm).

These FWHMs measured using the NEMA protocol, while providing a useful index of ultimate system performance, are not necessarily representative of clinical performance, because these spatial resolution studies can be acquired using longer imaging times and closer orbits than would be possible in a patient. Patient studies may require the use of lower resolution (higher efficiency) collimators than the one used in the NEMA measurement to obtain adequate image statistics. In addition, the filters used before backprojection for clinical studies cause more blurring than do the ramp filters used in NEMA spatial resolution measurements. The NEMA spatial resolution measurements fail to show the advantage of SPECT systems with two or three camera heads; double and triple head cameras will permit the use of higher resolution collimators for clinical studies than will single head cameras. Finally, the NEMA protocol is not applicable to, nor does it reflect, spatial resolution for iterative reconstruction SPECT, in particular, with system resolution, attenuation, and scatter compensations applied.

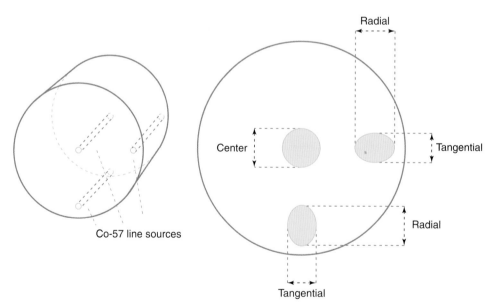

■ **FIGURE 19-12** NEMA phantom for evaluating the spatial resolution of a SPECT camera (left). The phantom is a 22-cm-diameter plastic cylinder, filled with water and containing three Co-57 line sources. One line source lies along the central axis and the other two are parallel to the central line source, 7.5 cm away. A SPECT study is acquired with a camera radius of rotation (distance from collimator to AOR) of 15 cm. The spatial resolution is measured from reconstructed transverse images, as shown on the right. Horizontal and vertical profiles are taken through the line sources and the FWHMs of these LSFs are determined. The average central resolution (FWHM of the central LSF) and the average tangential and radial resolutions (determined from the FWHMs of the two peripheral sources as shown) are determined. (Adapted by permission of the National Electrical Manufacturers Association, Performance Measurements of Scintillation Cameras, 2001.)

Spatial resolution deteriorates as the radius of the camera orbit increases. For this reason, brain SPECT produces images of much higher spatial resolution than does body SPECT. For optimal spatial resolution, the SPECT camera heads should orbit the patient as closely as possible. Body-contouring orbits (see above, "Design and Operation") provide better resolution than do circular orbits.

Comparison of SPECT to Conventional Planar Gamma Camera Imaging

In theory, SPECT should produce spatial resolution similar to that of planar gamma camera imaging. In clinical imaging using filtered backprojection, its resolution is usually slightly worse. The camera head is usually closer to the patient in conventional planar imaging than in SPECT. The spatial filtering used in SPECT to reduce statistical noise also reduces spatial resolution. The short time per view of SPECT may mandate the use of a lower resolution collimator to obtain adequate numbers of counts. On the other hand, iterative reconstruction SPECT is capable of having better resolution than planar, especially when compensation for system resolution is applied.

In planar nuclear imaging, radioactivity in tissues in front of and behind an organ or tissue of interest causes a reduction in contrast. Furthermore, if the activity in these overlapping structures is not uniform, the pattern of this activity distribution is superimposed on the activity distribution in the organ or tissue of interest. As such, it is a source of structural noise that impedes the ability to discern the activity distribution in the organ or tissue of interest. The main advantage of SPECT over conventional planar nuclear imaging is improved contrast and reduced structural noise produced by eliminating counts from the activity in overlapping structures. SPECT using iterative reconstruction can also partially compensate for the effects of the scattering of photons in the patient and collimator effects such as the decreasing spatial resolution with distance from the camera and collimator septal penetration. When attenuation is measured using sealed radioactive transmission sources or an x-ray CT scanner, SPECT can partially compensate for the effects of photon attenuation in the patient.

19.2.3 Quality Control in SPECT

Even though a technical quality control program is important in planar nuclear imaging, it is critical to SPECT. Equipment malfunctions or maladjustments that would not noticeably affect planar images can markedly degrade the spatial resolution of SPECT images and produce significant artifacts, some of which may mimic pathology. Upon installation, a SPECT camera should be tested by a medical physicist. Following acceptance testing, a quality control program should be established to ensure that the system's SPECT performance remains comparable to its performance at acceptance.

X and *Y* Magnification Factors and Multienergy Spatial Registration

The *X* and *Y* magnification factors, often called *X* and *Y* gains, relate distances in the object being imaged, in the *x* and *y* directions, to the numbers of pixels between the corresponding points in the resultant image. The *X* magnification factor is determined from an image of two point sources placed against the camera's collimator a known distance apart along a line parallel to the *x*-axis:

$$X_{mag} = \frac{\text{actual distance between centers of points sources}}{\text{number of pixels between centers of point sources}}.$$

The *Y* magnification factor is determined similarly but with the sources parallel to the *y*-axis. The *X* and *Y* magnification factors should be equal. If they are not, the projection images will be distorted in shape, as will be coronal, sagittal, and oblique images. (The transverse images, however, will not be distorted.) Multielement gamma camera (discussed in the previous chapter) do not suffer from such magnification errors, as detector element and total detector dimensions are identical between detectors, and Anger logic is not used for event positioning.

The multienergy spatial registration, described in the previous chapter, is a measure of the camera's ability to maintain the same image magnification, regardless of the energy of the x- or γ-rays forming the image. The multienergy spatial registration is not only important in SPECT when imaging radionuclides such as Ga-67 and In-111, which emit useful photons of more than one energy, but also because uniformity and AOR corrections, to be discussed shortly, determined with one radionuclide will only be valid for others if the multienergy spatial registration is correct. (As discussed in the previous chapter, multienergy spatial registration is not applicable to multielement gamma cameras).

Alignment of Projection Images to the Axis of Rotation (COR Calibration)

The AOR is an imaginary reference line about which the head or heads of a SPECT camera revolve. If a radioactive line source were placed on the AOR, each projection image would depict it as a vertical straight line near the center of the image; this projection of the AOR into the image is called the COR. The location of the COR in each projection image must be known to correctly calculate the three-dimensional activity distribution from the projection images. Ideally, the COR is aligned with the center, in the *x*-direction, of each projection image. However, there may be misalignment of the COR with the centers of the projection images. This misalignment may be mechanical; for example, the camera head may not be exactly centered in the gantry. It can also be electronic or a digital setting. The misalignment may be the same amount in all projection images from a single camera head, or it may vary with the angle of the projection image or along the AOR. There are actually four other possible misalignments of a SPECT detector besides *x*-direction shift: axial tilt (discussed later in this chapter), detector-to-detector axial shift, yoke swivel, and axial swivel with respect to the AOR.

If a COR misalignment is not corrected, it causes a loss of spatial resolution in the resultant transverse images. If the misalignment is large, it can cause a point source to appear as a tiny "doughnut" (Fig. 19-13). (These "doughnut" artifacts are not seen in clinical images; they are visible only in reconstructed images of point or line sources. The "doughnut" artifacts caused by COR misalignment are not centered in the image and so can be distinguished from the ring artifacts caused by non-uniformities.) gamma cameras manufacturers provide software to assess and correct the effects of

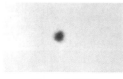
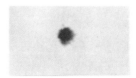
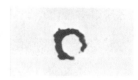

| Correct COR | 2 Pixel COR Error | 6 Pixel COR Error |

■ **FIGURE 19-13** Center-of-rotation (COR) misalignment in SPECT. Small misalignments cause blurring (center), whereas large misalignments cause point sources to appear as "tiny doughnut" artifacts (right). Such "tiny doughnut" artifacts would only be visible in phantom studies and are unlikely to be seen in clinical images.

COR misalignment. The COR alignment is assessed by placing a point source, several point sources, or a line source in the camera's FOV, acquiring a set of projection images, and analyzing these images using the SPECT system's computer. If a line source is used, it is placed parallel to the AOR.

The SPECT system's computer corrects the COR misalignment by shifting each clinical projection image in the x-direction by the proper number of pixels prior to filtered backprojection or iterative reconstruction. When a line source or multiple points along the AOR are used for calibration, a COR correction can be derived and applied separately for each transverse slice. If the COR misalignment varies with the camera head angle, instead of being constant for all projection images, it can only be corrected if the computer permits angle-by-angle corrections. Separate assessments of the COR correction must be made for different collimators and dual-head configurations (*e.g.*, 180° and 90°), and, on some systems, for different camera zoom factors and image formats (*e.g.*, 64^2 versus 128^2). The COR correction determined using one radionuclide will only be valid for other radionuclides if the multienergy spatial registration is correct.

Uniformity

The uniformity of the camera head or heads is important; non-uniformities that are not apparent in low count daily uniformity studies can cause significant artifacts in SPECT. The artifact caused by a non-uniformity appears in transverse images as a ring centered about the AOR (Fig. 19-14).

Multihead SPECT systems can produce partial ring artifacts when projection images are not acquired by all heads over a 360° arc. Clinically, ring artifacts are most apparent in high-count density studies, such as liver scans. However, ring artifacts may be most harmful in studies such as myocardial perfusion in which, due to poor counting statistics and large variations in count density, they may not be recognized and thus lead to misinterpretation.

The causes of non-uniformities were discussed in the previous chapter. As mentioned in that chapter, modern gamma cameras have digital circuits using lookup tables to correct the X and Y position signals from each interaction for systematic position-specific errors in event location assignment and the Z (energy) signal for systematic position-specific variations in scintillator light collection or CZT charge

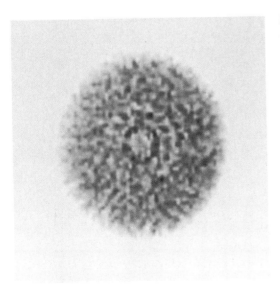

■ **FIGURE 19-14** Image of a cylinder filled with a uniform radionuclide solution, showing a ring artifact due to a non-uniformity. The artifact is the dark ring toward the center.

generation efficiency. However, these correction circuits cannot correct non-uniformity due to local variations in detection efficiency, such as dents or manufacturing defects in the collimators.

If not too severe, non-uniformities of this latter type can be largely corrected. A very high-count uniformity image is acquired. The ratio of the average pixel count to the count in a specific pixel in this image serves as a correction factor for that pixel. Following the acquisition of a projection image during a SPECT study, each pixel of the projection image is multiplied by the appropriate correction factor before COR correction and filtered backprojection or iterative reconstruction. For the high-count uniformity image, at least 30 million counts should be collected for 64^2 pixel images and 120 million counts for a 128^2 pixel format. These high-count uniformity images are typically acquired weekly to monthly. Correction images must be acquired for each camera head and collimator. For cameras from some manufacturers, separate intrinsic correction images must be acquired for each radionuclide. The effectiveness of a camera's correction circuitry and use of high-count flood correction images can be tested by acquiring a SPECT study of a large plastic cylindrical container or a SPECT performance phantom filled with a well-mixed solution of Tc-99m and examining the transverse images for ring artifacts. However, this testing will not assess parts of the collimator or camera face outside the projected image of the container or phantom.

Camera Head Tilt

The camera head or heads must be aligned with the AOR; for most types of collimators, this requires that faces of the heads be exactly parallel to the AOR. If they are not, a loss of spatial resolution and contrast will result from out-of-slice activity being backprojected into each transverse image slice, as shown in Figure 19-15. The loss of resolution and contrast in each transverse image slice will be less toward the center of the slice and greatest toward the edges of the image. If the AOR of the camera is aligned to be level when the camera is installed and there is a flat surface on the camera head that is parallel to the collimator face, a bubble level may be used to test for head tilt. Some SPECT cameras require the head tilt to be manually adjusted for each acquisition, whereas other systems set it automatically. The accuracy of the automatic systems should be periodically tested. A more reliable method than the bubble level is to place a point source in the camera FOV, centered in the axial (y) direction, but

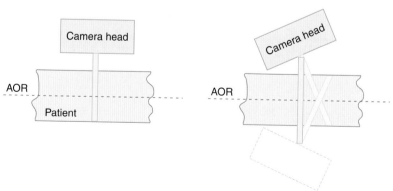

■ **FIGURE 19-15** Head-tilt. The camera head on the left is parallel to the AOR, causing the counts collected in a pixel of the projection image to be backprojected into the corresponding transverse image slice of the patient. The camera head on the right is tilted, causing counts from activity outside of a transverse slice (*along the grey diagonal lines of response*) to be backprojected into the transverse image slice (*orange colored vertical slice*).

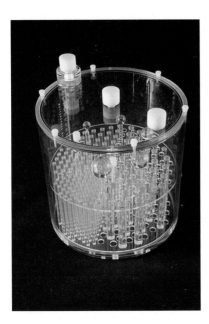

■ **FIGURE 19-16** Flangeless deluxe Jaszczak phantom for testing SPECT systems, a product of Data Spectrum Corporation. (Courtesy of Data Spectrum Corporation.) A soluble radioactive material, typically labeled with Tc-99m, is introduced into the phantom and mixed in the water until it is uniformly distributed. The acrylic plastic spheres and rods are not radioactive and are "cold" objects in the radioactive solution.

near the edge of the field in the transverse (x) direction. A series of projection images is then acquired. If there is head tilt, the position of the point source will vary in the y-direction from image to image. Head tilt can be evaluated from viewing a cine of the projection images.

SPECT Quality Control Phantoms

There are commercially available phantoms (Fig. 19-16) that may be filled with a solution of Tc-99m or other radionuclide and used to evaluate system performance. These phantoms are very useful for the semiquantitative assessment of spatial resolution, image contrast, and uniformity, although the small sizes of most such phantoms allow uniformity to be assessed only over a relatively small portion of the camera's face. They are used for acceptance testing of new systems and periodic testing, typically quarterly, thereafter. Table 19-1 provides a suggested schedule for a SPECT quality control program.

19.2.4   Dual Modality Imaging—SPECT/X-ray CT Systems

Several manufacturers provide imaging systems incorporating two gamma camera heads capable of planar imaging and SPECT and an x-ray CT system with a single patient bed. Some of these systems have very simple x-ray CT systems that provide x-ray CT information for attenuation correction of the SPECT information and image co-registration only, whereas others can produce diagnostic quality CT images.

The advantages and disadvantages of using an x-ray CT system for attenuation correction and image co-registration are the same as in the case of the PET/CT systems described later in this chapter. The x-ray CT system acquires the attenuation information much more quickly than does a system using radioactive sealed sources and the attenuation information has less statistical noise, but the linear attenuation coefficients for the energies of the γ-rays must be estimated from the CT attenuation information. The methods for doing this are similar to those used in PET/CT, which are discussed later in this chapter. Artifacts can occur when the calculation produces the wrong attenuation coefficient. This can be caused by high atomic number material in the

TABLE 19-1 RECOMMENDED SCHEDULE FOR ROUTINE QUALITY CONTROL TESTING OF A PLANAR OR SPECT GAMMA CAMERA

TEST	FREQUENCY	NOTES
Set and check energy discrimination window(s)	Before first use daily	Point (intrinsic) or planar (extrinsic) source of radionuclide
Extrinsic or intrinsic low-count uniformity images of all camera heads	Before first use daily	5–10 million counts, depending upon effective area of camera head
Cine review of projection images and/or review of sinogram[a] (S)	After each clinical SPECT study	Check for patient motion
Visual inspection of collimators for damage	Daily and when changing collimators	If new damage found, acquire a new high-count uniformity calibration image
High count-density extrinsic or intrinsic uniformity images of all camera heads (S)	Monthly	30 million counts for 64^2 images and 120 million counts for 128^2
Spatial resolution check with bar pattern	Weekly	Cycle week-to-week between 0°, 90°, 180° and 270° orientation of bar pattern
Center of rotation (S)	Weekly to monthly	Point or line source(s), as recommended by manufacturer
Efficiency of each camera head	Quarterly, semiannually, or annually	
Reconstructed cylindrical phantom uniformity (S)	Annually	Cylindrical phantom filled with Tc-99m solution
Point source reconstructed spatial resolution (S)	Annually	Point source
Reconstructed SPECT phantom (S)	Quarterly	Using a phantom such as the one shown in Figure 19-16
Pixel size check	Annually	Two point sources
Head-tilt angle check (S)	Quarterly	Bubble level or point source
Extrinsic uniformity images of all collimators not tested above	Annually	Planar source. High-count density images of all collimators used for SPECT
Multienergy spatial registration	Annually	Ga-67 point source
Count rate performance	Annually	Tc-99m source

The results of these tests are to be compared with baseline values, typically determined during acceptance testing. If the manufacturer recommends or an accrediting body specifies additional tests or more frequent testing, these recommendations or specifications should take precedence. For tests with multiple frequencies listed, it is recommended that the tests be performed initially at the higher frequency, but the frequency be reduced if the measured parameters prove stable. Tests labeled (S) need not be performed for cameras used only for planar imaging.
[a]A sinogram is an image containing projection data corresponding to a single transaxial image of the patient. Each row of pixels in the sinogram is the row, corresponding to that transaxial image, of one projection image.

patient, such as metal objects and concentrated contrast material. Furthermore, the SPECT and x-ray CT information are not acquired simultaneously and patient organ motion can result in the misregistrations of, and therefore artifacts in, SPECT image information, the same as in PET/CT (discussed later in this chapter).

A common use of SPECT/CT is myocardial perfusion imaging. In myocardial perfusion imaging, non-uniform attenuation, particularly by the diaphragm and, in women, the breasts, can cause apparent perfusion defects in the SPECT images. Attenuation correction using the CT information has been reported to improve diagnostic accuracy by compensating for these artifacts. However, spatial misregistration between the heart in the CT and SPECT images can cause artifacts (Goetze et al., 2007). General SPECT-only imaging is being supplanted by dual-modality imaging, due to the mainstreaming and thus proliferation of SPECT/CT systems. An important quality assurance step in SPECT/CT is to verify the alignment of the SPECT and CT image information in every clinical examination.

19.3 POSITRON EMISSION TOMOGRAPHY

PET generates images depicting the distribution of positron-emitting nuclides in patients. Nearly all PET systems manufactured today are coupled to x-ray CT systems, with a single patient bed passing through the bores of both systems, and are referred to as "PET/CT" systems. Figure 19-17 shows a PET/CT system. This section discusses PET imaging systems; their use in PET/CT systems is discussed later in this chapter.

In a typical PET system, several rings of detectors surround the patient. PET scanners use *annihilation coincidence detection* (ACD) instead of collimation to obtain projections of the activity distribution in the subject. The PET system's computer then reconstructs the transverse images from the projection data, as does the computer of an x-ray CT or SPECT system. Modern PET scanners are multislice devices, permitting the simultaneous acquisition of many transverse images over a preset axial distance. The clinical importance of PET today is largely due to its ability to image the radiopharmaceutical fluorine-18 fluorodeoxyglucose (FDG), a glucose analog used for locating malignant neoplasms, differentiating malignant neoplasms from benign lesions, staging patients with malignant neoplasms, monitoring the response to therapy for neoplasms,

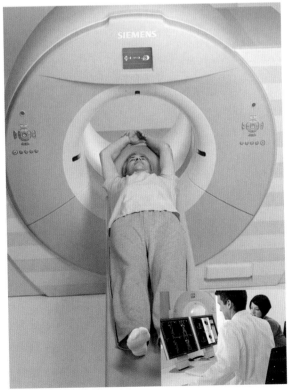

■ **FIGURE 19-17** A commercial PET/CT scanner. (© Siemens Healthineers 2019. Used with permission.)

differentiating severely hypoperfused but viable myocardium from scar, and other applications. However, other positron-emitting radiopharmaceuticals have been approved for use and their clinical use is increasing; these are discussed later in this chapter.

19.3.1 Design and Principles of Operation

Annihilation Coincidence Detection

Positron emission is a mode of radioactive transformation and was discussed in Chapter 15. Positrons emitted in matter lose most of their kinetic energy by causing ionization and excitation. When a positron has lost most of its kinetic energy, it interacts with an electron by *annihilation*, as shown on the left in Figure 19-18. The entire mass of the electron-positron pair is converted into energy equal to 1.02 MeV ($E = mc^2$, where c is the speed of light and m is the combined mass of the electron and positron), which appear as two 511-keV photons that are emitted in nearly opposite directions. In solids and liquids, positrons travel only very short distances (see Table 19-3) before annihilation.

If both photons from an annihilation interact with detectors and neither photon is scattered in the patient, the annihilation occurred near the line connecting the two interactions, as shown on the right in Figure 19-18. Circuitry within the scanner identifies pairs of interactions occurring at nearly the same time, a process called ACD. The circuitry of the scanner then determines the line in space connecting the locations of the two interactions, which is known as a *line of response* (LOR). Thus, ACD establishes the trajectories of detected photons, a function performed by collimation in SPECT systems. However, the ACD method is much less wasteful of photons than collimation. Additionally, ACD avoids the degradation of spatial resolution with distance from the detector that occurs when collimation is used to form projection images.

True, Random, and Scatter Coincidences

A *true coincidence* is the nearly simultaneous interaction with the detectors of emissions resulting from a single nuclear transformation. A *random coincidence* (also called an *accidental* or *chance coincidence*), which mimics a true coincidence, occurs when emissions from different nuclear transformations interact nearly simultaneously with the detectors (Fig. 19-19). A *scatter coincidence* occurs when one or both of the photons from a single annihilation are scattered, and both are detected (Fig. 19-19). A scatter coincidence is a true coincidence because both interactions result from a

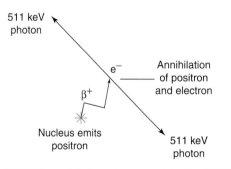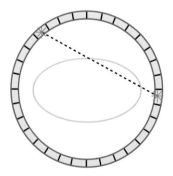

■ **FIGURE 19-18** Annihilation coincidence detection (ACD). When a positron is emitted by a nuclear transformation, it scatters through matter losing energy. After it loses most of its energy, it annihilates with an electron, resulting in two 511-keV photons that are emitted in nearly opposite directions (left). When two interactions are nearly simultaneously detected within a ring of detectors surrounding the patient (right), it is presumed that an annihilation occurred on the line connecting the interactions (*i.e.*, line of response). Thus, ACD, by determining the path of the detected photons, performs the same function for a PET scanner as does the collimator of a scintillation camera.

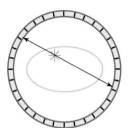 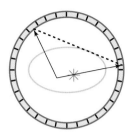 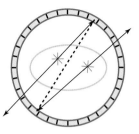

■ **FIGURE 19-19** True coincidence (left), scatter coincidence (center), and random (accidental) coincidence (right). A scatter coincidence is a true coincidence, because it is caused by a single nuclear transformation, but results in a count attributed to the wrong LOR (dashed line). The random coincidence is also attributed to the wrong LOR.

single positron annihilation. Random coincidences and scatter coincidences result in misplaced coincidences because they are assigned to LORs that do not intersect the actual locations of the annihilations. They are therefore sources of noise, whose main effects are to reduce image contrast and increase statistical noise.

Detection of Interactions

Scintillation crystals optically coupled to photomultiplier tubes (PMTs) or other light detectors are used as detectors in commercial PET systems today; the low intrinsic efficiencies of gas-filled and semiconductor detectors for detecting 511-keV photons make them impractical for use in PET. The signals from the PMTs or other light detectors are processed using pulse mode (the signals from each interaction are processed separately from those of other interactions) to create signals identifying the position in the detector, deposited energy, and time of each interaction. The energy signal is used for energy discrimination to reduce mispositioned events due to scattering and the time signal is used for coincidence detection and, in some PET systems, time-of-flight (ToF) determination (discussed later in this chapter).

In early PET scanners, each scintillation crystal was optically coupled to a single PMT. In this design, the size of the individual crystal largely determined the spatial resolution of the system; reducing the size (and therefore increasing the number of crystals) improved the resolution. It became increasingly costly and impractical to pack more and more smaller PMTs into each detector ring. Modern designs reduce the number of needed PMTs by combining multiple crystals together into a detector block, which in turn is coupled to a smaller number of PMTs; one such design is shown in Figure 19-20 whereby an 8×8 detector block is coupled to 4 PMTs (ratio of 16 crystals to 1 PMT). The relative magnitudes of the signals from the PMTs coupled to the detector block are then used to identify the location of the crystal within the detector block that had a photon interaction, as in a scintillation camera. (This method of event localization is known as Anger logic.) Today, many new PET systems use solid-state semiconductor devices instead of PMTs to collect light from the scintillation crystals; this is discussed later in this chapter.

The scintillation material must emit light very promptly to permit true coincident interactions to be distinguished from random coincidences and to minimize dead-time count losses at high interaction rates. Also, to maximize the counting efficiency, the material must have a high linear attenuation coefficient for 511-keV photons. A high conversion efficiency (fraction of deposited energy emitted as light or UV radiation) is also important; it permits more precise event localization in the detectors and better energy discrimination. For many years, most PET systems used crystals of bismuth germanate ($Bi_4Ge_3O_{12}$, abbreviated BGO). The light output of BGO is only 12% to 14% of that of NaI(Tl), but its greater density and average atomic number give it a much higher efficiency in detecting 511-keV annihilation photons. Light is emitted

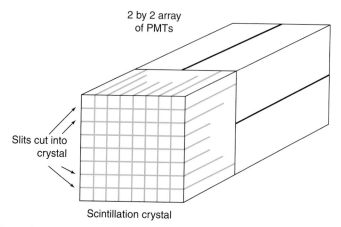

■ **FIGURE 19-20** A technique for coupling scintillation crystals to photomultiplier tubes (PMTs). The relative heights of the pulses from the four PMTs are used to determine the position of each interaction in the crystal. The thick (2 to 3 cm) crystal is necessary to provide a reasonable detection efficiency for the 511-keV annihilation photons. The slits cut in the scintillation crystal form light pipes, limiting the spread of light from interactions in the front portion of the crystal, which otherwise would reduce the spatial resolution. This design permits four PMTs to serve 64 detector elements.

rather slowly from BGO (decay constant of 300 ns), which contributes to dead-time count losses and random coincidences at high interaction rates. Several inorganic scintillators that emit light more quickly are replacing BGO. These include lutetium oxyorthosilicate (Lu_2SiO_4O, abbreviated LSO), lutetium yttrium oxyorthosilicate ($Lu_xY_{2-x}SiO_4O$, abbreviated LYSO), and gadolinium oxyorthosilicate (Gd_2SiO_4O, abbreviated GSO), all activated with cerium. Their attenuation properties are nearly as favorable as those of BGO and their much faster light emission produces better performance at high interaction rates, especially in reducing dead-time effects and in discriminating between true and random coincidences. A disadvantage of LSO and LYSO is that they are slightly radioactive; about 2.6% of naturally occurring lutetium is radioactive Lu-176, which has a half-life of 38 billion years, producing about 295 nuclear transformations per second in each cubic centimeter of LSO. NaI(Tl) was used as the scintillator in some less-expensive PET systems. The properties of BGO, LSO, LYSO, and GSO are contrasted with those of NaI(Tl) in Table 19-2.

The energy signals from the detectors are sent to energy discrimination circuits, which can reject events in which the deposited energy differs significantly from 511

TABLE 19-2 PROPERTIES OF SEVERAL INORGANIC SCINTILLATORS OF INTEREST IN PET

SCINTILLATOR	DECAY CONSTANT (ns)	PEAK WAVELENGTH (nm)	ATOMIC NUMBERS	DENSITY (g/cm³)	ATTENUATION COEFFICIENT 511 keV (cm⁻¹)	CONVERSION EFFICIENCY RELATIVE TO NAI
NaI(Tl)	250	415	11,53	3.67	0.343	100%
BGO	300	460	83,32,8	7.17	0.964	12%–14%
GSO(Ce)	56	430	64,14,8	6.71	0.704	41%
LSO(Ce)	40	420	71,14,8	7.4	0.870	75%

Decay constants, peak wavelengths, densities, and conversion efficiencies of BGO, GSO, and LSO. (Data from Ficke DC, Hood JT, Ter-Pogossian MM. A spheroid positron emission tomograph for brain imaging: a feasibility study. *J Nucl Med.* 1996;37(7):1219-1225.)

LYSO(Ce) has a decay constant, peak emission wavelength, and relative conversion efficiency similar to those of LSO(Ce), but its density and attenuation coefficient are less. Its density and attenuation coefficient vary with the proportion of yttrium to lutetium. (Data on LYSO from Chen J, Zhang L, Zhu RY. Large size LYSO crystals for future high energy physics experiments. *IEEE Trans Nucl Sci.* 2005;52(6):3133-3140.)

keV, to reduce the effect of photon scattering in the patient. However, some annihilation photons that have escaped the patient without scattering interact with the detectors by Compton scattering, depositing less than 511 keV. An energy discrimination window that encompasses only the photopeak rejects these interactions as well as photons that have scattered in the patient. The energy window can be set to encompass only the photopeak, with maximal rejection of scatter, but also reducing the number of valid interactions detected, or the window can include part of the Compton continuum, increasing the sensitivity, but also increasing the number of scattered photons detected.

The time signals of interactions not rejected by the energy discrimination circuits are used for coincidence detection. When a coincidence is detected, the circuitry or a computer in the scanner determines a line in space connecting the two interactions (LOR), as shown in Figure 19-18. The number of coincidences detected along each LOR is stored in the memory of the computer. Figure 19-21 compares the acquisition of projection data by SPECT and PET systems. Once data acquisition is complete, the computer uses the projection data to produce transverse images of the radionuclide distribution in the patient, as in x-ray CT or SPECT.

Timing of Interactions and Detection of Coincidences

To detect coincidences, the times of individual interactions in the detectors must be compared. However, interactions themselves cannot be directly detected; instead, the signals caused by interactions are detected. In scintillators, the emission of light after an interaction is characterized by a relatively rapid increase in intensity followed by a more gradual decrease. A timing circuit connected to each detector must designate one moment that follows each interaction by a constant time interval. The time signal is determined from the leading edge of the electrical signal from the PMTs or other light sensors connected to a detector crystal because the leading edge is steeper than the trailing edge. When the time signals from two detectors occur within a selected time interval called the *time window*, a coincidence is recorded. A typical time window for a system with BGO detectors is 12 ns. A typical time window for a system with LSO detectors, which emit light more promptly, is 4.5 ns.

True versus Random Coincidences

The rate of random coincidences between any pair of detectors is

$$R_{random} = \tau S_1 S_2,$$ [19-1]

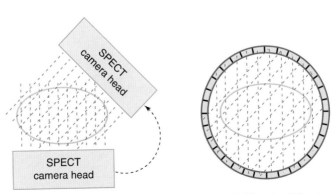

■ **FIGURE 19-21** Acquisition of projection data by a SPECT system (left) and a PET system (right), showing how each system collects data for two projections. However, the PET system collects data for all projections simultaneously, whereas the scintillation camera head of the SPECT system must move to collect data from each projection angle.

where τ is the coincidence time window and S_1 and S_2 are the actual count-rates of the detectors, often called *singles rates*. The time window is the designated time interval during which a pair of interactions in different detectors is considered to be a coincidence. Equation 19-1 shows that the rate of random coincidences decreases as the time window is shortened. However, there is a limit to how small the time window can be. The time window must accommodate the difference in arrival times of true coincidence photons from annihilations occurring in locations up to the edge of the device's FOV. For example, if the longest path for an unscattered annihilation photon crossing the FOV is 70 cm, the time window can be no shorter than

$$\Delta t = 0.7 \text{ m}/(3.0 \times 10^8 \text{ m/s}) = 2.33 \text{ ns,}$$

where 3.0×10^8 m/s is the speed of light. Furthermore, the time window must also be sufficiently long to accommodate the imprecision in the measured times of interactions. Scintillation materials that emit light promptly permit the use of shorter time windows and thus better discrimination between true and random coincidences.

Because the singles rates in individual detectors, ignoring dead-time count losses, are approximately proportional to the activity in the patient, Equation 19-1 shows that the rate of random coincidences is approximately proportional to the square of the activity in the patient. The true coincidence rate, ignoring dead-time count losses, is approximately proportional to the activity in the patient and so the ratio of random coincidences to true coincidences is approximately proportional to the administered activity. In this regard, increasing the administered activity as means to improve image statistics causes a net increase of random coincidences, which is counter to the desired objective.

Scatter Coincidences

As previously mentioned, a scatter coincidence occurs when one or both of the photons from an annihilation are scattered in the patient and both are detected (Fig. 19-19). The fraction of scatter coincidences is dependent upon the amount of scattering material and thus is less in head than in body imaging. Because scatter coincidences are true coincidences, reducing the activity administered to the patient, reducing the time window, or using a scintillator with faster light emission does not significantly reduce the scatter coincidence fraction. Scatter coincidences in PET imaging can be very high (reaching 60%–70% of the acquired coincidence data), particularly in larger cross sections of the body and when data is acquired in three dimensions (see next section). This is primarily due to the high Compton interaction cross section for 511 keV photons in body tissues and detector material as well as the dependence on only one of the two 511 keV photons to scatter before a scatter coincidence is recorded. Furthermore, the low light output from the scintillation crystals (*e.g.*, BGO and LSO versus NaI) results in a wider photopeak, which necessitates wider energy discriminator thresholds, thereby accepting more scattered coincidences. The energy discrimination circuits of the PET scanner can be used to reject some scatter coincidences. As was mentioned previously, energy discrimination to reduce scatter is less effective in PET than in SPECT, because many of the 511-keV annihilation photons interact with the detectors by Compton scattering, depositing less than their entire energies in the detectors. Using an energy window closely enveloping the photopeak will reject many annihilation photons that have not scattered in the patient.

Two- and Three-Dimensional Data Acquisition

In two-dimensional (slice) data acquisition, coincidences are detected and recorded only within each ring of detector elements or within a few adjacent rings of detector

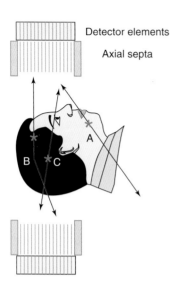

■ **FIGURE 19-22** Side view of PET scanner illustrating two-dimensional data acquisition. The axial septa prevent photons from activity outside the field-of-view **(A)** and most scattered photons **(B)** from causing counts in the detectors. However, many valid photon pairs **(C)** are also absorbed.

elements. PET scanners designed for two-dimensional acquisition have axial septa, thin annular collimators, typically made of tungsten, to prevent most radiation emitted by activity outside a transaxial slice from reaching the detector ring for that slice (Fig. 19-22). The fraction of scatter coincidences is greatly reduced in PET systems using two-dimensional data acquisition and axial collimation because of the geometry. Consider an annihilation occurring within a particular detector ring with the initial trajectories of the annihilation photons toward the detectors. If either of the photons scatters, it is likely that the new trajectory of the photon will cause it to miss the detector ring, thereby preventing a scatter coincidence. Furthermore, most photons from out-of-slice activity are absorbed by the axial septa.

In two-dimensional data acquisition, coincidences within one or more pairs of adjacent detector rings may be added to improve the sensitivity, as shown in Figure 19-23. The data from each pair of detector rings are added to that of the slice midway between the two rings. For example, if N is the number of a particular ring of detector elements, coincidences between rings $N - 1$ and $N + 1$ are added to the projection data for ring N. For further sensitivity, coincidences between rings $N - 2$ and

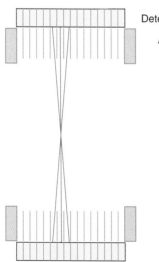

■ **FIGURE 19-23** Side view of PET scanner performing two-dimensional data acquisition, showing LORs for a single transverse image. Cross-ring coincidences have been added to those occurring within the ring of detector elements. This increases the number of coincidences detected, but causes a loss of axial spatial resolution that increases with distance from the axis of the scanner.

$N + 2$ can also be added to those of ring N. After the data from these pairs of detector rings are added, a standard two-dimensional reconstruction is performed to create a transverse image for this slice. Similarly, coincidences between two immediately adjacent detector rings, that is, between rings N and $N + 1$, can be used to generate a transverse image halfway between these rings. For greater sensitivity, coincidences between rings $N - 1$ and $N + 2$ can be added to these data. However, increasing the number of pairs of adjacent rings used in two-dimensional acquisition reduces the axial spatial resolution.

In three-dimensional (volume) data acquisition, axial septa are not used and coincidences are detected between many or all detector rings (Fig. 19-24). Three-dimensional acquisition greatly increases the number of true coincidences detected and may permit smaller activities to be administered to patients, compared to two-dimensional image acquisition. There are disadvantages to three-dimensional data acquisition. For the same administered activity, the greatly increased interaction rate increases the random coincidence fraction and the dead-time count losses. Furthermore, the scatter coincidence fraction is much larger and the number of interactions from activity outside the FOV is greatly increased. (Activity outside the FOV causes few true coincidences, but increases the rate of random coincidences detected and dead-time count losses.) Some PET systems are equipped with retractable axial septa, permitting them to perform two- or three-dimensional acquisition; however, all new PET systems are designed with only three–dimensional acquisition capabilities because of the advances in scatter rejection techniques that have been implemented by the various manufacturers of PET systems.

Figure 19-25 shows the efficiency of coincidence detection when two- or three-dimensional acquisition is used. In two-dimensional acquisition, the efficiency is nearly constant along the axial length of the detector rings. In three-dimensional acquisition, if coincidences are detected among all rings of detector elements, the coincidence detection efficiency increases linearly from the ends of the rings to the center. PET scans of extended lengths of patients are commonly accomplished by a discontinuous motion of the patient table through the system, with the table stopping for individual bed positions. Because of the greatly varying coincidence detection efficiency, a much greater overlap of bed positions is necessary when using three-dimensional acquisitions to make up for this degraded detection efficiency at the edges of the axial FOV.

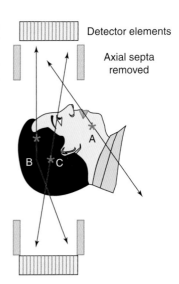

■ **FIGURE 19-24** Side view of PET scanner illustrating three-dimensional data acquisition. Without axial septa, interactions from activity outside the FOV **(A)** and scattered photons **(B)** are greatly increased, increasing the dead time, random coincidence fraction, and scatter coincidence fraction. However, the number of true coincidences **(C)** detected is also greatly increased.

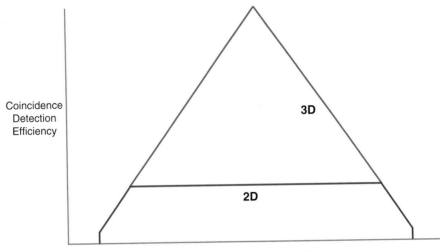

■ FIGURE 19-25 Efficiency of coincidence detection along axis of detector rings for two- and three-dimensional data acquisition. The three-dimensional acquisition example presumes that coincidences are detected among all rings of detector elements. The coincidence detection efficiency in two-dimensional acquisition is least if coincidences are detected only within individual rings of detector elements; it substantially increases when coincidences are also detected among adjacent rings, as shown in Figure 19-23.

Transverse Image Reconstruction

After the projection data are acquired, the data for each LOR are corrected for random coincidences, scatter coincidences, dead-time count losses, and attenuation (described below). Following these corrections, transverse image reconstruction is performed. For two-dimensional data acquisition, image reconstruction methods are similar to those used in SPECT. As in SPECT, either filtered backprojection or iterative reconstruction methods can be used. For three-dimensional data acquisition, special three-dimensional analytical or iterative reconstruction methods are required. These are beyond the scope of this chapter but are discussed in the suggested readings listed at the end of the chapter.

An advantage of PET over SPECT is that, in PET, the correction for non-uniform attenuation can be applied to the projection data before reconstruction. In SPECT, the correction for non-uniform attenuation is intertwined with and complicates the reconstruction process.

19.3.2 Data Correction

One of the advantages of PET imaging is its ability to produce images that accurately depict the distribution of radiopharmaceuticals in the body. Achieving this requires correction of the acquired data for several confounding factors that could bias the observed activity concentration in the resultant reconstructed image.

Normalization Correction

Modern PET scanners are composed of tens of thousands of individual detector elements that can have slightly variable performance (hyper or hypo sensitive detector element). This variability could, in turn, lead to differences in the number of detected events along an LOR, which ultimately will result in differences in measured activity concentration. Correction for this variability is known as normalization correction and is similar in principle to what is performed in gamma camera imaging. It is

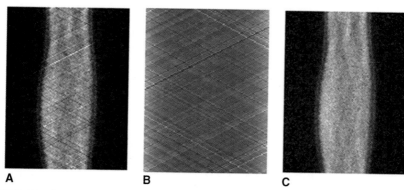

A   B   C

■ **FIGURE 19-26** Effect of normalization correction. The figure shows PET projection data of an object without normalization correction **(A)**, the normalization map **(B)**, and projection data of the object with normalization correction applied **(C)**.

performed by applying a normalization map to the acquired data. This is done by first illuminating all the detector elements in the PET scanner with a uniform source of radioactivity. Each coincident detector pair/LOR should then record the same number of detected events; a high number of detected events is required to decrease the statistical variability in detected events. Any difference in recorded events will be due to detector performance variations and will be captured in the normalization map. Correcting for the detector variability is then performed by multiplying the acquired data by the inverse of the normalization map. Figure 19-26 shows PET projection data of an object without normalization correction (A), the normalization map (B), and with normalization correction (C).

Randoms Correction

Although individual random coincidences cannot be distinguished from true coincidences, there are two methods to correct for random coincidences. The number of random coincidences along each LOR can be measured by adding a long time delay (much longer than the coincidence window) to one of the two timing signals used for coincidence detection, so that no true (or scatter) coincidences are detected. The coincidence rate in that delayed channel then provides an estimate of the random coincidences along that LOR. This method is known as randoms from delays. Alternatively, an estimate of the number of random coincidences may be calculated from the single event count-rates of the detectors, using Equation 19-1. This method is known as randoms from singles. In either case, the number of random coincidences is then subtracted from the number of true plus random coincidences for each LOR. While both correction methods are possible, the approach of randoms from singles is more accurate due to its reduced statistical noise in estimating the number of random coincidences (singles rate is higher than the coincidence rate).

Scatter Correction

Scatter coincidences result in a loss of image contrast due to mispositioning of the LOR along which the annihilation event occurred (Fig. 19-19), and misrepresentation of activity concentration in the reconstructed image. This, coupled with the fact that scatter coincidences represent the majority of recorded events in large patients and with data acquired in three-dimensional mode, necessitated the introduction of scatter correction techniques in PET imaging. Two main approaches are currently used. In the first approach, the distribution of scatter coincidences in individual projections is estimated from the reconstructed PET image as well as the attenuation image (see below on attenuation correction) while employing computer modeling of photon interaction physics. These scatter estimates are then subtracted from the projection profiles during image reconstruction to produce scatter-corrected PET images. This approach is also used in hybrid PET/CT systems (see Section 19.4) while replacing the PET attenuation image by the CT-based attenuation image, which works very well due to the decreased noise in CT compared to PET attenuation images. This approach also works well when all the activity is within the FOV but results in artifacts when some of this activity is located outside the FOV and results in scatter coincidences that cannot be accounted for by CT-based attenuation images. In a second approach, scatter coincidences along a projection profile can be estimated from events that fall outside the imaged object (only scatter events are detected outside an object). By fitting smoothly varying continuous functions (Gaussian and cosine functions have been used) to the tails of the projection profile (outside the imaged object) an estimate of the scatter coincidences can be derived, which can then be subtracted from the True plus Scatter coincidences profiles following randoms subtraction. While this method is simple and quick, it suffers from situations where the imaged object occupies the entire FOV (to projection tails to fit) or when complex scatter profiles exist that cannot be modeled with simple continuous functions. These methods of scatter correction do not compensate for the statistical noise caused by the random nature of the scatter.

Deadtime Correction

The scintillation detectors of a PET scanner exhibit deadtime and pulse pile-up effects at high count rates, which are reflected as an underestimation of activity concentration in the resultant reconstructed image. Examples of PET applications or situations that are adversely affected by deadtime effects include first-pass cardiac imaging and studies that require large amounts of administered activity to maintain adequate counting statistics throughout the acquisition due to short-lived radionuclides such as oxygen-15 ($T_{1/2}$ = 2 min) as well as in situations where large amounts of radioactivity are accumulated throughout the study time (such as in the bladder). Correction for deadtime and pileup rely on applying correction factors based on total system count rate performance or on an individual detector pair basis. In either case, these factors are derived from observing the deviation of the count rate performance from a linear response at varying activity levels while using different object sizes.

Decay Correction

PET imaging is characterized by relatively long imaging times due to its low counting efficiency. Current acquisition times are about 1–5 minutes per bed position, depending on the scanner model, the number of bed positions needed to cover the whole body, or the body part being imaged. Correction for the duration of the PET data acquisition time while the activity is decaying is necessary to ensure an accurate reflection of the activity concentration in the resultant image, especially when using radionuclides that have relatively short half-lives compared to the scan duration. The decay factor (DF), which describes the reduction in the number of recorded events for data acquired between time t and $t + \Delta t$ is

$$\text{DF} = e^{-(\lambda * t)} * \left[\frac{1 - e^{-(\lambda * \Delta t)}}{\lambda * \Delta t} \right], \qquad [19\text{-}2]$$

where λ is the decay constant of the radionuclide. From Equation 19-2, the DF is composed of two terms, the first describes the decay of a radionuclide measured at time t relative to time $t = 0$, and the second term describes the decay of a radionuclide during an interval t to $t + \Delta t$.

Correction for decay during the time interval Δt is then done by multiplying the observed counts during the time interval Δt by the inverse of the decay factor.

Attenuation Correction

A large fraction of the emitted 511 keV photons are attenuated in the patient, the overwhelming majority by Compton scattering interactions. Attenuation correction in PET imaging is the process that accounts for this attenuation in order to provide an accurate depiction of the activity concentration in the patient. Attenuation in PET differs from attenuation in SPECT because in PET both annihilation photons must escape the patient to cause a coincident event to be registered. The probability of both photons escaping the patient without interaction is the product of the probabilities of each escaping:

$$\left(e^{-\mu x}\right) \cdot \left(e^{-\mu(d-x)}\right) = e^{-\mu d}, \qquad [19\text{-}3]$$

where d is the total path length through the patient, x is the distance one photon must travel to escape, and $(d - x)$ is the distance the other must travel to escape (Fig. 19-27). Thus, the probability of both escaping the patient without interaction is independent of where on the line the annihilation occurred and is the same as the probability of a single 511-keV photon passing entirely through the patient along the same path. (Equation 19-3 was derived for the case of uniform attenuation, but this principle is also valid for non-uniform attenuation.)

Even though the attenuation coefficient for 511-keV annihilation photons in soft tissue ($\mu/\rho = 0.095$ cm²/g) is lower than those of photons emitted by most radionuclides used in SPECT ($\mu/\rho = 0.15$ cm²/g for 140 keV γ-rays), the average path length for both to escape the patient is much longer. For a 20-cm path in soft tissue, the chance of both annihilation photons of a pair escaping the tissue without interaction is only about 15%. Thus, attenuation is more severe in PET than in SPECT. The vast majority of the interactions with tissue are Compton scattering. Attenuation causes a loss of information and, because the loss is not the same for all LORs, causes artifacts in the reconstructed tomographic images. The loss of information also contributes to the statistical noise in the images.

■ **FIGURE 19-27** Attenuation in PET. The probability that both annihilation photons emitted along a particular LOR escape interaction in the patient is independent of the position on the LOR where the annihilation occurred.

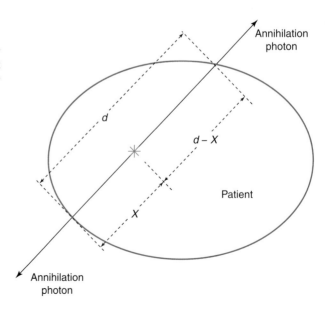

As in SPECT, both approximate methods and methods using radioactive sources to measure the attenuation have been used for attenuation correction in PET. Most of the approximate methods used a profile of the patient and presume a uniform attenuation coefficient within the profile.

Many older PET systems provided one or more retractable positron-emitting sources inside the detector ring between the detectors and the patient to measure the transmission of annihilation photons from the sources through the patient. As mentioned above, the probability that a single annihilation photon from a source will pass through the patient without interaction is the same as the probability that both photons from an annihilation in the patient traveling along the same path through the patient will escape interaction. These sources were usually configured as rods and were parallel to the axis of the scanner (Fig. 19-28). The sources revolved around the patient so that attenuation was measured along all LORs through the patient. These sources usually contained Ge-68, which has a half-life of 271 days and decays to Ga-68, which primarily decays by positron emission. Alternatively, a source containing a γ-ray–emitting radionuclide, such as Cs-137 (662-keV γ-ray), has been used for attenuation measurements instead of a positron-emitting radionuclide source. When a γ-ray–emitting radionuclide is used to measure the attenuation, the known position of the source and the location where a γ-ray is detected together determine a LOR for that interaction. In either case, the transmission data acquired using the external sources were used to correct the emission data for attenuation prior to transverse image reconstruction.

There are the advantages and disadvantages of attenuation correction from transmission measurements using radioactive sources. The transmission measurements increase the imaging time; slightly increase the radiation dose to the patient; and increase the statistical noise in the images. Also, spatial misregistration between the attenuation map and the emission data, most often caused by patient motion, can cause significant artifacts if the transmission data are not acquired simultaneously with the emission data.

Today, nearly every PET system manufactured is coupled to an x-ray CT system. These are called PET/CT systems. On such systems, the x-ray transmission information is used to correct the PET information for attenuation and so they are not provided with radioactive transmission sources for attenuation correction. PET/CT systems are discussed in detail later in this chapter.

19.3.3 Quantitation and Detrimental Factors

Quantitative Nature of PET Imaging

It is desirable, for research studies and many clinical studies, that each pixel value in a PET image be proportional to the number of nuclear transformations occurring

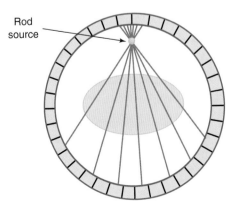

Rod source

■ **FIGURE 19-28** Rod source for attenuation correction in a dedicated PET system.

during imaging in the corresponding voxel of the patient. For example, in myocardial perfusion imaging, it is desirable that the count in each pixel depicting left ventricular myocardium be proportional to the concentration of radioactive tracer in the corresponding voxel in the patient's heart. PET, and PET/CT imaging with all data corrections described above, are considered quantitative imaging modalities, and the reconstructed voxel values can be calibrated in units of activity.

Scanner Calibration

Scanner calibration is the process of transforming the recorded counts following all data corrections to a corresponding activity concentration. This transformation is a global scale factor that is applied to all image voxel values. The scale factor is usually obtained by imaging a cylinder containing a known uniform radioactivity concentration. The ratio of the resultant reconstructed counts per pixel to the known activity concentration is the calibration factor after all data corrections are applied.

Standardized Uptake Value

Calibrated PET images in units of activity concentration can be further transformed into units of radiotracer uptake known as standardized uptake value (SUV) to correlate the activity concentration in a region of interest with the administered activity. Some physicians use the SUV to assist in characterizing tissues that accumulate the radiopharmaceutical, particularly in distinguishing benign from malignant lesions or in monitoring tumor therapy. It is defined as

$$ SUV = \frac{\text{activity concentration in a voxel or group of voxels}}{\text{activity administered}/\text{body mass}}, \qquad [19\text{-}4] $$

where either the administered activity or the activity concentration is corrected for radioactive decay from the time of dosage assay until imaging.

The SUV has units of density, for example, g/cm^3. Some institutions use lean body mass or body surface area instead of body mass in the denominator of this equation. Because the SUV is not based upon a physiological model, such as the Sokoloff model for glucose metabolism, it is regarded as an approximate or semiquantitative index of FDG uptake, which is a biomarker for glucose metabolism.

There are a number of factors, described below, that affect the magnitude of the measured SUV. Some of these factors, such as the time interval from the injection of the F-18 FDG to the PET imaging, that have a considerable effect on the magnitude of the SUV are chosen by the nuclear medicine laboratory performing the imaging and can vary from laboratory to laboratory. These factors should be considered in clinical decision-making based upon SUVs.

Factors Affecting Image Quantification

There are several factors that affect the quantitative accuracy of a PET image. These factors have been grouped into three categories: (1) technical factors, (2) biological factors, and (3) physical factors.

Technical Factors

Technical factors are those originating from the PET scanner itself and its support equipment. Examples of these factors include (1) error in the scanner calibration factor due to a systematic error in the dose calibrator used to assay the dose when calibrating the PET system; (2) residual activity in the syringe or administration system resulting in a lower net administered activity to the patient than anticipated and hence a lower SUV; (3) incorrect synchronization between the scanner time, the dose assay, and the administration time; this also includes inaccurate recording of these times; (4) paravenous administration of the radioactivity resulting in a lower effective administered activity reaching the areas of interest; and (5) inaccurate measurement of the patient body mass.

Biologic Factors

These factors are primarily dependent on the patient being imaged. Examples of these factors include (1) physiologic condition of the patient that could impact the biodistribution of the administered compound such as blood glucose level in the case of FDG imaging—a high blood glucose level results in a lower SUV measurement; similarly, inflammatory processes near areas of interest in the PET image will also result in an artificially biased SUV; (2) scan time post administration of the radiopharmaceutical (Given the dynamic nature of the radiopharmaceutical biodistribution in the body, it is necessary to consistently image the patient at a preset time.); (3) patient motion or breathing. Motion during the PET data acquisition or between the emission scan and the attenuation scan result in biased SUV measurements (see Section 19.5.5 on motion correction on advances in PET imaging), and (4) patient comfort during the uptake time of the radiopharmaceutical compound can have large effects on its biodistribution that could lead to biased SUV measurements.

Physical Factors

These factors are related to PET image acquisition and generation. Examples of these factors include (1) scan acquisition parameters. For example, short scan duration will result in higher image noise, which leads to an upward bias in SUV measurements; (2) image reconstruction parameters. For example, iterative reconstruction techniques require that reconstruction parameters be chosen such that the reconstruction reaches convergence in order to reflect an accurate activity concentration in the resultant image. Insufficient convergence will result in lower resolution and lower activity concentration, which leads to a lower SUV measurement in the resultant image; (3) limited resolution of the PET image, which causes *partial volume effects* (PVEs), is a reduction in the apparent activity concentration and hence SUV in smaller objects due to averaging of the actual activity concentration with that of surrounding tissues. Causes of the PVE are blurring due to the detector size; blurring by the tomographic reconstruction process (*e.g.*, the spatial filtering used in filtered backprojection or after iterative reconstruction), and the sizes of the pixels in the resultant images; (4) the region size and shape used to calculate the SUV, especially if the mean SUV in the region is desired; and (5) PET scanner quality control and assurance program that ensures all detectors and electronics are operating in an optimal condition. This would include an updated scanner calibration and normalization map, tuned PMT gains, and energy profiles, as well as coincidence timing resolution for each detector pair.

Each of these factors biases the SUV measurement and should thus be taken into consideration when making clinical decisions based on SUV. One approach to mitigate these effects is to harmonize their impact in longitudinal studies leaving any changes in SUV measurements to be truly reflective of radiopharmaceutical uptake in the region of interest. In multicenter clinical trials, such harmonization becomes further complicated by variations in imaging system performance and clinical practices, which necessitates further adherence to protocol design and analysis that might require the services of a centralized data analysis core to ensure standardization of scanner performance and outcome measurements.

19.3.4 Performance

Spatial Resolution

Modern whole-body PET systems achieve a spatial resolution slightly better than 5-mm FWHM of the LSF in the center of the detector ring when measured by the NEMA standard, *Performance Measurements of Positron Emission Tomographs* (National Electrical Manufacturers Association, NEMA NU 2-2007, Performance Measurements of Positron Emission Tomographs). The spatial resolution of PET scanners is limited by four primary factors: (1) the intrinsic spatial resolution of the detectors (R_d), (2) the distances traveled by the positrons before annihilation (R_r), (3) the fact that the annihilation photons are not emitted in exactly opposite directions from each other (R_c), and (4) the inaccuracy in determining the exact location of the interacting photon in the detector block (R_l). The intrinsic resolution of the detectors is the major factor determining the spatial resolution in current scanners. In older systems in which the detectors consisted of separate crystals each attached to a single PMT, the size of the crystals determines the resolution. In clinical imaging, spatial resolution is also reduced by organ motion, most commonly due to respiration.

The distance traveled by the positron before annihilation also slightly degrades the spatial resolution. This distance is determined by the maximal positron energy of the radionuclide and the density of the tissue and is known as the positron range. A radionuclide that emits lower energy positrons yields better resolution. Table 19-3 lists the maximal energies of positrons emitted by radionuclides commonly used in PET. Activity in denser tissue yields higher resolution than activity in less dense tissue such as lung tissue.

Although positrons lose nearly all of their momentum before annihilation, the positron and electron possess some residual momentum when they annihilate. Conservation of momentum predicts that the resultant photons will not be emitted in exactly opposite directions and is known as the non-collinearity effect. This causes a small loss of resolution, which increases with the diameter of the detector ring and is given by $R_c = 0.0022 \times D$ where D is the scanner diameter.

Most current PET detectors use block designs whereby signals from several PMTs are used to identify which detector element recorded an interaction; in these, an error in this exact identification within the detector block can occur, particularly when the

TABLE 19-3 PROPERTIES OF POSITRON-EMITTING RADIONUCLIDES COMMONLY USED IN PET

NUCLIDE	HALF-LIFE (min)	POSITRONS PER TRANSFORMATION	MAXIMAL POSITRON ENERGY (keV)	MAXIMAL POSITRON RANGE (mm)[a]	NOTES
C-11	20.4	1.00	960	4.2	
N-13	10.0	1.00	1,198	5.4	
O-15	2.0	1.00	1,732	8.4	
F-18	110	0.97	634	2.4	Most common use is F-18 fluorodeoxyglucose.
Rb-82	1.3	0.95	3,356	17	Produced by a Sr-82/Rb-82 generator.

The average positron range is much less than the maximal range, because positrons are emitted with a continuum of energies and because the paths of positrons in matter are not straight.
[a]In water from ICRU Report 37.

light output of the crystal is relatively low such as with BGO crystals. This uncertainty has decreased with newer detector materials, such as LSO or LYSO, that have higher light outputs, as well as with silicon photomultipliers (SiPMs) (described in Chapter 17).

The overall PET system resolution can then be obtained by combining each of these effects according to the following equation:

$$R_{\text{sys}}^2 = R_{\text{d}}^2 + R_{\text{r}}^2 + R_{\text{c}}^2 + R_{\text{l}}^2 .$$

The spatial resolution of a PET system is best in the center of the detector ring and decreases slightly (FWHM increases) with distance from the center. This occurs because of the considerable thickness of the detectors. Uncertainty in the depth of interaction causes uncertainty in the LOR for annihilation photons that strike the detectors obliquely. Photons emitted from the center of the detector ring can only strike the detectors "head-on," but many of the photons emitted from activity away from the center strike the detectors from oblique angles (Fig. 19-29). Some newer PET systems can estimate the depths of interactions in the detectors and have more uniform spatial resolution across a transverse image.

Efficiency in Annihilation Coincidence Detection

Consider a point source of a positron-emitting radionuclide in air midway between two identical detectors and assume that all positrons annihilate within the source. The true coincidence rate of the pair of detectors is

$$R_{\text{T}} = 2AG\varepsilon^2 , \qquad\qquad [19\text{-}5]$$

where A is the rate of positron emission by the source, G is the geometric efficiency of either detector, and ε is the intrinsic efficiency of either detector. (Geometric and intrinsic efficiency were defined in Chapter 17.) Because the rate of true coincidences detected is proportional to the square of the intrinsic efficiency, maximizing the intrinsic efficiency is very important in PET. For example, if the intrinsic efficiency of a single detector for a 511-keV photon is 0.9, 81% of the annihilation photon pairs emitted toward the detectors will have coincident interactions. However, if the intrinsic efficiency of a single detector is 0.1, only 1% of pairs emitted toward the detectors will have coincident interactions.

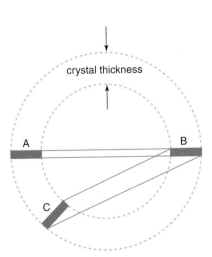

■ FIGURE 19-29 Cause of reduced spatial resolution with distance from center of PET scanner. Only three crystal segments in the detector ring are shown. For coincident interactions in detectors A and B, there is little uncertainty in the LOR. When coincidences occur in detectors B and C, there is greater uncertainty in the LOR. Using thinner crystals would reduce this effect, but would also reduce their intrinsic detection efficiency and thus the number of coincidences detected.

As mentioned previously, most PET systems today use crystals of high density, high atomic number scintillators such as BGO, LSO, LYSO, or GSO. These crystals are typically about two to three cm thick. For example, a 2-cm-thick crystal of LSO has an intrinsic efficiency of 82%, although energy discrimination reduces the fraction of detected photons used for coincidence detection below this value.

As mentioned above in "Two- and Three-Dimensional Data Acquisition," increasing the axial acceptance angle of annihilation photons greatly increases the efficiency. The efficiency of current commercial PET systems operated in two and three-dimensional mode is on the order of 0.1%–0.3% and 1%–2%, respectively.

Other factors that increase scanner efficiency include decreasing the scanner detector ring diameter as well as increasing the axial length of the detector ring, both of which result in capturing a larger fraction of the emitted annihilation photons. Most commercial PET scanners are designed to image the whole body (compared to brain), and as such the scanner diameter is limited by the size of the patient to be imaged. Most PET systems have scanner bores of about 60–80 cm (with detector-to-detector diameters of about 90–100 cm). A decrease in the size of the scanner bore could lead to patient claustrophobia, which in turn can cause patient discomfort and motion during the scan, which could result in image motion artifacts and errors in measured activity concentration and SUVs. Increasing the scanner axial extent is another approach to increasing scanner efficiency; however, it increases the cost of the system. Current PET scanners have axial extents of 15–30 cm, with one manufacturer providing a 194-cm system.

19.3.5 Quality Control in PET

Daily, typically before imaging the first patient, a scan is performed of a uniform positron-emitting source. This may be a line source or a cylindrical source. Ge-68 is a radionuclide commonly used in these sources; its daughter Ga-68, with which it is in secular equilibrium, emits positrons. This scan, typically displayed as detector maps or sinograms, will reveal poorly performing or inoperative detectors, detectors requiring normalization, and detectors with improperly set energy windows. Tomographic uniformity is periodically assessed using a cylindrical phantom with a uniform distribution of a positron-emitting radionuclide. If the daily or periodic uniformity scans reveal changes in detector efficiencies, a detector normalization calibration is performed to measure the efficiencies of all the detector LORs in the system and update the stored normalization factors. Periodically, an absolute activity calibration should also be performed if clinical measurements of activity concentration are to be performed. A medical physicist should perform a complete systems test and review the quality control program at least annually. This systems test assesses many parameters, including spatial resolution, statistical noise, count-rate performance, sensitivity, and image quality.

Acceptance Testing

Acceptance testing of a PET scanner is done upon the installation or relocation of the system. Acceptance testing procedures of PET systems are described by the NEMA NU2 standard. The most recent version of this standard is NU2-2018. The NEMA testing procedure for PET scanners includes assessments of the following parameters: (1) spatial resolution; (2) scatter fraction, count losses, and randoms; (3) sensitivity; (4) accuracy evaluating the correction for count losses and randoms; (5) image quality, accuracy, and corrections; (6) ToF resolution for systems with such a capability; and (7) co-registration accuracy between the PET and CT images for hybrid systems.

Detailed descriptions of each of these tests can be found in the NEMA NU2 standard and are beyond the scope of this chapter. The results of these tests should be compared to the manufacturer's specifications of the corresponding PET system.

Routine Testing and Frequency

Several professional and accreditation bodies have developed routine testing schedules for PET systems. Additionally, each manufacturer of PET systems recommends a set of tests to be performed routinely on its PET scanners. Table 19-4 lists the routine tests that should be conducted and their frequencies. The table also includes tests that should be done on the CT components of hybrid systems.

Most accreditation bodies require routine testing of PET systems using phantoms to evaluate PET image quality under conditions similar to those encountered in the

TABLE 19-4 ROUTINE TESTS FOR PET

TEST	DAILY	WEEKLY	QUARTERLY	SEMI-ANNUAL	ANNUAL
CT QC	X				
PET QC	X				
PET Update Gains and Coincidence Timing			X		
PET Normalization				X[a]	
PET Calibration				X[a]	
Preventive Maintenance and Inspection				X	
Source Replacement					X
PET Spatial Resolution					X
PET & CT Registration				X[b]	
PET Sensitivity					X[a]
PET Count Rate Performance					X[c]
PET Accuracy of Corrections					X
PET Image Contrast and Scatter/ Attenuation Evaluation				X	
PET Image Uniformity Assessment					X[d]
Image Display Monitor Evaluation					X
Emergency Buttons Testing					X
Synchronize System Clocks		X			
Additional Daily Tests[d]					
Restart Computers	X				
Manufacturer-Recommended CT Warm-up Cycle and Calibrations	X				
Archive Patient Data	X				
Clear Scheduler	X				
Clear Local, Network, and Film Queries	X				

Adapted with permission from American Association of Physicists in Medicine, Report No. 126—PET/CT Acceptance Testing and Quality Assurance (2019). Copyright © AAPM.
[a]Or if a detector module is replaced.
[b]Or after the gantry is opened.
[c]Or if the electronic boards are replaced.
[d]Philips recommends these tests to be done on a quarterly basis.

clinic. Most of these bodies specify the use of the PET American College of Radiology (ACR) phantom for this evaluation. The ACR phantom is composed of three sections, each to evaluate image contrast, uniformity, and spatial resolution. The top section, used to evaluate image contrast, contains four "hot" cylinders of different diameters (8, 16, 22, and 25 mm) with a uniform activity concentration relative to background and 3 cylinders (each of 25 mm diameter) with different material density (air, water, and Teflon). Maximum SUV measurements are used to calculate image contrast from the four "hot" cylinders. Mean and minimum SUV measurements are used to calculate scatter/attenuation from the Teflon, air, water, and background regions. These values are all measured on images reconstructed with all corrections applied (attenuation, scatter, random counts, dead time, etc.). The middle section, which is filled with a uniform activity concentration, is used to evaluate image uniformity, whereas the lower section contains six groups of plastic cylinders of varying diameters arranged in a pie shape and is used to evaluate image resolution. A detailed description of the PET ACR phantom testing can be found in the ACR PET Accreditation Program Testing Instructions. The AAPM TG 126 has also recently published a document on PET/CT acceptance testing and quality assurance.

19.4 DUAL MODALITY IMAGING—PET/CT, AND PET/MRI

Nuclear medicine tomographic imaging, whether SPECT or PET, of cancer, infections, and inflammatory diseases often reveals lesions with greater radionuclide concentrations than surrounding tissue, but often provides little information regarding their exact locations in the organs of the patients. Spatial co-registration of SPECT or PET images with images from another modality, such as x-ray CT or MRI, that provides a good depiction of anatomy can be very useful. This can be accomplished by imaging the patient using separate SPECT or PET and CT or MRI systems and aligning the resultant images using multimodality image registration software. However, it is difficult to align the patient on the bed of the second imaging system exactly the same as on the first system, which in turn makes it very difficult to accurately align the SPECT or PET data with the CT or MRI data.

As mentioned earlier in this chapter, another problem common to both SPECT and PET is the attenuation of the γ-rays, x-rays, or annihilation photons by the patient, causing a reduction in apparent activity toward the centers of transverse images and attenuation artifacts, particularly when attenuation is non-uniform. In both SPECT and PET, manufacturers have provided the capability to perform attenuation correction using sealed radioactive sources to measure the transmission through the patient from the various projection angles. As mentioned earlier, the use of radioactive sources for attenuation correction in SPECT was not met with universal acceptance, whereas the use of external sources for attenuation correction in PET was generally accepted. However, in PET, the use of radioactive sources for attenuation correction increased imaging times, reducing patient throughput.

To solve these problems, systems have been developed that incorporate a PET or SPECT system and a conventional x-ray CT system in a single gantry or in coupled gantries (Figs. 19-17 and 19-1A and B). The patient lies on a bed that passes through the bores of both systems. X-ray CT imaging is performed of the same length of the patient as the PET or SPECT imaging, either before or after the PET or SPECT image acquisition. Because the patient's position on the bed is the same during CT and PET or SPECT image acquisition, accurate co-registration of the CT and PET or SPECT information is usually possible. In the co-registered images, the PET or SPECT information is usually superimposed in color on grayscale CT images (Fig. 19-30).

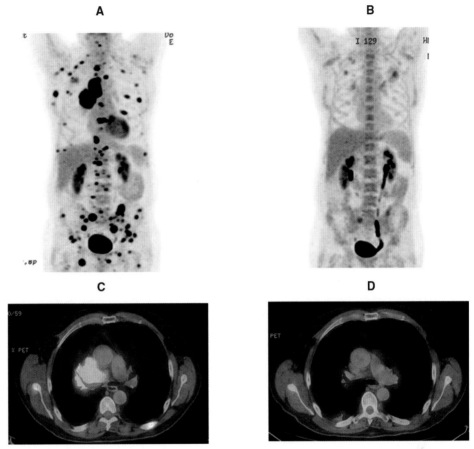

■ **FIGURE 19-30** Co-registered PET and CT images. (Courtesy of David K. Shelton, MD, Professor of Radiology, Emeritus, UC Davis Medical Center.)

Advantages of using x-ray CT systems instead of radioactive sources for attenuation correction are much quicker attenuation scans, permitting increased patient throughput and reducing the likelihood of patient motion; less statistical noise in the attenuation data due to the high x-ray flux from the CT; and higher spatial resolution attenuation data. However, there are disadvantages as well, which are discussed below.

Manufacturers have provided SPECT/CT and PET/CT systems with x-ray CT subsystems that are capable of producing diagnostic quality CT images and with less-expensive CT systems that are not capable of producing diagnostic quality CT images. If the x-ray CT subsystem is capable of diagnostic quality imaging, it may be used with low tube current, providing low radiation dose but non-diagnostic CT information for attenuation correction and anatomic localization only, or with high tube current, providing diagnostic quality CT images.

Nearly all PET systems sold today are integrated PET/x-ray CT systems, because of their ability to provide attenuation-corrected PET images co-registered to x-ray CT images with high patient throughput. Combined PET/MRI systems are also commercially available. PET/MRI systems are discussed later in this chapter.

19.4.1 Attenuation Correction in PET/CT

As mentioned above, the x-ray CT system provides information that can be used for attenuation correction of the PET information, replacing the positron-emitting rod sources formerly used for attenuation correction by PET systems. A modern x-ray CT system can provide the attenuation information, with very little statistical noise, in a fraction of a minute, in comparison with the many minutes required when positron-emitting rod sources were used.

An x-ray CT system measures the average linear attenuation coefficients, averaged over the x-ray energy spectrum, for individual volume elements (voxels) of the patient. However, linear attenuation coefficients for 511-keV annihilation photons are necessary for attenuation correction of PET information. Linear attenuation coefficients, measured using the x-rays from x-ray CT systems, are very different from those for 511-keV photons, and the ratio between the coefficients depends upon the material in the individual voxel. If the x-ray CT information is to be used for correction of the PET emission information, the linear attenuation coefficient for each voxel for 511-keV photons must be estimated from the linear attenuation coefficient (or, equivalently, the CT number) for that voxel for x-rays from the CT system.

The linear attenuation coefficient is the product of the density of a material and its mass attenuation coefficient. Table 19-5 lists the mass attenuation coefficients for 70-keV x-rays and 511-keV annihilation photons for several materials. The mass attenuation coefficients in the CT energy range vary greatly with the atomic number (Z) of the material because of the photoelectric effect. Although the interactions of the x-rays from an x-ray CT system with soft tissue and bodily fluids are mainly by Compton scattering, their interactions with higher atomic number materials such as bone mineral, x-ray contrast material, and metal objects in the body, are by both the photoelectric effect and Compton scattering. However, 511-keV annihilation photons almost entirely interact with all these materials by Compton scattering. As discussed in Chapter 3, the Compton scattering component of the linear attenuation coefficient for photons of a specific energy is determined by the number of electrons per volume, which in turn is largely determined by the density of the material.

The commonly used methods for estimating the linear attenuation coefficients for 511-keV photons from the CT numbers (defined in Chapter 10) are based upon making assumptions about the composition of the material in individual voxels using their CT numbers. One method for estimating the linear attenuation coefficients for 511-keV photons from the CT numbers is to divide the voxels into two groups: those with CT numbers less than a value such as 50 and those with CT numbers greater than this value (Carney et al., 2006). Voxels with CT numbers less than this value are assumed to contain only soft tissue, body fluids, gas, or a mixture of them, whereas voxels with CT numbers greater than this value are assumed to contain bone mineral and soft tissue. For each of these two groups, the linear attenuation coefficient for 511-keV photons is calculated from a linear equation relating these linear attenuation coefficients to the CT number. For voxels in the low CT number group:

$$\mu_{511\,keV} = (9.6 \times 10^{-5}\,cm^{-1}) \cdot (CT\ number + 1,000).$$

This equation will yield the correct linear attenuation coefficients for air (CT number $= -1,000, \mu_{511\,keV} = 0$) and water (CT number $= 0, \mu_{511\,keV} = 0.096\,cm^{-1}$) and approximately correct linear attenuation coefficients for most soft tissues. For voxels in the high CT number group, the linear attenuation coefficient for 511-keV photons is calculated from

$$\mu_{511\,keV} = m \cdot (CT\ number) + b,$$

where m and b are empirically determined constants that differ with the kV used by the x-ray CT system. In effect, the linear equation for the lower CT number voxels uses the CT number to determine the density of the soft tissue in a voxel, whereas the linear equation for the high CT number voxels uses the CT number to determine the ratio of mass of bone mineral to mass of soft tissue in a voxel. These methods for estimating the linear attenuation coefficients for 511-keV photons from CT numbers are successful when the assumptions about the composition of the material in a voxel are valid, but can fail badly when these assumptions are not correct.

Incorrect estimation of the linear attenuation coefficients for 511-keV photons can cause artifacts in the attenuation-corrected images. This commonly occurs when there is a material, such as metal or concentrated x-ray contrast material, that does not conform to the assumptions implicit in the method used to estimate attenuation coefficients for 511-keV photons from the x-ray CT data. If the attenuation coefficient for 511-keV photons is significantly overestimated, the artifact typically appears as a falsely elevated radionuclide concentration. Such artifacts are discussed below.

19.4.2 Artifacts in PET/CT Imaging

Most things that cause artifacts in CT imaging, such as implanted metal objects that cause star artifacts and patient motion, can in turn cause artifacts in attenuation-corrected PET/CT images. However, there are also artifacts, discussed below, that are not artifacts in the PET images or the CT images themselves but are caused by the interactions of the two image sets.

Spatial Misregistration Artifacts

Despite the fact that the patient lies in the same position during both the PET and x-ray CT scans, spatial misregistration of image information can still occur because the PET and x-ray CT image information are not acquired simultaneously. Misregistration most commonly occurs due to organ motion, particularly in or near the thorax, due to respiration. The x-ray CT imaging is commonly performed during a single breath-hold to produce images without the effects of respiratory motion, whereas PET imaging occurs during normal resting respiration. In particular, if the CT imaging is performed with breath-holding after full inspiration and the PET imaging is acquired during shallow breathing, F-18 FDG avid lesions located in the liver close

TABLE 19-5 COMPARISON OF MASS ATTENUATION COEFFICIENTS FOR SOME TISSUES AND MATERIALS

PHOTON ENERGY (keV)	MASS ATTENUATION COEFFICIENTS (cm²/g)			
	Skeletal Muscle	*Cortical Bone*	*Titanium*	*Iodine*
70	0.192	0.263	0.545	5.02
511	0.0951	0.0894	0.0811	0.0952

For x-rays of a typical energy (70 keV) produced by a CT scanner, the likelihood of the photoelectric effect has a large effect on mass attenuation coefficients and so they vary greatly with the atomic numbers of the material. However, for 511-keV annihilation photons, Compton scattering is by far the most likely interaction in these materials and the mass attenuation coefficient varies little with atomic number. Note that attenuation is determined by the linear attenuation coefficient, which is the product of the mass attenuation coefficient and the density of the material.
Data from Hubbell JH, Seltzer SM. Tables of X-Ray Mass Attenuation Coefficients and Mass Energy-Absorption Coefficients 1 keV to 20 MeV for Elements $Z = 1$ to 92 and 48 Additional Substances of Dosimetric Interest, NISTIR 5632, US Department of Commerce, May 1995.

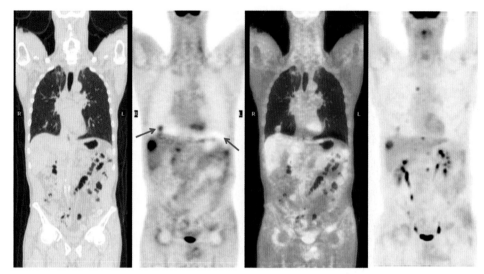

■ **FIGURE 19-31** PET/CT study showing diaphragmatic misregistration with superimposition of a hypermetabolic liver nodule over the right lung base on the fused PET-CT. Left to right: coronal CT, attenuation-corrected PET, fused attenuation corrected PET-CT, and attenuation-corrected PET maximum intensity projection images. CT shows no nodule in the right lung base, and attenuation-corrected PET and fused PET-CT images show a clear band above the diaphragm due to misregistration. (Images and interpretation courtesy of George M. Segall, MD, VA Palo Alto Health Care System.)

to the diaphragm or in the chest wall may appear to be in the lungs in the fused PET/CT images. Figure 19-31 shows a case of misregistration due to respiratory motion.

A partial solution to this problem is to acquire low-dose x-ray CT information for image co-registration and attenuation correction during normal resting breathing and, if needed, to acquire separate high-dose diagnostic quality CT images during breath holding at maximal inspiration. Another partial solution is to acquire the CT images with breath-holding at mid-inspiration or mid-expiration. Some systems allow respiratory gating to be performed during the PET acquisition. Respiratory gating can reduce respiratory motion artifacts and permit more accurate determination of tissue volumes and activity concentrations, but increases the acquisition time.

Attenuation Correction Artifacts

When x-ray CT information is used for attenuation correction of the PET information, incorrect estimation of linear attenuation coefficients for 511-keV photons can cause artifacts. As mentioned above under Attenuation Correction in PET/CT, material in the patient that does not meet the assumptions inherent in the method to estimate attenuation coefficients for 511-keV photons from x-ray CT data can cause significant errors in attenuation correction. If the attenuation coefficient for 511-keV photons is significantly overestimated, the artifact typically appears as a falsely elevated radionuclide concentration, which can mimic a lesion of clinical relevance. This can occur where there are metallic objects in the body, such as pacemakers, orthopedic devices, or body piercings, or concentrations of x-ray contrast material. Such an artifact is shown in Figure 19-32.

Voluminous metal objects, such as hip implants, in the patient, may not cause such attenuation artifacts displaying falsely elevated radionuclide concentration. Although the attenuation coefficient for 511-keV photons is greatly overestimated, there is no positron-emitting radionuclide in the metal object and so the attenuation correction and image reconstruction process has no signal to incorrectly overamplify.

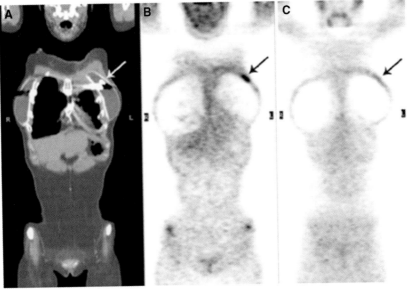

■ **FIGURE 19-32** Attenuation correction artifact caused by overestimation of attenuation by a metal object, in this case a body piercing. CT image **(A)** shows a streaking artifact at the location of the metal object on the left breast. Overestimation of attenuation causes the attenuation-corrected PET image **(B)** to display a falsely elevated concentration of F-18 FDG at the location of the metal object. Notice that that concentration of F-18 FDG is not elevated in the PET image **(C)** that is not attenuation corrected. (This research was originally published in JNM. Sureshbabu W, Mawlawi O. PET/CT imaging artifacts. *J Nucl Med Technol.* 2005;33(3):156-161. Copyright © 2020 SNMMI.)

As mentioned above, x-ray contrast material, commonly containing iodine (intravascular contrast material) or barium (contrast material for GI studies) can also cause errors in attenuation correction (Mawlawi et al., 2006; Otero et al., 2009). It appears that such material, unless concentrated in a particular location, is not likely to have clinically significant effects.

A focus of apparent enhanced uptake in the attenuation-corrected images can be confirmed or refuted by a review of the corresponding uncorrected images. Spatial misregistrations of CT and PET data can also cause errors in attenuation correction. Such an artifact appears at the level of the diaphragm (band of falsely-low pixel values) in the middle two images in Figure 19-31.

Truncation Artifacts

The radial FOVs of the CT and PET systems may differ significantly. Commonly, the PET system has a much larger radial FOV than the CT, although at least one manufacturer offers a system in which the PET and CT systems have equal FOVs. If part of a patient, for example, a patient of large girth or a patient imaged with the arms by his or her side, extends outside the FOV of the CT, there will be an error in the attenuation correction of the PET images because attenuation by the portion of the patient outside the CT's FOV is not considered.

19.4.3   PET/MRI Systems

Dual modality PET/MRI systems have recently been developed. These include small systems for imaging of animals and larger systems for imaging humans for research. As in PET/CT, the MRI system provides tomographic images with excellent depiction of anatomic detail, and the PET information is spatially co-registered with the MRI information. The MRI information is also used to estimate attenuation coefficients in each voxel of the patient for correction of the PET information for attenuation of the annihilation photons.

A problem that must be addressed in the design of PET/MRI imaging systems is that PMTs are adversely affected by magnetic fields, particularly very strong ones such as those produced by MRI magnets. Furthermore, PMTs are very bulky. Two methods have been used to address this problem. In one approach, the rings of PET detectors are inside the bore of the MRI system's main magnet. These detectors consist of scintillation crystals optically coupled to avalanche photodiodes or SiPMs, which are not affected by the strong magnetic field. (Avalanche photodiodes were briefly discussed in Chapter 17.) In the other approach, the PET system is at one end of the patient couch and the MRI system is at the other end of the patient couch, with the two systems being separated by a distance of about 2 m. In this latter approach, the PET detectors consist of scintillation crystals coupled to PMTs. A system with the PET detectors inside the MRI permits simultaneous image acquisition, whereas the other design requires sequential imaging.

19.4.4 Quality Control of Dual Modality Imaging Systems

There are three aspects to the quality control of dual-modality imaging systems. There is quality control testing of the SPECT or PET imaging system (discussed earlier in this chapter) as well as of the CT or MRI system. Lastly, there should be testing of the operation of the combined systems. The two major items to be tested are the accuracy of the spatial co-registration of the two modalities and the accuracy of the attenuation correction.

19.5 ADVANCES IN PET IMAGING

19.5.1 Time of Flight Imaging

The introduction of detector materials such as LSO and LYSO with fast scintillation light decay times has enabled an improved form of PET image acquisition/reconstruction known as ToF imaging. With ToF imaging, information about the detection (arrival) time of the annihilation photons is also recorded. This knowledge is subsequently used during image reconstruction to inform on where along a LOR an annihilation event occurred in the FOV of the scanner, as compared to conventional PET systems that do not have this capability. The knowledge about the arrival times has been shown to improve the resultant signal to noise ratio (SNR) of reconstructed PET images as described in the equations below:

$$\text{SNR}_{\text{TOF}} \cong \sqrt{\frac{D}{\Delta X}}\,\text{SNR}_{\text{Conv}} \quad \Delta X = \frac{\Delta t}{2}c,$$

where D is the diameter of the object being imaged, c is the speed of light, and Δt is the timing resolution for determining the arrival time of the annihilation photon.

These equations show that, as the timing resolution decreases (ability to better pinpoint the arrival time), the SNR of ToF imaging improves. Furthermore, these equations show that larger objects (patients) will benefit more from ToF imaging than smaller objects. The timing resolution of state-of-the-art PET scanners is on the order of 250–500 ps, with the manufacturers striving to reduce these values. With a 500 ps timing resolution, the arrival time can be converted to a positional error (Δx)

of 7.5 cm in the FOV of the scanner, whereas a 300 ps timing resolution reduces that error to 4.5 cm—a 40% reduction and an improvement of SNR by about 30%. If the timing resolution were decreased by a factor of 10 (to 25–50 ps) then there would be no need for image reconstruction, since the image could be directly generated as the data are acquired. This, however, would require a faster detector material than LSO or LYSO; several are currently under consideration.

The use of faster detectors (shorter decay time following scintillation) also has implications on scanner deadtime. Faster detectors such as LSO and LYSO greatly reduce deadtime effects, thereby allowing imaging procedures that necessitate a large amount of radioactivity in the FOV of the scanner as in the case of cardiac imaging or imaging in situations where the administered radiopharmaceutical accumulates in high concentrations.

19.5.2 Digital Detectors

A PET detector is composed of two components: the material that stops/detects the annihilation photons and an electronic device, coupled to the end of the detector material, which in turn transforms the light signal from the detected photon into an electrical signal including signal amplification and processing. Currently, the scintillators LSO and LYSO are the dominant detector materials used in PET imaging due to their high stopping powers for 511 keV annihilation photons and their fast scintillation times that can enable ToF imaging. With regard to the electronic device that transforms the light signal to an electrical signal, the PMT has been the dominant device used since the introduction of the first PET scanner. A PMT is an analog device that first transforms the incident light (from the scintillator/detector material) to an electrical pulse and then amplifies this signal for subsequent processing. Several limitations exist with such a process from losses in light absorption to non-uniformities in light conversion along the surface of the PMT. Additionally, given that PMTs are glass vacuum enclosures, there is a limitation on how small they can be manufactured as well as their ability to accurately pinpoint the location of where the light was emitted from the scintillation material, which limits the overall spatial resolution of PET images. Recently, detectors known as SiPMs have been introduced as a replacement to the PMTs. SiPMs, consisting of rectangular arrays of avalanche photodiodes operated in Geiger mode, were discussed in Chapter 17. The use of SiPMs greatly improves light absorption and conversion, better event timing, and potential improvement in spatial resolution due to the small size of SiPMs. Furthermore, their compact sizes and their lack of magnetic susceptibility make them ideal devices for use in PET/MR systems as compared to PMTs, which cannot be used in such an environment. Today, most state-of-the-art PET/CT scanners use LSO or LYSO crystals coupled to SiPMs. The detector material (scintillator) is usually configured in a rectangular block design with dimensions of 2–5 by 2–5 by 15–30 mm along the x, y, and z directions (with z being the height of the detector material). This finite size (along the x and y directions) places a physical lower limit on the spatial resolution of PET scanners and contributes to PVEs—a decrease in the measured activity concentration in a volume of interest that is smaller than the spatial resolution of the scanner. With PMTs, this effect is further exaggerated by the physical sizes of PMTs as well as their inability to accurately determine the exact location of the scintillation light. SiPMs, on the other hand, have smaller sizes and can be designed to match the physical detector sizes, thereby reducing this resolution limitation and hence PVE. There are two methods for optically coupling SiPMs to the scintillation crystals. If a SiPM channel (with thousands of photodiodes) matches the cross-sectional size of a

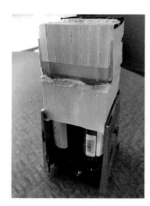
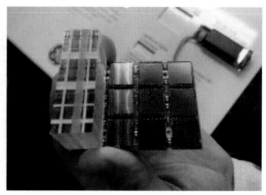

■ **FIGURE 19-33** Comparison of a conventional and digital detector of a PET scanner. Conventional PET detectors use glass PMT that are attached to scintillation crystals. Usually four such photomultipliers are attached to a block of scintillation crystals (left). Digital detectors use silicon PMT instead (right). The Silicon PMT chips are arranged in different configurations each containing a large number of individual channels.

scintillation crystal (*e.g.*, 4 × 4 mm crystal area and 4 × 4 mm SiPM channel), the channel with the largest signal identifies the location of an interaction and Anger logic is not needed for event localization. However, if the crystal sizes are smaller than the channel sizes, Anger logic can be used for event localization. Figure 19-33 shows a conventional and digital PET detector module, highlighting the difference in form factors of the two detectors.

19.5.3 Continuous Bed Motion

Whole-body PET imaging is usually performed today using a series of overlapping bed positions, with the patient and bed stationary during the acquisition at each bed position, to cover the desired extent of the patient; this type of acquisition is known as "step and shoot." The bed positions are usually overlapped (up to 50%) to compensate for the decrease in scanner sensitivity at the two ends of the axial FOV. Recently, PET data acquisition with continuous bed motion (CBM) has been introduced. With CBM, the patient is continuously translated through the scanner while the PET data is acquired. Several advantages are gained from CBM during PET data acquisition: (1) Image uniformity along the axial direction is improved compared to step and shoot given that every imaged section passes through the center of the scanner (which has the highest sensitivity). This advantage, however, diminishes with increasing bed overlap percentage. (2) More flexibility in imaging workflow. With CBM, imaging can be started and stopped at any location along the axial extent of the patient, while in step-and-shoot, one is limited to an integral number of bed positions. (3) The flexibility with the imaging workflow has implications on the CT radiation exposure to the patient. Since in step-and-shoot, one is limited to an integral number of bed positions, this could lead to imaging beyond the desired area.

19.5.4 Resolution Recovery

Several factors affect PET image resolution. These have been discussed in part in Section 19.3.4. Resolution recovery, better known as PSF reconstruction, in PET imaging is a method that compensates for these effects. Several approaches to determine the resolution loss due to these effects have been proposed. These approaches rely on analytical derivations, Monte Carlo simulations, or direct experimental measurements with the last approach being the common approach used on current PET systems. With PSF reconstruction, the effects of resolution loss are modeled as part of the iterative reconstruction process and have been shown to improve the spatial resolution of reconstructed PET images as well as contrast recovery and lesion detectability. One concern with PSF reconstruction, however, is its impact on PET image quantification. With PSF reconstruction an artificial increase in signal intensity (radioactivity concentration) might be seen at the edges of objects that could potentially bias SUV measurements. Several manufacturers provide PSF reconstruction as an option on their PET systems. Figure 19-34 shows a comparison of PET image reconstruction with ToF, PSF, and regularized reconstruction (described later in this section). The figure shows improvement of image quality as these advances in PET imaging are applied during image reconstruction.

19.5.5 Motion Compensation

Two of the main advantages of PET imaging are its superior spatial resolution in comparison to other nuclear medicine imaging and its ability to accurately quantify the radioactivity distribution in the resultant reconstructed images, which is important in clinical decision-making and research. These advantages, however, are challenged by many factors, chief amongst them being patient motion, particularly respiratory and cardiac motion. Patient motion effects on PET/CT image quantification are attributed to two factors. One is the mismatch between the PET and CT images and the second is the motion blur that occurs during the PET image acquisition. Mismatch between PET and CT images can occur due to the difference in imaging time between CT and PET. In CT the object of interest is captured in one phase/amplitude of its motion cycle (end-expiration for example), while in PET the resultant image represents the average location of that moving object (averaged over the whole excursion of lesion motion). This difference results in attenuation correction artifacts that lead to errors in quantification, given that the CT is used to correct for attenuation. Several techniques have been developed to address the mismatch and image blur, with various levels of success and adoption into routine clinical work primarily due to the complexity of the workflows to implement them. These techniques include 4D PET/CT and quiescent phase/amplitude gating.

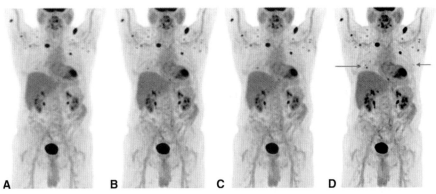

■ FIGURE 19-34 PET maximum intensity projection images with various applied data reconstruction improvements. Images with PSF reconstruction only **(A)**; with ToF and PSF **(B)**, with regularized reconstruction and PSF **(C)** and PSF, ToF and regularized reconstruction **(D)**. From left to right, the image quality improves with the addition of various advances in image reconstruction. The arrows clearly show small lesions that were not apparent on other reconstructions.

In 4D PET/CT, the motion cycle is divided into multiple bins and the corresponding PET data are acquired into each of these bins, essentially freezing the motion to that within the duration of each of the bins. Similarly, a CT scan is acquired for each of these bins and is then used to correct for attenuation of the corresponding PET bin. In this regard, the PET and CT images are matched and the PET images will have reduced motion blur, but at the expense of increased patient radiation dose from the multiple CT scans and increased noise since each PET image represents a fraction of the total imaging time. The latter, however, can be rectified by combining all the PET images into a single image through image registration during or following image reconstruction. Several software tools are currently available from manufacturers to achieve this objective. In quiescent gating, PET and CT image data are acquired only during one part of the motion cycle that has the least amount of movement (such as the end-expiration phase). In this case, the PET and CT data are matched and the PET images have reduced blur. Quiescent gating of PET data acquisition is currently available from manufacturers. Figure 19-35 shows PET maximum intensity projection images reconstructed without and with motion compensation using both of these software tools. The motion-compensated images show reduced tumor blur, which allows better visualization and lesion quantification.

19.5.6 Data-Driven Gating

Both motion compensation techniques (4D PET/CT and quiescent gating) require external hardware devices to record the motion cycle. Several such devices have been developed by various vendors based on different techniques (such as infrared cameras, strain gauges) all of which are relatively cumbersome to use, which has led to their infrequent use in routine clinical workflows. Recently, data-driven gating (DDG) techniques have been introduced to overcome this challenge. With DDG, no external devices are needed since the motion signal is derived from the PET data itself. Several approaches are currently under development and various manufacturers are in the process of making such approaches available on their commercial scanners. These approaches all depend on a high SNR to allow the extraction of the motion waveform from the background noise. In this regard, it is expected that scanners with high SNR will fare better with DDG than others. It is anticipated that with the elimination of

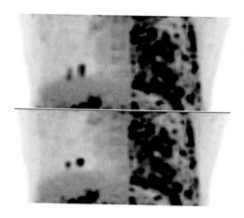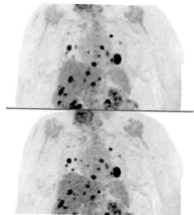

■ **FIGURE 19-35** PET maximum intensity projection image reconstructions without (top panel) and with (bottom panel) motion compensation using Qstatic (left) and HD-Chest (right). The motion compensated images (bottom panel) show improved lesion visibility, which leads to more accurate quantification.

external devices for recording the motion cycle, the motion compensation workflows will become much easier to use and will be adopted routinely in the PET clinic. In return, PET image quantification will be more accurate and patient management will be more precise.

19.5.7   Longer Axial Field of View

Traditionally, PET scanners have been designed as cylindrical structures with detectors covering the circumference of these structures and oriented towards the central axis of the cylinder. For a long time, commercial designs had diameters on the order of 80–100 cm, with lengths of about 15 cm, with detectors arranged in blocks or continuous modules around the circumference. Scanners with smaller diameters and longer extents are characterized by higher sensitivity—higher capability to capture the emitted annihilation photons at the expense of a tighter patient bore and higher cost. More recently, scanners with longer axial lengths have been introduced. By placing detector modules abutting next to one another, along the axial extent of the scanner, lengths of 20 to 26 cm are typical for commercial systems. One manufacturer has achieved 194 cm. This increase in axial extent has many advantages: it increases scanner throughput by reducing patient scan time, which improves the patient's experience, and it also increases scanner sensitivity, which can be traded for a reduced injected activity and hence a reduced patient radiation dose. It is important to note that the faster scan time comes from two primary gains, an increase in patient coverage as well as an increase in scanner sensitivity. With such scanners, a whole-body PET/CT scan can be performed in a couple of minutes, potentially transforming the use of PET imaging from a diagnostic tool to a screening tool. Other advantages of scanners with longer axial extents include the ability to perform multiple organ dynamic imaging, which enables the study of the biodistribution and pharmacokinetics of new radiopharmaceuticals and disease states with images representing true biological parameters (such as Ki, blood flow, receptor density) rather than semi-quantitative values such as SUVs.

19.5.8   Improved Image Reconstruction

Image reconstruction in PET has evolved throughout the years from the original 2D analytic techniques such as filtered backprojection to the more recent 3D iterative techniques such as ordered subset expectation maximization (OSEM), while incorporating several data corrections (such as attenuation, scatter, resolution recovery, etc.), during the iterative reconstruction (IR) process. With analytic techniques, the resultant image is generated directly from the acquired data while in IR techniques the resultant image is an estimate of the acquired data. Both 3D analytical and IR techniques are currently available on current PET and PET/CT systems with the latter being more routinely used in clinical whole-body PET imaging A major advantage of IR techniques are their ability to more accurately model the physics of the imaging process compared to analytical methods; however, these techniques are computationally expensive and require a longer time to reach convergence (solution). Additionally, IR techniques increase image noise with an increasing number of iterations. In this regard, most IR algorithms are terminated early at the expense of increased bias (underestimation) in the resultant image. To overcome this latter drawback, techniques that enforce desired resultant image properties (such as smoothness) during reconstruction have been introduced recently. Such techniques are known as regularized reconstruction (Fig. 19-34), which also include the maximum a posteriori

(MAP) reconstruction algorithm that could, in addition to constraining image noise, also include anatomical priors from other imaging modalities such as CT and MR to preserve edges in the resultant image.

Modeling data corrections during IR assumes that data correction maps are available. In PET/CT for example, attenuation correction maps are derived from the corresponding CT image and are used to correct for photon attenuation during the image reconstruction process. However, there are several situations where such CT attenuation maps might be compromised, such as in the case of metal artifacts, truncation, and contrast media, or in the case of PET/MR where such an attenuation map is not available altogether since MR images do not represent tissue attenuation. In this regard, new reconstruction algorithms, such as the maximum likelihood reconstruction of attenuation and activity (MLAA) that can approximate both the attenuation map and the resultant image, have been proposed and hold promise in addressing these challenges. More recently, artificial intelligence along with machine learning that uses deep learning algorithms have also been employed for PET image reconstruction. The performance of these techniques is currently being evaluated under various clinical conditions such as low count density (shorter scan times, low activity), and varying radiopharmaceutical biodistributions. Additionally, these approaches are also being considered to replace the reconstruction process altogether by just evaluating the acquired data and then predicting the resultant image from prior learned combination of acquired data and resultant images. Finally, as indicated before, the current trend towards improving the coincidence timing resolution of PET scanners (currently in the range of 200–250 ps) could potentially eliminate the whole process of image reconstruction since the image will be generated directly as the data is being acquired. With timing resolution in the order of 25–50 ps, the resultant error in the spatial positioning of the annihilation event origin will be on the order of about 5 mm, which is the current resolution of PET images.

19.6 CLINICAL ASPECTS, COMPARISON OF PET AND SPECT, AND DOSE

As mentioned in the first chapter of this textbook, nuclear medicine imaging produces images depicting function. The function depicted may be a mechanical function, such as the ability of the heart to contract, but very often is a physiological or biochemical function. However, a disadvantage is that the images may lack sufficient anatomic information to permit the determination of the organ or tissue containing a feature of interest. The fusion of nuclear medicine images with those from another modality, such as CT, providing a good depiction of anatomy can resolve this problem. Another disadvantage of imaging radiopharmaceuticals is that attenuation by the patient of the emitted photons can cause artifacts. CT attenuation information can be used to largely correct these artifacts.

19.6.1 F-18 Fluorodeoxyglucose and Other PET Radiopharmaceuticals

As discussed in the previous chapter, the utility of nuclear medicine is as much determined by the radiopharmaceutical as it is by the imaging device. For example, the success of the Anger scintillation camera was in part due to the development of many radiopharmaceuticals incorporating Tc-99m.

An advantage of PET is that there are positron-emitting radioisotopes of the common biochemical elements carbon, nitrogen, and oxygen, but these have short half-lives (20, 10, and 2 min, respectively). The use of radiopharmaceuticals incorporating them requires a nearby or on-site cyclotron and so their use has largely been restricted to research.

The widespread clinical adoption of PET and now PET/CT has been driven by the remarkable radiochemical (F-18)2-fluoro-2-deoxy-D-glucose (F-18 FDG). F-18 FDG is a glucose analog; it is transported by facilitated diffusion into cells that utilize glucose and phosphorylated, as is glucose. However, the phosphorylated F-18 FDG cannot proceed further along the metabolic path of glucose and therefore remains in the cells. Thus, F-18 accumulates in cells at a rate proportional to local extracellular concentration and glucose uptake. (Some cells have an enzyme that dephosphorylates glucose-6-phosphate and some F-18 FDG escapes these cells.) F-18 has a half-life of 110 min, permitting a cyclotron-equipped radiopharmacy to provide F-18 FDG throughout a metropolitan area or even over larger distances. FDG has shown clinical utility for differentiating Alzheimer's disease from other forms of dementia, identifying foci responsible for epileptic seizures, for differentiating hypoperfused myocardium from scar tissue, and for identifying loci of infections. However, its most common application today is in oncology, in which it is used to evaluate and assess the efficacy of treatment for the many forms of cancer that accumulate glucose. Nonetheless, F-18 FDG is only of limited use in some forms of cancer, notably prostate cancer.

The FDA has approved other PET radiopharmaceuticals such asfluorine-18 sodium fluoride for skeletal imaging, gallium-68 Dotatate (NetSpot) for neuroendocrine cancer, fluorine-18 Fluciclovine (Axumin) for prostate cancer, and rubidium-82 chloride for myocardial perfusion imaging; these are described in Chapter 16. Other PET radiopharmaceuticals are under study.

19.6.2 Radiation Doses

As mentioned in Chapter 16, the radiation doses from the administration of a radiopharmaceutical depend on the physiological behavior of the radiopharmaceutical, the physical half-life of the radionuclide, the activity administered, and the types and energies of the radiations emitted. Positrons deposit nearly all of their kinetic energies within millimeters of the sites of their emission. Much, but not all, of the energy of the annihilation photons escapes the patient. To keep the doses to patients sufficiently low, the radionuclides commonly used in PET have been restricted to ones with relatively short half-lives. The intravenous administration of 370 MBq (10 mCi) of F-18 FDG to an adult imparts an effective dose of about 7 mSv (Appendix F-2).

The radiation dose from a PET/CT or SPECT/CT examination includes that of the CT scan. In oncologic PET/CT, the CT scan is typically performed on a length of the body from just below the eyes to the symphysis pubis. The effective dose from this CT scan is relatively large because of the length of the body that is scanned. The CT scan can be a high x-ray tube current scan that produces images of diagnostic quality, or it can be a low dose scan that produces images only for attenuation correction and anatomic correlation. The effective dose from the former may be about 16 mSv, whereas that from the latter may be about 4 mSv (Brix et al., 2005). Innovations in CT such as automatic tube current modulation and iterative image reconstruction may reduce these doses.

19.6.3 Comparison of SPECT and PET

In single-photon emission imaging, the spatial resolution and the detection efficiency are primarily determined by the collimator. Both are ultimately limited by the compromise between collimator efficiency and collimator spatial resolution that is a

TABLE 19-6 COMPARISON OF SPECT AND PET

	SPECT	PET
Principle of projection data collection	Collimation.	Annihilation coincidence detection (ACD).
Transverse image reconstruction	Iterative methods or filtered backprojection.	Iterative methods or filtered backprojection.
Radionuclides	Any emitting x rays, γ-rays, or annihilation photons. Optimal performance for photon energies of 100–200 keV.	Positron emitters only.
Spatial resolution	Depends upon collimator and camera orbit.	Relatively constant across transaxial image, best at center.
	Within a transaxial image, the resolution in the radial direction is relatively uniform, but the tangential resolution is degraded toward the center.	Typically 4.5–5 mm FWHM at center.
	Typically about 10 mm FWHM at center for a 30 cm diameter orbit and Tc-99m.	
	Larger camera orbits produce worse resolution.	
Attenuation	Attenuation less severe. Radioactive attenuation correction sources or x-ray CT can correct for attenuation.	Attenuation more severe. Radioactive attenuation correction sources or x-ray CT can correct for attenuation.

consequence of collimated image formation. It is the use of ACD instead of collimation that makes the PET scanner much more efficient than the scintillation camera and also yields its superior spatial resolution.

In systems that use collimation to form images, the spatial resolution rapidly deteriorates with distance from the face of the imaging device. This causes the spatial resolution to deteriorate from the edge to the center in transverse SPECT images. In contrast, PET is not subject to this limitation and the spatial resolution in a transverse PET image is best in the center.

The cost of a dual-head SPECT system is typically a few hundred thousand dollars. The cost of a SPECT-CT system depends greatly on the capabilities of the CT system. As mentioned previously, some have slow low-dose CT systems that are not capable of producing diagnostic quality CT images, whereas others have multirow detector, subsecond rotation CT systems that can produce diagnostic-quality images. The cost of the latter system may be more than twice that of a SPECT system without CT. The cost of a PET/CT system is about twice that of a SPECT/CT system capable of diagnostic quality CT imaging. Table 19-6 compares SPECT and PET systems.

SUGGESTED READING AND REFERENCES

American College of Radiology. *PET Accreditation Program Testing Instructions.* Reston, Virginia: American College of Radiology; 2018. https://accreditationsupport.acr.org/support/solutions/articles/11000062800-phantom-testing-pet

Bax JJ, Wijns W. Editorial—fluorodeoxyglucose imaging to assess myocardial viability: PET, SPECT, or gamma camera coincidence imaging. *J Nucl Med.* 1999;40:1893-1895.

Boellaard R. Standards for PET image acquisition and quantitative data analysis. *J Nucl Med.* 2009;50 (suppl 1):11S-20S.

Boren EL Jr, Delbeke D, Patton JA, Sandler MP. Comparison of FDG PET and positron coincidence detection imaging using a dual-head gamma camera with 5/8-inch NaI(Tl) crystals in patients with suspected body malignancies. *Eur J Nucl Med Mol I.* 1999;26(4):379-387.

Brix G, Lechel U, Glatting G, Ziegler SI, Münzing W, Müller SP, Beyer T. Radiation exposure of patients undergoing whole-body dual-modality ^{18}F-FDG PET/CT examinations. *J Nucl Med.* 2005;46:608-613.

Carney JPJ, Townsend DW, Rappoport V, Bendriem B. Method for transforming CT images for attenuation correction in PET/CT imaging. *Med Phys.* 2006;33(4):976-983.

Chang LT. A method for attenuation correction in radionuclide computed tomography. *IEEE Trans Nucl Sci.* 1978;NS-25:638.

Cherry SR, Phelps ME. Positron emission tomography: methods and instrumentation. In: Sandler MP, et al., eds. *Diagnostic Nuclear Medicine.* 4th ed. Baltimore, MD: Lippincott Williams & Wilkins; 2003:61-83.

Delbeke D, Patton JA, Martin WH, Sandler MP. FDG PET and dual-head gamma camera positron coincidence detection imaging of suspected malignancies and brain disorders. *J Nucl Med.* 1999;40(1):110-117.

DePuey EG. Advances in SPECT camera software and hardware: currently available and new on the horizon. *J Nucl Cardiol.* 2012;19:551-581.

EANM Physics Committee: Sokole EB, Plachcínska A, Britten A with contribution from the EANM Working Group on Nuclear Medicine Instrumentation Quality Control: Georgosopoulou ML, Tindale W, Klett R. Routine quality control recommendations for nuclear medicine instrumentation. *Eur J Nucl Med Mol Imaging.* 2010;37:662-671.

Gelfand MJ, Thomas SR. *Effective Use of Computers in Nuclear Medicine.* New York, NY: McGraw-Hill; 1988.

Goetze S, Brown TL, Lavely WC, Zhang Z, Bengel FM. Attenuation correction in myocardial perfusion SPECT/CT: effects of misregistration and value of reregistration. *J Nucl Med.* 2007;48(7):1090-1095.

Groch MW, Ali A, Erwin WD, Fordham, EW. Focal plane dual head longitudinal tomography. In: Ahluwalia BD, ed. *Tomographic Methods in Nuclear Medicine: Physical Principles, Instruments and Clinical Applications.* Boca Raton, FL: CRC Press; 1988:123-150.

Groch MW, Erwin WD. SPECT in the year 2000: basic principles. *J Nucl Med Technol.* 2000;28:233-244.

Groch MW, Erwin WD, Bieszk JA. Single photon emission computed tomography. In: Treves ST, ed. *Pediatric Nuclear Medicine.* 2nd ed. New York, NY: Springer-Verlag; 1995:33-87.

Hendel RC, et al. The value and practice of attenuation correction for myocardial perfusion SPECT imaging: a joint position statement from the American Society of Nuclear Cardiology and the Society of Nuclear Medicine. *J Nucl Med.* 2002;43(2):273-280.

Hines H, Kayayan R, Colsher J, et al. NEMA recommendations for implementing SPECT instrumentation quality control. *J Nucl Med.* 2000;41:383-389.

Hudson HM, Larkin RS. Accelerated image reconstruction using ordered subsets of projection data. *IEEE Trans Med Imaging.* 1994;13:601-609.

IAEA human health series No. 6: quality assurance for SPECT systems. Vienna: International Atomic Energy Agency; 2009 (available on-line).

IAEA human health series No. 36: SPECT/CT atlas of quality control and image artefacts. Vienna: International Atomic Energy Agency; 2019 (available on-line).

Keyes JW Jr. SUV: standard uptake or silly useless value? *J Nucl Med.* 1995;36:1836-1839.

Kuhl DE, Edwards RQ. Image separation radioisotope scanning. *Radiology.* 1963;80:653-662.

Liu Y-H, Lam PT, Sinusas AJ, Wackers FJTh. Differential effect of 180° and 360° acquisition orbits on the accuracy of SPECT imaging: quantitative evaluation in phantoms. *J Nuclear Med.* 2002;43(8):1115-1124.

Macfarlane DJ, Cotton L, Ackermann RJ, et al. Triple-head SPECT with 2-[fluorine-18]fluoro-2-deoxy-D-glucose (FDG): initial evaluation in oncology and comparison with FDG PET. *Radiology.* 1995;194:425-429.

Masood Y, et al. Clinical validation of SPECT attenuation correction using x-ray computed tomography–derived attenuation maps: multicenter clinical trial with angiographic correlation. *J Nuclear Cardiol.* 2005;12(6);676-686.

Mawlawi O, Erasmus JJ, et al. Quantifying the effect of iv contrast media on integrated PET/CT: clinical evaluation. *AJR Am J Roentgenol.* 2006;186:308-319.

Meier JG, Erasmus JJ, Gladish GW, Peterson CB, Diab RH, Mawlawi OR. Characterization of continuous bed motion effects on patient breathing and respiratory motion correction in PET/CT imaging. *J Appl Clin Med Phys.* 2020;21(1):158-165.

National Electrical Manufacturers Association, NEMA NU 1-2007, Performance Measurements of Gamma Cameras.

National Electrical Manufacturers Association, NEMA NU 2-2007, Performance Measurements of Positron Emission Tomographs.

Nichols KJ. Editorial: how serious a problem for myocardial perfusion assessment is moderate misregistration between SPECT and CT? *J Nuclear Cardiol.* 2007;14(2):150-152.

Otero HJ, Yap JT, et al. Evaluation of low-density neutral oral contrast material in PET/CT for tumor imaging: results of a randomized clinical trial. *AJR Am J Roentgenol.* 2009;193:326-332.

Oturai PS, Mortensen J, Enevoldsen H, et al. gamma cameras ^{18}F-FDG PET in diagnosis and staging of patients presenting with suspected lung cancer and comparison with dedicated PET. *J Nucl Med.* 2004;45(8):1351-1357.

Patton JA, Turkington TG. SPECT/CT physical principles and attenuation correction. *J Nucl Med Technol.* 2008;36:1-10.

Phelps ME, Huang SC, Hoffman EJ, Selin C, Sokoloff L, Kuhl DE. Tomographic measurement of local cerebral glucose metabolic rate in humans with (F-18)2-fluoro-2-deoxy-D-glucose: validation of method. *Ann Neurol.* 1979;6:371-388.

Raff U, Kirch DL, Hendee WR. Seven-pinhole tomography in nuclear medicine. In: Ahluwalia BD, ed. *Tomographic Methods in Nuclear Medicine: Physical Principles, Instruments and Clinical Applications.* Boca Raton, FL: CRC Press; 1988:173-200.

Sokoloff L, Reivich M, Kennedy C, et al. The [14C] deoxyglucose method for the measurement of local cerebral glucose utilization: theory, procedure, and normal values in the conscious and anesthetized albino rat. *J Neurochem.* 1977;28:897-916.

Sureshbabu W, Mawlawi O. PET/CT imaging artifacts. *J Nucl Med Technol.* 2005;33:156-161.

Thie JA. Understanding the standardized uptake value, its methods, and implications for usage. *J Nucl Med.* 2004;45(9):1431-1434.

Tiepolt C, Beuthien-Baumann B, Hlises R, et al. 18F-FDG for the staging of patients with differentiated thyroid cancer: comparison of a dual-head coincidence gamma camera with dedicated PET. *Ann Nucl Med.* 2000;14(5):339-345.

Yester MV, Graham LS, eds. Advances in nuclear medicine: the medical physicist's perspective. Proceedings of the 1998 Nuclear Medicine Mini Summer School, American Association of Physicists in Medicine, June 21–23, 1998, Madison, WI.

Yutani K, Tatsumi M, Shiba E, Kusuoka H, Nishimura T. Comparison of dual-head coincidence gamma camera FDG imaging with FDG PET in detection of breast cancer and axillary lymph node metastasis. *J Nucl Med.* 1999;40(6):1003-1008.

Zaidi H, ed. *Quantitative Analysis in Nuclear Medicine Imaging.* New York, NY: Springer; 2006.

Zanzonico P. Routine quality control of clinical nuclear medicine instrumentation: a brief review. *J Nucl Med.* 2008;49:1114-1131.

Zhang H, Tian M, Oriuchi N, Higuchi T, Tanada S, Endo K. Oncological diagnosis using positron coincidence gamma camera with fluorodeoxyglucose in comparison with dedicated PET. *Br J Radiol.* 2002;75:409-416.

Zimny M, Kaiser HJ, Cremerius U, et al. F-18-FDG positron imaging in oncological patients: gamma camera coincidence detection versus dedicated PET. *Nuklearmedizin.* 1999;38(4):108-114.

SECTION

IV

Radiation Biology and Protection

CHAPTER 20

Radiation Biology

20.1 OVERVIEW

Rarely have beneficial applications and hazards to human health followed a major scientific discovery more rapidly than with the discovery of ionizing radiation. Soon after Roentgen's discovery of x-rays in 1895 and Becquerel's discovery of natural radioactivity in 1896, adverse biological effects from ionizing radiation were observed. Within months after their discovery, x-rays were being used in medical diagnosis and treatment. Unfortunately, the development and implementation of radiation protection techniques lagged behind the rapidly increasing use of radiation sources. Within the first 6 months of their use, several cases of erythema, dermatitis, and alopecia were reported among x-ray operators and their patients. Becquerel himself observed radiation-induced erythema on his abdomen from a vial of radium he carried in his vest pocket during a trip to London to present his discovery. Many years later, this effect was referred to as a "Becquerel burn." The first report of a skin cancer ascribed to x-rays was in 1902, to be followed 8 years later by experimental confirmation. However, it was not until 1915 that the first radiation protection recommendations were made by the British Roentgen Society, followed by similar recommendations from the American Roentgen Ray Society in 1922.

The study of the action of ionizing radiation on healthy and diseased tissue is the scientific discipline known as radiation biology. Radiation biologists seek to understand the nature and sequence of events that occur following the absorption of energy from ionizing radiation, the biological consequences of any damage that results, and the mechanisms that enhance, compensate for, or repair the damage. A century of radiobiologic research has amassed more information about the effects of ionizing radiation on living systems than is known about almost any other physical or chemical agent.

This chapter reviews the consequences of ionizing radiation exposure, beginning with the chemical basis by which radiation damage is initiated and its subsequent effects on cells, tissues and organ systems, and the whole body. This is followed by a review of the concepts and risks associated with radiation-induced carcinogenesis, hereditary effects, and the special concerns regarding radiation exposure of the fetus.

20.2 DETERMINANTS AND CLASSIFICATION OF THE BIOLOGIC RESPONSE OF RADIATION

20.2.1 Determinants of Biologic Response

Many factors contribute to producing the overall biologic response to radiation exposure. At the highest level, these variables can be thought of as those associated with the radiation source and those of the biological system being irradiated. The identification of these biologic effects depends on the method of observation and the time following irradiation. Radiation-related factors include the absorbed dose (quantity) and dose rate as well as the type and energy (quality) of the radiation. The radiosensitivity of a complex biologic system is determined by a number of variables. Some of these are inherent to the type of cells exposed while others relate to the cell's current biochemical, mitotic, and oxygen tension status as well as many other variables at the time of irradiation. Damage observed at the molecular or cellular level may or may not result in clinically detectable adverse effects. Furthermore, although some responses to radiation exposure appear instantaneously or within minutes to hours, others take weeks, years, or even decades to appear.

20.2.2 Classification of Biologic Effects

Biologic effects of radiation exposure can be classified as either *stochastic effects* or *tissue reactions (deterministic effects)*. A stochastic effect is one in which the probability of the effect occurring, rather than its severity, increases with dose. Radiation-induced cancer and hereditary effects are stochastic in nature. For example, the probability of radiation-induced leukemia is substantially greater after an exposure to 1 Gy than to 10 mGy, but there will be no difference in the severity of the disease if it occurs. Stochastic effects are believed not to have a dose threshold, because damage to a few cells or even a single cell could theoretically result in the production of the disease. Therefore, even minor exposures may carry some, albeit small, increased risk (*i.e.*, increased probability of radiation-induced cancer or a genetic effect). It is this basic, but unproven, model that *risk increases with dose and there is no threshold dose below which the magnitude of the risk goes to zero,* that is the basis of modern radiation protection programs, a goal of which is to keep exposures *as low as reasonably achievable* (see Chapter 21). Stochastic effects are regarded as the principal health risk from low-dose radiation, including exposures of patients and staff to radiation from diagnostic imaging procedures.

If the radiation dose to tissue is very high, the predominant biologic effect is cell killing, which presents clinically as degenerative changes in the exposed tissue. In this case, the effects are classified as *tissue reactions* (previously called deterministic effects), for which the severity of the injury, rather than its probability of occurrence, increases with dose. Tissue reactions differ from stochastic effects in that they require much higher doses to produce clinically observable effects and there is a *threshold* dose below which the effect does not occur or is subclinical. Skin erythema, fibrosis, and hematopoietic system damage are some of the tissue reactions that can result from large radiation exposures. As there is substantial individual variability in response to radiation, the "threshold dose" is just an approximation of the dose that would result in the specified effect. Many of these effects are discussed in the sections entitled "Response of Organ Systems to Radiation" and "The Acute Radiation Syndrome." Tissue reactions can be caused by severe radiation accidents and can be observed in healthy tissue that is unavoidably irradiated during radiation therapy. Although they have been observed following some lengthy, fluoroscopically guided interventional procedures (Koenig et al., 2001; Shope, 1996), they are unlikely to occur as a result of routine diagnostic imaging procedures or occupational exposure.

20.3 INTERACTION OF RADIATION WITH CELLS AND TISSUE

As discussed in Chapter 3, x- and γ-ray photon interactions in tissue, as well as radiations emitted during radionuclide decay, result in the production of energetic electrons. These electrons transfer their kinetic energy to surrounding matter via excitation, ionization, and thermal heating. Energy is deposited randomly and rapidly (in $<10^{-8}$ seconds [s]), and the secondary ionizations set many more low-energy electrons in motion, causing additional excitation and ionization along the path of the initial energetic electron. For example, a single 30 keV electron, set in motion following the photoelectric absorption of a single x-ray or γ-ray photon, can result in the production of over 1,000 low-energy secondary electrons (referred to as *delta rays*), each of which may cause additional excitation or ionization events in the tissue (Goodhead, 1994). This chain of ionizations ultimately gives rise to subexcitation electrons (*i.e.*, electrons with kinetic energies less than the first excitation potential of liquid water, 7.4 eV) that become thermalized as they transfer their remaining kinetic energy by vibrational, rotational, and collisional energy exchanges with the water molecules. Observable effects such as chromosome breakage, cell death, oncogenic transformation, and acute radiation sickness, all have their origin in radiation-induced chemical changes in important biomolecules.

20.3.1   Low Energy Electrons and Complex Damage

The delta rays and other lower-energy electrons, set in motion following an initial ionizing event, produce a unique ionization pattern in which closely spaced ionizations occur over a very short range (~4 to 12 nm) along the path of the primary ionization track. The energy deposition (~100 eV) along the shorter tracks referred to as *spurs*, whose diameters are approximately 4 to 5 nm, result in an average of three ionizing events. It is estimated that 95% of the energy deposition events from x-rays and γ-rays occur in spurs (Hall and Giaccia, 2018). Longer and less frequent pear-shaped tracks called *blobs* deposit more energy (~300 to 500 eV) and thus on average result in more ionization events (~12 ion pairs) over their path (~12 nm). High concentrations of reactive chemical species (such as free radicals—discussed below) are produced in these spurs and blobs and they increase the probability of molecular damage at these locations (Fig. 20-1A and B). If ionizing events occur near the DNA, whose diameter (~2 nm) is on the same order as that of these short ionization tracks, they can produce damage in multiple locations in the DNA in close proximity to one another. These lesions, initially referred to as *locally multiply damaged sites*, are more difficult for the cell to repair and may be repaired incorrectly, Figure 20-1C (Goodhead, 1994; Ward, 1988). Synonyms for this type of damage in common use today include *clustered damage, complex damage,* and *multiply damaged sites* (MDS).

While endogenous processes, such as oxidative metabolism, mainly produce isolated DNA lesions, the complex clustered damage, in which groups of several damaged nucleotides occur within one or two helical turns of the DNA, is a hallmark of ionizing radiation-induced DNA damage. However while the radiation-induced pattern of molecular damage is different from other oxidative events in the cell of endogenous and exogenous (*e.g.*, chemotherapy) origin, many of the functional changes produced in molecules, cells, tissues, and organs cannot be distinguished from damage produced by these other sources.

Repair of radiation damage occurs at molecular, cellular, and tissue levels. A complex series of enzymes and cofactors repair most radiation-induced DNA lesions within hours and, to the extent possible, damaged cells are often replaced within days following irradiation. However, the clinical manifestation of radiation-induced damage may appear over a period of time that varies from minutes to weeks and even years depending on the radiation dose, cell type, and the nature and scope of the damage. Only a fraction of the radiation energy deposited brings about chemical changes; the vast majority of the energy is deposited as heat. The heat produced is of little biologic significance compared with the heat generated by normal metabolic processes. For example, it would take more than 4,000 Gy, a supralethal dose, to raise the temperature of tissue by 1°C.

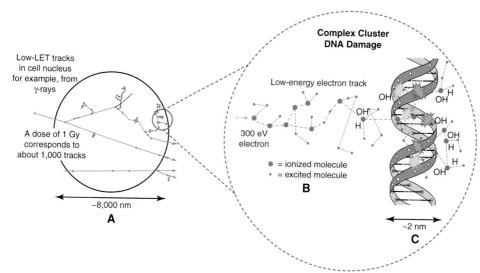

■ FIGURE 20-1 A. Low-LET radiation like x-rays and γ-rays is considered sparsely ionizing on average; however, a majority of the radiation energy is deposited in small regions (on the scale of nanometers) via denser clusters of ionizations from low-energy secondary electrons. This illustration depicts primary and secondary electron tracks producing clusters of ionization events. The calculated number of tracks is based on a cell nucleus with a diameter of 8 μm. The track size is enlarged relative to the nucleus to illustrate the theoretical track structure. **B.** A segment of the electron track is illustrated utilizing a Monte Carlo simulation of clustered damage produced by ionizations and excitations along the path of a low-energy (300 eV) electron. Excitation and ionization along with secondary electrons are shown until the electron energy drops below the ionization potential of water (~10 eV). **C.** DNA double helix drawn on the same scale as the ionization track. Complex clustered damage can result from closely spaced damage to the DNA sugar-phosphate backbone and bases from both direct ionizations and diffusion of OH radicals produced by the radiolysis of water molecules in close proximity (few nm) with the DNA (*i.e.*, indirect effect). Multiple damaged sites are shown as green, or orange, explosion symbols that denote DNA strand breaks, or damaged bases, respectively. In this example, the result is a complex double-strand break, consisting of three strand breaks and three damaged bases, all within ten base pairs along the DNA. This type of complex DNA lesion is more difficult for the cell to repair and can lead to cell death, impaired cell function, or transformations with oncogenic potential. (Reprinted with permission from Goodhead DT. Energy deposition stochastics and track structure: what about the target? *Radiat Prot Dosimetry*. 2006;122(1-4):3-15. Copyright © Oxford University Press.)

20.3.2 Free Radical Formation and Interactions

Radiation interactions that produce biologic changes are classified as either *direct* or *indirect*. The change is said to be due to direct action if a biologic macromolecule such as DNA, RNA, or protein becomes ionized or excited by an ionizing particle or photon passing through or near it. Indirect action refers to effects that are the result of radiation interactions within the medium (*e.g.*, cytoplasm) that create mobile, chemically reactive species that in turn interact with nearby macromolecules. Because approximately 70% of most cells in the body are composed of water, the majority (~70%) of radiation-induced damage from medical irradiation is caused by radiation interactions with water molecules. The physical and chemical events that occur when radiation interacts with a water molecule lead to the formation of a number of different highly reactive chemical species. Initially, water molecules are ionized to form H_2O^+ and free electrons (e^-). The e^- rapidly thermalizes and becomes hydrated, with a sphere of water molecules orienting around the e^- to form a hydrated or aqueous electron (e^-_{aq}). The e^-_{aq} then reacts with another water molecule to form a negative water ion $(H_2O + e^-_{aq} \rightarrow H_2O^-)$. These water ions are very unstable; each rapidly forms another ion and a *free radical*:

$$H_2O^+ + H_2O \rightarrow H_3O^+ + {}^\bullet OH \text{ (Hydroxyl Radical)}$$
$$H_2O^- \rightarrow OH^- + H\bullet \text{ (Hydrogen Radical)}$$

Free radicals are atomic or molecular species that have unpaired orbital electrons. They are denoted by a dot next to the chemical symbol of the element with the unpaired electron. Thus, free radicals can be radical ions (*e.g.*, H_2O^+ and H_2O^-), or electrically neutral ($^\cdot OH$, $H\cdot$). The hydrogen and hydroxyl radicals can be created by other reaction pathways, the most important of which is the radiation-induced excitation and disassociation of a water molecule (H_2O^* excitation $\rightarrow$ H· and $^\cdot OH$). The H^+ and OH^- ions do not typically produce significant biologic damage because of their extremely short lifetimes ($\sim 10^{-10}$ s) and their tendency to recombine to form water. Free radicals are extremely reactive chemical species that can undergo a variety of chemical reactions. Free radicals can combine with other free radicals to form nonreactive chemical species such as water (*e.g.*, H· + $^\cdot OH \rightarrow H_2O$), in which case no biologic damage occurs, or with each other to form other molecules such as hydrogen peroxide (*e.g.*, $^\cdot OH + ^\cdot OH \rightarrow H_2O_2$), which is toxic to the cell. However, for low linear energy transfer (LET) radiation like x- and γ-rays (see Chapter 3), the molecular yield of H_2O_2 is low and the majority of indirect effects are due to the interactions of the hydroxyl radicals with biologically important molecules.

The damaging effect of free radicals is enhanced by the presence of oxygen. Oxygen reacts with free radicals and reduces the probability of free radical recombination into nontoxic chemicals such as water or molecular hydrogen. Oxygen can combine with the hydrogen radical to form a highly reactive oxygen species (ROS) such as the hydroperoxyl radical (*e.g.*, H· + $O_2 \rightarrow HO_2\cdot$). Free radicals can act as strong oxidizing or reducing agents by combining directly with macromolecules. Free radicals can attack biomolecules (R) in a number of ways, including hydrogen abstraction (RH + $^\cdot OH \rightarrow R\cdot + H_2O$) and $^\cdot OH$ addition (R + $^\cdot OH \rightarrow ROH\cdot$). Chemical repair, restitution, of the damaged biomolecules can occur via radical recombination (*e.g.*, R· + H· $\rightarrow$ RH) or more commonly, by hydrogen donation from thiol compounds (RSH + R· $\rightarrow$ RH + RS·), producing the much less reactive or damaging thiyl radical. In the presence of oxygen, chemical repair is inhibited by the transformation of organic radicals into peroxyradicals (R· + $O_2 \rightarrow RO_2\cdot$). Because they are highly reactive, free radicals have limited lifetimes (less than 10^{-5} s) and very short diffusion distances, but they can diffuse sufficiently far in the cell (on the order of ~4 nm) to produce damage at locations other than their origin. Free radical–induced damage to DNA is the primary cause of biologic damage from low-LET radiation. While radiation exposure from medical imaging does result in some direct ionization of critical cellular targets, approximately two thirds of the total radiation damage is due to the free radical–mediated indirect effects of ionizing radiation.

Many enzymatic repair mechanisms exist within cells that are capable, in most cases, of returning the DNA to its preirradiated state. For example, if a break occurs in a single strand of DNA, the site of the damage is identified and the break may be repaired by rejoining the broken ends. If the damage is more complex or too severe or the cell repair mechanisms are compromised or overwhelmed by excessive radiation exposure, the damage to the DNA could persist. The clinical consequence of such DNA damage depends on a number of variables. For example, if the damage were to the DNA at a location that prevented the cell from producing albumin, the clinical consequences would be insignificant considering the number of cells remaining with the ability to produce this serum protein. If, however, the damage were to the DNA at a location that was responsible for controlling the rate of cell division (*e.g.*, in an oncogene or tumor suppressor gene), the clinical consequences could be the formation of a tumor or cancer. Heavily irradiated cells, however, often die during replication, thus preventing the propagation of seriously defective cells. Figure 20-2 summarizes the physical and biologic responses to ionizing radiation.

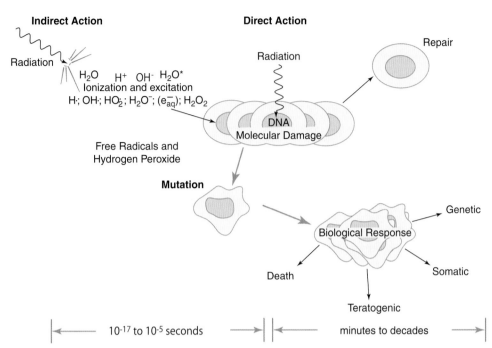

Indirect Action

Direct Action

■ **FIGURE 20-2** Physical and biologic responses to ionizing radiation. Ionizing radiation causes damage either directly by damaging the molecular target or indirectly by ionizing water, which in turn generates free radicals that attack molecular targets. The physical steps that lead to energy deposition and free radical formation occur within 10^{-5} to 10^{-6} s, whereas the biologic expression of the physical damage may occur from seconds to decades later.

Experiments with cells and animals have shown that the biologic effect of radiation depends not only on factors such as the dose, dose rate, environmental conditions at the time of irradiation, and radiosensitivity of the biologic system but also on the spatial distribution of the energy deposition at the molecular level (microdosimetry).

20.4 MOLECULAR AND CELLULAR RESPONSE TO RADIATION

Although all ionizing radiations are capable of producing similar types of biologic effects, the magnitude of the effect per unit dose differs. To evaluate the effectiveness of different types and energies of radiation and their associated LETs, experiments are performed that compare the dose required for the test radiation to produce the same specific biologic response produced by a particular dose of a reference radiation (typically, x-rays produced by a potential of 250 kV). The term relating the effectiveness of the test radiation to the reference radiation is called the *relative biological effectiveness* (RBE). The RBE is defined, for identical exposure conditions, as:

$$RBE = \frac{\text{Dose of 250-kV x-rays required to produce effect } Y}{\text{Dose of test radiation required to produce effect } Y}$$

The RBE is initially proportional to LET. As the LET of the radiation increases, so does the RBE (Fig. 20-3). The increase is attributed to the higher specific ionization (*i.e.*, ionization density) associated with high-LET radiation (*e.g.*, alpha particles) and its relative advantage in producing cellular damage (increased number and

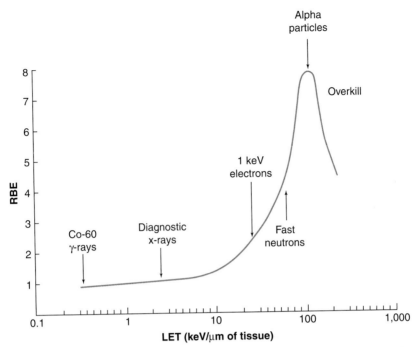

■ FIGURE 20-3 The RBE of a given radiation is an empirically derived value that, in general (with all other factors being held constant), increases with the LET of the radiation. However, beyond approximately 100 keV/μm, the radiation becomes less efficient due to overkill (*i.e.*, the maximal potential damage has already been reached), and the increase in LET beyond this point results in wasted dose.

complexity of clustered DNA lesions) compared with low-LET radiation (*e.g.*, x- and γ-rays). However, beyond approximately 100 keV/μm in tissue, the RBE decreases with increasing LET, because of the overkill effect. Overkill (or *wasted dose*) refers to the deposition of radiation energy in excess of that necessary to produce the maximal biologic effect. The RBE ranges from less than 1 to more than 20. For a particular type of radiation, the RBE depends on the biologic endpoint being studied. For example, chromosome aberrations, cataract formation, or acute lethality of test animals may be used as endpoints. Compared to high-energy γ-rays, the increased effectiveness of diagnostic x-rays in producing DNA damage is suggested not only by the differences in their microdosimetric energy deposition patterns but has also been demonstrated experimentally with an RBE of about 1.5 to 3. However, these differences do not necessarily imply (nor have epidemiological studies been able to confirm) an associated increase in cancer risk. The RBE also depends on the total dose, dose rate, fractionation, and cell type. Despite these limitations, the RBE is a useful radiobiologic tool that helps to characterize the potential damage from various types and energies of ionizing radiation. The RBE is an essential element in establishing the radiation weighting factors (w_R) discussed in Chapter 3.

Although all critical lesions responsible for cell killing have not been identified, it has been established that the radiation-sensitive targets are located in the nucleus and not in the cytoplasm of the cell. Cells contain numerous macromolecules, only some of which are essential for cell survival. For example, there are many copies of various enzymes within a cell; the loss of one particular copy would not significantly affect the cell's function or survival. However, if a key molecule, for which the cell has no replacement (*e.g.*, DNA), is damaged or destroyed, the result may be cell death. In the context of diagnostic x-ray exposure, cell death does not mean the acute physical

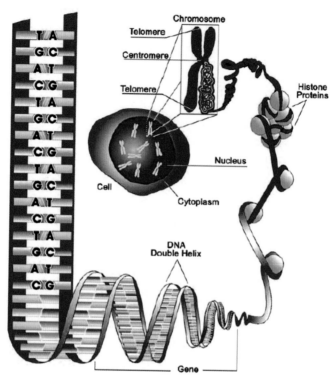

■ **FIGURE 20-4** DNA is a primary target for damage that results in radiation-induced cell and tissue effects. The schematic illustrates the many orders of chromatin packaging from "naked" DNA to give rise to the highly condensed metaphase chromosome. The double helical DNA is wrapped around histones to form nucleosomes that are packaged to produce chromatin fibers that ultimately become highly packed in the chromosomes visible at mitosis. A mitotic chromosome is characterized by the centromere, which binds the two homologous chromatids together into the chromosome. The tips of each chromosome arm contain the telomeres. A gene is a sequence of nucleotides in a given position in the chromosome that is the functional unit of hereditary information, sometimes coding for a specific protein or controlling the function of other genetic material. (Courtesy of REAC/TS).

destruction of the cell by radiation but rather a radiation-induced loss of mitotic capacity (*i.e.*, reproductive death). There is considerable evidence that damage to DNA (Fig. 20-4) is the primary cause of radiation-induced cell death.

20.4.1 Radiation-Induced DNA Damage and Response

Spectrum of DNA Damage

The deposition of energy (directly or indirectly) by ionizing radiation induces chemical changes in large molecules that may then undergo a variety of structural changes. These structural changes include (1) hydrogen bond breakage, (2) molecular degradation or breakage, and (3) intermolecular and intramolecular cross-linking. The rupture of the hydrogen bonds that link base pairs in DNA may lead to irreversible changes in the secondary and tertiary structure of the molecule that compromise genetic replication and transcription. Molecular breakages also may involve the sugar-phosphate polymers that are the backbones of the two helical DNA strands. They may occur as single-strand breaks (SSBs), double-strand breaks (DSBs) (in which both strands of the double helix break simultaneously at approximately the same nucleotide pair), base loss, base changes, or cross-links between DNA strands or between DNA and proteins (Fig. 20-5B). An SSB between the sugar and the phosphate can rejoin, provided there is no opportunity for the broken portion of the strands to separate. While the rejoining is not typically immediate, because the broken ends require the action of a series of enzymes (endonuclease, polymerase, ligase) to rejoin, the rejoining is fast and the repair typically occurs with high fidelity. The presence of oxygen potentiates the damage by causing peroxidation of a base, which then undergoes radical transfer to the sugar, causing damage that prevents rejoining.

A DSB can occur if two SSBs are juxtaposed or when a single, densely ionizing particle (*e.g.*, an alpha particle) produces a break in both strands. DNA DSBs are very genotoxic lesions that can result in chromosome aberrations. The genomic instability resulting from persistent or incorrectly repaired DSBs can lead to carcinogenesis through activation of oncogenes, inactivation of tumor suppressor genes, or loss of heterozygosity. SSBs (caused in large part by the OH radical) are more easily repaired than DSBs and are more likely to result from the sparse ionization pattern that is characteristic of low-LET radiation. For mammalian cells, an absorbed dose of one Gy from x-rays will cripple the mitotic capability of approximately half of the cells exposed. Each cell would experience approximately 40 DSBs, 1,000 SSBs, and 3,000 damaged bases. While DSBs and complex DNA damage are often associated with high-LET radiation, in reality, all ionizing radiation is capable of producing a substantial number of complex DSBs. In the case of low-LET radiations, used in diagnostic imaging, about a quarter to a third of the absorbed dose in tissue is deposited via low-energy secondary electrons with energies on the order of 0.1 to 5 keV. These low-energy electrons produce high ionization densities over very short tracks that are of the same scale as the DNA double helix. The result is an increased probability of complex DNA damage that may contain not only SSBs and DSBs but localized base damage as well. These complex DNA lesions are less likely to be repaired correctly than an isolated SSB, DSB, or base damage, which may lead to permanent DNA modifications or losses (Goodhead, 1988, 1994). The higher effectiveness of alpha particles in producing biological damage, in comparison to low-LET radiation, is not due to an increased yield of DNA damage but rather the ability of the higher ionization density to produce more complex DNA lesions (Brenner and Ward, 1992) (Fig. 20-5A). The ability to produce several MDS in proximity in the chromatin structure is referred to as regional multiply damaged sites (RMDS). These lesions are repaired more slowly, if at all, and may serve as a signal for gene induction for a longer time than following low-LET irradiation (Löbrich et al., 1996). In addition, the production of RMDS increases the probability that short double-stranded oligonucleotides will be released, making high fidelity repair without the loss of sequence information problematic. Figure 20-5 illustrates some of the common forms of damage to DNA.

When one considers radiation damage to DNA, it is important to keep in mind that cellular DNA is not "naked," but is highly organized, being wrapped around histones to form nucleosomes, which, in turn, are organized into chromatin fibers, which, ultimately, condense into the chromosomes that are visible at mitosis (Fig. 20-4). These increasing levels of complexity can also alter the radiation sensitivity of the DNA, as has been shown in studies that sequentially "simplified" the DNA structure from that in intact cells to isolated DNA.

Regardless of its severity or consequences, the loss or change of a base is considered a type of *mutation*. Although mutations can have serious implications, changes in the DNA are discrete and do not necessarily result in structural changes in the chromosomes. However, chromosome breaks produced by radiation do occur and can be observed microscopically during anaphase and metaphase, when the chromosomes are condensed. Radiation-induced chromosomal lesions can occur in both somatic

■ FIGURE 20-5 A. Ionization patterns for low- and high-LET radiations in DNA. **B.** Types of radiation-induced DNA damages. (Reprinted with permission from Japan Atomic Energy Agency, Dependence of Yield of DNA Damage Refractory to Enzymatic Repair on Ionization & Excitation of Density Radiation, 2007. Copyright © JAEA.)

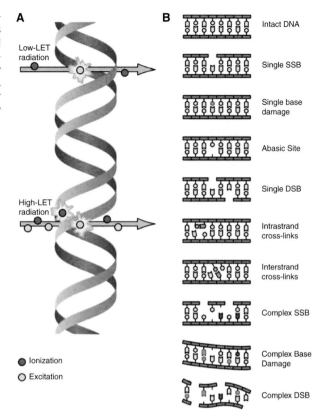

and germ cells and, if not repaired before DNA synthesis, may be transmitted during mitosis and meiosis. Chromosomal damage that occurs before DNA replication is referred to as *chromosome aberrations*, whereas that occurring after DNA synthesis is called *chromatid aberrations*. Unlike chromosomal aberrations, in chromatid aberrations, only one of the daughter cells will be affected if only one of the chromatids of a pair is damaged.

DNA Repair

Repair of DNA damage from the decay of naturally occurring and internally incorporated radionuclides (primarily C-14 and K-40) occurs constantly. Because these and other elements (stable and radioactive forms) are in physiological equilibrium (being constantly replenished by ingestion and inhalation), there are approximately 7,000 atoms undergoing radioactive decay each second in the average person. The damage done to DNA by this radiation is repaired rapidly and with high fidelity. Even in the absence of radiation, DNA damage is a relatively common event in the life of a cell. Mammalian cells experience many thousands of DNA lesions per cell per day as a result of a number of common cellular functions such oxidative damage induced by ROS during metabolism and DNA synthesis (*e.g.*, errors during base replication). It has been estimated that at least 10,000 oxidative DNA lesions are produced per cell per day by normal respiratory processes, and up to a million total DNA damages per cell per day by metabolic processes and environmental factors (Shrinivas et al., 2017). Yet the mutation rate is surprisingly low due to the effectiveness of the cell's response and the varied and robust DNA repair mechanisms operating within the cell. DNA damage induces several cellular responses that enable the cell either to repair or to cope with the damage. For example, the cell may activate cell cycle *checkpoints* (which arrest cell cycle progression) to allow for repair of damaged DNA or incompletely replicated chromosomes. In the case of potentially catastrophic DNA damage, the cell may initiate any of several cell death pathways (discussed below), effectively eliminating the damaged genetic material. The checkpoint and cell death responses (often known collectively as the DNA damage response [DDR]) utilize many of the same sensor molecules or complexes involved in DNA damage recognition and signal transduction. Many types of DNA repair mechanisms exist, including direct repair of a damaged nucleotide, base excision repair (BER), nucleotide excision repair (NER), SSB and DSB repair, and mismatch repair, each requiring its own set of enzymes (Fig. 20-6A). The repair of DNA damage depends on several factors, including the stage of the cell cycle and the type and location of the lesion.

There are specific endonucleases and exonucleases that, along with other proteins or complexes of proteins, are capable of repairing damage to the DNA. For example, most DNA base damage and SSBs are repaired by the BER pathway, involving enzymes that recognize the damage, enzymatic excision, use of the intact complementary DNA strand as the template on which to reconstruct the correct base sequence, and then a ligase to join DNA strands together (Fig. 20-6B). NER is the major pathway for the repair of bulky, helix-distorting lesions such as thymine dimers produced by exposure to ultraviolet radiation. While simple DNA lesions caused by metabolism and the actions of ROS are the primary substrates for the BER pathway, these lesions can also be recognized and repaired via the NER pathway. NER may play a more significant role in the repair of damage where significant distortions in the DNA structure occur. NER and BER processes are generally accurate and occur rapidly; approximately 90% of SSB and base damage are repaired within an hour after the initial damage. Even with DSBs, DNA rejoining is virtually complete within 24 hours (h) (Fig. 20-6C).

Since DNA DSBs (the simplest clustered lesion) are the most biologically important DNA damage caused by ionizing radiation, it is important to consider repair of DSBs in a bit more detail. DSBs can be repaired with high fidelity via homologous recombination repair (HRR) involving exchanges with homologous DNA strands (from sister chromatids after replication or from homologous chromosomes). More often DSBs are repaired by the error-prone nonhomologous end-joining (NHEJ) that involves end-to-end joining of broken strands (Fig. 20-7). Completely different sets of enzymes and repair processes are involved in HR and NHEJ (Fig. 20-8), and defects in a number of the enzymes, for example, ataxia telangiectasia mutated (ATM), components of the MRN complex, or ligase-4, result in increased radiosensitivity of individuals with those genetic defects.

Chromosomal Aberrations

HRR can preserve the genetic integrity of the chromosome while NHEJ repair results in loss of DNA fidelity. There is a strong force of cohesion between broken ends of chromatin material. Interchromosomal and intrachromosomal recombination may occur in a variety of ways, yielding many types of aberrations such as rings and dicentrics. Figure 20-9 illustrates some of the more common chromosomal aberrations and the consequences of replication and anaphasic separation. In some misrepair events, the two DSBs lead to a translocation (Fig. 20-9C). Translocations involve large scale rearrangements and can cause pre-carcinogenic alterations in cellular phenotype, but most do not impair cellular survival. Misrepair can also result in a dicentric chromosome aberration (Fig. 20-9D), which generally destroys the clonogenic viability of the cell.

The extent of the total genetic damage transmitted with chromosomal aberrations depends on a variety of factors, such as the cell type, the number and kind of genes deleted, and whether the lesion occurred in a somatic or in a gametic cell.

Summary of DNA Repair Mechanisms

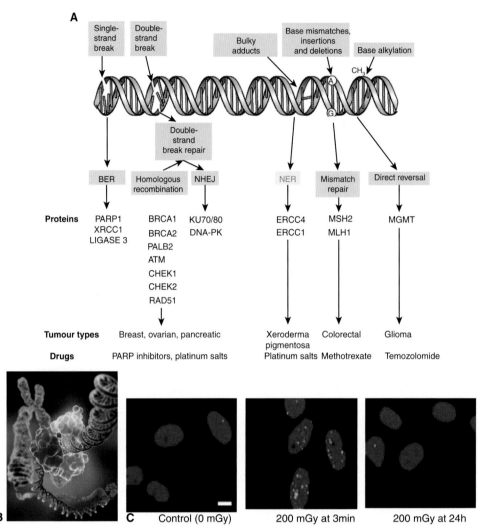

■ **FIGURE 20-6 A.** A summary of DNA repair processes. Each repair process is responsible for the repair of different types of DNA lesions. Some of the enzymes involved in each process are shown. Defects in some of these enzymes can lead to certain types of tumors or be targeted by certain drugs, as shown, for the treatment of cancers. (Reprinted with permission from Lord C, Ashworth A. The DNA damage response and cancer therapy. *Nature*. 2012;481:287-294. Copyright © Springer Nature.) **B.** Scientists have recently been able to visualize the complicated and dynamic structures of DNA ligase using a combination of x-ray crystallography and small-angle x-ray scattering techniques. These experiments revealed the crystal structure of the human DNA ligase I protein bound to a short DNA oligonucleotide. The ring-shaped structure in the center of the figure is the solvent-accessible surface of the protein. The extended, chromosomal DNA (long coils) is an artist's representation of the high-level organization of DNA structure. The figure illustrates the ring-shaped ligase protein sliding along the DNA searching for a break in the phosphodiester backbone of the DNA that is the substrate for the enzyme's DNA end-joining activity. The enzyme, DNA ligase, repairs millions of DNA breaks generated during the normal course of a cell's life, for example, linking together the abundant DNA fragments formed during replication of the genetic material in dividing cells. DNA ligase switches from an open, extended shape to a closed, circular shape as it joins DNA strands together. (Courtesy of Tom Ellenberger, DVM, PhD, Department of Biochemistry and Molecular Biophysics at Washington University School of Medicine, St. Louis, MO.) **C.** DSB induction and repair in primary human fibroblasts. Using immunofluorescence techniques, a fluorescent antibody-specific for γ-H2AX (a phosphorylated histone) forms discrete nuclear foci that can be visualized at sites of DSBs. DSB repair was evaluated at 3 min and 24 h after exposure to 200 mGy; repair was almost complete at 24 h. The length of the white scale bar shown in the unirradiated control panel equals 10 μm. (Reprinted with permission from Rothkamm K, Löbrich M. Evidence for a lack of DNA double-strand break repair in human cells exposed to very low x-ray doses. *Proc Natl Acad Sci U S A*. 2003;100:5057-5062. Copyright © National Academy of Sciences.)

Double Strand Break (DSB) Repair

Two main pathways

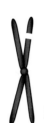
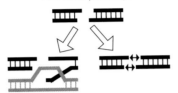

Homologous Recombination (HR)
- Uses sister chromatid or homologous chromosome
- Late S & G_2 phases
- Error-free

Non-homologous end joining (NHEJ)
- Ligation of DNA ends
- Repair without sister chromatid
- G_1 and early S phases
- Error-prone

■ **FIGURE 20-7** Comparison of the two pathways for repair of DNA double-strand breaks: homologous recombination (HR) and non-homologous end-joining (NHEJ). Because HR usually uses the sister chromatid for the repair, it can only occur in the late S or G_2 phases of the cell cycle, after DNA replication, but it is a highly accurate repair. On the other hand, the more common repair process, NHEJ, can occur at any time in the cell cycle but is an error-prone process that ligates the broken ends of DNA together, often resulting in loss of genetic information.

Chromosomal aberrations are known to occur spontaneously. In certain circumstances, the scoring of chromosomal aberrations in human lymphocytes has been used as a biologic dosimeter to estimate the dose of radiation received after accidental exposure. Lymphocytes are cultured from a sample of the patient's blood and then stimulated to divide, allowing a karyotype to be obtained. The cells are arrested at metaphase, and the frequency of rings and dicentrics are scored. Whole-body doses from penetrating radiation in excess of 250 mGy for acute exposure and

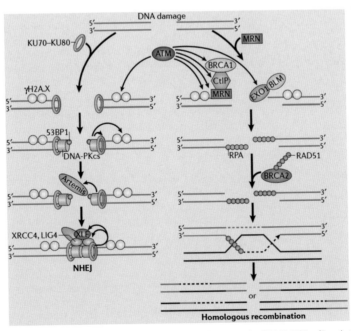

■ **FIGURE 20-8** Model of the key steps required for NHEJ and HR repair of DNA DSBs. (Reprinted with permission from Chowdhury D, Choi Y, Brault M. Charity begins at home: non-coding RNA functions in DNA repair. *Nat Rev Mol Cell Biol.* 2013;14:181-189. Copyright © Springer Nature.)

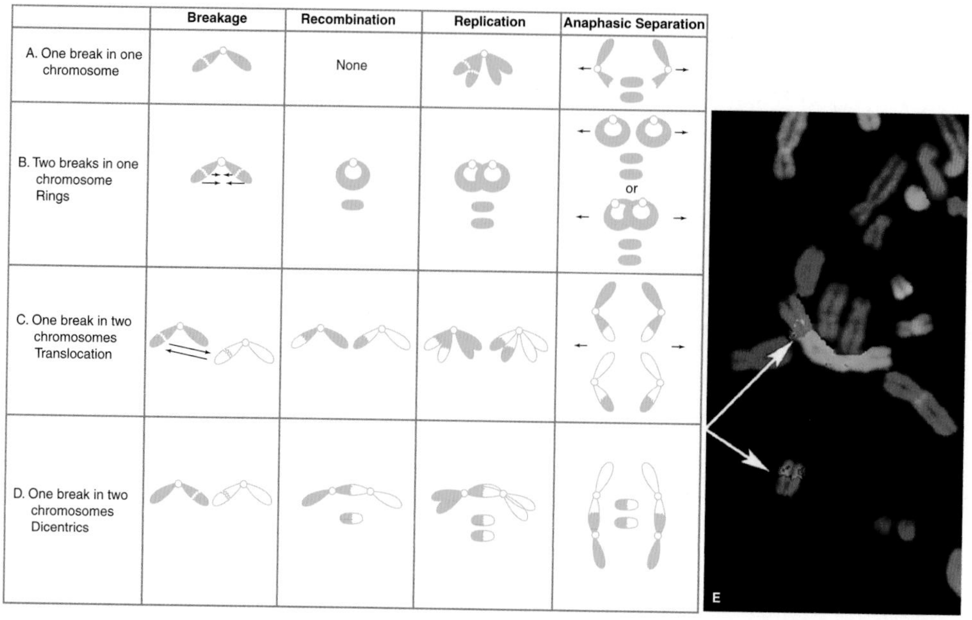

	Breakage	Recombination	Replication	Anaphasic Separation
A. One break in one chromosome		None		
B. Two breaks in one chromosome Rings				or
C. One break in two chromosomes Translocation				
D. One break in two chromosomes Dicentrics				

■ FIGURE 20-9 Examples of chromosomal aberrations and the effect of recombinations, replication, and anaphasic separation. **A.** A single break in one chromosome, which results in centric and acentric fragments. The acentric fragments are unable to attach to the mitotic spindle and are transmitted to only one of the daughter cells where they may remain in the cytoplasm. These fragments are eventually lost in subsequent divisions. **B.** Ring formation may result from two breaks in the same chromosome in which the two broken ends of the centric fragment recombine. The ring-shaped chromosome undergoes normal replication, and the two (ring-shaped) sister chromatids separate normally at anaphase—unless the centric fragment twists before recombination, in which case the sister chromatids will be interlocked and unable to separate. **C.** Translocation may occur when two chromosomes break and the acentric fragment of one chromosome combines with the centric fragment of the other and vice versa, or **(D)** the two centric fragments recombine with each other at their broken ends, resulting in the production of a dicentric. **E.** Metaphase spread, containing a simple dicentric interchange between chromosomes 2 and 8 visualized with multiplex fluorescence in situ hybridization (mFISH). This technique utilizes fluorescently labeled DNA probes with markers specific to regions of particular chromosomes, which allows for the identification of each homologous chromosome pair by its own color. The color is computer generated based on differences in fluorescence wavelength among probes. (Reprinted with permission from Cornforth MN, et al. Chromosomes are predominantly located randomly with respect to each other in interphase human cells. *J Cell Biol*. 2002;159(2):237-244. Copyright © Rockefeller University Press.)

400 mGy for chronic exposure can be detected with confidence limits that do not include zero. Although many chromosomal aberrations are unstable and gradually lost from circulation, this assay is generally considered the most sensitive method for estimating recent exposure (*i.e.*, within 6 months). More persistent, stable reciprocal translocations can be measured using fluorescence in situ hybridization (FISH). In this method, chromosomes are labeled with chromosome-specific fluorescent DNA probes, allowing translocations to be identified using fluorescent microscopy (Fig. 20-9E). Reciprocal translocations are believed to persist for a considerable period after the exposure, and this approach has been used as one of the methods to estimate the doses to survivors of the atomic bombs detonated in Hiroshima and Nagasaki decades ago.

20.4.2 Response to Radiation at the Cellular Level

There are a number of potential responses at the cellular level following radiation exposure. Depending on a variety of inherent and conditional biologic variables related to the cell and its environment (*e.g.*, cell type, oxygen tension, stage in the cell cycle at the time of exposure) as well as a number of physical factors related to the radiation exposure (*e.g.*, dose, dose rate, LET), a number of responses are possible such as delayed cell division, apoptosis, reproductive failure, genomic instability (delay expression of radiation damage), DNA mutations including pheno-typic (including potentially oncogenic) transformations, bystander effects (damage to neighboring unirradiated cells), and adaptive responses (irradiated cells become more radioresistant). Many of these effects are discussed in more detail below. While a wide variety of the biologic responses to radiation have been identified, the study of radiation-induced reproductive failure (also referred to as clonogenic cell death or loss of reproductive integrity) is particularly useful in assessing the relative biologic impact of various types of radiation and exposure conditions. The use of reproduc-tive integrity as a biologic effects marker is somewhat limited, however, in that it is applicable only to proliferating cell systems (*e.g.*, stem cells). For differentiated cells that no longer have the capacity for cell division (*e.g.*, muscle and nerve cells), cell death is often defined as loss of specific metabolic functions or functional capacity. One must also keep in mind that, with many of the assays described below, sensitiv-ity to detect changes may be limited at low radiation doses and dose rates, so data obtained at higher doses are often back-extrapolated, using various mathematical models discussed below, to low doses and dose rates.

Cell Survival Curves

Cells grown in tissue culture that are lethally irradiated may fail to show evidence of morphologic changes for long periods; however, reproductive failure eventually occurs. The most direct method of evaluating the ability of a single cell to proliferate is to wait until enough cell divisions have occurred to form a visible colony. Counting the number of *colonies* that arise from a known number of individual cells irradiated in vitro and cultured provides a way to easily determine the relative radiosensitivity of particular cell lines, the effectiveness of different types of radiation, or the effect of various environmental conditions. The loss of the ability to form colonies as a func-tion of radiation exposure can be described by cell survival curves.

Several mathematical models have been developed to describe the biological response to radiation. The shape of a cell survival curve reflects the relative radiosen-sitivity of the cell line and the random nature of energy deposition and subsequent biological effects. Survival curves are usually presented in graphical form, with the surviving fraction (SF) of cells plotted using a logarithmic scale on the *y*-axis, as a function of the radiation dose shown using a linear scale on the *x*-axis. In the *multitar-get model*, the response to radiation is defined by three parameters: the extrapolation number (n), the quasithreshold dose (D_q), and the D_0 dose (Fig. 20-10).

The D_0 describes the radiosensitivity of the cell population under study. The D_0 dose is the reciprocal of the slope of the linear portion of the survival curve, and it is the dose of radiation that produces, along the linear portion of the curve, a reduc-tion to 37% in the number of viable cells. Radioresistant cells have a higher D_0 than radiosensitive cells. A lower D_0 implies less survival per dose. The D_0 for mammalian cells ranges from approximately 1 to 2 Gy for low-LET radiation.

In the case of low-LET radiation, the survival curve of mammalian cells usu-ally is characterized by an initial "shoulder" before the linear portion of the curve on the semilogarithmic plot. The extrapolation number, which gives a measure of the "shoulder," is found by extrapolating the linear portion of the curve back to its intersection with the *y*-axis. The extrapolation number for mammalian cells ranges between 2 and 10; the larger the n, the larger the shoulder. D_q also defines the width of the shoulder region of the cell survival curve and is a measure of sublethal damage.

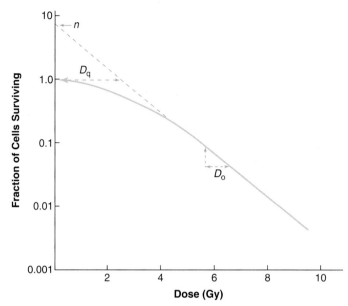

■ **FIGURE 20-10** Typical cell survival curve illustrating the portions of the curve used to derive the extrapolation number (n), the quasithreshold dose (D_q), and the D_0 dose.

Sublethal damage is a concept based on experiments that show that when the radiation dose is split into two or more fractions, with sufficient time between fractions, the cell survival increases after low-LET radiation. The presence of the shoulder in a cell survival curve is taken to indicate that more than one ionizing event ("hit"), on average, is required to kill a cell and the reappearance of the shoulder when a large dose is delivered in fractions indicates that the cells are capable of repairing sublethal damage between fractions.

The linear-quadratic (LQ) model is now the most often used to describe cell survival data where the SF is generally expressed as

$$SF\,(D) = e^{-\alpha D - \beta D^2}$$

where D is the dose in Gy, α is the coefficient of cell killing that is proportional to dose (i.e., the initial linear component on a log-linear plot) and β is the coefficient of cell killing that is proportional to the square of the dose (i.e., the quadratic component of the survival curve). The two constants (α and β) can be determined for specific tissues and cancers to predict dose response. As described previously, cell killing (i.e., loss of clonogenic viability) occurs via misrepaired or unrepaired chromosome damage such as dicentric aberrations that are formed when pairs of nearby DSBs wrongly rejoin to one another. The double helix can undergo a DSB as the result of two different mechanisms: (1) both DNA strands are broken by the same radiation track (or "event") and (2) each strand is broken independently, but the breaks are close enough in time and space to lead to a DSB. The linear (alpha) component of the survival curve represents the damage done by individual radiation particle tracks and is thus independent of dose rate. While the damage is partially repairable over time, α still represents the probability of cell death due to individual, noninteracting, particle tracks. This linear (single-hit kinetics) dose-response relationship dominates with high-LET radiation. The quadratic (beta) component of the survival curve represents the probability of cell death due to interactions between two or more individual particle tracks (i.e., dominates with low-LET radiation and follows multiple-hit kinetics) causing the curve to bend at higher doses and is sensitive to dose rate.

The LQ (or alpha-beta model, as many call it) is more commonly used than the previously described n-D_0 model, for several reasons: the LQ model is mechanistically based, it is more useful in radiotherapy for explaining fractionation effect differences between late responding normal tissues and early responding tissues or tumors, and the LQ model seems to fit most experimental data on human cell lines. The dose at which cell killing is equal from the linear (αD) and quadratic (βD^2) contributions is referred to as the α/β ratio. The α/β ratio is a measure of the curvature of the cell survival curve and, thus, a measure of the sensitivity of different cell types to fractionation of radiation dose, Figure 20-11. For example, late responding normal tissues such as spinal cord or lung that have smaller α/β ratios of 3 or 4 are preferentially "spared" by fractionation compared to tumors and early responding normal tissues (gut, skin, bone marrow) where the α/β ratio is larger (8 to 12), indicating less ability to repair (*i.e.*, more alpha component and less effect of fractionating the dose).

Modes of Radiation-Induced Cell Death

When irradiated cells fail to form a colony, it can be because of loss of proliferative capacity due to processes such as senescence, quiescence, or terminal differentiation, or because of cell death including mitotic catastrophe, apoptosis, autophagy, necroptosis, or necrosis, Most radiation-induced death in proliferating cells results from mitotic death/catastrophe that occurs when cells are unable to go through mitosis, generally because of chromosomal damage (discussed above). Those damaged cells may then exhibit demise by any of the other processes just mentioned. Nonproliferating cells may be lost through the regulated cell death processes of apoptosis, autophagy, or necroptosis, or unregulated necrosis. Each of those processes involves characteristic morphological changes in cells, as well as different pathways with distinct cascades of molecular events. Furthermore, cross-talk can occur among the different cell death pathways at various levels. Figure 20-12 diagrammatically compares morphological changes in cells undergoing apoptosis, autophagy, and necrosis. Figure 20-13 presents molecular cascades involved in apoptosis, necroptosis, and autophagy.

Apoptosis is a form of cell death that is characteristically different from cell necrosis in morphology and biochemistry, leading to the elimination of cells without releasing inflammatory substances into the surrounding area. Apoptosis results in cell shrinkage via nuclear condensation and extensive membrane blebbing, ultimately resulting in fragmentation of the cell into membrane-bound apoptotic

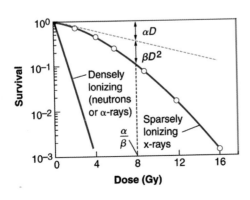

■ FIGURE 20-11 The LQ model. The experimental data are fitted to a LQ function. There are two components to cell killing: One is proportional to dose (αD); the other is proportional to the square of the dose βD^2. The dose at which the linear and quadratic components are equal is the ratio α/β. The LQ curve bends continuously but is a good fit to the experimental data for the first few decades of survival. (Reprinted with permission from Hall EJ, Giaccia AJ. *Radiobiology for the Radiologist.* 7th ed. Philadelphia, PA: Lippincott Williams and Wilkins; 2012.)

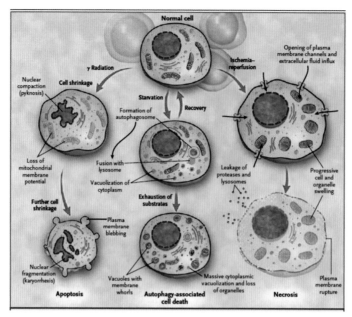

■ **FIGURE 20-12** Comparison of morphological changes in cells undergoing three different modes of radiation-induced cell death—apoptosis, autophagy, and necrosis. A particular mode of cell death may predominate depending on cell type, radiation quality, and dose, and other environmental factors. (Reprinted with permission from Hotchkiss RS, Strasser A, McDunn JE, Swanson PE. Cell death. *N Engl J Med.* 2009;361(16):1570-1583.)

bodies composed of cytoplasm and tightly packed organelles that are eliminated by phagocytosis. Hallmarks of apoptosis include the sequential activation of caspases (cysteine-dependent aspartate-directed proteases) from pro-caspases; interactions of pro- and anti-apoptotic members of the bcl-2 family of proteins, many working at the level of the mitochondria; cleavage of multiple proteins; and, ultimately, cleavage of DNA between nucleosomes to form characteristic fragments consisting of multiples of the amount of DNA in a nucleosome. Extrinsic apoptosis is initiated at the cell surface with activation of death receptors such as CD95 (Fas) receptor, dimerization and activation of the initiator, or upstream caspase, caspase-8, which, in turn, activates the downstream caspase-3, which activates endonucleases and other proteases

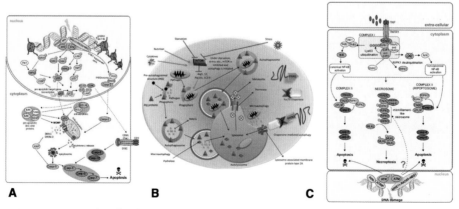

■ **FIGURE 20-13** Cascades of molecular events involved in apoptosis **(A)**, autophagy **(B)**, and necroptosis **(C)**. See text for explanations. (**A** and **C**: Reprinted with permission from Matt S, Hofmann TG. The DNA damage-induced cell death response: a roadmap to kill cancer cells. *Cell Mol Life Sci.* 2016;73:2829-2850. **B**: Reprinted from Hotchkiss RS, Strasser A, McDunn JE, Swanson PE. Cell death. *N Engl J Med.* 2009;361(16):1570-1583.)

to cleave DNA and many other cellular proteins. Intrinsic apoptosis is generally started at mitochondria where interactions of pro-apoptotic proteins, such as Bax and Bak, with anti-apoptotic Bcl-2 and Bcl-XL results in the release of cytochrome *c* from the mitochondria, formation of apoptosomes, activation of caspase-9, activation of caspase-3, and the cleavage of other cellular proteins and DNA. Radiation can induce apoptosis through DNA damage initiating the formation of pro-apoptotic proteins such as Noxa and Puma, which activate intrinsic apoptosis or upregulation of death receptors to begin extrinsic apoptosis pathways. This is an over-simplistic description of the processes, as there can be much cross-talk among pathways and regulation by other proteins, for example, p53 or XIAP (sex-linked inhibitor of apoptosis) at various steps.

Autophagy was initially recognized as a process by which cells that were starved of nutrients initiated a "self-digestion" of cellular components to obtain energy and thus promote survival. Autophagy can also remove damaged cellular molecules and components and can be activated by genotoxic stress, such as radiation-induced DNA damage. On the other hand, if cell damage is extensive, autophagy can result in cell death. As with apoptosis, at the molecular level autophagy involves complex sequences of protein changes and enzyme activations, with cross-talk among the cascades possible. Proteins of importance recognized in the autophagy cascades include Beclin, LC3, and a series of atg proteins. Ultimately, cells undergoing autophagy sequester the proteins or components to be digested into autophagosomes, which fuse with lysosomes containing the lytic enzymes. In cancer biology, autophagy can actually be a double-edged sword, in some cases removing excessively damaged cells or, in the case of therapy, being activated to kill cancer cells; on the other hand, if autophagy does not kill the cell, it may permit cell survival with damaged DNA to become, or allow continued growth of, a cancer cell.

Necroptosis, or regulated necrosis, is more recently recognized as a mode of programmed cell death, including genetically determined enzyme cascades in its molecular expression. Interestingly, necroptosis appears to involve protein ubiquitination steps, as well as the formation of a necroptosome, which includes several RIP (rest in peace) kinases. Although at this writing, necroptosis does not appear to be a large component of radiation-induced cell death, the relative importance of the various cell inactivation mechanisms, apoptosis, autophagy, senescence, etc. depends on many intrinsic and extrinsic factors including cell type, tissue environment, and radiation dose, dose rate, and type, to name a few.

When thinking about radiation-induced cell inactivation, it is also important to give consideration to the time between radiation exposure and the occurrence of the inactivation processes just described. Again, the picture is not simple, as it depends on cell type and environment as well as the cell inactivation mode. For example, the apoptosis process itself, as just described, occurs fairly rapidly, in many cases only requiring a half-hour or so from the first activation of upstream caspases to total cell demise into apoptotic bodies, but the time between initial damage induction, for example, DNA DSBs from irradiation, to the start of the apoptotic process is variable. In lymphocytes, in vitro, or in vivo, apoptosis is seen within hours after irradiation. However, in some cell types, for example, many cancer cells, the damaged cells and their progeny are capable of dividing as many as 4 or 5 times before apoptosis is initiated in many or all the progeny of the initially irradiated cells; this has been shown to require as long as a week. In another example, senescence, for example, in fibroblasts, may be activated immediately after irradiation, but the non-dividing cells may remain functional for up to weeks, before they may eventually be removed from the population by necrosis or apoptosis.

Factors Affecting Cellular Radiosensitivity

Cellular radiosensitivity can be influenced by a variety of factors that can enhance or diminish the response to radiation or alter the temporal relationship between the exposure and a given response. These factors can be classified as either *conditional* or *inherent*. Conditional radiosensitivities are those physical or chemical factors that exist before and/or at the time of irradiation. Some of the more important conditional factors affecting dose-response relationships are discussed in the following paragraphs, including dose rate, LET, and the presence of oxygen. Inherent radiosensitivity includes those biologic factors that are characteristics of the cells themselves, such as the mitotic rate, the degree of differentiation, and the stage in the cell cycle.

Conditional Factors

The rate at which a dose of low-LET radiation is delivered has been shown to affect the degree of biologic damage for a number of biologic endpoints including chromosomal aberrations, reproductive delay, and cell death. In general, high dose rates are more effective at producing biologic damage than low dose rates. The primary explanation for this effect is the diminished potential for repair of radiation damage. Cells have a greater opportunity to repair sublethal damage at low dose rates than at higher dose rates, reducing the amount of damage, and increasing the survival fraction. Figure 20-14 shows an example of the dose rate effect on cell survival.

Note that the broader shoulder associated with low-dose-rate exposure indicates its diminished effectiveness compared with the same dose delivered at a higher dose rate. This dose-rate effect is diminished or not seen with high-LET radiation primarily because the dense ionization tracks produce more complex, clustered DNA damage that cannot be repaired correctly. Therefore, for a given dose rate, high-LET radiation is considerably more effective in producing cell damage than low-LET radiation (Fig. 20-15).

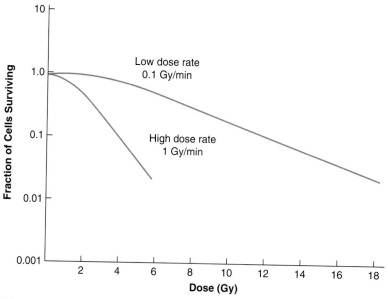

■ **FIGURE 20-14** Cell survival curves illustrating the effect of dose rate for low-LET radiation. Lethality is reduced because the repair of sublethal damage is enhanced when a given dose of radiation is delivered at a low versus a high dose rate.

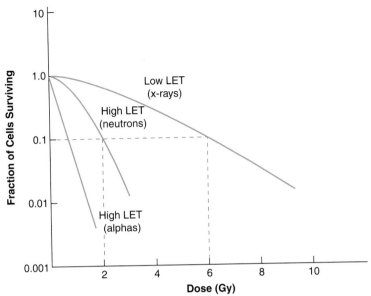

FIGURE 20-15 Cell survival curves illustrating the greater damage produced by radiation with high-LET. At 10% survival, high-LET neutron radiation is three times as effective as the same dose of low-LET radiation in this example.

For a given radiation dose of low-LET radiation, a reduction in radiation damage is also observed when the dose is *fractionated* over a period of time. This technique is fundamental to the practice of radiation therapy. The intervals between doses (hours to a few days) allow the repair mechanisms in healthy tissue to gain an advantage over the tumor by repairing some of the sublethal damage. Figure 20-16 shows an idealized experiment in which a dose of 10 Gy is delivered either all at once or in five

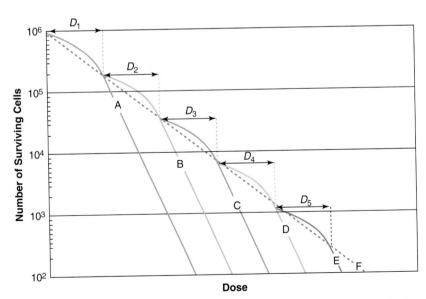

FIGURE 20-16 Idealized fractionation experiment depicting the survival of a population of 10^6 cells as a function of dose. Curve A represents one fraction of 10 Gy. Curve F represents the same total dose as in curve A delivered in equal fractionated doses (D_1 through D_5) of 2 Gy each, with intervals between fractions sufficient to allow for repair of sublethal damage. (Modified from Hall EJ. *Radiobiology for the Radiologist.* 5th ed. Philadelphia, PA: Lippincott Williams & Wilkins; 2000.)

fractions of 2 Gy with sufficient time between fractions for repair of sublethal damage. For low-LET radiation, the decreasing slope of the survival curve with decreasing dose rate (see Fig. 20-14) and the reoccurrence of the shoulder with fractionation (see Fig. 20-16) are clear evidence of repair.

The presence of oxygen increases the damage caused by low-LET radiation by inhibiting the recombination of free radicals to form harmless chemical species and by inhibiting the chemical restitution of damage caused by free radicals. This effect is demonstrated in Figure 20-17, which shows a cell line irradiated under aerated and hypoxic conditions with low or high-LET radiations. The relative effectiveness of radiation to produce damage at various oxygen tensions is described by the oxygen enhancement ratio (OER). The OER is defined as the dose of radiation that produces a given biologic response in the absence of oxygen divided by the dose of radiation that produces the same biologic response in the presence of oxygen. Increasing the oxygen concentration at the time of irradiation has been shown to enhance the killing of otherwise hypoxic (and thus radioresistant) cells that can be found in some tumors. The OER for mammalian cells in cultures is typically between 2.5 and 3 for *low*-LET radiation. High-LET damage is not primarily mediated through free radical production, and therefore the OER for high-LET radiation can be as low as 1.0.

Inherent Factors

In 1906, two French scientists, J. Bergonie and L. Tribondeau, performed a series of experiments that evaluated the relative radiosensitivity of rodent germ cells at different stages of spermatogenesis. From these experiments, some of the fundamental characteristics of cells that affect their relative radiosensitivities were established. The law of Bergonie and Tribondeau states that radiosensitivity is greatest for those cells that (1) have a high mitotic rate, (2) have a long mitotic future, and (3) are undifferentiated. With only a few exceptions (*e.g.*, lymphocytes), this law provides a reasonable characterization of the relative radiosensitivity of cells in vitro and in vivo. For example, the pluripotential stem /early progenitor cells in the bone marrow have a high mitotic rate, have a long mitotic future, are poorly differentiated, and are

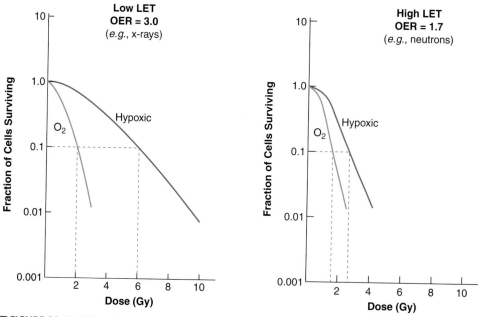

■ **FIGURE 20-17** Cell survival curves demonstrating the effect of oxygen during high (blue) and low (green) oxygen tension on the OER for high- and low-LET irradiation.

extremely radiosensitive compared with other cells in the body. On the other end of the spectrum, the fixed postmitotic neurons found in the central nervous system (CNS) are relatively radioresistant (Fig. 20-18). This classification scheme was refined in 1968 by Rubin and Casarett, who defined five cell types according to characteristics that affect their radiosensitivity (Table 20-1).

The stage of the cells in the reproductive cycle at the time of irradiation greatly affects their radiosensitivity. Figure 20-19 shows the phases of the cell reproductive cycle and several checkpoints that can arrest the cell cycle or interrupt the progression to allow for the integrity of key cellular functions to be evaluated and if necessary, repaired. Experiments indicate that, in general, cells exposed to low-LET radiation are most sensitive during mitosis (M phase) and the "gap" (G_2) between S phase and mitosis, less sensitive during the preparatory period for DNA synthesis (G_1), and least sensitive during late DNA synthesis (S phase). If one looks at full survival curves from cells irradiated during each cell cycle phase, it is clear that the sensitive M and G_2 phase cells have straighter curves, that is, less repair of radiation damage, while the late S phase cells have a broader shoulder, more repair. Consistent with these differences in repair ability, cells irradiated with high-LET radiation show much less cell cycle phase dependence, as the survival curves for cells in all phases of the cycle have minimal shoulders.

In addition to variations in radiation sensitivity through the cell cycle, there are differences in radiation-induced cell cycle arrest. As described in the legend to Figure 20-19, cell cycle checkpoints are critical times at which the cell monitors its integrity to ensure that it should proceed to the next phase of the cycle. These processes are carefully orchestrated at the molecular level by the interplay of proteins called cyclins and cyclin-dependent kinases (cdks) and are controlled by regulatory proteins including inhibitors of cdks (*INK4 and KIP family regulators and Cdk inhibitors*). Radiation can alter the function of these proteins, and thus, alter cell cycle checkpoint activity. Best known is the radiation-induced cell cycle arrest in the G_2

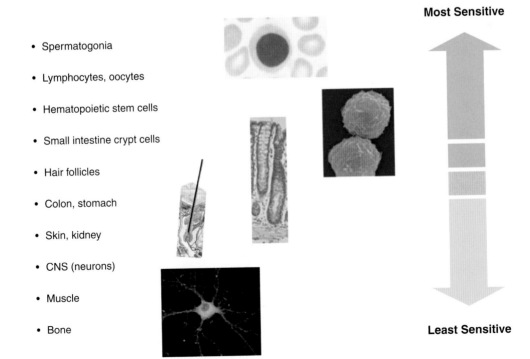

Most Sensitive

- Spermatogonia

- Lymphocytes, oocytes

- Hematopoietic stem cells

- Small intestine crypt cells

- Hair follicles

- Colon, stomach

- Skin, kidney

- CNS (neurons)

- Muscle

- Bone

Least Sensitive

■ **FIGURE 20-18** Relative radiosensitivity of tissues.

TABLE 20-1 CLASSIFICATION OF CELLULAR RADIOSENSITIVITY

CELL TYPE	CHARACTERISTICS	EXAMPLES	RADIOSENSITIVITY
VIM	Rapidly dividing; undifferentiated; do not differentiate between divisions	Type A spermatogonia Erythroblasts Crypt cells of intestines Basal cells of the epidermis	Most radiosensitive
DIM	Actively dividing; more differentiated than VIMs; differentiate between divisions	Intermediate spermatogonia Myelocytes	Relatively radiosensitive
MCT	Irregularly dividing; more differentiated than VIMs or DIMs	Endothelial cells Fibroblasts	Intermediate in radiosensitivity
RPM	Do not normally divide but retain the capability of division; differentiated	Parenchymal cells of the liver and adrenal glands Lymphocytes[a] Bone Muscle cells	Relatively radioresistant
FPM	Do not divide; differentiated	Some nerve cells Erythrocytes Spermatozoa	Most radioresistant

[a]Lymphocytes, although classified as relatively radioresistant by their characteristics, are in fact very radiosensitive.
VIM, vegetative intermitotic cells; DIM, differentiating intermitotic cells; MCT, multipotential connective tissue cells; RPM, reverting postmitotic cells; FPM, fixed postmitotic cells.
Data from: Rubin P, Casarett GW. Clinical radiation pathology as applied to curative radiotherapy. *Clin Pathol Radiat.* 1968;22:767-768.

phase because when it is prevented by genetic alterations or drugs such as caffeine, cells are sensitized to radiation. Also important for radiation sensitivity is the ability to arrest in the G_1 phase, which is highly dependent on cells having a functional p53 pathway (see bottom of Fig. 20-19). The tumor suppressor gene *TP53* (so named because it encodes a phosphorylated protein with a molecular weight of 53 kDa) operates predominantly at the G_1/S checkpoint. The p53 protein (discussed again in relation to radiation-induced carcinogenesis later in the chapter) induces cell-cycle arrest through the up-regulation of cyclin-dependent kinase inhibitors and thus allows for repair of DNA damage. The CIP/KIP (CDK interacting protein/Kinase inhibitory protein) family is one of two families (CIP/KIP and INK4) of mammalian cyclin-dependent kinase (CDK) inhibitors (CKIs) involved in regulating the cell cycle. The CIP/KIP family members also have a number of CDK-independent roles involving regulation of transcription, apoptosis, and the control of the cell's cytoskeleton. Thus the p53 protein activation of cyclin-dependent kinases can activate DNA repair mechanisms or, in the case of severe DNA damage, induce cell death via apoptosis.

Adaptive Response, Bystander Effect, and Genomic Instability

A number of other responses to radiation have been observed in vitro that raise interesting questions about the applicability of the LQ dose-response model for low-dose low-LET radiation used in medical imaging. An adaptive response to radiation has been demonstrated in which an initial exposure or "priming dose" reduced the effectiveness of a subsequent exposure. For example, it has been demonstrated in vitro with human lymphocytes that compared to controls not receiving a small initial exposure, a priming dose of 10 mGy significantly reduced the frequency of chromosomal aberrations in the cells exposed to several Gy a few hours later (Shadley et al., 1987). However, the magnitude of this adaptive response varies considerably with

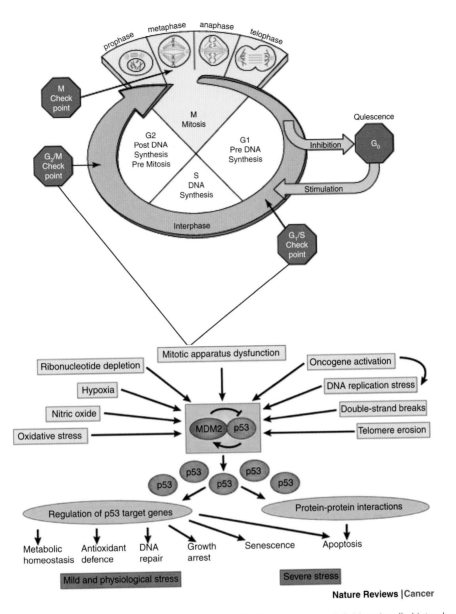

Nature Reviews | Cancer

■ **FIGURE 20-19** Phases of the cell's reproductive cycle. The time between cell divisions is called interphase. Interphase includes the period after mitosis but before DNA synthesis (G₁), which is the most variable in length of the phases; followed by S phase, during which DNA synthesis occurs; followed by G₂, all leading up to mitosis (M phase), the events of which are differentiated into prophase, metaphase, anaphase, and telophase. Much of the control of the progression through the phases of a cell cycle is exerted by specific cell cycle control genes at checkpoints. Checkpoints are critical control points in the cell cycle that have built-in stop signals that halt the cell cycle until overridden by external chemical signals to proceed. There are three major checkpoints in the cell cycle, G₁ checkpoint between G₁ and S phase (G₁/S), the G₂ checkpoint between G₂ and mitosis (G₂/M), and the M (metaphase) checkpoint. The G₁/S checkpoint is where the cell monitors its size, available nutrients, and the integrity of DNA (e.g., prevents copying of damaged bases, which would fix mutations in the genome) to assure all are adequate for DNA synthesis and progression on through the cell division cycle. In the absence of a proceed signal, the cell will enter a quiescent state G₀ (the state of most cells in the body) until it receives a stimulation signal to continue. Following DNA synthesis, the G₂/M checkpoint occurs at the end of the G₂ phase, during which DNA damage induced during replication, such as mismatched bases and double-stranded breaks, is repaired. The cell ensures that DNA synthesis (S-phase) has been successfully completed before triggering the start of mitosis, and at the metaphase (spindle) checkpoint the cell monitors spindle formation and ensures all chromosomes are attached to the mitotic spindle by kinetochores prior to advancing to anaphase. p53, the product of the tumor suppressor gene *TP53*, operates predominantly at the G₁/S checkpoint. The p53 pathway (inset) is vital to maintaining cell health, monitoring incoming stress from various sources such as oxidative stress, hypoxia, and DNA damage to name a few. Depending on the stressor, the response of the p53 pathway will change leading to cell cycle arrest, apoptosis, senescence, DNA repair, and metabolism adjustment.

dose and dose rate as well as among lymphocytes from different individuals and with other variables. Many other endpoints for adaptive response have been studied such as cell lethality, mutations, and defects in embryonic development for which the evidence for an adaptive response was highly variable. While many theories have been advanced to explain this phenomenon, there is still insufficient evidence to use these results to modify the dose-response relationship for human exposure to radiation.

The bystander effect is another fascinating phenomenon in which irradiated cells or tissues can produce alterations in nonirradiated cells or tissues. Sometimes also called the *abscopal* ("out-of-field") effect of radiation, the effect has been demonstrated in a variety of experiments. One of the earliest examples was the ability of plasma from patients who had received radiation therapy to induce chromosomal aberrations in lymphocytes from nonirradiated patients (Hollowell and Littlefield, 1968). Among the most compelling evidence for the bystander effect are in vitro experiments in which an α-particle microbeam, with the ability to irradiate a single cell, can produce a host of changes in neighboring unirradiated cells. Examples of induced changes in the unirradiated cells include DNA damage such as micronuclei formation, sister-chromatid exchanges, cell killing, as well as changes in a number of important proteins (*e.g.*, p53 and p21), genomic instability (discussed below), and even malignant transformation. Like adaptive response, the sequence of events following exposure is varied and complex and while many molecular mechanisms have been proposed to explain the bystander effects, the relationship of this phenomenon to low-dose, low-LET radiation effects characteristic of medical radiation exposure in humans is still an open question.

While the vast majority of unrepaired and misrepaired radiation-induced lesions are expressed as chromosomal damage at the first division, a fraction of cells can express chromosomal damage such as chromosomal rearrangements, chromatid breaks and gaps, and micronuclei over many cell cycles after they are irradiated. The biological significance and molecular mechanism surrounding this persistent *genomic instability* have been an area of active research for many years. Genomic instability has been demonstrated in vitro as delayed lethality in which cell cloning efficiency is reduced several generations after irradiation. Another interesting aspect is the differences in the types of mutations associated with radiation-induced genomic instability. Experiments have shown that the unirradiated progeny of the irradiated cells primarily demonstrate a de novo increase in lethal point mutations several generations after the initial irradiation. These mutations are more typical of spontaneous mutations than deletions and other mutations induced directly by ionizing radiation. There is evidence that suggests that errors induced during DNA repair may contribute to genomic instability. For example, experiments with cells deficient in the repair enzymes needed for NHEJ repair of radiation-induced DSBs demonstrate greater genomic instability than normal cells of the same type (Little, 2003). However, there are data to suggest that many other factors such as ROS, alterations in signal transduction pathways, centrosome defects, and other factors also play a role in radiation-induced genomic instability. Despite the many experimental models that have revealed different aspects of this phenomenon, the search for the relevance of radiation-induced genomic instability to radiation-induced cancer continues.

While radiation-induced responses such as genomic instability, adaptation, bystander effects, (as well as others which have not been discussed such as low-dose hypersensitivity) are fascinating in their own right, the results obtained are often restricted to specific experimental conditions and clear mechanistic understanding about these phenomena is still lacking. It has been suggested that these effects may alter the responses of cells and tissues to low doses of radiation, especially for carcinogenesis induction; however, at this time, they cannot be used reliably as modifying factors to predict the biological consequences of radiation exposure in humans. On the other hand, the nonlinear nature of these and other multicellular and tissue-level responses raises serious questions regarding the current paradigm of linear extrapolation of risk based on the individual cell and the target. An active area of current research focused on addressing these complex responses to radiation interactions is a multidimensional, systems-level approach that includes the integration of radiation epidemiology with radiobiological investigations.

20.5 TISSUE AND ORGAN SYSTEM RESPONSE TO RADIATION

The response of tissues and organ systems to radiation depends not only on the dose, dose rate, and LET of the radiation but also on the relative radiosensitivities of the cells that comprise both the functional parenchyma and the supportive stroma. In this case, the response is measured in terms of morphologic and functional changes of the tissues and organ systems as a whole rather than simply changes in cell survival and kinetics.

The response of an organ system after irradiation occurs over a period of time. The higher the dose, the shorter the interval before the physiologic manifestations of the damage become apparent (latent period), and the shorter the period of expression during which the full extent of the radiation-induced damage is evidenced. There are practical threshold doses below which no clinically significant changes are apparent. In most cases, the pathology induced by radiation is indistinguishable from pathology caused by other physical, chemical, or biological agents or (in some cases) even naturally occurring diseases of unknown etiology.

20.5.1 Characterization of Radiosensitivity

Classically, the characterization of a tissue or organ system as radioresistant or radiosensitive was thought to depend in large part on the radiosensitivity of cells that comprised the functional parenchyma, with cells of the supportive stromal tissue consisting mainly of cells of intermediate radiosensitivity. Therefore, when the parenchyma contains radiosensitive cell types (*e.g.*, stem/early progenitor cells in bone marrow or GI tract), the initial hypoplasia and concomitant decrease in functional integrity will be the result of damage to these radiosensitive cell populations, and functional changes are typically apparent within days or weeks after the exposure. However, if the parenchyma is populated by radioresistant cell types (*e.g.*, nerve or muscle cells), it was thought that damage to the functional layer occurred indirectly by compromise of the cells in the vascular stroma, and hypoplasia of the parenchymal cells is typically delayed several months. The relative radiosensitivity of various tissues and organs and the primary mechanism for radiation-induced parenchymal hypoplasia, as described initially by Rubin and Casarrett, is shown in Table 20-2.

However, it is now clear that cell killing alone cannot explain many tissue reactions (ICRP, 2012), as those reactions also depend on complex events including inflammatory, chronic oxidative, and immune reactions, as well as damage to the vasculature and the extracellular matrix (ECM). In general, early reactions, such as in skin and GI tract, involve killing of the stem/early progenitor cells that supply the mature functional cells in the tissue, as well as inflammatory reactions. On the other hand, late reactions, for example, in the lung, kidneys, and brain, involve complex and dynamic interactions between multiple cell types in the tissues and organs and include infiltrating immune cells, production of cytokines and growth factors, often in persistent, cyclic cascades, and chronic oxidative stress. Cytokines are a diverse

TABLE 20-2 RUBIN AND CASARETT CLASSIFICATION OF RELATIVE ORGAN AND TISSUE RADIOSENSITIVITY AND PRIMARY MECHANISM FOR RADIATION-INDUCED PARENCHYMAL HYPOPLASIA

ORGANS	RELATIVE RADIOSENSITIVITY	CHIEF MECHANISM OF PARENCHYMAL HYPOPLASIA
Lymphoid organs; bone marrow; testes and ovaries; small intestines	High	Destruction of parenchymal cells, especially the vegetative and differentiating cells
Skin and other organs with epithelial cell lining (cornea, lens, oral cavity, esophagus, GI organs, bladder, vagina, uterine cervix, uterus, rectum)	Fairly high	Destruction of radiosensitive vegetative and differentiating parenchymal cells of the epithelial lining
Growing cartilage; the vasculature; growing bones	Medium	Destruction of proliferating chondroblasts or osteoblasts; damage to the endothelium; destruction of connective tissue cells and chondroblasts or osteoblasts
Mature cartilage or bone; lungs; kidneys; liver; pancreas; adrenal gland; pituitary gland; thyroid; salivary glands	Fairly low	Hypoplasia secondary to damage to the fine vasculature and connective tissue elements
Muscle; brain; spinal cord	Low	Hypoplasia secondary to damage to the fine vasculature and connective tissue elements, with little contribution by the direct effect on parenchymal tissues

Note: Cells of the testes are more sensitive than ovaries. Skin radiosensitivity is particularly high around the hair follicles.
Adapted with permission from Rubin P, Casarett GW. Clinical radiation pathology as applied to curative radiotherapy. *Clin Pathol Radiat.* 1968;22:767-768.

group of soluble short-acting proteins, glycoproteins, and peptides produced by various immune and vascular cells that activate specific receptors and modulate the functions of many cells and tissues. Some cytokines may be membrane-bound or associated with ECM. Cytokines released by the vascular endothelium of irradiated tissues are implicated in the acute phase response to ionizing radiation and other inflammatory stimuli. Examples of radiation-induced cytokines include tumor necrosis factor (TNF3)-α, Interleukin (IL)-1, transforming growth factor (TGF)-β, and stem cell factor. Although many of these cytokines and growth factors, when induced by radiation, increase tissue damage, for example, the role of TGF-β in pneumonitis

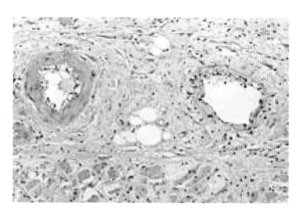

■ **FIGURE 20-20** Histopathology showing radiation-induced arteriole fibrosis (left). (From Zaharia M, Goans RE, Berger ME, et al. Industrial radiography accident at the Yanango hydroelectric power plant. In: Ricks RC, et al., eds. *The Medical Basis for Radiation Accident Preparedness, the Clinical Care of Victims.* New York, NY: The Parthenon Publishing Group; 2001:267-281.)

is well documented, some growth factors can be radioprotective in some tissues, *e.g.*, basic fibroblast growth factor protects microvasculature and IL-1 is a radioprotector of hematopoietic cells (Hall and Giaccia, 2018).

Important components of late responses also reflect damage to vasculature and development of fibrosis, caused by premature senescence and accelerated post-mitotic differentiation leading to excessive collagen production by mesenchymal cells such as fibroblasts. Late radiation effects on the vasculature include fibrosis, proliferation of myointimal cells, and hyaline sclerosis of arterioles, the effect of which is a gradual narrowing of the vessels and reduction in the blood supply to the point that the flow of oxygen and nutrients is insufficient to sustain the cells comprising the functional parenchyma (Fig. 20-20). Importantly, these multiple interactions of the elements of tissue reactions change and evolve over time.

20.5.2 Healing

Healing of tissue damage produced by radiation occurs by means of cellular *regeneration* (repopulation) and *replacement* (Fig. 20-21). Regeneration refers to repopulation of the damaged cells in the organ by cells of the same type, thus recovering the lost functional capacity. Replacement refers to the development of fibrotic scar tissue, in which case the functionality of the organ system is compromised. The types of response and the degree to which they occur are functions of the dose, the volume of tissue irradiated, and the relative radiosensitivity and regenerative capacity of the cells that comprise the organ system. In so far as repopulation at the cellular level occurs within days after irradiation (Trott, 1991), fractionation of the dose (*e.g.*, multiple fluoroscopically guided interventional procedures separated by days or weeks) allows for cellular repair and cellular repopulation and typically results in less extensive tissue damage than if the same total dose were to be delivered all at once. If the exposures are excessive, the ability of the cells to affect any type of healing may be lost, resulting in tissue fibrosis and necrosis.

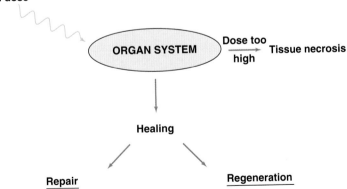

FIGURE 20-21 Schematic diagram of organ system response to radiation.

20.5.3 Specific Organ System Responses

This section focuses on radiation-induced changes to the skin, reproductive organs, and eyes. Effects on the hematopoietic, gastrointestinal, and cardiovascular systems and the CNS are addressed in the context of the acute radiation syndrome (ARS). Additional information on radiation effects on these and other tissues and organ systems can be found in several textbooks and review publications listed at the end of the chapter under sections for suggested reading and references (*e.g.*, Hall and Giaccia, 2018; ICRP, 2011; Mettler and Upton, 2008).

Skin

While radiation-induced skin damage is a relatively rare event, it is still the most commonly encountered tissue reaction (deterministic effect) following high-dose fluoroscopically guided interventional procedures. Acute radiation-induced skin changes were recognized soon after the discovery of x-rays and were reported in the literature as early as 1896 (Codman, 1902; Daniel, 1896). The first evidence of adverse biological effects of ionizing radiation appeared in the form of erythema and acute radiation dermatitis. In fact, before the introduction of the roentgen as the unit of radiation exposure, radiologists and radiation therapists evaluated the intensity of x-rays by using a quantity called the "skin erythema dose," which was defined as the dose of x-rays necessary to cause a certain degree of erythema within a specified time. This quantity was unsatisfactory for a variety of reasons, not least of which was that the response of the skin from radiation exposure is quite variable. Malignant skin lesions from chronic radiation exposure were reported as early as 1902 (Frieben, 1902).

The reaction of skin to high dose radiation (often referred to as the *cutaneous radiation syndrome*) has been studied extensively, and the degree of damage has been found to depend not only on the radiation quantity, quality, and dose rate but also on the location and extent of the exposure. Radiation-induced skin injuries can be severe and debilitating, and, in some cases, the dose has been high enough to cause chronic ulceration and necrosis requiring surgical intervention and a course of care lasting years.

While radiation oncologists are well versed in the potential for skin injury from radiotherapy, many physicians (including radiologists) are unfamiliar with the appearance, time course, and doses necessary to produce clinically significant skin damage. There are usually no immediate clinical signs and symptoms from high skin doses and, when initial symptoms do develop (*e.g.*, erythema, xerosis, pruritus), with the exception of prompt erythema, they are often delayed by weeks and may require months or even more than a year for full expression. Primary care physicians evaluating their patients may fail to consider the patient's past radiologic procedure as a potential cause of their symptoms. Fortunately, serious skin injuries are rare and, with the exception of prolonged fluoroscopically guided interventional procedures and very rare cases where excessive doses have been received from CT, it is highly unlikely that the radiation doses from carefully performed (*i.e.*, optimized) diagnostic examinations will be high enough to produce any of the effects discussed below.

Skin damage is a consequence of acute radiation-induced oxidative stress resulting in a cascade of inflammatory responses, reduction and impairment of functional stem/early progenitor cells, endothelial cell changes, and epidermal cell death via apoptosis and necrosis. The most sensitive structures in the skin include the germinal epithelium, sebaceous glands, and hair follicles. The cells that make up the germinal epithelium, located between the dermis and the epidermis, have a high mitotic rate and continuously replace sloughed epidermal cells. Complete turnover of the epidermis normally occurs within approximately 4 to 6 weeks. Skin reactions to radiation exposure have a threshold of approximately 1 Gy below which no effects are seen. At higher doses, radiation can interfere with normal maturation, reproduction, and repopulation of germinative epidermal cell populations. At very high doses, the mitotic activity in the germinal cells of the sebaceous glands, hair follicles, basal cell layer, and intimal cells of the microvasculature can be compromised.

A generalized erythema can occur within hours following an acute dose of 2 Gy or more of low-LET radiation and will typically fade within a few hours or days. This inflammatory response, often referred to as *early transient erythema*, is largely caused by increased capillary dilatation and permeability secondary to the release of vasoactive amines (*e.g.*, histamine). Higher doses produce earlier and more intense erythema. A later wave of erythema can reappear as early as 2 weeks after a high initial exposure or after repeated lower exposures (*e.g.*, 2 Gy/d as in radiation therapy), reaching a maximal response about the third week, at which time the skin may be edematous, may be tender, and may often exhibit a burning sensation. This secondary or *main erythema* is believed to be an inflammatory reaction secondary to the release of proteolytic enzymes from damaged epithelial basal cells as well as reflecting the loss of those epithelial cells. The oxidative stress resulting from a burst of radiation-induced free radicals is known to up-regulate numerous pathways pertinent to vascular damage, including adhesion molecules, proinflammatory cytokines, smooth muscle cell proliferation, and apoptosis. A third or *late erythema* wave may also be seen between 8 and 52 weeks after exposure. The dermal ischemia present at this stage produces erythema with a bluish or mauve tinge.

Temporary hair loss (epilation) can occur in approximately 3 weeks after exposure to 3 to 6 Gy, with regrowth beginning approximately 2 months later and complete within 6 to 12 months. After large doses, 40 Gy over a period of 4 weeks or 20 Gy in a single dose, intense erythema followed by an acute radiation dermatitis and moist desquamation occurs and is characterized by edema, dermal hypoplasia, inflammatory cell infiltration, damage to vascular structures, and permanent hair loss. Moist desquamation, which implies total destruction of the epidermis, is a clear predictor of late delayed injuries, particularly telangiectasia. Provided the vasculature and germinal epithelium of the skin have not been too severely damaged, reepithelialization occurs within 6 to 8 weeks, returning the skin to normal within 2 to 3 months. If these structures have been damaged but not destroyed, healing may occur, although the skin may be atrophic, hypo- or hyper-pigmented, and easily damaged by minor physical trauma. Recurring lesions and infections at the site of irradiation are common in these cases, and necrotic ulceration can develop. Chronic radiation dermatitis can also be produced by repeated low-level exposures (10 to 20 mGy/d) where the total dose approaches 20 Gy or more. In these cases, the skin may become hypertrophic or atrophic and is at increased risk for the development of skin neoplasms (especially squamous cell carcinoma). Erythema will not result from chronic exposures in which the total dose is less than 6 Gy.

The National Cancer Institute (NCI) has defined four grades of radiation-induced skin toxicity where Grade 1 is the least severe and Grade 4 is the most severe. The range or "band" of doses associated with each grade and the anticipated skin damage as well as the temporal character of the response is shown in Table 20-3. Figure 20-22 illustrates several grades of radiation-induced skin reactions from exposure to diagnostic and interventional imaging procedures.

Skin contamination with radioactive material can produce skin reactions. The extent of the reaction will depend on the quantity of radioactive material, characteristics of the radionuclide including the types and energy of the radiations emitted, the half-life, the region of the skin that was contaminated, and how long the contamination remained on the skin. Even in the absence of direct skin contamination mishandling of radionuclides with high-energy beta particle emissions such as Y-90 (used in the treatment of non-Hodgkin lymphoma as Y-90 Zevalin, a CD20-directed radiotherapeutic antibody) is likely to elicit skin reactions (*e.g.*, see Cremones et al., 2006).

20.5 Tissue and Organ System Response to Radiation

TABLE 20-3 TISSUE REACTIONS FROM A SINGLE-DELIVERY RADIATION DOSE TO THE SKIN OF THE NECK, TORSO, PELVIS, BUTTOCKS, OR ARMS[a,b]

SINGLE-SITE ACUTE SKIN- DOSE RANGE (GY)[c-e]	NCI (2006) SKIN REACTION GRADE	APPROXIMATE TIME OF ONSET OF EFFECTS[e,f]			
		Prompt <2 wk	Early 2–8 wk	Mid Term 6–52 wk	Long >40 wk
0–2	Not applicable		No observable effects expected at any time		
2–5	1	Transient erythema	Epilation	Recovery from hair loss	None expected
5–10	1–2	Transient erythema	Erythema, epilation	• Recovery • At higher doses: prolonged erythema, permanent partial epilation	• Recovery • At higher doses: dermal atrophy induration
10–15	2–3	Transient erythema	• Erythema, epilation • Possible dry or moist desquamation • Recovery from desquamation	• Prolonged erythema • Permanent epilation	• Telangiectasia[g] • atrophy induration • Skin likely to be weak; atrophic
>15	3–4	• Transient erythema • After very high doses: edema and acute ulceration, long-term surgical intervention likely to be required	• Erythema, epilation • Moist desquamation	• Dermal atrophy • Secondary ulceration due to failure of moist desquamation to heal, surgical intervention likely to be required • At higher doses: dermal necrosis, surgical intervention likely to be required	• Telangiectasia[g] • Dermal atrophy induration • Possible late skin breakdown • Wound might be persistent and progress into a deeper lesion • Surgical intervention likely to be required

[a]This table applies to the normal range of patient radiosensitivities in the absence of mitigating or aggravating physical or clinical factors.
[b]This table does not apply to the skin of the scalp.
[c]Skin dose refers to actual skin dose (including backscatter). This quantity is *not* air kerma at the reference point ($K_{a,r}$).
[d]Skin dosimetry based on $K_{a,r}$ or P_{KA} is unlikely to be more accurate than ±50%.
[e]The dose range and approximate time period are not rigid boundaries. Also, signs and symptoms can be expected to appear earlier as the skin dose increases.
[f]Abrasion or infection of the irradiated area is likely to exacerbate radiation effects.
[g]Refers to radiation-induced telangiectasia. Telangiectasia associated with an area of initial moist desquamation or the healing of ulceration may be present earlier.
Data from: *Radiation Dose Management for Fluoroscopically-Guided Interventional Procedures.* NCRP Report No. 168. Bethesda, MD: National Council on Radiation Protection; 2010.

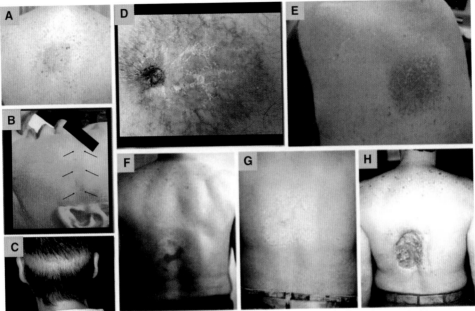

■ **FIGURE 20-22** Examples of radiation-induced effects on skin. **A.** National Cancer Institute (NCI) skin toxicity grade 1: Two fluoroscopically guided procedures were performed through overlapping skin ports in a 65-year-old man. Note enhanced reaction in the overlap zone. The first procedure was performed 6 weeks before and the second procedure, 2 weeks before this photograph was obtained (From Balter S, Hopewell JW, Miller DL, et al. Fluoroscopically guided interventional procedures: a review of radiation effects on patients' skin and hair. *Radiology.* 2010;254(2):326-341). **B.** Technologist error resulted in a 2-year-old child being accidentally exposed to radiation from 151 CT slice acquisitions without the table indexing and thus all were through almost the same 3 mm tissue plane. Within several hours after the failed CT scan, a line of erythema developed across the patient's face in the same distribution (arrows). Peak skin and brain dose within the slice were estimated to be 7.2 Gy and 5.2 Gy, respectively. CT scan parameters were set at 300 mAs and 120 kV. (Photo courtesy of Dr. Fred Mettler, dose estimates courtesy of Drs. Jerrold T. Bushberg and J. Anthony Seibert.). **C.** Patient with temporary hair loss in the region of four MDCT perfusion studies and two angiographies of the head within 15 days of admission for suspected stroke. Epilation appeared on day 37 after the first perfusion study and lasted for 51 days. Peak skin dose estimates for each of the MDCT procedures was ~1.93 Gy. (Reprinted with permission from Imanishi Y, Fukui A, Niimi H., et al. Radiation-induced temporary hair loss as a radiation damage only occurring in patients who had the combination of MDCT and DSA. *Eur Radiol.* 2005;15:41–46. Copyright © Springer Nature.) **D.** A 62-year-old man with a history of 2 previous cardiac catheterizations approximately 5 years prior. Lesion that had been developing for over a year presents as an NCI skin toxicity grade 3 chronic radiodermatitis at the site of beam entry. The lesion is an 8" × 6" well-demarcated erythematous atrophic plaque with telangiectasias and ulceration. (Reprinted with permission from Spiker, A et al. Fluoroscopy-induced chronic radiation dermatitis. *AJR* 2012:1861–1863. Copyright © Elsevier.) **E.** Dry desquamation (poikiloderma) at one month in a patient receiving approximately 11 Gy calculated peak skin dose. (Reprinted with permission from Chambers C, Fetterly K, Holzer R, et al. Radiation safety program for the cardiac catheterization laboratory. *Catheter Cardiovasc Interv.* 2011;77. Copyright © Wiley.). **F–H.** NCI skin toxicity grade 4. A 40-year-old male who underwent multiple coronary angiography and angioplasty procedures. The photographs show the time sequence of a major radiation injury. (Reprinted with permission from Shope TB. Radiation-induced skin injuries from fluoroscopy. *RadioGraphics* 1996;16:1195–1199. Copyright © Radiological Society of North America.) **(F)** Six to eight weeks postexposure (prolonged erythema with a mauve central area, suggestive of ischemia). The injury was described as "turning red about 1 month after the procedure and peeling a week later." By 6 weeks, it had the appearance of a second-degree burn; **(G)** sixteen to twenty-one weeks postexposure (depigmented skin with a central area of necrosis); and **(H)** eighteen to twenty-one months postexposure (deep necrosis with atrophic borders). Skin breakdown continued over the following months with progressive necrosis. The injury eventually required a skin graft. While the magnitude of the skin dose received by this patient is not known, from the nature of the injury it is probable that the dose exceeded 20 Gy. This sequence is available on the FDA Web site. (National Council on Radiation Protection and Measurements. *Radiation Dose Management for Fluoroscopically-Guided Interventional Procedures.* NCRP Report No. 168. Bethesda, MD: National Council on Radiation Protection; 2010.)

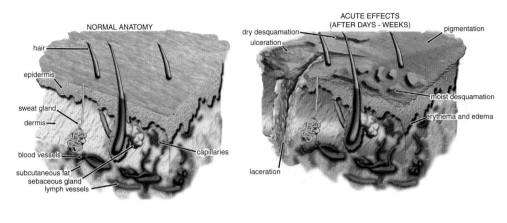

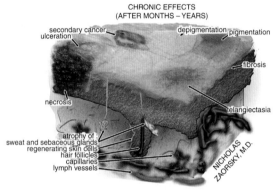

I

■ **FIGURE 20-22** (*Continued*) **I.** A three-dimensional view depicting the spectrum of radiation-induced effects on skin as shown in the previous photos (**A–H**) and discussed in the text. (Courtesy of Nicholas Zaorsky, MD.)

For all endpoints, the higher the dose and dose rate (beyond the threshold for effects) the shorter the latency, and the more severe the effect will be when fully evolved. However, it is important to recognize that the dose ranges shown in Table 20-3 are not to be interpreted as clear demarcations between various skin reactions and their associated dose. There are a number of factors that may cause the individual patient to be more or less sensitive to radiation exposure. Biologic factors, such as diabetes mellitus, systemic lupus erythematosus, scleroderma, or mixed connective tissue disease, and homozygosity for ataxia-telangiectasia (A-T), have increased sensitivity and potential for severe skin reactions. Other physical and biological variables that can substantially modify the severity of radiation-induced skin damage include high previous radiation dose to the same area being exposed, medications known to be radiosensitizers (particularly some chemotherapy agents), the size of the exposure area, anatomical location, fractionation, and patient health (Table 20-4).

Reproductive Organs

In general, the gonads are very radiosensitive. The testes contain cell populations that range from the most radiosensitive germ cells (*i.e.*, spermatogonia) to the most radioresistant, mature spermatozoa. The other cell populations with progressively greater differentiation during the 10-week maturation period (*i.e.*, primary and secondary spermatocytes and spermatids) are of intermediate radiosensitivity compared to the germ cells and mature sperm. The primary effects of radiation on the male reproductive system are reduced fertility, temporary sterility, and permanent sterility (azoospermia) (Clifton and Bremner, 1983). Temporary and permanent sterility can occur after acute doses of approximately 500 mGy and 6 Gy, respectively. The

TABLE 20-4 PHYSICAL AND BIOLOGICAL MODIFIERS OF RADIATION-INDUCED SKIN DAMAGE

FACTOR	EXAMPLES	COMMENT
Location of irradiated skin	Relative radiosensitivity: anterior aspect of the neck > flexor surfaces of the extremities > trunk > back > extensor surfaces of extremities > nape of the neck > scalp > palms of the hands > soles of feet	See Figure 20-22C demonstrating focal scalp epilation.
Size of the exposed area	Smaller lesions heal faster due to cell migration from skin margin surrounding the exposure area thus accelerating wound closure.	Benefit only significant for relatively small lesions. Not typically a factor for medical exposures where field sizes are larger
Dose fractionation	Dry Desquamation Threshold: Single exposure ~14 Gy; 3 fractions in 3 d ~27 Gy	Repair of sublethal damage to DNA is completed within ~24 h, however, repopulation can take days, weeks, or even months to complete.
Patient-related	Increased radiosensitivity examples: smoking, poor nutritional status, compromised skin integrity, light-colored skin, obesity, DNA repair defects, prior irradiation on the same area, UV exposure	DNA repair defect examples: ataxia-telangiectasia, Fanconi anemia, Bloom syndrome, and xeroderma pigmentosum. Other diseases, *e.g.*, scleroderma, hyperthyroidism, diabetes mellitus. Patients are more prone to sunburns and should minimize sun exposure following radiation-induced skin injury.
Drugs	Some drugs are known to increase radiosensitivity, *e.g.*, actinomycin D, doxorubicin, bleomycin, 5-fluorouracil and methotrexate.	Some chemotherapeutic agents, (*e.g.*, doxorubicin, etoposide, paclitaxel, epirubicin), antibiotics (*e.g.*, cefotetan), statins (*e.g.*, simvastatin), and herbal preparations can produce an inflammatory skin reaction at the site of prior irradiation (*radiation recall*) weeks to years after exposure at the same location.

Date from: Balter S, Hopewell JW, Miller DL, et al. Fluoroscopically guided interventional procedures: a review of radiation effects on patients' skin and hair. *Radiology*. 2010;254(2):326-341.

duration of temporary sterility is dose dependent, with recovery beginning at 1 and as long as 3.5 years after doses of 1 and 2 Gy, respectively. However, following exposure (and provided the dose is not excessive), there will be a window of fertility before the onset of sterility, as long as mature sperm are available. Chronic exposures of 20 to 50 mGy/wk can result in permanent sterility when the total dose exceeds 2.5 to 3 Gy. The reduced threshold for effect following chronic versus acute exposure is unusual (*i.e.*, an inverse fractionation effect) and is believed to be due to stem cells progressing into radiosensitive stages (Lushbaugh and Ricks, 1972). Reduced fertility due to decreased sperm count (oligospermia) and motility (asthenozoospermia) can occur 6 weeks after a dose of 150 mGy. These effects are not related to diagnostic examinations, because acute gonadal doses exceeding 100 mGy are unlikely.

The ova within ovarian follicles (classified according to their size as small, intermediate, or large) are sensitive to radiation. The intermediate follicles are the most radiosensitive, followed by the large (mature) follicles and the small follicles, which are the most radioresistant. Therefore, after a radiation dose as low as 1.5 Gy, fertility may be temporarily preserved owing to the relative radioresistance of the mature follicles, and this may be followed by a period of reduced fertility. Fertility will recur provided the exposure is not so high as to destroy the relatively radioresistant small primordial follicles. The dose that will produce permanent sterility is age dependent, with higher doses (~10 Gy) required to produce sterility prior to puberty than in pre-menopausal women over 40 years old (~2 to 3 Gy).

Another concern regarding gonadal irradiation is the induction of genetic mutations and their effect on future generations. This subject is addressed later in the chapter.

Ocular Effects

The lens of the eye contains a population of radiosensitive cells that can be damaged or destroyed by radiation. Insofar as there is no removal system for these damaged cells, they can accumulate to the point at which they cause vision-impairing cataracts. A unique aspect of cataract formation is that, unlike senile cataracts that typically develop in the anterior pole of the lens, radiation-induced cataracts are caused by abnormal differentiation of damaged epithelial cells that begin as small opacities (abnormal lens fibers) in the anterior subcapsular region and migrate posteriorly. Even at relatively minor levels of visual acuity loss, these posterior subcapsular cataracts can impair vision by causing glare or halos around lights at night. While the degree of the opacity and the probability of its occurrence increase with the dose, the latent period is inversely related to dose. High-LET radiation is more efficient for cataractogenesis by a factor of 2 or more. There have been several recent studies of mechanistic models of radiation-induced cataractogenesis. Also, more recent epidemiological studies have included several additional occupational exposure populations and longer periods of observation for previously studied populations. These studies have raised concerns regarding the previous scientific consensus that regarded radiation-induced cataracts as a tissue reaction with dose thresholds for detectable opacities of 2 Gy for acute and 5 Gy for chronic exposures, respectively. The view that cataractogenesis is a tissue reaction, exhibiting a dose threshold below which lens opacities would not develop, served as the basis for ICRP and NCRP previously recommending an occupational dose limit to the lens of the eye of 150 mSv/y (ICRP, 1991, 2007a; NCRP, 1993). However, studies of A-bomb survivors who were young at the time of exposure and followed for longer periods than previous studies and other exposed populations such as workers involved in the cleanup around the Chernobyl nuclear reactor accident site and radiologic technologists in the United States (Gabriel, 2008) suggest that, if there is a threshold for cataract development, it is likely to be substantially lower than previously believed (Ainsbury et al., 2009; ICRP, 2011). These data, and the presumption that subclinical but detectable opacities will, if given enough time, eventually progress to impair vision led the ICRP to conclude that the threshold for acute and chronic exposure may be more on the order of 0.5 Gy (ICRP, 2011). Furthermore, some suggest that the dose-response may be more accurately described by a linear no-threshold stochastic (rather than a tissue reaction) model. ICRP's recent review of the scientific evidence regarding the risk of radiation-induced cataract has led the commission to propose a much more conservative occupational equivalent dose limit for the lens of the eye (20 mSv/y averaged over 5 years, with no single year exceeding 50 mSv).

Cataracts among early radiation workers were common because of the extremely high doses resulting from long and frequent exposures from poorly shielded x-ray equipment and the absence of any substantial shielding of the eyes. Today, radiation-induced cataracts are much less common; however, there is concern that for radiation workers receiving higher lens exposures in a medical setting (typically from interventional fluoroscopic procedures) there may be a risk for clinically significant lens opacities over an occupational lifetime. Considering the mounting evidence of a substantially lower threshold for radiation-induced cataracts, the current U.S. regulatory limit of 150 mSv/y to the lens of the eye may need to be reevaluated. However, the proposed ICRP limit is almost a factor of 10 lower than current limits and lower than the whole-body dose limit in the United States of 50 mSv/y. Similarly, the NCRP has recommended an occupational dose limit for the lens of the eye of 50 mGy/y (NCRP, 2016), although the U.S. national regulations have not yet been revised. Adoption of ICRP or NCRP recommendations by regulatory bodies would present new challenges for radiation protection in health care settings, especially for those involved in performing fluoroscopically guided interventional procedures. In any case, the use of eye protection in the form of leaded glasses and/or ceiling mounted lead acrylic shielding is imperative for workers whose careers will involve long-term exposure to scattered radiation.

Summary

There is general agreement that acute doses below 100 mGy will not result in any functional impairment of tissues or organ systems. This can also be considered generally applicable to the risk of clinically significant lenticular opacities with the caveat that the existence of a true threshold for radiation-induced cataracts remains uncertain. The previous discussion has been limited to tissues and organ systems that are often the focus of concerns for patients and for staff performing diagnostic and interventional fluoroscopic procedures. A more complete discussion of these and other organ and tissue reactions to radiation exposure can be found in the ICRP report devoted to this subject (ICRP, 2012). A summary from this report of threshold doses (defined as ~1% incidence in morbidity) in tissues and organs in adults exposed to acute, fractionated or protracted, and chronic irradiation is reproduced in Table 20-5. Additional information, including a systematic review of epidemiologic evidence related to radiogenic cataracts, was performed by the NCRP (NCRP, 2016).

20.6 WHOLE-BODY RESPONSE TO RADIATION: THE ACUTE RADIATION SYNDROME

As previously discussed, the body consists of cells of differing radiosensitivities and a large radiation dose delivered acutely yields greater cellular damage than the same dose delivered over a protracted period. When the whole body (or a large portion of the body) is subjected to a high acute radiation dose, there are a series of characteristic clinical responses known collectively as the *acute radiation syndrome* (ARS). The ARS is an organismal response quite distinct from isolated local radiation injuries such as epilation or skin ulcerations.

The ARS refers to a group of subsyndromes occurring in stages over a period of hours to weeks after the exposure as the injuries to various tissues and organ systems are expressed. These subsyndromes result from the differing radiosensitivities of these organ systems. In order of their occurrence with increasing radiation dose, the ARS is divided into the hematopoietic, gastrointestinal, and neurovascular syndromes. These syndromes are identified by the organ system in which the damage is primarily responsible for the clinical manifestation of the disease. The ARS can occur when a high radiation dose is (1) delivered acutely, (2) involves exposure to the whole body (or at least a large portion of it), and (3) is from external penetrating radiation, such as x-rays, γ-rays, or neutrons. Accidental internal or external contamination with radioactive material is unlikely to result in a sufficiently acute dose to produce the ARS in the organ systems. However, as the widely publicized death of Alexander Litvinenko in 2006 from Po-210 (an alpha emitter) poisoning demonstrated, ARS can be observed when internal contamination with large quantities of highly radiotoxic material (~2 GBq in this case) are widely distributed in the body. Mr. Litvinenko died

TABLE 20-5 THRESHOLD DOSES IN TISSUES AND ORGANS IN ADULTS EXPOSED TO ACUTE, FRACTIONATED OR PROTRACTED, AND CHRONIC RADIATION EXPOSURE[a]

EFFECT	ORGAN/TISSUE	TIME TO DEVELOP EFFECT	ACUTE EXPOSURE (Gy)	HIGHLY FRACTIONATED (2 Gy PER FRACTION) OR EQUIVALENT PROTRACTED EXPOSURES (Gy)[B]	ANNUAL (CHRONIC) DOSE RATE FOR MANY YEARS (Gy/y)
Temporary sterility	Testes	3–9 wk	~0.1	NA	0.4
Permanent sterility	Testes	3 wk	~6	<6	2.0
Permanent sterility	Ovaries	<1 wk	~3	6.0	>0.2
Depression of hematopoiesis	Bone marrow	3–7 d	~0.5	~10–14 Gy	>0.4
Xerostomia	Salivary glands	1 wk	NA	<20	NA
Dysphasia, stricture	Esophagus	3–8 mo	NA	55	NA
Dyspepsia, ulceration	Stomach	2 y	NA	50	NA
Stricture	Small intestine	1.5 y	NA	45	NA
Stricture	Colon	2 y	NA	45	NA
Anorectal dysfunction	Rectum	1 y	NA	60	NA
Hepatomegaly, ascites	Liver	2 wk to 3 mo	NA	<30–32	NA
Main phase of skin reddening	Skin (large areas)	1–4 wk	<3–6	30	NA
Skin burns	Skin (large areas)	2–3 wk	5–10	35	NA
Temporary hair loss	Skin	2–3 wk	~4	NA	NA
Late atrophy	Skin (large areas)	>1 y	10	40	NA
Telangiectasia at 5 y	Skin (large areas)	>1 y	10	40	NA
Cataract (visual impairment)	Eye	>20 y	~0.5	~0.5	~0.5 divided by years of duration[c]
Acute pneumonitis	Lung	1–3 mo	6–7	18	NA
Edema	Larynx	4–5 mo	NA	70	NA
Renal failure	Kidney	>1 y	7–8	18	NA
Fibrosis/necrosis	Bladder	>6 mo	15	55	NA

Stricture	Ureters	>6 mo	NA	55–60	NA
Fracture	Adult bone	>1 y	NA	50	NA
Fracture	Growing bone	<1 y	NA	25	NA
Necrosis	Skeletal muscle	Several years	NA	55	NA
Endocrine dysfunction	Thyroid	>10 y	NA	>18	NA
Endocrine dysfunction	Pituitary	>10 y	NA	≤10	NA
Paralysis	Spinal cord	>6 mo	NA	55	NA
Necrosis	Brain	>1 y	NA	55–60	NA
Cognitive defects	Brain	Several years	1–2	<20	NA
Cognitive defects infants <18 mo	Brain	Several years	0.1–0.2	NA	NA

Note: Protracted doses at a low dose rate of around 10 mGy/min are approximately isoeffective to doses delivered in 2 Gy fractions at high dose rate for some tissues, but this equivalence is dependent on the repair half-time of the particular tissue. Further details can be found in ICRP (2011) report references Joiner and Bentzen (2009), Bentzen and Joiner (2009), and van der Kogel (2009). Most values rounded to nearest Gy; ranges indicate area dependence for skin and differing medical support for bone marrow.

[a]Defined as 1% incidence in morbidity.

[b]Derived from fractionated radiotherapeutic exposures, generally using 2 Gy per fraction. For other fraction sizes, the following formula can be used, where D is total dose (number of fractions multiplied by d), d is dose per fraction (2 Gy in the case of D_1, and a new value of d in the case of D_2), and the ratio α/β can be found in the appropriate section of the ICRP (2011) report: $D_1[1 + 2/(\alpha/\beta)] = D_2[1 + d_2/(\alpha/\beta)]$.

[c]The values quoted for the lens assume the same incidence of injury irrespective of the acute or chronic nature of the exposure, with more than 20 years' follow-up. It is emphasized that great uncertainty is attached to these values.

NA, not available.

Adapted with permission from Stewart FA, et al. ICRP publication 118: ICRP statement on tissue reactions and early and late effects of radiation in normal tissues and organs—threshold doses for tissue reactions in a radiation protection context. *Ann ICRP.* 2012;41(1-2):1-322. Copyright © Sage Publications.

approximately 3 weeks after the poisoning from the complications of profound pancytopenia that is characteristic of severe hematopoietic damage.

20.6.1 Sequence of Events

The clinical manifestation of each of the subsyndromes occurs in a predictable sequence of events that includes the *prodromal, latent, manifest illness,* and, if the dose is not fatal, *recovery* stages (Fig. 20-23).

The onset of prodromal symptoms is dose dependent and can begin within minutes to hours after the exposure. As the whole-body exposure increases above a threshold of approximately 0.5 to 1 Gy, the prodromal symptoms, which (depending on dose) can include anorexia, nausea, lethargy, fever, vomiting, headache, diarrhea, and altered mental status, begin earlier and are more severe. Table 20-6 summarizes some of the clinical findings, probability of occurrence, and time of onset that may be anticipated during the prodromal phase of ARS as a function of whole-body dose.

The time of onset and the severity of these symptoms were used during the initial phases of the medical response to the Chernobyl (Ukraine) nuclear reactor accident in 1986 to triage patients with respect to their radiation exposures. The prodromal symptoms subside during the latent period, whose duration is shorter for higher doses and may last for up to 4 weeks for modest exposures less than 1 Gy. The latent period can be thought of as an "incubation period" during which the organ system damage is progressing. The latent period ends with the onset of the clinical expression of organ system damage, called the *manifest illness stage,* which can last

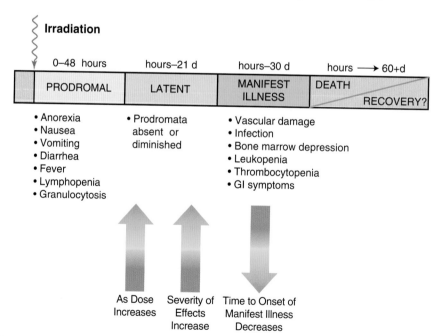

■ FIGURE 20-23 ARS follows a clinical pattern that can be divided into three phases: (1) an initial or prodromal phase that presents as non-specific clinical symptoms, such as nausea, vomiting, and lethargy (hematological changes may also occur during this period); (2) the latent phase, during which the prodromal symptoms typically subside; and (3) the manifest illness phase, during which the underlying organ system damage is expressed. The type, time of onset, and severity of prodromal symptoms are dose dependent. The duration of the latent period, as well as the time of onset and severity of the manifest illness phase, and ultimate outcome are all, to a variable extent, dependent upon total dose, uniformity of the exposure, and individual radiation sensitivity. As a rule, higher doses shorten the time of onset and duration of all three phases and increase the severity of the prodromal and the manifest illness phases.

TABLE 20-6 **CLINICAL FINDINGS DURING PRODROMAL PHASE OF ARS**

Symptoms and Medical Response	ARS DEGREE AND THE APPROXIMATE DOSE OF ACUTE WHOLE BODY EXPOSURE				
	Mild (1–2 Gy)	Moderate (2–4 Gy)	Severe (4–6 Gy)	Very Severe (6–8 Gy)	Lethal (>8 Gy)[a]
Vomiting Onset	2 h after exposure or later	1–2 h after exposure	Earlier than 1 h after exposure	Earlier than 30 min after exposure	Earlier than 10 min after exposure
Incidence, %	10–50	70–90	100	100	100
Diarrhea	None	None	Mild	Heavy	Heavy
Onset			3–8 h	1–3 h	Within minutes or 1 h
Incidence, %			<10	>10	Almost 100
Headache	Slight	Mild	Moderate	Severe	Severe
Onset			4–24 h	3–4 h	1–2 h
Incidence, %			50	80	80–90
Consciousness	Unaffected	Unaffected	Unaffected	May be altered	Unconsciousness (may last seconds to minutes)
Onset					Seconds/minutes
Incidence, %					100 (at <50 Gy)
Body temperature	Normal	Increased	Fever	High fever	High fever
Onset		1–3 h	1–2 h	<1 h	<1 h
Incidence, %		10–80	80–100	100	100
Medical response	Outpatient observation	Observation in a general hospital, treatment in specialized hospital if needed	Treatment in a specialized hospital	Treatment in a specialized hospital	Palliative treatment (symptomatic only)

[a]With intensive medical support and marrow resuscitative therapy, individuals may survive for 6 to 12 months with whole-body doses as high as 12 Gy.
ARS, acute radiation syndrome.
Adapted with permission from *Diagnosis and Treatment of Radiation Injuries*. Safety Report Series No. 2. Vienna, Austria: International Atomic Energy Agency, World Health Organization; 1998; Koenig KL, Goans RE, Hatchett RJ, et al. Medical treatment of radiological casualties: current concepts. *Ann Emerg Med*. 2005;45:643-652. Copyright © Elsevier.

for approximately 2 to 4 weeks or in some cases even longer. This stage is the most difficult to manage from a therapeutic standpoint, because of the overlying immunoincompetence that results from damage to the hematopoietic system. Therefore, treatment during the first 6 to 8 weeks after the exposure is essential to optimize the chances for recovery. If the patient survives the manifest illness stage, recovery is likely; however, the patient will be at higher risk for cancer and, to a much lesser extent, his or her future progeny may have an increased risk of genetic abnormalities.

20.6.2 Hematopoietic Syndrome

Although increasing evidence indicates that hematopoietic stem cells, located in the stem cell niche in the bone marrow, are more radiation resistant, the early progenitor cells are very radiosensitive. However, with the exception of lymphocytes, their mature counterparts in circulation are relatively radioresistant. Hematopoietic tissues are located at various anatomic sites throughout the body; however, posterior radiation exposure maximizes damage because the majority of the active bone marrow is located in the spine and posterior region of the ribs and pelvis. The hematopoietic syndrome is the primary acute clinical consequence of an acute radiation dose between 0.5 and 10 Gy. Healthy adults with proper medical care almost always recover from doses lower than 2 Gy, whereas doses greater than 8 Gy are almost always fatal unless advanced therapies such as the use of colony-stimulating factors or bone marrow transplantation are successful. Growth factors such as granulocyte-macrophage colony-stimulating factor and other glycoproteins that induce bone marrow hematopoietic progenitor cells to proliferate and differentiate into specific mature blood cells have shown promise in the treatment of severe stem cell depletion. Even with effective stem cells therapy, however, it is unlikely that patients will survive doses in excess of 12 Gy because of irreversible damage to the gastrointestinal tract and the vasculature. In the absence of medical care, the human $LD_{50/60}$ (the dose that would be expected to kill 50% of an exposed population within 60 days) is approximately 3.25 to 4.5 Gy to the bone marrow. The $LD_{50/60}$ may extend to 6 to 7 Gy with supportive care such as the use of transfusions and antibiotics and may be as high as 6 to 8 Gy with effective use of hematopoietic growth factors in an intensive care setting (MacVittie and Farese, 2013). In contrast to whole body high-dose penetrating radiation exposures, radiation exposure during some accident scenarios may result in inhomogeneous exposures for which the potential for spontaneous hematopoietic regeneration from unirradiated or only mildly irradiated stem cells is much greater. The probability of recovering from a large radiation dose is reduced in patients who are compromised by trauma or other serious comorbidities. The severe burns and trauma received by some of the workers exposed during the Chernobyl nuclear accident resulted in a lower $LD_{50/60}$ than would have been predicted from their radiation exposures alone. In addition, patients with certain inherited diseases that compromise DNA repair, such as A-T, Fanconi anemia, and Bloom syndrome, are known to have an increased sensitivity to radiation exposure.

The prodromal symptoms associated with the hematopoietic syndrome can occur within a few hours after exposure and may consist of nausea, vomiting, headache, and diarrhea. If these symptoms appear early and severe diarrhea occurs within the first 2 days, the radiation exposure may prove to be fatal. The prodromal and latent periods may each last for weeks. Although the nausea and vomiting may subside during the latent period, patients may still feel fatigued and weak. During this period, damage to the stem/early progenitor cells reduces their number and thus their ability to maintain normal hematologic profiles by replacing the circulating blood cells that eventually die by senescence. The kinetics of this generalized pancytopenia are accelerated

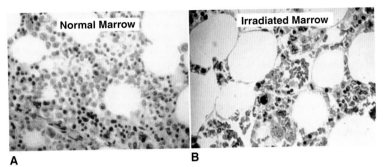

■ **FIGURE 20-24 A.** Normal bone marrow stem cells. **B.** Pyknotic stem cell damage following a bone marrow dose of approximately 2 Gy. (Adapted from *Medical Management of Radiological Casualties.* Online 3rd ed. Bethesda, MD: Armed Forces Radiobiology Research Institute; June 2010. http://www.usuhs.mil/afrri/outreach/pdf/3edmmrchandbook.pdf)

with higher (acute) exposures. An example of radiation-induced stem cell damage following a bone marrow dose of 2 Gy is shown in Figure 20-24. Figure 20-25 illustrates the time course of the hematological consequences of bone marrow doses of 1 and 3 Gy.

The initial rise in the neutrophil count is presumably a stress response in which neutrophils are released from extravascular stores. The decline in the lymphocyte

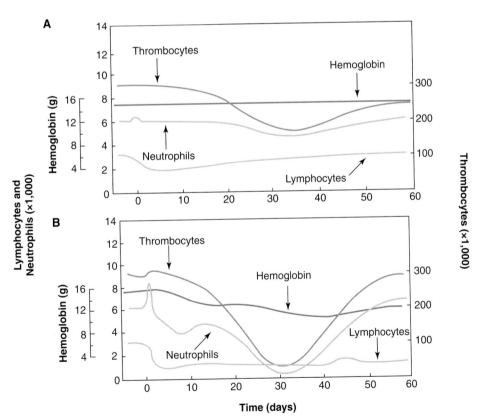

■ **FIGURE 20-25** Hematological changes following an acute bone marrow dose of 1 Gy **(A)** and 3 Gy **(B)**. One Gy causes a transient and 3 Gy an extended period of neutropenia, and thrombocytopenia. The lymphopenia is a consequence of radiation-induced apoptosis in some types of lymphocytes. (Adapted from *Medical Management of Radiological Casualties.* Online 3rd ed. Bethesda, MD: Armed Forces Radiobiology Research Institute; June 2010. http://www.usuhs.mil/afrri/outreach/pdf/3edmmrchandbook.pdf)

count occurs within hours after exposure and is a crude early biologic marker of the magnitude of exposure. The threshold for a measurable depression in the blood lymphocyte count is approximately 0.25 Gy; an absolute lymphocyte count lower than 1,000/mm^3 in the first 48 h indicates a severe exposure.

The clinical manifestation of bone marrow depletion peaks 3 to 4 weeks after the exposure as the number of cells in circulation reaches its nadir. Hemorrhage from platelet loss and opportunistic infections secondary to severe neutropenia are the potentially lethal consequences of severe hematopoietic compromise. Overall, the systemic effects that can occur from the hematopoietic syndrome include mild to profound immunologic compromise, sepsis, hemorrhage, anemia, and impaired wound healing.

20.6.3 Gastrointestinal Syndrome

At higher doses, the clinical expression of the gastrointestinal syndrome becomes the dominant component of the radiation response, the consequences of which are more immediate and severe and overlap with those of the hematopoietic syndrome. At doses greater than 12 Gy, this syndrome is primarily responsible for lethality. Its prodromal stage includes severe nausea, vomiting, watery diarrhea, and cramps occurring within hours after the exposure, followed by a much shorter latent period (5 to 7 days). The manifest illness stage begins with the return of the prodromal symptoms that are often more intense than during their initial presentation. The intestinal dysfunction is the result of the severe damage to the intestinal mucosa. Severely damaged crypt stem cells lose their reproductive capacity. As the mucosal lining ages and eventually sloughs, the differentiated cells in the villi are not adequately replaced by cells from the progenitor compartment in the crypt. The denuding of bowel villi, in turn, causes a host of pathophysiological sequelae. The breakdown of the mucosal barrier allows for the entry of luminal contents such as antigens, bacterial products, and digestive enzymes into the intestinal wall ultimately resulting in a radiation-induced intestinal mucositis. The net result is a greatly diminished capacity to regulate the absorption of electrolytes and nutrients and, at the same time, a portal is created for intestinal flora to enter the systemic circulation. These changes in the gastrointestinal tract are compounded by equally drastic changes in the bone marrow. The most potentially serious effect is the severe decrease in circulating white cells at a time when bacteria are invading the bloodstream from the gastrointestinal tract.

Overall, intestinal pathology includes mucosal ulceration and hemorrhage, disruption of normal absorption and secretion, alteration of enteric flora, depletion of gut lymphoid tissue, and disturbance of gut motility. The systemic effects of acute radiation enteropathy include malnutrition resulting from malabsorption; vomiting and abdominal distention from paralytic ileus; anemia from gastrointestinal bleeding; sepsis resulting from an invasion of intestinal bacteria into the systemic circulation; and dehydration and acute renal failure from fluid and electrolyte imbalance. The patient may not become profoundly pancytopenic, because death will likely occur before radiation-induced damage to the bone marrow causes a significant decrease in cell types with longer life spans (*e.g.*, platelets and red cells). Lethality from the gastrointestinal syndrome is essentially 100%. Death occurs within 3 to 10 days after the exposure if no medical care is given or as long as 2 weeks afterward with intensive medical support.

It is important to appreciate that even at doses within the hematopoietic syndrome dose range (2 to 10 Gy), damage to the gastrointestinal tract is occurring. It is responsible for many of the prodromal symptoms and contributes to the toxicity of the radiation-induced myelosuppression that is the signature of the hematopoietic component of the ARS. While a whole-body dose of 6 Gy does not result in the full gastrointestinal sequelae described above, damage to the mucosal barrier causes cytokines and other inflammatory mediators to be released into the circulation. In addition, sepsis resulting from the entry of bacteria from the bowel into the systemic circulation during a period of progressive neutropenia is an important cause of death from doses in the hematopoietic syndrome dose range.

20.6.4 Neurovascular Syndrome

Death occurs within 2 to 3 days after supralethal doses in excess of 50 Gy. Doses in this range result in cardiovascular shock with a massive loss of serum and electrolytes into extravascular tissues. The ensuing circulatory problems of edema, increased intracranial pressure, and cerebral anoxia cause death before damage to other organ systems and tissues can become clinically significant.

The stages of the neurovascular syndrome are extremely compressed. Patients may experience transitory incapacitation or unconsciousness. The prodromal period may include a burning sensation of the skin that occurs within minutes, followed by nausea, vomiting, confusion, ataxia, and disorientation within 1 h. There is an abbreviated latent period (4 to 6 h), during which some improvement is noted, followed by a severe manifest illness stage. The prodromal symptoms return with even greater severity, coupled with respiratory distress and gross neurologic changes (including tremors and convulsions) that inevitably lead to coma and death. Many other aspects of this syndrome are not understood because human exposures to supralethal radiation are rare. Experimental evidence suggests that the initial hypotension may be caused by a massive release of histamine from mast cells, and the principal pathology may result from massive damage to the microcirculation (Park et al., 2016).

20.6.5 Summary of Clinical Features during the Manifest Illness Phase of the Acute Radiation Syndrome

Table 20-7 summarizes the clinical features of the ARS within several dose ranges with respect to hematological changes, manifestations of clinical symptoms, latency, as well as the medical response, and the probability of survival. The previously discussed relationships among various elements of the ARS are summarized in Figure 20-26.

20.7 RADIATION-INDUCED CARCINOGENESIS

20.7.1 Introduction

Most of the radiation-induced biologic effects discussed thus far are detectable within a relatively short time after the exposure. Ionizing radiation can, however, cause damage whose expression is delayed for years or decades. The ability of ionizing radiation to increase the risk of cancer years after exposure has been well established. Cancer, unfortunately, is not a rare disease; indeed, it is the second most likely cause of death, after cardiovascular disease, in the United States. According to recent statistics on cancer in the United States from the American Cancer Society (ACS, 2020), the lifetime probability of developing an invasive cancer is 39.4% (40.1% male and 38.7% female) and the probability of dying from cancer is about half that, 19.8% (21.3%

TABLE 20-7 CLINICAL FEATURES DURING THE MANIFEST ILLNESS PHASE OF ARS

	DEGREE OF ARS AND APPROXIMATE DOSE OF ACUTE WHOLE-BODY EXPOSURE				
	Mild (1–2 Gy)	Moderate (2–4 Gy)	Severe (4–6 Gy)	Very Severe (6–8 Gy)	Lethal (>8 Gy)
Onset of signs	>30 d	18–28 d	8–18 d	<7 d	<3 d
Lymphocytes, G/L[a]	0.8–1.5	0.5–0.8	0.3–0.5	0.1–0.3	0.0–0.1
Platelets, G/L[a]	60–100	30–60	25–35	15–25	<20
Percent of patients with cytopenia	10%–25%	25%–40%	40%–80%	60%–80%	80%–100%[b]
Clinical manifestations	Fatigue, weakness	Fever, infections, bleeding, weakness, epilation	High fever, infections, bleeding, epilation	High fever, diarrhea, vomiting, dizziness and disorientation, hypotension	High fever, diarrhea, unconsciousness
Lethality, %	0–1	0–50	20–70	50–100	100
Onset	6–8 wk	6–8 wk	4–8 wk	1–2 wk	1–2 wk
Medical response	Prophylactic	Special prophylactic treatment from days 14–20; isolation from days 10–20	Special prophylactic treatment from days 7–10; isolation from the beginning	Special treatment from the first day; isolation from the beginning	Symptomatic only

[a]G/L, SI units for concentration and refers to 10⁹ per liter.

[b]In very severe cases, with a dose greater than 50 Gy, death precedes cytopenia.

Adapted with permission from *Diagnosis and Treatment of Radiation Injuries.* Safety Report Series No. 2. Vienna, Austria: International Atomic Energy Agency, World Health Organization; 1998; Koenig KL, Goans RE, Hatchett RJ, et al. Medical treatment of radiological casualties: current concepts. *Ann Emerg Med.* 2005;45:643-652. Copyright © Elsevier.

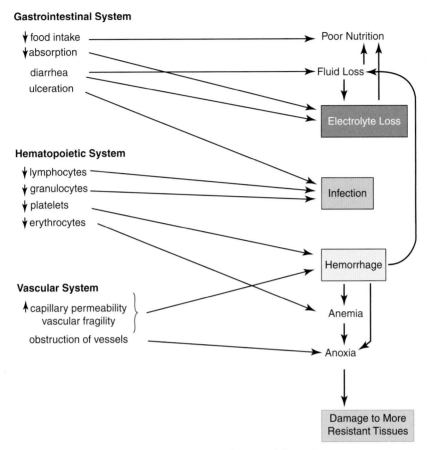

■ **FIGURE 20-26** Relationships among various elements of the ARS.

male and 18.3% female). Incidence rates are defined as the number of people per 100,000 who are diagnosed with cancer during a given time period (typically provided as an annual age-adjusted rate per 100,000). The National Center for Health Statistics recommends that the U.S. 2000 standard population be used when calculating and comparing age-adjusted rates for specific population groups. If one compares age-adjusted rates from different populations, the same standard population must be used for the comparison. The annual cancer incidence and mortality age-adjusted rates, for the U.S. population, are approximately 436 and 156 per 100,000, respectively, with males having a higher incidence rate (471 per 100,000) than females (413 per 100,000) (CDC, 2020). Subsequent sections of this chapter address estimates of radiation-induced cancer (incidence and mortality). To help place these numbers in perspective, the baseline lifetime risk of cancer incidence, mortality, and average years of life lost are shown in Table 20-8. As previously discussed, ICRP tissue weighting factors (w_T) were developed to account for inherent differences in tissue sensitivity to "detriment" caused by radiation exposure. Part of the detriment values are based on average years of life lost, which, even in the absence of additional radiation exposure, can vary between sexes and by type of cancer by almost a factor of two (*e.g.*, prostate and breast cancer).

Although the etiologies of most cancers are not well defined, diet, lifestyle, genetic, and environmental conditions appear to be among the most important factors affecting specific cancer risks. For example, the total cancer incidence among

TABLE 20-8 BASELINE LIFETIME RISK ESTIMATES OF CANCER INCIDENCE AND MORTALITY

	INCIDENCE		MORTALITY	
CANCER SITE	*Males*	*Females*	*Males*	*Females*
Solid cancer[a]	45,500	36,900	22,100 (11)	17,500 (11)
Stomach	1,200	720	670 (11)	430 (12)
Colon	4,200	4,200	2,200 (11)	2,100 (11)
Liver	640	280	490 (13)	260 (12)
Lung	7,700	5,400	7,700 (12)	4,600 (14)
Breast	—	12,000	—	3,000 (15)
Prostate	15,900	—	3,500 (8)	—
Uterus	—	3,000	—	750 (15)
Ovary	—	1,500	—	980 (14)
Bladder	3,400	1,100	770 (9)	330 (10)
Other solid cancer	12,500	8,800	6,800 (13)	5,100 (13)
Thyroid	230	550	40 (12)	60 (12)
Leukemia	830	590	710 (12)	530 (13)

Note: Number of estimated cancer cases or deaths in a population of 100,000 (no. of years of life lost per death).
[a]Solid cancer incidence estimates exclude thyroid and non-melanoma skin cancers.
Reprinted with permission from *Health Risks from Exposure to Low Levels of Ionizing Radiation: BEIR VII, Phase 2*. Committee to Assess Health Risks from Exposure to Low Levels of Ionizing Radiation, Board of Radiation Effects, Research Division on Earth and Life Studies, National Research Council of the National Academies. National Academy of Sciences, Washington, DC: National Academies Press; 2006.

populations around the world varies by only a factor of 2 or so, but the incidences of specific cancers can vary by a factor of 200 or more!

Cancer is the most important delayed somatic effect of radiation exposure. However, radiation is a relatively weak carcinogen at low doses (*e.g.*, occupational and diagnostic exposures), which together with its high natural incidence and mortality makes radioepidemiological investigations at low doses very challenging. While moderate doses of radiation cause well-documented effects, most studies have not detected significantly increased risks in populations at the doses typically encountered in diagnostic imaging. In fact, the body's robust capacity to repair radiation damage means that the possibility of no increased risk at low doses is, by no means certain; however, it cannot be ruled out either. The effectiveness of different DNA repair systems was previously discussed. The determinants of radiation-induced cancer risk are discussed in greater detail later in the chapter.

Molecular Biology and Cancer

Cancer arises from abnormal cell division. Cells in a tumor are believed to descend from a common ancestral cell that at some point (typically decades before a tumor results in clinically noticeable symptoms) lost its control over normal reproduction. The malignant transformation of such a cell can occur through the accumulation of mutations in specific classes of genes. Mutations in these genes are a critical step in the development of cancer.

Any protein involved in the control of cell division may also be involved in cancer. However, two classes of genes, *tumor suppressor genes*, and *protooncogenes*, which respectively inhibit and encourage cell growth, play major roles in triggering cancer. Tumor suppressor genes such as the *TP53* gene (Fig. 20-19, inset), in its nonmutated or "wild-type state," promotes the expression of certain proteins. One of these halts the cell cycle and gives the cell time to repair its DNA before dividing. Alternatively, if the damage cannot be repaired, the p53 protein pushes the cell into apoptosis. The loss of normal function of the p53 gene product may compromise DNA repair mechanisms and lead to tumor development. Defective *TP53* genes can cause abnormal cells to proliferate and as many as 50% of all human tumors have been found to contain *TP53* mutations.

Protooncogenes code for proteins that stimulate cell division. Mutated forms of these genes, called *oncogenes*, can cause the stimulatory proteins to be overactive, resulting in excessive cell proliferation. For example, mutations of the *RAS* protooncogenes (*H-RAS*, *N-RAS*, and *K-RAS*) are found in about 25% of all human tumors. The RAS family of proteins plays a central role in the regulation of cell growth and the integration of regulatory signals. These signals govern processes within the cell cycle and regulate cellular proliferation. Most mutations result in abrogation of the normal enzymatic activity of RAS, which causes a prolonged activation state and unregulated stimulation of RAS signaling pathways that either stimulate cell growth or inhibit apoptosis.

Stages of Cancer Development

Cancer is thought to occur as a multistep process in which the initiation of damage in a single cell leads to a preneoplastic stage followed by a sequence of events that permit the cell to successfully proliferate. All neoplasms and their metastases are thought to be derivatives or clones of a single cell and are characterized by unrestrained growth, irregular migration, and genetic diversity. For the purpose of setting radiation protection standards, it is assumed that there is no threshold dose for the induction of cancer because even a single ionization event could theoretically lead to molecular changes in the DNA that result in malignant transformation and ultimately cancer. However, the probability of cancer development is far lower than would be expected from the number of initiating events. For example, a whole-body dose of 3 mGy of low-LET radiation (equivalent to the average annual background in the United States) generates multiple DNA lesions (including on average, three SSBs and five to eight damaged bases) in every cell (BEIR, 2006). However, cancer may never arise because a host of defense mechanisms are initiated following radiation-induced damage to prevent cancer development (*e.g.*, activation of DNA repair systems; free radical scavenging; cell cycle checkpoint controls; induced apoptosis, mitotic failure, etc.). Additionally, all of the subsequent steps required for expression of the malignant potential of the cell may not occur.

Cancer formation can be thought of (albeit in a greatly oversimplified way) as occurring in three stages: (1) *initiation*, (2) *promotion*, and (3) *progression*. During initiation, a somatic mutational event occurs that is misrepaired. This initial damage can be produced by radiation or any of a variety of other environmental or chemical carcinogens. During the promotion stage, the preneoplastic cell is stimulated to divide. A promoter is an agent that by itself does not cause cancer but, once an initiating carcinogenic event has occurred, promotes or stimulates the cell containing the original damage. Unlike many carcinogens, radiation may act as an initiator and a promoter. Some hormones act as promoters by stimulating the growth of target tissues. For example, estrogen and thyroid-stimulating hormone may act as promoters of breast cancer and thyroid cancer, respectively. The final stage is progression, during which the transformed cell produces a number of phenotypic clones, not all of which are neoplastic. Eventually, one phenotype acquires the selective advantage of evading the host's defense mechanisms, thus allowing the development of a tumor and possibly metastatic cancer. Radiation may also enhance progression by immunosuppression resulting from damage to lymphocytes and macrophages that are essential to the humoral antibody response.

Although the three-stage model has been highly useful for mechanistic under-standing and development of mathematical models of cancer progression, it is now recognized that as cells evolve progressively to a neoplastic state, they acquire a succession of hallmark capabilities (Hanahan and Weinberg, 2000, 2011) such that the multistep carcinogenic process involves the acquisition of a number of traits that enable cells to become tumorigenic and ultimately malignant. Hanahan and Weinberg originally described six "Hallmarks of Cancer" (Hanahan and Weinberg, 2000): sustaining proliferative signaling, evading growth suppressors, resisting cell death, enabling replicative immortality, inducing angiogenesis, and activating invasion and metastasis (Fig. 20-27A). In addition to the six Hallmarks of Cancer, Hanahan and Weinberg (2011) enumerate two enabling characteristics—genome instability, which

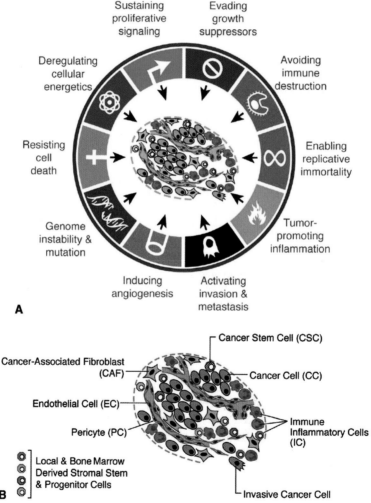

■ **FIGURE 20-27** The "Hallmarks of Cancer." **A.** This illustration depicts the original six "Hallmarks of Cancer" described in 2000 by Hanahan and Weinberg as well as the two emerging hallmarks (deregulating cellular energetics and avoiding immune destruction) and enabling characteristics (genome instability and mutation and tumor-promoting inflammation) they added subsequently. (**A:** Reprinted with permission from Hanahan D, Weinberg RA. Hallmarks of cancer: the next generation. *Cell*. 2011;144(5):646-674. Copyrighyt © Elsevier.) Radiation could play a role in many or all of these processes involved in carcinogenesis. **B.** In addition to the cancer cells, a tumor is composed of multiple cell types that interact to produce the tumor microenvironment that has a critical role in cancer development as well as response to treatments, including radiation. (**B:** Modified with permission from Hanahan D, Weinberg RA. Hallmarks of cancer: the next generation. Cell. 2011;144(5):646-674. Copyrighyt © Elsevier.)

generates the genetic diversity that expedites hallmark acquisition, and inflammation, which fosters hallmark functions—and two emerging hallmarks: energy metabolism and evading immune destruction (Fig. 20-27A). Furthermore, it is clear that tumors are not just a collection of cancer cells but are complex tissues, composed of multiple interacting cell types. The stromal cells include fibroblasts and the endothelial cells and pericytes of the vasculature, as well as immune inflammatory cells (Fig. 20-27B). Together, these various cell types create a tumor microenvironment, which not only is critical for cancer development but also can influence the response of a tumor to treatments, including radiation (Barcellos-Hoff and Brooks, 2001).

Environmental Risk Factors

Environmental factors implicated in the promotion of cancer include tobacco, alcohol, diet, sexual behavior, air pollution, and bacterial and viral infections. Support for the role of environmental factors comes from observations such as the increased incidence of colon and breast cancer among Japanese immigrants to the United States compared with those living in Japan. Among the best known and striking modifiers of cancer risk is smoking. For men, the relative risk (RR) of developing lung cancer is 20 to 40 times greater in smokers than nonsmokers. In addition, agents that compromise the immune system, such as the human immunodeficiency virus, increase the probability of successful progression of a preneoplastic cell into cancer. There are a number of chemical agents that, when given alone, are neither initiators nor promoters, but when given in the presence of an initiator will enhance cancer development. Many of these agents are present in cigarette smoke, which may in part account for its potent carcinogenicity. Environmental exposure to nonionizing radiation, such as radiofrequency radiation from cellular telephones and their base stations or magnetic field exposures from power lines, has been an area of intense research in the last few decades. While reports of possible associations between sources of nonionizing radiation and cancer have received considerable media attention, the evidence of any causal connection is weak and inconsistent and no biologically plausible mechanism of action has been identified.

A number of national and international agencies and organizations such as the World Health Organization's International Agency for Research on Cancer (IARC) and the National Toxicology Program (NTP) (an inter-agency program within the U.S. Department of Health and Human Services) report on the carcinogenic potential of various physical and chemical agents. Each organization has its own rules and classification schemes, which often lead to confusion in the public and the media regarding the potential health impact of a substance that appears in one of these reports. Periodically, the NTP publishes an update of its *Report on Carcinogens* (RoC). This report, now in its 14th edition (NTP, 2016), identifies substances that are considered to have carcinogenic potential in humans. The NTP lists more than 245 substances, which are classified into one of two categories: "known to be carcinogenic in humans," of which there are 62 in the current report including benzene, smoking tobacco, vinyl chloride, asbestos, several viruses and of course, ionizing radiation; and another 186 agents that are classified as "reasonably anticipated to be human carcinogens" including exogenous progesterone used for contraception, chemotherapeutic agents adriamycin and cisplatin, as well as naturally occurring contaminants such as aflatoxin, formed by certain fungi on crops.

Risk Expressions

One way of expressing the risk from radiation (or any other agent) in an exposed population is in terms of its *relative risk* (RR). RR is the ratio of the disease (*e.g.*, cancer) incidence in the exposed population to that in the general (unexposed) population;

thus, a RR of 1.2 would indicate a 20% increase over the spontaneous rate that would otherwise have been expected in a population. The *excess relative risk* (ERR) is simply RR − 1; in this case, 1.2 − 1 = 0.2. While the RR of a specific cancer following some exposure is informative about the magnitude of the increased risk relative to its natural occurrence, it does not provide a sense of perspective of the risk in terms of the overall health impact the risk represents. For example, a study showing that a particular exposure resulted in a 300% increase (*i.e.*, RR of 4) in the incidence of a very rare cancer with a natural incidence of 2 per 100,000 means that the cancer risk is now 8 per 100,000. When compared to the total incidence of cancer in the population of approximately 43,000 per 100,000, a 300% increase of a rare disease does not seem as significant a potential health threat. *Absolute risk* (AR) is another way of expressing risk, as the number of excess cancer cases per 100,000 in a population. In radiation epidemiology, it may be expressed as a rate such as the number of excess cases per 10^4 or 10^5 people per Sv per year (*e.g.*, #/10^4/Sv/y). For example, for a cancer with a radiation-induced AR of 4/10^4/Sv/y (or 4×10^{-4} Sv^{-1} y^{-1}) and a minimum latency period of about 10 years, the risk of developing cancer within the next 40 years from a dose of 0.1 Sv would be 30 years × 0.1 Sv × 4×10^{-4} Sv^{-1} y^{-1} = 12 per 10,000 or 0.12%. In other words, if 10,000 people (with the same age and gender distribution as in the general population) each received a dose of 0.1 Sv, 12 additional cases of cancer would be expected to develop in that population over the subsequent 40 years. The previous example is also characterized as the risk at an *attained age* of 50 from exposure at 10 years of age. *Excess Absolute Risk* (EAR), also referred to as *attributable risk*, is the difference between two ARs and is commonly used in radiation epidemiology expressed as the EAR per unit dose. Thus if the AR in a population exposed to 1 Sv was 95×10^{-5} y^{-1} and 20×10^{-5} y^{-1} in the unexposed population, the EAR would be (95 per 100,000 per year) − (20 per 100,000 per year) = 75×10^{-5} y^{-1} Sv^{-1}.

20.7.2 Modifiers of Radiation-Induced Cancer Risk

Radiation-induced cancers can occur in most tissues of the body and are indistinguishable from those that arise from other causes. The probability of developing a radiation-induced cancer depends on several physical and biological factors. Physical factors include the radiation quality (*e.g.*, LET), total dose, and, in some instances, the rate at which the dose was received (*e.g.*, acute versus chronic). Research on the biological factors that may influence the carcinogenic effectiveness of radiation has been undertaken in numerous biomolecular, cellular, animal, and epidemiological studies. The influence of radiation quality, dose fractionation, age at exposure, tumor type, and gender on radiation-induced cancer risks following exposure and the influence of genetic susceptibility to cancer will be discussed briefly below. Many of these topics will be revisited in the context of specific results from major epidemiological investigations of radiation-induced cancer discussed later in this chapter.

Radiation Quality

The RBE of radiation as a function of LET for a variety of biological endpoints (*e.g.*, double-strand DNA breaks, clonogenic potential of cells in culture) was discussed earlier in this chapter. The high ionization density of high-LET radiation is more effective in producing DNA damage that is less likely to be faithfully repaired than damage produced by low-LET radiation. Consequently, for a given absorbed dose, the probability of inducing a cancer-causing mutation is higher for high-LET radiation, but so is the probability of cell killing. Although the RBE values and their modifying factors for radiocarcinogenesis are not known with great certainty, high-LET radiation (*e.g.*, α-particles) has been shown to produce more cancers of the lung, liver, thyroid, and bone than an equal dose of low-LET radiation in human populations. The uncertainty in α-particle risk is substantial, with a median value of 14.1 and a 90% CI from 5 to 40 (EPA, 2011), and similarly factors of about 5 for solid cancers and 9 for leukemias in more recent reviews (NCRP, 2015). The EPA, ICRP, and the NCRP recommend risk coefficients for α-particles that are based on an RBE of 20. RBE values obtained from epidemiological studies vary greatly. For example, studies of the patients injected with thorium-232 dioxide (a primordial alpha-emitting radionuclide with a half-life of billions of years) as a diagnostic contrast agent (Thorotrast) for cerebral angiography from about 1930 to the mid-1950s, found an RBE of approximately 20 for liver cancer, but an RBE of only about 1 for leukemia.

It has been demonstrated that for certain biological endpoints, such as the efficiency of producing dicentrics in human lymphocytes, that low-energy photons are more effective than high-energy photons (Fig. 20-28). Presumably, this is a result of the higher LET of lower energy secondary electrons (*e.g.*, 30 keV electron LET ~ 1 keV/μm) compared to that of higher energy electrons (*e.g.*, 500 keV electron LET ~ 0.2 keV/μm) and the resultant increase in complex DNA damage generated by ionization and excitation events of these low-energy electrons near the ends of their tracks.

While there is experimental and theoretical evidence supporting higher RBEs of low-photon and low-electron energies, epidemiological support for such an effect is lacking. In fact, risk coefficients for x-rays derived from studies of medically irradiated cohorts are in some cases lower than what has been observed for the A-bomb survivors. However, there are a number of potential confounders that may have prevented

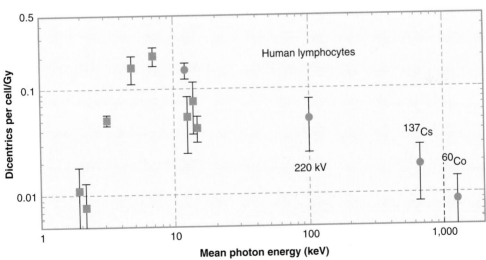

■ **FIGURE 20-28** Efficacy of producing dicentric chromosomes per unit dose in human peripheral blood lymphocytes as a function of photon energy. Data points and standard errors of the number of dicentrics per cell per Gy for monoenergetic photons at low and high energies (*x*-axis) Squares are for monoenergetic photons; circles are x-ray spectra or γ-rays. (*Source:* Sasaki MS, Kobayashi K, Hieda K, et al. Induction of chromosome aberrations in human lymphocytes by monochromatic x-rays of quantum energy between 4.8 and 14.6 keV. *Int J Radiat Biol.* 1989;56:975-988; Sasaki MS. Primary damage and fixation of chromosomal DNA as probed by monochromatic soft x-rays and low-energy neutrons. In: Fielden EM, O'Neil P, eds. *The Early Effects of Radiation on DNA.* Vol. H54. NATO ASI Series, Berlin: Springer-Verlag; 1991:369–384; BEIR VII National Research Council. *Health Risks from Exposure to Low Levels of Ionizing Radiation: BEIR VII, Phase 2 Committee to Assess Health Risks from Exposure to Low Levels of Ionizing Radiation.* Washington, DC: Board of Radiation Effects, Research Division on Earth and Life Studies, National Academy of Sciences; 2006.)

the detection of an elevated risk if it were present. Thus any difference in carcinogenic risk, per unit dose, from low-energy x-rays compared to that of higher energy photons remains to be determined (BEIR, 2006; ICRP, 2003a, 2003b; NCRP, 2018c).

Dose Rate and Fractionation

It has long been recognized that the biological effectiveness of the radiation-induced damage to cells and tissues generally decreases at lower dose rates. This effect is due at least in part to the ability of cells to repair damage during low dose-rate exposure or between exposures in the case of fractionated exposures. The effect of fractionating large doses to increase the probability of cellular repair has been well characterized *in vitro* and has been shown to reduce the incidence of carcinogenesis in some cases such as leukemia. Currently, a dose and dose-rate effectiveness factor (DDREF) is used to convert high-dose-rate risk estimates to estimates for exposure at low dose rates for the purposes of radiation protection. Given the need to avoid image blur due to cardiac and pulmonary motion, most diagnostic examinations are acquired with breath-hold, at a high dose rate, and in less than 100 ms. For example, a typical chest x-ray is acquired in 7 ms with a skin entrance dose rate of ~1.4 Gy/min, and one slice of CT scan of the abdomen is acquired in ~1/2 s at a dose rate of ~12.2 Gy/min. These values exceed even typical radiation therapy dose rates where conventional fractionated treatments deliver 1.8–2 Gy per fraction delivered over a period of 2–10 minutes (min). However, at the low total doses associated with diagnostic examinations and occupational exposures, dose rate may not affect cancer risk (Kocher et al., 2018).

Age at Exposure, Gender, Tumor Type, and Latency

Latency (the period between exposure and clinical expression of disease) and the risk of radiation-induced cancers vary with the type of cancer and age at the time of exposure. For example, the risk of ovarian cancer from an acute exposure at age 10 is approximately three times greater than if the exposure occurred at age 50. For whole-body exposure, females on average have a 40% higher risk of radiogenic cancer than do males. This is due in large part to the high risks for radiation-induced breast, ovarian, and lung cancer in women and the substantially lower risks for radiation-induced testes and prostate cancer in men. Breast cancer occurs almost exclusively in women, and AR estimates for lung cancer induction by radiation are (unlike the normal incidence) approximately twice as high for women than for men. However, for some specific cancers, the radiation-induced cancer risk is lower for women than for men (*e.g.*, liver cancer ~50% lower risk in females than males). The organs at greatest risk for radiogenic cancer induction and mortality are breast and lung for women and lung and colon for men. The minimal latent period is 2 to 3 years for leukemia, with a period of expression (*i.e.*, the time interval required for the full expression of the radiogenic cancer increase) proportional to the age at the time of exposure, ranging from approximately 12 to 25 years. Latent periods for solid tumors range from 5 to 40 years, with a period of expression for some cancers longer than 50 years.

Genetic Susceptibility

Mutations in one or more specific genes, while rare, are known to increase susceptibility to developing cancer. Over the last few decades, extensive efforts have been made to identify specific gene mutations that act as sources of genetic susceptibility to cancer. Increasing numbers of observational studies investigating the association between specific gene variants and cancer risk have been published. This effort has been greatly accelerated by the mapping of the human genome and the results from related advances aimed at identifying the quantity, type, location, and frequency of genetic variants in human genes. Advances in sequencing technology have allowed results to be obtained much faster and less expensively than before and continue to contribute to the understanding of the genetic susceptibility to cancer and to advance the goal of improved, individualized gene therapy.

While there are still many unanswered questions, the ability of specific inherited gene mutations to substantially increase the risk of developing specific cancers (i.e., high penetrance genes) has been well documented. For example, women with inherited mutations in the breast cancer susceptibility genes 1 or 2 (*BRCA1* or *BRCA2*) and a family history of multiple cases of breast cancer carry a lifetime risk of breast cancer that is approximately 5 times higher than for women in the general population, (i.e., 60% and 12%, respectively) (NCI, 2011).

A-T, a rare, recessive genetic disorder of childhood, occurs in 1–2 of every 100,000 people. Patients with the ataxia-telangiectasia mutation (ATM) have trouble walking as children (ataxia) and have small red spider-like veins (telangiectasia). These patients are at substantially higher risk of infection and of developing cancer (especially leukemias and lymphomas) than the general population. These patients are also hypersensitive to ionizing radiation exposure because of defective DNA repair mechanisms. The product of the *ATM* gene plays a central role in the recognition and repair of double-strand DNA breaks and the activation of cell cycle checkpoints. A-T patients exhibit unusual susceptibility to injury by radiation and often suffer more severe reactions to radiotherapy than do other radiotherapy patients. While physicians who treat A-T patients limit their x-ray exposures to the extent possible, they do recommend diagnostic x-ray imaging procedures when needed, if there are no appropriate alternative procedures that do not use ionizing radiation.

There are still many open questions regarding these single gene human genetic disorders and their influence on cancer risks. One such question is to what extent radiation exposure modifies the cancer risk in patients with these inherited mutations. The BEIR VII committee concluded that, while there is evidence to suggest that many of the known, strongly expressing, cancer-prone human genetic disorders are likely to show an elevated risk of radiation-induced cancer, the rarity of these disorders in the population will not significantly distort current population-based cancer risk estimates. Their view was that the more practical issue associated with these high penetrance genes was their impact on the risk of second cancers in such patients following radiotherapy.

20.7.3 Epidemiologic Investigations of Radiation-Induced Cancer

Although the dose-response relationship for cancer induction at high dose (and dose rate) has been fairly well established for several cancers, the same cannot be said for low doses like those resulting from typical diagnostic and occupational exposures. Insufficient data exist to determine accurately the risks of low-dose radiation exposure to humans. Animal and epidemiologic investigations indicate that the risks of low-level exposure are small, but how small is still (despite decades of research) a matter of great debate in the scientific community. Nevertheless, there is general agreement that above cumulative doses of 100 to 150 mSv (acute or protracted exposure), direct epidemiological evidence from human populations demonstrates that exposure to ionizing radiation likely increases the risk of some cancers.

The populations that form the bases of the epidemiologic investigation of radiation bioeffects come from four principal sources: (1) the Life Span Study (LSS) cohort of survivors of the atomic bomb explosions in Hiroshima and Nagasaki, (2) patients with medical exposure during treatment of a variety of neoplastic and nonneoplastic diseases, (3) persons with occupational exposures, and (4) populations with high natural background exposures (Fig. 20-29).

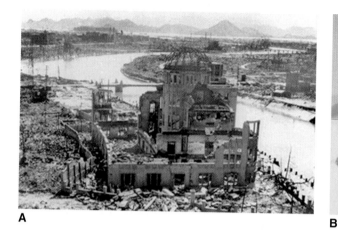

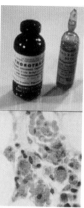

A

B

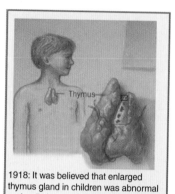

1918: It was believed that enlarged thymus gland in children was abnormal and radiation was suggested to shrink it.

C

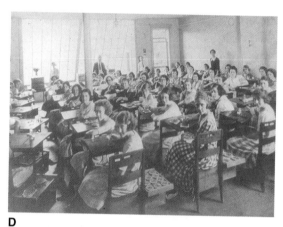

D

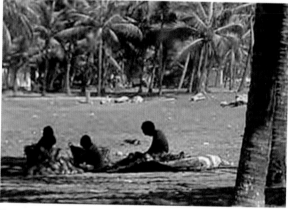

E

■ **FIGURE 20-29** Sources of data on exposure of humans to radiation. The most important source of epidemiological data is the LSS of the Japanese atomic bomb survivors, who received acute doses of radiation, over a range of doses up to 2 Gy, beyond which errors in dose reconstruction and mortality from complications of the ARS provided limited radioepidemiological information. The studies of cancer mortality in the LSS began in 1950 and have formed the basis of radiation protection guidelines ever since. **A.** There was widespread destruction following the detonation of the atomic bomb in Hiroshima, Japan at 8:15 AM on August 6, 1945. The building shown was the former Hiroshima Prefecture Industrial Promotion Hall, where special products of Hiroshima were exhibited and various gatherings were held. Located just under the hypocenter, blast pressure was vertically exerted on the building and only the dome-shaped framework and part of the outer wall remained. **B.** From 1931 to the mid-1950s, Thorotrast, a colloidal suspension of radioactive thorium dioxide (top panel), was commonly used as a diagnostic contrast agent for cerebral angiography. Thorotrast (containing thorium, a long-lived alpha emitter) remains in the body, accumulates in the liver, and results in liver cancer and leukemia. Thorotrast-laden macrophages in the bone marrow shown at 1,000× (bottom panel). (Reprinted with permission from Graham SJ, et al. Whole-body pathologic analysis of a patient with Thorotrast-induced myelodysplasia. *Health Phys.* 1992;63(1):20-26. Copyright © Wolters Kluwer.) **C.** Radiation has also been used in the past to treat benign medical conditions with unfortunate consequences such as the increase in thyroid cancer in children who were unnecessarily irradiated to reduce the size of the thymus gland. During a review of children with thyroid cancer, Dr. Fitzgerald noticed that nine out of the first ten patients he reviewed had had a history of thymic radiation. Drs. Duffy and Fitzgerald's report, *Cancer of the thyroid in children,* in the *Journal of Endocrinology* in 1950 was the first demonstration of an association between radiation treatment and thyroid cancer. **D.** In the 1920s, bone cancer was linked with the ingestion of large quantities of radium by young women who painted dials on watches and clocks with radium-laden paints. The type of bone cancer (osteogenic sarcoma) is rare, but it occurred with an alarming incidence in radium-dial painters and its location (often in the mandible) is an extremely unusual location for this type of cancer. **E.** Several areas of the world have high natural background due to being at high elevation or having high concentrations of naturally occurring radioactive material in the ground. High concentrations of radioactive thorium-containing monazite sands are found in the coastal belt of Karunagappally, Kerala, India. The median outdoor radiation levels are more than 4 mGy/y and, in some locations, as high as 70 mGy/y. A cohort of all 385,103 residents in Karunagappally was established in the 1990s to evaluate the health effects of living in a high background radiation area. Studies to date however have not shown any excess cancer risk from this chronic exposure to γ-radiation (Adapted from Nair RR, Rajan B, Akiba S, et al. Background radiation and cancer incidence in Kerala, India-Karanagappally cohort study. *Health Phys.* 2009;96:55-66; Boice JD Jr, Hendry JH, Nakamura N, et al. Low-dose-rate epidemiology of high background radiation areas. *Radiat Res.* 2010;173:849-854.)

It is very difficult to detect a small increase in the cancer rate due to radiation exposure at low doses (less than ~100 mSv) because radiation is a relatively weak carcinogen, the natural incidence of many types of cancer is high and the latent period for most cancers is long (NCRP, 2018c). To rule out statistical fluctuations, a very large irradiated population is required. To be able to detect a relative cancer risk of 1.2 with a statistical confidence of 95% (*i.e.*, $p < 0.05$) when the spontaneous incidence is 2% in the population (typical of many cancers), a study population in excess of 10,000 is required. More than 1 million people would be required to identify a RR of 1.01 (*i.e.*, a 1% cancer rate increase) in this same population! A simplified hypothetical example that demonstrates the limited statistical power faced by many epidemiological studies of radiation exposure at low doses was provided in an ICRP report on low-dose extrapolation of radiation-related cancer risk (ICRP, 2006). Statistical power calculations were performed to assess the population size needed for 80% power to detect an excess risk at the 5% significance level in which baseline cancer risk, for an unspecified and hypothetical subset of cancers, is known to be 10%, and the "unknown" radiation-related excess risk is actually 10% at 1 Gy and proportional to dose between 0 and 1 Gy. As shown in Table 20-9, the population size necessary to be able to detect an increased risk at doses typical of many diagnostic imaging exams (organ dose less than 10 mGy) would require a very large population and enormous resources to accomplish. As pointed out by ICRP, the calculation is unrealistically optimistic since, as one can never be that sure of the baseline rate in any exposed population, it may be necessary to estimate the baseline rate by including an equal number of nonexposed subjects (*i.e.*, twice the population size would be required to have equal power for detecting the difference). Confounding factors take on much greater importance when excess risks are low, and spurious results can occur by chance alone, which results in exaggerated estimates of risk, only to be amplified and distorted further by some in the media. Commenting on this problem, the ICRP stated, "At low and very low radiation doses, statistical and other variations in baseline risk tend to be the dominant sources of error in both epidemiological and

TABLE 20-9 STATISTICAL POWER CALCULATIONS FOR A HYPOTHETICAL STUDY IN WHICH THE BASELINE RISK, FOR AN UNSPECIFIED SUBSET OF CANCER SITES, IS KNOWN TO BE 10%, AND THE UNKNOWN RADIATION-RELATED EXCESS RISK IS 10% AT 1 Gy AND PROPORTIONAL TO DOSE BETWEEN 0 AND 1 Gy

RADIATION DOSE	EXCESS RISK	TOTAL RISK	POPULATION SIZE *N*
1 Gy	10%	20%	80
100 mGy	1%	11%	6,390
10 mGy	0.1%	10.1%	620,000
1 mGy	0.01%	10.01%	61.8 million

N, the population size needed for 80% power to detect the excess risk at the 5% significance level.
Adapted with permission from International Commission on Radiological Protection. Low-dose extrapolation of radiation-related cancer risk. ICRP publication 99. *Ann ICRP*. 2006;35:1-140. Copyright © Sage Publications.

experimental carcinogenesis studies, and estimates of radiation-related risk tend to be highly uncertain because of a weak signal-to-noise ratio and because it is difficult to recognize or to control for subtle confounding factors. At such dose levels, and with the absence of bias from uncontrolled variation in baseline rates, positive and negative estimates of radiation-related risk tend to be almost equally likely on statistical grounds, even under the LNT theory. Also, by definition, statistically significant positive or negative findings can be expected in about one in 20 independent studies when the underlying true excess risk is close to zero. Thus, even under the LNT theory, the smaller the dose, the more likely it is that any statistically significant finding will be a purely chance occurrence and that it will be consistent with either beneficial effects of radiation (hormesis) or a grossly exaggerated risk (Land, 1980). A result predictable under both of two opposing hypotheses supports neither of them against the other. Thus, for example, failure of epidemiological studies to demonstrate a statistically significant excess cancer risk associated with exposures of the order of 1 mGy does not imply that there is no risk, although it does suggest that any such risk is small relative to baseline cancer rates" (ICRP, 2006).

Considering the limitations (both practical and inherent) to epidemiological investigations (which are by nature, observational, not experimental), there is no such thing as a perfect epidemiological study. Some epidemiologic investigations have been complicated by such factors as failure to adequately control exposure to other known carcinogens or an inadequate period of observation to allow for the full expression of cancers with long latent periods. Other studies suffer from inadequate design, resulting in problems such as small study size or biased selection of case and control populations or poor assessment of estimated exposure. Exposure assessment that relies on data that are incomplete, inaccurate, or surrogates for the actual exposure of interest can lead to flawed conclusions. In retrospective studies, in particular, the use of questionnaires that relied on people's recollections to estimate exposure can be particularly problematic, especially if there is a high likelihood of recall bias among cases compared to controls. For example, the case subjects may have more reliable memories than the control subjects because they have been searching for a plausible explanation of the cause of their disease. These methodological issues notwithstanding, epidemiology has made invaluable contributions to public health, especially in cases where the exposures, such as in smoking, resulted in widespread adverse public health consequences. The situations where epidemiological investigations have the most difficulty are where the risks are small compared to the normal incidence of the disease and where exposures in cases and controls are difficult to quantify. Table 20-10 summarizes details of some of the principal epidemiologic

TABLE 20-10 SUMMARY OF MAJOR EPIDEMIOLOGIC INVESTIGATIONS THAT FORM THE BASIS OF CURRENT CANCER DOSE-RESPONSE ESTIMATES IN HUMAN POPULATIONS

POPULATION AND EXPOSURE	EFFECTS OBSERVED	STRENGTHS AND LIMITATIONS
A-bomb survivors: The LSS of the Japanese A-bomb survivors have provided detailed epidemiological data from a study of this population for about 50 y. Three cohorts currently being studied are: (1) A cancer (and non-cancer) incidence and mortality study of ~105,000 residents of Hiroshima and Nagasaki (1950) with doses ranging from 0 (e.g., not in the city at the time of the bombing) to 4 Gy (42% received a dose between 5 and 100 mGy); and (3) F1 generation children of those exposed (~77,000). The cancer incidence and mortality assessment through 1998 have been completed. Mean organ doses have been calculated for 12 organs. Risk estimates were revised in 2006 by the National Academy of Sciences/National Research Council Committee on the Biological Effects of Ionizing Radiation. Their reanalysis of the scientific data on low-dose radiation health effects was undertaken in light of a reassessment of the doses received by the Japanese atomic-bomb survivors, referred to as the DS02 dose estimate, (Young, 2005), additional information on non-targeted effects of radiation (e.g., bystander effect, low-dose hypersensitivity), as well as an additional decade of follow-up of the A-bomb survivors.	A-bomb survivor data demonstrates an undeniable increase in cancer for doses >100 mSv (some say 50 while others say 200 mSv). Excess risks of most cancer types have been observed, the major exceptions being chronic lymphocytic leukemia, multiple myeloma, non-Hodgkin's lymphoma, and pancreatic, prostate, and gallbladder cancers. A total of 853 excess solid cancers from a total of 17,488 cases are thought to have been induced by radiation exposure. Table 20-11 lists, for each dose category, the observed and expected numbers of cancers, the excess number of cancers, and the percent of cancers that can be attributed to radiation exposure (attributable fraction). The small but statistically significant increase in the 5–100 mGy exposure group is of particular interest in medical imaging as it is similar to organ dose experienced in many diagnostic imaging studies. In more than 50 y of follow-up of the 105,427 atomic-bomb survivors, the percent of cancers attributed to their radiation exposure is 10.7%. Estimates of the site-specific solid cancer risks are shown in Figure 20-30. The influence of sex and age at the time of exposure, and the risk as a function of attained age following exposure can be very significant and examples of their influence are shown in Figure 20-31.	The analysis of the data from the atom-bomb survivors' cohort is the single most important factor that has influenced current radiation-induced cancer risk estimates. The population is large and there is a wide range of doses from which it is possible to determine the dose-response and the effects of modifying factors such as age on the induction of cancer. Data at high doses are limited; thus the analysis only included individuals in whom the doses were 2 Gy or less. The survivors were not representative of a normal Japanese population insofar as many of the adult males were away on military service while those remaining presumably had some physical condition preventing them from active service. In addition, the children and the elderly perished shortly after the detonation in greater numbers than did young adults, suggesting the possibility that the survivors may represent a hardier subset of the population. Another important uncertainty is the transfer of site-specific cancer risk estimates to the U.S. population, based on results obtained on the LSS population, for cancers with substantially different baseline incidence rates.

(Continued)

TABLE 20-10 SUMMARY OF MAJOR EPIDEMIOLOGIC INVESTIGATIONS THAT FORM THE BASIS OF CURRENT CANCER DOSE-RESPONSE ESTIMATES IN HUMAN POPULATIONS (Continued)

POPULATION AND EXPOSURE	EFFECTS OBSERVED	STRENGTHS AND LIMITATIONS
Ankylosing spondylitis: This cohort consists of ~14,000 patients treated with radiotherapy to the spine for ankylosing spondylitis throughout the United Kingdom between 1935 and 1954. Although individual dose records were not available for all patients, estimates were made ranging from 1 to 25 Gy to the bone marrow and other various organs.	Mortality has been reported through 1982, at which point 727 cancer deaths had been reported. Excess leukemia rates were reported from which an absolute risk of 80 excess cases/Gy/y per million was estimated.	This group represents one of the largest bodies that has provided data on radiation-induced leukemia in humans for which fairly good dose estimates exist. Control groups were suboptimal, however, and doses were largely unfractionated. In addition, only cancer mortality (not incidence) was available for this cohort.
Postpartum mastitis study: This group consists of ~600 women, mostly between the ages of 20 and 40 y, treated with radiotherapy for postpartum acute mastitis in New York in the 1940s and 1950s for which ~1,200 non-exposed women with mastitis and siblings of both groups of women served as controls. Breast tissue doses ranged from 0.6 to 14 Gy.	Forty-five year follow-up identified excess breast cancer in this population as compared with the general female population of New York.	A legitimate objection to using the data from this study to establish radiation-induced breast cancer risk factors is the uncertainty as to what effect the inflammatory changes associated with postpartum mastitis and the hormonal changes due to pregnancy have on the risk of breast cancer.
Radium dial painters: Young women who ingested radium (Ra-226 and Ra-228 with half-lives of ~1,600 and 7 y, respectively) while licking their brushes (containing luminous radium sulfate) to a sharp point during the application of luminous paint on dials and clocks in the 1920s and 1930s. Over 800 were followed.	Large increase in osteogenic sarcoma. Osteogenic sarcoma is a rare cancer (incidence, ~5 per 10^6 population). RR in the population was >100×. No increase was seen below doses of 5 Gy, but a sharp increase was noticed thereafter.	One of only a few studies that analyzed the radiocarcinogenic effectiveness of internal contamination with high-LET radiation in humans.
Thorotrast: Several populations were studied in which individuals were injected intravascularly with an x-ray contrast medium, Thorotrast, used between 1931 and 1950. Thorotrast contains 25% by weight radioactive colloidal Th-232 dioxide. Th-232 is an alpha emitter with a half-life of ~14 billion y.	Particles were deposited in the reticuloendothelial systems. An increase was noted in the number of cancers, particularly liver cancer (angiosarcoma, bile duct carcinomas, and hepatic cell carcinomas) and leukemia. Evaluation of the data resulted in estimates of alpha radiation-induced liver cancer risk of $\sim 8 \times 10^{-2}$ per Gy, which appears to be linear with dose. Alpha RBE ~20. An increase in leukemia was also seen; however, the RBE was much lower (~1).	Dose estimates are fairly good. However, the extent to which the chemical toxicity of the Thorotrast may have influenced the risk is not known. Thorotrast administration resulted in chronic alpha particle irradiation from radionuclides in the thorium decay series. Organs of deposition of Th-232 and from the daughter products of radon-220 in the lungs and of radium-224 and its decay products in the skeletal system.

Source: Adapted and updated from the National Academy of Sciences/National Research Council Committee on the Biological Effects of Ionizing Radiation. *The Health Effects of Exposure to Low Levels of Ionizing Radiation (BEIR V).* Washington, DC: NAS/NRC; 1990.

TABLE 20-11 SOLID CANCERS CASES BY DOSE CATEGORY

DOSE CATEGORY[a]	SUBJECTS	OBSERVED	BACKGROUND[b]	FITTED EXCESS[b]	ATTRIBUTABLE FRACTION (%)
<0.005	60,792	9,597	9,537	3	0
0.005–0.1	27,789	4,406	4,374	81	1.8
0.1–0.2	5,527	968	910	75	7.6
0.2–0.5	5,935	1,144	963	179	15.7
0.5–1	3,173	688	493	206	29.5
1–2	1,647	460	248	196	44.2
2–4[c]	564	185	71	111	61
Total	**105,427**	**17,448**	**16,595**	**853**	**10.7**

[a]Weighted colon dose in Gy.
[b]Note: Estimates of background and fitted excess cases are based on an ERR model with a linear dose response with effect modification by gender, age at exposure, and attained age.
[c]Note that the most reliable epidemiological data in the LSS include doses up to 2 Gy, beyond which, due to errors in dose reconstruction and mortality from complications of the ARS, limited radioepidemiological information is provided.
Reprinted with permission from Preston DL, Shimizu Y, Pierce DA, et al. Studies of mortality of atomic bomb survivors. Report 13: Solid cancer and noncancer disease mortality: 1950–1997. *Radiat Res.* 2003;160:381-407. © 2020 Radiation Research Society.

investigations on which current dose-response estimates are based. Several excellent overviews on radiation epidemiology and perspective on the relative strength of the evidence supporting current risk estimates for radiation-induced cancers and future challenges are available in the literature and are highly recommended (Boice, 2006, 2011; NCRP, 2016, 2018a; UNSCEAR, 2008).

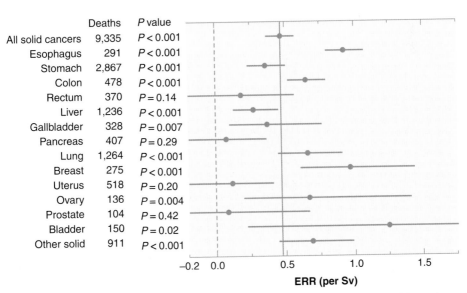

■ **FIGURE 20-30** Estimates of the site-specific solid cancer mortality ERR with 90% confidence intervals. Except for gender-specific cancers (breast, ovary, uterus, and prostate), the estimates are averaged over gender. The dotted vertical line at 0 corresponds to no excess risk, while the solid vertical line indicates the gender-averaged risk for all solid cancers. Some cancer sites such as brain, testes, cervix, oral cavity, and kidney are not included. (Reprinted with permission from Preston DL, Shimizu Y, Pierce DA, et al. Studies of mortality of atomic bomb survivors. Report 13: Solid cancer and noncancer disease mortality: 1950-1997. *Radiat Res.* 2003;160:381-407. © 2020 Radiation Research Society.)

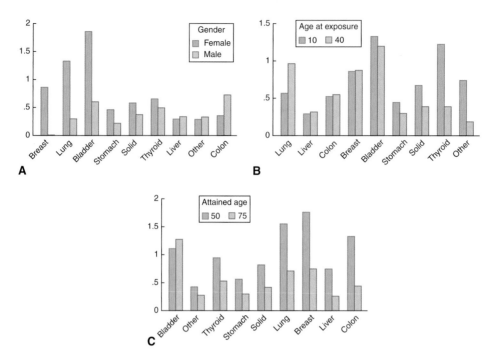

■ **FIGURE 20-31** Comparison of gender **(A)**, age-at-exposure **(B)**, and attained-age **(C)** effects on standardized $ERR_{1\,Gy}$ for selected sites and incidence of all solid cancers in the LSS. The ERR estimates for the "Other" category are based on the results of analyses of the 5,396 cancer cases not included in the sites explicitly considered here. The gender-specific estimates correspond to the fitted ERR per Gy at age 70 for a person exposed at age 30. The age-at-exposure specific estimates are gender-averaged ERR estimates at age 70 after exposure at age 10 (red bar) or age 40 (green bar). Attained-age-specific estimates are gender averaged ERR estimates at ages 50 (red bar) and 75 (green bar) after exposure at age 30. Within each panel, the sites are ordered based on the magnitude of the ratio of the effect pairs. (Reprinted with permission from Preston DL, et al. Solid cancer incidence in atomic bomb survivors: 1958–1998. *Radiat Res*. 2007;168:1. © 2020 Radiation Research Society.)

20.7.4 Estimates of Radiation-Induced Cancer Risks from Low-Dose, Low-LET Radiation

Several national and international scientific organizations periodically report on the state of scientific knowledge regarding the carcinogenic risk and other biological effects of ionizing radiation. Recent reports from these organizations include the United Nations Scientific Committee on the Effects of Atomic Radiation (UNSCEAR, 2006, 2008, 2009, 2011) reports; the National Research Council, Committee on the Biological Effects of Ionizing Radiations (BEIR VII) report entitled *Health Effects of Exposure to Low Levels of Ionizing Radiation* (BEIR, 2006); the U.S. Environmental Protection Agency's report on *Radiogenic Cancer Risk Models and Projections for the U.S. Population* (EPA, 2011); as well as reports focused on specific radiation health and radiation protection related topics by the NCRP, ICRP, and others. While there are some differences in the interpretation of specific aspects in the scientific literature among these various expert bodies, it is fair to say that there is general agreement on the most important aspects of radiation-induced risks, including the magnitude of the risk for the general population and its uncertainty at low doses. General points of agreement that are consistent with the results from the A-bomb survivor LSS include (1) risk varies according to cancer site; (2) risk is greater when exposures occur at younger ages; (3) risk is greater for females than males; (4) solid cancer risk is consistent with a linear function of dose when all cancers are combined; (5) leukemia risk is consistent with a nonlinear function of dose; (6) except for leukemia for which there is a fairly well-defined risk interval following exposure, the risk remains elevated for 50+ years after exposure; and (7) there is no convincing epidemiological evidence of radiation causing genetic (inherited) effects. Inasmuch as there is not a major divergence of opinion expressed in the reports cited above, information on radiation-induced cancer risks and genetic effects will be presented based on the analysis and perspectives contained in the BEIR VII committee report.

20.7.5 BEIR VII Report

The *BEIR VII* report was an update of their previous 1990 report (BEIR V) on the same topic and a report focused on risk from radon exposure (BEIR VI), published in 1999. The primary objective of the BEIR VII report was to provide a comprehensive reassessment of the health risks resulting from exposures to low-dose, low-LET radiation in humans. The report provided updated risk estimates based on a review of the relevant scientific evidence from epidemiology and the vast array of data from laboratory experiments that included everything from long-term animal studies to molecular mechanisms of radiation-induced damage and response. In particular, additional epidemiological data were available from the continued health surveillance of the LSS cohort Japanese atomic bomb survivors (with mortality data through 1997) and their improved dose estimates for this LSS cohort as well. For the purpose of the report, the BEIR VII committee defined "low dose" as less than 100 mGy and "chronic exposure" as dose rates less than 0.1 mGy/min (irrespective of the total dose). The report provided risk estimates of cancer incidence and mortality from radiation in the U.S. population as well as population and organ-specific risk estimates adjusted for gender, age at exposure, and time interval following exposure including lifetime risks. Heritable effects and risk from in utero radiation exposure were also considered. For most cancer risk estimates, the BEIR VII committee relied on the most recent cancer incidence and mortality data from the A-bomb survivor LSS. For breast and thyroid cancer, the committee used a pooled analysis of data from the LSS and studies of medically exposed persons.

20.7.6 Modeling of Epidemiological Data

Within the context of the limitations of epidemiology described earlier, scientists have developed dose-response models to predict the risk of cancer in human populations from exposure to low levels of ionizing radiation. While the data from the LSS are without doubt the most robust data set from which cancer risk estimates can be made, their use requires answers to several important questions such as (1) how can the effects demonstrated at high dose and high dose rate be compared to low dose and low dose rate exposures typical of most medical, occupational, and environmental exposures; (2) what is the effect of age at time of exposure on risk estimates; (3) how well do the risk estimates based on exposure in the Japanese population translate to what might be expected in the U.S. population and (4) how representative is a population exposed in 1945 in a war-torn country with nutritional and other deficiencies to a modern healthy population of today?

Dose-Response Models

Several models have been proposed to characterize dose-response relationships of radiation exposure in humans. The shapes of the dose-response curves have been characterized as *linear non-threshold* (LNT), *linear-quadratic* (LQ), and *threshold* (Fig. 20-32). The two LNT extrapolations represent the high dose and dose rate

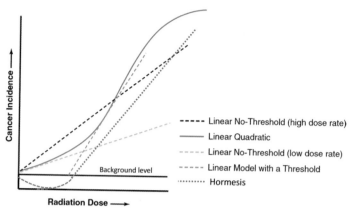

FIGURE 20-32 Possible dose-response relationship for radiation-induced cancer. See text for discussion.

(black) and low dose rate (orange) components of the dose-response data. The LQ dose-response curve (red) demonstrates reduced effectiveness for radiogenic cancer induction at lower dose and greater effectiveness at higher dose that eventually flattens out, reflecting doses associated with substantial cell killing.

In addition to the experimental evidence previously mentioned, there is also epidemiological evidence for a threshold for some cancers (*e.g.*, blue dashed line in Fig. 20-32). For example, a threshold model provides the best fit for the osteogenic sarcoma risk among dial painters who had substantial internal radium contamination (discussed previously in this chapter). Other cancers, for which the evidence for radiation-induced risk is consistent with a threshold, include bone, soft tissue sarcoma, rectum, and non-melanoma skin cancer. The hormesis curve (green) in Figure 20-32 illustrates a hypothesis, proposed by some arguing there is evidence to suggest that low levels of radiation are beneficial because of the activation of processes, for example, DNA repair or up-regulation of anti-oxidant defenses, that protect against radiation-induced cancer. Also, there are anatomic sites for which there is no convincing evidence for a radiation-induced increase in cancer risk (*e.g.*, prostate, pancreas, testes, cervix).

However, even though there is evidence for some types of radiation exposure in specific tissues for a threshold dose below which no radiogenic cancer risk is evident, the evidence supporting this model is not sufficient to be accepted for general use in assessing cancer risk from radiation exposure. Both the ICRP (ICRP, 2006) and the BEIR VII committee concluded that, although there are alternatives to linearity, there is no strong evidence supporting the choice of another form of the dose-response relationship. The NCRP (2018a) recently reexamined available radioepidemiological studies and concluded the following that captures the essence of the consensus view in this regard: "While the ongoing development of science requires a constant reassessment of prior and emerging evidence to assure that the approach to radiation protection is optimal, though not necessarily perfect, NCRP concludes that, based on current epidemiologic data, the LNT model (with the steepness of the dose–response slope perhaps reduced by a DDREF [dose and dose-rate effectiveness] factor) should continue to be utilized for radiation protection purposes. This is in accord with the judgment by other national and international scientific committees … that no alternative dose–response relationship appears more pragmatic or prudent for radiation protection purposes than the LNT model."

Figure 20-33, adapted from BEIR VII, shows the point estimates (orange dots) of ERRs of solid cancer incidence (averaged over gender and standardized to represent individuals exposed at age 30 who have attained age 60) for specific dose intervals

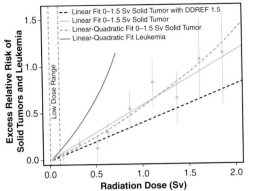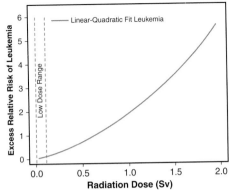

■ **FIGURE 20-33** Dose-response models of ERR for solid cancer and leukemia from cancer incidence data of Japanese A-bomb survivors. (Adapted from *Health Risks from Exposure To Low Levels of Ionizing Radiation: BEIR VII, Phase 2.* Committee to Assess Health Risks from Exposure to Low Levels of Ionizing Radiation, Board of Radiation Effects, Research Division on Earth and Life Studies, National Research Council of the National Academies. National Academy of Sciences, Washington, DC: National Academies Press; 2006.)

from the A-bomb survivor LSS. Vertical lines represent the 95% confidence intervals around each point estimate. The orange solid line and the green dashed line are linear and LQ dose-response models (respectively) for ERR of solid tumors, estimated from all subjects with doses in the range 0 to 1.5 Sv. The LQ dose-response function was discussed previously in the context of cell survival curves. Here the probability of an effect (cancer induction in this case) is proportional to the sum of two coefficients, one that is proportional to dose (αD) and one that is proportional to square of the dose (βD^2). Just as with the cell survival curves, the linear and quadratic components represent the response to low dose and high dose and dose rate effects, respectively. The degree of curvature is the ratio of the quadratic and linear coefficients. These coefficients can be estimated for different cancers reflecting their unique dose-response relationships.

As discussed previously, the biological effectiveness of the radiation-induced damage to cells and tissues generally decreases at lower dose and lower dose rates. This effect is due, at least in part, to the ability to repair damage during low dose exposure or between exposures in the case of a higher total dose delivered in smaller dose fractions. A DDREF has been used to adjust risk estimates from exposures at high dose and high dose rate for use at much lower doses typically encountered in occupational and public settings within a system of radiation protection. The BEIR VII committee applied a DDREF of 1.5 to adjust the response observed in the high dose range making it roughly equivalent to the line representing the LNT low-dose response (black dashed line in Fig. 20-33). This line represents an extension of the linear portion (i.e., zero-dose tangent) of the LQ model (seen more clearly as the low-dose LNT line in Fig. 20-32). The value of the DDREF was derived based on a 95% confidence interval of a Bayesian statistical analysis of the solid cancer incidence data from the A-bomb survivor LSS, as well as the results from selected laboratory animal data. The BEIR VII committee, however, noted the uncertainty in their estimate of a DDREF because of the substantial inconsistency and imprecision in the animal data and because the DDREF estimate was particularly sensitive to the selection of the dose range used for estimation, the particular studies chosen for analysis, and the approach used for estimating curvature that is presumed to be the same across all studies. While it would be equally correct to use the LQ fit to the solid cancer risk data, the BEIR VII committee chose to use the DDREF-adjusted linear dose-response model for cancer risk estimates with the exception of leukemia, for which the LQ model was a better fit. In the absence of a superior dose-response model, the decision was made because it was simple to apply and is widely used by other organizations for this purpose, albeit with a somewhat different DDREF value (*e.g.*, DDREF of 2 was chosen by UNSCEAR and ICRP). Note that in the low-dose range of interest in medical imaging and occupational exposure to radiation (less than 100 mSv), the difference between the linear fit to the solid tumor data (incorporating a DDREF 1.5—black dashed line) and the LQ fit to the same data (green dashed line) is relatively small compared to the 95% confidence intervals. The red lines in the left and right panels of Figure 20-33 show the ERR for leukemia, which best fit a LQ dose-response model. The left panel shows the ERR for leukemia plotted on the same ERR scale as the solid cancer risk data up to approximately 0.7 Sv while the panel on the right shows the same dose-response up to 2 Sv on a broader ERR scale. One can appreciate the greater ERR per unit dose (*i.e.*, the degree of curvature) observed for this cancer.

Multiplicative and Additive Risk Models (Transport of Risk between Populations)

Previous estimates of radiation-induced cancer have employed both the *multiplicative* and the *additive* risk models. The multiplicative risk-projection model (also referred to as the *relative risk* model) is based on the assumption that the excess cancer risk increases in proportion to the baseline cancer rate. Thus, the multiplicative risk model predicts that, after the latent period (*e.g.*, 10 years), the excess risk is a multiple of the natural age-specific risk for the specific cancer and population in question (Fig. 20-34A). The alternative *additive* (or *absolute*) risk model (expressed in terms of EAR) is based on the assumption that, following the latent period, the

■ **FIGURE 20-34** Comparison of multiplicative and additive risk models. Radiation-induced risk increments are seen after a minimal latent period (ℓ); X is age at exposure. **A.** In the multiplicative risk model, the excess risk is a multiple of the natural age-specific cancer risk for a given population, which increases with age. **B.** The additive risk model is shown in which a fixed incremental increased risk is added to the spontaneous disease incidence, which is assumed to be constant over the remaining lifetime. The multiplicative risk model predicts the greatest increment in incidence at older ages.

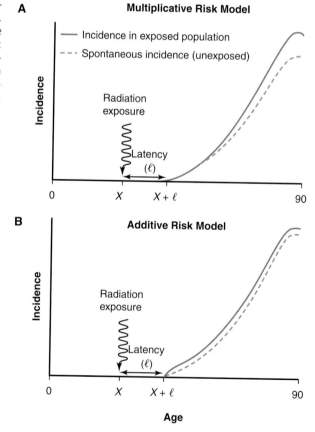

excess cancer rate is constant and independent of the spontaneous population and age-specific natural cancer risk (see Fig. 20-34B). While neither of these two simple models appears adequate to completely describe the risk of radiation-induced cancer, the multiplicative risk model is consistent with the scientific evidence that radiation acts predominantly as an initiator, rather than a promoter, of carcinogenesis. In addition, the copious epidemiological evidence, which indicates that exposure of children to radiation carries a greater risk than exposures later in life, further supports its role as an initiator rather than a promoter. The multiplicative risk model was used by the BEIR VII Committee for deriving tissue-specific solid cancer risk estimates as a function of gender, age at the time of exposure, and time elapsed since exposure.

The multiplicative and additive risk-projection models can be used to transport risk calculated from one population to another dissimilar population. This is a critical issue, insofar as the LSS of the Japanese A-bomb survivors serves as the foundation of many radiation risk estimates and radiation protection regulations. The problem is especially important for U.S. population-based radiation risk estimates because the natural incidence of several types of cancer in the United States and Japan are very dissimilar. For example, the incidence of breast cancer in the United States is 3 times that of Japan while the incidences of liver and stomach cancer are 7.5 and 10 times higher, respectively, in Japan than in the United States (Table 20-12). The previous BEIR committee (BEIR V) based its estimates on multiplicative risk transport, where it is assumed that the excess risk due to radiation is proportional to baseline cancer risks. BEIR VII took a hybrid approach using the multiplicative risk model for some cancers (*e.g.*, thyroid); the AR model for others (*e.g.*, breast); and, for most, a weighted average between the values calculated using the absolute and multiplicative risk models.

20.7.7 Age- and Gender-Specific Radiation Risk Estimates

A summary of the BEIR VII preferred estimates of lifetime attributable risk of solid cancer (incidence and mortality) along with their 95% confidence intervals for different exposure scenarios is shown in Table 20-13. Tables of lifetime attributable cancer incidence and mortality risk by age at exposure and cancer site are provided in the BEIR VII report.

The risks in these tables are expressed as the number of additional cases per 100,000 per 100 mGy to the specified tissue. From this information, organ-specific

TABLE 20-12 BASELINE CANCER INCIDENCE RATES IN UNITED STATES AND JAPAN (FEMALES)[a]

	UNITED STATES	JAPAN
All	280	185
Stomach	3.5	34
Colon	22	17
Liver	1.3	9.8
Lung	34	12
Breast	89	30
Bladder	5.9	2.6

[a]Incidence rates per 100,000 women.
Source: Correa CN, Wu X-C, Andrews P, et al., eds. *Cancer Incidence in Five Continents*. Vol. VIII. Lyon, France: IARC Scientific Publications No. 155; 2002.

TABLE 20-13 BEIR VII PREFERRED ESTIMATES OF LIFETIME ATTRIBUTABLE RISK OF SOLID CANCER INCIDENCE AND MORTALITY WITH 95% CONFIDENCE INTERVALS[a]

EXPOSURE SCENARIO	INCIDENCE		MORTALITY	
	Men	*Women*	*Men*	*Women*
0.1 Gy to population of mixed ages	800 (400–1,590)	1,310 (690–2,490)	410 (200–830)	610 (300–1,230)
0.1 Gy at age 10	1,330 (660–2,660)	2,530 (1,290–4,930)	640 (300–1,390)	1,050 (470–2,330)
0.1 Gy at age 30	600 (290–1,290)	1,000 (500–2,020)	320 (150–650)	490 (250–950)
0.1 Gy at age 50	510 (240–1,100)	680 (350–1,320)	290 (140–600)	420 (210–810)
1 mGy/y throughout life	550 (280–1,100)	970 (510–1,840)	290 (140–580)	460 (230–920)
10 mGy/y from ages 18 to 65	2,600 (1,250–5,410)	4,030 (2,070–7,840)	1,410 (700–2,860)	2,170 (1,130–4,200)

[a]Cancer incidence and mortality per 100,000 exposed persons. 95% Confidence intervals shown in parentheses.
Source: BEIR. *Health Risks from Exposure to Low Levels of Ionizing Radiation: BEIR VII, Phase 2.* Committee to Assess Health Risks from Exposure to Low Levels of Ionizing Radiation, Board of Radiation Effects, Research Division on Earth and Life Studies, National Research Council of the National Academies. National Academy of Sciences, Washington, DC: National Academies Press; 2006.

risk estimates can be derived. For example, if a 10-year-old girl received a 20 mGy breast dose from a chest CT exam, the lifetime risk of being diagnosed with breast cancer as a result of the exam would be:

From Table 20-14, the radiation-induced breast cancer risk at age 10 is 712 cases per 100,000 per 100 mGy. Thus the risk would be calculated as (712) (20 mGy/100 mGy) = 142 per 100,000 or approximately 1 in 700.

If the same dose were received by a 50-year-old woman, the risk would drop by approximately a factor of 10 (~1 in 7,000). It is important to understand that the risk coefficients presented in these tables have large uncertainties and there are many other risk factors for breast cancer (discussed below). Furthermore, the evidence that radiation causes breast cancer at 100 mSv is equivocal and this uncertainty is even greater for doses less than 20 mSv, implying that the statistical uncertainty of risk estimates at these low doses is large and the possibility of no increase in risk cannot be excluded. Nevertheless, they can be used to provide a perspective of the magnitude of the risk engendered from the dose received for a particular exam in a given patient population. A number of such risks estimates have been made in recent years for a variety of imaging studies. The result from one such study evaluating the change in dose and risk with age of exposure for CT exams of the head and abdomen is shown in Figure 20-35. As discussed in Chapter 21, the use of medical imaging using ionizing radiation has increased dramatically in the last 20 years. There has been a growing awareness of the potential for overutilization of this technology and the attendant radiation risk to patients (Brenner and Hall, 2007; Fazel et al., 2009). This issue is of particular concern regarding the pediatric patient population, which has inherently higher cancer risks from a given dose and (depending on the imaging study) may receive higher organ doses than adults for the same procedure (Brenner et al., 2001;

20.7 Radiation-Induced Carcinogenesis

TABLE 20-14 LIFETIME ATTRIBUTABLE RISK OF SITE-SPECIFIC CANCER INCIDENCE

NUMBER OF CASES PER 100,000 PERSONS EXPOSED TO A SINGLE DOSE OF 0.1 Gy

CANCER SITE	Age at Exposure (y)										
	0	5	10	15	20	30	40	50	60	70	80
Men											
Stomach	76	65	55	46	40	28	27	25	20	14	7
Colon	336	285	241	204	173	125	122	113	94	65	30
Liver	61	50	43	36	30	22	21	19	14	8	3
Lung	314	261	216	180	149	105	104	101	89	65	34
Prostate	93	80	67	57	48	35	35	33	26	14	5
Bladder	209	177	150	127	108	79	79	76	66	47	23
Other	1,123	672	503	394	312	198	172	140	98	57	23
Thyroid	115	76	50	33	21	9	3	1	0.3	0.1	0.0
All solid	2,326	1,667	1,325	1,076	881	602	564	507	407	270	126
Leukemia	237	149	120	105	96	84	84	84	82	73	48
All cancers	2,563	1,816	1,445	1,182	977	686	648	591	489	343	174
Women											
Stomach	101	85	72	61	52	36	35	32	27	19	11
Colon	220	187	158	134	114	82	79	73	62	45	23
Liver	28	23	20	16	14	10	10	9	7	5	2
Lung	733	608	504	417	346	242	240	230	201	147	77
Breast	1,171	914	712	553	429	253	141	70	31	12	4
Uterus	50	42	36	30	26	18	16	13	9	5	2
Ovary	104	87	73	60	50	34	31	25	18	11	5
Bladder	212	180	152	129	109	79	78	74	64	47	24
Other	1,339	719	523	409	323	207	181	148	109	68	30
Thyroid	634	419	275	178	113	41	14	4	1	0.3	0.0
All solid	4,592	3,265	2,525	1,988	1,575	1,002	824	678	529	358	177
Leukemia	185	112	86	76	71	63	62	62	57	51	37
All cancers	4,777	3,377	2,611	2,064	1,646	1,065	886	740	586	409	214

Source: Adapted from BEIR VII Table 12 D-1, BEIR. *Health Risks from Exposure to Low Levels of Ionizing Radiation: BEIR VII, Phase 2.* Committee to Assess Health Risks from Exposure to Low Levels of Ionizing Radiation, Board of Radiation Effects, Research Division on Earth and Life Studies, National Research Council of the National Academies, National Academy of Sciences. Washington, DC: National Academies Press; 2006.

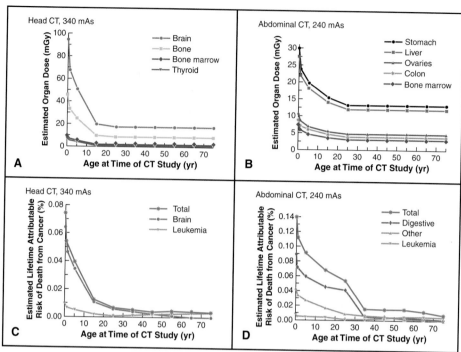

FIGURE 20-35 Estimated organ doses and lifetime cancer risk with age of exposure for CT exams of the head and abdomen. **A and B** show estimated radiation doses for selected organs from a single CT scan of the head or the abdomen. As discussed in Chapter 10, for a given mAs, pediatric doses are typically larger than adult doses, because there is less self-shielding of organs during the tube rotation. Exposure parameters and other aspects of imaging studies should be optimized for each patient. However, it is especially important for children due to their increased risk of radiogenic cancer and often higher organ doses. Optimization of imaging procedures in this context includes not only the technical factors related to the image acquisition but also (and often most importantly) the appropriateness of the requested examination to resolve the particular clinical question. Panels **C and D** show the corresponding estimated lifetime percent cancer mortality risk attributable to the radiation from a single CT scan; the risks (both for selected individual organs and overall) have been averaged for male and female patients. One can appreciate that even though doses are higher for the head CT scans, the risks are higher for abdominal scans because organs exposed are more sensitive than the brain to radiation-induced cancer. It should be noted that the mAs (and resultant doses) used in these examples are from the source cited below and are higher than typical doses for similar exams performed with image acquisition parameters optimized for smaller patients. Contrary to current practice, these data assume that no tube current adjustment for patient size has been applied, which of course would substantially reduce the dose (and thus risk) in the pediatric population. (Reprinted with permission from Brenner DJ, Hall EJ. Computed tomography—an increasing source of radiation exposure. *N Engl J Med.* 2007;357:2277-2284. Copyright © Massachusetts Medical Society.)

Brody et al., 2007). Efforts to educate physicians and patients about these issues continue and will no doubt be necessary for many years to come. Optimization of imaging procedures in this context includes not only the technical factors related to image acquisition, which determine the radiation dose to the patient, but also (and often most importantly) the appropriateness of the requested examination to resolve the particular clinical question.

As discussed in more detail in Chapter 21, the American College of Radiology (ACR) promulgates appropriateness use criteria (AUC) (https://www.acr.org/Clinical-Resources/ACR-Appropriateness-Criteria) as evidence-based guidelines to assist referring physicians and other providers in making the most appropriate imaging or treatment decision for a specific clinical condition (*i.e.*, implementing the principle of Justification). Several institutions have begun to institute clinical decision support (CDS) software or applications incorporated as part of order entry systems to assist physicians/clinicians in determining the most appropriate type of imaging exam (*e.g.*, applying ACR appropriateness criteria scores) for a patient with specific symptoms or disease. The pressure in some cases from parents who may insist on a CT exam for the child being evaluated for relatively minor head injury adds to this problem. The use of clear evidence-based guidelines and appropriateness criteria for medical imaging procedures is an important quality care goal and their implementation in an emergency department setting when evaluating pediatric patients is especially important (American College of Radiology, 2020; Kuppermann et al., 2009).

Estimates of the total cancer incidence and mortality risk as a function of sex and age at exposure are presented graphically in Figure 20-36. The increased cancer risk associated with exposure to radiation of children and infants is easily appreciated. Compared to the risk to adults, the risk for a 12-month-old infant is three to four times higher. The increased risk of radiation exposure in females compared to males at all ages is also shown; however, the magnitude of the difference decreases with age. It is important to appreciate that this overall increase in cancer risk is not the same for all organs nor at all ages. For some organs there does not appear to be an increase in risk with younger age at exposure (*e.g.*, bladder) and for at least one (lung) there is a decrease in risk with younger age at exposure (Table 20-15).

20.7.8 Population Radiation Risk Estimates

Population-averaged radiation-induced cancer incidence and mortality risk estimates, calculated from data provided in the BEIR VII report, are shown in Table 20-16.

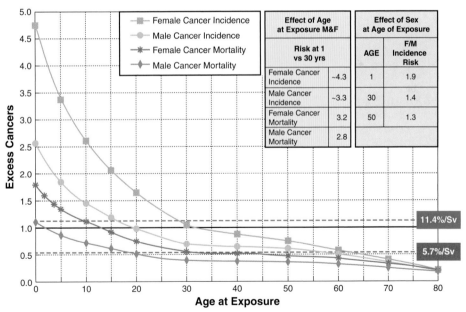

■ **FIGURE 20-36** Lifetime radiation cancer incidence and mortality as a function of sex and age at exposure. Excess cancer cases per 1,000 following a whole-body dose of 10 mSv (multiply by 10 to convert to percent per Sv). The table insets show the relative effect on cancer incidence and mortality for exposures at ages 1 and 30 years old (left) and the relative increased radiogenic cancer risk for females compared to males as a function of exposure at 1, 30, and 50 years old (right). The population-averaged cancer incidence of 11.4% per Sv (green line) and mortality 5.7% per Sv (red line) as calculated from the BEIR VII data are superimposed over the age and sex-specific risk estimates. (Adapted with permission from *Health Risks from Exposure to Low Levels of Ionizing Radiation: BEIR VII, Phase 2*. Committee to Assess Health Risks from Exposure to Low Levels of Ionizing Radiation, Board of Radiation Effects, Research Division on Earth and Life Studies, National Research Council of the National Academies. National Academy of Sciences, Washington, DC: National Academies Press; 2006.)

TABLE 20-15 COMPARISON OF CARCINOGENESIS RISKS AT AGE-AT-EXPOSURE FOR CHILDREN VERSUS ADULTS

CANCER SITE	MORE	NO DIFFERENCE	LESS	NO SUFFICIENT DATA	LEVEL OF EVIDENCE
Esophagus				X	
Stomach (mortality)	ERR	EAR			Moderate
Small intestine[a]				X	
Colon					
(incidence)	EAR	ERR			Weak
(mortality)	EAR & ERR				
Rectum[a]				X	
Pancreas[a]				X	
Liver		X			Weak
Lung			X[b]		Moderate
Skin non-melanoma	X				Moderate
Breast	X				Strong
Uterus				X	
Cervix[a]				X	
Ovary				X	
Prostate[a]				X	
Kidney				X	
Bladder		X			Moderate
Brain	X				Strong
Thyroid	X				Strong
Parathyroid				X	
Hodgkin's lymphoma[a]				X	
Non-Hodgkin's lymphoma				X	
Myeloma				X	
Leukaemia non-CLL	X				Strong
Myelodysplasia	X				Weak

[a]These tumors are not definitely shown to be increased by radiation exposure.
[b]The limited data on radon and lung cancer indicate approximately the same risk after exposure at pre-adult and adult ages.
ERR, excess relative risk; EAR, excess absolute risk.
Reprinted with permission from *Sources, Effects and Risks of Iionizing Radiation*: UNSCEAR 2013 Report, Volume II, Scientific Annex B: Effects of radiation exposure of children. Copyright © United Nations.

The risk estimates in ICRP Publication 103 (ICRP, 2007a) are based on essentially the same radiation-induced cancer incidence and mortality data available to the BEIR VII Committee. While the ICRP methodology to developing their risk estimates in ICRP 103 was different from that of the BEIR Committee, they are in general agreement with those in the BEIR VII report. As mentioned earlier, the ICRP risk estimates were made for the purpose of radiation protection (see Chapter 3) and are not directly comparable to the BEIR VII cancer risk estimates. The current ICRP risk estimates of

TABLE 20-16 THE U.S. POPULATION AVERAGED RADIATION-INDUCED CANCER INCIDENCE AND MORTALITY RISK ESTIMATES IN PERCENT PER Sv

	INCIDENCE	MORTALITY
Female	13.7	6.6
Male	9.0	4.8
U.S. population average	11.4	5.7

Source: Calculated from *Health Risks from Exposure to Low Levels of Ionizing Radiation: BEIR VII, Phase 2.* Committee to Assess Health Risks from Exposure to Low Levels of Ionizing Radiation, Board of Radiation Effects, Research Division on Earth and Life Studies, National Research Council of the National Academies. National Academy of Sciences, Washington, DC: National Academies Press; 2006.

radiation-induced "detriment"[1] (*e.g.,* cancer and genetic effects) at low dose are 4.2% per Sv for a population of adult workers and 5.7% per Sv for the whole population (which includes more radiosensitive subpopulations, such as children). The majority of this detriment is assigned to a cancer risk of 4.1% and 5.5% per Sv for adult workers and the general population, respectively. Even though the definitions and methodology of calculating radiation-induced cancer risk are different for the ICRP and the BEIR VII committee, the ICRP population estimate of cancer detriment from radiation exposure (5.5% per Sv) corresponds fairly well to BEIR VII lifetime attributable cancer mortality projections averaged for the U.S. population (5.7% per Sv).

To estimate the risk to the general population from radiation exposure at low exposure levels, the approximate values of 11% and 6% per Sv, respectively, for cancer incidence and mortality can be used. As mentioned earlier, the lifetime probabilities of developing or dying from cancer in the United States (averaged for both sexes) are approximately 41% and 22%, respectively. According to the linear risk-projection model, an acute exposure of 100 people to 100 mSv would add approximately 1 additional cancer case to the 41 normally expected to occur over the lifetime of a group with an age and sex distribution similar to the general population (Fig. 20-37).

Of course, there would be no way of identifying which person had the additional cancer (if it occurred at all) that was caused by the radiation exposure and, given the small number of individuals exposed, the natural variation associated with the average incidence of cancer would be larger than one. The number of exposed individuals and the dose in the example above were chosen to provide a simple example of the LNT dose-response relationship. However, it would be very unusual for such a group to receive such a large whole-body dose at one time. Using a more realistic dose from an (albeit unlikely) exposure scenario, one could imagine an accidental release of radioactive material into the environment exposing a population of 10,000 to 10 mSv in 1 year (*i.e.,* ten times the annual public exposure limit in the United States). The LNT model would project 11 additional cancer cases (approximately one half of which would be fatal) over the lifetime of the population. This represents an increase of less than 0.3% above the spontaneous cancer incidence rate. UNSCEAR and ICRP, however, argue against using collective dose to predict future cancer deaths when the average dose to the population is small and below the doses where excess risks have been convincingly demonstrated. An additional perspective on cancer risks is

---

[1]The total harm to health experienced by an exposed group and its decendants as a result of the group's exposure to a radiation source. Detriment is a multidimensional concept. Its principal components are the stochastic quantities: probability of attributable fatal cancer, weighted probability of attributable non-fatal cancer, weighted probability of severe heritable effects, and length of life lost if the harm occurs.

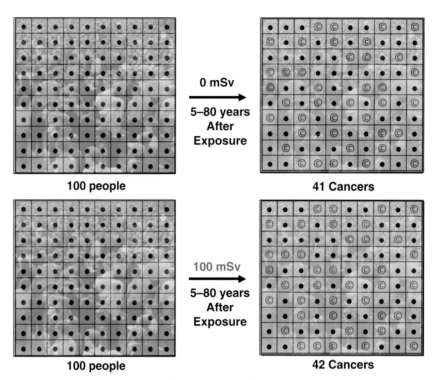

■ **FIGURE 20-37** Cancer incidence for two identical groups of 100 people with age and sex distributions similar to the general population. An acute exposure to 100 mSv for each person in one group would be expected to add approximately 1 additional cancer case (occurring anytime after a latent period of approximately 5 years) to the 41 normally expected to occur in the identical unexposed group over the group's lifetime.

presented in Table 20-17, which compares adult cancers with respect to their spontaneous and radiation-induced incidence.

20.7.9 CT Examinations and Future Cancer Risk

Evaluations of both benefit and risk are important in the use of radiation for medical imaging. Study results on potential risks associated with medical exposures are subject to significant uncertainties including, but not limited to, partial body (or organ) irradiations, lack of historical exposure data, limited organ dosimetry for organs other than the target organ, and potential biases because radiologic procedures are often administered for an existing health condition (diagnosed or undiagnosed) (NCRP, 2018a). Recent epidemiologic studies (Mathews et al., 2013; Pearce et al., 2012) have involved populations who had received computed tomography (CT) scans during childhood to young adulthood when risk might be greater because CT doses were relatively high and young people may be more radiosensitive to cancer induction than adults. However, information on organ doses from CT examinations in the 1980s and 1990s is sparse and individual doses have been reconstructed from surveys and not from any individual parameters. In such studies, there is a critical need to avoid serious biases that render findings difficult to interpret or misleading. In particular, there is a fundamental requirement to disentangle radiation effects from the reasons why the CT examination was given. Just such potential specific biases, confounding by indication (triggered by conditions that predispose to cancer) and reverse causation (preexisting, but as yet undetected malignancy as the reason for the CT scan), are extremely important deficiencies of several CT studies (*e.g.*, Mathews et al., 2013;

TABLE 20-17 SPONTANEOUS INCIDENCE AND SENSITIVITY OF VARIOUS TISSUES TO RADIATION-INDUCED CANCER

SITE OR TYPE OF CANCER	SPONTANEOUS INCIDENCE	RADIATION SENSITIVITY
Most Frequent Radiation-Induced Cancers		
Female breast	Very high	High in children and young women
Thyroid	Low	Very high in children, especially in females, but very low in adults
Lung (bronchus)	Very high	Moderate
Leukemia	Moderate	Very high
Alimentary tract	High	Moderate
Less Frequent Radiation-Induced Cancers		
Pharynx	Low	Moderate
Liver and biliary tract	Low	Moderate
Lymphomas	Moderate	Moderate
Kidney and bladder	Moderate	Low
Brain and nervous system	Low	Low
Salivary glands	Very low	Low
Bone	Very low	Low
Skin	High	Low
Magnitude of Radiation Risk Uncertain		
Larynx	Moderate	Low
Nasal sinuses	Very low	Low
Parathyroid	Very low	Low
Ovary	Moderate	Low
Connective tissue	Very low	Low
Radiation Risk Not Demonstrated		
Prostate	Very high	Absent?
Uterus and cervix	Very high	Absent?
Testis	Low	Absent?
Mesothelium	Very low	Absent?
Chronic lymphocytic leukemia	Low	Absent?

Source: Modified from Committee on Radiological Units, Standards, and Protection. *Medical Radiation: A Guide to Good Practice*. Chicago, IL: American College of Radiology; 1985.

Pearce et al., 2012) that initially seemed to indicate associations between CT studies and an increased risk of certain types of cancer. In addition, these studies suffer from weak dosimetry so the results have limited reliability for evaluating potential risks (NCRP, 2018a). Subsequent evaluations (Journy et al., 2015; Krille et al., 2015) attempted to adjust for the indication for the CT studies, whether suspected cancer or other cancer-predisposing factors, and found no significant excess risk observed in relation to CT exposures, thus emphasizing the importance of such considerations when performing these analyses.

There are several ongoing studies of the associations between pediatric CT examinations and subsequent cancer outcomes, including cohorts in Australia, Canada, and the EPI-CT study in Europe. Among other things, these studies will need improvements in the dosimetry compared to existing reports, including use of individual organ/tissue doses, more accurate characterization of historical CT doses, and accounting for all past CT examinations or other medical examinations with relatively high doses (NCRP, 2018a). Appropriate incorporation of minimum latency periods for cancer induction, typically 2 y for leukemia and 5 or 10 y for solid cancers, is also essential. For the results of the EPI-CT (or other) epidemiological study to be considered meaningful, the impact of all of the potential sources of biases and missing sources of data are carefully assessed (Bosch de Basea et al., 2015). However, owing to limitations in existing individual medical records, that may not be possible.

While there are no dose limits for patients undergoing CT examinations, evaluation of doses is still an important aspect of radiation protection programs. Dose metrics suitable for comparison with published diagnostic reference levels and achievable doses should be assessed, as discussed in Chapter 21. The definition, use, and limitations of effective dose, often in units of millisieverts (mSv), as a dose descriptor were presented in Chapter 3. CT effective doses are often on the order of about 1–10 mSv, depending on procedure and patient variables.

Effective dose estimates are only valid for prospective radiological protection purposes and should not be used for retrospective dose assessments, epidemiologic evaluations, or the estimation of a specific individual's risk (ICRP, 2007a; NCRP, 2018b). Effective dose may be used as a general indicator (*i.e.*, order of magnitude) of radiation risk for exposure to radiation for diagnostic or interventional procedures (Harrison et al., 2016; Martin, 2008). The effective dose concept can also be helpful in framing the generally small radiation risk associated with CT procedures that are both justified (anticipated benefit greater than the corresponding risk) and optimized (doses utilized are not higher than those required for producing images of diagnostic quality). For example, based on ICRP approaches to radiation protection (ICRP, 2007a), the current nominal risk coefficients for stochastic effects (mainly cancer) after exposure to radiation at low dose rate (*i.e.*, ~ 5% per Sv) would suggest a justified CT procedure that delivered an effective dose of 10 mSv to a population of patients might only increase that population's risk by ~0.05% above the natural background rate of fatal cancer in that population. In other words, for any one person, the risk of radiation-induced cancer is much, much smaller than the natural risk of cancer (FDA, 2020).

Communicating with staff, patients, and the public on both benefits and risks associated with medical imaging procedures is challenging, but necessary (Dauer et al., 2018; McCollough et al., 2015; Thornton et al., 2015). To assist in communications, the NCRP (NCRP, 2020) has suggested a classification scheme for use of effective dose as just such a qualitative indicator of radiation detriment for balancing against potential medical benefits, utilizing the following descriptors: *negligible* (<0.1 mSv), *minimal* (0.1–1 mSv), *minor* (>1–10 mSv), *low* (>10–100 mSv), and acceptable in the context of the expected benefit (>100 mSv). In this construct, most justified CT examinations could be described qualitatively as a *minimal* or *minor* radiation detriment risk to be balanced with likely individual benefit. There are now several radiation "risk" calculators that are available to assist in estimating nominal radiation dose from CT protocols (and other radiation imaging procedures) and in developing language to help describe the possible effects of the radiation appropriate for the subject populations that take into account factors such as age and gender (ASRT, 2018; Duke, 2019; NCICT, 2020; RADAR, 2019; UW, 2008). The World Health Organization has developed an excellent publication that focuses on communication between the medical care team (including imaging professionals and the providers, referring physicians) and pediatric patients and their families (WHO, 2016).

In addition, the NCRP has developed guidance and suggested language to be used for communicating radiation imaging risks that can be very helpful when responding to patient inquiries or as part of research-informed consent dialogues (NCRP, 2020). An example of the type of language that could be considered for a typical CT scan with an estimated dose of about 10 mSv could be as follows:

> *"The amount of radiation involved in this study is small but may slightly increase your risk of getting cancer later in life. Scientists are not certain about the actual cancer risk at these low doses, and there may be no risk at all. Any increase in risk may be about 1 chance in 2,000 or less. For comparison, your risk of developing cancer at some time in your life, even if you do not receive this additional radiation (and associated medical benefit) is about 40% (4 chances in 10, which is the same as about 800 in 2,000). By having this CT study your risk of developing cancer at some time in your life may only increase to about 801 in 2,000."*

Medical professionals are encouraged to consult additional resources with regard to CT dose, benefit, and risk offered by the ACR (e.g., https://www.acr.org/Clinical-Resources/Radiology-Safety/Radiation-Safety); the Radiological Society of North America (https://www.radiologyinfo.org/); and specific information on pediatric CT doses by the Image Gently Alliance (https://www.imagegently.org/Procedures/Computed-Tomography).

20.7.10 Cancer Risk for Selected Organs and Tissues

Leukemia

Leukemia is a relatively rare disease, with an incidence in the general U.S. population of approximately 1 in 10,000 per year. However, genetic predisposition to leukemia can dramatically increase the risk. For example, an identical twin of a leukemic child has a one in three chance of developing leukemia. Although it is rare in the general population, leukemia is one of the most frequently observed radiation-induced cancers. Leukemia may be acute or chronic, and it may take a lymphocytic or myeloid form. With the exception of chronic lymphocytic leukemia and viral-induced leukemia, increases in all forms of leukemia have been detected in human populations exposed to radiation and in animals experimentally irradiated.

Within a few years after the detonation of the A-bombs, an increase in the incidence of leukemia was apparent in the survivor population. This evidence, together with subsequent studies of medically and occupationally exposed cohorts, indicates that excess leukemia cases can be detected as soon as 1 to 2 years after exposure and reach a peak approximately 12 years after the exposure. The incidence of leukemia is influenced by age at the time of exposure. The younger the person is at the time of exposure, the shorter are the latency period and the period of expression (Fig. 20-38).

Although the incidence of radiation-induced leukemia decreases with age at the time of exposure, the interval of increased risk is prolonged. The BEIR VII committee's preferred model for leukemia risk is an LQ function of dose and, like models for solid cancers, leukemia risk is expressed as a function of age at exposure. However, the unique temporal wave-like character of the elevated risk for leukemia makes it more useful to express risk as a function of time since exposure rather than attained age (Fig. 20-39).

Another unique feature of the risk model is that there was no need to apply a DDREF as the estimates are already based on a LQ function of dose. The BEIR VII preferred model for leukemia estimates an excess lifetime risk from an exposure to 0.1 Gy for 100,000 persons with an age distribution similar to that of the U.S. population to be approximately 70 and 100, for females and males, respectively (i.e., ~1% per Sv).

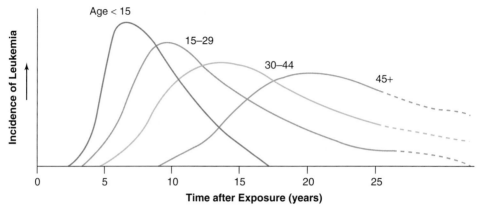

■ **FIGURE 20-38** Effect of age at the time of exposure on the incidence of leukemia (all forms except chronic lymphocytic leukemia) among the A-bomb survivors. (Reprinted with permission from Ichuimaru M, et al. *Incidence of Leukemia in Atomic-Bomb Survivors, Hiroshima and Nagasaki 1950 to 1971, by Radiation Dose, Years After Exposure, Age, and Type of Leukemia.* Technical Report RERF 10-76. Hiroshima, Japan: Copyright © Radiation Effects Research Foundation; 1976.)

Thyroid Cancer

Distinct from the previously discussed cancer risk estimates, the preferred BEIR VII models for thyroid and breast cancers are based on pooled analyses of the LSS data and medically irradiated cohorts. Spontaneous and radiation-induced thyroid cancer shows a greater difference by gender than most cancers, with women having a risk approximately two to three times as great as that for men (presumably because of hormonal influences on thyroid function). Persons of Jewish and North African ancestry also appear to be at greater risk than the general population. Thyroid cancer

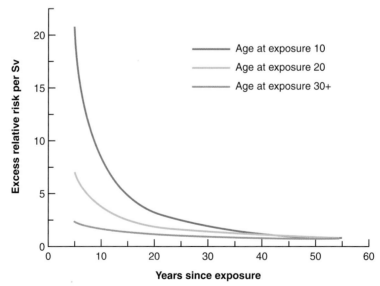

■ **FIGURE 20-39** Age-time patterns in radiation-associated risks for leukemia mortality. Curves are sex-averaged estimates of the risk at 1 Sv for people exposed at age 10 (red line), age 20 (orange line), and age 30 or more (blue line). (Adapted with permission from *Health Risks from Exposure to Low Levels of Ionizing Radiation: BEIR VII, Phase 2.* Committee to Assess Health Risks from Exposure to Low Levels of Ionizing Radiation, Board of Radiation Effects, Research Division on Earth and Life Studies, National Research Council of the National Academies. National Academy of Sciences, Washington, DC: National Academies Press; 2006.)

accounts for only approximately 2% of the yearly total cancer incidence. In addition, the mortality is low, resulting in only approximately 0.2% of all cancer deaths each year. Even though there is a large RR for thyroid cancer from radiation exposure in childhood, the ARs (even in children and young adults) are lower than for breast, colon, and lung cancers. There is also a rapid decrease in radiogenic cancer risk with age at exposure, with the lifetime AR per Gy for thyroid cancer at age 40 and beyond lower than the risk to all but a few other organs and tissues. Most studies do not indicate any elevation in risk when exposure occurs in adulthood.

The majority of radiation-induced thyroid neoplasms are well-differentiated papillary adenocarcinomas, with a lower percentage being of the follicular form. Because of improved diagnostic procedures and the fact that radiation-induced thyroid cancers do not usually include the anaplastic and medullary types, the associated mortality rate is very low ($\sim 5/10^6$ per year for all races and both genders). The dose-response data for thyroid cancer fit a linear pattern. The latency period for benign nodules is approximately 5 to 35 years, and for thyroid malignancies, approximately 10 to 35 years. While recent studies of the risk of radiation-induced thyroid cancer have taken different modeling approaches to estimate the risk (BEIR VII, 2006; EPA, 2011; NCRP, 2008), the results differ by less than a factor of 2 and all estimates had a range representing the 95% confidence interval that were a factor of 4 or more from their point estimate.

The relative effectiveness of producing radiogenic thyroid cancer from internally deposited radionuclides has been shown to be approximately 60% to 100% as effective as external irradiation from x-rays. A comprehensive update of a previous NCRP report on radiation effects on the thyroid (NCRP, 2008), found that for the same absorbed dose, I-131 and I-125 were no more than 30% to 60% as effective as external radiation in causing thyroid cancer with the higher effectiveness applicable to radioiodine exposure in children. However, the report concluded that other radionuclides including I-123 and Tc-99m were equally effective (per unit thyroid dose) as external radiation in causing thyroid cancer.

Irradiation of the thyroid may produce other responses, such as hypothyroidism and thyroiditis. Threshold estimates for adult populations range from 2 Gy for external irradiation to 50 Gy for internal (low-dose-rate) irradiation. Lower threshold estimates exist for children. Approximately 10% of persons with thyroid doses of 200 to 300 Gy from radioactive iodine will develop symptoms of thyroiditis and/or a sore throat, and higher doses may result in thyroid ablation.

Due to the considerable ability of the thyroid gland to concentrate iodine, the thyroid dose from radioiodine in elemental or ionic form is typically 1,000 times greater than in other organs in the body. The relatively large thyroid dose per unit activity administered explains why thyroid cancer is a major concern following exposure to radioiodine, especially in children. The Chernobyl nuclear plant accident released large quantities of radioiodine that resulted in a substantial increase in the incidence of thyroid cancer among children living in heavily contaminated regions. The cows concentrated the radioiodine in their milk by eating contaminated foliage, which was further concentrated in the thyroid glands of people who consumed the milk. The thyroid dose to children was higher because they consume more milk and their thyroid glands had higher concentrations of radioiodine than in adult thyroid glands. Decreased dietary levels of stable iodine dramatically increase radioiodine uptake by the thyroid. It appears that dietary iodine deficiency was an important factor in the elevated occurrence of thyroid cancer observed in children exposed to radioiodine from the Chernobyl disaster. The increase so far has been almost entirely papillary carcinoma, which is the most common malignant tumor of the thyroid in adults, adolescents, and children. There has been no increase in thyroid cancer in cohorts made up of adults at the time of the accident, consistent with the absence of a thyroid cancer excess among patients treated with I-131 NaI for Graves disease and other thyroid disorders. In addition, no other cancers have shown an increased incidence thus far, and no increase has been detected in the incidence of birth defects.

Breast Cancer

For women exposed to ionizing radiation during mammography, the potential for an increase in the risk of breast cancer is of particular concern. The high prevalence and morbidity of breast cancer in the female population and the often differing professional opinions about the risk and benefits of screening mammography only serve to exacerbate these concerns. Breast cancer is the most commonly diagnosed cancer among women regardless of race or ethnicity. According to NCI, one out of every eight women (12.5%) in the United States develops breast cancer with approximately 268,600 new cases of invasive breast cancer and 48,100 cases of non-invasive (in situ) breast cancer expected to be diagnosed in women each year (ACS, 2019). The lifetime breast cancer mortality risk for women is approximately 2.6% with significant variation by race and ethnicity (*e.g.*, annual mortality rates for Black, White and Asian/Pacific Islanders and Hispanic populations are 28.4, 20.3, 14.0, and 11.5 per 100,000 respectively) (Henley, 2020). Other etiologic factors in the risk of breast cancer include age at first full-term pregnancy, family history of breast cancer, and estrogen levels in the blood. Women who have had no children or only one child are at greater risk for breast cancer than women who have had two or more children. In addition, reduced risks are associated with women who conceived earlier in life and who nursed a child by breast for a longer period of time. A familial history of breast cancer can increase the risk twofold to fourfold, with the magnitude of the risk increasing as the age at diagnosis in the family member decreases. As shown previously for Japan and the United States, there is also considerable racial and geographic variation in breast cancer risk. Several investigations have suggested that the presence of estrogen, acting as a promoter, is an important factor in the incidence and latency associated with spontaneous and radiation-induced breast cancer.

The BEIR VII Committee utilized a pooled analysis of data on A-bomb survivors and medically exposed persons to evaluate the breast cancer risk for low-LET radiation. The data fit a linear dose-response model, with a dose of approximately 800 mGy required to double the natural incidence of breast cancer. The data from acute and fractionated (but high dose rate) exposure studies indicate that fractionation of the dose does not reduce the risk of breast cancer induced by low-LET radiation. There is some evidence that protracted exposure to radiation in children reduces the risk of radiation-induced breast cancer compared with acute or highly fractionated exposures (Preston et al., 2002). The latent period ranges from 10 to 40 years, with younger women having longer latencies. In contrast to leukemia, there is no identifiable window of expression; therefore the risk seems to continue throughout the life of the exposed individual. The lifetime attributable risk of developing breast cancer in a population of women with an age distribution similar to that of the U.S. general population is $310/10^5/0.1$ Gy. The risk is very age dependent, being approximately 13 times higher for exposure at age 5 ($914/10^5/0.1$ Gy) than at age 50 ($70/10^5/0.1$ Gy) (BEIR VII, 2006). Using the age-specific values in the BEIR VII report, the lifetime attributable risks of developing breast cancer for females receiving a breast dose of 20 mGy from a chest CT at age 10, 30, or 50 are approximately 0.14%, 0.05%, and 0.014%, respectively.

Use of the automatic tube current modulation (TCM) capability of modern scanners has substantially lowered the dose and subsequent cancer risk, especially for younger patients. The following example illustrates the benefit of TCM compared to fixed mA for chest CT in 50-, 30-, and 10-year-old patients. In this example, we will assume a nominal breast dose of 15 mGy for a chest CT scan of a 50-year-old woman using fixed mA. In the absence of any other changes except decreasing body habitus at a younger age, the breast dose might increase to 20 and 25 mGy for similar exams in the 30- and 10-year-old patients, respectively. As seen in Table 20-18, the increase in future cancer risk in the 10-year-old is 17 times that of the 50-year-old due to the combined effects of both increased dose and greater risk per unit dose associated with the 10-year-old's scan. With TCM activated, the dose to 50-year-old women might increase somewhat but the dose (and associated risk) reductions in the other two age groups relative to that for the 50-year-old patient is substantial. It can also be appreciated that while the relative reduction in risk can be dramatic as shown in the example above, the change to the baseline breast cancer risk at the age of exposure is much less so. Thus, while the difference in dose reduction techniques illustrated above has only a minor influence on the cancer risk for an individual patient, considering the high utilization of CT in the United States and elsewhere, the overall public health impact could be quite important. Further discussion of the effect of TCM on dose reduction can be found in Chapter 10 and the literature (Angel et al., 2009).

Improvements in quality assurance and the introduction of digital mammography have resulted in a substantial reduction in dose to the breast (see Chapter 8). Women participating in large, controlled mammographic screening studies have been shown to have a decreased risk of mortality from breast cancer. The American Cancer Society, the American College of Obstetricians and Gynecologists, and the ACR currently recommend annual mammography examinations for women beginning at age 40. This section started with noting that there has been concern over radiation risks associated with mammographic screening examinations. It is reassuring that the risk of radiation-induced breast cancer decreases substantially with age at exposure and, despite the models used for risk estimation, there is no consistent epidemiologic evidence for significant risks for exposures once a woman has passed the menopausal ages. Further, the exposures for mammographic images are substantially below the levels for which significantly increased risks have been detected.

Lung Cancer

The lung is another organ in which there has been considerable debate about the dose-response for cancer and whether there is a sex-specific risk for radiation-induced

TABLE 20-18 EFFECT OF AGE AND TCM ON BREAST DOSE AND LIFETIME ATTRIBUTABLE CANCER RISK (LAR) FROM CHEST CT

AGE	CT mA (FIXED/ TCM)	BREAST DOSE (mGy)	LAR BEIR VII PER 10⁵ PER 0.1 Gy	LIFETIME RISK AT AGE (%)	LAR FROM CT AT AGE (%)	LIFETIME RISK + LAR FROM CT AT AGE (%)	RISK RATIO AGE/50	RISK RATIO FIXED mA/TCM AT AGE
10	Fixed	25	712	12.3	0.178	12.478	17.0	2.50
	TCM	10	712	12.3	0.071	12.371	5.1	
30	Fixed	20	253	12.3	0.051	12.351	4.8	1.33
	TCM	15	253	12.3	0.038	12.338	2.7	
50	Fixed	15	70	10.9	0.011	10.911	1.0	0.75
	TCM	20	70	10.9	0.014	10.914	1.0	

TCM, tube current modulation.

cancer. The LSS of the Japanese atomic bomb survivors has found an increased risk of lung cancer from radiation and also indicates that the risk is nearly three times greater in women than in men (Cahoon et al., 2017; Ozasa et al., 2012). On the other hand, studies on tuberculosis patients in Canada and Massachusetts who received frequent chest x-rays to monitor lung collapse therapy have not shown any increased risk for lung cancer, although in some cases the lung doses exceeded those in the Japanese A-bomb population (Fig. 20-40) (Davis et al., 1989; Howe, 1995). The reasons for the differences in these dose responses for lung cancer has been unclear, although one possibility is the differences in the dose rate (Fry, 1996) since the A-bomb survivors received their dose in a single, instantaneous, large exposure, while the TB patients received multiple smaller doses over extended periods of time. A recent study evaluated five occupational cohorts within the Million Person Study (MPS) of Low-Dose Health Effects and the Canadian fluoroscopy cohort of tuberculosis patients (Boice et al., 2019). In this large study, having 15,065 lung cancers among the 443,684 subjects, the combined cohorts provided little evidence for a radiation dose-response among males or females and little evidence that either chronic or fractionated radiation exposures increased the risk of lung cancer. These findings are supported by other epidemiologic studies from other countries that also fail to find a statistically meaningful increase in lung cancer risk. Additional studies are ongoing, including a large study of medical workers and a new follow-up of the Canadian TB patients, which could provide additional insight on the RR for lung cancer under different radiation situations and in different populations.

20.7.11   Non-cancer Radiation Effects

Studies of some radiotherapy patient populations have demonstrated increased risks for diseases other than cancer, particularly cardiovascular disease. There is

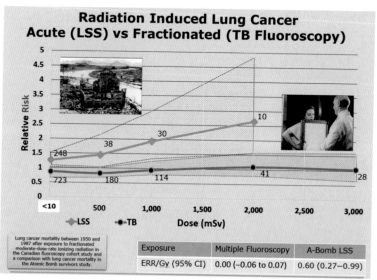

■ **FIGURE 20-40** Relative risk (RR) of radiation-induced lung cancer in the LSS population and Canadian TB patients. The A-bomb survivors (LSS population) received their lung doses virtually instantaneously, while the TB patients were exposed to multiple, small, thorax-localized doses from frequent chest fluoroscopic exams to monitor lung collapse therapy, such that, in some cases, the total lung doses exceeded those received by the A-bomb survivors. (Data from Howe GR. Lung cancer mortality between 1950 and 1987 after exposure to fractionated moderate-dose-rate ionizing radiation in the Canadian Fluoroscopy Cohort Study and a comparison with lung cancer mortality in the Atomic Bomb survivors study. *Radiat Res*. 1995;142:295-304.)

also evidence of an increase in cardiovascular disease at much lower doses among A-bomb survivors; however, there is no statistically significant increase at doses below 0.5 Sv (ICRP, 2012). This evidence notwithstanding, there is no direct evidence for an increased risk of cardiovascular disease or other non-cancer effects at the low doses associated with typical occupational exposures and diagnostic imaging procedures and, thus far, the data are inadequate to quantify this risk if it exists.

20.8 HEREDITARY EFFECTS OF RADIATION EXPOSURE

Conclusive evidence of the ability of ionizing radiation to produce genetic effects was first obtained in 1927 with the experimental observations of radiation-induced genetic effects in fruit flies (Muller, 1927). Extensive laboratory investigations since that time (primarily large-scale studies in mice; Russell et al., 1958) have led scientists to conclude that (1) radiation is a mutagenic agent; (2) most mutations are harmful to the organism; (3) radiation does not produce unique mutations; (4) chronic radiation exposure produces fewer heritable effects in offspring than the same dose delivered acutely; and (5) radiation-induced genetic damage can theoretically occur (like cancer) from a single mutation and appears to be linearly related to dose (i.e., LNT dose-response model). However, it is reassuring that no human study has demonstrated transgenerational effects following parental exposure. Specifically, the studies of over 70,000 children, of A-bomb survivors and the children of cancer survivors treated with radiotherapy, find no evidence for increased risks of malformations, neonatal deaths, stillbirths, chromosomal abnormality, or gene changes that could be related to the exposure to radiation of fathers and mothers (Signorello et al., 2010; Winther et al., 2009). Although genetic effects were initially thought to be the most significant biologic effect of ionizing radiation, it is clear that, for doses associated with occupational and medical exposure, the risks are small compared with the spontaneous incidence of genetic anomalies and are secondary to their carcinogenic potential.

20.8.1 Epidemiologic Investigations of Radiation-Induced Hereditary Effects

Epidemiologic investigations have failed to demonstrate radiation-induced hereditary effects, although mutations of human cells in culture have been shown. For a given exposure, the mutation rates found in the progeny of irradiated humans are significantly lower than those previously identified in insect populations. The largest population studied is the A-bomb survivors and their progeny. Based on current risk estimates, failure to detect an increase in radiation-induced mutations in this population is not surprising considering how few are predicted in comparison to the spontaneous incidence. Screening of 28 specific protein loci in the blood of 27,000 children of A-bomb survivors resulted in only two mutations that might have been caused by radiation exposure of the parents.

Earlier studies of survivors' children to determine whether radiation exposure caused an increase in sex-linked lethal gene mutations that would have resulted in increased prenatal death of males or alteration of the gender birth ratio were negative. Irradiation of human testes has been shown to produce an increase in the incidence of translocations in spermatogonial stem cells, although no additional chromosomal aberrations have been detected in children of A-bomb survivors. A large cohort study of more than 90,000 U.S. radiologic technologists (RTs) examined the risk of childhood cancer (less than 20 years) among more than 100,000 offspring born between

1921 and 1984 to the technologists (Johnson et al., 2008). Parental occupational radiation exposure of the testis or ovary prior to conception was estimated from work history data, dosimetry records, and estimates from the literature for exposure before 1960. Despite the size of the study population, no convincing evidence of an increase in radiation exposure–related risk of childhood cancer in the offspring of RTs was found. The result from several recent studies evaluating the potential for trans-generational effects in the children of cancer survivors treated with radiotherapy has also been consistently negative (Signorello et al., 2010; Tawn et al., 2011; Winther et al., 2009).

20.8.2 Estimating Genetic Risk

The *genetically significant dose* is an index of the presumed genetic impact of radiation-induced mutation in germ cells in an exposed population. The sensitivity of a population to radiation-induced genetic damage can be measured by the *doubling dose*, defined as the dose required per generation to double the spontaneous mutation rate. The spontaneous mutation rate is approximately 5×10^{-6} per locus and 7 to 15×10^{-4} per gamete for chromosomal abnormalities. The doubling dose for humans is estimated to be approximately 1 Gy per generation; however, this represents an extrapolation from animal data. The BEIR VII committee estimated that an exposure of 10 mGy to the parental generation would cause 30 to 47 additional genetic disorders per 1 million births in the succeeding generation, as a result of increases in the number of autosomal dominant and (to a much lesser degree) sex-linked dominant mutations.

Variations in exposure to natural background do not contribute significantly to a population's genetic risk. Even a dose of 100 mGy would only be estimated to produce about 400 additional genetic disorders per 1 million live births in the first generation (0.4%/Gy), compared with the normal incidence of approximately 1 in 20 or 5% (some estimates are 1 in 10). Therefore, the 100-mGy dose would cause an increase in the spontaneous rate of genetic disorders of less than 0.8%.

While the estimates of cancer risk attributable to radiation exposure published in authoritative reports from the BEIR committees, UNSCEAR, NCRP, and ICRP, have not changed greatly in the past three decades, new data and risk modeling have resulted in a substantial reduction in the estimated radiation-induced risk of heritable disease. According to a review by the ICRP, previous estimates of radiation-induced genetic effects from experiments in mice, and the study of genetic data from A-bomb survivors likely overestimated the risk of heritable disease from radiation exposure (ICRP, 2006). Taking into consideration substantial advances in the understanding of human genetic diseases and the process of germ line mutagenesis after radiation exposure, the ICRP substantially reduced the proportion of detriment ascribed to the potential heritable effects of radiation exposure. The ICRP currently estimates the genetic risks, up to the second generation, to be about 0.2% per Gy. The change in the ICRP estimates of the relative contribution to the total detriment from cancer and heritable effects is shown in Table 20-19. For the population at large, the contribution of heritable effects attributed by ICRP to the total detriment from radiation exposure has been reduced from 23% in 1990 to 3.5% in 2006. This has, of course, also been reflected in a similar reduction to the tissue weighting factor for the gonads from 0.2 to 0.08.

Typical diagnostic and occupational radiation exposures, although increasing the dose to the gonads of those exposed, would not be expected to result in any significant genetic risk to their progeny. Although delaying conception after therapeutic

TABLE 20-19 DETRIMENT-ADJUSTED NOMINAL RISK COEFFICIENTS FOR STOCHASTIC EFFECTS AT LOW DOSE RATE (UNIT, % Sv⁻¹)

EXPOSED	CANCER		HERITABLE		TOTAL	
	1990	*2007*	*1990*	*2007*	*1990*	*2007*
All	6.0	5.5	1.3	0.2	7.3	5.7
Adult	4.8	4.1	0.8	0.1	5.6	4.2

doses of radiation to reduce the probability of transmission of genetic damage to offspring is sometimes recommended, it is not a commonly recommended practice for the relatively low gonadal doses from most diagnostic imaging procedures.

20.9 RADIATION EFFECTS IN UTERO

Developing organisms are highly dynamic systems that are characterized by rapid cell proliferation, migration, and differentiation. Thus, the developing embryo is extremely sensitive to ionizing radiation, as would be expected based on Bergonie and Tribondeau's early characterization of cellular radiosensitivity. The response after exposure to ionizing radiation depends on many factors including (1) total dose, (2) dose rate, (3) radiation quality, and (4) the stage of development at the time of exposure. Together, these factors determine the likelihood of potential consequences (if any) of in utero radiation exposure, including such effects as prenatal or neonatal death, congenital abnormalities, growth impairment, reduced intelligence, genetic aberrations, and an increase in future risk of cancer. A comprehensive review of preconception and prenatal radiation exposure health effects and protective guidance has been developed by the NCRP (NCRP, 2013) and should be consulted when necessary by the medical professionals.

2.9.1 Radiation Effects and Gestation

The gestational period can be divided into three stages: a relatively short *preimplantation* stage, followed by an extended period of *major organogenesis*, and finally the *fetal growth* stage, during which differentiation is complete and growth occurs. Each of these stages is characterized by different responses to radiation exposure, owing principally to the relative radiosensitivities of the tissues at the time of exposure.

Preimplantation

The preimplantation stage begins with the union of the sperm and egg and continues through day 9 in humans, when the zygote becomes embedded in the uterine wall. During this period, the two pronuclei fuse, cleave, and form the morula and blastula.

The conceptus is very sensitive during the preimplantation stage, and susceptibility to the lethal effects of irradiation is a concern. However, for doses less than 100 mGy, the risks are very low. Embryos exhibit a so-called *all-or-nothing response* to radiation exposure at this stage of development, in which, if the exposure is not lethal, the damaged cells are repaired or replaced to the extent that there is unlikely to be any additional radiation-induced risk of congenital abnormalities beyond those which would occur for other reasons. Several factors, including repair capability, lack of cellular differentiation, and the relatively hypoxic state of the embryo, are thought to contribute to its resistance to radiation-induced abnormalities. During the first few divisions, the cells are undifferentiated and lack predetermination for a particular organ system. If radiation exposure were to kill some cells at this stage, the remaining cells could continue the embryonic development without gross malformations because they are indeterminate. However, any misrepaired chromosomal damage at this point may be expressed at some later time. When cells become specialized and are no longer indeterminate, loss of even a few cells may lead to anomalies, growth retardation, or prenatal death. The periods most sensitive to the induction of chromosomal aberrations following radiation exposure in humans are at 12 h after conception, when the two pronuclei fuse to the one-cell stage, and again at 30 and 60 h when the first two divisions occur. Chromosomal aberrations from radiation exposure at the one-cell stage could result in loss of a chromosome in subsequent cell divisions that would then be uniform throughout the embryo. Most chromosomal loss at this early stage is lethal. Loss of a sex chromosome in female embryos may result in Turner syndrome, although there is no evidence that this has occurred following radiation exposure.

A woman may not know she is pregnant during the preimplantation period, the time at which the conceptus is at greatest risk of lethal effects. Animal experiments have demonstrated an increase in the spontaneous abortion (prenatal death) rate after doses as low as 50 to 100 mGy delivered during the preimplantation period. After implantation, doses in excess of 250 mGy are required to induce prenatal death. The risk of spontaneous abortion following a dose of 10 mGy to the conceptus is approximately 1%, compared to the naturally occurring rate, which is reported to be between 30% and 50% (Brent and Gorson, 1972; Jacobsen, 1968; Roux et al., 1993). The LD_{50} for stages from the zygote to expanded blastocysts is in the range of 1 Gy (ICRP, 2003a).

Organogenesis

Embryonic malformations occur more frequently during the period of major organogenesis (second to eighth week after conception). The initial differentiation of cells to form certain organ systems typically occurs on a specific gestational day. For example, neuroblasts (stem cells of the CNS) appear on the 18th gestational day, the forebrain and eyes begin to form on Day 20, and primitive germ cells are evident on Day 21. Each organ system is not at equal risk during the entire period of major organogenesis. In general, the greatest probability of a malformation in a specific organ system (the so-called *critical period*) exists when the radiation exposure is received during the period of peak differentiation of that system. This may not always be the case, however, because damage can occur to adjacent tissue, which has a negative effect on a developing organ system. Some anomalies may have more than one critical period. For example, cataract formation has been shown to have three critical periods in mice.

The only organ system (in humans or laboratory rodents) that has shown an association between malformations and low-LET radiation doses less than 250 mGy is the CNS. Embryos exposed early in organogenesis exhibit the greatest intrauterine growth retardation, presumably because of cell depletion. *In utero* exposure to doses greater than 100–200 mGy from the Hiroshima atomic bomb resulted in a significant increase in the occurrence of microcephaly.

In general, radiation-induced teratogenic effects are less common in humans than in animals. This is primarily because, in humans, a smaller fraction of the gestational period is taken up by organogenesis (about $\frac{1}{15}$ of the total, compared with $\frac{1}{3}$ for mice). Nevertheless, the development of the CNS in humans takes place over a much longer gestational interval than in experimental animals, and therefore the CNS is more likely to be a target for radiation-induced damage. An important distinguishing characteristic of teratogenic effects in humans is the concomitant effects on the CNS and/or fetal growth. All cases of human in utero irradiation that have resulted in gross malformations have been accompanied by CNS abnormalities or growth retardation or both. The response of each organ to the induction of radiation-induced malformations is unique. Such factors as gestational age; radiation quantity, quality, and dose rate; oxygen tension; the cell type undergoing differentiation and its relationship to surrounding tissues; and other factors influence the outcome.

Fetal Growth Stage

The fetal growth stage in humans begins after the end of major organogenesis (Day 50) and continues until term. During this period the occurrence of radiation-induced prenatal death and congenital anomalies is, for the most part, negligible, unless the exposures are exceptionally high and in the therapeutic range. Anomalies of the nervous system and sense organs are the primary radiation-induced abnormalities observed during this period, which coincides with their relative growth and development. Much of the damage induced at the fetal growth stage may not be manifested until later in life as behavioral alterations or reduced intelligence (e.g., IQ). Figure 20-35 summarizes the relative sensitivity for radiation-induced in utero effects during different gestational periods.

20.9.2 Epidemiologic Investigations of Radiation Effects In Utero

Teratogenic Effects

Two groups that have been studied for teratogenic effects of in utero irradiation are the children of the A-bomb survivors and children whose mothers received medical irradiation (diagnostic and/or therapeutic) during pregnancy. The predominant effects that were observed included microcephaly and mental and growth retardation. Eye, genital, and skeletal abnormalities occurred less frequently. Excluding the mentally retarded, individuals exposed in utero[2] at Hiroshima and Nagasaki between the 8th and 25th week after conception demonstrated poorer IQ scores and school performance than did unexposed children. No such effect was seen in those exposed before the 8th week or after the 25th week. The decrease in IQ was dose dependent (~25 points/Gy), with an apparent threshold at approximately 100 mGy below which, if there was any effect, it was considered negligible (Otake and Schull, 1998). Dose-dependent adverse effects were also observed on intelligence and school performance, with the greatest sensitivity between the 8th and 15th weeks post conception(at the time of rapid neuronal production and migration), and a lesser effect between the 16th and 25th weeks when glial cell proliferation and synaptogenesis occur (BEIR V, 1990). The greatest sensitivity for radiation-induced mental retardation is seen between the 8th and 15th weeks, during which the risk for severe mental retardation (SMR) to the fetus is approximately 44% per Gy with a threshold for SMR of approximately 200 to 300 mGy (ICRP, 2003a).

Microcephaly was observed in children exposed in utero at the time of the atomic bomb detonations. For those exposed before the 16th week, the incidence of microcephaly was proportional to the dose, from about 100–200 mGy up to 1.5 Gy, above which the decreased occurrence was presumably due to the increase in fetal mortality (UNSCEAR, 1986). Similar effects have been reported after in utero exposure

---

[2]All the time periods pertaining to the children who were irradiated in utero at Hiroshima and Nagasaki are given in weeks postconception, as reported in the relevant references. To convert to weeks of gestation, add two weeks (e.g., 8th to 15th week postconception would be 10th to 17th week of gestation).

during medical irradiation of the mother. Twenty of twenty-eight children irradiated in utero as a result of pelvic radium or x-ray therapy were mentally retarded, among which sixteen were also microcephalic (Goldstein and Murphy, 1929). Other deformities, including abnormal appendages, hydrocephaly, spina bifida, blindness, cataracts, and microphthalmia have been observed in humans exposed in utero to high (radiotherapy) doses.

Although each exposure should be evaluated individually, the prevailing scientific opinion is that there are thresholds for most congenital abnormalities. Doses lower than 100 mGy to perhaps 200 mGy are generally thought to carry negligible risk compared with the reported occurrence of congenital anomalies (4% to 6%) in liveborn children. **Recommendation of therapeutic abortion for fetal doses less than 100 mGy, regardless of the gestational age, would not usually be justified** (NCRP, 2013). At one time, radiation was widely used to induce therapeutic abortion in cases where surgery was deemed inadvisable. The standard treatment was 3.5 to 5 Gy given over 2 days, which typically resulted in fetal death within 1 month. However, in diagnostic imaging, even several abdominal/pelvic CT scans or dozens of chest CT scans would not expose the fetus to doses in excess of 100 mGy. In fact, in most instances, fetal irradiation from diagnostic procedures rarely exceeds 50 mGy (see Appendix E-8), which has not been shown to place the fetus at any significantly increased risk for congenital malformation or growth retardation.

Carcinogenic Effects

According to the U.S. National Cancer Institute, a newborn male and female have 0.25% and 0.22% probability of developing cancer by age 15, respectively (*i.e.*, 1 in 400 males and 1 in 450 in females, respectively) (NIH, 2009). The majority of these cancers are leukemia and CNS neoplasms.

A correlation between childhood leukemia and solid tumors and *in utero* diagnostic radiation was reported by Stewart in 1956 in a retrospective study of childhood cancer in Great Britain (often referred to as the "Oxford Survey of Childhood Cancers" [OSCC]; Stewart et al., 1958). This observation was supported by several similar case-control studies of children born between the late 1940s and early 1980s reporting a RR of approximately 1.4 for childhood cancer based on interviewing mothers of children with and without cancer (Doll and Wakeford, 1997; UNSCEAR, 1996; Wakeford and Little, 2003). However, no childhood leukemias and only one childhood cancer were observed among survivors of the atomic bombs who were irradiated in utero. Absence of a positive finding in the A-bomb survivors could have been predicted on a statistical basis, owing to the relatively small sample size, but the much higher fetal dose compared with diagnostic radiography points to an inconsistency in the studies (1 childhood cancer observed versus 8.8 predicted based on fetal dose). These positive studies have been criticized based on a variety of factors, including the influence of the preexisting medical conditions for which the examinations were required, the lack of individual dosimetry and the possibility of recall bias in that mothers with children who died of cancer may have had more reliable memories of their prenatal exposures than mothers who did not have such a traumatic experience.

Doll and Wakeford reviewed the scientific evidence and concluded that irradiation of the fetus in utero (particularly in the last trimester) does increase the risk of childhood cancer; that the increase in risk is produced by doses on the order of 10 mGy; and that the excess risk is approximately 6% per Gy (Doll and Wakeford, 1997). If these estimates are correct, they represent a notable exception to the previously mentioned limit on the general sensitivity of radioepidemiological studies to detect cancer from acute exposures less than approximately 100-mGy. This may reflect the combined effect of a low background incidence of, and an increased fetal radiosensitivity to, childhood cancer.

However, the reported association with prenatal x-ray and childhood cancer is not uniformly accepted as causal (ICRP, 2003a). The argument against causality is that the Oxford survey reported the same risk (odds ratio) for each childhood malignancy, including leukemia, lymphoma, CNS, Wilms tumor, or neuroblastoma. Such commonality of risks has never been reported in any radiation study, even among atomic bomb survivors exposed in childhood. The biological implausibility of the case-control studies is indicated by the high risks seen for Wilms tumor and neuroblastoma, which are embryonic malignancies and not likely to be induced following pelvimetry examinations occurring shortly before birth. High dose exposures among children and newborns have not been correlated with increases in Wilms tumor or neuroblastoma. In addition, no cohort study has reported an increase in childhood leukemia following prenatal x-rays, even a large series of over 30,000 exposed mothers followed in the United Kingdom. This finding is further supported by animal studies that also failed to demonstrate an increased risk of leukemia following in utero exposures. Summarizing their view of the increased RR reported in the OSCC, the ICRP stated, "Although the arguments fall short of being definitive because of the combination of biological and statistical uncertainties involved, they raise a serious question of whether the great consistency in elevated RRs, including embryonal tumors and lymphomas, may be due to biases in the OSCC study rather than a causal association" (ICRP, 2003a). Thus the cancer risk associated with *in utero* exposure and the often-cited risk estimate of 6% per Gy for childhood cancer remain controversial.

This controversy notwithstanding, it is instructive to place the possibly increased risk of childhood cancer from medical x-rays into perspective by evaluating the magnitude of the potential risk from common diagnostic imaging procedures. Recall that the baseline risk of a male developing a malignancy through age 15 years is 1/400. If a two-view chest x-ray delivered 2 μGy to the conceptus (and employing the conservative assumption of a causal association between exposure and increased cancer risk at low dose of 6% per Gy), the probability of developing cancer during childhood from the exposure would be less than 1 in 8.3 million! Even a chest CT, which might deliver a dose to the conceptus that is on the order of 100 times greater than a chest x-ray (i.e., 200 μGy), still results in a small additional statistical risk of approximately 1/83,000 (0.0012%) of developing a childhood cancer. Using the 6%/Gy risk coefficient suggested by Doll, the doubling dose for childhood malignancies induced by radiation in utero would be on the order of 35 to 40 mGy. However, current estimates of the risk coefficient, based on further study of atomic bomb survivors, are on the order of 0.6%/Gy and may be lower than the risk following exposures in early childhood (Preston et al., 2008).

The lifetime risk of cancer is also believed to be elevated following radiation exposure in utero. ICRP considers the risk to be of the same order of magnitude as the estimated increased risk from radiation exposure during childhood compared to exposures as adults. The Commission's 2006 report states that it *"considers that it is prudent to assume that lifetime cancer risk following* in utero *exposure will be similar to that following irradiation in early childhood, i.e., at most, about three times that of the population as a whole"* (ICRP, 2006). However, the most recent data from the in utero exposed atomic bomb survivors indicate an increased risk of cancer later in life that is much lower than the incidence seen for survivors exposed under the age of 6 years (Preston et al., 2008). While there is little doubt about the relative increase in cancer risk (compared with adult populations) from childhood exposures of some organs and tissues early in life (*e.g.*, breast, thyroid), the magnitude of the increase and the applicability of these data for all radiogenic cancers (and for in utero exposures) remains open to debate. A summary of fetal effects from low-level radiation exposure is shown in Table 20-20.

U.S. regulatory agencies limit occupational radiation exposure of the fetus (for women who have chosen to declare their pregnancies in writing) to no more than 5 mSv during the gestational period, provided that the dose rate does not substantially exceed 0.5 mSv in any 1 month. If twice the maximally allowed dose were received, the statistical probability of developing cancer during childhood from the exposure would be approximately 1 in 1,600. Table 20-21 presents a comparison of the risks of radiation exposure with other risks encountered during pregnancy. It is clear from these data that, although unnecessary radiation exposure should be minimized, its risk at levels associated with occupational and diagnostic exposures is nominal when compared with other potential risk factors.

20.9.3 Risks from In Utero Exposure to Radionuclides

Radiopharmaceuticals may be administered to pregnant women if the diagnostic information to be obtained outweighs the risks associated with the radiation dose. The principal risk in this regard is the dose to the fetus. Radiopharmaceuticals can be divided into two broad categories: those that cross the placenta and those that remain on the maternal side of the circulation. Radiopharmaceuticals that do not cross the placenta irradiate the fetus by the emission of penetrating radiation (mainly γ-rays and x-rays). Early in the pregnancy, when the embryo is small and the radiopharmaceutical distribution is fairly uniform, the dose to the fetus can be approximated by the dose to the ovaries. Estimates of early-pregnancy fetal doses from commonly used radiopharmaceuticals are listed in Appendix F-4A. Radiopharmaceuticals that cross the placenta may be distributed in the body of the fetus or be concentrated locally if the fetal target organ is mature enough. A classic (and important) example of such a radiopharmaceutical is radioiodine.

Radioiodine rapidly crosses the placenta, and the fetal thyroid begins to concentrate radioiodine around the 11th to 12th-week postconception. The ability of the fetal thyroid to concentrate iodine remains relatively low until the 22nd week, after which it increases progressively and eventually exceeds that of the mother. The biologic effect on the fetal thyroid is activity dependent and can result in hypothyroidism or ablation if the dose administered to the mother is high enough. For I-131, estimates of dose to the fetal thyroid range from 230 to a maximum of 580 mGy/MBq (851 to 2,146 rad/mCi) for gestational ages between 3 and 5 months. Total body fetal dose ranges from 0.072 mGy/MBq (0.266 rad/mCi) early in pregnancy to a maximum of 0.27 mGy/MBq (1 rad/mCi) near term. Table 20-22 presents the fetal thyroid dose from various radioiodines and Tc-99m.

20.9.4 Summary

Radiation exposure of the embryo at the preimplantation stage usually leads to an all-or-nothing phenomenon (*i.e.*, either fetal death and resorption or normal fetal risk). During the period of organogenesis, the risk of fetal death decreases substantially, whereas the risk of congenital malformation coincides with the peak developmental periods of various organ systems. Exposures in excess of 1 Gy are associated with a high incidence of CNS abnormalities. During the fetal growth stage in utero, exposure poses little risk of congenital malformations; however, growth retardation,

TABLE 20-20 FETAL EFFECTS FROM LOW-LEVEL RADIATION EXPOSURE

EFFECT	MOST SENSITIVE PERIOD AFTER CONCEPTION Weeks (Days)	THRESHOLD DOSE AT WHICH AN EFFECT WAS OBSERVED (mGy)		ABSOLUTE INCIDENCE[a]	COMMENTS
		Animal Studies	Human Studies		
Prenatal death	0–1 (0–8)	Preimplantation 50–100 / Postimplantation 250	ND	ND	If the conceptus survives, it is thought to develop fully, with no radiation damage.
Growth retardation	1–8 (8–56)	10	200	ND	A-bomb survivors who received 200 mGy were 2–3 cm shorter and 3 kg lighter than controls and had, on average, head circumferences 1 cm smaller.
Organ malformation[b]	2–8 (14–56)	250	250	ND	Coincides with period of peak organ system development
Microcephaly (MC)	2–15 (14–105)	100	ND	5%–10%	MC can appear without SMR between 0–7 wk (see text)
Severe mental retardation (SMR)	8–15 (56–105)	ND	200–300	4%	At 8–15 wk 95% CI (2.2%–5.7%). No increase in absolute incidence was observed for exposure in the first 7 weeks or after the 25th wk.
	16–25 (112–175)	ND	600–900	0.9%	At 16–25 wk 95% CI (0%–1.8%)
Reduction of IQ	8–15 (56–105)	ND	100	2.5 IQ pts	Effects from a dose of 100 mGy or less were statistically unrecognizable. At 8–15 wk 2.5 pts 95% CI (1.8–3.3). At 16–25 wk 2.1 pts 95% CI (1.2–3.1).
Childhood cancer	2–term (14–term)	No threshold observed	No threshold observed	0.06–0.6[c]	Leukemia is the most common type of childhood cancer. Magnitude of the risk is controversial.

[a]Absolute incidence is defined as the percentage of exposed fetuses in which an effect is expected to be observed with an equivalent dose of 100 mGy.

[b]Organ malformation is defined as malformation of an organ outside the CNS. Data regarding the most sensitive period after conception are from animal studies.

[c]The baseline risk of childhood cancer up to age 15 for unexposed fetuses is approximately 0.25% (1 in 400).

IQ, intelligence quotient; ND, no data or inadequate data; CI, confidence interval; wk, weeks; d, days.

Source: Adapted and modified from McCollough CH, Schueler BA, Atwell TD, et al. Radiation exposure and pregnancy: when should we be concerned? *Radiographics.* 2007;27:909–917; International Commission on Radiological Protection. Biological effects after prenatal irradiation (embryo and fetus). ICRP Publication 90. *Ann ICRP.* 2003a;33(1/2):1–201.

TABLE 20-21 EFFECT OF RISK FACTORS ON PREGNANCY-OUTCOME

EFFECT	APPROXIMATE NUMBER OCCURRING FROM NATURAL CAUSES	RISK FACTOR	ESTIMATED EXCESS OCCURRENCES FROM RISK FACTORS
Radiation Risks			
Childhood Cancer			
Cancer incidence in children (0–15)	~3/1,000	Radiation dose of 10 mGy received before birth	0.06/1,000 to 0.6/1,000
Abnormalities		Radiation dose of 10 mGy received during specific periods after conception:	
Small head size	40/1,000	4–7 wk	5/1,000
Small head size	40/1,000	8–11 wk	9/1,000
Mental retardation	4/1,000	8–15 wk	BT
Non-radiation Risks			
Occupation			
Stillbirth or spontaneous abortion	200/1,000	Work in high-risk occupations	90/1,000
Alcohol Consumption			
Fetal alcohol syndrome	1–2/1,000[a]	2–4 drinks/d	100/1,000
Fetal alcohol syndrome	1–2/1,000[a]	More than 4 drinks/d	200/1,000
Fetal alcohol syndrome	1–2/1,000[a]	Chronic alcoholic (>10 drinks/d)	350/1,000
Perinatal infant death	23/1,000	Chronic alcoholic (>10 drinks/d)	170/1,000
Smoking			
Perinatal infant death	23/1,000	<1 pack/d	5/1,000
Perinatal infant death	23/1,000	≥1 pack/d	10/1,000

[a]There is a naturally occurring syndrome that has the same symptoms as a fetal alcohol syndrome that occurs in children born to mothers who have not consumed alcohol.
BT, below threshold for established effects.
Source: Adapted from U.S. Nuclear Regulatory Commission. *Instruction Concerning Prenatal Radiation Exposure.* Regulatory Guide 8.13, Rev. 2.

abnormalities of the nervous system, and the risk of childhood cancer can be increased depending on the fetal dose. Growth retardation after *in utero* fetal doses in excess of 200 mGy has been demonstrated. Fetal doses from most diagnostic x-ray and nuclear medicine examinations are typically much lower than 50 mGy (see Appendices E-8 and F-4A) and have not been demonstrated to produce any significant impact on fetal growth and development. A number of epidemiologic studies have evaluated the association between in utero radiation exposure and child-hood neoplasms. Although these studies show conflicting results and remain open to varying interpretations, a reasonable estimate of the excess risk of childhood can-cer from in utero irradiation is approximately 0.6% to 6% per Gy. Figure 20-41 and Table 20-20 summarize the relative incidence of radiation-induced health effects at various stages in fetal development.

TABLE 20-22 ABSORBED DOSE mGy/MBq (rad/mCi) IN FETAL THYROID FROM RADIONUCLIDES GIVEN ORALLY TO MOTHER

FETAL AGE (Mo)	IODINE-123	IODINE-125	IODINE-131	TECHNETIUM-99^m
3	2.7 (10)	290 (1,073)	230 (851)	0.032 (0.12)
4	2.6 (10)	240 (888)	260 (962)	
5	6.4 (24)	280 (1,036)	580 (2,146)	
6	6.4 (24)	210 (777)	550 (2,035)	0.15 (0.54)
7	4.1 (15)	160 (592)	390 (1,443)	
8	4.0 (15)	150 (555)	350 (1,295)	
9	2.9 (11)	120 (444)	270 (1,000)	0.38 (1.40)

Source: Watson EE. Radiation absorbed dose to the human fetal thyroid. In: Watson EE, Schlaske-Stelson A, eds. *5th International Radiopharmaceutical Dosimetry Symposium.* Oak Ridge, TN. May 7–10, 1991. Oak Ridge, TN: Oak Ridge Associated Universities; 1992.

While there has been a justifiable concern both in public opinion and among health care providers regarding the potential for overutilization of x-rays in medical imaging, the concern regarding radiation exposure during pregnancy is often disproportionate to the actual risks involved. In one study evaluating perceptions of teratogenic risk with the use of medical x-rays, approximately 6% of primary care physicians and gynecologists suggested that therapeutic abortion would be appropriate for women having undergone an abdominal CT scan (Ratnapalan, 2004). Pregnant patients have also been shown to greatly overestimate the radiation-related risk to the fetus (Cohen-Kerem et al., 2006). The risk of *in utero* radiation exposure can be placed in perspective by considering the probability of birthing a healthy child after a given dose to the conceptus (Table 20-23).

Clearly, even a conceptus dose of 100 mGy does not significantly affect the risks associated with pregnancy. Fetal doses from diagnostic examinations rarely, if ever, justify therapeutic abortion; however, some patients may receive one or more high-dose interventional exams or radiation therapy where the fetal doses are significant. Each case should be evaluated individually, and the risks should be explained to the patient. Many professional organizations including the NCRP, ICRP, the American College of Radiology (ACR), and the American College of Obstetricians and Gynecologists (ACOG) have issued policy statements regarding the use of therapeutic abortion and the relatively low risk of diagnostic imaging procedures resulting in radiation exposure of the fetus. The ACR policy states, "*The interruption of pregnancy is rarely justified because of radiation risk to the embryo or fetus from a radiologic examination*" (ACR, 2005). The ACOG policy, which was revised in 2004, states, "*Women should be counseled that x-ray exposure from a single diagnostic procedure does not result in harmful fetal effects. Specifically, exposure to less than 5 rad [50 mGy] has not been associated with an increase in fetal anomalies or pregnancy loss*" (ACOG, 2004).

Every effort should be made to optimize radiation exposure of the patient and to reduce or avoid fetal exposure whenever possible. However, considering the relatively small risk associated with diagnostic examinations, postponing clinically necessary examinations or scheduling examinations around the patient's menstrual cycle to avoid irradiating a potential conceptus are unwarranted measures. Nevertheless, every fertile female patient should be asked whether she might be pregnant before diagnostic examinations or therapeutic procedures using ionizing radiation are performed. If the patient is pregnant and alternative diagnostic or therapeutic procedures are inappropriate, the risks and benefits of the procedure should be discussed with the patient.

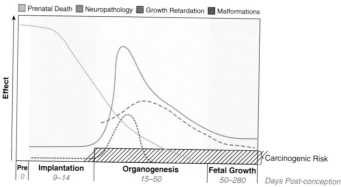

■ **FIGURE 20-41** Relative sensitivity for radiation-induced effects during different stages of fetal development. (Data from Mettler FA, Upton AC. *Medical effects of ionizing radiation*. 3rd ed. Philadelphia, PA: Saunders, Co., 2008.)

20.10 RADIATION RISK COMMUNICATIONS

Radiation risk communication is a key component of good practice in medical imaging. Much of the following discussion is based on concepts presented in an excellent document mentioned previously on communicating radiation risks to pediatric patients developed by an expert group assembled by the WHO (WHO, 2016) and in NCRP Report No. 185 (NCRP, 2020).

A major goal of radiation risk communication in medicine is to ensure that patients and their families and/or caregivers receive information about radiation exposures from a procedure in a way that they can understand readily (Dauer et al., 2011; McCollough et al., 2015). They need sufficient and straightforward information to

TABLE 20-23 PROBABILITY OF BIRTHING HEALTHY CHILDREN

DOSE TO CONCEPTUS mGy[a]	CHILD WITH NO MENTAL RETARDATION (%)	CHILD WITH NO BIRTH DEFECT (%)	CHILD WILL NOT DEVELOP CANCER (%)[b,c]	CHILD WILL NOT DEVELOP CANCER OR HAVE MENTAL RETARDATION OR BIRTH DEFECT (%)[c]
0	99.6	96	99.77	95.40
1.0	99.6	96	99.76	95.39
2.5	99.6	96	99.75	95.38
5	99.6	96	99.74	95.37
10	99.6	96	99.71	95.34
100	99.6	96	99.17	94.82

[a]Refers to equivalent dose above natural background. Dose assumed to be delivered during the most sensitive period of gestation (mental retardation: 8–15 weeks post-conception; malformation: 2–7 weeks post-conception).
[b]Assumes conservative risk estimates, and it is possible that there is no added radiation-induced cancer risk. Childhood (0–15 years) cancer risk from fetal irradiation of 6%/Gy. *Source*: Doll R, Wakeford R. Risk of childhood cancer from fetal irradiation *Br J Radiol*. 1997;70:130-139; Wakeford R, Little MP. Risk coefficients for childhood cancer after intrauterine irradiation: a review. *Int J Radiat Biol*. 2003;79:293-309; International Commission on Radiological Protection. Pregnancy and medical radiation. ICRP Publication 84. *Ann ICRP*. 2000;30(1):iii-viii, 1-43.
[c]Precision displayed is only for the purpose of showing the magnitude of the potential change in risk as a function of dose and should not be interpreted as a measure of precision with which these outcomes can be predicted.
Source: Adapted and modified from Wagner LK, Hayman LA. Pregnancy in women radiologists. *Radiology*. 1982;145:559-562; International Commission on Radiological Protection. Pregnancy and medical radiation. ICRP Publication 84. *Ann ICRP*. 2000;30(1):iii-viii, 1-43.

understand the imaging being performed, why it is necessary, and the benefits and risks involved. The risks inherent in the disease and/or patient's clinical condition also have to be considered when discussing the need to perform an imaging procedure.

Outside the radiation fields in medicine, the level of awareness on the part of other health professionals about radiation doses and associated risks in medical imaging can be low. However, referring medical practitioners should have sufficient background, education, and resources to understand and then communicate clearly and effectively about the benefits and risks of imaging procedures with their patients when making a referral for a radiation procedure. Radiologists play an important role in providing that information. Also, it is important for referrers and other health professionals to identify the communication needs and preferred communication styles of their patients, the families, and caregivers. Each patient and family may be different—their specific cultural background, as well as their personal health history may require individually adapted risk communication (Guillerman, 2014), and the radiologist may need to work with the referring practitioner to provide information appropriate to the situation. Effective and balanced communication of radiation risks requires sufficient knowledge to support the benefit-risk dialogue. For example, it is important to communicate that risks can be controlled and benefits maximized by selecting an appropriate procedure and using methods to reduce patient exposure without reducing clinical effectiveness.

There are many challenges in expressing radiation risk to patients and their families. Estimation of risk from ionizing radiation is technically complex, and presenting quantitative or qualitative information about possible radiation effects in a comprehensible manner can be difficult. Patients may have read reports in the popular press about the health effects of medical radiation exposure, but many have little understanding of the scientific concepts involved in radiation exposure. Depending on the bias inherent in either the exaggerated reporting or the underreporting about scientific research by the media, patients may have formed opinions about the benefits and potential harm of medical radiation before coming to their physicians. Even when presented with factual information in simple language, patients' decisions may be influenced by their individual perception of the risk and their overall level of tolerance of risks.

Messages that may convey useful information to a patient include the following:

- low-level background radiation is part of the Earth's natural environment;
- the degree of risk associated with exposure to low-level ionizing radiation is thought to be very low;
- scientists disagree about the precise magnitude of this risk; and
- any risk from radiation must be balanced against the benefits provided by the activity producing the radiation (Slovic et al., 1981).

It is generally recommended that risk be communicated as AR, as opposed to RR (Fagerlin et al., 2011; Politi et al., 2007). For example, if a baseline disease incidence is 6%, and the intervention (e.g., treatment) reduces disease incidence to 3%, the AR of the disease is reduced from 6% to 3%; however, the RR of the disease is reduced by 50%. Emphasizing the RR could misrepresent the benefit of the intervention (e.g., treatment) to the patient. There is debate over whether statistical information is better understood when presented as percentages or frequencies. People with low numeracy skills often are more comfortable with frequencies (e.g., "1 out of 10" as opposed to "10 %") (Fagerlin et al., 2011). Graphic material, especially pictographs, can be of substantial assistance when presenting risk information (Fagerlin et al., 2011;

Fahey et al., 2011), and summary tables can help in explaining protocols with numerous risks and benefits (Fagerlin et al., 2011).

Although the inclusion of quantitative dose information is reasonable, it can be more helpful to express radiation dose and risk in ways that put the information in perspective and enable patients to make a judgment about whether or not the radiation risk is acceptable to them (Reiman, 2013). Informing the patient that there is no conclusive evidence for an increased risk of cancer with low doses of radiation (*i.e.*, <100 mGy) can assist in providing perspective. Dose benchmarks, reference doses from common or everyday experiences associated with radiation exposure, for which typical E are known, may be used as analogies in explaining the radiation dose expected from a procedure. For example, the E passengers receive during a one-way, non-stop airplane flight from New York City to Los Angeles (~0.025 mSv) might be used as a benchmark (EPA, 2018; FAA, 2019). Thus, when explaining the dose from a posteroanterior chest radiograph (~0.02 mSv) (FDA, 2016; HPS, 2000) one might say that the radiation dose incurred would be equivalent to that received during a one-way flight from New York City to Los Angeles. Other analogies might be average background radiation in the United States (~3 mSv/y) or radiation from the number of days spent at high altitude [*e.g.*, Denver (11.8 mSv/y)] (ISIS, 2019; NCRP, 1987).

The "background equivalent radiation time" has been proposed as a radiation dose unit that members of the public might understand better than millirem or millisievert (Cameron, 1991). Normalizing the radiation dose from a radiological study to the average annual E received from natural background sources in the United States at sea level (3 mSv), and multiplying by 1 y, results in a unit of time that may be converted into days, weeks, months, or years, whichever is most convenient. Conversion to background equivalent time is the method of benchmark comparison used in the sections on radiogenic risks in the NCI informed consent template (NCI, 2013). Using background radiation (or background equivalent time) is informative. However, like the airplane example above, this analogy alone is insufficient to justify the acceptability of dose without further explanation. Otherwise, merely equating the proposed radiation exposure in a protocol with the natural (*i.e.*, background radiation) involves accepting the premise that "if it is natural, it must be good" without further support of that premise. An additional potentially misleading feature of comparing patient radiation doses to equivalent natural background exposures is that background radiation involves whole-body exposure whereas diagnostic radiation exposures more often involve localized exposures.

Another approach is to use one radiation study as a dose benchmark for another radiation study, but this approach requires caution. Consider the example of comparing CT procedures with standard radiographs. Although the statement that "A CT scan of the abdomen gives the same radiation dose as 250 chest x rays" may be quantitatively correct, it depends on the patient's perception of the dose and risk of a chest x-ray. If patients do not have a basis for making a judgment about the risk of chest x-rays, they may come to incorrect conclusions about the risk of CT scans (Reiman, 2013).

Many radiologists may be involved in developing research protocols in human subjects that include exposure to ionizing radiation or in reviewing such protocols as members of Institutional Review Boards (IRBs). Much of the information just discussed regarding risk communications applies to discussions of radiation with potential research subjects and writing of informed consent documents. Several recent publications provide more detailed discussions of radiation risk communications with patients, their families, and caregivers; with other non-radiation specialists; and with research subjects and IRBs, as well as examples of language and effective communication approaches (NCRP, 2020; WHO, 2016).

SUGGESTED READING AND REFERENCES

ACOG Committee on Obstetric Practice. Guidelines for diagnostic imaging during pregnancy. ACOG Committee opinion no. 299, September 2004 (replaces no. 158, September 1995). *Obstet Gynecol.* 2004;104:647-651.

Ainsbury EA, et al. Radiation cataractogenesis: a review of recent studies. *Radiat Res.* 2009;172:1-9.

Alliance for Radiation Safety in Pediatric Imaging. Image gently. http://www.pedrad.org/associations/5364/ig/. Accessed August 1, 2011.

American Cancer Society. *Breast Cancer Facts & Figures 2019-2020.* Atlanta: American Cancer Society, Inc.; 2019.

American Cancer Society. *Lifetime Risk of Developing or Dying From Cancer.* Atlanta, GA: American Cancer Society; 2020. https://www.cancer.org/cancer/cancer-basics/lifetime-probability-of-developing-or-dying-from-cancer.html

American College of Radiology. *ACoR 04–05 Bylaws.* Reston, VA: American College of Radiology; 2005.

American College of Radiology. The Image Gently Alliance. 2020. https://www.imagegently.org/

Amundson S, et al. Low-dose radiation risk assessment. Report of an International Workshop on Low Dose Radiation Effects held at Columbia University Medical Center, New York, April 3–4, 2006. *Radiat Res.* 2006;166:561-565.

Angel E, Yaghmai N, Jude CM, et al. Monte Carlo simulations to assess the effects of tube current modulation on breast dose for multidetector CT. *Phys Med Biol.* 2009;54:497-512.

ASRT. *X-ray Risk.* Albuquerque, NM: American Society of Radiologic Technologists; 2018. http://www.xray-risk.com/index.php

Balter S, Hopewell JW, Miller DL, et al. Fluoroscopically guided interventional procedures: a review of radiation effects on patients' skin and hair. *Radiology.* 2010;254(2):326-341.

Barcellos-Hoff MH, Brooks AL. Extracellular signaling through the microenvironment: a hypothesis relating carcinogenesis, bystander effects, and genomic instability. *Radiat Res.* 2001;156(5 Pt 2):618-627.

BEIR V National Research Council. *Health Effects of Exposure to Low Levels of Ionizing Radiation:* Washington, DC: The National Academies Press; 1990. https://doi.org/10.17226/1224

BEIR VII National Research Council. *Health Risks from Exposure to Low Levels of Ionizing Radiation: BEIR VII, Phase 2 Committee to Assess Health Risks from Exposure to Low Levels of Ionizing Radiation.* Washington, DC: Board of Radiation Effects, Research Division on Earth and Life Studies, National Academy of Sciences; 2006.

Bernstein JL, Thomas DC, Shore RE, et al. Radiation-induced second primary breast cancer and BRCA1 and BRCA2 mutation carrier status: a report from the WECARE Study. *Eur J Cancer.* 2013;49(14):2979-2985.

Boice JD Jr. Ionizing radiation. In: Schottenfeld D, Fraumeni JF Jr, eds. *Cancer Epidemiology and Prevention.* 3rd ed. New York, NY: Oxford University Press; 2006.

Boice JD Jr. Lauriston S. Taylor lecture: Radiation epidemiology: the golden age and future challenges. *Health Phys.* 2011;100:59-76.

Boice JD Jr, Miller RW. Childhood and adult cancer after intrauterine exposure to ionizing radiation. *Teratology.* 1999;59(4):227-233.

Boice JD, Ellis ED, Golden AP, Zablotska LB, Mumma MT, Cohen SS. Sex-specific lung cancer risk among radiation workers in the million-person study and patients TB-fluoroscopy. *Int J Radiat Biol.* 2019. doi: 10.1080/09553002.2018.1547441.

Boice JD Jr, Hendry JH, Nakamura N, et al. Low-dose-rate epidemiology of high background radiation areas. *Radiat Res.* 2010;173:849-854.

Bosch de Basea M, Pearce MS, Kesminiene A, et al. EPI-CT: design, challenges and epidemiologic methods of an international study on cancer risk after paediatric and young adult CT. *J Radiol Prot.* 2015;35(3):611-628.

Brenner DJ, Hall EJ. Computed tomography—an increasing source of radiation exposure. *N Engl J Med.* 2007;357:2277-2284.

Brenner DJ, Ward JF. Constraints on energy deposition and target size of multiply-damaged sites associated with DNA double-strand breaks. *Int J Radiat Biol.* 1992;61:737.

Brenner DJ, Doll R, Goodhead DT, et al. Cancer risks attributable to low doses of ionizing radiation: assessing what we really know. *Proc Natl Acad Sci USA.* 2003;100:13761-13766.

Brenner D, Elliston C, Hall E, et al. Estimated risks of radiation-induced fatal cancer from pediatric CT. *AJR Am J Roentgenol.* 2001;176(2):289-296.

Brent RL. Saving lives and changing family histories: appropriate counseling of pregnant women and men and women of reproductive age, concerning the risk of diagnostic radiation exposures during and before pregnancy. *Am J Obstetr Gynecol.* 2009;200(1):4-24.

Brent RL, Gorson RO. Radiation exposure in pregnancy. *Curr Probl Radiol.* 1972;2:1.

Brody AS, Frush DP, Huda W, et al.; American Academy of Pediatrics Section on Radiology. Radiation risk to children from computed tomography. *Pediatrics.* 2007;120(3):677-682.

Cahoon EK, Preston DL, Pierce DA, et al. Lung, laryngeal and other respiratory cancer incidence among Japanese atomic bomb survivors: an updated analysis from 1958 through 2009. *Radiat Res.* 2017;187:538-548.

Cameron JR. A radiation unit for the public. *Phys Soc.* 1991;20(2):2.

Centers for Disease Control and Prevention; United States Cancer Statistics (USCS). 2020. https://www.cdc.gov/cancer/uscs/index.htm

Chambers C, Fetterly K, Holzer R, et al. Radiation safety program for the cardiac catheterization laboratory. *Catheter Cardiovasc Interv.* 2011;77:546-556.

Chowdhury D, Choi YE, Brault ME. Charity begins at home: non-coding RNA functions in DNA repair. *Nat Rev Mol Cell Biol.* 2013;14(3):181-189.

Clifton DK, Bremner WJ. The effect of testicular x-irradiation on 6872 spermatogenesis in man. A comparison with the mouse. *J Androl.* 1983;4:387-392.

Cohen-Kerem R, Nulman I, Abramow-Newerly M, et al. Diagnostic radiation in pregnancy: perception versus true risks. *J Obstet Gynaecol Can.* 2006;28:43-48.

Correa CN, Wu X-C, Andrews P, et al., eds. *Cancer Incidence in Five Continents.* Vol. VIII. Lyon, France: IARC Scientific Publications No. 155; 2002.

Court Brown WM, Doll R, Hill RB. Incidence of leukaemia after exposure to diagnostic radiation in utero. *Br Med J.* 1960;2(5212):1539-1545.

Cremonesi M, Ferrari M, Paganelli G, et al. Radiation protection in radionuclide therapies with 90Y-conjugates: risks and safety. *Eur J Nucl Med Mol Imaging.* 2006;33:1321-1327. https://doi.org/10.1007/s00259-006-0151-1

Dauer LT, Brooks AL, Hoel DG, et al. Review and evaluation of updated research on the health effects associated with low-dose ionising radiation. *Radiat Prot Dosimetry.* 2010;140(2):103-136.

Dauer LT, Chu BP, Zanzonico PB, eds. *Dose, Benefit, and Risk in Medical Imaging.* New York, NY: CRC Press; 2019.

Dauer LT, Thornton RH, Hay JL, Balter R, Williamson MJ, St Germain J. Fears, feelings and facts: interactively communicating benefits and risks of medical radiation with patients. *Am J Roent.* 2011;196(4):756-761.

Davis FG, Boice JD Jr, Hrubec Z, Monson RR. Cancer mortality in a radiation-exposed cohort of Massachusetts tuberculosis patients. *Cancer Res.* 1989;49:6130-6136.

De Santis M, Di Gianantonio E, Straface G, et al. Ionizing radiations in pregnancy and teratogenesis. A review of the literature. *Reprod Toxicol.* 2005;20:323-329.

Dekaban AS. Abnormalities in children exposed to x-irradiation during various stages of gestation: tentative time table of radiation injury to human fetus. *J Nucl Med.* 1968;9:471-477.

Doll R, Wakeford E. Risk of childhood cancer from fetal irradiation. *Br J Radiol.* 1997;70:130-139.

Double EB, Mabuchi K, Cullings HM, et al. Long-term radiation-related health effects in a unique human population: lessons learned from the atomic bomb survivors of Hiroshima and Nagasaki. *Disaster Med Public Health Prep.* 2011;5(suppl 1):S122-S133.

Duke. *IRB Protocol Radiation Risk Statements.* Durham, NC: Duke University Medical Center; 2019. https://vmw-oesoapps.duhs.duke.edu/radsafety/consents/irbcf_asp/default.asp

FAA. *Galactic Radiation Received in Flight.* Washington, DC: Federal Aviation Administration; 2019. http://jag.cami.jccbi.gov/cariprofile.asp

Fagerlin A, Zikmund-Fisher BJ, Ubel PA. Helping patients decide: ten steps to better risk communication. *J Natl Cancer Inst.* 2011;103(19):1436-1443.

Fahey FH, Treves ST, Adelstein SJ. Minimizing and communicating radiation risk in pediatric nuclear medicine. *J Nucl Med.* 2011;52:1240-1251.

Fazel R, Krumholz HM, Wang Y, et al. Exposure to low-dose ionizing radiation from medical imaging procedures. *N Engl J Med.* 2009;361(9):849-857.

Frieben H. Demonstration eines Cancroid des rechten Handruckens, das sich nach langdauernder Einwirkung von Rontgenstrahlen entwickelt hatte. *Fortschr Rontgenstr.* 1902;6:106-111.

Fry RJ. Effects of low doses of radiation. *Health Phys.* 1996;70:823-827.

Fry RJM, Boice JD Jr. Radiation carcinogenesis. In: Souhami RL, Tannock I, Hohenberger P, Horiot JC, eds. *Oxford Textbook of Oncology.* 2nd ed. New York, NY: Oxford Press; 2002:167-184.

Gabriel C. Risk of cataract after exposure to low doses of ionizing radiation: a 20-year prospective cohort study among US radiologic technologists. *Am J Epidemiol.* 2008;168(6):620-631.

Goldstein L, Murphy DP. Etiology of ill-health in children born after postconceptional maternal irradiation. *Am J Roentgenol.* 1929;22:322-331.

Goodhead DT. Spatial and temporal distribution of energy. *Health Phys.* 1988;55:231-240.

Goodhead DT. Initial events in the cellular effects of ionizing radiations: clustered damage in DNA. *Int J Radiat Biol.* 1994;65:7-17.

Graham SJ, et al. Whole-body pathologic analysis of a patient with thorotrast-in-induced myelodysplasia. *Health Phys.* 1992;63(1): 20-26.

Granel F, Barbaud A, Gillet-Terver MN, et al. Chronic radiodermatitis after interventional cardiac catheterization: four cases [in French]. *Ann Dermatol Venereol.* 1998;125:405-407.

Guillerman RP. From "Image Gently" to image intelligently: a personalized perspective on diagnostic radiation risk. *Pediatr Radiol.* 2014;44(3):S444-S449.

Hall EJ, Giaccia AJ. *Radiobiology for the Radiologist.* 8th ed. Philadelphia, PA: Lippincott Williams & Wilkins; 2018.

Hall EJ, Metting N, Puskin J, et al. Low dose radiation epidemiology: what can it tell us? *Radiat Res.* 2009;172:134-138.

Hanahan D, Weinberg RA. The hallmarks of cancer. *Cell.* 2000;100:57-70.

Hanahan D, Weinberg RA. Hallmarks of cancer: the next generation. *Cell.* 2011;144:646-674.

Harrison JD, Balnov M, Martin CJ, et al. Use of effective dose. *Ann ICRP.* 2016;45(1 suppl):215-224.

Health Physics Society (HPS). *Doses from Medical X-Ray Procedures.* McLean, VA: Health Physics Society; 2000. https://hps.org/physicians/documents/Doses_from_Medical_X-Ray_Procedures.pdf

Henley SJ, Thomas CC, Lewis DR, et al. Annual report to the Nation on the Status of Cancer, part II: progress toward Healthy People 2020 objectives for 4 common cancers. *Cancer* 2020. https://acsjournals.onlinelibrary.wiley.com/doi/epdf/10.1002/cncr.32802

Henry FA, et al. Fluoroscopy-induced chronic radiation dermatitis: a report of three cases. *Dermatol Online J.* 2009;15(1):1-6.

Hollowell JG Jr, Littlefield LG. Chromosome damage induced by plasma of x-rayed patients: an indirect effect of x-ray. *Proc Soc Exp Biol Med.* 1968;129:240-244.

Hotchkiss RS, Strasser A, McDunn JE, Swanson PE. Cell death. *N Engl J Med.* 2009;361(16):1570-1583.

Howe GR. Lung cancer mortality between 1950 and 1987 after exposure to fractionated moderate-dose-rate ionizing radiation in the Canadian Fluoroscopy Cohort Study and a comparison with lung cancer mortality in the Atomic Bomb survivors study. *Radiat Res.* 1995;142:295-304.

Howlader N, Noone AM, Krapcho M, et al., eds. *SEER Cancer Statistics Review, 1975–2008.* Bethesda, MD: National Cancer Institute; 2011. http://seer.cancer.gov/csr/1975_2008/. Based on November 2010 SEER data submission, posted to the SEER web site.

International Agency for Research on Cancer. *IARC Monographs on the Evaluation of Carcinogenic Risks to Humans.* Vol. 75: Ionizing Radiation, Part 1: X- and Gamma (γ)—Radiation, and Neutrons. Lyon, France: IARC; 2000.

International Atomic Energy Agency. *Cytogenetic Dosimetry: Applications in Preparedness for and Response to Radiation Emergencies.* Vienna: International Atomic Energy Agency; 2011.

International Commission on Radiological Protection. 1990 Recommendations of the International Commission on Radiological Protection. ICRP Publication 60. *Ann ICRP.* 1991;21(1-3):1-201.

International Commission on Radiological Protection. Genetic susceptibility to cancer. ICRP publications 79. *Ann ICRP.* 1998;28(1-2):1-157.

International Commission on Radiological Protection. Pregnancy and medical radiation. ICRP Publication 84. *Ann ICRP.* 2000;30(1):iii-viii, 1-43.

International Commission on Radiological Protection. Biological effects after prenatal irradiation (embryo and fetus). ICRP Publication 90. *Ann ICRP.* 2003a;33(1/2):1-201.

International Commission on Radiological Protection. Relative biological effectiveness (RBE), quality factor (Q), and radiation weighting factor (wR). ICRP Publication 92. *Ann ICRP.* 2003b;33(4);1-117.

International Commission on Radiological Protection. Low-dose extrapolation of radiation-related cancer risk. ICRP Publication 99. *Ann ICRP.* 2006;35:1-140.

International Commission on Radiological Protection. The 2007 recommendations of the International Commission on Radiological Protection. ICRP Publication 103. *Ann ICRP.* 2007a;37:1-332.

International Commission on Radiological Protection. Radiological protection in medicine. ICRP Publication 105. *Ann ICRP.* 2007b;37(6):1-63.

International Commission on Radiological Protection. ICRP reference 4825-3093-1464. Statement on Tissue Reactions Approved by the Commission on April 21, 2011. 2011.

International Commission on Radiological Protection. ICRP statement on tissue reactions/early and late effects of radiation in normal tissues and organs—threshold doses for tissue reactions in a radiation protection context. ICRP Publication 118. *Ann ICRP.* 2012;41(1/2):1-322.

ISIS. *Table 7: Background Radiation in Denver: Average Annual Dose Equivalent of Ionizing Radiation and Risk.* Washington, DC: Institute for Science and International Security; 2019. http://isis-online.org/risk/tab7

Jacobsen L. *Low-Dose X-irradiation and Teratogenesis.* Copenhagen: Munksgaard; 1968.

Johnson KJ, Alexander BH, Doody MM, et al. Childhood cancer in the offspring born in 1921–1984 to US radiologic technologists. *Br J Cancer.* 2008;99:545-550.

Joiner M, van der Kogel A. *Basic Clinical Radiobiology.* 4th ed. London: Hodder Arnold; 2009.

Journy N, Rehel J-L, LePointe HD, et al. Are the studies on cancer risk from CT scans biased by indication? Elements of answer from a large-scale cohort study in France. *Br J Cancer.* 2015;112:185-193.

Khandia R, et al. Comprehensive review of autophagy and its various roles in infectious, non-infectious, and lifestyle diseases: current knowledge and prospects for disease prevention, novel drug design, and therapy. *Cells.* 2019;8:674.

Kocher DC, Apostoaei AI, Hoffman FO, Trabalka JR. Probability distribution of dose and dose-rate effectiveness factor for use in estimating risks of solid cancers from exposure to low-let radiation. *Health Phys.* 2018;114(6):602-622.

Koenig TR, Wolff D, Mettler FA, Wagner LK. Skin injuries from fluoroscopically guided procedures: part 1, characteristics of radiation injury. *AJR Am J Roentgenol.* 2001;177(1):3-11.

Krille L, Dreger S, Schindel R, et al. Risk of cancer incidence before the age of 15 years after exposure to ionising radiation from computed tomography: results from a German cohort study. *Radiat Environ Biophys.* 2015;54:1-12.

Kuppermann N, Holmes JF, Dayan PS, et al.; Pediatric Emergency Care Applied Research Network (PECARN). Identification of children at very low risk of clinically-important brain injuries after head trauma: a prospective cohort study. *Lancet.* 2009;374(9696):1160-1170.

Levine A, Oren M. The first 30 years of p53: growing ever more complex. *Nat Rev Cancer.* 2009;9:749-758.

Little JB. Genomic instability and bystander effects: a historical perspective. *Oncogene.* 2003;22:6978-6987.

Löbrich M, Cooper PK, Rydberg B. Non-random distribution of DNA double-strand breaks induced by particle irradiation. *Int J Radiat Biol.* 1996;70:493.

Lord CJ, Ashworth A. The DNA damage response and cancer therapy. *Nature.* 2012;481(7381):287-294.

Lushbaugh CC, Ricks RC. Some cytokinetic and histopathologic considerations of irradiated male and female gonadal tissues. *Front Radiat Ther Oncol.* 1972;6:228-248.

MacVittie TJ, Farese AM. Chapter 14: Evidenced-based support for the treatment of a potentially lethal hematopoietic acute radiation subsyndrome. In: Christensen DM, Sugarman SL, O'Hara FM Jr, eds. *The Medical Basis for Radiation-Accident Preparedness: Medical Management Proceedings of the Fifth International REAC/TS Symposium on the Medical Basis for Radiation-Accident Preparedness and the Biodosimetry Workshop,* September 2011, Miami, FL. ISBN 978-0-9890502-0-3. 2013.

Martin CJ. The application of effective dose to medical exposures. *Radiat Prot Dosim.* 2008;128(1):1-4.

Mathews JD, Forsythe AV, Brady Z, et al. Cancer risk in 680000 people exposed to computed tomography scans in childhood or adolescence: data linkage study of 11 million Australians. *Br Med J.* 2013;346:f2360.

McCollough CH, Bushberg JT, Fletcher JG, Eckel LJ. Answers to common questions about the use and safety of CT scans. *Mayo Clin Proc.* 2015;90(10):1380-1392.

McCollough CH, Schueler BA, Atwell TD, et al. Radiation exposure and pregnancy: when should we be concerned? *Radiographics.* 2007;27:909-917.

Mettler FA, Upton AC. *Medical Effects of Ionizing Radiation.* 3rd ed. Philadelphia, PA: W.B. Saunders Co.; 2008.

Muller HJ. Artificial transmutation of the gene. *Science.* 1927;66:84-87.

Nair RR, Rajan B, Akiba S, et al. Background radiation and cancer incidence in Kerala, India-Karanagappally cohort study. *Health Phys.* 2009;96:55-66.

National Cancer Institute (NCI). *PDQ® Cancer Information Summary. Genetics of Breast and Ovarian Cancer (PDQ®)—Health Professional.* Bethesda, MD; 2011. Date last modified June 23, 2011. http://www.cancer.gov/cancertopics/pdq/genetics/breast-and-ovarian/healthprofessional. Accessed July 15, 2011.

National Cancer Institute (NCI). *Consent form Template for Adult Cancer Trials: Version date May 12, 2013.* Bethesda, MD: National Cancer Institute; 2013. http://ctep.cancer.gov/protocolDevelopment/docs/Informed_Consent_Template.docx

National Council on Radiation Protection and Measurements. *Ionizing Radiation Exposures of the Population of the United States.* NCRP Report No. 93. Bethesda, MD: National Council on Radiation Protection and Measurements; 1987.

National Council on Radiation Protection and Measurements. *Limitation of Exposure to Ionizing Radiation.* NCRP Report No. 116. Bethesda, MD: National Council on Radiation Protection and Measurements; 1993.

National Council on Radiation Protection and Measurements. *Radiation Protection Guidance for Activities in Low-Earth Orbit.* NCRP Report No. 132. Bethesda, MD: National Council on Radiation Protection and Measurements; 2000.

National Council on Radiation Protection and Measurements. *Extrapolation of Radiation-Induced Cancer Risks from Nonhuman Experimental Systems to Humans.* NCRP Report No. 150. Bethesda, MD: National Council on Radiation Protection and Measurements; 2005.

National Council on Radiation Protection and Measurements. *Risk to the Thyroid from Ionizing Radiation.* NCRP Report No. 159. Bethesda, MD: National Council on Radiation Protection and Measurements; 2008.

National Council on Radiation Protection and Measurements. *Radiation Dose Management for Fluoroscopically-Guided Interventional Procedures.* NCRP Report No. 168. Bethesda, MD: National Council on Radiation Protection; 2010.

National Council on Radiation Protection and Measurements. *Preconception and Prenatal Radiation Exposure: Health Effects and Protective Guidance.* NCRP Report No. 174. Bethesda, MD: National Council on Radiation Protection; 2013.

National Council on Radiation Protection and Measurements. *Uncertainties in the Estimation of Radiation Risks and Probability of Disease Causation.* NCRP Report No. 171. Bethesda, MD: National Council on Radiation Protection; 2015.

National Council on Radiation Protection and Measurements. *Guidance on Radiation Dose Limits for the Lens of the Eye.* NCRP Commentary No. 26. Bethesda, MD: National Council on Radiation Protection; 2016.

National Council on Radiation Protection and Measurements. *Implications of Recent Epidemiologic Studies for the Linear-Nonthreshold Model and Radiation Protection.* NCRP Commentary No. 27. Bethesda, MD: National Council on Radiation Protection; 2018a.

National Council on Radiation Protection and Measurements. NCRP Report No. 180. *Management of Exposure to Ionizing Radiation: Radiation Protection Guidance for the United States 2018.* Bethesda, MD: National Council on Radiation Protection; 2018b.

National Council on Radiation Protection and Measurements. *Evaluation of the Relative Effectiveness of Low-Energy Photons and Electrons in Inducing Cancer in Humans.* NCRP Report No. 181. Bethesda, MD: National Council on Radiation Protection; 2018c.

National Council on Radiation Protection and Measurements. *Evaluating and Communicating Radiation Risks for Studies Involving Human Subjects: Guidance for Researchers and Institutional Review Boards.* NCRP Report No. 185. Bethesda, MD: National Council on Radiation Protection; 2020.

National Council on Radiation Protection and Measurements (NCRP). Commentary No. 23. *Radiation Protection for Space Activities: Supplement to Previous Recommendations.* Bethesda, MD: National Council on Radiation Protection and Measurements; 2014.

NCICT. National Cancer Institute Dosimetry System for Computed Tomography. 2020. https://ncidose.cancer.gov/#ncict

NIH. *Probability of Developing or Dying of Cancer Software, Version 6.4.1.* Statistical Research and Applications Branch, National Cancer Institute; 2009. http://srab.cancer.gov/devcan

NTP. *Report on Carcinogens.* 14th ed. Research Triangle Park, NC: U.S. Department of Health and Human Services, Public Health Service, National Toxicology Program; 2016.

Otake M, Schull WJ, Fujikoshi Y, Yoshimaru H. *Effect on School Performance of Prenatal Exposure to Ionizing Radiation in Hiroshima: A Comparison of T65DR and DS86 Dosimetry Systems.* Technical Report No. 2-88. Hiroshima: Radiation Effects Research Foundation; 1988.

Ozasa K, Shimizu Y, Suyama A, et al. Studies of the mortality of atomic bomb survivors, Report 14, 1950–2003: an overview of cancer and noncancer diseases. *Radiat Res.* 2012;177:229-243.

Park KR, Monsky WL, Lee CG, et al. Mast cells contribute to radiation-induced vascular hyperpermeability. *Radiat Res.* 2016;185(2):182-189. doi: 10.1667/rr14190.1.

Pearce MS, Salotti JA, Little MP, et al. Radiation exposure from CT scans in childhood and subsequent risk of leukemia and brain tumours: a retrospective cohort study. *Lancet.* 2012;380(9840):499-505.

Politi MC, Han PKJ, Col NF. Communicating the uncertainty of harm and benefits of medical interventions. *Med Decis Making.* 2007;27(5):681-695.

Preston DL, Cullings H, Suyama A, et al. Solid cancer incidence in atomic bomb survivors exposed in utero or as young children. *J Natl Cancer Inst.* 2008;100(6):428-436.

Preston DL, et al. Solid cancer incidence in atomic bomb survivors: 1958–1998. *Radiat Res.* 2007;168:1.

Preston DL, Mattsson A, Holmberg E, Shore R, Hildreth NG, Boice JD Jr. Radiation effects on breast cancer risk: a pooled analysis of eight cohorts. *Radiat Res.* 2002;158:220-235.

Preston DL, Pierce DA, Shimizu Y, et al. Effect of recent changes in atomic bomb survivor dosimetry on cancer mortality, risk estimates. *Radiat Res.* 2004;162:377-389.

Preston DL, Shimizu Y, Pierce DA, et al. Studies of mortality of atomic bomb survivors. Report 13: Solid cancer and noncancer disease mortality: 1950–1997. *Radiat Res.* 2003;160:381-407.

RADAR. *RADAR Medical Procedure Radiation Dose Calculator and Consent Language Generator.* Nashville, TN: Radiation Dose Assessment Resource; 2019. http://www.doseinfo-radar.com/RADARDoseRisk-Calc.html

REAC/TS. *The Medical Basis for Radiation-Accident Preparedness: Medical Management.* Kindle Edition. Oak Ridge Associated Universities.

Reiman RE. Informed consent in human research: what to say and how to say it. *Health Phys.* 2013;104(2 suppl 1):S17-S22.

Roux C, Horvath C, Dupuis R. Effects of preimplantation low-dose radiation on rat embryos. *Health Phys.* 1993;45:993-999.

Russell WL, Russell LB, Kelly EM. Radiation dose rate and mutation frequency. *Science*. 1958;128:1546-1550.

Sasaki MS. Primary damage and fixation of chromosomal DNA as probed by monochromatic soft x-rays and low-energy neutrons. In: Fielden EM, O'Neil P, eds. *The Early Effects of Radiation on DNA*. Vol. H54. NATO ASI Series. Berlin: Springer-Verlag; 1991:369-384.

Sasaki MS, Kobayashi K, Hieda K, et al. Induction of chromosome aberrations in human lymphocytes by monochromatic x-rays of quantum energy between 4.8 and 14.6 keV. *Int J Radiat Biol*. 1989;56:975-988.

Schull WJ, Neel JV. Atomic bomb exposure and the pregnancies of biologically related parents. A prospective study of the genetic effects of ionizing radiation in man. *Am J Public Health Nations Health*. 1959;49(12):1621-1629.

Shadley JD, Afzal V, Wolff S. Characterization of the adaptive response to ionizing radiation induced by low doses of x rays to human lymphocytes. *Radiat Res*. 1987;111:511-517.

Shope TB. Radiation-induced skin injuries from fluoroscopy. *RadioGraphics*. 1996;16:1195-1199.

Shrieve L. *Human Radiation Injury*. Philadelphia, PA: Wolters Kluwer Health/Lippincott Williams & Wilkins; 2011.

Shrinivas SA, Shanta SH, Prajakta BB. DNA: damage and repair mechanisms in humans. *Glob J Pharm Sci*. 2017;3(2):555613.

Signorello LB, Mulvihill JJ, Green DM, et al. Stillbirth and neonatal death in relation to radiation exposure before conception: a retrospective cohort study. *Lancet*. 2010;376:624-630.

Slovic R, Fischhoff B, Lichtenstein S. Informing the public about the risks from ionizing radiation. *Health Phys*. 1981;41(4):589-598.

Stewart A, Webb J, Hewitt D. A survey of childhood malignancies. *Br Med J*. 1958;30:1495-1508.

Tawn EJ, Rees GS, Leith C, et al. Germline minisatellite mutations in survivors of childhood and young adult cancer treated with radiation. *Int J Radiat Biol*. 2011;87:330-340.

Thornton RH, Dauer LT, Shuk E, et al. Patient perspectives and preferences for communication of medical imaging risks in a cancer care setting. *Radiology*. 2015;275(2):545-552.

U.S. Environmental Protection Agency (EPA). EPA radiogenic cancer risk models and projections for the U.S. population, EPA 402-R-11–001, April 2011. *Fed Reg*. 2011;76(104).

U.S. Environmental Protection Agency (EPA). *Radiation Protection: Calculate Your Radiation Dose*. Washington, DC: U.S. Environmental Protection Agency; 2018. https://www.epa.gov/radiation/calculate-your-radiation-dose

U.S. Food and Drug Administration (FDA). *Radiation-Induced Skin Injuries from Fluoroscopy*. Rockville, MD: U.S. Food and Drug Administration; 1995. http://www.fda.gov/Radiation-EmittingProducts/RadiationEmittingProductsandProcedures/MedicalImaging/MedicalX-Rays/ucm116682.htm. Accessed July 11, 2011.

U.S. Food and Drug Administration (FDA). Title 21 – Chapter I – Subchapter D – Part 361.1 Radioactive Drugs for Certain Research Uses. 21CFR361.1 last updated 4/1/16. Washington, DC: U.S. Food and Drug Administration; 2016. http://www.accessdata.fda.gov/scripts/cdrh/cfdocs/cfcfr/CFRSearch.cfm?FR=361.1

U.S. Food and Drug Administration (FDA). *What Are Radiation Risks from CT?* Rockville, MD: U.S. Food and Drug Administration; 2020. https://www.fda.gov/radiation-emitting-products/medical-x-ray-imaging/what-are-radiation-risks-ct

United Nations Scientific Committee on the Effects of Atomic Radiation (UNSCEAR). *UNSCEAR 2006 Report to the General Assembly with Scientific Annexes, Effects of Ionizing Radiation*. Vol. 1: Report and Annexes A and B, 2008. Vol. 2: Annexes C, D, and E, 2009, 2011, New York, NY: United Nations. https://www.unscear.org/docs/publications/2013/UNSCEAR_2013_Report_Vol.II.pdf

United Nations Scientific Committee on the Effects of Atomic Radiation (UNSCEAR). *Sources and Effects of Ionizing Radiation. 1996 Report to the General Assembly with Scientific Annex*. New York, NY: United Nations; 1996. https://www.unscear.org/docs/publications/1996/UNSCEAR_1996_Report.pdf

United Nations Scientific Committee on the Effects of Atomic Radiation (UNSCEAR). *UNSCEAR 2013 Report to the General Assembly with Scientific Annexes, Effects of Ionizing Radiation*. Vol II: Scientific Annex B. New York, NY: United Nations; 2013. https://www.unscear.org/docs/reports/2013/UNSCEAR2013Report_AnnexB_Children_13-87320_Ebook_web.pdf

United Nations Scientific Committee on the Effects of Atomic Radiation (UNSCEAR). *Genetic and Somatic Effects of Ionizing Radiation*. UNSCEAR 1986 Report to the General Assembly, with annexes. United Nations sales publication E.86.IX.9. New York, NY: United Nations; 1986. https://www.unscear.org/docs/publications/1986/UNSCEAR_1986_Annex-C.pdf

Upton AC, Odell TT Jr, Sniffen EP. Influence of age at time of irradiation on induction of leukemia and ovarian tumors in RF mice. *Proc Soc Exp Biol Med*. 1960;104:769-772.

UW Dose Risk Tool. University of Washington; 2008. http://staff.washington.edu/aalessio/doserisk2/

20.10 Radiation Risk Communications

Wagner LK, Lester RG, Saldana LR. *Exposure of the Pregnant Patient to Diagnostic Radiations: A Guide to Medical Management.* 2nd ed. Madison, WI: Medical Physics Publishing; 1997.

Wakeford R, Little MP. Risk coefficients for childhood cancer after intrauterine irradiation: a review. *Int J Radiat Biol.* 2003;79:293-309.

Ward JF. DNA damage produced by ionizing radiation in mammalian cells: identities, mechanisms of formation, and repairability. *Prog Nucleic Acid Res Mol Biol.* 1988;35:95-125.

Ward JF. The complexity of DNA damage: relevance to biological consequences. *Int J Radiat Biol.* 1994;66:427-432.

West CM, Martin CJ, Sutton DG, et al. 21st L H Gray Conference: the radiobiology/radiation protection interface. *Br J Radiol.* 2009;82(977):353-362.

Winther JF, Boice JD Jr, Fredericksen K, et al. Radiotherapy for childhood cancer and risk for congenital malformations in offspring: a population-based cohort study. *Clin Genet.* 2009;75:50-56.

World Health Organization (WHO). *Communicating Radiation Risks in Paediatric Imaging.* Geneva, Switzerland: WHO Press; 2016. https://www.who.int/ionizing_radiation/pub_meet/radiation-risks-paediatric-imaging/en/. Accessed June 30, 2020.

Young R, Kerr G. *Report of the joint US-Japan working group. Reassessment of the atomic bomb radiation dosimetry for Hiroshima and Nagasaki: dosimetry system DS02.* Radiation Effects Research Foundation; 2005.

IAEA: Radiation Protection of Patients. https://rpop.iaea.org/RPOP/RPoP/Content/index.htm

20.10 Radiation Risk Communications

CHAPTER 21

Radiation Protection

It is incumbent upon all individuals who use radiation in medicine to strive for an optimal compromise between its clinical utility and the risk from radiation doses to patients, staff, and the public. Federal and state governments and even some large municipalities have agencies that promulgate regulations regarding the safe use of radiation and radioactive material. Radiation protection programs are designed and implemented to ensure compliance with these regulations. To a large degree, the success of radiation protection programs depends on the development of procedures for the safe use of radiation and radioactive material and the education of staff about radiation safety principles, the risks associated with radiation exposure and contamination, and the procedures for safe use. This chapter discusses the application of radiation protection principles (also known as health physics) in diagnostic x-ray and nuclear imaging, image-guided interventional procedures, and therapy with radioactive material.

21.1 SOURCES OF EXPOSURE TO IONIZING RADIATION

Much of the data referenced below on sources of exposure to radiation is from National Council on Radiation Protection and Measurements (NCRP) reports 94, 160, and 184 (NCRP, 1987, 2009, 2019) which have consolidated information on population exposure from both naturally occurring and artificially produced sources of exposure to radiation. According to the NCRP Report No. 160, the average annual per capita effective dose, exclusive of doses to patients from external beam radiation therapy, from exposure to ionizing radiation in the United States in 2006 was approximately 6.2 millisievert (mSv). These averages apply to the entire population of the United States. Approximately half of this, about 3.1 mSv, was from naturally occurring sources, whereas about 48%, 3.0 mSv, was from medical exposure of patients. Only about 2%, 0.14 mSv, was from other sources, such as consumer products and activities and occupational exposure. A decade later, in its Report No. 184, NCRP updated the information on the medical radiation exposure of patients in the United States, finding a 15% to 20% reduction, from 2006 to 2016, in the average dose to the U.S. population from medical imaging procedures, likely due to advances in technology as well as campaigns to increase awareness of medical imaging doses and to optimize patient doses. Doses to individuals from these sources vary considerably with a variety of factors discussed below.

21.1.1 Ubiquitous Background Exposure

Naturally occurring sources of radiation include (1) cosmic rays, (2) cosmogenic radionuclides, and (3) primordial radionuclides and their radioactive decay products. Cosmic radiation includes both the primary extraterrestrial radiation that strikes the Earth's atmosphere and the secondary radiations produced by the interaction of primary cosmic rays with the atmosphere. Primary cosmic rays predominantly consist of extremely penetrating high-energy (mean energy ~10 GeV) particulate radiation, approximately 80% of which is high-energy protons. Almost all primary cosmic radiation collides with our atmosphere before reaching the ground, producing showers of secondary particulate radiations (*e.g.*, electrons and muons) and electromagnetic radiation. The average per capita effective dose from cosmic radiation is approximately 0.33 mSv per year or approximately 11% of natural background radiation. However, the range of individual exposures is considerable. The majority of the population of the United States is exposed to cosmic radiation near sea level where the outdoor effective dose rate is approximately 0.3 mSv per year. However, smaller populations receive much more than this amount (*e.g.*, Colorado Springs, CO, at 1,840 m, ~0.82 mSv per year). Exposures increase with altitude, approximately doubling every 1,500 m, as there is less atmosphere to attenuate the cosmic radiation. Cosmic radiation is also greater at the Earth's magnetic poles than at the equator, as charged particles encountering the Earth's magnetic field are forced to travel along the field lines to either the North or the South Pole. Structures provide some protection from cosmic radiation; the indoor effective dose rate is approximately 20% lower than outdoors.

Some of the secondary cosmic ray particles collide with stable atmospheric nuclei producing "cosmogenic" radionuclides (*e.g.*, $^{14}_{7}N[n, p]^{14}_{6}C$). Although many cosmogenic radionuclides are produced, they contribute very little (~0.01 mSv per year or <1%) to natural background radiation. The majority of the effective dose caused by cosmogenic radionuclides is from carbon 14.

The radioactive materials that have been present on the Earth since its formation are called *primordial radionuclides.* Primordial radionuclides with physical half-lives comparable to the age of the Earth (~4.5 billion years) and their radioactive decay products are the largest sources of terrestrial radiation exposure. The population radiation dose from primordial radionuclides is the result of external radiation exposure, inhalation, and incorporation of radionuclides in the body. Primordial radionuclides with half-lives less than 10^8 years have decayed to undetectable levels since their formation, whereas those with half-lives greater than 10^{10} years do not significantly contribute to background radiation levels because of their long physical half-lives (*i.e.*, slow rates of decay). Most radionuclides with atomic numbers greater than lead decay to stable isotopes of lead through a series of radionuclide decays called *decay chains.* The radionuclides in these decay chains have half-lives ranging from seconds to many thousands of years. Other primordial radionuclides, such as potassium 40 (K-40, $T\frac{1}{2}$ = 1.28 × 10^9 years), decay directly to stable nuclides. The decay chains of uranium 238 (U-238), $T\frac{1}{2}$ = 4.51 × 10^9 years (uranium series), and thorium 232 (Th-232), $T\frac{1}{2}$ = 1.41 × 10^{10} years (thorium series), produce several dozen radionuclides that together with K-40 are responsible for most of the external terrestrial average effective dose of 0.21 mSv per year or approximately 7% of natural background. Individuals may receive much higher or lower exposures than the average, depending on the local concentrations of terrestrial radionuclides. The range in the United States is approximately 0.1 to 0.4 mSv per year. There are a few regions of the world where terrestrial radionuclides are highly concentrated. For example, as discussed in Chapter 20, monazite sand deposits, containing high concentrations of radionuclides from the Th-232 decay series, are found along certain beaches in India. The external radiation levels on these black sands range up to 70 mGy per year (Nair et al., 2009), which is more than 300 times the average level from terrestrial sources in the United States.

The short-lived alpha particle–emitting decay products of radon 222 (Rn-222) are believed to be the most significant source of exposure from the inhalation of naturally occurring radionuclides. Radon 222, a noble gas, is produced in the U-238 decay chain by the decay of radium 226 (Ra-226). Rn-222 decays by alpha emission, with a half-life of 3.8 days, to polonium 218 (Po-218), followed by several other alpha and beta decays, eventually leading to stable lead-206 (Pb-206). When the short-lived daughters of radon are inhaled, most of the dose is deposited in the tracheobronchial region of the lung. Radon concentrations in the environment vary widely. There are both seasonal and diurnal variations in radon concentrations. Radon gas emanates primarily from the soil in proportion to the quantity of natural uranium deposits; its dispersion can be restricted by structures, producing much higher indoor air concentrations than found outdoors in the same area. Radon gas dissolved in domestic water supplies can be released into the air within a home during water usage, particularly when the water is from a well or another groundwater source. Weatherproofing of homes and offices and other energy conservation measures typically decrease ventilation by outside air, resulting in higher indoor radon concentrations.

The radiation from exposure to Rn-222 and its daughters in the United States results in an average effective dose of approximately 2.1 mSv per year or approximately 68% of natural background. The dose from the inhalation of radon decay products is primarily to the bronchial epithelium. In order to convert the absorbed dose from the alpha particles to an effective dose, a tissue weighting factor (w_T) of 0.08 is applied along with a radiation weighting factor (w_R) of 20 to account for increased risk from exposure to high LET radiation.

The average indoor air concentration of Rn-222 in homes in the United States is approximately 46 Bq/m^3 (1.24 pCi/L); however, levels can exceed 2.75 kBq/m^3 (75 pCi/L) in poorly ventilated structures with high concentrations of U-238 in the soil. Outdoor air concentrations are approximately three times lower, 15 Bq/m^3 (0.41 pCi/L). The U.S. Environmental Protection Agency (EPA, 2020) recommends taking action to reduce radon levels in homes exceeding 147 Bq/m^3 (4 pCi/L), whereas other countries have somewhat different action levels (*e.g.*, the United Kingdom and Canada have higher action levels, 200 Bq/m^3 [5.4 pCi/L]). Although Rn-222 accounts for about two thirds of the natural radiation effective dose, it can be easily measured, and exposures can be reduced when necessary.

The third-largest source of natural background radiation is from the ingestion of food and water containing primordial radionuclides (and their decay products), of which K-40 is the most significant. K-40 is a naturally occurring isotope of potassium (~0.01%). Skeletal muscle has the highest concentration of potassium in the body. K-40 produces an average effective dose of approximately 0.15 mSv per year or approximately 5% of natural background. Th-232 and U-238 and their decay products are found in food and water and result in an average annual effective dose of approximately 0.13 mSv.

Long-lived radionuclides released to or created in the environment from the atmospheric testing of nuclear weapons (450 detonations between 1945 and 1980) consist mainly of carbon 14, tritium (H-3), cesium 134 and 137 (Cs-134, Cs-137), strontium 90, plutonium, and transplutonium elements. A large fraction of these radionuclides have since decayed and/or have become progressively less available for biologic uptake and as a result, the average annual effective dose is less than 10 µSv (NCRP, 1987).

21.1.2   Medical Exposure of Patients

The single greatest controllable source of radiation exposure in the US population (and that of many other developed countries) is medical imaging. The majority of the exposure is from x-ray imaging (primarily from diagnostic radiology), with a smaller contribution from nuclear medicine due to the lower number of examinations

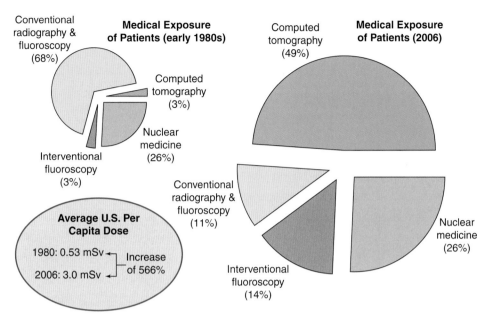

FIGURE 21-1 Average annual per capita effective doses in the United States from medical imaging procedures, showing the large increase from 1980 to 2006. (From National Council on Radiation Protection and Measurements. *Exposure of the Population in the United States and Canada from Natural Background Radiation*. NCRP Report No. 94. Bethesda, MD: National Council on Radiation Protection and Measurements; 1987; National Council on Radiation Protection and Measurements. *Ionizing Radiation Exposure of the Population of the United States*. NCRP Report No. 160. Bethesda, MD: National Council on Radiation Protection and Measurements; 2009.) Updated estimates from 2016 show a slight decrease in contribution from medical imaging procedures, reflecting new technology and as a result of an emphasis on dose optimization. (Reprinted with permission from National Council on Radiation Protection and Measurements. *Medical Radiation Exposure of Patients in the United States*. NCRP Report No. 184. Bethesda, MD: National Council on Radiation Protection and Measurements; 2019. http://NCRPonline.org.)

performed per year. Doses from individual medical imaging procedures are summarized in Appendices E and F. NCRP Report No. 160 (NCRP, 2009) showed that the average annual effective dose to the U.S. population from the medical use of radiation (not including radiation therapy) had increased from about 1980 to 2006, by more than a factor of five (0.53 to 3 mSv), representing ~97% of the total from artificial radiation sources and nearly half of the total average annual effective dose from all sources. Of course, there had been significant advances in medical imaging technology and its use from 1980 to 2006. The report identified the increased utilization of CT and nuclear medicine imaging procedures as the two most significant factors that led to the increase in the average dose from the medical use of radiation (Fig. 21-1). In 2006, while CT and nuclear medicine procedures collectively accounted for only ~21% of all medical imaging procedures using ionizing radiation, they delivered ~75% of the collective effective dose. The CT and nuclear medicine procedures that contributed the most to this dose were CT of the abdomen and the pelvis and [99m]Tc- and ^{201}Tl myocardial perfusion imaging, which together accounted for more than half of the effective dose to the population from medical imaging. Conversely, conventional radiographic and fluoroscopically guided non-cardiac interventional procedures, which accounted for ~75% of the imaging procedures, resulted in only ~11% of the collective effective dose[1] (Table 21-1A).

---

[1]Collective effective dose (S) in units of person-Sv, is the product of the mean effective dose for a population and the number of persons. The U.S. population used for NCRP 184 was 323 million in 2016. The report used the current ICRP Publication 103 tissue weighting factors.

21.1 Sources of Exposure to Ionizing Radiation

TABLE 21-1 RADIATION EXPOSURE TO US POPULATION IN 2006 AND 2016— MEDICAL EXPOSURES (EXCLUDING RADIATION THERAPY)

	Number of procedures	Percentage	Collective Effective Dose (person-Sv) ICRP 1990w_T (S60)	Percentage	Average Individual Effective Dose (mSv) ICRP 1990 w_T (E_{US}60)	Percentage
Data from NCRP (2009)			2006			
CT[a]	62	16.5%	438,000	49.5%	1.46	50.0%
Nuclear Medicine	21% / 17	4.5%	222,000	74.6% / 25.1%	0.73	25.0%
Cardiac Interventional Fluoroscopy	4.6	1.2%	68,000	7.7%	0.23	7.9%
Radiography	281	74.6%	97,000	11.0%	0.3	10.3%
Fluoroscopy Guided Noncardiac Interventional	12	3.2%	60,200	6.8%	0.2	6.8%
TOTALS	376.6	100%	885,200	100%	2.92	100%
Data from NCRP (2019)			2016			
CT[a]	74	20.0%	46,900	62.1%	1.45	62.2%
Nuclear Medicine	13.5	3.6%	133,000	17.6%	0.41	17.6%
Cardiac Interventional Fluoroscopy	4.1	1.1%	42,000	5.6%	0.13	5.6%
Radiography	275	74.2%	71,000	9.4%	0.22	9.4%
Fluoroscopy Guided Noncardiac Interventional	4	1.1%	40,000	5.3%	0.12	5.2%
TOTALS	371	100%	755,000	100%	2.33	100%

[a]For CT the values are for procedures. The estimated number of scans in 2006 and 2016 were 67 and 84 million, respectively.
[b]Value adjusted from NCRP Report No. 160 (NCRP, 2009) due to an extrapolation that was likely an overestimate.

While much of this increase was almost certainly beneficial for patients as it prevented many unnecessary exploratory surgeries, identified early-stage cancers, allowed for effective intervention in stroke patients, etc., the concerns centered around those scans that may not have been necessary and those that could have been accomplished at lower doses to the patients. In response to this increase in patient exposure, several initiatives were put into place by the radiology community, the two most significant of which were centered around dose optimization and appropriate utilization of imaging services. Optimization means adjusting the quality and quantity of the radiation to the body habitus of the patient to use only the dose necessary for producing a study from which a diagnosis can be made with confidence. The term ALADA (As Low As Diagnostically Acceptable) has been cited in the literature by some who wish to distinguish it from the radiation protection concept of ALARA (As Low As Reasonably Achievable) over the concern that the dose (rather than the diagnostic utility of the image) may become the overriding metric of quality (Fernandes et al., 2016). While this is not the intent of ALARA and it certainly can be applied to medicine if correctly interpreted, some see the distinction useful to keep the right balance on the elements that most affect patient care. There has also been a renewed focus on the utilization of appropriateness criteria for evaluating which imaging procedures are best suited to the specific patient and clinical question at hand. Both of these concepts are expanded upon in Section 21.4.1 under the general radiation safety principles of justification and optimization.

A recent estimate of medical radiation exposure of patients in the United States, NCRP Report 184 (NCRP, 2019), based on data from 2016 (10 years after the previous assessment) indicated that the annual number of diagnostic and interventional radiologic examinations that had been reported for 2006 (377 million) was essentially unchanged. There had actually been an increase in the annual number of CT scans performed per year over that period; however, there were decreases in other imaging procedures (*e.g.*, nuclear medicine; fluoroscopy). After taking into account the population increase of 24 million, the overall annual individual (per capita) effective dose from diagnostic and interventional medical procedures was shown to have decreased from 2.9 mSv in 2006 to 2.3 mSv in 2016. Similarly, the U.S. annual collective effective dose had decreased from 885,000 to 755,000 person-sievert[2] (Table 21-1B).

21.1.3 Consumer Products and Activities

This category includes a variety of sources, most of which are consumer products. The largest contribution in this category is from tobacco products. Two alpha-emitting radionuclides, Pb-210 and Po-210 (which occur naturally from the decay of Ra-226), have been measured in both tobacco leaves and cigarette smoke. It has been estimated that a one-pack-a-day smoker increases his or her annual effective dose by approximately 0.36 mSv. The NCRP estimated the average annual effective dose to an exposed individual is 0.3 mSv and, based on a smoking population of 45 million in the United States, this resulted in an average annual effective dose to the entire population of 0.045 mSv, which is about 35% of the effective dose from all consumer products and activities.

Many building materials contain radioisotopes of uranium, thorium, radium, and potassium. These primordial radionuclides and their decay products are found in higher concentrations in such materials as brick, concrete, clay, and granite, and thus structures and household items made from these materials will cause higher exposures than those made from other materials. The typical annual effective dose received by a member of the public from glazed ceramics amounts to 7–50 µSv from external radiation, together with an increase of 3–5 Bq/m^3 in indoor radon concentration. By contrast, porcelain tiles give rise to an annual effective dose of 3–150 µSv from external radiation and an increase in radon concentration of 10–46 Bq/m^3. The average annual per capita effective dose is estimated to be approximately 0.035 mSv from these types of sources.

Air travel can substantially add to an individual's cosmic ray exposure. For example, a 5-h transcontinental flight in a commercial jet aircraft will result in an equivalent dose of approximately 0.025 mSv. The average annual per capita effective dose to passengers from commercial air travel is estimated to be approximately 0.034 mSv.

There are many other less important sources of enhanced natural radiation exposure, such as mining and agricultural activities (primarily from fertilizers containing members of the uranium and thorium decay series and K-40); combustible fuels, including coal and natural gas (radon); and consumer products, including smoke alarms (americium-241), gas lantern mantles (thorium), and dental prostheses, certain ceramics, and optical lenses (uranium). These sources contribute less than 12% of the average annual effective dose from consumer products and activities.

21.1.4 Occupational and Other Sources of Exposure

Occupational exposures are received by some people employed in medicine, including veterinary medicine, by aircraft crew in commercial aviation, by workers in some

---

[2]Effective dose per individual in the U.S. population (E_{US103}), computed by dividing collective effective dose E_{US103} using ICRP Publication 103 tissue weighting factors by the total number of individuals in the U.S. population (323 million in 2016) whether exposed to the specific source or not.

industrial and commercial activities; by workers in the commercial nuclear power industry, by workers in some educational and research institutions, and by some individuals in the military, some in governmental agencies, and some in U.S. Department of Energy facilities. Since most individuals are not occupationally exposed to radiation and the majority of those who are exposed typically receive fairly low annual doses, the contribution to the average annual per capita effective dose to the population from occupational exposure is very low, 0.005 mSv (<0.1%). However, among those occupationally exposed to radiation, the average annual effective dose was 1.1 mSv.

In 2006, medical personnel, whose occupational exposures were monitored, received an average annual effective dose of approximately 0.75 mSv (NCRP, 2009). This average is somewhat lower than might be expected because the doses to many staff members are quite low (*e.g.*, radiology supervisors and radiologists who perform few if any fluoroscopic procedures). For example, occupational doses to radiologists not routinely performing interventional procedures have been declining in recent years and an average annual effective dose of approximately 0.1 to 0.2 mSv is common (Linet et al., 2010). Similarly, full-time technologists working in large hospitals performing mostly CT and radiography examinations will typically have annual effective doses of approximately 0.5 to 1 mSv. However, the medical staff involved in fluoroscopically guided interventional procedures will typically have much higher occupational exposures. The actual doses received by the staff will depend on a number of factors including their roles in the procedures (*i.e.*, performing or assisting), the number of procedures performed, the type and difficulty (which determines the lengths) of the cases, as well as the availability and use of radiation protection devices and techniques. Annual doses recorded by the dosimeters worn at the collar (outside the lead apron) in the range of 5 to 15 mSv are typical for personnel routinely performing these procedures. In reality, these are only partial body exposures (*i.e.*, to the head and extremities), because the use of radiation-attenuating aprons greatly reduces the exposure to most of the body. Adjusting their measured exposures to account for the shielding provided is discussed in the following section on dosimetry. After adjusting for shielding, the effective dose is typically reduced by a factor of 3 or more compared to that recorded on the collar dosimeter.

For most routine nuclear medicine procedures, the effective doses to the technologists are typically less than 1 μSv per procedure, putting typical annual exposures in the range 2 to 3 mSv. However, for positron emission tomography (PET) procedures, an effective dose of 1 to 5 μSv per procedure has been reported (Guillet et al., 2005). Nuclear medicine technologists whose routine workload also includes dose preparation and imaging of patients for PET may have annual effective doses in the range of 10 to 15 mSv.

Airline crew members are estimated to receive an additional average annual effective dose of approximately 3.1 mSv; some receive effective doses of more than twice this value. It is interesting to note that the average annual effective dose to airline crew exceeds the annual effective doses of many diagnostic radiology personnel.

The contribution to the annual effective dose of members of the public (those not working in the industry) from activities related to commercial nuclear power production is minimal, approximately 0.5 μSv. Population radiation exposure from nuclear power production occurs from all phases of the fuel cycle, including uranium mining and processing, uranium enrichment, manufacturing of uranium fuel, reactor operations, and radioactive waste disposal.

21.1.5 Summary

The average annual effective dose to the US population from all radiation sources is obtained by dividing the annual collective effective dose by the size of the US population. The result in 2006 was approximately 6.2 mSv per year or approximately 17 µSv per day for all people in the United States from all sources, exclusive of radiation therapy. It is interesting to note that, although nuclear power, fallout from atomic weapons, and a variety of consumer products receive considerable attention in the popular media, they, in fact, cause only a small fraction of the average population exposure to radiation.

The average annual effective dose is somewhat misleading for categories such as the medical use of radiation, in that many people in the population are neither occupationally nor medically exposed yet are included in the average. Figure 21-2 presents a summary of the average annual effective dose for the US population from the radiation sources previously discussed.

21.2 PERSONNEL DOSIMETRY

The radiation exposure of some people must be monitored for both safety and regulatory purposes. Such assessments may need to be made over periods of several minutes to several months. There are three main types of individual radiation recording devices called *personnel dosimeters* used in diagnostic radiology and nuclear medicine: (1) *film badges* (usage has significantly declined, but still in use), (2) *dosimeters using*

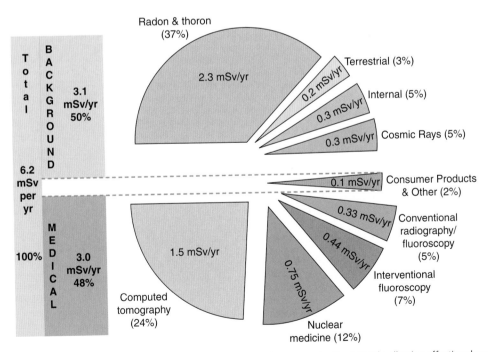

■ **FIGURE 21-2** Percent contributions of various sources of exposure to the annual collective effective dose (1,870,000 person-Sv) and the average annual effective dose per person in the US population (6.2 mSv) in 2006. Percentages have been rounded to the nearest 1%. (Adapted with permission from National Council on Radiation Protection and Measurements. *Ionizing Radiation Exposure of the Population of the United States.* NCRP Report No. 160. Bethesda, MD: National Council on Radiation Protection and Measurements; 2009. http://NCRPonline.org.)

storage phosphors (*i.e.*, thermoluminescent dosimeters [TLDs] or optically stimulated luminescence dosimeters [OSLs]), and (3) *electronic personal dosimeters*, each with advantages and disadvantages.

Ideally, one would like to have a single personnel dosimeter capable of meeting all of the dosimetry needs in medical imaging. The ideal dosimeter would respond instantaneously, distinguish among different types of radiation, and accurately measure the dose and dose equivalent from each form of ionizing radiation, with energies from several keV to MeV, independent of the angle of incidence. In addition, the dosimeter would be small, lightweight, rugged, easy to use, inexpensive, and unaffected by environmental conditions (*e.g.*, temperature, humidity, pressure) and nonionizing radiation sources. Unfortunately, no such dosimeter exists; however, most of these characteristics can be satisfied to some degree by selecting the dosimeter best suited for a particular application.

21.2.1 Film Badges

A film badge consists of a small sealed packet of radiation-sensitive film, similar to dental x-ray film, placed inside a special plastic holder that can be clipped to clothing. Although film badges are mostly historical in use, some locations and vendors still utilize these simple badges for occupational dose monitoring. Radiation striking the emulsion causes a darkening of the developed film. The amount of darkening increases with the absorbed dose to the film emulsion and is measured with a densitometer. The film emulsion contains grains of silver bromide, resulting in a higher effective atomic number than tissue; therefore, the dose to the film is not equal to the dose to tissue. However, with the selective use of several metal filters over the film (typically lead, copper, and aluminum), the relative optical densities of the film underneath the metal filters can be used to identify the approximate energy range of the radiation and to calculate the dose to soft tissue. Film badges typically have an area where the film is not covered by a metal filter or plastic and thus is directly exposed to the radiation. This "open window" is used to detect medium- and high-energy beta radiation that would otherwise be attenuated (Fig. 21-3).

Most film badges can record doses from about 100 µSv to 15 Sv (10 mrem to 1,500 rem) for photons and from 500 µSv to 10 Sv (50 mrem to 1,000 rem) for beta radiation. The film in the badge is usually replaced monthly and sent to the commercial supplier for processing. The developed film is usually kept by the vendor, providing a permanent record of radiation exposure.

Film badges are small, lightweight, inexpensive, and easy to use. However, exposure to excessive moisture or temperature can damage the film emulsion, making dose estimates difficult or impossible. As with film-screen image receptors in radiography, film-based dosimeters have all but disappeared in most countries.

21.2.2 Thermoluminescent and Optically Stimulated Luminescent Dosimeters

Some dosimeters contain storage phosphors in which a fraction of the electrons, raised to excited states by ionizing radiation, become trapped in excited states. When these trapped electrons are released, either by heating or by exposure to light, they fall to lower energy states with the emission of light. The amount of light emitted can be measured and indicates the radiation dose received by the phosphor material.

TLDs, discussed in Chapter 17, are excellent personnel and environmental dosimeters. The most commonly used TLD material for personnel dosimetry is lithium

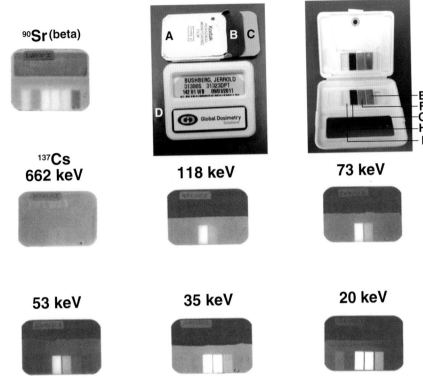

■ **FIGURE 21-3** A film pack **(A)** consists of a light opaque envelope **(B)** containing the film **(C)**. The film pack is placed in the plastic film badge **(D)** sandwiched between two sets of metal filters containing strips of **(E)** lead, **(F)** copper, aluminum, **(G)** and **(H)** polyethylene (plastic) filters. Film badges typically have an area where the film pack is not covered by a filter or the plastic of the badge and thus is directly exposed to the radiation. This "open window" area **(I)** is used to detect medium- and high-energy beta radiation that would otherwise be attenuated. The relative darkening of the developed film (filter pattern) provides a crude but useful assessment of the energy of the radiation. The diagram shows typical filter patterns from exposure to a high-energy beta emitter (Sr-90), a high-energy γ emitter (Cs-137), and x-rays with effective energies from 20 to 118 keV.

fluoride (LiF). LiF TLDs have a wide dose-response range of 100 μSv to 10 Sv and are reusable (Fig. 21-4). These dosimeters can be used over a long time interval (up to 6 months if necessary) before being returned to the vendor for analysis. The energy response is 0.8 to 5 MeV (E_{max}) for beta radiation and 20 keV to 6 MeV for x-ray and gamma (γ)-ray radiation.

Another advantage of LiF TLDs is that their effective atomic number is close to that of the tissue; therefore, the dose to a LiF chip is close to the tissue dose over a wide energy range. TLDs do not provide a permanent record, because heating the chip to read the exposure removes the deposited energy. TLDs are routinely used in nuclear medicine as extremity dosimeters; a finger ring containing a chip of LiF worn on the hand is expected to receive the highest exposure during radiopharmaceutical preparation and administration. Figure 21-5 shows a finger ring dosimeter and a LiF chip.

Dosimeters using OSL are now widely available as an alternative to TLDs. The principle of OSL is similar to that of TLDs, except that the release of trapped electrons and light emission are stimulated by laser light instead of by heat. Crystalline aluminum oxide activated with carbon (Al_2O_3:C) is commonly used. Like LiF TLDs, these OSL dosimeters have a broad dose-response range and are capable of detecting doses as low as 10 μSv. As in film dosimeters, the Al_2O_3 has a higher effective atomic

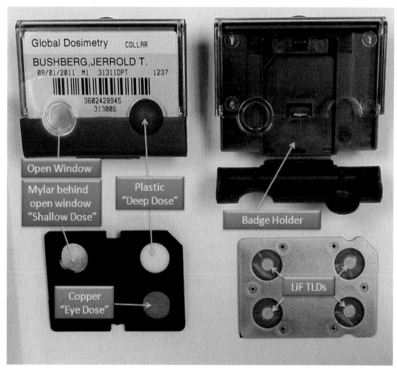

■ **FIGURE 21-4** TLD dosimeter with four LiF TLDs. The filters in this dosimeter are made of Mylar (7 mg/cm²), copper (300 mg/cm²), and polypropylene plastic (1,000 mg/cm²), representing the specified depths for determination of dose to the skin ("shallow dose") at a depth of 0.007 cm, lens of the eye at a depth of 0.3 cm, and deep dose at a depth of 1.0 cm, respectively.

number than soft tissue and so an OSL dosimeter has filters over the sheet of OSL material that are used to estimate dose to soft tissue, as in film badges. However, OSL dosimeters have certain advantages over TLDs in that they can be reread several times and an image of the filter pattern can be produced to differentiate between static (*i.e.*, in a fixed position with respect to a radiation source during exposure) and dynamic (*i.e.*, normal) exposure. TLDs or OSL dosimeters are the dosimeters of choice when longer dose assessment intervals (*e.g.*, quarterly) are required.

■ **FIGURE 21-5** A small chip of LiF (right) is sealed in a finger ring (underneath the identification label). In nuclear medicine, the ring is worn with the LiF chip on the palmar surface such that the chip would be facing a radiation source held in the hand.

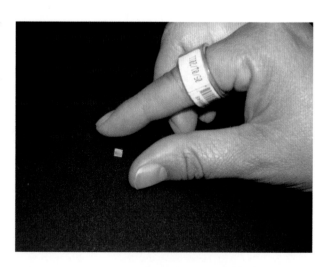

21.2.3 Direct Ion Storage Dosimeters

Direct ion storage dosimeters use a non-volatile analog memory cell, surrounded by a gas-filled ion chamber, is used to record radiation exposure (Fig. 21-6) for photons initially, and now including betas in the latest technology. The initial interactions of the x-ray and γ-ray photons and betas occur in the wall material or thin windows, and secondary electrons ionize the gas of the chamber. The positive ions are attracted to a central negative electrode, resulting in a reduction in electrical charge and voltage that is proportional to the dose received by the dosimeter. The dose recorded by the dosimeter can be read at any time by connecting it to the USB port of any computer with Internet access. The advantages of this technology include a broad dose (0.001 mSv to 40 Sv) and photon energy (6 keV to 9 MeV) response ranges. These devices provide for unlimited real-time dose readings by the user without the need for a special reader, online management of dosimeter assignment and dosimetry reports, and elimination of the periodic distribution and collection of dosimeters as well as the delay and cost associated with returning the dosimeters for processing by the dosimetry vendor. Disadvantages include the initial cost of the dosimeters, more costly replacement of lost dosimeters, and the need for users to upload dosimetry information periodically.

21.2.4 Practical Aspects of Dosimeter Use

Nearly every medical facility obtains non–self-reading TLD or OSL dosimeters, from a commercial vendor monthly or quarterly. One or more control dosimeters are shipped with each batch. At the beginning of a wear period, typically at the beginning

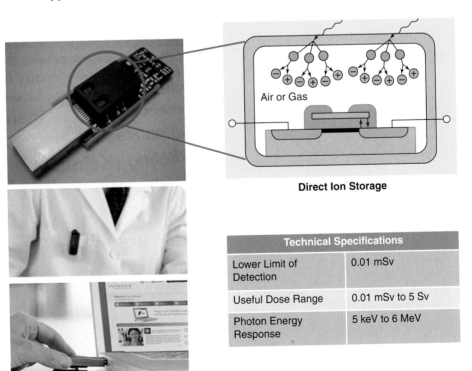

Direct Ion Storage

Technical Specifications	
Lower Limit of Detection	0.01 mSv
Useful Dose Range	0.01 mSv to 5 Sv
Photon Energy Response	5 keV to 6 MeV

■ **FIGURE 21-6** Direct ion storage dosimeter.

of a month, the new dosimeters are issued to staff and the used dosimeters from the previous wear period are collected and returned to the dosimeter vendor for reading. At least one control dosimeter from the same batch is included in the shipment. Control dosimeters are stored in an area away from radiation sources. The vendor subtracts the reading from the control dosimeter from the readings of the dosimeters that were used. An exposure report is usually available online through the vendor's password-protected portal in about 2 weeks. However, reporting of unusual exposures or exposures over regulatory limits can be expedited. The dosimetry report lists the "shallow" dose, corresponding to the skin dose, the "eye" dose corresponding to the dose to the lens of the eye, and the "deep" dose, corresponding to penetrating radiations.

21.2.5 Placement of Dosimeters on the Body

A dosimeter is typically worn on the part of the torso that is expected to receive the largest radiation exposure or is most sensitive to radiation damage. Most radiologists, x-ray technologists, and nuclear medicine technologists wear a dosimeter at the waist or shirt-pocket level. A pregnant radiation worker typically wears an additional dosimeter at waist level (behind the lead apron, if one is worn) to assess the fetal dose. During fluoroscopy, a dosimeter is typically placed at collar level in front of the lead apron to measure the dose to the thyroid and lens of the eye as most of the body is shielded from exposure. Alternatively, a dosimeter can be placed at the collar level in front of the radiation-protective apron, and a second dosimeter can be worn on the torso underneath the apron. The "double badge" method allows for the estimation of the effective dose equivalent (H_E).

21.2.6 Estimating Effective Dose and Effective Dose Equivalent for Staff Wearing Protective Aprons

Protective aprons shield the torso and upper legs during diagnostic and interventional x-ray imaging procedures. Methods recommended by the NCRP that take this shielding into account allow for an effective dose and effective dose equivalent to be estimated. When a single dosimeter is worn at collar level outside the apron, the NCRP recommends that effective dose equivalent (H_E) be calculated from the dose recorded by the collar dosimeter (H_N) using Equation 21-1:

$$H_E = 0.18\, H_N. \qquad\qquad [21\text{-}1]$$

When a dosimeter is worn at collar level outside the protective apron and another dosimeter is worn underneath the apron at the waist or chest, the recommended method for calculating H_E is to use H_N and the dose (H_W) recorded by the dosimeter worn under the lead apron in Equation 21-2:

$$H_E = 1.5\, H_W + 0.04\, H_N. \qquad\qquad [21\text{-}2]$$

These and similar equations for estimating the effective dose can be found in NCRP Report No. 122 (NCRP, 1995).

21.2.7 Electronic Personal Dosimeters

The major disadvantage to film, thermoluminescent, and OSL dosimeters is that the accumulated dose is not immediately displayed. Electronic personal dosimeters (EPDs) measure radiation exposure and can be read immediately on a digital display. There is a wide range of EPDs options from full-featured devices with event recording capabilities (Fig. 21-7) to others that simply display the accumulated dose (Fig. 21-8). These dosimeters typically use solid-state electronics and either Geiger-Mueller (GM) tubes or radiation-sensitive semiconductor diodes to measure and display radiation dose in a range from approximately 10 µSv to 100 mSv. EPDs typically include alarm functions to alert the wearer when a dose threshold is exceeded. EPDs should also be considered as supplemental dosimeters when high doses are expected, such as during cardiac catheterization or manipulation of large quantities of radioactivity. Table 21-2 summarizes the characteristics of the various personnel monitoring devices discussed above. Additional information specific to staff and patient radiation protection and monitoring during fluoroscopy is reviewed along with other x-ray imaging procedures in Section 21.6. Radiation dosimetry and other protection issues specific to Nuclear Medicine are discussed in Section 21.7.

21.2.8 Problems with Personnel Dosimetry

Common problems associated with dosimetry include dosimeters being left in radiation fields when not worn, contamination of a dosimeter with radioactive material, lost and damaged dosimeters, and the wearing of dosimeters improperly or not at all when working with radiation sources. If a dosimeter is positioned so that the body is between it and the radiation source, attenuation will cause a significant underestimation of the true exposure. Most personnel do not remain in constant

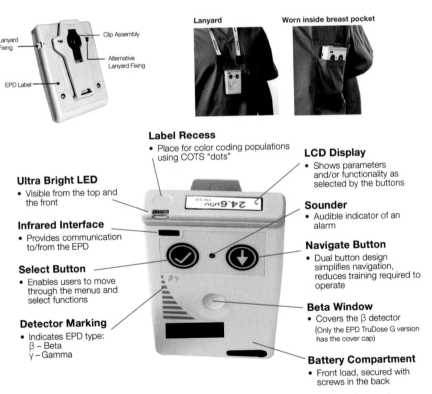

■ FIGURE 21-7 Full-featured integrated electronic personal dosimeter including Bluetooth communications capability; high sensitivity a low as 0.05 µSv/h; real-time event recording; electromagnetic interference shielding; wide dose range from 1.0 µSv to ≥10 Sv; wide photon energy range capability 17 keV to 6 MeV and thresholds alarm settings. (Thermo Scientific™ EPD TRUDOSE™ © Thermo Fisher Scientific Inc.)

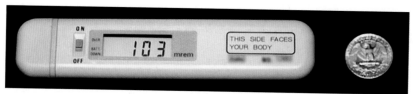

■ **FIGURE 21-8** A simpler direct read digital pocket dosimeter.

geometry with respect to the radiation sources they use. Consequently, the dosimeter measurements are usually representative of the individual's average exposure. For example, if a dosimeter is worn properly and the radiation field is multidirectional or the wearer's orientation toward it is random, then the mean exposure over a period of time will tend to be a good approximation (±10% to 20%) of the individual's true exposure.

21.2.9 Environmental Dosimetry

Placing environmental TLD or OSL in public spaces near the radiopharmacy, PET/CT imaging facilities, and any other areas for which there is a concern or perception that radiation exposure may be high in an uncontrolled space adjacent to controlled area is a recommended practice. These dosimeters are typically exchanged quarterly. While there are typically only background levels recorded on these dosimeters, they provide a relatively inexpensive independent record demonstrating that individuals working adjacent to these areas, who would not typically be wearing dosimetry, were not exposed to radiation in excess of regulatory limits for the public.

TABLE 21-2 SUMMARY OF PERSONNEL MONITORING METHODS

METHOD	MEASURES	USEFUL RANGE (X- AND γ-RAY)	PERMANENT RECORD	USES AND COMMENTS
Film badge	Beta; γ- and x-ray	0.1–15,000 mSv[a] (beta) 0.5–10,000 mSv[a]	Yes	Have been replaced by OSL and TLD in most applications for routine personnel monitoring diagnostic radiology and nuclear medicine
TLD	Beta; γ- and x-ray	0.01–10⁴ mSv[a]	No	Widely used for personnel dosimetry and for phantom and patient dosimetry
OSL	Beta; γ- and x-ray	0.01–10⁶ mSv[a]	No[b]	Widely used for personnel dosimetry and for phantom and patient dosimetry Advantage over TLD includes the ability to reread the dosimeters and distinguish between dynamic and static exposures
Electronic Personal Dosimeter (EPD)	γ- and x-ray	Digital 0–10⁴ mSv[a]	No[c]	Special monitoring (e.g., cardiac cath); permits direct (i.e., real-time) reading of exposure

[a]Multiply mSv by 100 to obtain mrem.
[b]OSL dosimeters are typically retained and can be reread by the manufacturer for approximately 1 year.
[c]Some EPD manufacturers provide wireless transfer of recorded data that can be retained.
OSL, optically stimulated luminance; TLD, thermoluminescent dosimeter.

21.3 RADIATION DETECTION EQUIPMENT IN RADIATION SAFETY

A variety of portable radiation detection instruments, the characteristics of which are optimized for specific applications, are used in radiology and nuclear medicine. The portable GM survey meter and portable ionization chamber survey meter satisfy most of the requirements for radiation protection measurements in nuclear medicine. X-ray machine evaluations require specialized ion chamber or solid-state diode instruments capable of recording exposure, exposure rates, and exposure durations. All portable radiation detection instruments should be calibrated at least annually. A small radioactive check source can be used to verify an instrument's response to radiation.

21.3.1 Geiger-Mueller Survey Instruments

One of the main advantages of GM survey instruments and their probes is that they react quickly during surveys to detect the presence and provide semiquantitative estimates of the intensities of radiation fields. Measurements from GM survey meters typically are in units of counts per minute (cpm) rather than mR/h, because the GM detector does not duplicate the conditions under which exposure is defined. In addition, the relationship between count rate and exposure rate with most GM probes is a complicated function of photon energy. If a GM survey meter is calibrated to indicate exposure rate (most commonly performed using a sealed source containing Cs-137 [662 keV γ-rays]), one should refer to the detector's energy response curve before making quantitative measurements of photons whose energies significantly differ from the energy for which it was calibrated. However, with specialized energy–compensated probes, GM survey instruments can provide approximate measurements of exposure rate (typically in mR/h) over a wide range of photon energies, although with reduced sensitivity. The theory of operation of GM survey instruments was presented in Chapter 17.

A common application of GM survey meters is to perform surveys for radioactive contamination in nuclear medicine. A survey meter coupled to a thin window ($\sim$1.5 to 2 mg/cm^2), large surface area GM probe (called a "pancake" probe) is ideally suited for contamination surveys (see Fig. 17-7). Thin window probes can detect alpha ($>$3 MeV), beta ($>$45 keV), and x- and γ ($>$6 keV) radiations.

These detectors are extremely sensitive to charged particulate radiations with sufficient energy to penetrate the window but are much less sensitive to x- and γ radiations. These detectors will easily detect natural background radiation ($\sim$50 to 100 cpm at sea level). These instruments have long dead-times resulting in significant count losses at high exposure (count) rates. For example, a typical dead time of 100 μs will result in an $\sim$20% loss at 100,000 cpm. Some GM survey instruments will saturate in high-radiation fields and read zero, which, if unrecognized, could result in significant overexposures. Portable GM survey instruments are best suited for low-level contamination surveys and should not be used in high-radiation fields or when accurate measurements of exposure rate are required unless specialized energy–compensated probes or other techniques are used to account for these inherent limitations.

21.3.2 Portable Ionization Chamber Survey Meters

Portable ionization chamber survey meters are used when accurate measurements of radiation exposure rates from x- and γ-rays are required (see Fig. 17-6). These ionization chambers approximate the conditions under which the roentgen is defined (see Chapter 3). They have many applications, including assessment of radiation fields near brachytherapy or radionuclide therapy patients, surveys of radioactive material packages, evaluation of the adequacy of radiation shielding, and measuring radiation fields during incidents in which people may be exposed to high levels of γ radiation. The main advantages of ion chamber survey meters are that they have linear responses over wide ranges of exposure rates and photon energies and that the quantities that they indicate, exposure rate or air kerma rate, are very useful in quickly deterring if an unsafe radiation exposure environment exists. The principles of operation of ion chambers are discussed in Chapter 17.

The ion chambers of some survey meters are filled with ambient air, whereas others have sealed ion chambers. Some of those with sealed chambers are pressurized to increase the sensitivity. The main advantage of measurements with ionization chamber bases instruments is that they are sufficiently accurate ($\pm 10\%$) for the photon energy and exposure rates likely to be encountered in medical imaging or therapy environments. For example, a typical portable ion chamber survey meter will experience only an ~5% loss for exposure rates approaching ~0.44 Gy/h (~50 R/h). Specialized detectors are required to measure higher exposure rates.

All instruments have limitations and susceptibilities that users should be aware of, and ion chambers are no exception. A decrease in sensitivity can occur in the presence of low energy photons due to attenuation by the wall of the ion chamber and, only if the wall surrounds the ion chamber. The magnitude of the loss in sensitivity depends on the thickness of the material around the ion chamber and the energy of the photons (*e.g.*, 30% under response at 20 keV is typical). Most portable ionization chamber survey meters respond slowly to rapidly changing radiation exposure rates. The lower the exposure rate, the longer the time necessary for the instrument to equilibrate and display its most accurate reading (*i.e.*, response time). For example, typical response time for a portable handheld ion chamber in fields at the lower end of its range, ~88 µGy/h (~1 mR/h), is ~8 s while at fields near the maximum of its range, ~0. 44 Gy/h (~50 R/h), the response time drops to ~2 s. Some ionization chambers have a cover over one end of the detector, which serves as a buildup cap to establish electronic equilibrium for accurate measurement of higher-energy x- and γ-rays; it can be removed to improve the accuracy when measuring low-energy x- and γ-rays. Removing the cap also permits assessment of the contribution of beta particles to the radiation field. The slow response time and limited sensitivity of these detectors preclude their use as low-level contamination survey instruments or to locate a lost low-activity radiation source. These instruments must be allowed to warm up and stabilize before accurate measurements can be obtained. Some are also affected by orientation and strong magnetic fields (*e.g.*, MRI scanners).

21.4 FUNDAMENTAL PRINCIPLES AND METHODS OF EXPOSURE CONTROL

21.4.1 Principles of Justification, Optimization, and Limitation as Applied to Medical Imaging and Therapy

The International Commission on Radiological Protection (ICRP) has formulated a set of principles that apply to the practice of radiation protection (ICRP, 2007a, 2007b, 2007c):

- The principle of justification: Any decision that alters the radiation exposure situation, for example, by introducing a new radiation source or by reducing existing exposure, should do more good than harm, that is, yield an individual or societal benefit that is higher than the detriment it causes.

- The principle of optimization of protection: Optimization of protection should ensure the selection of the best protection option under the prevailing circumstances, that is, maximizing the margin of good over harm. Thus, optimization involves keeping exposures ALARA, considering economic and societal factors.
- The principle of limitation of maximum doses: In planned situations, the total dose to any individual from all the regulated sources should not exceed the appropriate regulatory limits.

While the ICRP recommends that the first two principles apply to medical exposure of patients, they do not recommend that the limitation of maximal doses be applied to patient dose from medical imaging or interventional procedures or during emergency situations.

Often the most appropriate way to reduce dose is to not perform an imaging procedure that is not medically warranted. This is key to the application of the principle of justification in medical imaging. The ICRP has identified three levels of justification for a radiological practice in medicine, including medical imaging (ICRP, 2007a, 2007b, 2007c). At the first and most general level, the proper use of radiation in medicine is accepted as doing more good than harm to society; that is, this general level of justification is taken for granted. At the second level, a specified imaging procedure with a specified objective is defined and justified (e.g., chest x-rays for patients showing relevant symptoms) to judge whether the radiological procedure will improve the diagnosis or will provide information necessary to properly treat the patient. At the third level, the application of the procedure to an individual patient should be justified (i.e., the particular application should be judged to do more good than harm to the individual patient). Once a particular procedure has been justified at these levels, then the dose should be optimized for the medical purpose for which it is being performed.

When applied to medical imaging, both the ALARA and the ICRP optimization principles imply using the lowest dose necessary to produce an examination result of appropriate diagnostic quality or, in the case of an image-guided intervention, to achieve the goals of the intervention. Therefore, reducing the examination dose to the point where important diagnostic information is lost or that results in the exam needing to be repeated is counterproductive and increases rather than decreases the overall risk to the patient. This is, in essence, the ALADA concept mentioned earlier.

The American College of Radiology (ACR) promulgates appropriateness criteria as evidence-based guidelines to assist referring physicians and other providers in making the most appropriate imaging or treatment decision for a specific clinical condition (i.e., implementing the principle of Justification). Several institutions have incorporated clinical decision support (CDS) software or applications as part of order entry systems to assist physicians and other clinicians in determining the most appropriate type of imaging exam (e.g., applying ACR appropriateness criteria scores) for a patient with specific symptoms or disease. Studies have shown this produced a significant improvement in imaging study appropriateness scores at some larger medical facilities (Huber et al., 2018, Ip et al., 2012, Sistrom et al., 2014). Implementation of a CDS is discussed in Chapter 5.

21.4.2 Methods of Exposure Control

There are four principal methods by which radiation exposure to persons can be minimized: (1) reducing the time (period) of exposure, (2) increasing distance from the radiation source, (3) shielding the source of the radiation, and

(4) controlling contamination of radioactive material. Although these methods are widely used in radiation protection programs, their application to medical imaging is addressed below.

Time

Although it is obvious that reducing the time spent near a radiation source will reduce one's radiation exposure, techniques to minimize the time in a radiation field are not always recognized or practiced. First, not all sources of radiation produce constant exposure rates. Diagnostic x-ray machines typically produce high exposure rates during brief time intervals. For example, a typical chest x-ray produces an entrance skin exposure of ~0.175 mGy (~20 mR) in less than $1/100$ of a second, an exposure rate of 12.6 Gy/h (1,440 R/h). In this case, exposure is minimized by not activating the x-ray tube when staff are near the radiation source. Nuclear medicine procedures, however, typically produce lower exposure rates for extended periods of time. The time spent near a radiation source can be minimized by having a thorough understanding of the tasks to be performed and the appropriate equipment to complete them in a safe and timely manner. Similarly, radiation exposure to staff and patients can be reduced during fluoroscopy if the operator is proficient in the procedure to be performed, resulting in less x-ray beam-on time.

Distance

The exposure rate from a source of radiation decreases with increasing distance from the source, even in the absence of an attenuating material. In the case of a point source of radiation (*i.e.*, a source whose physical dimensions are much less than the distance from which it is being measured), the exposure rate decreases by the inverse square of the distance between the measurement location and the source. This principle is called *the inverse square law* (ISL) and is the result of the geometric relationship between the surface area (*A*) and the radius (*r*) of a sphere: $A = 4\pi r$. Thus, if one considers an isotropic point radiation source at the center of the sphere, the surface area over which the radiation is distributed increases as the square of the distance from the source (*i.e.*, the radius). If the exposure rate from a point source is X_1 at distance d_1, at another distance d_2 the exposure rate X_2 will be

$$X_2 = X_1 (d_1/d_2)^2.$$

[21-3]

For example, if the exposure rate at 20 cm from a source is 792 μGy/h (90 mR/h), doubling the distance will reduce the exposure by $(1/2)^2 = 1/4$ to 198 μGy/h (22.5 mR/h); increasing the distance to 60 cm decreases the exposure by $(1/3)^2 = 1/9$ to 88 μGy/h (10 mR/h) (Fig. 21-9).

This relationship is only valid for point sources (*i.e.*, sources whose dimensions are small with respect to the distances d_1 and d_2). Thus, this relationship would not be valid near (*e.g.*, <1 m from) a patient injected with radioactive material. In this case, the exposure rate decreases less rapidly than 1/(distance)^2.

This rapid change in radiation intensity with distance is familiar to all who have held their hand over a heat source, such as a stovetop or candle flame. There is only a fairly narrow range over which the infrared (thermal, non-ionizing) radiation felt is comfortable. A little closer and the heat is intolerable; a little further away and the heat is barely perceptible. Infrared radiation, like all electromagnetic radiation, follows the inverse square law. The intensity of light, sound, and gravity also obeys the ISL law, as do other quantities.

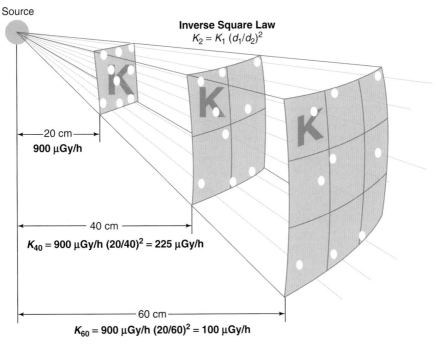

Source

Inverse Square Law
$$K_2 = K_1 (d_1/d_2)^2$$

20 cm
900 μGy/h

40 cm
$$K_{40} = 900 \text{ μGy/h } (20/40)^2 = 225 \text{ μGy/h}$$

60 cm
$$K_{60} = 900 \text{ μGy/h } (20/60)^2 = 100 \text{ μGy/h}$$

■ **FIGURE 21-9** The inverse square law, showing the decreasing air kerma rate with distance from a point source.

Scattered radiation from a patient, x-ray tabletop, or shield is also a source of personnel radiation exposure. For diagnostic energy x-rays, a good rule of thumb is that at 1 m from a patient at 90° to the incident beam, the radiation intensity is approximately 0.1% to 0.15% (0.001 to 0.0015) of the intensity of the beam incident upon the patient for a 400 cm² x-ray field area on the patient (typical field area for fluoroscopy). All personnel should stand as far away from the patient as practicable during x-ray imaging procedures and behind a shielded barrier or out of the room, whenever possible. The NCRP recommends that personnel should stand at least 2 m from the x-ray tube and the patient during radiography with mobile equipment (NCRP, 1989b).

Due to the higher photon energies emitted from most of the radionuclides used in nuclear medicine, it is often not practical to shield the technologist from the radiation emitted from the patient during a nuclear medicine exam (see "Shielding"). Distance is the primary dose reduction technique. The majority of nuclear medicine technologist's annual whole-body radiation dose is received during patient imaging. Imaging rooms should be designed to allow a large distance between the imaging table and the computer terminal where the technologist spends most of the time during image acquisition and processing.

Shielding

Shielding is used in diagnostic radiology and nuclear medicine to reduce exposures of patients, staff, and the public. The decision to utilize shielding, and its type, thickness, and location for a particular application, are functions of the photon energy, intensity and geometry of the radiation sources, exposure limits at various locations, and other factors. The principles of attenuation of x- and γ-rays are reviewed in Chapter 3.

Shielding may be installed in a wall, floor, or ceiling of a room; this is commonly done for rooms containing x-ray imaging machines and PET/CT and SPECT/CT systems, and sometimes rooms housing patients who have been administered large activities of radiopharmaceuticals. Shielding may be in the walls of a cabinet used to store radioactive sources, around a work area, such as the dose preparation area in a nuclear medicine radiopharmacy. Shielding containers or enclosures may be used for individual sources such as an x-ray tube or a vial or syringe containing radioactive material. Shielding is incorporated behind the image receptors of fluoroscopes and radiographic machines and in the gantries of CT devices. Shielding is also worn as personal protective equipment (PPE) in the form of protective aprons, leaded glasses, and thyroid collars during fluoroscopy. Additional movable shielding is available in the form of freestanding and ceiling-mounted (often transparent lead acrylic) shields in fluoroscopic procedure rooms.

The maximum energy of x-rays from machines used for diagnostic and interventional imaging typically does not exceed ~140 keV and the average energy of the x-ray spectrum is much less. The annihilation photons used in PET have energies of 511 keV and require the use of a high atomic number material for shielding such as lead to enhance photoelectric absorption thus reducing the thickness of the shielding compared to lower density materials. The energy of the γ-rays emitted by the other radionuclides used in nuclear medicine are typically less than 365 keV, although some radionuclides emit higher-energy γ-rays of low abundance. In general, placing shielding closer to a source of radiation does not reduce the thickness needed, but does reduce the mass of shielding necessary by reducing the area requiring shielding.

Design of Medical Imaging Facilities

Shielding is an important radiation safety consideration during the design phase of a medical facility whether it is an entire medical center, a radiology or interventional cardiology or nuclear medicine department, or a PET/CT imaging suite. For example, the weight of shielding, particularly for PET/CT facilities, must be supported by the building structure. Placing rooms, that would otherwise require heavy shielding, such as the PET/CT imaging room or PET uptake rooms, against the outside or corner walls of a building can substantially reduce the amount of shielding needed. Locating such rooms on the ground floor of a building obviates the need to install shielding below. Siting rooms of low occupancy, such as supply storage rooms, adjacent to imaging rooms can also reduce shielding requirements. The radiopharmacy should be located near injection and imaging rooms. Also, it is important to treat the location of nuclear medicine patient waiting areas (often occupied by patients containing radioactive material) as a source of radiation from which exposure to others should be kept ALARA.

21.5   STRUCTURAL SHIELDING OF IMAGING FACILITIES

The purpose of radiation shielding of rooms containing x-ray machines is to limit radiation exposures of employees and members of the public to acceptable levels. Several factors must be considered when determining the amount and type of radiation shielding. Personnel exposures may not exceed limits established by regulatory agencies. Furthermore, personnel radiation exposures must be kept ALARA.

Methods and technical information for the design of shielding for diagnostic and interventional x-ray rooms are found in NCRP Report No. 147, *Structural Shielding Design for Medical X-Ray Imaging Facilities* (NCRP, 2004). The recommended quantity for shielding design calculations is *air kerma* (K), with the unit of Gy; typical annual amounts of air kerma in occupied areas are commonly expressed in mGy. The recommended radiation protection quantity for the limitation of exposure of people to sources of ionizing radiation is *effective dose* (E), defined as the sum of the weighted equivalent doses to specific organs or tissues (the equivalent dose to each organ or tissue being multiplied by a corresponding tissue weighting factor, w_T), expressed in Sv (see Chapter 3 for definition); for protection purposes, typical levels of E are expressed in mSv.

Areas to be protected by shielding are designated as *controlled* and *uncontrolled areas*; a controlled area is an area to which access is controlled for the purpose of radiation protection and in which the occupational exposure of personnel to radiation is under the supervision of a person responsible for radiation protection. Controlled areas, such as procedure rooms and control booths, may contain the x-ray and nuclear medicine imaging devices or are usually in the immediate vicinity. The workers in controlled areas are usually radiologic technologists, nurses, radiologists, and other physicians trained in the use of ionizing radiation and whose radiation exposures are typically individually monitored. Uncontrolled areas for radiation protection purposes are most other areas in the hospital or clinic, such as offices adjacent to x-ray rooms.

Shielding design goals, P, are amounts of air kerma delivered over a specified time at a stated reference point that is used in the design and evaluation of barriers constructed for the protection of employees and members of the general public from a medical x-ray or radionuclide imaging source or sources. Shielding design goals are stated in terms of K (mGy) at a reference point beyond a protective barrier (*e.g.*, 0.3 m for a wall, a conservative assumption of the distance of closest approach). Because of conservative assumptions, achieving the design goals will ensure that the respective annual recommended values for E are not exceeded. The relationship between E and K is complex and depends on several factors, including the x-ray energy spectrum and the posture (*e.g.*, standing or sitting) of the exposed individual. Because E cannot be directly measured, it is impractical to use it for a shielding design goal, and therefore, shielding design goals P are stated in terms of K.

There are different shielding design goals for controlled and uncontrolled areas. Radiation workers, typically employees, have significant potential for exposure to radiation in the course of their jobs, and as a result, are subject to routine monitoring by personal dosimeters. On the other hand, many people in uncontrolled areas have not voluntarily chosen to be irradiated and may not be aware that they are being irradiated. NCRP Report No. 147 recommends that the shielding design goal P for controlled areas be 5 mGy per year and that for uncontrolled areas be 1 mGy per year. These are equivalent to shielding design goals, P, of 0.1 mGy per week for controlled areas, and 0.02 mGy per week for uncontrolled areas.

There are also air-kerma design goals for stored radiographic film and loaded film-screen cassettes to avoid film fogging. A shielding design goal, P, less than 0.1 mGy is recommended for the period in which radiographic film is stored. Since loaded screen-film cassettes and CR cassettes awaiting use are more sensitive to radiation, a P not to exceed 0.5 µGy for the period of storage (on the order of a few days) is recommended.

These shielding design methods are based upon conservative assumptions that will result in the actual air kerma transmitted through each barrier being much less than the applicable shielding design goal. These assumptions include (1) neglecting the attenuation of the primary x-ray beam by the patient (the patient typically attenuates the x-ray beam by a factor of 10 to 100); (2) assuming perpendicular incidence of the radiation on the barrier, which has the greatest transmission through the barrier; (3) ignoring the presence of other attenuating materials in the path of the radiation; (4) assuming a large x-ray beam field size for scattered radiation levels; and (5) assuming high occupancy factors for uncontrolled areas.

Shielding designed by these methods will keep the effective doses or effective dose equivalents received by workers in these areas much less than a tenth of the current occupational dose limits in the United States, will keep the dose to an embryo or fetus of a pregnant worker much less than 5 mGy over the duration of gestation, and will keep the effective doses to members of the public and employees, who are not considered radiation workers, less than 1 mSv per year.

21.5.1   Sources of Exposure

The sources of exposure that must be shielded in a diagnostic or interventional x-ray room are *primary radiation*, *scattered radiation*, and *leakage radiation* (Fig. 21-10).

Scatter and leakage radiation are together called *secondary* or *stray radiation*. Primary radiation, also called the *useful beam,* is the radiation passing through the open area defined by the collimator of the x-ray source. The amount of primary radiation depends on the output of the x-ray tube (determined by the kV, mGy/mAs, and mAs) per examination, the average number of examinations performed during a week, the fraction of time the x-ray beam is directed toward any particular barrier, the distance to the point to be protected, and the presence (or absence) of a primary barrier built into the imaging equipment. Scattered radiation arises from the interaction of the useful beam with the patient, causing a portion of the primary x-rays to be redirected. For radiation protection purposes scatter is considered as a separate radiation source with essentially the same photon energy spectrum (and penetrability) as the primary beam. In general, the exposure from scattered radiation at 1 m from the patient is approximately 0.1% to 0.15% of the incident exposure to the patient for typical diagnostic x-ray energies with a 20 cm × 20 cm (400 cm²) field area. The scattered radiation is proportional to the field size and can be calculated as a fraction of the reference field area. For CT applications, the rectangular collimation over a smaller volume will have a distinct scattered radiation distribution and is considered separately, as discussed below. Leakage is the radiation that emanates from the x-ray

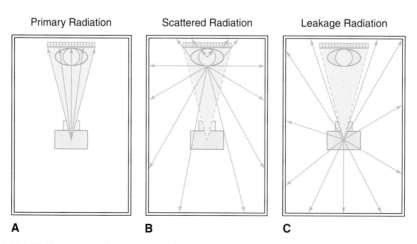

■ **FIGURE 21-10** The sources of exposure in a diagnostic x-ray room. **A.** Primary radiation emanating from the focal spot. **B.** Scattered radiation emanating from the patient. **C.** Leakage radiation emanating from the x-ray tube housing (other than the collimated primary radiation).

tube housing other than the useful beam. Because leakage radiation passes through the shielding of the housing, its effective energy is very high (only the highest energy photons are transmitted). The exposure due to leakage radiation is limited by FDA regulations to 0.88 mGy/h (100 mR/h) at 1 m from the tube housing when the x-ray tube is operated at the maximum allowable continuous tube current (usually 3 to 5 mA) at the maximum rated tube potential, typically 150 kV.

The primary and secondary radiation exposure of an individual in an adjacent area to be protected depends primarily on (1) the amount of radiation produced by the source; (2) the distance between the patient and the radiation source; (3) the amount of time a given individual spends in an adjacent area; (4) the amount of protective shielding between the source of radiation and the individual; and (5) the distance between the source of radiation and the individual.

21.5.2 Types of Medical X-ray Imaging Facilities

General purpose radiographic installations produce intermittent radiographic exposures using tube potentials of 50 to 150 kV, with the x-ray beam directed toward the patient and the image receptor. Depending on the type of procedures, a large fraction of the exposures will be directed towards the floor or to an upright image receptor, and sometimes to other barriers (as in cross-table lateral image acquisitions). Barriers that can intercept the unattenuated primary beam are considered primary barriers. A protected control area for the technologist is required, with the ability to observe and communicate with the patient. The viewing window of the control booth should be of similar attenuation as the wall and large enough to allow unobstructed viewing. The configuration of the room should not depend on the control area shielding as a primary barrier, and in no situation should there be an unprotected direct line of sight from the patient or x-ray tube to the x-ray machine operator or loaded CR cassettes, regardless of the distance from the radiation sources. Also, the switch that energizes the x-ray tube should be installed so that the operator cannot stand outside of the shielded area and activate the switch.

Fluoroscopic imaging systems are typically operated over a range of 60 to 120 kV. Since the image receptor is designed to also be a primary barrier, only secondary radiation barriers need to be considered in the shielding design. In some cases, a radiographic and fluoroscopic combined unit is installed, and the shielding requirements are based on the combination of the workloads of both units. In this case, the radiographic room issues discussed above must also be considered.

Interventional facilities include angiography and vascular interventional, neuroangiography, and cardiovascular and electrophysiology imaging suites. Like other fluoroscopic rooms, the walls, floors, and ceilings of interventional suites are considered to be secondary radiation barriers. However, they may have multiple x-ray tubes and the procedures often require long fluoroscopy times and include cine and digital fluorography image sequences that have large workload factors and so the rooms may require more shielding than general fluoroscopy rooms.

A dedicated chest radiography installation has the x-ray tube directed at the image receptor assembly on a particular barrier all of the time. Since the receptor can be used at various heights above the floor, the area behind the image receptor from the finished floor to a height of 2.1 m (7 ft) must be considered to be a primary barrier. All other areas in this room are secondary barriers, and any portion of the wall that the primary beam cannot be directed toward can also be considered a secondary barrier.

Mammography employs a very low kV in the range of 25 to 35 kV, and the breast support provides the primary barrier for the incident radiation. Thus, radiation barriers protect from secondary radiation only and given the low x-ray energies and the small volume of tissue irradiated, often all that is needed in a permanent mammography room is the installation of a second layer of gypsum wallboard. Doors for mammography rooms might need special consideration because wood attenuates much less than typical gypsum wallboard; a metal door may be advisable. For operator safety, mammography systems have transparent lead acrylic barriers to protect the control area.

CT uses a collimated x-ray fan beam intercepted by the patient and by the detector array; thus, only secondary radiation reaches protective barriers. The x-ray tube voltage used for most scans is 120 kV, over a range of 80 to 140 kV. As mentioned in Chapter 10, modern wide-beam multirow detector CT scanners (MDCTs) make more efficient use of the radiation produced by the x-ray tubes than did the now-obsolete single detector row scanners. MDCTs can perform extensive scanning without exceeding their heat limits, allowing more procedures per day, more contrast phases per procedure, and scans that cover more patient anatomy. Although the amount of scattered radiation per equivalent scan is not significantly more than that produced by a single-row scanner, a large number of scans per day can require a greater thickness of shielding for walls, and perhaps even additional shielding of floors and ceilings. Secondary scatter emanating from the scanner is not isotropic, as there are much higher radiation levels along the axis of the patient table than in the direction of the gantry (see Fig. 21-14). Assuming an isotropic scatter distribution is conservative in terms of the amount of shielding for the various barriers in a room, it provides flexibility for future CT scanner installations when different orientations are considered.

Mobile radiography and fluoroscopy systems (used in situations in which patients cannot be transported to fixed imaging systems or used in operating rooms or intensive care units) present a challenge for protecting nearby individuals. For bedside radiography, protection is chiefly accomplished by maintaining a distance from the source of radiation and keeping the primary beam directed away from anyone nearby. For mobile fluoroscopy, all individuals within 2 m of the patient should wear protective aprons, and if available, protective mobile shielding should be positioned between the patient and attending personnel. If a mobile system is routinely used in a particular room, there should be an evaluation of doses to adjacent areas to determine if additional shielding is necessary.

A *bone mineral densitometry x-ray system* typically uses a well-collimated scanning beam and, due to the low beam intensity and correspondingly low x-ray scatter, such a scanner will not produce scattered radiation levels above 1 mGy per year at 1 m for a busy facility, which is the shielding design goal for a fully occupied, uncontrolled area (NCRP, 2004). While structural shielding is not required in most situations, most states require a shielding evaluation demonstrating that fact to be submitted. The control console should be placed as far away as practicable to minimize exposure to the operator.

Dental and veterinary x-ray facilities require special consideration depending on the scope and unique attributes of the procedures. The NCRP has published reports that describe shielding and radiation protection requirements for these facilities. For these and all other applications and future developments, sources of ionizing radiation should be evaluated by a qualified expert in order to determine the type and nature of the shielding required in the facility.

21.5.3 Shielding Materials

X-ray shielding is accomplished by interposing an attenuating barrier between the source(s) of radiation and the area to be protected in order to reduce the exposures to below acceptable limits. The thickness of shielding needed to achieve the desired attenuation depends on the shielding material selected. Lead is the most commonly used material because of its high-attenuation properties and relatively low cost. Commercially available thicknesses of lead sheet are commonly specified in nominal weight per area (in pounds per square foot), with corresponding thicknesses specified in inches and millimeters, as shown in Figure 21-11. The actual masses per area are considerably less than the nominal values. The least thickness commonly installed is 2 lb/ft² equal to 1/32 inch or 0.79 mm; there are little cost savings from using a lesser thickness. Other thicknesses and relative costs are compared in the figure. For typical shielding installations, the lead sheet is glued to a sheet of gypsum wallboard and installed with nails or screws on wood or metal studs. Where the edges of two lead sheets meet, continuity of shielding must be ensured by overlapping lead, as well as for gaps and inclusions in the wall (*e.g.*, electrical junction boxes and switches).

Other shielding materials are also used, such as gypsum wallboard, concrete, glass, leaded glass, and leaded acrylic. Gypsum wallboard (sheetrock) is used for wall construction in medical facilities, and a nominal 5/8 inch thickness (14 mm minimum) is most often used. While there is little protection provided at higher energies, significant attenuation occurs at the low x-ray energies used for mammography. Because of possible non-uniformity of the gypsum sheets, it is prudent to specify an extra layer (*e.g.*, two sheets of wallboard) when using this material for shielding. Concrete is a common construction material used in floors, wall panels, and roofs, and is usually specified as standard-weight (147 lb/ft³, 2.4 g/cm³) or lightweight (115 lb/ft³, 1.8 g/cm³). The concrete density must be known to determine the thickness needed to provide the necessary attenuation. When concrete is poured on a ribbed-profile steel deck, the thickness is not constant, and the minimum concrete thickness should be used for attenuation specifications. Glass, leaded glass, and leaded acrylic are transparent shielding materials. Ordinary plate glass may be used when protection requirements are low; its attenuation may be increased by laminating two or more 6-mm glass sections. More common and useful are leaded glass

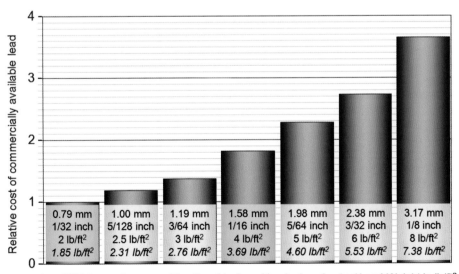

Lead Thickness in mm and fractional inches; Nominal *and actual* Lead Weight in lb/ft²

■ **FIGURE 21-11** Relative cost of commercially available lead (Adapted with permission from National Council on Radiation Protection and Measurements. *Structural Shielding Design for Medical X-Ray Imaging Facilities.* NCRP Report No. 147. Bethesda, MD: National Council on Radiation Protection and Measurements; 2004, rev 2005. http://NCRPonline.org.). Lead is commercially sold by nominal weight in pounds per square foot (lb/ft²). Equivalent thickness in inches and millimeters are also stated. The height of each bar is the relative cost of lead sheet compared to 2 lb/ft², normalized to a value of 1.

(glass with a high lead content) and leaded acrylic (impregnated with lead during manufacturing) that are specified in various thicknesses of lead equivalence, such as 0.5, 0.8, 1.0, and 1.5 mm.

21.5.4 Computation of X-ray Imaging Shielding Requirements

Terminology

As stated above, the shielding design goals, P, are 0.1 mGy/wk for controlled areas and 0.02 mGy/wk for uncontrolled areas. The distance from the radiation source to the nearest approach to the barrier of the sensitive organs of a person in the occupied area must be chosen; the point of closest approach to the barrier is assumed to be 0.3 m for a wall, 1.7 m above the floor below, and, for transmission through the ceiling, at least 0.5 m above the floor of the room above, as shown in Figure 21-12.

The occupancy factor, T, for an area is defined as the average fraction of time that the maximally exposed individual is present while the x-ray beam is on. The maximally exposed individuals will usually be employees of the facility, or residents or employees of an adjacent facility. Recommended values for T are listed in Table 21-3, for use when information about actual occupancy for a specific situation is not known. The occupancy factor modifies the shielding design goal allowable at a given point by $1/T$; in other words, the attenuation of a barrier must lower the radiation to a level given by the ratio P/T.

The *workload* (W) is the time integral of the x-ray tube current in milliampere-minutes over a period of 1 week (mA-min/wk). In NCRP Report No. 147, a normalized average workload per patient, W_{norm}, is also described; it includes multiple exposures depending on the type of radiographic exam and clinical goal. The total workload per week, W_{tot}, is the product of W_{norm} and the average number of patients per week (N).

Unlike earlier shielding methods that assumed a single, fixed high kV value for the workload, the *workload distribution* described in NCRP Report No. 147 is a function of the kV, which is spread over a wide range of operating potentials for extremity examinations (*e.g.*, about 1/3 of the total exams in a general radiographic room) at

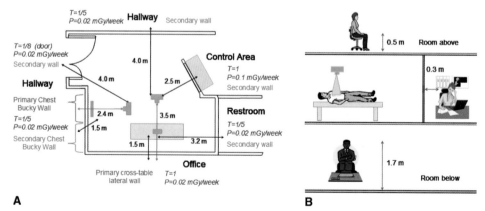

A   **B**

■ **FIGURE 21-12 A.** Floor plan of a general-purpose radiographic room shows the location of the x-ray source, orientation and location of the x-ray beam for various acquisitions, and the adjacent areas with typical occupancy factors, T; shielding design goals, P; and an indication of primary and secondary barriers. Distances to each barrier are determined for the primary beam, leakage radiation from the x-ray tube, and scattered radiation from the patient. For secondary radiation, the closest distance is used. **B.** The elevation diagram provides information to determine the distances to adjacent areas above and below the x-ray room to be shielded. The floor-to-floor heights in multi-story buildings must be known.

TABLE 21-3 SUGGESTED OCCUPANCY FACTORS FOR ADJACENT AREAS

OCCUPANCY LEVEL	LOCATION	OCCUPANCY FACTOR (T)
Full	Administrative or clerical offices; laboratories, pharmacies, and other work areas fully occupied by an individual; receptionist areas, attended waiting rooms, children's indoor play areas, adjacent x-ray rooms, film-reading areas, nurse's stations, x-ray control rooms	1
Partial	Rooms used for patient examinations and treatments	1/2
	Corridors, patient rooms, employee lounges, staff restrooms	1/5
	Corridor doors	1/8
Occasional	Public toilets, unattended vending areas, storage rooms, outdoor areas with seating, unattended waiting rooms, patient holding areas	1/20
	Outdoor areas with only transient pedestrian or vehicular traffic, unattended parking lots, vehicular drop-off areas (unattended), attics, stairways, unattended elevators, janitor's closets	1/40

Reprinted with permission from National Council on Radiation Protection and Measurements. *Structural Shielding Design for Medical X-Ray Imaging Facilities.* NCRP Report No. 147. Bethesda, MD: National Council on Radiation Protection and Measurements; 2004, rev 2005. http://NCRPonline.org.

50 to 60 kV, abdominal exams at 70 to 80 kV, and chest exams at greater than 100 kV (with reduced tube current-time product). Workload distributions are specific for a given type of radiological installation, including radiographic room (all barriers, chest bucky, floor, or other barriers), fluoroscopy tube (R&F room), radiographic tube (R&F room), chest room, mammography room, cardiac angiography, and peripheral angiography. For shielding design, the magnitude of the workload is less important than the distribution of the workload as a function of kV, since attenuation properties of the barriers have a strong kV dependence.

The *use factor* (U) is the fraction of the primary beam workload that is directed toward a given primary barrier and will depend on the type of radiographic room and the orientation of the equipment. In a dedicated chest room, the primary barrier has $U = 1$, since the x-ray beam is always directed toward the wall-mounted chest receptor, and all other walls are secondary radiation barriers. In a general radiographic room, U must be estimated for the types of procedures and the amount of time the x-ray beam will be used for a specific orientation. Most often, the x-ray beam is pointed at the floor for acquiring images with patients on the table, occasionally pointed at a wall for a cross-table acquisition, and pointed at a chest receptor stand for a combined room. For a general radiographic room, a survey of clinical sites (NCRP Report No. 147) yielded, for radiography not using a vertical chest receptor, $U = 0.89$ for the floor, $U = 0.09$; for the cross-table lateral wall, and $U = 0.02$ for an unspecified wall; for procedures using a vertical chest receptor stand, $U = 1$ for the chest receptor stand; and $U = 0$ for the ceiling and the control area barrier in that same room. For fluoroscopy and mammography, the primary beam stop is the image receptor assembly, so $U = 0$ and only secondary radiation must be considered.

The *primary barrier*, found in radiographic, dedicated chest, and radiographic-fluoroscopic rooms, is designed to attenuate the primary beam to the shielding design goal. Unshielded primary air kerma at the point to be protected per week is dependent on the average number of patients per week (N), the use factor (U) for that barrier, the primary air kerma per patient at 1 m, and the distance to the point (inverse square law correction is applied).

The *secondary barrier* is designed to attenuate the unshielded secondary air kerma from leakage and scatter radiation to the shielding design goal (or less). All walls not considered primary barriers are secondary barriers. Scattered radiation from the patient increases with the intensity and area of the useful beam and is a function of the scattering angle. The total contribution from unshielded secondary air kerma, proportional to W_{tot}, is calculated from the clinical workload distributions, determined at 1 m, and modified by the inverse square law to the distance of the point to be protected, similar to that described for primary radiation. In certain orientations such as lateral acquisitions, the distance from the scattering source (the patient) will be different than the distance from the leakage radiation source (the x-ray tube) to the point to be protected.

Example Shielding Calculation

Room diagrams of a radiographic room are shown in Figure 21-12, with distances in meters from each of the radiation sources (primary, x-ray tube leakage, and scatter from the patient), as well as adjacent areas that are defined in terms of T, P, and primary or secondary barriers.

There are many complexities involved in calculating the necessary attenuation of the primary and secondary barriers to achieve the shielding design goals that are beyond the scope of this book. Many of the details regarding workloads, workload distributions, normalized workloads per patient (W_{norm}), field size area, attenuation of primary radiation by the image receptor, and other nuances are incorporated into shielding thickness charts found in NCRP Report No. 147, which display the required shielding thicknesses for the various barriers as a function of $N \times T/(P \times d^2)$, where, as stated previously, N is the number of patients per week, T is the occupancy factor (see Table 21-3), P is the shielding design goal in mGy/wk, and d is the distance in meters from the radiation source to the point to be protected. In abbreviated notation, this is NT/Pd^2. These charts, which assume specific normalized workloads per patient (W_{norm}) as described in NCRP Report No. 147, are provided for radiographic and radiographic/fluoroscopic rooms for both lead and concrete shielding materials. If the site-normalized workload per patient (W_{site}) is different, then the values of NT/Pd^2 are scaled by W_{site}/W_{norm}. Primary beam use factors U are identified by specific curves in each chart for primary barriers.

Three of these charts are shown in Figure 21-13 for a radiographic room, considering (A) no primary beam preshielding, (B) primary beam preshielding, and (C) secondary radiation. The required lead thickness in millimeters is a function of NT/Pd^2. The term "preshielding" refers to the attenuation of the primary beam by the image receptor. The graphs for primary beam preshielding consider the attenuation of the image receptor in the radiographic table or wall-mounted cassette holder due to the grid, cassette, and support structures, equivalent to 0.85 mm lead, and for cross-table laterals, attenuation due to the grid and cassette, equivalent to 0.3 mm lead. Note the decreased requirement for lead thickness with primary beam preshielding (*e.g.*, for the chest bucky wall barrier and $NT/Pd^2 = 1,000$, without preshielding the thickness is 1.95 mm lead and with preshielding is 1.13 mm lead, as shown in Fig. 21-13A and B, respectively).

For determination of barrier thicknesses using NT/Pd^2 methods, scale drawings of the room, including elevation drawings, location of the equipment, designations of adjacent areas as controlled or uncontrolled, occupancy factors of adjacent areas,

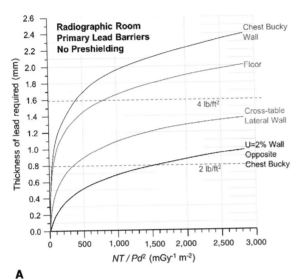

A

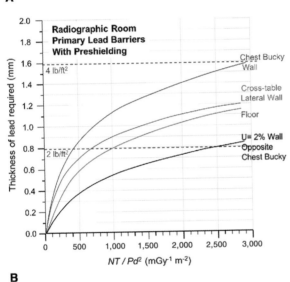

B

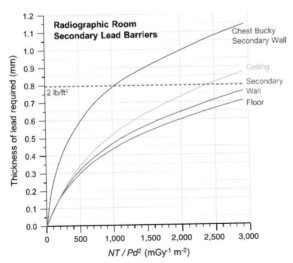

C

■ **FIGURE 21-13** Required lead barrier thickness for a radiographic room as a function of NT/Pd^2, using $W_{norm} = 0.6$ mA min patient^{-1} for the chest bucky and 1.9 mA min/patient for the floor and other barriers. **A.** No preshielding for primary barriers. **B.** Preshielding for primary barriers. **C.** Secondary lead barriers. In each of the graphs, the horizontal dotted lines indicate the common lead thicknesses of 0.79 and 1.58 mm, corresponding to 2 and 4 lb/ft^2 lead sheet. (Adapted with permission from National Council on Radiation Protection and Measurements. *Structural Shielding Design for Medical X-Ray Imaging Facilities.* NCRP Report No. 147. Bethesda, MD: National Council on Radiation Protection and Measurements; 2004, rev 2005. http://NCRPonline.org.)

and distances to adjacent areas are necessary, in addition to the average number of patients, N, per week. Charts are selected according to room type and shielding materials. For example, using the diagrams in Figure 21-12, if $N = 120$ patients per week for a general radiographic room, then NT/Pd^2 can be calculated for each barrier and the required lead thickness is determined from the graph. For the chest bucky wall primary radiation barrier with $T = 0.2$, $P = 0.02$ mGy/wk, and $d = 2.4$ m, $NT/Pd^2 = 120 \times 0.2/(0.02 \times 2.4^2) = 208$ and, using the blue curve labeled chest bucky wall, the lead thickness required is about 1.3 mm to achieve the shielding design goal. Therefore, the primary barrier to be installed is specified as 4 lb/ft^2 (1.6 mm) over the indicated area, which is from the finished floor to a height of 2.1 m (7 ft), with lateral margins around the image receptor of at least 0.5 m (e.g., a leaded drywall sheet 4 ft wide).

Shielding for secondary barriers is determined in a similar manner; however, because the total amount of secondary radiation emanates from a variety of locations and distances, the calculations can be very complex. A conservative approach is to assume that all of the secondary radiation in the room emanates from the closest distance to the barrier, which would increase the shielding thickness. Thus, for the wall adjacent to the chest wall bucky designated as a secondary barrier, the closest distance is 1.5 m, and $NT/Pd^2 = 120 \times 0.2/(0.02 \times 1.5^2) = 533$. From Figure 21-13C, the thickness of lead (using the chest bucky secondary wall curve) is about 0.6 mm, and therefore the secondary barrier is specified as 2 lb/ft^2, installed continuously and seamlessly with the adjacent primary radiation barrier. For the control area barrier with $T = 1$, $P = 0.1$ mGy/wk, $d = 2.5$ m, $NT/Pd^2 = 120 \times 1/(0.1 \times 2.5^2) = 192$, and using the curve labeled "secondary wall," the lead thickness is 0.15 mm, so 2 lb/ft^2 of lead is specified. For the control area window, leaded acrylic is often used and would be specified as having an equivalent attenuation as the surrounding wall of 2 lb/ft^2 or 0.8 mm lead. Note that in these situations, the conservative approach ensures more than adequate protection for individuals in adjacent areas and allows for increased room workload in the future. The shielding for each other radiation barrier, including doors, the floor, and the ceiling, is similarly calculated and specified.

In walls, the shielding (e.g., leaded drywall, leaded doors, leaded acrylic, and sheet lead) is usually installed from the finished floor to a height of 2.1 m (7 ft) with overlapping lead at the seams of at least 1 cm, and lead backing at electrical outlets and other access points (electrical junction boxes, plumbing, etc.) into the wall to ensure continuous protection. Attachment screws used for mounting leaded drywall do not need lead backing (the steel that displaces the lead combined with the length of the screw provides adequate attenuation), but care must be taken to ensure that the screws that penetrate the lead sheet remain in place to maintain shielding integrity.

Surveys after Shielding Installation

After installation of shielding, a radiation protection survey should be performed by a qualified expert to ensure the adequacy of the installed shielding. The survey should verify that the barriers are contiguous and free of voids and defects and provide sufficient attenuation to meet the relevant shielding design goal divided by the occupancy factor (P/T). Visual inspection during installation should be part of the evaluation, followed by transmission measurements using a γ-ray source of suitable energy (e.g., Tc-99m) and a detector with high sensitivity and fast response (e.g., GM survey meter). Alternatively, the x-ray source in the room can be used to generate a primary beam and secondary radiation, and measurements performed with a suitable high-sensitivity integrating survey meter.

Computed Tomography Scanner Shielding

For a CT scanner, all walls in the room are secondary barriers, because the detector array within the gantry is the primary radiation barrier. The scatter distribution emanating from the scanner is highly directional, being highest along the scanner axis (Fig. 21-14). Because most CT scans are acquired at 120 and 140 kV with a highly filtered beam, the scattered radiation is highly penetrating. Three methods can be used to determine the shielding requirements, one based upon $CTDI_{vol}$, another based upon typical dose length product (DLP) values per acquisition, and the third based on the measured scatter distribution isodose maps provided by the manufacturer. For instance, using typical values for DLP, the scatter intensity (air kerma in mGy/acquisition) at 1 m is estimated for head and body scans, and then multiplied by the number of acquisitions (much greater than the number of patients due to multiple acquisitions being performed of many patients) expected over a typical work week for an 8-h shift (the busiest shift if the scanner is operated over extended hours). This is the total unshielded peak air kerma at 1 m from the gantry. For each barrier, the distance from the gantry to the calculation point beyond the barrier is determined, and the inverse square law is applied. A thickness of shielding is then determined to

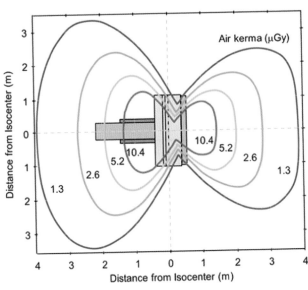

■ **FIGURE 21-14** Secondary (scatter and leakage) radiation distributions for a 32-cm-diameter PMMA phantom, 40-mm collimation, 64-channel MDCT, 140 kV, 100 mA, 1 s scan. Actual secondary radiation levels must be scaled to the techniques used for the acquisition. **A.** Horizontal isodose scatter distribution at the height of the isocenter. **B.** Elevational isodose scatter distribution; the distribution is vertically symmetric above and below the level of the table.

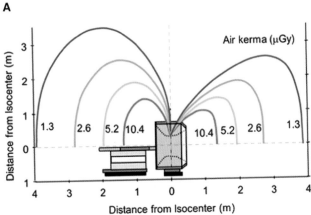

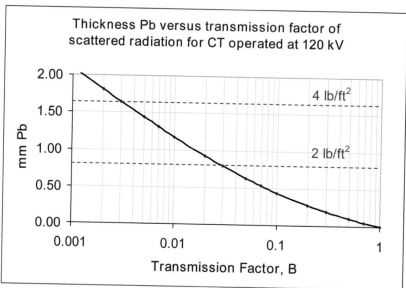

■ FIGURE 21-15 Lead thickness as a function of transmission factor for secondary radiation from a CT scanner operated at 120 kV. (Reprinted with permission from National Council on Radiation Protection and Measurements. *Structural Shielding Design for Medical X-Ray Imaging Facilities*. NCRP Report No. 147. Bethesda, MD: National Council on Radiation Protection and Measurements; 2004, rev 2005. http://NCRPonline.org.)

reduce the radiation level to the design goal modified by the inverse of the occupancy factor (P/T) by the use of specific transmission charts (Fig. 21-15).

Example Barrier Calculation for a CT Scanner

A CT scanner performs 125 head procedures/wk and 150 body procedures/wk using a tube voltage of 120 kV and produces a scatter air kerma of 63.8 mGy/wk at 1 m from the gantry isocenter. A barrier that is 3.3 m (11 ft) from the gantry isocenter to an uncontrolled corridor with $P = 0.02$ mGy/wk and an occupancy factor $T = 0.2$ requires a transmission factor to reduce the radiation to a level less than $P/T = 0.02/0.2 = 0.1$ mGy/wk. At 3.3 m, the unshielded air kerma is $63.8/3.3^2 = 5.86$ mGy/wk, and the transmission factor through the lead must, therefore, be less than $0.1/5.86 = 0.017$. Consulting Fig. 21-15, this transmission factor requires a minimum of 1.0 mm lead. This is greater than 2 lb/ft, so 4 lb/ft² is specified for this barrier. The shielding for other barriers of the CT scanner room is calculated similarly. For the floors and ceilings, a transmission chart with varying thicknesses of concrete should be used; if the thickness of concrete is insufficient, a sheet of lead should be installed above or below the concrete.

For multirow detector array scanners with collimator widths of 40 mm (and in some cases greater, up to 160 mm), the amount of scatter per gantry rotation for a specific kV and mAs will typically be much higher than that of a single-slice scanner. However, because of the increased axial coverage per rotation, the total mAs per scan will be a fraction of the single-slice scanner's, on the order of two to four times lower, and thus, the amount of scatter per scan will be comparable. On the other hand, the acquisition speed allows a larger number of patients to be scanned, which can significantly increase the total amount of scatter that must be considered for shielding calculations. It is therefore prudent to determine the shielding for the peak patient workloads expected over a given work shift (8 h is typical, but in some cases, this can be up to 12 h on the job) to ensure adequate protection from secondary radiation in adjacent areas. Dose-reducing features on CT scanners, such as automatic tube current modulation, may reduce shielding requirements.

PET/CT and SPECT/CT Shielding

Most PET today is performed using the radiopharmaceutical F-18 fluorodeoxyglu-cose (FDG). In PET imaging with F-18 FDG, the radiopharmaceutical is adminis-tered to a patient, the patient rests for a period of about 45 to 90 min to allow uptake by cells and washout from other physiologic compartments, the patient urinates to remove activity from the bladder, and then the patient is imaged. The installation of shielding must be considered for the room containing the PET/CT system and for the uptake rooms where patients rest after radiopharmaceutical administration and before imaging. It is common for a PET/CT facility to have three uptake rooms per PET/CT system because a modern PET/CT system can scan about three patients an hour. Required shielding depends upon the patient workload, the activity adminis-tered per patient, the uses of areas near the PET/CT room and uptake rooms, and the distances to these nearby occupied areas. Because of the high energies (511 keV) of annihilation photons, the shielding thicknesses can be very large, and consideration must be given to whether the building can support the weight of the shielding. The amount of shielding needed can be minimized by placing the PET/CT and uptake rooms on the lowest floor (no shielding needed below) or on the top floor (no shield-ing needed above) and against an exterior wall or walls, thereby reducing or elimi-nating the need for shielding of one or two walls. Placing the uptake rooms adjacent to each other also reduces the weight of shielding needed. The amount of needed shielding can be further reduced by designing the area so that areas of low occupancy (*e.g.*, storage rooms, mechanical and electrical equipment rooms, and bathrooms) are immediately adjacent to the uptake and PET/CT rooms. The shielding design meth-ods for PET/CT facilities are described in AAPM Report No. 108, *PET and PET/CT Shielding Requirements* (AAPM, 2006).

The shielding design for a PET/CT or a SPECT/CT facility must also consider the radiation from the x-ray CT system. In most PET/CT installations, the thick shielding for the annihilation photons is more than sufficient for the lower-energy secondary radiation from the x-ray CT system. SPECT imaging rooms are often not shielded; for a SPECT/CT, a shielding calculation should be performed for the x-ray CT sys-tem and shielding should be installed if needed. In some SPECT/CT scanners, a cone-beam detector is utilized to acquire the CT projection data and will have scatter distributions that might require specific considerations when determining the bar-rier thickness. If a nuclear medicine imaging room is near a PET/CT room or a PET uptake room, shielding of greater thickness than needed for the protection of people may be required so that the high-energy photons emanating from patients do not interfere with imaging procedures in the nearby room.

21.6 RADIATION PROTECTION IN DIAGNOSTIC AND INTERVENTIONAL X-RAY IMAGING

21.6.1 Personnel Protection in Medical X-ray Imaging

During CT, radiographic, and remote fluoroscopic procedures, medical staff are seldom in the room with the patient while x-rays are being produced, although there may be exceptions for pediatric and critically ill patients and those who are incapable of following instructions. During most procedures, staff are pro-tected from radiation by the structural shielding installed in the walls of the room. However, physicians and assisting staff are in the room for most procedures uti-lizing fluoroscopy, particularly angiographic and interventional procedures, and

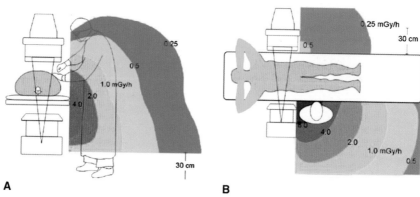

A   **B**

■ **FIGURE 21-16** Dose rates from scattered radiation during fluoroscopy, with the x-ray beam in PA **(A)** and lateral **(B)** orientations. These diagrams show the decrease in dose rate with distance from the location where the x-ray beam enters the patient. When the x-ray tube is beneath the patient **(A)**, the highest scatter intensity is to the lower part of the operator's body. When the x-ray beam has a lateral angulation **(B)**, the scatter intensity is much less on the side of the patient toward the image receptor. (Reprinted from Schueler BA. Operator shielding: How and why. *Tech Vasc Interv Radiol.* 2010;13(3):167-171. Copyright © 2010, with permission from Elsevier. doi: 10.1053/j.tvir.2010.03.005.)

during some CT-guided diagnostic and interventional procedures. Figure 21-16 shows the varying intensity of stray radiation, primarily scattered x-rays from the patient, during fluoroscopy. Understanding the spatial pattern of stray radiation can help staff to reduce the doses by where they stand during the procedure and how they position movable shielding. In particular, when the x-ray beam is in a lateral angulation, the stray radiation intensity is much higher on the side of the patient toward the x-ray source than on the side toward the image receptor. The x-ray doses to the heads and arms of staff tend to be least when the x-ray tube is beneath the patient.

Several items protect staff during a fluoroscopic or radiographic imaging procedure. The first and foremost is the *protective apron* worn by all individuals who must work in the room when the x-ray tube is operated, Figure 21-17A. Lead equivalent thicknesses from 0.25 to 0.50 mm are typical. Usually, the lead apron is in the form of a rubber material to provide flexibility and handling ease. Care must be taken to place aprons on supportive hangers when not in use to prevent excessive folding,

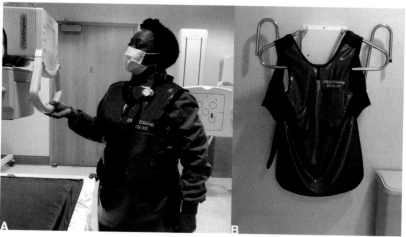

■ **FIGURE 21-17 A.** Technologist wearing 0.5-mm-equivalent lead apron thyroid collar and TLD dosimeter in a radiographic imaging suite. **B.** Hanger for storage of lead apron when not in use.

which may lead to tears in the shielding material over time, Figure 21-17B. Aprons protect the torso of the body and the upper legs and are available in designs with only frontal shielding or with wrap-around shielding, the latter being important when the back is exposed to the scattered radiation for a considerable portion of the time. Greater than 90% of the scattered radiation incident on the apron is attenuated by the 0.25-mm thickness at standard x-ray energies (*e.g.*, tube voltage <100 kV). Aprons of 0.35 and 0.50 mm lead equivalents give greater protection (up to 95% to 99% attenuation) but weigh 50% to 100% more than the 0.25-mm lead equivalent aprons. Since the k-absorption edge of lead is at 88 keV and the average energy of typical diagnostic x-rays is about 35 to 40 keV, materials in the middle range of atomic numbers (Z) such as tin and barium are more efficient per unit weight in absorbing those x-rays than is lead. Several types of non-lead and lead composite aprons for shielding personnel from diagnostic x-rays are available (Murphy et al., 1993; Zuguchi et al., 2008). The shielding capabilities of the lighter aprons are commonly specified in mm lead equivalent, but such a specification is valid only for a specific x-ray energy spectrum. These lighter aprons are typically adequate for x-rays generated at tube potentials up to 120 kV, but their effectiveness compared to conventional lead aprons declines at tube potentials above about 100 kV. For long fluoroscopic procedures, the weight of the apron may become a limiting factor in the ability of the physician and the attending staff to complete the case without substitutions. Some apron designs, such as skirt-vest combinations, place much of the weight on the hips instead of the shoulders. The areas not covered by the apron include the arms, lower legs, the head and neck, and the back (except for wrap-around aprons).

Aprons also do not protect the thyroid gland or the eyes. Accordingly, there are *thyroid shields* and *leaded glasses* that can be worn by the personnel in the room. The leaded thyroid shield wraps around the neck to provide attenuation similar to that of a lead apron. Leaded glasses attenuate the incident x-rays to a lesser extent, typically 30% to 70%, depending on the content (weight) of the lead. Unfortunately, their weight is a major drawback. Normal, everyday glasses provide only limited protection, typically much less than 20% attenuation. During fluoroscopy, the operator commonly looks at the display monitor while x-rays are produced, and the x-rays typically strike his or her head from the side and below. Therefore, the protective glasses or goggles should provide shielding on the sides, or the glasses should be of wrap-around designs. Whenever the hands must be near the primary beam, *protective gloves* of 0.5-mm thick lead (or greater) should be considered when their use does not interfere with the dexterity required to carry out the procedure.

In high workload angiographic and interventional laboratories, *ceiling-mounted, table-mounted, and mobile radiation barriers* are often used (Fig. 21-18). These devices are placed between the location where the x-ray beam intercepts the patient and the personnel in the room. The ceiling-mounted system is counterbalanced and easily positioned. Leaded glass or leaded acrylic shields are transparent and usually provide greater attenuation than the lead apron.

Only people whose presence is necessary should be in the imaging room during imaging. All such people must be protected with lead aprons or portable shields. In addition, no persons, especially individuals who are pregnant or under the age of 18 years, should routinely hold patients during examinations. Mechanical supporting or restraining devices must be available and used whenever possible. In no instance should the holder's body be in the useful beam, and it should be as far away from the primary beam as possible.

■ **FIGURE 21-18** Shielding used with a C-arm fluoroscope. The optimal position of the movable ceiling-mounted transparent shield is approximately perpendicular to and in contact with the patient. A table-mounted shield (seen in front and to the left of the operator) protects the lower part of his body. The operator is looking at the display monitors and scattered radiation striking his face is from the side and below. (Reprinted with permission from National Council on Radiation Protection and Measurements. *Radiation Dose Management for Fluoroscopically-Guided Interventional Medical Procedures.* NCRP Report No. 168. Bethesda, MD: National Council on Radiation Protection and Measurements; 2010. http://NCRPonline.org.)

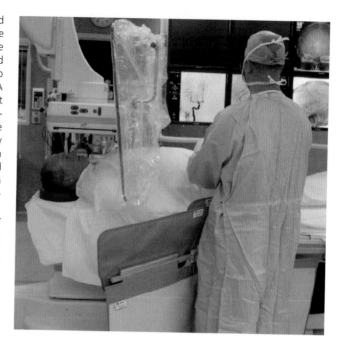

21.6.2 Environmental or Area Monitoring Dosimetry

In some instances, for example, public spaces adjacent to PET/CT and any areas for which there is a concern or perception that radiation dose is high in an uncontrolled space near a controlled area, the use of environmental or area monitoring may be appropriate. Such monitoring can employ TLDs or OSLDs mounted on walls or in areas where public individuals or workers in uncontrolled spaces have significant occupancy. These can be periodically (*e.g.*, monthly or quarterly) exchanged and read out to provide average dose rates over deployment periods. This information can be used for ongoing trending as well as program auditing and verification.

Tube Voltage and Beam Filtration

An important goal in diagnostic imaging is to achieve an optimal balance between image quality and dose to the patient. *Increasing the kV* will result in a greater transmission (and therefore less absorption) of x-rays through the patient. Even though the air kerma (or exposure) per mAs increases as the kV is increased, an accompanying reduction in the mAs to produce a similar signal to the image receptor will decrease the incident exposure to the patient. Unfortunately, there is a concomitant reduction in image contrast due to the higher effective energy of the x-ray beam. Within limits, this compromise is acceptable. Therefore, patient exposure can be reduced by using a higher kV and lower mAs. However, in procedures such as angiography and CT angiography in which contrast material is to be visualized and not soft tissue, greater beam filtration and lower kV can dramatically improve the contrast to noise ratio, which can result in a lower dose to the patient for these applications.

Filtration of the polychromatic x-ray energy spectrum can significantly reduce exposure by selectively attenuating the low-energy x-rays in the beam that would otherwise be absorbed in the patient with little or no contribution to image formation. These low-energy x-rays mainly impart dose to the skin and shallow tissues where the beam enters the patient. As the beam filtration is increased, the beam becomes "hardened" (the average photon energy increases) and the dose to the patient *decreases* because fewer low-energy photons are in the incident beam. The amount of filtration that can be added is limited by the increased x-ray tube loading necessary to offset the reduction in tube output, and the decreased contrast that occurs with excessive beam hardening. Except for mammography, a moderate amount of beam filtration does not significantly decrease subject contrast. The *quality* (effective energy) of the x-ray beam is assessed by measuring the HVL. Adequate filtration helps to avoid or minimize skin injuries from prolonged fluoroscopically guided interventional procedures. State and federal regulations require the HVL of the beam to exceed a minimum value. Always consult the appropriate regulatory authority for the requirements in your area.

Field Area, Organ Shielding, and Geometry

Restriction of the field size by collimation to just the necessary volume of interest is an important dose reduction technique. While it does not significantly reduce the entrance dose to the area in the primary beam, it reduces the volume of tissue in the primary beam and thus the energy imparted to the patient. It also reduces the amount of scatter and thus the radiation doses to adjacent organs. From an image quality perspective, the scattered radiation incident on the detector is also reduced, thereby improving image contrast and the signal-to-noise ratio.

When possible, particularly radiosensitive organs of patients undergoing radiographic examinations should be protected from the primary x-ray beam. This is best done by careful collimation of the beam and using projections (for chest radiographs, PA instead of AP) that reduce doses to organs such as the thyroid and breasts. For instance, when imaging a limb (such as a hand), a lap apron should be provided to the patient. However, when performing abdominal exams, gonadal shielding should not be used routinely as in the past, for the following reasons: (1) improvements in technology and reduced absorbed dose to the pelvic organs; (2) use of gonadal shielding can interfere with automatic exposure control sensors and cause an increase in dose; (3) heritable genetic effects have never been demonstrated with any statistical significance in humans; (4) gonadal shielding does not completely shield the gonads in the majority of patients because of normal variations in patient anatomy; (5) a substantial portion of gonadal dose to the ovaries is delivered by scattered radiation that is not attenuated by the shielding; and (6) shielding may obscure portions of anatomic structures that may prevent identification of important information on radiographs. Proposals to revise state and local regulations and guidance are now being considered in light of recent publications and findings. Other organs that may benefit from shielding if they must be in the primary beam include the lenses of the eyes and breast tissue in female children and young women. Care must be taken regarding proper placement of organ-specific shielding; distracted technologists have been known to place it on the x-ray receptor side of the patient instead of the x-ray tube side. And particularly, care also must be taken to ensure that gonadal and other organ-specific shielding does not block an active sensor for the automatic exposure control system.

Patient shielding should not be utilized in CT as the dose to organs and tissues outside the primary beam is mostly due to internal scatter, which would not be reduced by the external shielding (AAPM, 2019). In addition, the use of such shielding in CT may interfere significantly with automatic tube current modulation, as well as introduce image artifacts and general degradation of image quality.

Increasing the distance from the x-ray source to the patient (source-to-object distance [SOD]) helps reduce dose. As this distance is increased, a reduced beam divergence limits the volume of the patient being irradiated, thereby reducing the integral dose. Increasing this distance also reduces entrance dose due to the inverse square law. The exposure due to tube leakage is also reduced since the distance from the tube to the patient is increased, although this is only a minor consideration. With C-arm fluoroscopic systems that have fixed source-to-image receptor distances, patient dose is reduced by increasing the SOD as much as possible and moving the patient as close to the image receptor as possible. Federal regulations (21 CFR 1020.32[g]) specify a minimum patient (or tabletop) to focal spot distance of 20 cm. Furthermore, maintaining at least 30 cm is strongly recommended to prevent excessive radiation exposure.

X-ray Image Receptors

Digital radiography devices using photostimulable storage phosphor (PSP) plates or flat-panel thin-film transistor array image receptors have wide exposure latitudes. Post-acquisition image scaling (adjustments to brightness and contrast) and processing modify the image for optimal viewing. Thus, these detectors can compensate (to a large degree) for under- and overexposure and can reduce retakes caused by inappropriate radiographic techniques. However, underexposed images may contain excessive quantum mottle, hindering the ability to discern contrast differences, and overexposed images result in needless exposure to the patient. In terms of quantum mottle and noise digital flat-panel detectors have higher detection efficiencies, equivalent to 400- to 600-speed screen-film receptors while CR (PSP) detectors are equivalent to a 200-speed receptor due to lower detective quantum efficiency. For compensation and equivalent image noise, technique factors for CR receptors are typically two times higher than corresponding TFT flat-panel detectors. Techniques for extremity imaging with digital radiographic receptors should deliver somewhat higher exposure levels to achieve reduced noise and allow for edge-enhancement techniques to improve the sharpness of the images. In pediatric imaging, there are many examinations and corresponding technique protocols that allow low-dose, high-speed imaging; however, there are also situations requiring high spatial resolution and high signal-to-noise ratio, which, in turn, require higher dose. The flexibility of the digital detector response can be used to advantage in these situations to achieve optimal image quality at appropriate patient doses.

Screen-film radiographic image receptors, now obsolete, had an inherent safety feature. If the film processor was operating properly and the kV was adequate, using an excessive quantity of radiation to produce an image resulted in an overly dark film. On the other hand, when digital image receptors are used for radiography, fluoroscopy, and CT, excessive incident radiation may not have an adverse effect on image quality, and unnecessarily high exposures to patients may go unnoticed. Routine monitoring of the exposures to the digital image receptors in radiography, particularly in mobile radiography in which automatic exposure control is commonly not possible, is therefore necessary as a quality assurance measure. One solution is the implementation of the international exposure index standard for digital radiography, IEC-62494-1 (Seibert and Morin, 2011), described in Chapter 7. This standard requires the imaging device vendor to estimate the radiation dose incident on the detector for a given exam (*e.g.*, chest, abdomen, extremity) as an Exposure Index, EI, and to compare it to an accepted target Exposure Index, EIT, for that same exam. For immediate feedback to the technologist, a Deviation Index, DI, is generated as: DI = 10 log[EI/EIT], where negative DI values indicate underexposure, positive DI values indicate overexposure, and a DI value of 0 indicates the ideal exposure. The standard requires specific EIT values for each exam to be deemed appropriate as determined by the radiologist and to be recorded as such into the digital radiography database. Each of these values is included in the DICOM metadata for systems conforming to the standard. Acceptable DI values should be within -3.0 (underexposure of 50%) to $+3.0$ (overexposure of 100%). This range is based upon the recent experience of sites implementing the standard, and outliers should be considered for retakes. The review of DI values is an important quality assurance undertaking to identify under- and overexposures in radiography, and to take corrective steps to avoid inappropriate doses to patients.

Fluoroscopy

Fluoroscopy imparts a moderate fraction of the cumulative effective dose delivered in medical imaging (~18% of the total in 2006 and ~11% of the total in 2016), (NCRP, 2009, 2019), but imparts some of the largest tissue doses to individual patients. Even though the fluoroscopic techniques are quite modest (*e.g.*, 1 to 3 mA continuous tube current at 75 to 85 kV or higher mA, short exposure pulsed fluoroscopy at 3.25 to 15 frames per second in the United States), a fluoroscopic examination can require several minutes and, in some difficult cases, can exceed hours of "on" time. For example, a procedure using 2 mA at 80 kV for 10 min of fluoro time (1,200 mAs) delivers an air kerma of 60 mGy at 1 m (assuming 50 µGy/mAs for 80 kV at 1 m). If the focal spot is 30 cm from the skin, the patient entrance air kerma is $(100/30)^2$ × 60 mGy ~ 670 mGy! In the United States, fluoroscopic patient entrance air kerma (exposure) rates at 30 cm from the x-ray source for C-arm systems and at 1 cm above the table for systems with the x-ray tube fixed under the table are limited to a maximum of 87.4 {~88} mGy/min (10 R/min) for systems with automatic exposure rate control (AERC) and to 44 mGy/min (5 R/min) for systems without AERC. Some systems have a high air-kerma-rate fluoroscopic ("turbo") mode delivering up to 175 mGy/min (20 R/min) output at this reference point, a factor of five to ten times greater than the typical fluoro levels. This capability, which requires continuous manual activation of a switch by the operator and produces a continuous audible signal, must be used very judiciously. Cineangiography studies can deliver high dose rates of 175 to 610 mGy/min (20 to 70 R/min) at high frame rates (15 to 30 frames/s) but typically with short acquisition times. The patient entrance air-kerma rate depends on the angulation of the beam through the patient, with the air-kerma rate increasing with the thickness of the body traversed by the beam (*e.g.*, the air kerma rate is greater for lateral projections than for anteroposterior [AP] or posteroanterior [PA] projections).

Severe x-ray–induced skin injuries to patients have been reported following prolonged fluoroscopically guided interventional procedures, such as percutaneous transluminal coronary angioplasty, radiofrequency cardiac catheter ablation, vascular embolization, transjugular intrahepatic portosystemic shunt placement, and other percutaneous endovascular reconstructions (Koenig et al., 2001). The cumulative skin doses in difficult cases or from a series of procedures of a single area of the body can exceed 10 Gy, which can lead to severe radiation-induced skin injuries (see Specific Organ System Responses—Skin in Chapter 20). Figure 20-18 shows severe skin injuries following several fluoroscopically guided interventional procedures. Such injuries may not become fully apparent until many weeks, months, or even more than a year after the procedure. It is recommended that each medical facility determine the procedures that may impart doses that exceed the threshold for skin injury. Prior to each such procedure, it is recommended that each patient be screened for factors that may decrease the dose threshold for skin injury; these include large radiation exposures to the same part of the body from fluoroscopically guided interventional procedures or radiation therapy; some drugs, primarily chemotherapeutic agents; some hereditary diseases affecting DNA repair; and possibly other diseases such as connective tissue disorders, diabetes mellitus, and hyperthyroidism (Balter et al., 2010; Koenig et al., 2001; NCRP, 2010a). While large radiation doses may be unavoidable in difficult cases, care should be taken during all examinations to employ techniques that will minimize radiation exposure.

Chapter 9 discusses the metrics of patient dose that are displayed by fluoroscopes. Fluoroscopes manufactured since June 10, 2006, display the cumulative air kerma at a reference point (for C-arm fluoroscopes, this reference point is in the center of the x-ray beam, 15 cm from the isocenter of rotation, toward the x-ray source, or at another location defined by the manufacturer), typically the kerma-area product or dose-area product, and the cumulative fluoroscopy time. Older systems may display only the cumulative fluoro time. Studies have shown that cumulative air kerma and kerma area product correlate better with peak skin dose than does the total fluoro time (Fletcher et al., 2002; Miller et al., 2003). Today, in addition to reference point air kerma ($K_{a,r}$) and Kerma Area Product (KAP), also designated P_{KA}, major fluoroscope manufacturers offer additional dose information; two vendors display the air kerma for the current projection and two provide skin dose maps. Such advanced dose information is very useful to the fluoroscope operator during an interventional procedure, but the format of this information is not standardized, which limits the ability to transfer it, store it, and use it later. "Gafchromic" films that self-develop can be placed between the patient and support table to provide a post-examination map of skin dose. Dosimeters may be placed on the patients' skin to measure skin dose. In any dose-monitoring system, the real-time display of accumulated patient dose provides the physician with the ability to modify the procedure, if necessary, to reduce the likelihood of radiation-induced skin injuries.

Modern fluoroscopes have many features to protect the patient from unnecessary radiation and radiation injuries, in addition to the dose information displays mentioned immediately above. These include spacers installed in front of the x-ray source to prevent the patient from being dangerously close to the source. On some systems, particularly mobile ones, these spacers are easily removable. They should only be removed when necessary and, if they are removed, care must be taken to maintain an appropriate source-to-patient's-skin distance. Many modern fluoroscopes provide virtual collimation, which allows adjustment of the x-ray beam collimator without irradiating the patient. All fluoroscopes manufactured in the United States since mid-2006 continuously display the last image produced ("last image hold"), so clinicians can study an image without irradiating the patient. And most fluoroscopes sold today provide "fluoro store," whereby the last several seconds of fluoroscopy can be replayed and stored for later viewing. Fluoro store can replace high dose image recording, such as cine runs, in some situations in which higher random noise in the images can be tolerated.

Physicians using or directing the use of fluoroscopic systems should be trained and credentialed to ensure they understand the technology of fluoroscopy machines, particularly the dose implications of the different modes of operation; the biological effects of x-rays; and the techniques used to minimize patient and personnel exposure. In addition, physicians should be familiar with radiation control regulations.

NCRP Report No. 168 is an excellent resource for all radiation protection aspects of fluoroscopically guided interventional procedures, including the management of radiation exposure to patients and staff (NCRP, 2010a). Also, the ICRP has generated useful guidance for interventional fluoroscopy and cardiology, including considerations for pediatric patients, that should be consulted (ICRP, 2010, 2013a, 2013b).

Patient and Staff Safety for Fluoroscopically Guided Diagnostic and Interventional Procedures

It is important to protect both patients and staff from the radiation from fluoroscopically guided diagnostic and interventional procedures. A key principle in fluoroscopic radiation protection is that many of the actions taken to reduce radiation exposure to the patient also reduce radiation exposure to staff. Except for relatively rare remotely controlled fluoroscopes, clinical staff are in the room with the patient during procedures and are exposed to radiation. As in all x-ray imaging procedures, there is concern about the risk of possible stochastic effects, particularly cancer, for both patients and staff. However, for some complex and prolonged fluoroscopically guided procedures, there is also the risk of radiation-induced tissue reactions to the skin and underlying tissues of the patient. And there are indications that staff may be at increased risk of radiation-induced lenticular opacities (ICRP, 2012).

It is useful to group fluoroscopically guided procedures into two categories—those very unlikely to cause radiation-induced tissue reactions (also called deterministic effects) to patients, and those for which there is a real risk of such injuries. The latter are referred to as *potentially high radiation dose procedures*; a definition of such a procedure, adapted from NCRP Report No. 168, is—a *procedure for which* more than 5% of cases of that procedure result in a reference point air kerma, $K_{a,r}$ exceeding 3 Gy or an air kerma-area product, P_{KA}, exceeding 300 Gy cm². The dose metric P_{KA} is a reasonable indicator of the total radiation energy delivered to the patient and therefore enables the comparison of procedures and protocols from the perspective of the risk of stochastic radiation effects. However, on most fluoroscopes today, the best dose metric for assessing the risk of tissue reactions to the skin and underlying tissues of the patient is $K_{a,r}$. Some new fluoroscopes provide improved dose metrics such as peak skin dose (the maximal skin dose), skin dose maps, or air kerma to specific zones on the skin.

The following discussion of radiation safety for fluoroscopically guided interventions is an abbreviated one; additional information is presented in Chapter 9 and more complete discussions can be found in references such as NCRP Report No. 168. To protect a patient, some actions should be taken before a procedure, during a procedure, and after a procedure. Protocols should be established for common procedures, such as coronary artery angiography and interventions and vascular embolization.

Before a procedure, there should be an assessment of risk factors for radiation skin injury. These were discussed above and include previous large radiation exposures to the same part of the body from fluoroscopy or radiation oncology; some drugs, mostly chemotherapeutic agents; and some diseases, particularly some rare DNA repair disorders. Obesity and large body habitus are a risk factor because body attenuation causes increased x-ray output and much larger skin doses. The patient's skin should be visually examined for areas of previous radiation skin injury from fluoroscopy or radiation therapy. Patients at greater risk for skin injury should be assigned to the most dose efficient fluoroscope. Plans should be made to avoid areas on the skin that previously received large doses. And during the pre-procedure time-out, the technical settings on the fluoroscope should be confirmed to be correctly set per the appropriate protocol, skin areas to be avoided with the primary beam should be reviewed, and the patient table should be adjusted to maintain source-to-skin distance from the x-ray tube.

The following is a list of measures to be taken during a procedure to protect the patient:

- Keep the patient as far from the x-ray source as is practicable. When the x-ray tube is beneath the patient, this is done by raising the patient table, but not so high as to impede the procedure.

- Select the lowest acceptable dose mode and fluoro pulse rate. (On some systems, fluoro pulse rate is not directly selectable and is combined in another control or selection.)
- Select the lowest acceptable digital magnification setting.
- Remove the anti-scatter grid for small patients, for small body parts, and when the image receptor is far from the patient.
- Minimize the distance between the image-receptor and the patient.
- Collimate the x-ray beam aggressively. Use "virtual collimation," which requires no radiation, to adjust the collimator.
- Minimize beam-on time. The operator's foot should be off the pedal when he or she is not looking at the display monitor. The operator should only activate fluoroscopy to see motion. If nothing is moving in the image, the operator's foot should be off the pedal. When the operator needs to study the image, he or she should briefly tap the pedal to create an image and then study the static image displayed by the last-image-hold feature.
- Minimize image recording. In cine and DSA, limit the number of imaging acquisition runs, duration of runs, and frame rate. Use fluoro-store as a low dose alternative when you can tolerate the increased random noise.
- Be aware that steeper beam angles increase the dose, due to the greater thickness of the body along the x-ray beam axis.
- Use more than one beam angle ("dose spreading") if the dose to an area on the skin is approaching an amount that may cause injury. Large changes in beam angle and tight collimation are needed to avoid x-ray field overlap on the skin, and so it may be advisable to plan for dose spreading before beginning a procedure.
- Implement precautions to ensure, in steep oblique and lateral projections, that the patient's arm is not accidentally in the x-ray beam. Having an arm in the beam has been a contributing factor for some terrible tissue injuries. A supporting staff member such as a nurse can be assigned to this task.
- Assign a staff member to notify the operator when specified dose metric thresholds are reached. These notifications should be made at clinically appropriate times and not during critical maneuvers. For the metric reference point air kerma ($K_{a,r}$), recommended notification values are 3 Gy and every Gy thereafter (NCRP, 2010a). If a more advanced dose metric is displayed, such as reference point air kerma for a specific skin zone, these notifications may be applied to the dose metric for each skin zone. The operator should verbally acknowledge each notification. If the procedure uses a biplane fluoroscopy system (two x-ray tubes and two image receptors), the notifications should be performed for both systems.

There are also actions to be taken after a procedure to protect the patient. The metrics of dose to the patient should be reviewed and recorded. If the dose metrics indicate that the patient received a substantial radiation dose, the patient should be informed, counseled on possible skin effects that might occur, and instructed to inform the interventional service if they arise. A substantial radiation dose level may be defined as an estimated skin dose of 3 Gy or a $K_{a,r}$ of 5 Gy (NCRP, 2010a). Arrangements should also be made for appropriate clinical follow-up. This should include implementing precautions to avoid a skin biopsy if a skin injury becomes manifest.

The following is a list of actions to be taken by staff to protect themselves:

- Wear appropriate radiation protective apparel. This typically includes either a radiation protective apron or skirt-vest combination. The latter may be preferable because it reduces the weight on the wearer's spine. It is common to also wear a thyroid shield and radiation protective eyewear. Radiation protective glasses should have side shields to protect from radiation from the side because the operator is looking at the image display monitor while x-rays are being generated.

- When the x-ray beam is at an oblique or lateral angle, be aware that the scatter intensity is much higher on the x-ray tube side of the patient.
- Increase distance from where the x-ray beam intercepts the patient, particularly during high dose rate parts of the procedure, such as cine or DSA image recording. A simple step back by the operator and other tableside staff can reduce dose by half or more. Support staff in the room should stand well back from the patient whenever they can. When support staff need to approach the patient, they should notify the operator, wait until the operator states that radiation is off, and then notify the operator when they are clear of the patient.
- Use appropriate shielding. This typically includes a ceiling-mounted moveable transparent leaded shield and tableside scatter shielding. Appropriate positioning of the ceiling-mounted shield is important. Radiation-attenuating pads can be placed on the patient to absorb scatter from the patient. It is preferable for ancillary staff members who are not tableside to each have a free-standing mobile radiation shield to stand behind.
- Staff should keep their hands out of the primary x-ray beam, unless absolutely necessary. If they must be in the beam, it should be for as short a duration as possible. If the hands must be in the beam, it is preferable that they be in the beam on the x-ray beam exit side, as the intensity of the beam exiting the patient is just a few percent of the intensity of the beam on the beam-entrance side of the patient. Wearing a lead glove while a hand is in the beam may make things worse, particularly if the lead glove shadows a sensor for the automatic exposure control system; this may cause the x-ray output to greatly increase.
- Wear dosimeters correctly. There are two common practices. In one, a dosimeter is worn outside the radiation protective apparel at the collar or neck level, and another dosimeter is worn on the front of the torso underneath the protective apparel. In the other, a single dosimeter is worn outside the radiation protective apparel at the collar or neck level.
- Many of the patient and staff radiation protection principles discussed above are illustrated in Fig. 21-19A and B, respectively.

Computed Tomography

As mentioned earlier in this chapter, the average annual effective dose to the population of the United States from medical imaging increased by more than a factor five from about 1980 until 2006, and about half of this effective dose in 2006 was from CT imaging. Data from a decade later showed that the previous increase in the average annual dose to the population of the United States from CT had not significantly changed since 2006 indicating a flatting of the utilization curve (NCRP, 2019). In 2001, it was reported in the medical literature that at least some medical facilities in the United States were using adult technique factors for the CT examinations of children and even infants (Paterson et al., 2001); it has been estimated that this practice could increase risk of cancer to these patients by a factor of 10 compared to adult patients (Brenner et al., 2001). As previously mentioned, professional societies, advisory bodies such as the ICRP and NCRP, and governmental agencies continue to support efforts to "right-size" or optimize the dose to patients from medical imaging, especially pediatric patients.

In CT, many operator-selectable parameters determine the patient dose. These include the kV and mA applied to the x-ray tube, time per x-ray tube rotation, detector-table motion pitch, beam filter, and axial scan length. As mentioned in

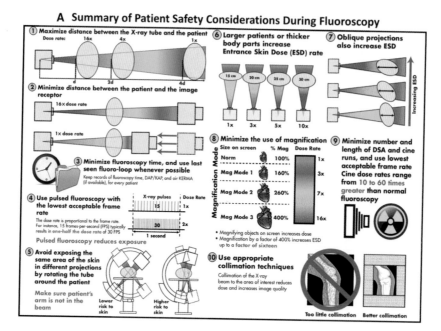

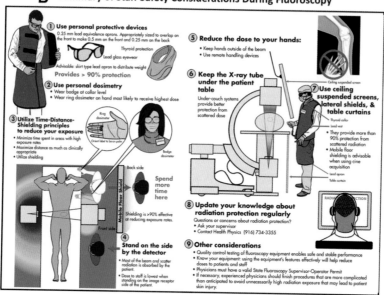

■ **FIGURE 21-19 A.** Summary of Patient Safety Considerations During Fluoroscopy. **B.** Summary of Staff Safety Considerations During Fluoroscopy.

Chapter 10, these are not usually individually selected by a technologist for each patient procedure but are instead specified in organ- and procedure-specific protocols, such as "chest (routine)," "three-phase liver," and "brain (CTA)." A technologist selects the appropriate protocol for a patient and clinical indication, although the technologist may have to modify the technique in the protocol for patient-specific circumstances. Modern CT scanners provide the capability to protect protocols with passwords, which should be restricted to only a few individuals. Such use of passwords can protect protocols from inadvertent or deliberate but unauthorized modification.

Most radiographic images, other than those acquired with mobile machines, are acquired utilizing automatic exposure control. However, older CT scanners used a fixed kV and mAs selected by the technologist, regardless of the size of the patient, unless the CT technologist changed them. The fixed techniques in CT for a given protocol often led to unnecessarily high mAs values for thinner patients, particularly infants and young children. A way to avoid this unnecessary radiation dose to the patient is to train the CT technologists to reduce the mAs (and perhaps the kV) for thinner patients. A technique chart can be devised for each such CT scanner showing kV and mAs values for different diameter patients as a guide to achieving good image quality at proper dose levels. Table 21-4 shows the dose reductions that can be achieved if the CT protocols (mAs values) are adjusted to the patient's size.

Nearly all scanners today have the ability to modulate the tube current as a function of patient body habitus, tube rotation angle, and axial position on the patient, to compensate for the attenuation variations along the beam path through the patient. Nearly all CTs use the localizer images (scout scan or topogram) to determine the mA, and some also measure the amount of transmitted radiation during the scan itself. Automatic tube current modulation can markedly reduce exposure, particularly to smaller and average size patients, without decreasing image quality. However, each implementation of automatic tube current modulation requires information to be provided to the CT regarding the amount of random noise in the resultant images that can be tolerated by the interpreting physicians. The various CT manufacturers specify this differently (*e.g.*, for one manufacturer, a parameter called "noise index" and the reconstructed slice thickness must be selected, whereas for another manufacturer, a parameter called the "reference mAs" and a setting of "weak," "average," or "strong" must be selected). This information is commonly stored in the organ and procedure-specific CT protocols and can vary among protocols.

TABLE 21-4 DOSE REDUCTION POTENTIAL IN CT

PATIENT DIAMETER (cm)	PERCENT (mAs)	mAs
14	0.3	1
16	0.6	2
18	1.2	4
20	2.2	7
22	4.2	13
24	7.9	24
26	15	45
28	28	85
30	53	160
32	100	300
34	188	564
36	352	1,058
38	661	1,983
40	1,237	3,712

Note: If a CT technique of 120 kV and 300 mAs delivers good image quality (low noise images) for a 32-cm-diameter patient, the same image quality (signal to noise ratio [SNR]) can be achieved by reducing the mAs to the levels indicated for patients smaller than 32, and increasing the mAs for patients larger than 32 cm. The large mA values for very large diameters are not possible; alternatively, a higher kV could be used. Large patients have greater amounts of abdominal fat that results in improved conspicuity of organ boundaries, and a lesser SNR might be tolerable.

Another innovation in CT that has led to a significant reduction in doses to patients is iterative image reconstruction, discussed in Chapter 10. It addresses random noise more effectively than filtered backprojection and can produce images of equal quality with significantly lower radiation doses. Iterative reconstruction methods do not directly reduce dose; instead, they allow CT parameters that control dose to be set to values that reduce dose. Artificial intelligence methods are poised to provide an even greater step in addressing random noise by using machine learning algorithms that have recently been approved for clinical use by the FDA (Higaki et al., 2020).

Yet another innovation is automatic kilovoltage selection, which automatically adjusts the x-ray tube potential based upon patient body habitus, as indicated by the localizer scan. This feature can be turned on or off in individual scanning protocols. When used, it reduces dose to smaller and thinner patients and increases the conspicuity of contrast material in patients.

Two indices of dose to a patient displayed by modern CT scanners are the $CTDI_{vol}$ and the DLP, the DLP being the $CTDI_{vol}$ multiplied by the scanned length of the patient (see Chapter 11). For scans of a significant length, the $CTDI_{vol}$ is approximately the average dose that would be imparted to a cylindrical acrylic phantom from the scan being given to the patient. Therefore, the $CTDI_{vol}$ and DLP provide information about the amount of radiation being given to a specific patient but do not reflect the actual doses to the patient. To address the issues of the discrepancy between the size of the patient and the size of the CTDI phantom leading to under- or overestimating dose to the patient, the American Association of Physicists in Medicine (AAPM) developed a methodology "Size Specific Dose Estimate" (SSDE), which adjusts the indicated $CTDI_{vol}$ provided by the scanner to the SSDE value (in mGy) according to the equivalent diameter of the patient relative to the CTDI phantom diameter (AAPM, 2011a). This provides a more accurate estimate of the dose to the patient.

Modern CT scanners display the $CTDI_{vol}$ and DLP before and after each scan and have the ability to send this dose information to a PACS or other digital information system after a scan, either as a secondary capture image with the study or as a DICOM Radiation Dose Structured Report (RDSR). If automatic tube current modulation is used, the $CTDI_{vol}$ and DLP displayed before a scan may not be identical to those displayed after the scan. The display of these dose metrics before a scan provides the technologist the ability to assess the approximate magnitude of the radiation exposure before performing a scan. The RDSR has a full description of the procedure with radiation dose metrics and includes many details not found in the DICOM metadata associated with the images; however, because the RDSR is a separate DICOM object, reading or storing the information as a RDSR is a separate DICOM transaction. To ensure compatibility in dose reporting, the non-profit organization, Integrating the Healthcare Enterprise's (IHE) Radiation Exposure Monitoring integration profile should be specified when purchasing new imaging systems (IHE integration profiles are discussed in Chapter 5).

CT scanners that comply with the National Electrical Manufacturers Association (NEMA) XR 25 Computed Tomography Dose Check standard have the capability of displaying notifications and alerts when the $CTDI_{vol}$ or DLP of a CT study about to be performed is expected to exceed preset values. A "notification value" is the dose metric of an individual scan or series of a study that causes a notification warning to be displayed. An "alert value" is the cumulative dose metric of the entire study already acquired plus that for the scan or series about to be performed that causes a warning to be displayed. By setting notification and alert values, the technologist is warned if the scan he or she is planning to acquire exceeds the user-configured level of dose.

The alert value is intended to be set to avoid significant patient injury. The FDA has recommended that the alert value be set at $CTDI_{vol} = 1$ Gy. This is an unusually (and likely unnecessarily) high dose for a CT procedure—about one half the level that could result in skin erythema. If an alert is displayed for an alert value of 1 Gy, it is highly likely that something is wrong, and the technologist should review the acquisition parameters for an error. If the alert cannot be resolved, radiologist approval should be obtained before proceeding, except in a dire emergency. The notification level could be set to a diagnostic reference level (DRL) (describing in more detail below); however, that would result in numerous notifications, particularly for larger and obese patients. The AAPM has recommended that the notification level be set higher than the relevant diagnostic reference level so that notifications are issued only for doses that are "higher than usual," thereby warning the technologist that an acquisition parameter may be set incorrectly. The notification values recommended by AAPM are shown below (AAPM, 2011b). This document also contains recommendations for notification levels for pediatric CT examinations.

EXAMINATION	$CTDI_{vol}$ (mGy)
Adult head	80
Adult torso	50
Brain perfusion	600
Cardiac—retrospective gating	150
Cardiac—prospective gating	50

Dose Optimization in CT

An essential step to optimizing radiation dose in CT imaging is to review and optimize the CT protocols. This topic was discussed in Chapter 10 and is a substantial and complicated task worthy of further study (Demb et al., 2017). The bullet points provided below should only be considered an overview of this topic.

- Many protocols (*e.g.*, 3 phase liver protocol) specify scan before the administration of intravenous contrast material and one or more scans after the administration. Eliminating one or more phases from a protocol will greatly reduce patient dose.
- Thin slices are usually noisier and, in some cases, may require a higher mA. One should consider whether high axial spatial resolution is diagnostically necessary. One might overcome the noise of thin slices by calculating thicker slices but at intervals smaller than the slice thickness (*i.e.*, overlapping). However, thin slices exhibit sharper anatomic boundaries and less partial volume effect and so benefit from higher tissue contrast, which can partially compensate for the higher statistical noise (ICRP, 2007a).
- Tissues with inherently high tissue contrast may be acquired at low dose without loss of diagnostic value. These include lung and bone. A renal stone CT examination, for example, could be acquired at a much lower dose than a liver examination and a lung nodule follow-up protocol requires much less dose than a routine chest protocol.
- Patients who are obese generally require greater dose. However, a factor that balances this effect is that adipose tissue better delineates soft tissues, which causes acceptable contrast to be more easily achieved in abdominal and pelvic scans of obese patients than in thinner patients. A kV of 140 could be selected for the most obese patients.
- Create separate abdominal protocols for obese patients.

- Lower kV can increase the visibility of contrast material in angiography or brain perfusion imaging. The k-absorption edge of iodine—where its attenuation coefficient reaches a maximum—is at about 30 keV. Improved images and lower patient dose may be achieved with a tube voltage of 100 kV instead of 120 kV in angiography. A tube voltage of 80 kV is commonly used in brain perfusion imaging. Reduced kV can also be employed in lung perfusion scans for pulmonary embolism.
- Scan only the z-axis length you need.
- When possible, avoid radiation directly to the eyes.
- Vary tube current according to contrast phase. You may be able to use a lower mA for non-contrast phases.
- Compare your protocols with optimized protocols for the same model of CT. Sample CT protocols are available from the CT manufacturer, AAPM, and other sources. (See the Image Wisely Web site.)
- Look to see that protocols of similar body parts have similar dose indices, taking into consideration that some indications require less relative noise.
- Use iterative reconstruction, if available.
- Use automatic tube current modulation (see below) for procedures for which it will reduce dose. Most procedures, and particularly scans of the neck, chest, abdomen, and pelvis, should use it. (Not all procedures, *e.g.*, brain perfusion imaging, benefit from it.)
- Ensure body imaging protocols that do not use automatic mA modulation require technique adjustment for patient body habitus.
- Create low-dose protocols (*e.g.*, low-dose chest protocol, low-dose kidney stone protocol, low-dose abdominal aortic aneurism protocol) for use when indicated, particularly for follow-up examinations.
- Most automatic mA modulation systems have a maximum allowable mA setting. Ensure this is set to a reasonable value, beyond which you increase the kV.
- Ensure the $CTDI_{vol}$ for brain perfusion CT does not exceed 0.5 Gy.
- Record the $CTDI_{vol}$ and DLP for a patient of average size in each protocol document. You may need to average the values from several patients.
- Compare these dose indices from individual scan protocols with DRLs and achievable doses.

For cardiac CT protocols, substantial dose reduction can be achieved by the following strategies:

- Minimize the scan range.
- Use heart rate reduction.
- Prospective triggering results in lower dose than does retrospective gating.
- If using retrospective gating, employ ECG-gated mA modulation.
- Reduce tube voltage whenever possible to 100 kV or even 80 kV.

Miscellaneous Considerations

Careful identification of the patient and, for female patients of reproductive age, determination of pregnancy status are necessary before an examination is performed. For higher-dose studies (*e.g.*, fluoroscopy and multiphase CT examinations) of the abdomen or pelvis, a pregnancy test within 72 h before the examination should be performed in addition to the usual screening for pregnancy, unless the possibility of pregnancy is eliminated by certain premenarche in a child, certain postmenopausal state, or documented hysterectomy or tubal ligation.

A significant reduction in population dose can be achieved by eliminating screening exams that only rarely detect pathology. Standing-order x-rays, such as presurgical chest exams for hospital admissions or surgeries not involving the chest, are inappropriate. Frequent screening examinations are often not indicated without a specific reason or a reasonable amount of time elapsed (*e.g.*, years) from the previous exam. A good example is the "yearly" dental x-ray. While yearly exams are appropriate for some patients, a 2-year interval between x-ray examinations in non–cavity-prone adult patients with a healthy mouth is appropriate. Another opportunity for significant patient dose reduction in dentistry is the use of high-speed film (*e.g.*, E-speed film) or digital image receptors. Many dental offices still use slower D-speed films that require approximately twice the exposure (and thus patient dose). Periodic screening mammography examinations are not appropriate for women younger than 35 to 40 years old unless there is a familial history of breast cancer or other indication. However, as the probability of cancer increases with age, and the fact that survival is drastically enhanced by early detection have led some professional medical groups to recommend yearly screening mammograms for the general population of women 40 to 50 years old. A review of the recommendations by several organizations and professional societies can be found at the CDC's Web site (CDC, 2020).

Each radiology department should have a program to monitor examinations that must be repeated. The frequency of repeat exams due to faulty technique, improper position, or patient motion is primarily determined by the skill and diligence of the x-ray technologists. Training institutions often have higher repeat rates, mainly attributed to lack of experience. The largest numbers of studies that must be repeated are commonly from mobile exams, in which positioning difficulty causes the anatomy of interest to be improperly represented on the image, and lack of automatic exposure control increases the likelihood of inadequate dose to the image receptor.

Programmed techniques for examinations are commonly available on radiographic equipment and can eliminate the guesswork in many radiographic situations (of course, provided that the techniques are properly set up). The use of photostimulable phosphor imaging plates or direct digital image receptors (Chapter 7) can significantly reduce the number of exams that must be repeated because of improper radiographic technique. The examinations with the highest retake rates are commonly portable chests; lumbar spines; thoracic spines; kidneys, ureters, and bladders; and abdomens. Continuous monitoring of retakes and inadequate images and identification of their causes are important components of a quality assurance program, so that appropriate action may be taken to improve quality. Many errors are eliminated by a quality control program that periodically tests the performance of the x-ray equipment, image receptors, and post-processing/image quality.

Diagnostic Reference Levels, Achievable Doses, and Reference Levels

A DRL is a particular value of a metric of dose, such as entrance air kerma in radiography or $CTDI_{vol}$ in CT, from a common diagnostic imaging procedure, to be used as an investigational level in a quality assurance program to identify possibly excessive doses to patients (ACR, 2018; ICRP, 2017). A dose value from an imaging procedure that exceeds a DRL should be investigated but would not be presumed as excessive until so determined by an investigation. An achievable dose is a particular value of a metric of dose from a common diagnostic imaging procedure that may serve a goal for dose optimization efforts (ACR, 2018; ICRP, 2017).

DRLs and achievable doses are typically determined from a study of a dose metric from many institutions and imaging systems. A DRL is typically set at the seventy-fifth percentile of the set of data from the study, meaning that three fourths of the measurements in the data set were less than the DRL. An achievable dose is typically set at the median value of the dose distribution from the study.

DRLs and achievable doses may be based upon measurements made with a phantom, such as CTDI measurements made using the FDA CT body or head phantom, or they may be based upon dose metrics, such as $CTDI_{vol}$ and DLP, from clinical imaging of patients. There are advantages and disadvantages, discussed below, to each approach. Some sources of data for DRLs and achievable doses are also described below.

In the United States, the Nationwide Evaluation of x-ray Trends (NEXT) Program, conducted jointly by the US Food and Drug Administration, the Conference of Radiation Control Program Directors, and most state radiation regulatory agencies, periodically performs measurements of doses from x-ray imaging devices. NEXT studies have been of phantom-based dose measurements.

As mentioned in Chapter 11, the automated collection of dose information, using standard DICOM and IHE protocols, from clinical procedures and its collection by dose registries may facilitate the timely creation and updating of reference levels and the comparison of dose metrics from clinical procedures with reference levels. The ACR maintains a national dose index registry (ACR, 2019, 2020) that enables facilities to compare their CT dose indices to regional and national values and take appropriate dose optimization steps as appropriate. Recently, DRLs and ADs for common CT procedures, based upon data from the ACR Dose Index Registry, have become available (Kanal et al., 2017).

There are shortcomings to the use of reference levels as a quality assurance tool. Reference levels for dose measurements made using phantoms may not fully test an imaging device and imaging protocol. For example, the cylindrical FDA CT dose phantoms have shapes very different from patients and do not assess the effect of automatic tube current modulation. On the other hand, using DRLs and achievable doses determined from actual patient studies involves uncertainty due to factors such as patient body size. The studies used to determine reference levels may lag current technology and uses; furthermore because the studies used to determine reference levels are costly of resources, there are many clinical imaging protocols for which there are no appropriate reference levels. Lastly, comparisons of dose metrics to DRLs identify high outliers; a dose metric that is less than a reference level does not imply that the protocol or procedure is fully optimized.

Nonetheless, reference levels are a useful tool in identifying imaging protocols, equipment, and practices imparting unnecessarily high doses to patients.

The ACR maintains a practice parameter that summarizes current national DRLs and achievable doses (ACR, 2018). Because of the ongoing evolution of radiological equipment and associated optimization developments, the most recent ACR, DRLs, and ADs should be consulted for evaluating each modality and protocol (ACR, 2018). European governmental agencies are another source of reference levels. Reference levels may also be provided by studies reported in the professional literature (*e.g.*, Hausleiter et al., 2009). Guidance on the use of DRLs for optimization in medical imaging has been developed by both the NCRP (NCRP, 2012) and ICRP (ICRP, 2017).

Attempts have been made to extend the concept of DRLs to fluoroscopically guided interventional procedures; the investigational levels from these are commonly called "reference levels." As is the case for DRLs, these are commonly set at the seventy-fifth percentile of the dose metrics from a sample of procedures from a number of institutions. The establishment of such reference levels is complicated because such procedures are less standardized than common diagnostic procedures, and because of variations in the difficulty of individual patient procedures, the body habitus of the patients, and the skill of the interventionalists.

21.7 RADIATION PROTECTION IN NUCLEAR MEDICINE

21.7.1 Minimizing Time of Exposure to Radiation Sources

Nuclear medicine procedures typically produce low exposure rates for extended periods of time. For example, the typical exposure rate at 1 m from a patient after the injection of 740 MBq (20 mCi) of technetium 99m methylenediphosphonate (Tc-99m MDP) for a bone scan is ~8.8 µGy/h (~1 mR/h), which, through radioactive decay and urinary excretion, will be reduced to ~4.4 µGy/h (~0.5 mR/h) at 2 h after injection, when imaging typically begins. Therefore, knowledge of both the exposure rate and how it changes with time is important in minimizing personnel exposure. Table 21-5 shows the typical exposure rates at 1 m from adult nuclear medicine patients after the administration of commonly used radiopharmaceuticals.

The time spent near a radiation source can be minimized by having a thorough understanding of the tasks to be performed and the appropriate equipment to complete them in a safe and timely manner. For example, elution of a Mo-99/Tc-99m generator and subsequent radiopharmaceutical preparation requires several steps with a high-activity source. It is important to have practiced these steps with a non-radioactive source to learn how to manipulate the source proficiently and use the dose measurement and preparation apparatus.

21.7.2 Minimizing Exposure with Distance from Radiation Sources

Other than very low-activity sealed sources (*e.g.*, a 370-kBq [10 µCi] Co-57 marker), unshielded radiation sources should not be manipulated by hand. The use of tongs or other handling devices to increase the distance between the source and the hand substantially reduces the exposure rate. Table 21-6 lists the exposure rates from radionuclides commonly used in nuclear medicine and the 100-fold exposure rate reduction achieved simply by increasing the distance from the source from 1 to 10 cm.

Radiation exposure rates in the nuclear medicine laboratory can range from over 874 mGy (10 R/h), (*e.g.*, contact exposure from an unshielded vial containing

---

TABLE 21-5 TYPICAL EXPOSURE RATE AT 1 m FROM AN ADULT NUCLEAR MEDICINE PATIENT AFTER RADIOPHARMACEUTICAL ADMINISTRATION

STUDY	RADIO-PHARMACEUTICAL	ACTIVITY MBq (mCi)	EXPOSURE RATE AT 1 m µGy/h (mR/h)
Thyroid cancer therapy	I-131 (NaI)	7,400 (200)	~27.3 (3.1)
Tumor imaging	F-18 (FDG)	370 (10)	~44.0 (5.0)
Cardiac-gated imaging	Tc-99m RBC	740 (20)	~7.9 (0.9)
Bone scan	Tc-99m MDP	925 (25)	~10.6 (1.2)
Tumor imaging	Ga-67 citrate	111 (3)	~3.5 (0.4)
Liver-spleen scan	Tc-99m sulfur colloid	148 (4)	~1.8 (0.2)
Myocardial perfusion imaging	Tl-201 chloride	111 (3)	~0.9 (0.1)

Exposure rate measurements courtesy of M. Hartman, University of California, Davis.

TABLE 21-6 EFFECT OF DISTANCE ON EXPOSURE WITH COMMON RADIONUCLIDES USED IN NUCLEAR MEDICINE

RADIONUCLIDE 370 MBq (10 mCi)	EXPOSURE RATE[a] mGy/h[b] (R/h) AT 1 cm	EXPOSURE RATE[a] mGy/h[b] (R/h) AT 10 cm
Ga-67	65.5 (7.5)	0.65 (0.075)
Tc-99m	54.1 (6.2)	0.54 (0.062)
I-123	143 (16.3)	1.43 (0.163)
I-131	190 (21.8)	1.90 (0.218)
Xe-133	46.3 (5.3)	0.46 (0.053)
Tl-201	39.3 (4.5)	0.39 (0.045)
F-18	494 (56.6)	4.9 (0.57)

[a]Calculated from the Γ_{20}.
[b]Air kerma rate.

approximately 37 GBq [1 Ci] of Tc-99m generator eluate or a therapeutic dosage of approximately 11 GBq [300 mCi] of I-131) to natural background. The air kerma rate at any distance from a small container of a particular radionuclide can be calculated using the air-kerma-rate constant (Γ_δ), of the radionuclide. The air-kerma-rate constant for a photon-emitting radionuclide is defined by the ICRU as:

$$\Gamma_\delta = \frac{l^2 \dot{K}_{air\delta}}{A},$$ [21-4]

where $\dot{K}_{air\delta}$ is the air kerma rate due to photons of energy greater than δ, at a distance l from a point source of the nuclide having an activity A. The air-kerma-rate constant has units of m^2 Gy/Bq s. For convenience, the air-kerma-rate constant is sometimes expressed in m^2 µGy/GBq h.

Because very low energy photons are significantly attenuated in air and other intervening materials, air-kerma-rate constants usually ignore photons below a specified energy. For example, Γ_{20} represents the air-kerma-rate constant for photons ≥ 20 keV.

EXAMPLE: An unshielded vial containing 3.7 GBq of Tc-99m pertechnetate is left on a lab bench. For Tc-99m, Γ_{20} = 14.6 m^2 µGy/GBq h What would be the air kerma (K_{air}) if a technologist were standing 0.5 m from such a source for 30 min?

SOLUTION

$$\dot{K}_{Air} = (14.6 \text{ m}^2 \text{ µGy/GBq h}) (3.7 \text{ GBq}) (0.5 \text{ h})/(0.5 \text{ m})^2 = 108 \text{ µGy}$$

Multiplying the air kerma in µGy by 0.1142 mR/µGy will convert it to exposure in units of mR; thus 108 µGy is equivalent to (108 µGy × 0.1142 mR/µGy) = 12.3 mR.

The air-kerma-rate constant is replacing the older *exposure rate constant* (expressed in units of R cm^2/mCi h). The exposure rate in R/h of the specified radionuclide is calculated as

$$\text{Exposure rate (R/h)} = \Gamma_x A/l^2,$$ [21-5]

where Γ_x is the exposure rate constant R cm^2/mCi h for photons of energy greater than x, A is the activity in mCi, and l is the distance in centimeters from a point source of radioactivity.

One can multiply the exposure rate constant in R cm^2/mCi h by 23.69 to convert to the air-kerma-rate constant in µGy m^2/GBq h. This conversion assumes that the photon energy cutoffs (*i.e.*, δ and x) are the same.

21.7.3 Shielding in Nuclear Medicine

Tungsten, lead, leaded-glass, and leaded acrylic shields are used in nuclear medicine to reduce the radiation exposure from vials and syringes containing radioactive material. Table 21-7 shows exposure rate constants and lead HVLs for radionuclides commonly used in nuclear medicine.

TABLE 21-7 EXPOSURE RATE CONSTANTS (Γ_{20} AND Γ_{30})^a AND HALF VALUE LAYERS (HVL) OF LEAD FOR RADIONUCLIDES OF INTEREST TO NUCLEAR MEDICINE

RADIONUCLIDE	$\Gamma_{20}{}^{b,c}$	$D_{20}{}^d$	$\Gamma_{30}{}^c$	HVL IN PB (cm)^{e,f}
C-11, N-13, O-15	139 (5.85)	153.10	5.85	0.39
Co-57	13.2 (0.56)	14.51	0.56	0.02
Co-60	303 (12.87)	333.41	12.87	1.2
Cr-51	4.24 (0.18)	4.66	0.18	0.17
Cs-137/Ba-137m	76.5 (3.25)	84.19	3.25	0.55
F-18	135 (5.66)	148.44	5.66	0.39
Ga-67	17.7 (0.75)	19.43	0.75	0.1
I-123	38.4 (1.63)	42.23	0.86	0.04
I-125	34.6 (1.47)	38.08	0.26	0.002
I-131	51.3 (2.18)	56.47	2.15	0.3
In-111	75.4 (3.20)	82.90	2.0	0.1
Ir-192	108.6 (4.61)	119.43	4.61	0.60
Mo-99/Tc-99m^g	34.6 (1.47)	38.08	1.43	0.7
Rb-82	134 (5.65)	159	5.65	0.7
Tc-99m	14.6 (0.62)	16.06	0.60	0.03
Tl-201	10.6 (0.45)	11.66	0.45	0.02
Xe-133	12.5 (0.53)	13.73	0.53	0.02

^{a}(Γ_{20} and Γ_{30}) calculated from the absorption coefficients of Hubbell and Seltzer (1995) and the decay data table of Kocher (1981): Hubbell JH, Seltzer SM. Tables of x-ray mass attenuation coefficients and mass energy-absorption coefficients 1 keV to 20 MeV for elements $Z = 1$ to 92 and 48 additional substances of dosimetric interest. NISTIR 5632, National Institute of Standards and Technology, May 1995 and Kocher DC. Radioactive decay data tables. DOE/TIC-11026, Technical Information Center, U.S. Department of Energy, 1981.
^{b}Air kerma rate constant, 20 keV photon energy cutoff, in µGy m^2/GBq h.
^{c}(R cm/mCi h): Multiply by 23.69 to obtain air kerma rate constant in µGy m^2/GBq h.
^{d}Equivalent dose rate µSv m^2/GBq h.
^{e}The first HVL will be significantly smaller than subsequent HVLs for those radionuclides with multiple photon emissions at significantly different energies (e.g., Ga-67) because the lower-energy photons will be preferentially attenuated in the first HVL.
^{f}Some values were adapted from Goodwin PN. Radiation safety for patients and personnel. In: *Freeman and Johnson's Clinical Radionuclide Imaging*. 3rd ed. Philadelphia, PA: WB Saunders; 1984:370. Other values were calculated by the authors.
^{g}In equilibrium with Tc-99m.

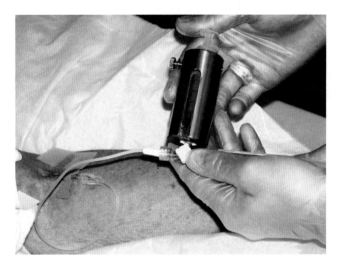

■ **FIGURE 21-20** A butterfly needle and three-way stopcock connected to a syringe with normal saline and a syringe shield containing the syringe with the radiopharmaceutical for injection. The barrel of the syringe shield is made of a high-Z material (*e.g.*, lead or tungsten) with a leaded glass window so that the syringe scale and the contents of the syringe can be seen.

Syringe shields (Fig. 21-20) are used to reduce personnel exposure from syringes containing radioactivity during dose preparation and administration to patients. Syringe shields can reduce hand exposure from Tc-99m by as much as 100-fold.

Leaded glass or acrylic shields are used in conjunction with solid lead shields in radiopharmaceutical preparation areas. Radiopharmaceuticals are withdrawn from vials surrounded by thick lead containers (called "lead pigs") into shielded syringes behind the leaded glass shield in the dose preparation area (Fig. 21-21).

People handling radionuclides should wear laboratory coats, disposable gloves, finger ring TLD dosimeters, and body dosimeters. The lead aprons utilized in diagnostic radiology are of limited value in nuclear medicine because, in contrast to their effectiveness in reducing exposure from low-energy scattered x-rays, they do not attenuate enough of the higher energy photons emitted by Tc-99m (140 keV) to be practical (Table 21-8).

Radioactive material storage areas are shielded to minimize exposure rates. Mirrors mounted on the back walls of high-level radioactive material storage areas are often used to allow retrieval and manipulation of sources without direct exposure to the head and neck. Beta radiation is best shielded by low atomic number (Z) material (*e.g.*, plastic or glass), which provides significant attenuation while minimizing bremsstrahlung x-ray production. For high-energy beta emitters (*e.g.*, P-32), the low Z shield can be further shielded by lead to attenuate bremsstrahlung. With the exception of PET facilities, which are commonly shielded to protect people in surrounding areas from the 511-keV annihilation radiation, SPECT/CT imaging rooms, and possibly rooms for administering therapeutic radiopharmaceuticals such as Lu-177 dotatate, most nuclear medicine laboratories do not have shielded walls within or surrounding the department. However, there may be situations, such as a patient waiting area adjacent to an office, where shielding is advisable.

21.7.4 Contamination Control and Surveys

Contamination is simply uncontained radioactive material located where it is not wanted. Contamination control methods are designed to prevent radioactive material from coming into contact with people and to prevent its spread to other work surfaces. Protective clothing and handling precautions to control contamination are similar to the "universal precautions" that are taken to protect hospital personnel from pathogens. In most cases, disposable plastic gloves, laboratory coats, and closed-toe

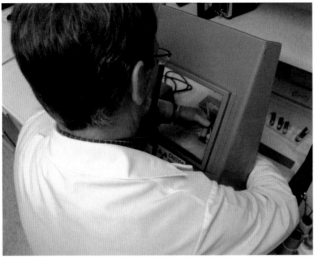

A

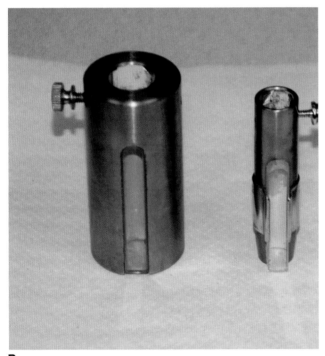

B

■ **FIGURE 21-21 A.** Dose preparation workstation. The technologist is placing a syringe containing a radiopharmaceutical into a syringe shield. Protection from radiation exposure is afforded by working behind the lead "L-shield" with a 1.8-mm lead equivalent glass window that reduces the radiation exposure from Tc-99m by approximately 100. The technologist is wearing a lab coat and disposable gloves to protect his skin and clothing from contamination. A film badge is worn on the lab coat to record body exposure and a TLD finger ring dosimeter is worn inside the glove with the TLD chip facing the source to record the extremity exposure. **B.** A much thicker syringe shield is required for PET radiopharmaceuticals to attenuate the 511 keV annihilation photons (left) compared to the typical syringe shields used for shielding the 140 keV photons from Tc-99m (right).

TABLE 21-8 EXPOSURE REDUCTION ACHIEVED BY A 0.5-mm LEAD EQUIVALENT APRON FOR VARIOUS RADIATION SOURCES

SOURCE	ENERGY (keV)	EXPOSURE REDUCTION WITH 1 APRON	NO. OF APRONS TO REDUCE EXPOSURE BY 90% (*i.e.*, 1 TVL)	WEIGHT (lb)
Scattered x-rays	10–30	>90%	~1	~15
Tc-99m	140	~70%	~2	~30
Cs-137	662	~6%	~36	~540

shoes offer adequate protection. One advantage of working with radioactive material, in comparison to other hazardous substances, is that small quantities can be easily detected. Personnel and work surfaces must be routinely surveyed for contamination. Non-radioactive material work areas near radioactive material use areas (*e.g.*, reading rooms and patient exam areas) should be posted as "clean areas" where radioactive materials are prohibited. Work surfaces where unsealed radioactive materials are used should be covered by plastic-backed absorbent paper that is changed when contaminated or worn. Volatile radionuclides (*e.g.*, I-131 and Xe-133 gas) should be stored in a fume hood with 100% exhaust to the exterior of the building to prevent airborne contamination and subsequent inhalation. Personnel should discard gloves into designated radioactive waste receptacles after working with radioactive material and monitor their hands, shoes, and clothing for contamination periodically. All personnel should wash their hands after handling radioactive materials and especially before eating or drinking to minimize the potential for internal contamination. If the skin becomes contaminated, the best method of decontamination is washing with soap and warm water. The skin should not be decontaminated too aggressively to avoid creating abrasions that can enhance internal absorption. External contamination is rarely a serious health hazard; however, internal contamination can lead to significant radiation exposure. Good contamination control techniques help prevent inadvertent internal contamination.

The effectiveness of contamination control is monitored by periodic GM meter surveys (after handling unsealed radioactive material, whenever contamination is suspected, before lunch, at the end of each workday) and wipe tests (typically weekly) of radionuclide use areas. Wipe tests are performed by wiping surfaces using small pieces of filter paper or cotton-tipped swabs to check for removable contamination at various locations throughout the nuclear medicine laboratory. These wipe test samples (sometimes called "swipes"), typically performed over an area of about 100 cm^2, are usually counted in a NaI(Tl) γ well counter. Areas that are demonstrated to have swipes in excess of about 200–1,000 or greater disintegrations per minute (dpm) over an area of 100 cm^2, depending on local regulations and practices, are considered to be contaminated. The contaminated areas should be promptly decontaminated followed by additional wipe tests to confirm the effectiveness of decontamination efforts. Careful and deliberate GM meter surveys are also performed throughout the department at the end of the day to detect areas of contamination. A common action level is twice the background radiation level. In addition, exposure rate measurements (with a portable ion chamber survey meter) are made near areas that could produce high exposure rates (*e.g.*, radioactive waste and material storage areas).

21.7.5 Laboratory Safety Practices

The following are other laboratory safety practices to minimize the potential for personnel or facility contamination. Examples of these radiation safety practices are shown in Figure 21-22.

- Label each container of radioactive material with a "Caution—Radioactive Material" label and the radionuclide, measurement or calibration date, activity, and chemical form.
- Wear laboratory coats or other protective clothing at all times in areas where radioactive materials are used.
- Wear disposable gloves at all times while handling radioactive material.
- Have available GM probes and scintillator probes with associated meters that are calibrated.

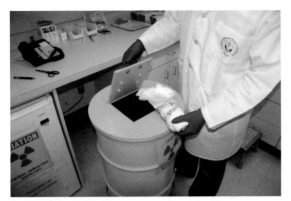

A

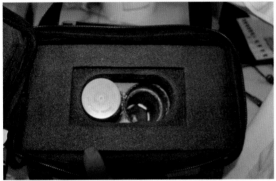

B

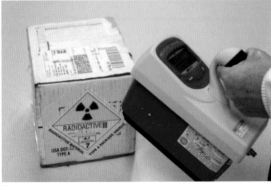

C

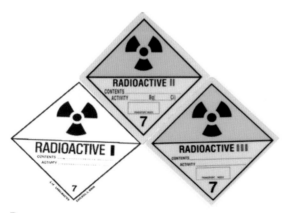

D

■ **FIGURE 21-22** Routine radiation safety practices in nuclear medicine. **A.** Disposal of radioactive waste into a shielded container and proper posting of caution radioactive material signs. **B.** Unit dosages of radiopharmaceuticals come from a commercial radiopharmacy in lead shielded tubes that are cushioned for transport. **C.** Package survey with ion chamber survey meter to verify the shielding of the radioactive material is intact. **D.** Package labels state the radionuclides, the activity, and the maximum exposure rates expected at one meter from the package surface.

21.7 Radiation Protection in Nuclear Medicine

- Either after each procedure or before leaving the area, monitor hands and clothing for contamination in a low-background area using an appropriate survey instrument. In many high-volume use areas, *e.g.*, radiopharmacy, hand and foot monitors should be installed near the entrances/exits to encourage proper personal contamination monitoring.
- Use syringe shields for the reconstitution of radiopharmaceutical kits and administration of radiopharmaceuticals to patients, except when their use is contraindicated (*e.g.*, recessed veins, infants). In these and other exceptional cases, use other protective methods, such as remote delivery of the dose. Using a butterfly needle to obtain venous access will allow the use of a syringe shield in difficult cases.
- Wear personnel monitoring devices, if required, at all times while in areas where radioactive materials are used or stored. When not being worn to monitor occupational exposures, personnel monitoring devices shall be stored in the workplace in a designated low-background area.
- Wear an extremity dosimeter, if required, when handling radioactive material. This should be worn on the hand likely to receive the larger radiation exposure.
- Dispose of radioactive waste only in designated, labeled, and properly shielded receptacles.
- Shield sources of radioactive material to reduce exposure to people.
- After the delivery of a package of radioactive material, survey the package to ensure the source shielding has not been damaged in transport and that the package is not leaking or contaminated.
- Do not eat, drink, store food, smoke, or apply cosmetics in any area where radioactive material is stored or used.
- Perform Xe-133 ventilation studies in a room with negative pressure with respect to the hallway. (Negative pressure will occur if the room air exhaust rate substantially exceeds the supply rate. The difference is made up by air flowing from the hallway into the room, preventing the escape of the xenon gas.) Xe-133 exhaled by patients undergoing ventilation studies should be exhausted into a Xe trap. Xe traps have large shielded activated charcoal cartridges, which adsorb xenon on the large surface areas presented by the charcoal, thus slowing its migration through the cartridge and allowing significant decay to occur before it is exhausted to the environment.
- Report serious spills or accidents to the radiation safety officer (RSO) or health physics staff.

21.7.6 Ordering, Receiving, and Unpacking Radioactive Materials

National (10 CFR Part 20) and local radiation safety regulations (*e.g.*, those of agreement states) and guidelines/model procedures (see appendix P, NRC, 2016) have specific requirements for ordering, receiving, and opening radioactive materials. It is important to authorize, through a designee (*e.g.*, RSO), each order of radioactive material and ensure that the requested materials and quantities are authorized by the license for use by the requesting authorized user (AU) and that possession limits are not exceeded. Carriers should be instructed to deliver radioactive packages directly to a specified area. Additionally, the security of radioactive material must be considered for all receiving areas. Licensees must ensure that the type and quantity of the radioactive material possessed are in accordance with the license conditions. Packages must be secured and radiation exposure from such packages should be minimized.

Precautions for safely opening packages containing radioactive materials should include the use of gloves to prevent hand contamination, visual inspection of the package to identify possible damage, monitoring the external surfaces of a labeled (*i.e.*, radioactive white I, yellow II, or yellow III label per US Department of Transportation regulation) package for radioactive contamination and radiation levels, checking the integrity of the final source container, and a check to ensure that the material received is the material that was ordered by the user. In the US, licensees must monitor the external surface of each package for radioactive contamination (*e.g.*, by swipe sampling) within 3 hours of receipt if it is received during normal working hours, or not later than 3 hours from the beginning of the next working day if it is received after working hours.

Facilities that may prepare for shipment, ship, or transport of radioactive materials, including radioactive waste, must develop, implement, and maintain safety programs for the transport of radioactive material to ensure compliance with all US Nuclear Regulatory Commission (NRC) (*e.g.*, 10 CFR 30 and 71) and US Department of Transportation (DOT) regulations (*e.g.*, 49 CFR Parts 171–178). Most packages of licensed material for medical use contain quantities of radioactive material that require particular packaging (*i.e.*, DOT Type A packages). Many packages shipped by medical facilities (*e.g.*, unused radiopharmaceutical dosages) frequently meet the "Excepted Package for Limited Quantities" criteria as described by DOT (49 CFR 173.421) and are therefore excepted from certain DOT requirements, provided certain other less restrictive requirements are met. Most national and local regulations require specific training and/or certifications for shipping radioactive material.

21.7.7   Radioactive Material Spills

Urgent first aid takes priority over decontamination after an accident, and personnel decontamination takes priority over facility decontamination efforts. Keep in mind the following actions immediately following the discovery of a spill of radioactive material (S.W.I.M): **s**top the spill, **w**arn others about the spill, **i**solate the area, and **m**itigate (clean from the outside in). Report serious spills or accidents to the RSO or health physics staff. Individuals in the immediate area should be alerted to a spill and remain until they can be monitored with a GM survey instrument to ensure that they have not been contaminated. Radioactive material spills should be contained with absorbent material and the area isolated and posted with warning signs indicating the presence of radioactive contamination. Disposable shoe covers and plastic gloves should be donned before beginning decontamination. Decontamination should be performed from the perimeter of the spill toward the center to limit the spread of contamination. Decontamination is usually accomplished by simply absorbing the spill and cleaning the affected areas with detergent and water. A meter survey and wipe test should be used to verify successful decontamination. Personnel participating in decontamination should remove their protective clothing and be surveyed with a GM survey instrument to assure that they are not contaminated. If the spill involves volatile radionuclides or if other conditions exist that suggest the potential for internal contamination, bioassays should be performed by the radiation safety staff. Common bioassays for internal contamination include external counting with a NaI(Tl) detector (*e.g.*, thyroid bioassay for radioiodine) and measurement of radioactivity in urine (*e.g.*, tritium bioassay).

21.7.8   Protection of the Patient in Nuclear Medicine

Sometimes nuclear medicine patients are administered the wrong radiopharmaceutical or the wrong activity. Depending upon the activity, dose, and other specifics, these accidents may meet the regulatory criteria for what are referred to as *medical events* (see Chapter 16), which have prescriptive reporting and quality improvement requirements. The following event has occurred at several institutions: a patient referred for a whole-body bone scan (typically 740 MBq [20 mCi] of Tc-99m MDP) has been mistakenly administered up to 370 MBq (10 mCi) of I-131 sodium iodide for a whole-body thyroid cancer survey (thyroidal dose for 370 MBq and 20% uptake is ~100 Gy [10,000 rad]). The cause has often been a verbal miscommunication. In another case, a mother who was nursing an infant was administered a therapeutic dose of I-131 sodium iodide without being instructed to discontinue breast-feeding, resulting in an estimated dose of 300 Gy (30,000 rad) to the infant's thyroid. The following precautions, most of which are mandated by the U.S. Nuclear Regulatory Commission (NRC), are intended to reduce the frequency of such incidents.

Each syringe or vial that contains a radiopharmaceutical must be conspicuously labeled with the name of the radiopharmaceutical or its abbreviation. Each syringe or vial shield must also be conspicuously labeled unless the label on the syringe or vial is visible. It is prudent to also label each syringe or vial containing a dosage of a radiopharmaceutical with the patient's name. The patient's identity must be verified, whenever possible by two means (*e.g.*, by having the patient recite his or her name and birth date). The possibility that a female adolescent or a woman is pregnant or nursing an infant by breast must be ascertained before administering the radiopharmaceutical. In the case of activities of I-131 sodium iodide exceeding 30 µCi and therapeutic radiopharmaceuticals, pregnancy should be ruled out by a pregnancy test within 72 h before the procedure, certain premenarche in a child, certain postmenopausal state, or documented hysterectomy or tubal ligation.

Before the administration of activities exceeding 1.1 MBq (30 µCi) of I-131 in the form of sodium iodide and any radionuclide therapy, a written directive must be prepared by a nuclear medicine physician, designated as an AU for such administrations, identifying the patient, the radionuclide, the radiopharmaceutical, the activity to be administered, and the route of administration. The written directive must be consulted at the time of administration and the patient's identity should be verified by two methods. Although not required by the NRC, similar precautions should be taken when reinjecting autologous radiolabeled blood products to prevent transfusion reactions and the transmission of pathogens.

21.7.9 Cessation/Interruption of Breast-Feeding

In some cases, women who are nursing infants by breast at the time of nuclear medicine examinations may need to be counseled to discontinue breast-feeding until the radioactivity in breast milk has been reduced to a safe level. Table 21-9 contains recommendations for the period of cessation of breast-feeding after the administration of radiopharmaceuticals to mothers (Mitchell et al., 2019). In addition to reducing or preventing dose to the infant from breast milk, cessation may also help minimize breast dose. For example, ceasing breast-feeding 4–6 weeks before I-131 therapy allows time for lactation to stop before administration of the dose and minimizes breast dose from tissue uptake of I-131.

Radiation doses from activity ingested by a nursing infant have been estimated for the most common radiopharmaceuticals used in diagnostic nuclear medicine (Stabin and Breitz, 2000). In many cases, no interruption in breast-feeding is needed to maintain a radiation dose to the infant well below 1 mSv. Only a brief interruption (hours to days) of breast-feeding was advised for other Tc-99m radiopharmaceuticals: macroaggregated albumin, pertechnetate, red blood cells, white blood cells, as well as I-123 metaiodobenzylguanidine, and Tl-201. Another alternative would be to suggest pumping milk and storing it before the scan. If a woman can pump a day

TABLE 21-9 RECOMMENDED DURATION OF INTERRUPTION OF BREAST-FEEDING FOLLOWING RADIOPHARMACEUTICAL ADMINISTRATION TO A PATIENT TO LIMIT THE EDE TO A NURSING INFANT OR CHILD TO ≤1 mSv[a]

RADIOPHARMACEUTICAL	ADMINISTERED ACTIVITY MBq (mCi)	DURATION OF INTERRUPTION OF BREAST-FEEDING
Tc-99m DTPA, MDP, PYP, RBC, or GH	740 (20)	None
Tc-99m sestamibi or tetrofosmin	1,110 (30)	None
Tc-99m disofenin	300 (8)	None
Tc-99m MAG3	370 (10)	None
Tc-99m sulfur colloid	444 (12)	None
I-123 OIH	74 (2)	None
Tc-99m sodium pertechnetate	185 (5)	4 h
Tc-99m MAA	148 (4)	12 h
F-18 FDG[b]	740 (20)	12 h[b]
I-123 NaI	14.8 (0.4)	24 h
I-123 MIBG	370 (10)	48 h
Tc-99m WBC	185 (5)	48 h
In-111 WBC	18.5 (0.5)	1 wk
Tl-201 chloride	111 (3)	96 h
Ga-67 citrate	185 (5)	Discontinue[c]
I-131 NaI	1 (0.027)	Discontinue[c]

"None" means that interruption of breast-feeding need not be recommended, given criterion of a limit of 1 mSv effective dose to infant and these administered activities. However, even this low dose may be reduced by a 12 to 24-h interruption of breast-feeding.

[a]Adapted from NUREG 1556, Vol. 9, Rev. 3, Program-Specific Guidance About Medical Use Licenses, Appendix U, U.S. Nuclear Regulatory Commission, January 2016; as well as The Academy of Breastfeeding Medicine (Mitchell, 2019). (See Romney BM, Nickloff EL, Esser PD, et al. Radionuclide administration to nursing mothers: mathematically derived guidelines. *Radiology.* 1986;160:549-554; for derivation of milk concentration values for radiopharmaceuticals.)

[b]Minimal F-18 FDG in breast milk (*J Nucl Med.* 2001;42(8):1238-1242). Waiting 6 half-lives (12 h) lowers the exposure to the infant from the mother.

[c]Discontinuance is based not only on the long duration recommended for cessation of breast-feeding but also on the high dose the breasts themselves would receive during the radiopharmaceutical breast transit. (Stabin MG, Breitz HB. Breast milk excretion of radiopharmaceuticals: mechanisms, findings, and radiation dosimetry. *J Nucl Med.* 2000;41(5):863-873.)

DTPA, diethylenetriaminepentaaceticacid; MAA, macroaggregated albumin; disofenin is an iminodiacetic acid derivative; FDG, fluorodeoxyglucose; MIBI, methoxyisobutylisonitrile; MDP, methylene diphosphonate; PYP, pyrophosphate; RBC, red blood cells; WBC, white blood cells; OIH, orthoiodohippurate; MIBG, metaiodobenzylguanidine; GH, glucoheptonate; MAG3, mercaptoacetyltriglycine.

or two of milk before a Tc-99m scan there would essentially be no radiation dose to the child from breast milk while nursing. Complete cessation is suggested for Ga-67 citrate and I-131; however, a prior recommendation for cessation following I-123 NaI administration was based on 2.5% contamination with I-125, which is no longer applicable (Siegel, 2002).

The NRC requires written instructions be given to nursing mothers if the sum the internal and external doses (referred to as the total effective dose equivalent or TEDE, see "Summing Internal and External Doses" below) to a nursing infant could exceed 1 mSv (Code of Federal Regulations Title 10 Part 35.75). The instructions include guidance on the interruption or discontinuation of breast-feeding, and information on the potential consequences, if any, of failure to follow the guidance.

21.7.10 Radionuclide Therapies

Treatment of thyroid cancer and hyperthyroidism with I-131 sodium iodide are proven and widely utilized forms of radionuclide therapy. NaI-131 is manufactured in liquid and capsule form. I-131 in capsules is incorporated into a waxy or crystalline matrix or bound to a gelatin substance, all of which reduce the volatility of the I-131. In recent years, advances in monoclonal antibody and chelation chemistry technology have produced a variety of radioimmunotherapeutic agents, many labeled with I-131. I-131 decays with an 8-day half-life and emits high-energy beta particles and γ-rays. These decay properties, together with the facts that I-131 can be released as a gas under certain conditions, can be absorbed through the skin, and concentrates in the thyroid, necessitate several radiation protection precautions during the preparation and administration of therapeutic quantities of I-131.

Following administration, I-131 is secreted or excreted in all body fluids including urine, saliva, and perspiration. In some cases, the patient may need to be hospitalized as a radiation safety precaution or because of comorbidities (criteria for hospitalization are discussed below). If a patient is to be hospitalized, before I-131 is administered, surfaces of the patient's room likely to become contaminated, such as the floor, bed controls, mattress, light switches, toilet, and telephone, are covered with plastic or absorbent plastic-backed paper to prevent contamination. In addition, the patient's meals are served on disposable trays. Containers are placed in the patient's room to dispose of used meal trays and to hold contaminated linens for decay. Radiation safety staff will measure exposure rates at the bedside, at the doorway, and in neighboring rooms. In some cases, immediately adjacent rooms must be posted off-limits to control radiation exposure to other patients and nursing staff. These measurements are posted, together with instructions to the nurses and visitors including maximal permissible visiting times. Nursing staff are required to wear dosimeters and are trained in the radiation safety precautions necessary to care for these patients safely. Visitors are required to wear disposable shoe covers or to remain outside the room, and staff members wear both shoe covers and disposable gloves to prevent contamination. Visiting times are limited and patients are instructed to stay in their beds during visits and avoid direct physical contact with visitors to keep radiation exposure and contamination to a minimum. Visitors and staff are usually restricted to non-pregnant adults. After the patient is discharged, the health physics or nuclear medicine staff decontaminates the room and verifies through wipe tests and GM surveys that the room is sufficiently decontaminated. Federal or state regulations may require thyroid bioassays of staff technologists and physicians directly involved with dose preparation or administration of large activities of I-131. Additional radiation protection guidance for nuclear medicine therapy is provided by the ICRP in Publication 140, *Radiological Protection in Therapy with Radiopharmaceuticals* (ICRP, 2019).

Phosphorus-32 as sodium phosphate is used for the treatment of polycythemia vera and some leukemias, and palliation of pain from cancerous metastases in bone; P-32 in colloidal form is used to treat malignant effusions and other diseases. Strontium-89 chloride, samarium-153 lexidronam, and radium-223 dichloride are used to treat intractable pain from metastatic bone disease. The primary radiation safety precaution for these radionuclide therapies is contamination control. For example, the wound and bandages at the site of an intra-abdominal instillation of P-32 should be checked regularly for leakage. The blood and urine will be contaminated, and universal precautions should be observed. Exposure rates from patients treated with pure beta emitters like P-32 are not significant. Likewise, the exposure rates from patients treated with Sr-89 and Y-90 are insignificant compared to the risk of contamination.

Iodine-131, yttrium-90, and lutetium-177, bound to monoclonal antibodies or peptides, are used to treat several cancers that exhibit particular antigens (*e.g.*, non-Hodgkin's lymphomas, or neuroendocrine cancers). The precautions for therapy with I-131 antibodies are similar to those for therapies using I-131 sodium iodide. Similarly, the precautions for therapies with Y-90 antibodies are similar to those in the previous paragraph. Recent therapeutic advances include the use of targeted alpha-emitting radionuclides (*e.g.*, Ra-223, At-211, Bi-213, and Ac-225), and while external dose rates from such patients are typically very low, careful contamination control and appropriate alpha surveying and monitoring are important considerations.

Lu-177 dotatate is used for the treatment of some neuroendocrine cancers and at least one other Lu-177 therapeutic agent is in clinical trials. Lu-177 dotatate is usually administered by a slow intravenous infusion in 4 dosages, eight weeks apart. An amino acid solution is also administered, starting at least 30 min before each Lu-177 administration and continuing for a few hours after the Lu-177 administration. Lu-177 is in the patients' excreta, particularly urine. Such administrations require a room, prepared in advance to control contamination, and a nearby toilet. Precautions should be taken to prevent the spread of contamination; these include a survey of the room after each administration. Because Lu-177 emits γ-rays, precautions also should be taken to minimize exposures to clinical staff providing care to the patient, and possibly to people in nearby areas.

Intra-arterial treatment of hepatocellular carcinoma and liver metastases now includes selective internal radiation therapy with Y-90 microspheres, administered by direct infusion into hepatic artery branches that supply the tumors. The microspheres are administered through a catheter, using fluoroscopic imaging guidance, typically in an interventional radiology imaging suite. The most important radiation safety concerns are proper administration to patients and contamination control in the healthcare setting. Microspheres should be treated as unsealed sources of radiation, and comprehensive plans should be in place to reduce the risk of or respond effectively to, contamination. A hazard with Y-90 microspheres is that, if spilled, they can spread widely, particularly if they become dry.

21.7.11 Patient Release Criteria

The NRC regulations (Title 10 CFR Part 35.75) require that patients receiving therapeutic radionuclides be hospitalized until or unless it can be demonstrated that the TEDE to any other individual from exposure to the released patient is not likely to exceed 5 mSv. Guidance on making this determination can be found in NRC Regulatory Guide 8.39, Revision 1, "Release of Patients Administered Radioactive Materials." Additional guidance and methodologies are provided by the NCRP in Report 155, "Management of Radionuclide Therapy Patients" (NCRP, 2006). These documents describe methods for calculating doses to other individuals and contain tables of activities not likely to cause doses exceeding 5 mSv. For example, patients may be released from the hospital following I-131 therapy when the activity in the patient is at or below 1.2 GBq (33 mCi) or when the dose rate at 1 m from the patient is at or below 70 µSv/h, or the patient is provided and acknowledges specific radiation precautions necessary to ensure doses to others are not likely to exceed 5 mSv and agrees to comply with them (NCRP, 2006).

To monitor the activity of I-131 in a patient, an initial exposure measurement is obtained at 1 m from the patient soon after the administration of the radiopharmaceutical. This exposure rate is proportional to the administered activity. Exposure rate measurements are repeated daily until the exposure rate associated with 1.2 GBq

(33 mCi) is obtained. The exposure rate from 33 mCi in a patient will vary with the mass of the patient. The activity remaining in the patient can be estimated by comparing initial and subsequent exposure rate measurements made at a fixed, reproducible geometry. The exposure rate equivalent to 1.2 GBq (33 mCi) remaining the patient ($X_{1.2}$) is

$$X_{1.2} = \frac{(1.2 \text{ GBq}) X_0}{A_0},$$

where X_0 is the initial exposure rate (~15 min after radiopharmaceutical administration) and A_0 is the administered activity (GBq).

For example, a thin patient is administered 5.55 GBq (150 mCi) I-131, after which an exposure rate measurement at 1 m reads 323 µGy/h (37 mR/h). The patient can be discharged when the exposure rate at 1 m falls below:

$$X_{1.2} = \frac{(1.2 \text{ GBq})(37 \text{ mR/h})}{5.5 \text{ GBq}} = 8.0 \text{ mR/h}.$$

Once below 1.2 GBq (33 mCi), assuming a stable medical condition, the patient may be released. If the TEDE to any other individual is likely to exceed 1 mSv (0.1 rem), the NRC requires the licensee to provide the released individual, or the individual's parent or guardian, with radiation safety instructions. These instructions must be provided in writing and include recommended actions that would minimize radiation exposure to, and contamination of, other individuals. The NCRP has developed guidelines for patient release in Report No. 155 (NCRP, 2006) and professional societies, such as the American Thyroid Association (Sisson et al., 2011), have developed radionuclide-specific recommendations that are available to the imaging physicist as useful methods. An example set of radiation safety precautions for home care following radioiodine therapy is shown in Appendix I. These precautions also apply to patient therapy with less than 1.2 GBq (33 mCi) of I-131 for hyperthyroidism. On the rare occasions when these patients are hospitalized for medical or radiation safety reasons (*e.g.*, small children at home), contamination control procedures similar to thyroid cancer therapy with I-131 should be observed.

21.7.12 Radioactive Waste Disposal

Minimizing radioactive waste is an important element of radioactive material use. Most radionuclides used in nuclear medicine have short half-lives that allow them to be held until they have decayed. As a rule, radioactive material is held for at least 10 half-lives and then surveyed in an area of low radiation background with an appropriate radiation detector (typically a GM survey instrument with a pancake probe) to confirm the absence of any detectable radioactivity before being discarded as nonradioactive waste. Disposal of decayed radioactive waste in the nuclear medicine department is made easier by segregating the waste into short half-life (*e.g.*, F-18 and Tc-99m), intermediate half-life (*e.g.*, Ga-67, In-111, I-123, Xe-133, Tl-201), and long half-life (*e.g.*, P-32, Cr-51, Sr-89, I-131) radionuclides.

Small amounts of radioactive material may be disposed of into the sanitary sewer system if the material is water-soluble and the total amount does not exceed regulatory limits. Records of all radioactive material disposals must be maintained for inspection by regulatory agencies. Radioactive excreta from patients receiving diagnostic or therapeutic radiopharmaceuticals are exempt from these disposal regulations and thus may be disposed into the sanitary sewer. The short half-lives and large dilution in the sewer system provide a large margin of safety with regard to environmental contamination and public exposure.

Many solid waste and medical waste disposal facilities have radiation detection systems to monitor incoming waste shipments. It is prudent for hospitals to take measures to ensure that radioactive patient waste such as diapers are not inadvertently placed into non-radioactive waste containers. Many hospitals have radiation waste monitoring systems and housekeepers take solid waste containers past them to ensure no significant amount of radioactive materials are present before discarding the waste into dumpsters.

21.8 REGULATORY AGENCIES AND RADIATION EXPOSURE LIMITS

21.8.1 Regulatory Agencies

Several regulatory agencies have jurisdiction over various aspects of the use of radiation in medicine. The regulations promulgated under their authority carry the force of law. These agencies can inspect facilities and records, levy fines, suspend activities, and issue and revoke radiation use authorizations.

The U.S. NRC regulates *special nuclear* material (plutonium and uranium enriched in the isotopes U-233 and U-235), *source* material (thorium, uranium, and their ores), and *by-product* material used in the commercial nuclear power industry, research, medicine, and a variety of other commercial activities. Under the terms of the Atomic Energy Act of 1954, which established the Atomic Energy Commission whose regulatory arm now exists as the NRC, the agency was given regulatory authority only for special nuclear, source, and by-product material. The term by-product material originally referred primarily to radioactive by-products of nuclear fission in nuclear reactors, that is, fission products and radioactive materials produced by neutron activation. However, the federal Energy Policy Act of 2005 modified the definition of by-product material to include material made radioactive by use of a particle accelerator. Thus, accelerator-produced radioactive materials (*e.g.*, cyclotron-produced radionuclides such as F-18, Tl-201, I-123, and In-111) are subject to NRC regulation.

Most states administer their own radiation control programs for radioactive materials and other radiation sources. These states have entered into agreements with the NRC, under the Atomic Energy Act of 1954, to promulgate and enforce regulations similar to those of the NRC and are known as "agreement states." These agreement states conduct the same regulatory oversight, inspection, and enforcement actions that would otherwise be performed by the NRC. In addition, the agencies of the agreement states typically regulate all sources of ionizing radiation, including diagnostic and interventional x-ray machines and linear accelerators used in radiation oncology.

While NRC and agreement state regulations are not identical, many essential aspects are common to all of these regulatory programs. Workers must be informed of their rights and responsibilities, including the risks inherent in utilizing radiation sources and their responsibility to follow established safety procedures. The NRC's regulations are contained in Title 10 (Energy) of the Code of Federal Regulations (CFR). The most important sections for medical use of radionuclides are the "Standards for Protection against Radiation" (Part 20) and "Medical Use of By-Product Material" (Part 35). Part 20 contains the definitions utilized in the radiation control regulations and requirements for radiation surveys; personnel monitoring (dosimetry and bioassay); radiation warning signs and symbols; and shipment, receipt, control, storage, and disposal of radioactive material. Part 20 also specifies the maximal permissible doses to radiation workers and the public; environmental release limits; and documentation and notification requirements after a significant radiation accident or event, such as the loss of a brachytherapy source or the release of a large quantity of radioactive material to the environment.

Part 35 lists the requirements for the medical use of by-product material. Some of the issues covered in this section include the medical use categories, training requirements, precautions to be followed in the medical use of radiopharmaceuticals, testing and use of dose calibrators, and requirements for the reporting of medical events involving specified errors in the administrations of radiopharmaceuticals to patients. The NRC also issues regulatory guidance documents, which provide the licensee with methods acceptable to NRC for satisfying the regulations. The procedures listed in these documents may be adopted completely or in part with the licensee's own procedures, which will be subject to NRC review and approval.

The FDA regulates the development and manufacturing of radiopharmaceuticals as well as the manufacturing of medical x-ray equipment. Its regulations regarding the manufacture of medical x-ray imaging equipment contain extensive design and performance requirements for the equipment. Although this agency does not directly regulate the end-user (except for mammography), it does maintain a strong involvement in both the technical and regulatory aspects of human research with radioactive materials (FDA, 2010) and other radiation sources and publishes guidance documents in areas of interest including radiologic health, design, and use of x-ray machines, radiopharmaceutical development, and specific regulations on mammographic imaging (FDA, 2020). FDA regulations, specifically 21 CFR 803, require the reporting of serious injuries and deaths that a medical device has or may have caused or contributed to.

The DOT regulates the shipping and transportation of radioactive materials. The U.S. Department of Labor (OSHA) promulgates worker-safety standards, including for radioactive material use. The Federal Policy for the Protection of Human Subjects, incorporated in the regulations of many federal agencies, promulgates requirements for research involving human subjects that are conducted, supported, or regulated by one of these agencies. It requires review and approval of the research by an institutional review board and that the subjects give informed consent to their participation. The U.S. Environmental Protection Agency (EPA) develops risk assessment techniques as well as requirements for waste disposal and land cleanup. Other regulations and recommendations related to medical radiation use programs are promulgated by other federal, state, and local agencies. Many States consider guidance from the Conference on Radiation Control Program Directors (CRCPD) when developing local regulations, thereby resulting in cooperation and consistency in addressing radiation protection issues between Federal agencies and local agencies. Often, x-ray regulations are promulgated at the State level (with the additional rules on mammography coming from the FDA) and several States specifically designate definitions of Qualified Medical Physicists.

21.8.2 Advisory Bodies

Several advisory organizations exist that periodically review the scientific literature and issue recommendations regarding various aspects of radiation protection. While their recommendations do not constitute regulations and thus do not carry the force of law, they are usually the origin of most of the regulations adopted by regulatory agencies and are widely recognized as "standards of good practice." Many of these recommendations are voluntarily adopted by the medical community even in the absence of a specific legal requirement. The two most widely recognized advisory bodies are the NCRP and the ICRP. The NCRP is a non-profit corporation chartered by Congress to collect, analyze, develop, and disseminate, in the public interest, information and recommendations about radiation protection, radiation measurements, quantities, and units. In addition, it is charged with working to stimulate cooperation and effective utilization of resources regarding radiation protection with other organizations including the ICRP. The ICRP is similar in scope to the NCRP; however, its international membership brings to bear a variety of perspectives on radiation health issues. The dose limits of the countries in the European Union are based upon its recommendations, with guidance provided by the International Atomic Energy Agency (IAEA). The IAEA also manages an international online resource for health professionals on the radiation protection of patients (IAEA, 2020), including several specific guidance documents for radiation safety in radiology and nuclear medicine applications. The NCRP and ICRP have published over 300 monographs containing recommendations on a wide variety of radiation health issues that serve as the reference documents from which many regulations are crafted. The United Nations Scientific Committee on the Effects of Atomic Radiation (UNSCEAR) reports to the United Nations General Assembly and assesses global levels and effects of ionizing radiation providing widely available evaluations of the scientific basis for radiation protection.

Several professional societies have developed practical specific recommendations and guidance in the area of radiation protection of patients and staff that should be consulted by practicing medical physicists, for example, American Association of Physicists in Medicine (AAPM), American Brachytherapy Society (ABS), American College of Radiology (ACR), American Thyroid Association (ATA), American Society for Radiation Oncology (ASTRO), Health Physics Society, Radiological Society of North America (RSNA), Radiation Research Society (RRS), Society of Interventional Radiology (SIR), and Society of Nuclear Medicine and Molecular Imaging (SNMMI) among others. In addition, ongoing collaboration between radiology equipment vendors, imaging physicists, and the radiology community serves an important role in overall improvements in medical imaging radiation protection, for example, Medical Imaging & Technology Alliance (MITA) a division of the National Electrical Manufacturer's Association (NEMA), and the International Electrotechnical Commission (IEC).

21.8.3 NRC "Standards for Protection against Radiation"

As mentioned above, the NRC has established "Standards for Protection against Radiation" (10 CFR 20) to protect radiation workers and the public. The regulations incorporate a twofold system of dose limitation: (1) the doses to individuals shall not exceed limits established by the NRC, and (2) all exposures shall be kept ALARA, social and economic factors being taken into account. The regulations adopt a system recommended by the ICRP, which permits internal doses (from ingested or inhaled radionuclides) and doses from radiation sources outside the body to be summed, with a set of limits for the sum.

21.8.4 Summing Internal and External Doses

There are significant differences between external and internal exposures. The dose from an internal exposure continues after the period of ingestion or inhalation until the radioactivity is eliminated by radioactive decay or biologic removal. The exposure may last only a few minutes, for example, in the case of the radionuclide O-15 ($T\frac{1}{2} = 122$ s), or may last the lifetime of the individual, as is the case for the ingestion of long-lived Ra-226. The *committed dose equivalent* ($H_{50,T}$) is the dose equivalent to a tissue or organ over the 50 years following the ingestion or inhalation of radioactivity. The committed effective dose equivalent (CEDE) is a weighted average of the committed dose equivalents to the various tissues and organs of the body:

$$\text{CEDE} = \sum w_T H_{50,T}. \qquad [21\text{-}6]$$

The NRC adopted the quantity *effective dose equivalent* and the tissue weighting factors (w_T) from ICRP Publication 26 (1977) and the annual limits on intake (ALIs) of radionuclides by workers (discussed below) from ICRP Publication 30 (1978–1988), which predate those in the most current ICRP recommendations (ICRP Publication 103, see Chapter 3: Effective Dose).

To sum the internal and external doses to any individual tissue or organ, the deep dose equivalent (indicated by a dosimeter worn by the exposed individual) and the committed dose equivalent to the organ are added. The sum of the external and internal doses to the entire body, called the total effective dose equivalent (TEDE), is the sum of the deep dose equivalent and the CEDE.

21.8.5 Occupational Dose Limits

The NRC's radiation dose limits are intended to limit the risks of stochastic effects, such as cancer and genetic effects, and to prevent deterministic effects, such as cataracts, skin damage, sterility, and hematologic consequences of bone marrow depletion (deterministic and stochastic effects are discussed in Chapter 20). To limit the risk of stochastic effects, the sum of the external and internal doses to the entire body, the TEDE, may not exceed 0.05 Sv (5 rem) in a year. To prevent deterministic effects, the sum of the external dose and committed dose equivalent to any individual organ except the lens of the eye may not exceed 0.5 Sv (50 rem) in a year. The current regulatory dose limit to the lens of the eye is still 0.15 Sv (15 rem) in a year (Fig. 21-23). As discussed in Chapter 20, the ICRP recently reviewed the scientific evidence regarding the risk of radiation-induced cataract and proposed a much more conservative occupational equivalent dose limit for the lens of the eye (20 mSv per year averaged over 5 years, with no single year dose >50 mSv). Similarly, the NCRP has recommended an occupational dose limit for the lens of the eye of 50 mGy per year (NCRP, 2016), although the national regulations have not yet been revised.

The dose to the fetus of a declared pregnant radiation worker may not exceed 5 mSv (0.5 rem) over the entire gestational period and should not substantially exceed 500 µSv (50 mrem) in any 1 month. Table 21-10 lists the most important ICRP and NRC radiation dose limits.

21.8.6 Annual Limits on Intake and Derived Air Concentrations

In practice, the committed dose equivalent and CEDE are seldom used in protecting workers from ingesting or inhaling radioactivity. Instead, the NRC has established annual limits on intake (ALIs), which limit the inhalation or ingestion of radioactive material to activities that will not cause radiation workers to exceed any of the limits in Table 21-10. The ALIs are calculated for the "standard person" and expressed in units of microcuries. ALIs are provided for the inhalation and oral ingestion pathways for a wide variety of radionuclides, some examples of which, relevant to nuclear medicine, are shown in Table 21-11.

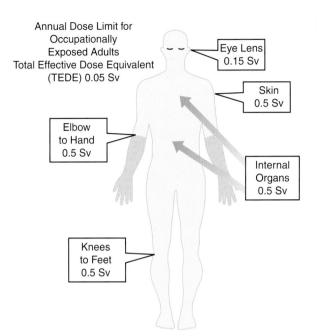

Annual Dose Limit for
Occupationally
Exposed Adults
Total Effective Dose Equivalent
(TEDE) 0.05 Sv

Eye Lens
0.15 Sv

Skin
0.5 Sv

Elbow
to Hand
0.5 Sv

Internal
Organs
0.5 Sv

Knees
to Feet
0.5 Sv

Annual Occupational Dose Limits for Adults
NRC 10CFR20

■ **FIGURE 21-23** NRC's occupational radiation dose limits.

Exposure to airborne activity is also regulated via the derived air concentration (DAC), which is that concentration of a radionuclide that, if breathed under conditions of light activity for 2,000 h (the average number of hours worked in a year), will result in the ALI; DACs are expressed in units of µCi/mL. Table 21-11 lists DACs and ALIs for volatile radionuclides of interest in medical imaging. In circumstances in which either the external exposure or the internal deposition does not exceed 10% of its respective limits, the summation of the internal and external doses is not required to demonstrate compliance with the dose limits; most nuclear medicine departments will be able to take advantage of this exemption.

21.8.7 As Low as Reasonably Achievable Principle

Dose limits to workers and the public are regarded as upper limits rather than as acceptable doses or thresholds of safety. In fact, the majority of occupational exposures in medicine and industry result in doses far below these limits. In addition to the dose limits specified in the regulations, in the United States, all licensees are required to employ good health physics practices and implement radiation safety programs to ensure that radiation exposures to workers and members of the public are kept *ALARA*, taking societal and economic factors into consideration. The ALARA doctrine is the driving force for many of the policies, procedures, and practices in radiation laboratories and represents a commitment by both employee and employer to minimize radiation exposure to staff and the public. For example, the *L*-shield in the nuclear pharmacy may not be specifically required by a regulatory agency; however, its use has become common practice in nuclear medicine departments and represents a "community standard" against which the department's practices will be evaluated.

The ALARA principle is equivalent to the ICRP's principle of optimization of protection, stated in Section 21.4. While the NRC's regulations only apply the ALARA

TABLE 21-10 NUCLEAR REGULATORY COMMISSION REGULATORY REQUIREMENTS (NRC REGULATIONS, 10 CFR 20) AND INTERNATIONAL COMMISSION ON RADIOLOGICAL PROTECTION RECOMMENDATIONS (ICRP 2007) FOR MAXIMUM PERMISSIBLE DOSE

LIMITS[a]	MAXIMUM PERMISSIBLE ANNUAL DOSE LIMITS	
	ICRP 2007 mSv	*NRC mSv (rem)*
Occupational Limits		
Effective dose (total effective dose equivalent)	20/y averaged over 5 y; 50 in any 1 y	50 (5)
Equivalent dose (Dose equivalent) to any individual organ (except lens of the eye) including the skin, hands, feet	500	500 (50)
Equivalent dose (Dose equivalent) to the lens of the eye	20/y averaged over 5 y; 50 in any 1 y	150 (15)[b]
Minor (<18 years old)	Public limits	10% of adult limits
Equivalent dose (Dose equivalent) to an embryo or fetus[c]	1 in 9 mo	5 (0.5) in 9 mo
Non-occupational (public) Limits	1	1.0 (0.1)
Effective dose (total effective dose equivalent)	1	1 (0.1)
Effective dose (total effective dose equivalent) to medical caregivers (*e.g.*, at home with I-131 therapy patient)	5 per episode; 20/y maximum	5 (0.5)
Dose equivalent in an unrestricted area	NA	0.02 (0.002) in any 1 h[d]

[a]These limits are exclusive of natural background and any dose the individual receives for medical purposes; inclusive of internal committed dose equivalent and external effective dose equivalent (*i.e.*, total effective dose equivalent). As explained in the text, ICRP and NRC use different (although similar) dose quantities. In this column, the first quantity is the ICRP quantity and the NRC quantity is in parentheses.
[b]Note that NCRP has recommended that the annual dose limit for occupational exposures for the lens of the eye be reduced to 50 mGy. NCRP. Guidance on Radiation Dose Limits for the Lens of the Eye. NCRP Commentary No. 26. 2016. National Council on Radiation Protection and Measurements.
[c]Applies only to a conceptus of a worker who declares her pregnancy. If the limit exceeds 4.5 mSv (450 mrem) at declaration, the conceptus dose for the remainder of gestation is not to exceed 0.5 mSv (50 mrem).
[d]This means the dose to an unrestricted area (irrespective of occupancy) shall not exceed 0.02 mSv (2 mrem) in any 1 h. This is not a restriction of the instantaneous dose rate to 0.02 mSv/h (2 mrem/h). ICRP. The 2007 Recommendations of the International Commission on Radiological Protection. ICRP Publication 103. *Ann ICRP.* 2007;37:1-332.

principle to the radiation doses of workers and members of the public, the ICRP and many other advisory bodies, professional societies, and governmental agencies recommend the application of the ALARA principle to the radiation doses received by patients in diagnostic and interventional imaging.

21.9 PREVENTION OF ERRORS

A goal of radiation protection programs is to reduce the likelihood and severity of accidents involving radiation and radioactive materials. Although this pertains to the protection of staff, patients, and members of the public, this section focuses on the protection of the patient. However, the principles discussed apply to all of these categories of people.

TABLE 21-11 EXAMPLES OF DACs[a] AND ALIs[b] FOR OCCUPATIONALLY EXPOSED WORKERS (NRC REGULATIONS: 10 CFR 20)

RADIONUCLIDE	DAC (µCi/mL)[c]	ALI (µCi)[a] INGESTION
I-125	3×10^{-8}	40
I-131	2×10^{-8}	30
Tc-99m	6×10^{-5}	8×10^4
Xe-133 (gas)	1×10^{-4}	N/A

[a]DAC is derived air concentration.
[b]ALI is annual limit on intake.
[c]Multiply µCi/mL (or µCi) by 37 to obtain kBq/mL (or kBq).
N/A, not applicable.

21.9.1 Error Prevention Culture

Error prevention is certainly not a field exclusive to medical radiation protection or even medicine in general. Most of the principles have been developed in other industries such as aviation and nuclear power. The report, *To Err Is Human*, by the Institute of Medicine (Kohn et al., 2000) focused national attention on errors in the delivery of care to patients. There has been national media attention regarding the delivery of excessive doses to patients by CT (Bogdanich, 2009) and the professional literature has reported the delivery of unnecessarily high doses to children and infants from CT due to the use of adult technique factors (Paterson et al., 2001). Methods for the prevention of errors in the delivery of care to patients are only briefly discussed in this section.

Efforts in error prevention can be prospective, to avoid errors in the future or retrospective, in response to an error or "near miss" that has occurred, with the goal of preventing a recurrence. The efforts directed toward the prevention of a particular error should be in proportion to the severity of the consequences of the error and the likelihood of the error. Methods for the prevention of errors include the development of written procedures and training of staff initially, periodically thereafter, and in response to incidents or changes in procedures. Policies and procedures may incorporate the use of a "time out" in which the staff about to perform a clinical procedure jointly verify that the intended procedure is to be properly performed on the intended patient; the use of written or computerized checklists to ensure that essential actions are not omitted; checks of critical tasks by a second person; requiring that certain critical communications be in writing; employing readback in verbal communications, whereby the person hearing information repeats it aloud; and measures to avoid distractions and interruptions during critical tasks (from the aviation concept, "sterile cockpit"), such as prohibiting unnecessary conversations unrelated to a task. In developing procedures, it is advisable to consider what errors might occur, procedures developed at other institutions and errors that have occurred in the past. The incorporation of engineered safety features, such as interlocks that prevent unsafe actions, and automated checks, such as the dose notifications and alerts provided by newer CT scanners, help avoid accidents due to human errors. The Joint Commission (TJC) has included similar recommendations in a universal protocol to prevent error prior to surgery, which is one of a number of its national patient safety goals (TJC, 2020).

When an error or a "near-miss" occurs, an analysis should be performed to determine the causes and to devise actions to reduce the likelihood of a recurrence and possibly, the severity of a recurrence. These analyses attempt to identify the most basic correctable causes, called "root causes." Methods for such root cause analyses may be found in several texts. The actions implemented to avoid a recurrence should be designed with the root causes in mind.

Safety culture is a set of attributes of an organization, such as radiology or nuclear medicine department, that are believed to reduce the likelihood of errors. There are varying, but similar definitions or descriptions by various organizations focusing on safety. Safety culture may be defined as the behavior and practices resulting from a commitment by leaders and individuals to emphasize safety over competing goals to protect patients, staff, and the public. The following list of traits of a safety culture was adapted from an NRC policy statement (NRC, 2012):

- Leaders demonstrate a commitment to safety in their decisions and behaviors.
- All individuals take personal responsibility for safety.
- Issues potentially impacting safety are promptly identified, evaluated, and corrected commensurate with their significance.
- Work activities are planned and conducted so that safety is maintained.
- Opportunities to learn about ways to ensure safety are sought out and implemented.
- A work environment is maintained in which people feel free to raise safety concerns.
- Communications maintain a focus on safety.
- Trust and respect permeate the organization.
- Workers avoid complacency and continuously challenge, in a spirit of cooperation, conditions and activities in order to identify discrepancies that might result in an error.

21.9.2 The Joint Commission

The Joint Commission (TJC), formerly the Joint Commission on Accreditation of Healthcare Organizations, is a not-for-profit organization that accredits thousands of hospitals and other health care facilities in the United States. Most state governments have conditioned receipt of Medicaid reimbursement on accreditation by TJC or a similar organization.

TJC defines a *sentinel event* as "an unexpected occurrence involving death or serious physical or psychological injury, or the risk thereof." A sentinel event does not necessarily indicate that a medical error has occurred. However, each sentinel event should be promptly investigated, and action taken if warranted.

TJC defines as a sentinel event prolonged fluoroscopy with a cumulative dose exceeding 15 Gy to a single field, "a single field" being a location on the skin onto which the x-ray beam is directed. The issue here is the magnitude of the dose to that portion of the skin that receives the maximal dose. The maximal dose may result from using several different x-ray beam projections whose beam areas on the patient's skin overlap in a specific location to produce a region of highest radiation dose. It may also result from two or more procedures days or even months apart.

TJC issues sentinel event alerts (SEAs) that identify serious unanticipated incidents in a health care setting that could or did harm patients. TJC expects accredited facilities to consider the information in a SEA when evaluating similar processes and consider implementing relevant suggestions contained in the SEA or reasonable alternatives. TJC has revised a SEA, *Radiation Risks of Diagnostic Imaging, and Fluoroscopy* (TJC, 2019). It warns that health care organizations must seek new ways to reduce exposure to repeated doses of harmful radiation from these diagnostic procedures. The SEA urges greater attention to the risk of long-term damage and cumulative harm that can occur if a patient is given repeated doses of diagnostic radiation. TJC suggests that health care organizations can reduce risks due to avoidable diagnostic radiation by raising awareness among staff and patients of the increased risks associated with cumulative doses and by providing the right test and the right dose through effective processes, safe technology, and a culture of safety. The actions suggested include the following:

- Use of imaging techniques other than CT or fluoroscopy, such as ultrasound or MRI, and collaboration between radiologists and referring physicians about the appropriate use of diagnostic imaging
- Adherence to the ALARA principle, as well as guidelines from the Society for Pediatric Radiology, American College of Radiology and the RSNA, for imaging for children and adults
- Assurance by radiologists that the proper dosing protocol is in place for the patient being treated and review of all dosing protocols either annually or every 2 years
- Expansion of the RSO's role to explicitly include patient safety as it relates to radiation and dosing, as well as education on proper dosing and equipment usage for all qualified medical personnel who prescribe diagnostic radiation or use diagnostic radiation equipment
- Use of a diagnostic medical physicist in designing and altering CT scan protocols; centralized quality and safety performance monitoring of all diagnostic imaging equipment that may emit high amounts of cumulative radiation; testing imaging equipment initially and annually or every 2 years thereafter; and designing a program for quality control, testing (including daily functional tests), and preventive maintenance activities
- Investing in technologies that optimize or reduce patient dose

21.10 MANAGEMENT OF RADIATION SAFETY PROGRAMS

The goals of a radiation safety program were discussed in the introductory paragraph of this chapter. They include maintaining the safety of staff, patients, and members of the public; compliance with regulations of governmental agencies; and preparedness for emergencies involving radiation and/or radioactive material. In particular, the radiation doses of staff and members of the public must not exceed regulatory limits and should conform to the ALARA principle (equivalent to the ICRP's principle of optimization), as described earlier in this chapter. Although there are no regulatory limits to the radiation doses that patients may receive as part of their care, the doses to patients should be optimized. The methods for achieving these goals are described in the other sections of this chapter.

A license from a state regulatory agency, or the US NRC, is required to possess and use radioactive materials in medicine. The license lists the radioactive materials that may be used, the amounts that may be possessed, and the uses that are allowed. The licenses for most institutions list the physicians permitted to use and supervise the use of radioactive material, including diagnostic AUs (10 CFR 35.100 and 35.200, or equivalent) and AUs for procedures requiring written directives (10 CFR 35.300 and 35.1000, or equivalent). Licenses also contain requirements, in addition to the regulations of the state regulatory agency or NRC, regarding procedures and record-keeping requirements for radioactive material receipt, transportation, use, and disposal. Radioactive material use regulations require "cradle-to-grave" control of all radiation sources. Many model procedures can be found in NRC's NUREG 1556, Vol. 9, Rev. 3, *Program-Specific Guidance About Medical Use Licenses* (NRC, 2016).

21.10.1 Radiation Safety Officer

Each medical institution using radioactive material must designate a person, called the RSO, who is responsible for the day-to-day oversight of the radiation safety program and is named on the institution's radioactive material license. The RSO must have appropriate training and qualifications for the role (see 10 CFR 35.50, or equivalent). At a smaller institution, the RSO may be a physician or a consultant. A larger institution may have a person whose main duty is to be the RSO. At very large institutions, the RSO is assisted by additional health physics or medical health physics staff.

21.10.2 Radiation Safety Program Elements

An institution with complex uses of radiation and radioactive material will have a radiation safety committee that oversees the radiation safety program. A radiation safety committee typically meets quarterly and approves policies and procedures, periodically reviews the program, and reviews corrective actions after adverse incidents involving radiation or radioactive material. The radiation safety committee is comprised of the RSO, representatives from departments with substantial radiation and radioactive material use (*e.g.*, nuclear medicine, radiology, cardiology, radiation oncology, and nursing), and a member representing hospital management.

A radiation safety program should include an audit program to ensure compliance with regulatory requirements, accepted radiation safety practices, and institutional procedures. The audit program should evaluate people's knowledge and performance of radiation safety–related activities in addition to reviewing records. This is best accomplished by observing people while they perform tasks related to radiation safety. Personnel dosimetry reports should be reviewed when they arrive from the dosimetry vendor and larger or unusual doses should be investigated. The radiation safety program should ensure the training of staff in regulatory requirements, good radiation safety practices, and institutional procedures; training should be provided initially, periodically thereafter, and as needed, for example, following incidents, changes in regulations, or changes in uses of radiation or radioactive material. A review should be performed of the radiation safety program at least annually, with the findings presented to the radiation safety committee and executive management. The radiation safety program should be "risk-informed," that is, the efforts devoted to radiation safety regarding a particular use should be in proportion to the risks associated with that use.

A diagnostic medical physicist is essential to the radiation safety program of a medical facility performing radiological imaging. A diagnostic medical physicist has expertise in the diagnostic and interventional applications of x-rays, γ-rays, ultrasonic radiation, radiofrequency radiation, and magnetic fields; the equipment associated with their production, use, measurement, and evaluation; the doses of radiation to patients from these sources; the quality of images resulting from their use; and health physics associated with their production and use. Usually, it is the responsibility of a diagnostic medical physicist for testing imaging equipment initially, annually, and after repairs or modifications that may affect the radiation doses to patients or the quality of the images. The diagnostic medical physicist should also participate in the creation and evaluation of the organization's technical quality assurance programs, safety programs (*e.g.*, radiation safety and MRI safety) regarding diagnostic and interventional imaging, and optimization of clinical imaging protocols. Diagnostic medical physicists commonly design the structural shielding for rooms containing radiation-producing equipment and perform shielding evaluations, based upon measurements of transmitted radiation, after the installation of the shielding. Another task occasionally performed is the estimation of the radiation dose to the embryo or fetus after a pregnant patient received an examination before her pregnancy was known or when a procedure on a pregnant patient is being considered. The RSO may be a diagnostic medical physicist. In larger facilities, the radiation safety program may also be implemented by a senior medical health physicist who has expertise in ionizing, non-ionizing radiation protection, radiation biology, and radiation protection. A qualified medical health physicist will be board certified and have extensive knowledge of safety and regulatory aspects of the use of radiation for both diagnostic and therapeutic purposes as well as the use of equipment to perform appropriate radiation measurements. There should be close collaboration and support between diagnostic medical physics and medical health physics teams on many aspects of the radiation safety program.

Another task of a radiation safety program is to respond to adverse incidents or regulatory violations. When such an incident or violation is identified, an analysis of the causes should be performed and actions to prevent a recurrence should be implemented. In some cases, such as a medical event involving a patient, serious injury or death of a patient involving medical equipment, or a person receiving a radiation dose exceeding a regulatory limit, notification of the pertinent state or federal regulatory agency may be required. When such an incident occurs, action to protect the patient, staff, or other people should take priority over meeting regulatory requirements.

21.11 IMAGING OF PREGNANT AND POTENTIALLY PREGNANT PATIENTS

The risks of ionizing radiation to the embryo and fetus must be considered when imaging female patients of childbearing age using ionizing radiation and performing nuclear medicine procedures, especially those involving the administration of I-131 sodium iodide and other therapies using radiopharmaceuticals. These risks vary with the radiation dose and the stage of gestation and have been discussed in Chapter 20. Each department performing imaging or treatments with ionizing radiation should have policies and procedures regarding this issue.

In general, the pregnancy status of a patient of childbearing age should be determined prior to an imaging examination or treatment involving ionizing radiation. Pregnancy status should be determined for female patients from about 12 to 50 years of age. The measures to determine whether a patient is pregnant depend upon the radiation dose that an embryo or fetus would receive. For most examinations, a technologist asks the patient whether she could be pregnant, inquiring about the last menstruation, and documents this information on a form. For a patient who is a minor, it is best to obtain this information in a private setting without the parents or a guardian present. For some procedures that would or might impart doses to an embryo or fetus exceeding 100 mSv, such as possibly prolonged fluoroscopically guided procedures and multi-phase diagnostic CT examinations of the abdomen or pelvis, a pregnancy test should also be obtained within 72 hours before the examination or procedure, unless the examination is medically urgent or the possibility of pregnancy can be eliminated by factors such as a documented hysterectomy. Pregnancy tests should always be obtained before radiopharmaceutical therapies and other administrations of I-131 sodium iodide. Pregnancy tests can produce false-negative results and should not preclude questioning the patient regarding the possibility of pregnancy. Some examinations can be performed without regard to pregnancy due to the very low dose that an embryo or fetus would receive if the patient were pregnant. These include mammograms and diagnostic x-ray imaging of the head, arms and hands, and lower legs and feet.

Occasionally imaging is considered for a patient who is known to be pregnant or suspected of being pregnant. In this case, the radiation dose and potential risks to the embryo or fetus should be estimated and presented to the imaging physician. Consideration should be given to whether the examination or procedure can be delayed until after the pregnancy, alternative examinations or procedures that would not involve ionizing radiation, or that would deliver less radiation to the embryo or fetus, and ways to modify the examination to reduce the radiation dose to the embryo or fetus. However, care should be taken to ensure that modifications to reduce the radiation dose do not cause an inadequate examination that must be repeated. The imaging physician must obtain informed consent from the patient.

Occasionally it is discovered after an examination or treatment with ionizing radiation was performed, that the patient was pregnant at the time of the examination or treatment. In this case, fetal age, the radiation dose to the embryo or fetus, and the potential effects on the embryo or fetus should be estimated. The dose estimation is commonly performed by a diagnostic medical physicist. The patient is then counseled by a physician. In most cases, the risks to the embryo or fetus are small in comparison with the other risks of gestation. The NCRP does not recommend medical intervention with a pregnancy even be considered for estimated doses to the embryo or fetus that do not exceed 100 mSv; if the dose exceeds 100 mSv, decisions would be guided by the fetal age and individual circumstances (NCRP, 2013). All x-ray imaging examinations, in which the embryo or fetus is not close to the area being imaged, impart doses much less than 100 mSv to the embryo or fetus and most x-ray examinations of the abdomen and pelvis, including single-phase diagnostic CT examinations, impart doses less than 100 mSv. More detailed guidance regarding the pregnant or possibly pregnant patient is available in ACR (2018), Dauer et al. (2012), NCRP (2013), and Wagner et al. (1997).

21.12 MEDICAL EMERGENCIES INVOLVING IONIZING RADIATION

Medical institutions should be prepared to respond to emergencies involving radiation and radioactive materials. These may include incidents within the institution, such as spills of radioactive material, contamination of personnel with radioactive material, and medical events involving errors in the administration of radioactive material to patients; these also include external incidents, such as transportation accidents involving shipments of radioactive material, accidents at nuclear facilities, and radiological or nuclear terrorism, which could result in contaminated and injured people arriving at medical facilities. Serious accidents involving substantial radiation exposure or contamination are rare. Hence, most health care providers are unfamiliar with (and may have unjustified fear of) treating patients who have been exposed to radiation or contaminated with radioactive material. Radiologists and other health care professionals familiar with the properties of radiation, its detection, and biological effects (*e.g.*, radiation oncologists, radiation therapists, health and medical physicists, and nuclear medicine and radiology technologists) may be called upon to assist in such emergencies and should be prepared to provide guidance and technical assistance to medical staff managing such patients; they should also assist the medical institution's emergency planner in preparing for such emergencies. The overarching goal in these incidents is to ensure that critically ill or injured patients are not denied effective medical care due to unfounded concerns of medical personnel about risk from providing care to the patients.

21.12.1 Potential Sources of Radiation Exposure and Contamination

Radiation Accidents

Incidents have occurred in which people have been injured by inadvertently coming into contact with objects or material that they did not realize contained large quantities of radioactive material. Small metal capsules containing high-intensity γ-emitting radioactive sources are commonly used for industrial radiography. Failure to realize or report the loss of such sources has resulted in a number of severe radiation injuries to individuals who found the sources but did not recognize the danger. In two cases, stolen radioactive sources once used for cancer therapy were opened, causing widespread contamination and injury to people (Juarez Mexico in 1983 and 1984, Goiânia Brazil in 1987).

A nuclear reactor accident, in which an accidental prompt-critical power excursion caused a steam explosion (Chernobyl in Ukraine in 1986), killed workers and emergency responders and released massive amounts of fission products to the environment (UNSCEAR, 2020). In 2011, a tsunami following a massive earthquake off the coast of Japan caused the loss of core cooling of multiple reactors at the Fukushima Daiichi nuclear power facility. Even though the reactors shut down during the earthquake (stopping further fissioning of the fuel in the reactors), there was still a tremendous amount of heat being produced by the decay of the fission products already created. This led to the core melting in the three reactors in operation at the time and large releases of radioactive material to the atmosphere and the Pacific Ocean and, due to meteorological conditions, a fraction was dispersed over eastern mainland Japan. The rapid accident progression prompted "precautionary evacuation" (within days) of the population living close to the plant (mainly within the 20-km zone) and subsequent "deliberate evacuation" (within weeks up to few months) of people living further afield in areas where the deposition density of radioactive material was high. These actions, along with restrictions on certain food and drink items, likely resulted in a significant reduction in doses (UNSCEAR, 2014). However, there are ongoing difficulties in the post-accident cleanup, both at the plant and in contaminated areas, and challenges associated with the selection, implementation, and communication of appropriate cleanup levels.

Radiological and Nuclear Terrorism

There is concern that radioactive material or an improvised nuclear device (an improvised nuclear weapon, less likely but potentially much more devastating) could be used as a weapon of terrorism. A hidden radioactive source referred to as a radiation exposure device could be used to expose people to large doses of radiation. Victims of such a device might exhibit the signs and symptoms of the acute radiation syndrome and possibly also localized radiation skin injuries. Alternatively, a large activity of radioactive material could be dispersed in a populated area. A device to do this is referred to as a radiological dispersal device (RDD). An RDD that uses a chemical explosion to accomplish the dispersion is called a "dirty bomb." An RDD, to be effective, would require a large activity of radioactive material with a relatively long half-life and that emits abundant penetrating radiation and/or has a high radiotoxicity if ingested or inhaled. Radionuclides having these qualities and which are commonly used in very large activities are Co-60 ($T\frac{1}{2}$ = 5.27 years, 1.17 and 1.33 MeV γ-rays), Sr-90 ($T\frac{1}{2}$ = 28.8 years, no γ-rays, very high-energy beta rays), Cs-137 ($T\frac{1}{2}$ = 30.1 years, 662 keV γ-rays), Ir-192 ($T\frac{1}{2}$ = 73.8 days, 296 to 612 keV γ-rays), and Am-241 ($T\frac{1}{2}$ = 433 years, 59.5 keV γ-rays, alpha particles). A dirty bomb detonation could result in a few or dozens of casualties with trauma and radioactive contamination and a much larger number of uninjured people with radioactive contamination. Attack on or sabotage of a nuclear power facility or shipments of large quantities of radioactive material could also cause widespread contamination; attacks of this nature have the potential to release a much larger quantity of radioactive material. In recent years, many countries have greatly increased the security of nuclear facilities and of sources containing large activities of radioactive material (including those in hospitals and research facilities) to prevent or discourage radiological terrorism.

The detonation of an improvised or stolen nuclear weapon in a city is much less likely than other forms of terrorism because the construction of such a device requires several kilograms of plutonium or highly enriched uranium and considerable technical expertise, and access to nuclear weapons is tightly controlled. However, with the proliferation of nuclear weapons and nuclear weapons technology, such an attack may become more likely in the future. The successful use of such a device in a major metropolitan area would be devastating, with an area around the weapon demolished by the blast and prompt thermal radiation. If the weapon were detonated at ground level or a low altitude, there would be extensive radioactive fallout in a pattern determined by surface and higher-altitude winds. A large number of casualties would be created rapidly by the blast wave, collapses of structures, injuries from shrapnel and falling objects, prompt thermal radiation, fires caused by the explosion, and prompt radiation consisting of x- and γ-rays and neutrons from the detonation. Delayed radiation injuries, particularly the acute radiation syndrome from exposure to γ-rays from radioactive fallout and cutaneous injuries from beta radiation from fallout on the skin, would also occur to some people in the fallout zone. The mass casualties, widespread infrastructure failure, and initial inability to operate in the fallout zone would greatly impede the response to the incident.

Each medical facility has or should have a plan for responding to radiation emergencies of varying types and scopes. In particular, the emergency department should be expected to receive and treat injured patients with radioactive contamination. Radioactive contamination has only very rarely been an immediate health threat to patients and almost never to medical staff. Treatment of severe injuries or life-threatening medical conditions should take priority over decontamination, although very simple and quick measures, such as removal of the patients' clothing and wiping exposed skin with mild soap, tepid water, and a damp cloth, will likely remove most of the contamination. Standard protective clothing commonly worn by emergency department staff is sufficient to protect them from radioactive contamination. Periodic surveys with a GM detector and methods similar to common infection prevention techniques will prevent significant contamination with radioactive material (Fig. 21-24).

Concern for radiation exposure or radioactive material contamination should not prevent the use of any of a hospital's diagnostic and treatment capabilities, including the use of medical imaging facilities and operating rooms. Most contamination can be prevented and any contamination that does occur can be managed and would not render any of these facilities inoperable or unsuitable for other critically ill patients.

Following a large-scale emergency involving radiation and/or radioactive material, it is possible that many people, perhaps some with radioactive contamination, but without serious injuries or medical conditions requiring emergency treatment,

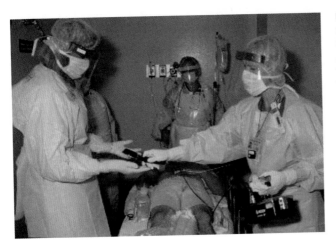

■ **FIGURE 21-24** Standard protective clothing commonly worn by ED staff and periodic surveys with a GM survey meter protect staff from contamination with radioactive material.

will arrive at medical centers seeking care. The medical centers' plans should include measures to prevent emergency departments from becoming overwhelmed by these people. Each community should prepare to establish decontamination centers away from hospitals. However, each medical center should prepare to promptly establish a triage (see Table 20-6), monitoring, and decontamination center away from the emergency department and to divert to this center people not requiring emergency care. More detailed information on developing a radiological emergency response plan, staff training, and sources of expert consultation is widely available (ACR, 2006; Bushberg et al., 2007; HPS, 2011; NCRP, 2001, 2005, 2009, 2010b; REAC/TS, 2020; REMM, 2020).

21.12.2 Decontamination of Individuals

External radioactive contamination is the contamination of a person's clothing, skin, and perhaps other parts of the body surface with radioactive material. An incident involving external radioactive contamination may be as simple as a single nuclear medicine or research laboratory worker who has spilled radioactive material on a small part of his or her body or it could involve dozens or hundreds of people, some injured and many contaminated, arriving at a medical center after a radiological terrorist incident.

Decontamination is commonly performed by removing contaminated clothing and washing the contaminated area with soap and water, taking care not to spread contamination to other parts of the body or onto other people, and to ensure that people do not inhale or ingest the radioactive material. If the radioactive material is not water-soluble, another solvent may be needed. Uncontaminated wounds should be protected by waterproof dressings during decontamination. Thermal burns of the skin should be decontaminated by gentle rinsing with sterile saline solution but should not be scrubbed to avoid further injury. The progress of decontamination is assessed by surveys using a portable radiation survey meter. Decontamination is performed until the amount of remaining radioactive contamination approaches background levels or until decontamination efforts cease to reduce the amount of remaining contamination. If large numbers of people are contaminated, a greater amount of residual contamination may have to be accepted. Decontamination efforts should not abrade the skin to avoid the absorption of radioactive material through the injured skin.

Contaminated wounds are decontaminated by flushing with sterile saline and mild scrubbing. Excision of viable tissue to remove radioactive contamination should be performed only after consulting with an expert.

Personnel with external radioactive contamination, particularly on the upper parts of their bodies, may also have internal contamination. Radioactive contamination of a person should never delay critical medical care.

21.12.3 Treatment for Internal Radioactive Contamination

The term *internal contamination* refers to radioactive material in the body. It may enter the body by inhalation, by ingestion, through a wound, by injection, or, for some radioactive material, by absorption through the skin. It may result from an accident, poor contamination control in the workplace, a terrorist act or an act of war, or an administration error in nuclear medicine.

Effective treatment of internal contamination varies with the radionuclide, its chemical and physical form, and, in some cases, its route into the body. In general, treatment is more effective the sooner it is begun after the radioactive material is introduced into the body. Hence, it may be best to begin treatment before definitive information is available. NCRP Report No. 161, *Management of Persons Contaminated with Radionuclides*, provides detailed guidance on the treatment of internal contamination (NCRP, 2008).

An accident in nuclear medicine or a research laboratory or a nuclear reactor accident with a release of fission products can cause internal contamination with radioactive iodine. Radioactive iodine is sequestered by the thyroid gland and retained with a long biological half-life. The most effective treatment is to administer nonradioactive iodine to block thyroidal uptake of the radioactive iodine. This treatment is most effective the sooner it is begun, becoming much less effective with time after an intake. Table 21-12 provides guidance for the treatment of internal contamination with radioactive iodine.

The amount of internal contamination and the effectiveness of treatment may be assessed by bioassays. Bioassays are usually either measurements of radiation from the body (*e.g.*, thyroid counts using a thyroid probe or whole-body counts using a whole-body counter) or assays of excreta, usually urine.

21.12.4 Treatment of the Acute Radiation Syndrome

The acute radiation syndrome, discussed in Chapter 20 (see Tables 20-6 and 20-7), is typically caused by the irradiation of the entire body or a large portion of the body to a very large dose of penetrating radiation, such as x-rays, γ-rays, or neutrons. An acute dose of x- or γ-rays to the bone marrow exceeding 0.5 Gy is usually necessary to cause the syndrome; an acute dose of about 3.5 Gy will kill about half of exposed individuals without medical care, and an acute dose exceeding 10 Gy will kill nearly all individuals even with medical care. The lethality is increased by skin burns or trauma. The most significant adverse effects, for individuals receiving doses that they may survive, are injury to the lining of the gastrointestinal tract and the red bone marrow, causing a loss of electrolytes, the entry of intestinal flora into the body, and depression or even elimination of white blood cells, increasing the risk of infection.

The dose received by an individual can be crudely estimated by the severity of the prodromal phase, particularly the time to emesis. It can be more accurately estimated by the kinetics of circulating white blood cells, particularly lymphocytes, and by a cytogenetic assay of circulating lymphocytes, which requires a blood sample to be sent to a specialized laboratory. Treatment involves reverse isolation, support of electrolytes, support of bone marrow recovery by the administration of cytokines, perhaps the administration of irradiated red blood cells and platelets, prophylactic

TABLE 21-12 GUIDANCE FOR KI ADMINISTRATION: THRESHOLD THYROID RADIOACTIVE EXPOSURES AND RECOMMENDED DOSAGES OF KI FOR DIFFERENT RISK GROUPS

	PREDICTED THYROID GLAND EXPOSURE (cGy)[a]	KI DOSE (mg)	NUMBER OR FRACTION OF 130 mg TABLETS	NUMBER OR FRACTION OF 65 mg TABLETS	MILLILITERS (mL) OF ORAL SOLUTION, 65 mg/mL[b]
Adults over 40 y	≥500	130	1	2	2 mL
Adults over 18 through 40 y	≥10	130	1	2	2 mL
Pregnant or lactating women	≥5	130	1	2	2 mL
Adolescents, 12 through 18 y[c]	≥5	65	½	1	1 mL
Children over 3 y through 12 y	≥5	65	½	1	1 mL
Children 1 mo through 3 y	≥5	32	Use KI oral solution[d]	½	0.5 mL
Infants birth through 1 mo	≥5	16	Use KI oral solution[d]	Use KI oral solution[d]	0.25 mL

[a]A centigray (cGy) is a hundredth of a gray (Gy) and is equal to one rad.
[b]See the Home Preparation Procedure for Emergency Administration of Potassium Iodide Tablets to Infants and Small Children at the URL below.
[c]Adolescents approaching adult size (≥150 lbs) should receive the full adult dose (130 mg).
[d]Potassium iodide oral solution is supplied in 1 oz (30 mL) bottles with a dropper marked for 1, 0.5, and 0.25 mL dosing. Each mL contains 65 mg of potassium iodide.
Data from NAS: National Research Council. *Distribution and Administration of Potassium Iodide in the Event of a Nuclear Incident.* Washington, DC: National Academies Press; 2004. http://www.fda.gov/Drugs/EmergencyPreparedness/BioterrorismandDrugPreparedness/ucm072248.htm

treatment with antibiotics, and treatment of infections (Waselenko et al., 2004). If surgery is needed for injuries, it should either be performed in the first 2 days after the exposure or be delayed until the hematopoietic system recovers.

SUGGESTED READING AND REFERENCES

ACR–AAPM–SPR Practice Parameter for Diagnostic Reference Levels and Achievable Doses in Medical X-ray Imaging, 2018. https://www.acr.org/-/media/ACR/Files/Practice-Parameters/diag-ref-levels.pdf?la=en. Accessed August 17, 2020.

American Association of Physicists in Medicine. AAPM Task Group 108: PET and PET/CT shielding requirements. *Med Phys.* 2006;33(1):4-15.

American Association of Physicists in Medicine. Size-specific dose estimates (SSDE) in pediatric and adult body CT examinations. Report of AAPM Task Group 204. 2011a. https://www.aapm.org/pubs/reports/RPT_204.pdf. Accessed May 13, 2020.

American Association of Physicists in Medicine. AAPM Dose Check Guidelines version 1.0. April 27, 2011b. http://www.aapm.org/pubs/CTProtocols/documents/NotificationLevelsStatement_2011-04-27.pdf. Accessed October 1, 2011.

American Association of Physicists in Medicine. AAPM Professional Policy Position Statement on the use of patient gonadal and fetal shielding (PP 32-A). 2019. https://www.aapm.org/org/policies/details.asp?id=468&type=PP. Accessed June 13, 2020.

American College of Radiology. *Disaster Preparedness for Radiology Professionals, Response to Radiological Terrorism: A Primer for Radiologists.* version 3. Radiation Oncologists and Medical Physicists; 2006. www.acr.org

American College of Radiology. ACR-SPR practice parameter for imaging pregnant or potentially pregnant adolescents and women with ionizing radiation. Revised 2018 (Resolution 39). https://www.acr.org/-/media/ACR/Files/Practice-Parameters/Pregnant-Pts.pdf

American College of Radiology. Validation of adult relative radiation levels using the ACR Dose Index Registry: report of the ACR Appropriateness Criteria Radiation Exposure Subcommittee. *J Am Coll Radiol.* 2019;16(2):236-239.

American College of Radiology. Dose Index Registry. 2020. https://www.acr.org/Practice-Management-Quality-Informatics/Registries/Dose-Index-Registry

Balter S, Hopewell JW, Miller DL, Wagner LK, Zelefsky MJ. Fluoroscopically guided interventional procedrues: a review of radiation effects on patients' skin and hair. *Radiology.* 2010;254(2):326-341.

Bogdanich W. Radiation overdoses point up dangers of CT scans. *New York Times*, October 15, 2009.

Brateman L. The AAPM/RSNA physics tutorial for residents: radiation safety considerations for diagnostic radiology personnel. *RadioGraphics.* 1999;19:1037-1055.

Brenner DJ, Hall EJ. Computed tomography: an increasing source of radiation exposure. *N Engl J Med.* 2007;357(22):2277-2284.

Brenner DJ, Elliston CD, Hall EJ, Berdon WE. Estimated risks of radiation-induced fatal cancer from pediatric CT. *AJR.* 2001;176:289-296.

Bushberg JT, Leidholdt EM Jr. Radiation protection. In: Sandler MP, et al., eds. *Diagnostic Nuclear Medicine.* 4th ed. Philadelphia, PA: Lippincott Williams & Wilkins; 2001.

Bushberg JT, Kroger LA, Hartman MB, et al. Nuclear/radiological terrorism: emergency department management of radiation casualties. *J Emerg Med.* 2007;32(1):71-85.

CDC Breast Cancer Screening Guidelines for Women. https://www.cdc.gov/cancer/breast/pdf/BreastCancerScreeningGuidelines.pdf?s_cid=cs_3605#:~:text=average%20risk&text=Women%20aged%2040%20to%2044,should%20get%20mammograms%20every%20year. Accessed June 22, 2020.

Dauer LT. Chapter 20—Management of therapy patients. In: Bailey DL, Humm JL, Todd-Pokropek A, van Aswegen A, eds. *Nuclear Medicine Physics Handbook.* Vienna: International Atomic Energy Agency; 2014.

Dauer LT, Chu BP, Zanzonico PB, eds. *Dose, Benefit, and Risk in Medical Imaging.* New York, NY: CRC Press; 2019.

Dauer LT, Thornton RH, Miller DL, et al.; SIR, CIRSE. Radiation management for interventions using fluoroscopic or computed tomographic guidance during pregnancy: a joint guideline of the Society of Interventional Radiology and the Cardiovascular and Interventional Radiology Society of Europe with Endorsement by the Canadian Interventional Radiology Association. *J Vasc Interv Radiol.* 2012:23:19-32.

Demb J, Chu P, Nelson T, et al. Optimizing radiation doses for computed tomography across institutions: dose auditing and best practices. *JAMA Intern Med.* 2017;177(6):810-817.

EPA. What is EPA's action level for radon and what does it mean? 2020. https://www.epa.gov/radon/what-epas-action-level-radon-and-what-does-it-mean. Accessed June 20, 2020.

Fernandes K, Levin T, Miller T, Schoenfeld AH, Amis ES Jr. Evaluating an image gently and image wisely campaign in a multihospital health care system. *J Am Coll Radiol.* 2016;13:1010-1017.

Fletcher DW, Miller DL, Balter S, Taylor MA. Comparison of four techniques to estimate radiation dose to skin during angiographic and interventional radiology procedures. *J Vasc Interv Radiol.* 2002;13:391-397.

Guillet B, et al. Technologist radiation exposure in routine clinical practice with ^{18}F-FDG PET. *J Nucl Med Technol.* 2005;33:175-179.

Hausleiter J, Meyer T, Hermann F, et al. Estimated radiation dose associated with cardiac CT angiography. *JAMA.* 2009;301(5):500-507.

Higaki T, Nakamura Y, Zhou J, et al. Deep learning reconstruction at CT: phantom study of the image characteristics. *Acad Radiol.* 2020;27(1):82-87.

HPS. *Emergency Department Management of Radiation Casualties.* Health Physics Society; 2011. http://hps.org/hsc/responsemed.html

Huber TC, Krishmnaraj A, Patrie J, Gaskin CM. Impact of a commercially available clinical decision support program on provider ordering habits. *J Am Coll Radiol.* 2018;15(7):951-957.

International Atomic Energy Agency. IAEA radiation protection of patients. 2020. https://www.iaea.org/resources/rpop

International Commission on Radiological Protection. ICRP Publication 102: managing patient dose in multi-detector computed tomography (MDCT). *Ann ICRP.* 2007a;37(1):1-79.

International Commission on Radiological Protection. Radiation protection in medicine. ICRP Publication 105. *Ann ICRP.* 2007b;37(6):1-61.

International Commission on Radiological Protection. The 2007 Recommendations of the International Commission on Radiological Protection. ICRP Publication 103. *Ann ICRP.* 2007c;37:1-332.

International Commission on Radiological Protection. Radiological protection in fluoroscopically guided procedures outside the imaging department. ICRP Publication 117. *Ann ICRP.* 2010;40(6):1-105.

International Commission on Radiological Protection. ICRP statement on tissue reactions and early and late effects of radiation in normal tissues and organs—threshold doses for tissue reactions in a radiation protection context. ICRP Publication 118. *Ann ICRP.* 2012;41(1-2):1-325.

International Commission on Radiological Protection. Radiological protection in cardiology. ICRP Publication 120. *Ann ICRP.* 2013a;42(1):1-128.

International Commission on Radiological Protection. Radiological protection in pediatric diagnostic and interventional radiology. ICRP Publication 121. *Ann ICRP.* 2013b;42(2):1-66.

International Commission on Radiological Protection. Diagnostic reference levels in medical imaging. ICRP Publication 135. *Ann ICRP.* 2017;46(1):1-140.

International Commission on Radiological Protection. Radiological protection in therapy with radiopharmaceuticals. ICRP Publication 140. *Ann ICRP.* 2019;48(1):1-106.

Ip IK, Schneider LI, Hanson R, et al. Adoption and meaningful use of computerized physician order entry with an integrated clinical decision support system for radiology: ten-year analysis in an urban teaching hospital. *J Am Coll Radiol.* 2012;9(2):129-136.

Jaju PP, Jaju SP. Cone-beam computed tomography: time to move from ALARA to ALA-DA. *Imaging Sci Dent.* 2015;45:263-265.

Kanal KM, Butler PF, Sengupta D, Bhargavan-Chatfield M, Coombs LP, Morin RL. U.S. diagnostic reference levels and achievable doses for 10 adult CT examinations. *Radiology.* 2017;284(1):120-133. doi: 10.1148/radiol.2017161911.

Koenig TR, Wolff D, Mettler FA, Wagner LK. Skin injuries from fluoroscopically guided procedures, part 1: characteristics of radiation injury. *Am J Roentgenol.* 2001;177(1):3-11.

Kohn LT, Corrigan JM, Donaldson MS, eds.; Committee on Quality of Health Care in America, Institute of Medicine. *To Err Is Human: Building a Safer Health System.* Washington, DC: National Academies Press; 2000. Accessed January 30, 2004.

Linet MS, Kwang PK, Miller DL, Kleinerman RA, Simon S, Berrington de Gonzalez A. Historical review of cancer risks in medical radiation workers. *Radiat Res.* 2010;174(6):793-808.

Miller DL, Balter S, Cole PE, et al. Radiation doses in interventional radiology procedures: the RAD-IR study. Part II: skin dose. *J Vasc Interv Radiol.* 2003;14:977-990.

Miller DL, Vano E, Bartel G, et al. Occupational radiation protection in interventional radiology: a joint guideline of the cardiovascular and Interventional Society of Europe and the Society of Interventional Radiology. *Cardiovasc Interv Radiol.* 2010;33:230-239.

Mitchell KB, Fleming MM, Anderson PO, Geisbrandt JB; the Academy of Breastfeeding Medicine. ABM Clinical Protocol #31: radiology and nuclear medicine studies in lactating women. *Breastfeed Med.* 2019;14(5):290-294.

Murphy PH, Wu Y, Glaze SA. Attenuation properties of lead composite aprons. *Radiology.* 1993;186: 269-272.

Nair RR, Rajan B, Akiba S, et al. Background radiation and cancer incidence in Kerala, India-Karanagappally cohort study. *Health Phys.* 2009;96:55-66.

NAS: National Research Council. *Distribution and Administration of Potassium Iodide in the Event of a Nuclear Incident.* Washington, DC: National Academies Press; 2004.

National Council on Radiation Protection and Measurements. *Exposure of the Population in the United States and Canada from Natural Background Radiation.* NCRP Report No. 94. Bethesda, MD: National Council on Radiation Protection and Measurements; 1987.

National Council on Radiation Protection and Measurements. *Exposure of the U.S. Population from Diagnostic Medical Radiation.* NCRP Report No. 100. Bethesda, MD: National Council on Radiation NCRP Protection and Measurements; 1989a.

National Council on Radiation Protection and Measurements. *Radiation Protection for Medical and Allied Health Personnel.* NCRP Report No. 105. Bethesda, MD: National Council on Radiation Protection and Measurements; 1989b.

National Council on Radiation Protection and Measurements. *Limitation of Exposure to Ionizing Radiation.* NCRP Report No. 116. Bethesda, MD: National Council on Radiation Protection and Measurements; 1993.

National Council on Radiation Protection and Measurements. *Use of Personal Monitors to Estimate Effective Dose Equivalent and Effective Dose to Workers for External Exposure to Low-LET Radiation.* NCRP Report No. 122. Bethesda, MD: National Council on Radiation Protection and Measurements; 1995.

National Council on Radiation Protection and Measurements. *Management of Terrorist Events Involving Radioactive Material.* NCRP Report No. 138. Bethesda, MD: National Council on Radiation Protection and Measurements; 2001.

National Council on Radiation Protection and Measurements. *Structural Shielding Design for Medical X-ray Imaging Facilities.* NCRP Report No. 147. Bethesda, MD: National Council on Radiation Protection and Measurements; 2004.

National Council on Radiation Protection and Measurements. *Key Elements of Preparing Emergency Responders for Nuclear and Radiological Terrorism.* NCRP Commentary No. 19. Bethesda, MD: National Council on Radiation Protection and Measurements; 2005.

National Council on Radiation Protection and Measurements. *Management of Radionuclide Therapy Patients.* NCRP Report No. 155. Bethesda, MD: National Council on Radiation Protection and Measurements; 2006.

National Council on Radiation Protection and Measurements. *Management of Persons Contaminated with Radionuclides.* NCRP Report No. 161. Bethesda, MD: National Council on Radiation Protection and Measurements; 2008.

National Council on Radiation Protection and Measurements. *Ionizing Radiation Exposure of the Population of the United States.* NCRP Report No. 160. Bethesda, MD: National Council on Radiation Protection and Measurements; 2009.

National Council on Radiation Protection and Measurements. *Radiation Dose Management for Fluoroscopically-Guided Interventional Medical Procedures.* NCRP Report No. 168. Bethesda, MD: National Council on Radiation Protection and Measurements; 2010a.

National Council on Radiation Protection and Measurements. *Responding to a Radiological or Nuclear Terrorism Incident: A Guide for Decision Makers.* NCRP Report No. 165. Bethesda, MD: National Council on Radiation Protection and Measurements; 2010b.

National Council on Radiation Protection and Measurements. *Reference Levels and Achievable Doses in Medical and Dental Imaging: Recommendations for the United States.* NCRP Report No. 172. Bethesda, MD: National Council on Radiation Protection and Measurements; 2012.

National Council on Radiation Protection and Measurements. *Preconception and Prenatal Radiation Exposure: Health Effects and Protective Guidance.* NCRP Report No. 174. Bethesda, MD: National Council on Radiation Protection and Measurements; 2013.

National Council on Radiation Protection and Measurements. *Guidance on Radiation Dose Limits for the Lens of the Eye.* NCRP Commentary No. 26. Bethesda, MD: National Council on Radiation Protection and Measurements; 2016.

National Council on Radiation Protection and Measurements. *Management of Exposure to Ionizing Radiation: Radiation Protection Guidance for the United States.* NCRP Report No. 180. Bethesda, MD: National Council on Radiation Protection and Measurements; 2018.

National Council on Radiation Protection and Measurements. *Medical Radiation Exposure of Patients in the United States.* NCRP Report No. 184. Bethesda, MD: National Council on Radiation Protection and Measurements; 2019.

National Council on Radiation Protection and Measurements. *Evaluating and Communicating Radiation Risks for Studies Involving Human Subjects: Guidance for Researchers and Institutional Review Boards.* NCRP Report No. 185. Bethesda, MD: National Council on Radiation Protection and Measurements; 2020.

Paterson A, Donald P, Frush DP, Donnelly LF. Helical CT of the body: are settings adjusted for pediatric patients? *Am J Roentgenol.* 2001;176:297-301.

Proceedings of the Thirty-third Annual Meeting of the National Council on Radiation Protection and Measurements. The effects of pre- and postconception exposure to radiation. *Teratology.* 1999;59(4).

Radiation Emergency Assistance Center/Training Site (REAC/TS). Oak Ridge Institute for Science and Education (ORISE) positions the U.S. Department of Energy (DOE); 2020. http://orise.orau.gov/reacts/

Radiation Emergency Medical Management (REMM). Department of Health and Human Services; 2020. http://www.remm.nlm.gov/

Schueler BA, Vrieze TJ, Bjarnason H, et al. An investigation of operator exposure in interventional radiology. *RadioGraphics.* 2006;26:1533-1541.

Seibert JA, Morin RL. The standardized exposure index for digital radiography: an opportunity for optimization of radiation dose to the pediatric population. *Pediatr Radiol.* 2011;41(5):573-581.

Siegel JA. *Guide for Diagnostic Nuclear Medicine.* Reston, VA: Society of Nuclear Medicine; 2002.

Sisson JC, Freitas J, McGougall IR, et al. Radiation safety in the treatment of patients with thyroid diseases by radioiodine 131I: practice recommendations of the American Thyroid Association. *Thyroid.* 2011;21(4):335-346.

Sistrom CL, Weilburg JB, Rosenthal DI, Dreyer KJ, Thrall JH. Use of imaging appropriateness criteria for decision support during radiology order entry: the MGH experience. In: Lau L, Ng K, eds. *Radiological Safety and Quality: Paradigms in Leadership and Innovation.* Dordrecht: Springer; 2014.

Stabin MG, Breitz HB. Breast milk excretion of radiopharmaceuticals: mechanisms, findings, and radiation dosimetry. *J Nucl Med.* 2000;41(5):863-873.

The Joint Commission. 2020 National Patient Safety Goals. https://www.jointcommission.org/en/standards/national-patient-safety-goals/

The Joint Commission. *Sentinel Event Alert, Radiation Risks of Diagnostic Imaging.* Issue 47. Revised February 2019.

Title 10 (Energy) of the Code of Federal Regulations (CFR). Part 20: Standards for Protection Against Radiation.

Title 10 (Energy) of the Code of Federal Regulations (CFR). Part 35: Medical Use of By-product Material.

UNSCEAR. *Effects and Risks of Ionizing Radiation: United Nations Scientific Committee on the Effects of Atomic Radiation.* 2013 Report. Volume 1. Annex A. Levels and effects of radiation exposure due to the nuclear accident after the 2011 great east-Japan earthquake and tsunami. New York, NY: United Nations; 2014.

UNSCEAR. *The Chernobyl Accident.* New York, NY: United Nations; 2020. https://www.unscear.org/unscear/en/chernobyl.html

US Environmental Protection Agency. Federal Guidance Report No. 14: Radiation Protection Guidance for Diagnostic and Interventional X-ray Procedures. Washington, DC: Interagency Working Group on Medical Radiation, US Environmental Protection Agency; 2014.

US Food & Drug Administration. Guidance for Industry and Researchers. The Radioactive Drug Research Committee: Human Research without an Investigational New Drug Application. 2010. https://www.fda.gov/media/76286/download

US Food & Drug Administration. Mammography Quality Standards Act and Program. 2020. https://www.fda.gov/radiation-emitting-products/mammography-quality-standards-act-and-program

U.S. Nuclear Regulatory Commission, NUREG 1556, Vol. 9, Rev. 3, Program-Specific Guidance About Medical Use Licenses Washington, DC; January 2016.

US Nuclear Regulatory Commission. Safety Culture Policy Statement, NUREG/BR-0500. Rev. 1. Washington, DC: US Nuclear Regulatory Commission; 2012.

Wagner LK, Archer BR. *Minimizing Risks from Fluoroscopic X-Rays; Bioeffects, Instrumentation and Examination, a Credentialing Program for Physicians.* 4th ed. Houston, TX: Partners in Radiation Management; 2004.

Wagner LK, Lester RG, Saldana LR. *Exposure of the Pregnant Patient to Diagnostic Radiations.* 2nd ed. Madison, WI: Medical Physics Publishing; 1997.

Waselenko JK, MacVittie TJ, Blakely WF, et al. Medical management of the acute radiation syndrome: recommendations of the Strategic National Stockpile Radiation Working Group K. *Ann Intern Med.* 2004;140(12):1037-1051.

Williams MB, Krupinski EA, Strauss KJ, et al. Digital radiography image quality: image acquisition. *J Am Coll Radiol.* 2007;4:371-388.

Zuguchi M, Chida K, Taura M, Inaba Y, Ebata A, Yamada S. Usefulness of non-lead aprons in radiation protection for physicians performing interventional procedures. *Radiat Prot Dosimetry.* 2008;131(4):531-534.

Appendices

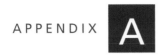
Fundamental Principles of Physics

A.1 PHYSICS LAWS, QUANTITIES, AND UNITS

A.1.1 Laws of Physics

Physics is the study of the physical environment around us—from the smallest quarks to the galactic dimensions of black holes and quasars. Much of what is known about physics can be summarized in a set of laws that describe physical reality. These laws are based on reproducible results from physical observations that are consistent with theoretical predictions. A well-conceived law of physics is applicable in a wide range of circumstances. A physical law that states that the force exerted by gravity on an individual on the surface of the Earth is 680 N is a poor example, because it is a description of a single situation only. Newton's law of gravity, however, describes the gravitational forces between any two bodies at any distance from each other and is an example of a well-conceived, generally usable law.

A.1.2 Vector Versus Scalar Quantities

For some quantities, such as force, velocity, acceleration, and momentum, direction is important, in addition to the magnitude. These quantities are called *vector* quantities. Quantities that do not incorporate direction, such as mass, time, energy, electrical charge, and temperature, are called *scalar* quantities.

A vector quantity is represented graphically by an arrow whose length is proportional to the magnitude of the vector. A vector quantity is represented by boldface type, as in the equation $\mathbf{F} = m\mathbf{a}$, where $\mathbf{F}$ and $\mathbf{a}$ are vector quantities and m is a scalar quantity.

In many equations of physics, such as $\mathbf{F} = m\mathbf{a}$, a vector is multiplied by a scalar. In vector-scalar multiplication, the magnitude of the resultant vector is the product of the magnitude of the original vector and the scalar; however, the direction of the vector is not changed by the multiplication. If the scalar has units, the multiplication may also change the units of the vector. Force, for example, has different units than acceleration. Vector-scalar multiplication is shown in Figure A-1.

Two or more vectors may be added. This addition is performed graphically by placing the tail of one vector against the head of the other, as shown in Figure A-2. The resultant vector is that reaching from the tail of the first to the head of the second. The order in which vectors are added does not affect the result. A special case occurs when one vector has the same magnitude but opposite direction of the other; in this case, the two vectors cancel, resulting in no vector.

A.1.3 International System of Units

As science has developed, many disciplines have devised their own specialized units for measurements. An attempt has been made to establish a single set of units to be

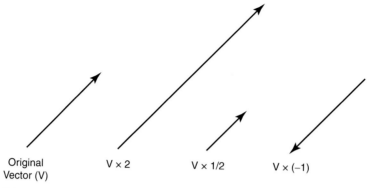

■ **FIGURE A-1** Vector-scalar multiplication.

used across all disciplines of science. This set of units, called the *Systeme International* (SI), is gradually replacing the traditional units. The SI establishes a set of seven base units—the kilogram, meter, second, ampere, kelvin, candela, and mole—whose magnitudes are carefully described by standards laboratories. Two supplemental units, the radian and steradian, are used to describe angles in two and three dimensions, respectively. All other units, called *derived units*, are defined in terms of these fundamental units. For representing quantities much greater than or much smaller than an SI unit, the SI unit may be modified by a prefix. Commonly used prefixes are shown in Table A-1. A more complete list of prefixes is provided in Appendix C along with physical constants, geometric formulae, conversion factors, and radiologic data for elements 1 through 100.

A.2   CLASSICAL PHYSICS

A.2.1   Mass, Length, and Time

Mass is a measure of the resistance a body has to acceleration. It should not be confused with weight, which is the gravitational force exerted on a mass. The SI unit for mass is the kilogram (kg). The SI unit for length is the meter (m) and for time is the second (s).

■ **FIGURE A-2** Vector addition.

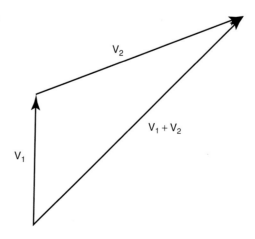

TABLE A-1 COMMONLY USED PREFIXES FOR UNITS

PREFIX	MEANING	PREFIX	MEANING
centi (c)	10^{-2}		
milli (m)	10^{-3}	kilo (k)	10^{+3}
micro (μ)	10^{-6}	mega (M)	10^{+6}
nano (n)	10^{-9}	giga (G)	10^{+9}
pico (p)	10^{-12}	tera (T)	10^{+12}
femto (f)	10^{-15}	peta (P)	10^{+15}

A.2.2 Velocity and Acceleration

Velocity, a vector quantity, is the rate of change of position with respect to time:

$$\mathbf{v} = \Delta \mathbf{x}/\Delta t. \qquad \text{[A-1]}$$

The magnitude of the velocity, called the *speed*, is a scalar quantity. The SI unit for velocity and speed is the meter per second (m/s). *Acceleration*, also a vector quantity, is defined as the rate of change of velocity with respect to time:

$$\mathbf{a} = \Delta \mathbf{v}/\Delta t. \qquad \text{[A-2]}$$

The SI unit for acceleration is the meter per second per second (m/s^2).

A.2.3 Forces and Newton's Laws

Force, a vector quantity, is a push or pull. The physicist and mathematician Isaac Newton proposed three laws regarding force and velocity:

1. Unless acted upon by external force, an object at rest remains at rest and an object in motion remains in uniform motion. That is, an object's velocity remains unchanged unless an external force acts upon the object.

2. For every action, there is an equal and opposite reaction. That is, if one object exerts a force on a second object, the second object also exerts a force on the first that is equal in magnitude but opposite in direction.

3. A force acting upon an object produces an acceleration in the direction of the applied force:

$$F = m\mathbf{a}. \qquad \text{[A-3]}$$

The SI unit for force is the newton (N): 1 N is defined as 1 kg-m/s². There are four types of forces: *gravitational*, *electrical*, *magnetic*, and *nuclear*. These forces are discussed later.

A.2.4 Energy

Kinetic Energy

Kinetic energy, a scalar quantity, is a property of moving matter that is defined by the following equation:

$$E_k = \frac{1}{2}mv^2, \qquad \text{[A-4]}$$

where E_k is the kinetic energy, m is the mass of the object, and v is the speed of the object. (Einstein discovered a more complicated expression that must be used for objects with speeds approaching the speed of light.) The SI unit for all forms of energy is the joule (J): 1 J is defined as 1 kg-m²/s².

Potential Energy

Potential energy is a property of an object in a force field. The force field may be a gravitational force field. If an object is electrically charged, it may be an electrical force field caused by nearby charged objects. If an object is very close to an atomic nucleus, it may be influenced by nuclear forces. The potential energy (E_p) is a function of the position of the object; if the object changes position with respect to the force field, its potential energy changes.

Conservation of Energy

The total energy of an object is the sum of its kinetic and potential energies:

$$E_{total} = E_k + E_p. \qquad \text{[A-5]}$$

Aside from friction, the total energy of the object does not change. For example, consider a brick held several feet above the ground. It has a certain amount of gravitational potential energy by virtue of its height, but it has no kinetic energy because it is at rest. When released, it falls downward with a continuous increase in kinetic energy. As the brick falls, its position changes and its potential energy decreases. The sum of its kinetic and potential energies does not change during the fall. One may think of the situation as one in which potential energy is converted into kinetic energy.

A.2.5 Momentum

Momentum, like kinetic energy, is a property of moving objects. However, unlike kinetic energy, momentum is a vector quantity. The momentum of an object is defined as follows:

$$\mathbf{p} = m\mathbf{v}, \qquad \text{[A-6]}$$

where $\mathbf{p}$ is the momentum of an object, m is its mass, and $\mathbf{v}$ is its velocity. The momentum of an object has the same direction as its velocity. The SI unit of momentum is the kilogram-meter per second (kg-m/s). It can be shown from Newton's laws that, if no external forces act on a collection of objects, the total momentum of the set of objects does not change. This principle is called the law of conservation of momentum.

A.3 ELECTRICITY AND MAGNETISM

A.3.1 Electricity

Electrical Charge

Electrical charge is a property of matter. Matter may have a positive charge, a negative charge, or no charge. The charge on an object may be determined by observing how it behaves in relation to other charged objects. The *coulomb* (C) is the SI derived unit of electric charge. It is defined in terms of two SI base units as the charge transported by a steady current of one ampere in one second. The smallest magnitude of charge is that of the electron. There are approximately 10^{19} electron charges per coulomb.

A fundamental law of physics states that electrical charge is conserved. This means that, if charge is neither added to nor removed from a system, the total amount of charge in the system does not change. The signs of the charges must be considered in calculating the total amount of charge in a system. If a system contains two charges of the same magnitude but of opposite sign—for example, in a hydrogen atom, in which a single electron (negative charge) orbits a single proton (positive charge)—the total charge of the system is zero.

Electrical Forces and Fields

The force (**F**) exerted on a charged particle by a second charged particle is described by the equation:

$$\mathbf{F} = kq_1q_2/r^2,$$ [A-7]

where q_1 and q_2 are the charges on the two particles, r is the distance between the two particles, and k is a constant. The direction of the force on each particle is either toward or away from the other particle; the force is attractive if one charge is negative and the other positive, and it is repulsive if both charges are of the same sign.

An electrical field exists in the vicinity of electrical charges. To measure the electrical field strength at a point, a small test charge is placed at that point and the force on the test charge is measured. The electrical field strength (**E**) is then calculated as follows:

$$\mathbf{E} = \mathbf{F}/q,$$ [A-8]

where **F** is the force exerted on the test charge and q is the magnitude of the test charge. Electrical field strength is a vector quantity. If the test charge q is positive, **E** and **F** have the same direction; if the test charge is negative, **E** and **F** have opposite directions.

An electrical field may be visualized as lines of electrical field strength existing between electrically charged entities. The strength of the electrical field is depicted as the density of these lines. Figure A-3 shows the electrical fields surrounding a point charge and between two parallel plate electrodes.

An *electrical dipole* has no net charge but does possess regional distribution of positive and negative charge. When placed in an electrical field, the dipole tends to align with the field because of the torque exerted on it by that field (attraction by unlike charges, repulsion by like charges). The electrical dipole structure of certain natural and man-made crystals is used in ultrasound imaging devices to produce and detect sound waves, as described in Chapter 16.

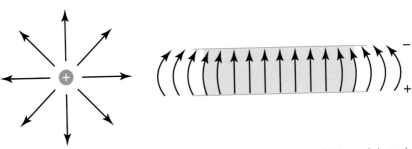

■ **FIGURE A-3** Electrical fields around a point charge (left) and between two parallel charged electrodes (right).

Electrical Forces on Charged Particles

When a charged particle is placed in an electrical field, it experiences a force that is equal to the product of its charge q and the electrical field strength $\mathbf{E}$ at that location:

$$\mathbf{F} = q\mathbf{E}.$$

If the charge on the particle is positive, the force is in the direction of the electrical field at that position; if the charge is negative, the force is opposite to the electrical field. If the particle is not restrained, it experiences an acceleration:

$$\mathbf{a} = q\mathbf{E}/m,$$

where m is the mass of the particle.

Electrical Current

Electrical current is the flow of electrical charge. Charge may flow through a solid, such as a wire; through a liquid, such as the acid in an automobile battery; through a gas, as in a fluorescent light; or through a vacuum, as in an x-ray tube. Current may be the flow of positive charges, such as positive ions or protons in a cyclotron, or it may be the flow of negative charges, such as electrons or negative ions. In some cases, such as an ionization chamber radiation detector, there is a flow of positive charges in one direction and a flow of negative charges in the opposite direction. Although current is often the flow of electrons, the direction of the current is defined as the flow of positive charge (Fig. A-4). The SI unit of current is the *ampere* (A): 1 A is 1 C of charge passing a point in an electric circuit per second.

■ **FIGURE A-4** Direction of electrical current. **A.** A situation is shown in which electrons are flowing to the left. **B.** Positive charges are shown moving to the right. In both cases, the direction of current is to the right. **C.** Although the electrons in an x-ray tube pass from cathode to anode, current technically flows in the opposite direction.

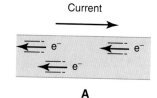

A

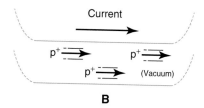

B

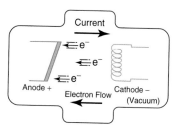

C

Electrical Potential Difference

Electrical potential, more commonly called *voltage*, is a scalar quantity. Voltage is the difference in the electrical potential energy of an electrical charge at two positions, divided by the charge:

$$V_{ab} = (E_{pa} - E_{pb})/q, \qquad [A-9]$$

where E_{pa} is the electrical potential energy of the charge at location a, E_{pb} is the electrical potential energy of the same charge at location b, and q is the amount of charge. It is meaningless to specify the voltage at a single point in an electrical circuit; it must be specified in relation to another point in the circuit. The SI unit of electrical potential is the volt (V): 1 V is defined as 1 J/C, or 1 kg m²/s²-C.

Potential is especially useful in determining the final kinetic energy of a charged particle moving between two electrodes through a vacuum, as in an x-ray tube. According to the principle of conservation of energy (Eq. A-5), the gain in kinetic energy of the charged particle is equal to its loss of potential energy:

$$E_{k\text{-final}} - E_{k\text{-initial}} = E_{p\text{-initial}} - E_{p\text{-final}}. \qquad [A-10]$$

Assuming that the charged particle starts with no kinetic energy ($E_{k\text{-initial}} = 0$) and using Equations A-9, and A-10, the final kinetic energy becomes

$$E_{k\text{-final}} = qV, \qquad [A-11]$$

where q is the charge of the particle and V is the potential difference between the two electrodes.

For example, the final kinetic energy of an electron (charge $= 1.602 \times 10^{-19}$ C) accelerated through an electrical potential difference of 100 kV is

$$E_{k\text{-final}} - qV\ (1.602 \times 10^{-19}\ \text{C})\ (100\ \text{kV}) = 1.602 \times 10^{-14}\ \text{J}.$$

The joule is a rather large unit of energy for subatomic particles. In atomic and nuclear physics, energies are often expressed in terms of the *electron volt* (eV). One electron volt is the kinetic energy developed by an electron accelerated across a potential difference of 1 V. One electron volt is equal to 1.602×10^{-19} J.

For example, the kinetic energy of an electron, initially at rest, that is accelerated through a potential difference of 100 kV is

$$E_k = qV = (1\ \text{electron charge})\ (100\text{kV}) = 100\ \text{keV}.$$

One must be careful not to confuse the units of potential difference (V, kV, and MV) with units of energy (eV, keV, and MeV).

Electrical Power

Power is defined as the rate of the conversion of energy from one form to another with respect to time:

$$P = \Delta E / \Delta t. \qquad [A-12]$$

For an example, an automobile engine converts chemical energy in gasoline into kinetic energy of the automobile. The amount of energy converted into kinetic energy per unit time is the power of the engine. The SI unit of power is the watt (W): 1 W is defined as 1 J/s.

When electrical current flows between two points of different potential, the potential energy of each charge changes. The change in potential energy per unit charge is the potential difference (V), and the amount of charge flowing per unit time is the current (i). Therefore, the electrical power (P) is equal to

$$P = iV, \qquad [A-13]$$

where i is the current and V is the potential difference. Because 1 V = 1 J/C and 1 A = 1 C/s, 1 W = 1 A-V:

$$(1 \text{ A})(1 \text{ V}) = (1 \text{ C/s})(1 \text{ J/C}) = 1 \text{ J/s} = 1 \text{ W}.$$

For example, if a potential difference of 12 V applied to a heating coil produces a current of 1 A, the rate of heat production is

$$P = iV = (1 \text{ A})(12 \text{ V}) = 12 \text{ W}.$$

Direct and Alternating Current

Electrical power is normally supplied to equipment as either *direct current* (DC) or *alternating current* (AC). DC power is provided by two wires connecting the equipment to a power source. The power source maintains a constant potential difference between the two wires (Fig. A-5A). Many electronic circuits require DC, and chemical batteries produce DC.

AC power is usually provided as *single-phase* or *three-phase* AC. Single-phase AC is supplied using two wires from the power source. The power source produces a potential difference between the two wires that varies sinusoidally with time (see Fig. A-5B). Single-phase AC is specified by its amplitude (the maximal voltage) and its frequency (the number of cycles per unit time). Normal household and building power is single-phase 117-V AC. Its actual peak amplitude is 1.4 × 117 V, or 165 V.

AC power is usually supplied to buildings and to heavy-duty electrical equipment as *three-phase* AC. It uses three or four wires between the power source and the equipment. When present, the fourth wire, called the *neutral wire*, is maintained at ground potential (the potential of the earth). The power source provides a sinusoidally varying potential on each of the three wires with respect to the neutral wire. Voltages on these three wires have the same amplitudes and frequencies; however, each is a third of a cycle *out of phase* with respect to the other two, as shown in Figure A-5C. Each cycle is assigned a total of 360°, and therefore each cycle in a three-phase circuit is 120° out of phase with the others.

AC is produced by electric generators and used by electric motors. The major advantage of AC over DC is that its amplitude may be easily increased or decreased using devices called *transformers*, as described later. AC is converted to DC for many electronic circuits.

Ground potential is the electrical potential of the earth. One of the two wires supplying single-phase AC is maintained at ground potential, as is the neutral wire used in supplying three-phase AC. These wires are maintained at ground potential by connecting them to a metal spike driven deep into the earth.

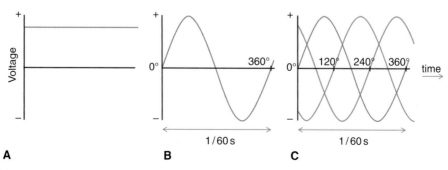

■ **FIGURE A-5 A.** Direct current. **B.** Single-phase AC. **C.** Three-phase AC, comprised of three single-phase AC sources, each separated by 120° over the repeating 360° cycle.

Conductors, Insulators, and Semiconductors

When a potential difference is applied across a conductor, it causes an electrical current to flow. In general, increasing the potential difference increases the current. The quantity *resistance* is defined as the ratio of the applied voltage to the resultant current:

$$R = V/i. \qquad \text{[A-14]}$$

The SI unit of resistance is the ohm (Ω): 1 Ω is defined as 1 volt per ampere.

Current is defined as the flow of positive charge. In solid matter, however, current is caused by the movement of negative charges (electrons) only. Based on the amount of current generated by an applied potential difference, solids may be roughly classified as conductors, semiconductors, or insulators. Metals, especially silver, copper, and aluminum, have very little resistance and are called conductors. Some materials, such as glass, plastics, and fused quartz, have very large resistances and are called insulators. Other materials, such as selenium, silicon, and germanium, have intermediate resistances and are called *semiconductors.*

The band theory of solids explains the conduction properties of solids. The outer-shell electrons in solids exist in discrete energy bands. These bands are separated by gaps; electrons cannot possess energies within the gaps. For an electron to be mobile, there must be a nearby vacant position in the same energy band into which it can move. In conductors, the highest energy band occupied by electrons is only partially filled, so the electrons in it are mobile. In insulators and semiconductors, the highest occupied band is completely filled and electrons are not readily mobile.

The difference between insulators and semiconductors is the width of the forbidden gap between the highest occupied band and the next higher band; in semiconductors, the gap is about 1 eV, whereas in insulators, it is typically greater than 5 eV. At room temperature, thermal energy temporarily promotes a small fraction of the electrons from the valence band into the next higher band. The promoted electrons are mobile. Their promotion also leaves behind vacancies in the valence band, called *holes,* into which other valence band electrons can move. Because the band gap of semiconductors is much smaller than that of insulators, a much larger number of electrons exist in the higher band of semiconductors, and the resistance of semiconductors is therefore less than that of insulators. Reducing the temperature of insulators and semiconductors increases their resistance by reducing the thermal energy available for promoting electrons from the valence band.

For certain materials, including most metallic conductors, the resistance is not greatly affected by the applied voltage. In these materials, the applied voltage and resultant current are nearly proportional:

$$V = iR. \qquad \text{[A-15]}$$

This equation is called Ohm's law.

A.3.2   Magnetism

Magnetic Forces and Fields

Magnetic fields can be caused by moving electrical charges. This charge motion may be over long distances, such as the movement of electrons through a wire, or it may be restricted to the vicinity of a molecule or atom, such as the motion of an unpaired electron in a valence shell. The basic features of magnetic fields can be illustrated by the bar magnet. First, the bar magnet, made of an iron ferromagnetic material, has a unique atomic electron orbital packing scheme that gives rise to an intense magnetic field due to the constructive addition of magnetic fields arising from *unpaired* spin-ning electrons in different atomic orbital shells. The resultant "magnet" has two poles and experiences a force when placed in the vicinity of another bar magnet or external magnetic field. By convention, the pole that points north under the influence of the earth's magnetic field is termed the *north pole*, and the other is called the *south pole*. Experiments demonstrate that like poles of two magnets repel each other and unlike poles attract. When a magnet is broken in two, each piece becomes a new magnet, with a north and a south pole. This phenomenon continues on to the atomic level. Therefore, the simplest magnetic structure is the magnetic *dipole*. In contrast, the simplest electrical structure, the isolated point charge, is unipolar.

Magnetic fields may be visualized as lines of magnetic force. Because magnetic poles exist in pairs, the magnetic field lines have no beginning or end and, in fact, circle upon themselves. Figure A-6A shows the magnetic field surrounding a bar magnet. A current-carrying wire also produces a magnetic field that circles the wire, as shown in Figure A-6B. Increasing the current flowing through the wire increases the magnetic field strength. The *right-hand rule* allows the determination of the mag-netic field direction by grasping the wire with the thumb pointed in the direction of the current (opposite the electron flow). The fingers will then circle the wire in the direction of the magnetic field. When a current-carrying wire is curved in a loop, the resultant concentric lines of magnetic force overlap and augment the total local magnetic field strength inside the loop, as shown in Figure A-6C. A coiled wire, called a *solenoid*, results in even more augmentation of the magnetic lines of force within the coil, as shown in Figure A-6D. The field strength depends on the number of turns in the coil over a fixed distance. An extreme example of a solenoid is found

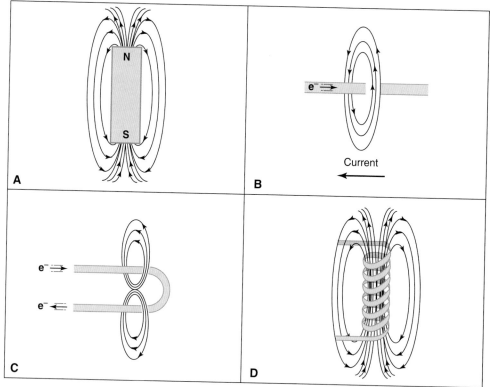

■ **FIGURE A-6** Magnetic field descriptions: surrounding a bar magnet **(A)**, around a wire **(B)**, about a wire loop **(C)**, and about a coiled wire **(D)**.

in most magnetic resonance scanners; in fact, the patient resides inside the solenoid during the scan. A further enhancement of magnetic field strength can be obtained by applying a greater current through the wire or by placing a ferromagnetic material such as iron inside the solenoid. The iron core in this instance confines and augments the magnetic field. The solenoid is similar to the bar magnet discussed previously; however, the magnetic field strength may be changed by varying the current. If the current remains fixed (*e.g.*, DC), the magnetic field also remains fixed; if the current varies (*e.g.*, AC), the magnetic field varies. Solenoids are also called *electromagnets*.

Current loops behave as magnetic dipoles. Like the simple bar magnet, they tend to align with an external magnetic field, as shown in Figure A-7. An electron in an atomic orbital is a current loop about the nucleus. A spinning charge such as the proton also may be thought of as a small current loop. These current loops act as magnetic dipoles and tend to align with external magnetic fields, a tendency that gives rise to the macroscopic magnetic properties of materials (discussed further in Chapter 12).

The SI unit of magnetic field strength is the *tesla* (T). An older unit of magnetic field strength is the *gauss* (G): 1 T is equal to 10^4 G. By way of comparison, the earth's magnetic field is approximately 0.05 to 0.1 mT whereas magnetic fields used for magnetic resonance imaging typically range from 1.5 T to 3.0 T and up to 7.0 T.

Magnetic Forces on Moving Charged Particles

A magnetic field exerts a force on a moving charge, provided that the charge crosses the lines of magnetic field strength. The magnitude of this force is proportional to (1) the charge; (2) the speed of the charge; (3) the magnetic field strength, designated B; and (4) the direction of charge travel with respect to the direction of the magnetic field. The direction of the force on the moving charge can be determined through the

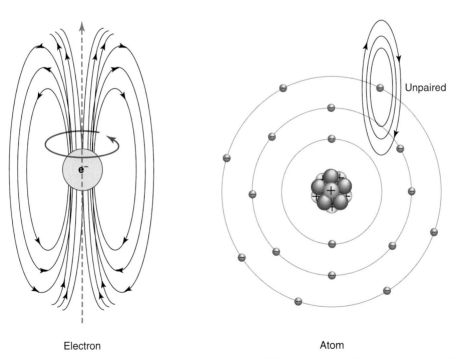

Electron   Atom

■ **FIGURE A-7** A spinning charge has an associated magnetic field, such as the electron (left). An unpaired electron in an atomic orbital produces a magnetic field (right). Each produces magnetic dipoles that will interact with an external magnetic field.

use of the right-hand rule. It is perpendicular to both the direction of the charge's velocity and the lines of magnetic field strength. Because an electrical current consists of moving charges, a current-carrying wire in a magnetic field will experience a force (a torque). This principle is used in devices such as electric motors.

Electromagnetic Induction

In 1831, Michael Faraday discovered that a *moving* magnet induces an electrical current in a nearby conductor. His observations with magnets and conducting wires led to the findings listed here. The major ideas are illustrated in Figure A-8.

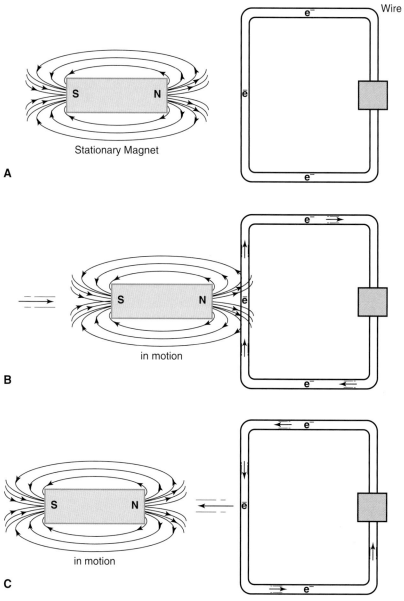

■ **FIGURE A-8** Faraday experiments: changing magnetic fields and induction effects. **A.** A stationary magnetic field is depicted, with no electron flow occurring. **B.** The magnetic field is moving towards the wire loop, resulting in the induction of an electromotive force that results in electron flow in a clockwise direction. **C.** The magnetic field is moving away from the position indicated in **(B)**, resulting in the reverse, counterclockwise flow of electrons in the wire loop.

1. A *changing* magnetic field induces a voltage (electrical potential difference) in a nearby conducting wire and causes a current to flow. An identical voltage is induced whether the wire moves with respect to the magnetic field position or the magnetic field moves with respect to the wire position. A *stationary* magnetic field *does not* induce a voltage in a stationary wire.

2. A stronger magnetic field results in a stronger induced voltage. The voltage is proportional to the number of magnetic field lines cutting across the wire conductor per unit time. If the relative speed of the wire or the magnet is increased with respect to the other, the induced voltage will be larger because an increased number of magnetic field lines will be cutting across the wire conductor per unit time.

3. A 90° angle of the wire conductor relative to the magnetic field will provide the greatest number of lines to cross per unit distance, resulting in a higher induced voltage than for other angles.

4. When a solenoid (wire coil) is placed in a magnetic field, the magnetic field lines cut by each turn of the coil are additive, causing the resultant induced voltage to be directly proportional to the number of turns of the coil.

The direction of current flow caused by an induced voltage is described by Lenz's law (Fig. A-9): *An induced current flows in a direction such that its associated magnetic field opposes the magnetic field that induced it.* Lenz's law is an important concept that describes self-induction and mutual induction.

Self-Induction

A time-varying current in a coil wire produces a magnetic field that varies in the same manner. By Lenz's law, the varying magnetic field induces a potential difference across the coil that opposes the source voltage. Therefore, a rising and falling source voltage (AC) creates an *opposing* falling and rising induced voltage in the coil. This phenomenon, called *self-induction*, is used in autotransformers that provide a variable incremental voltage.

Mutual Induction

A *primary* wire coil carrying AC produces a time-varying magnetic field. When a *secondary* wire coil is located under the influence of this magnetic field, a time-varying potential difference across the secondary coil is similarly induced, as shown in Figure A-9. The amplitude of the induced voltage, V_s, can be determined from the following equation, known as the law of transformers:

$$\left(\frac{V_p}{N_p} \right) = \left(\frac{V_s}{N_s} \right), \tag{A-16}$$

where V_p is the voltage amplitude applied to the primary coil, V_s is the voltage amplitude induced in the secondary coil, N_p is the number of turns in the primary coil, and N_s is the number of turns in the secondary coil. With a predetermined number of "turns" on the primary and secondary coils, this *mutual inductance* property can increase or decrease the voltage in electrical circuits. The devices that provide this change of voltage (current changes in the opposite direction) are called *transformers*. Further explanation of their use in x-ray generators is covered in Chapter 6.

Electric Generators and Motors

The electric generator utilizes the principles of electromagnetic induction to convert mechanical energy into electrical energy. It consists of a coiled wire mounted

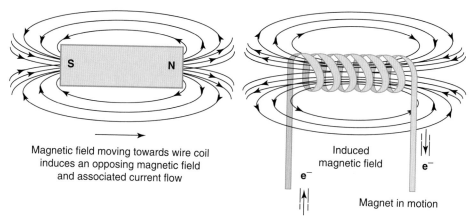

Magnetic field moving towards wire coil induces an opposing magnetic field and associated current flow

Induced magnetic field

e⁻ e⁻

Magnet in motion

■ **FIGURE A-9** Lenz's law, demonstrating mutual induction between a moving magnetic field and a coiled wire conductor.

on a rotor between the poles of a strong magnet, as shown in Figure A-10A. As an external mechanical energy source rotates the coil (*e.g.*, hydroelectric turbine generator), the wires in the coil cut across the magnetic force lines, resulting in a sinusoidally varying potential difference, the polarity of which is determined by the wire approaching or receding from one pole of the magnet. The generator serves as a source of AC power.

The electric motor converts electrical energy into mechanical energy. It consists of a coil of wires mounted on a freely rotating axis (rotor) between the poles of a fixed magnet, as shown in Figure A-10B. When AC flows through the coil, an increasing and decreasing magnetic field is generated, the coil acting as a magnetic dipole. This dipole tends to align with the external magnetic field, causing the rotor to turn. As the dipole approaches alignment, however, the AC and thus, the magnetic field of the rotor reverse polarity, causing another half-turn rotation to achieve alignment. The alternating polarity of the rotor's magnetic field causes a continuous rotation of the coil wire mounted on the rotor as long as AC is applied.

Magnetic Properties of Matter

The magnetic characteristics of materials are determined by atomic and molecular structures related to the behavior of the associated electrons. Three categories of magnetic properties are defined: diamagnetic, paramagnetic, and ferromagnetic. Their properties arise from the association of moving charges (electrons) and magnetic fields.

Diamagnetic Materials

Individual electrons orbiting in atomic or molecular shells represent a current loop and give rise to a magnetic field. The various electron orbits do not fall in any preferred plane, so the superposition of the associated magnetic fields results in a net magnetic field that is too small to be measured. When these atoms or molecules are placed in a changing magnetic field, however, the electron motions are altered by the induced electromotive force to form a reverse magnetic field *opposing* the applied magnetic field. *Diamagnetic materials*, therefore, cause a depletion of the applied magnetic field in the local micromagnetic environment. An example of a diamagnetic material is calcium, and its magnetic properties are described in Chapter 12.

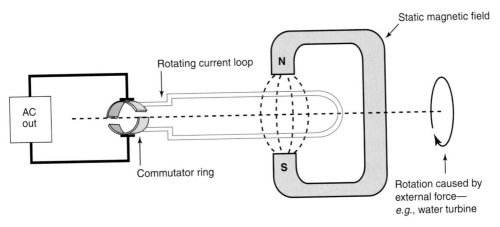

The rotating current wire loop in the static magnetic field creates an induced current occuring with an alternating potential difference.

A

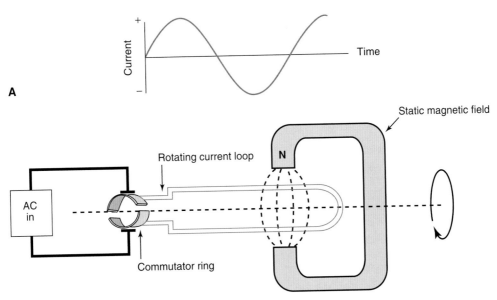

B Induced rotation of the current loop is caused by the variable magnetic field within current loop associated with the applied alternating current interacting with the static magnetic field.

■ **FIGURE A-10** Electrical and mechanical energy conversion: electric generators **(A)** and electric motors **(B)**.

Paramagnetic Materials

Based on the previous discussion, it would seem likely that all elements and molecules would behave as diamagnetic agents. In fact, all have diamagnetic properties, but some have additional properties that overwhelm the diamagnetic response. Electrons in atomic or molecular orbitals orient their magnetic fields in such a way as to cancel in pairs; however, in those materials that have an *odd* number of electrons, one electron is unpaired, exact cancellation cannot occur, and a magnetic field equivalent to one electron orbital results. Depending on orbital structures and electron filling characteristics, *fractional* unpaired electron spins can also occur, resulting in variations in the magnetic field strength. When placed in an external magnetic field, the magnetic field of the material caused by the unpaired electron aligns with the applied field. *Paramagnetic materials*, having unpaired electrons, locally *augment* the micro-magnetic environment. The overall magnetic properties of the atom result from these paramagnetic effects as well as the diamagnetic effects discussed earlier, with the paramagnetic characteristics predominating. An example of a paramagnetic material is gadolinium, an element used in magnetic resonance imaging contrast agents, as described in Chapters 12 and 13.

Ferromagnetic Materials

Iron, nickel, and cobalt can possess intrinsic magnetic fields and will react strongly in an applied magnetic field. These *ferromagnetic materials* are transition elements that have an unorthodox atomic orbital structure: electrons will fill the outer orbital shells before the inner orbitals are completely filled. The usual spin cancellation of the electrons does not occur, resulting in an unusually high atomic magnetic moment. While they are in a random atomic (elemental) or molecular (compound) arrangement, cancellation of the dipoles occurs and no intrinsic magnetic field is manifested; however, when the individual magnetic dipoles are non-randomly aligned by an external force (*e.g.*, a strong electrical field), a constructive enhancement of the individual atomic magnetic moments gives rise to an intrinsic magnetic field that reacts strongly in an applied magnetic field. Permanent magnets are examples of a permanent *non-random* arrangement of local "magnetic domains" of the transition elements. Ferromagnetic characteristics dominate over paramagnetic and diamagnetic interactions. These materials become dangerous in the vicinity of a strong magnetic field, and must be carefully identified and avoided in an around magnetic resonance imaging scanners, as explained in the MR safety section of Chapter 13.

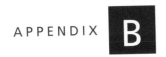

APPENDIX B

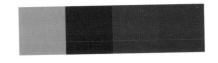

SI and Derived Units, Physical Constants, Prefixes, Definitions and Conversion Factors, Geometry, and Roman and Greek Symbols Used in Medical Physics

TABLE B-1 SI BASE UNITS

BASE QUANTITY		BASE UNIT	
Name	Typical Symbol	Name	Symbol
time	t	second	s
length	l, x, r, etc.	meter	m
mass	m	kilogram	kg
electric current	I, i	ampere	A
thermodynamic temperature	T	kelvin	K
amount of substance	n	mole	mol
luminous intensity	I_v	candela	cd

Reprinted from Bureau International des Poids et Mesures, The International System of Units (SI), 9th edition 2019. (CC BY 4.0) Available at: https://www.bipm.org/utils/common/pdf/si-brochure/SI-Brochure-9.pdf

TABLE B-2 THE 21 SI UNITS WITH SPECIAL NAMES AND SYMBOLS

DERIVED QUANTITY	SPECIAL NAME OF UNIT	UNIT EXPRESSED IN TERMS OF BASE UNITS[a]	UNIT EXPRESSED IN TERMS OF OTHER SI UNITS
plane angle	radian[b]	rad = m/m	
solid angle	steradian[c]	sr = m²/m²	
frequency	hertz[d]	Hz = s⁻¹	
force	newton	N = kg m s⁻²	
pressure, stress	pascal	Pa = kg m⁻¹ s⁻²	
energy, work, amount of heat	joule	J = kg m² s⁻²	Nm
power, radiant flux	watt	W = kg m² s⁻³	J/s
electric charge[a]	coulomb	C = A s	
electric potential difference[e]	volt	V = kg m² s⁻³ A⁻¹	W/A
capacitance	farad	F = kg⁻¹ m⁻² s⁴ A²	C/V
electric resistance	ohm	Ω = kg m² s⁻³ A⁻²	V/A

(Continued)

TABLE B-2 THE 21 SI UNITS WITH SPECIAL NAMES AND SYMBOLS *(Continued)*

DERIVED QUANTITY	SPECIAL NAME OF UNIT	UNIT EXPRESSED IN TERMS OF BASE UNITS[a]	UNIT EXPRESSED IN TERMS OF OTHER SI UNITS
electric conductance	siemens	$S = kg^{-1} m^2 s^3 A^2$	A/V
magnetic flux	weber	$Wb = kg\ m^2 s^{-2} A^{-1}$	Vs
magnetic flux density	tesla	$T = kg\ s^{-2} A^{-1}$	Wb/m²
inductance	henry	$H = kg\ m^2 s^{-2} A^{-2}$	Wb/A
Celsius temperature	degree Celsius[f]	$°C = K$	
luminous flux	lumen	$lm = cd\ sr^g$	cd sr
illuminance	lux	$lx = cd\ sr\ m^{-2}$	lm/m²
activity referred to a radionuclide[d,h]	becquerel	$Bq = s^{-1}$	
absorbed dose, kerma	gray	$Gy = m^2 s^{-2}$	J/kg
dose equivalent	sievert[i]	$Sv = m^2 s^{-2}$	J/kg

[a]Under the 2019 redefinition of the SI base units, which took effect on May 20, 2019, the elementary charge (*i.e.*, the charge of the proton or electron and other fundamental particles) was defined as exactly $1.602176634 \times 10^{-19}$ coulombs. Thus the coulomb is the charge of exactly $1/(1.602176634 \times 10^{-19})$ elementary charges, which is approximately $6.2415090744 \times 10^{18}$ elementary charges.
The intention was to reflect the underlying physics of the corresponding quantity equations although for some more complex derived units this may not be possible.
[b]The radian is the coherent unit for plane angle. One radian is the angle subtended at the centre of a circle by an arc that is equal in length to the radius. It is also the unit for phase angle. For periodic phenomena, the phase angle increases by 2π rad in one period. The radian was formerly an SI supplementary unit, but this category was abolished in 1995.
[c]The steradian is the coherent unit for solid angle. One steradian is the solid angle subtended at the centre of a sphere by an area of the surface that is equal to the squared radius. Like the radian, the steradian was formerly an SI supplementary unit.
[d]The hertz shall only be used for periodic phenomena and the becquerel shall only be used for stochastic processes in activity referred to a radionuclide.
[e]Electric potential difference is also called "voltage" in many countries, as well as "electric tension" or simply "tension" in some countries.
[f]The degree Celsius is used to express Celsius temperatures. The numerical value of a temperature difference or temperature interval is the same when expressed in either degrees Celsius or in kelvin.
[g]In photometry the name steradian and the symbol sr are usually retained in expressions for units.
[h]Activity referred to a radionuclide is sometimes incorrectly called radioactivity.
[i]The special name sievert is also used from the radiation protection quantity effective dose as specified by the International Commission on Radiological Protection (ICRP).
Adapted from Bureau International des Poids et Mesures, The International System of Units (SI), 9th edition 2019. (CC BY 4.0) Available at: https://www.bipm.org/utils/common/pdf/si-brochure/SI-Brochure-9.pdf

TABLE B-3 SELECTION OF COHERENT DERIVED UNITS IN THE SI EXPRESSED IN TERMS OF BASE UNITS

DERIVED QUANTITY	TYPICAL SYMBOL OF QUANTITY	DERIVED UNIT EXPRESSED IN TERMS OF BASE UNITS
area	A	m^2
volume	V	m^3
speed, velocity	v	$m\ s^{-1}$
acceleration	a	$m\ s^{-2}$
wavenumber	σ	m^{-1}
density, mass density	ρ	$kg\ m^{-3}$
surface density	ρ_A	$kg\ m^{-2}$
specific volume	v	$m^3\ kg^{-1}$
current density	j	$A\ m^{-2}$
magnetic field strength	H	$A\ m^{-1}$
amount of substance concentration	c	$mol\ m^{-3}$
mass concentration	ρ, γ	$kg\ m^{-3}$
luminance	L_v	$cd\ m^{-2}$

Reprinted from Bureau International des Poids et Mesures, The International System of Units (SI), 9th edition 2019. (CC BY 4.0) Available at: https://www.bipm.org/utils/common/pdf/si-brochure/SI-Brochure-9.pdf

TABLE B-4 SI DERIVED UNITS[a]

DERIVED QUANTITY	NAME OF COHERENT DERIVED UNIT	SYMBOL	DERIVED UNIT EXPRESSED IN TERMS OF BASE UNITS
moment of force	newton meter	$N\ m$	$kg\ m^2\ s^{-2}$
surface tension	newton per meter	$N\ m^{-1}$	$kg\ s^{-2}$
angular velocity, angular frequency	radian per second	$rad\ s^{-1}$	s^{-1}
angular acceleration	radian per second squared	rad/s^2	s^{-2}
heat flux density, irradiance	watt per square meter	W/m^2	$kg\ s^{-3}$
heat capacity, entropy	joule per kelvin	$J\ K^{-1}$	$kg\ m^2\ s^{-2}\ K^{-1}$
specific heat capacity, specific entropy	joule per kilogram kelvin	$J\ K^{-1}\ kg^{-1}$	$m^2\ s^{-2}\ K^{-1}$
specific energy	joule per kilogram	$J\ kg^{-1}$	$m^2\ s^{-2}$
thermal conductivity	watt per meter kelvin	$W\ m^{-1}\ K^{-1}$	$kg\ m\ s^{-3}\ K^{-1}$
energy density	joule per cubic meter	$J\ m^{-3}$	$kg\ m^{-1}\ s^{-2}$
electric field strength	volt per meter	$V\ m^{-1}$	$kg\ m\ s^{-3}\ A^{-1}$
electric charge density	coulomb per cubic meter	$C\ m^{-3}$	$A\ s\ m^{-3}$
surface charge density	coulomb per square meter	$C\ m^{-2}$	$A\ s\ m^{-2}$
electric flux density, electric displacement	coulomb per square meter	$C\ m^{-2}$	$A\ s\ m^{-2}$

(*Continued*)

TABLE B-4 SI DERIVED UNITS[a] (Continued)

DERIVED QUANTITY	NAME OF COHERENT DERIVED UNIT	SYMBOL	DERIVED UNIT EXPRESSED IN TERMS OF BASE UNITS
permittivity	farad per meter	$F\ m^{-1}$	$kg^{-1}\ m^{-3}\ s^4\ A^2$
permeability	henry per meter	$H\ m^{-1}$	$kg\ m\ s^{-2}\ A^{-2}$
exposure (x- and γ-rays)	coulomb per kilogram	$C\ kg^{-1}$	$A\ s\ kg^{-1}$
absorbed dose	gray	Gy	$m^2\ s^{-2}$
radiance	watt per square meter steradian	$W\ sr^{-1}\ m^{-2}$	$kg\ s^{-3}$

It is important to emphasize that each physical quantity has only one coherent SI unit, even though this unit can be expressed in different forms by using some of the special names and symbols. The converse, however, is not true, because in general several different quantities may share the same SI unit. For example, specific energy and absorbed dose are derived quantities that are both expressed in SI base units of $m^2\ s^{-2}$. It is therefore important not to use the unit alone to specify the quantity.

[a]Names and symbols include SI coherent derived units with special names and symbols.

Adapted from Bureau International des Poids et Mesures, The International System of Units (SI), 9th edition 2019. (CC BY 4.0) Available at: https://www.bipm.org/utils/common/pdf/si-brochure/SI-Brochure-9.pdf

TABLE B-5 PHYSICAL CONSTANTS

SYMBOL	CONSTANT	VALUE	SI UNITS
c	Velocity of light in vacuum	2.997925×10^8	$m\ s^{-1}$
e	Elementary charge	1.602177×10^{-19}	C
F	Faraday constant	9.64853×10^4	$C\ mol^{-1}$
g	Standard acceleration of free fall	9.80665	$m\ s^{-2}$
h	Planck's constant	6.626070×10^{-34}	$J\ s$
		4.1357×10^{-15}	$eV\ s$
k_B	Boltzmann's constant	1.380649×10^{-23}	$J\ K^{-1}$
		8.617343×10^{-5}	$eV\ K^{-1}$
m_e	Electron rest mass	9.109383×10^{-31}	kg
$m_e c^2$	Electron rest energy	8.187105×10^{-14}	J
		5.10999×10^5	eV
m_p	Proton rest mass	1.672622×10^{-27}	kg
N_A	Avogadro's number	6.022141×10^{23}	mol^{-1}
r_e	Classical electron radius	2.817940×10^{-15}	m
R	Gas constant	8.31446	$J\ mol^{-1}\ K^{-1}$
u	Mass unit (^{12}C standard)	1.660539×10^{-27}	kg
uc^2	Mass unit (energy units)	9.31494×10^8	eV
ε_0	Electrical permittivity of free space	8.85419×10^{-12}	$C^2\ N^{-1}\ m^{-2}$
λ_C	Compton wavelength of electron	2.42631×10^{-12}	m
μ_B	Bohr magneton	9.274010×10^{-24}	$J\ T^{-1}$
μ_0	Magnetic permeability of space	$4\pi \times 10^{-7}$	$T\ m\ A^{-1}$
		$\approx 12.566 \times 10^{-7}$	
μ_N	Nuclear magneton	5.050784×10^{-27}	$J\ T^{-1}$
m_n	Neutron rest mass	1.674929310227	kg
γ	Gyromagnetic ratio of proton	42.5764	$MHz/\ T^{-1}$

TABLE B-6 **PREFIXES**

PREFIXES	
yotta (Y)	10^{24}
zetta (Z)	10^{21}
exa (E)	10^{18}
peta (P)	10^{15}
tera (T)	10^{12}
giga (G)	10^{9}
mega (M)	10^{6}
kilo (k)	10^{3}
hecto (h)	10^{2}
deca (da)	10^{1}
deci (d)	10^{-1}
centi (c)	10^{-2}
milli (m)	10^{-3}
micro (µ)	10^{-6}
nano (n)	10^{-9}
pico (p)	10^{-12}
femto (f)	10^{-15}
atto (a)	10^{-18}
zepto (z)	10^{-21}
yocto (y)	10^{-24}

TABLE B-7 **DEFINITIONS AND CONVERSION FACTORS**

ANGLE 1 radian	$360°/2\pi \approx 57.2958°$
CURRENT 1 ampere 1 ampere	1 C/s 6.241×10^{18} electrons/s
ENERGY 1 electron volt (eV) 1 calorie	1.6022×10^{-19} J 4.187 J
LENGTH 1 inch 1 inch 1 Angstrom	25.4 mm 2.54 cm 10^{-10} m
MAGNETIC FLUX DENSITY 1 Gauss	10^{-4} T
MASS 1 pound 1 kg	0.45359 kg 2.02046 pound
POWER 1 watt (W)	J/s

(Continued)

TABLE B-7 DEFINITIONS AND CONVERSION FACTORS *(Continued)*

RADIOLOGIC UNITS	
1 roentgen (R)	2.58×10^{-4} C/kg
1 roentgen (R)	8.76 mGy air kerma
1 mGy air kerma	114.2 mR
1 gray (Gy)	100 rad
1 sievert (Sv)	100 rem
1 curie (Ci)	3.7×10^{10} becquerel (Bq)
1 becquerel (Bq)	1 disintegration s^{-1} (dps)
TEMPERATURE	
°C (Celsius)	$5/9 \times (°F - 32)$
°F (Fahrenheit)	$9/5 \times (°C + 32)$
°K (Kelvin)	$°C + 273.16$
VOLUME	
1 US gallon	3.7854 L
1 liter (L)	$1,000 \text{ cm}^3$

TABLE B-8 GEOMETRY

Area of circle	πr^2
Circumference of circle	$2 \pi r$
Surface area of sphere	$4 \pi r^2$
Volume of sphere	$(4/3) \pi^3$
Area of triangle	$(1/2) \text{ base} \times \text{height}$

TABLE B-9 ROMAN AND GREEK SYMBOLS USED IN MEDICAL PHYSICS[a]

SYMBOLS	
Roman Symbols	
a	area
A	ampere (SI unit of current)
A	age; aperture function; atomic mass number
A_Q	quantum detection efficiency
A_r	atomic weight
A_s	Swank factor
B	backscatter factor; barrier transmission; broad beam transmission factor; field strength; image brightness
B	magnetic field strength
c	dose conversion coefficient; speed of electromagnetic waves—speed of light; speed of sound
C	coulomb (SI unit of charge)
C	contrast; contour
$C_{a,100}$	CT kerma index
C_w	weighted CT kerma index
d	distance; width

TABLE B-9 ROMAN AND GREEK SYMBOLS USED IN MEDICAL PHYSICS[a] *(Continued)*

SYMBOLS

d'	detectability
d_{FID}	focus to image receptor distance
D	absorbed dose; density; diffusion coefficient of water
D_{max}	maximum optical density
D_v	directional derivative of a function in the direction **v**
e	charge on an electron ($=1.602 \times 10^{-19}$ C)
E	effective dose; energy; energy fluence; retinal illumination
E_K	K atomic absorption edge
E_s	binding energy of an electron shell
f	frequency; function; input to a system
f_D	Doppler frequency
f_N	Nyquist frequency
F	coherent form factor; field area
g	average fraction of energy transferred to charged particles that is lost to photons when the charged particles are slowed down in the same medium as they were released; output of a system; gain; gradient; acceleration due to gravity
g_I	speed function
G	Gaussian filter; gradient amplitude
h	Planck's constant
H	transfer function/system response function
$H*(d)$	ambient dose equivalent
$H'(d, \Omega)$	directional dose equivalent
$H_p(d)$	personal dose equivalent
I	electron current; intensity; mean excitation energy
$\mathbf{I}$	nuclear spin
J	joule (SI unit of energy)
k	Boltzmann constant; proportionality constant from Coulomb's law; signal to noise ratio
k	wave number
K	kerma
K_i	incident air kerma
$\dot{K_i}$	incident air kerma rate
K_{scat}	scatter kerma
K_{sec}	secondary kerma
kVp	peak kilovoltage
ℓ	azithumal quantum number (orbital angular momentum quantum number)
L	aperture length; luminance
L_Δ	linear energy transfer (LET)
m	magnetic quantum number; magnification; mass; noise
m_0	rest mass
M	atomic mass; demagnification; moment
M_{opt}	optical modulation transfer function

(Continued)

TABLE B-9 ROMAN AND GREEK SYMBOLS USED IN MEDICAL PHYSICS[a] *(Continued)*

SYMBOLS	
n	bit depth; number; principal quantum number; refractive index
n	noise
n_i	initial principal quantum number
n_f	final principal quantum number
N	number of neutrons in an atom; number
$\bar{N}$	unit normal vector to contour C
N_A	Avogadro's number
N_a	number of interaction centers (atoms) per unit volume
N_{am}	number of atoms per unit mass
N_0	number of x-ray quanta
p	projection; luminous flux to photon conversion factor
$\boldsymbol{p}$	angular momentum
P	power; power rating; target dose; wave amplitude
P_{It}	current–exposure time product
P_{KA}	air kerma–area product
P_{KL}	air kerma–length product
Q	charge; heat capacity; quality; quantity
r	grid ratio
r_0	"classical radius of the electron"
R	radiant energy; reflection coefficient; relaxation rate; voltage ripple
s	signal; spin quantum number
S	incoherent scattering function; scatter factor; sensitivity; signal; stopping power; survival
S_{ion}	ionizational mass stopping power
$\bar{\bar{S}}_g^w$	ratio of average stopping powers
Sv	sievert (unit of equivalent dose and unit of effective dose)
t	time; exposure time; thickness
t_e	exposure time
T	tesla (SI unit of magnetic flux density)
T	modulation transfer function; occupancy; temperature; thickness; threshold; time; transmission; transmission coefficient
$<T>$	expectation value of energy converted to secondary electrons
$T_{1/2}$	half-time, half-life ($T_p 1/2$ physical; $T_b 1/2$ biological)
T_1	time constant for spin-lattice relaxation
u	spatial frequency
U	unsharpness; field; use factor
v	velocity
V	volume
w	weighting coefficient/factor
w_i	normalized weight inaction of element i
W	workload
$\bar{W}_{air}$	mean energy spent in air to form an ion pair in dry air

TABLE B-9 ROMAN AND GREEK SYMBOLS USED IN MEDICAL PHYSICS[a] (Continued)

SYMBOLS	
x	thickness
X	exposure
Z	acoustic impedance; atomic number; nuclear charge
Greek Symbols	
α	(subscript) radiation emitted for transition between neighboring electron shells; frequency dependent amplitude attenuation coefficient. In nuclear medicine it would refer to an alpha particle (*i.e.*, helium nucleus)
α_E	Ernst angle
β	(subscript) radiation emitted for a transition between non-neighboring electron shells. In nuclear medicine it would refer to a beta particle emitted from the nucleus of a radionuclide during decay
γ	film gamma; gyromagnetic ratio. In nuclear medicine it would refer to a γ ray emitted from the nucleus of a radionuclide during decay
Γ	greyscale characteristic. In nuclear medicine (with subscript x) is would refer to the Specific Gamma Ray Dose (or Exposure) Constant of a radionuclide expressed in Dose (or Exposure) per unit time per unit activity. The x is the cutoff energy for x- and γ-rays considered in the calculation
ε_{tr}	energy transferred
$\bar{\varepsilon}_T$	energy imparted to a tissue
η	orthogonal dimension; quantum detection efficiency
θ	angle; azimuth angle; projection angle
θ_D	Doppler angle
λ	decision variable; wavelength
κ	compressibility; curvature of the contour C
μ	linear attenuation coefficient ($N_a\sigma$); unified atomic mass unit
μ	nuclear magnetic moment
μ_0	rest mass of electron
ν	frequency; photon frequency
ξ	areal density; lateral dimension within aperture plane
ρ	density
ρ_o	undisturbed mass density of a medium
σ	cross-sectional area; standard deviation
σ^2	variance
τ	cross section for a photon to interact
Φ	number of photons per unit area; fluence
Ψ	energy fluence (energy per unit area)
ω	fluorescent yield; frequency; resonance frequency
ω_o	Larmor frequency
Ω	solid angle

[a]Be aware that some of the symbols typically used in medical physics differ from those used in the SI system of units (*e.g.*, SI uses the symbol *H* to represent the magnetic field strength while in the field medical physics *H* is commonly used to represent the transfer function and *B* is used to represent the magnetic field strength).

TABLE B-10 **THE GREEK ALPHABET**

GREEK NAME	CAPITAL	LOWERCASE	GREEK NAME	CAPITAL	LOWERCASE
Alpha	A	α	Nu	N	ν
Beta	B	β	Xi	Ξ	ξ
Gamma	Γ	γ	Omicron	O	o
Delta	Δ	δ	Pi	Π	π
Epsilon	E	ε	Rho	P	ρ
Zeta	Z	ζ	Sigma	Σ	σ
Eta	H	η	Tau	T	τ
Theta	Θ	θ	Upsilon	Y	μ
Iota	I	ι	Phi	Φ	φ
Kappa	K	κ	Chi	X	χ
Lambda	Λ	λ	Psi	Ψ	ψ
Mu	M	μ	Omega	Ω	ω

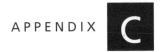

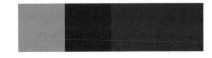

Radiologic Data for Elements 1–100

Appendix C: Radiologic Data for Elements 1–100

TABLE C-1 RADIOLOGIC DATA FOR ELEMENTS 1–100

Z	SYM	ELEMENT	DENSITY (g/cm³)	AT MASS (g/mol)	K-EDGE (keV)	L-EDGES: L_I (keV)	L-EDGES: L_{II} (keV)	L-EDGES: L_{III} (keV)	Ka_1 (keV)	Ka_2 (keV)	Kb_1 (keV)	Kb_2 (keV)
1	H	Hydrogen	8.988E−05	1.008	0.0136	2	2	2	2	2	2	2
2	He	Helium	0.0001785	4.003	0.0246	2	2	2	2	2	2	2
3	Li	Lithium	0.534	6.939	0.0550	2	2	2	0.052	0.052	2	2
4	Be	Beryllium	1.85	9.012	0.115	2	2	0.006	0.109	0.109	2	2
5	B	Boron	2.34	10.811	0.188	2	2	0.005	0.183	0.183	2	2
6	C	Carbon	2.267	12.011	0.282	2	2	0.005	0.277	0.277	2	2
7	N	Nitrogen	0.0012506	14.007	0.397	2	2	0.004	0.393	0.393	2	2
8	O	Oxygen	0.001429	15.999	0.533	2	2	0.008	0.525	0.525	2	2
9	F	Fluorine	0.001696	18.998	0.692	2	2	0.015	0.677	0.677	2	2
10	Ne	Neon	0.0008999	20.179	0.874	2	2	0.026	0.848	0.848	0.858	0.858
11	Na	Sodium	0.971	22.99	1.080	0.06	2	0.039	1.041	1.041	1.071	1.071
12	Mg	Magnesium	1.738	24.312	1.309	0.062	0.08	0.056	1.253	1.253	1.302	1.302
13	Al	Aluminum	2.698	26.982	1.840	0.118	0.076	0.075	1.487	1.486	1.557	1.557
14	Si	Silicon	2.3296	28.086	2.143	0.153	0.101	0.100	1.740	1.739	1.836	1.836
15	P	Phosphorus	1.82	30.974	2.471	0.193	0.130	0.129	2.014	2.013	2.139	2.139
16	S	Sulfur	2.067	32.064	2.824	0.237	0.164	0.163	2.308	2.307	2.464	2.464
17	Cl	Chlorine	0.003214	35.453	3.203	0.286	0.204	0.202	2.622	2.620	2.816	2.816
18	Ar	Argon	0.0017837	39.948	3.607	0.340	0.247	0.245	2.958	2.956	3.19	3.19
19	K	Potassium	0.862	39.102	4.034	0.403	0.296	0.293	3.314	3.311	3.59	3.59
20	Ca	Calcium	1.54	40.08	4.486	0.462	0.346	0.342	3.692	3.688	4.013	4.013
21	Sc	Scandium	2.989	44.958	4.965	0.529	0.400	0.396	4.090	4.086	4.461	4.461
22	Ti	Titanium	4.54	47.9	5.463	0.626	0.460	0.454	4.511	4.505	4.932	4.932
23	V	Vanadium	6.11	50.942	5.987	0.694	0.519	0.511	4.952	4.944	5.427	5.427
24	Cr	Chromium	7.15	51.996	6.537	0.768	0.582	0.572	5.415	5.405	5.947	5.947
25	Mn	Manganese	7.44	54.938	7.112	0.846	0.649	0.638	5.899	5.888	6.49	6.49

26	Fe	Iron	7.874	55.847	7.712	0.929	0.721	0.708	6.404	6.391	7.058	7.058
27	Co	Cobalt	8.86	58.933	8.339	1.016	0.797	0.782	6.930	6.915	7.649	7.649
28	Ni	Nickel	8.912	58.71	8.993	1.109	0.878	0.861	7.478	7.461	8.265	8.265
29	Cu	Copper	8.96	63.54	9.673	1.208	0.965	0.945	8.048	8.028	8.905	8.93
30	Zn	Zinc	7.134	65.37	10.386	1.316	1.057	1.034	8.639	8.616	9.572	9.6581
31	Ga	Gallium	5.907	69.72	11.115	1.426	1.155	1.134	9.252	9.231	10.271	10.3661
32	Ge	Germanium	5.323	72.59	11.877	1.536	1.259	1.228	9.887	9.856	10.983	11.1011
33	As	Arsenic	5.776	74.922	12.666	1.662	1.368	1.333	10.544	10.509	11.727	11.8641
34	Se	Selenium	4.809	78.96	13.483	1.791	1.485	1.444	11.222	11.181	12.496	12.6521
35	Br	Bromine	3.122	79.909	14.330	1.923	1.605	1.559	11.924	11.878	13.292	13.4701
36	Kr	Krypton	0.003733	83.8	15.202	2.067	1.732	1.680	12.650	12.598	14.113	14.3151
37	Rb	Rubidium	1.532	85.47	16.106	2.217	1.866	1.806	13.396	13.336	14.962	15.1851
38	Sr	Strontium	2.64	87.62	17.037	2.372	2.008	1.940	14.166	14.098	15.836	16.0851
39	Y	Yttrium	4.469	88.905	17.997	2.535	2.155	2.079	14.958	14.882	16.737	17.0151
40	Zr	Zirconium	6.506	91.22	18.985	2.698	2.305	2.227	15.770	15.692	17.662	17.9631
41	Nb	Niobium	8.57	92.906	20.002	2.867	2.464	2.370	16.615	16.521	18.623	18.9471
42	Mo	Molybdenum	10.22	95.94	21.048	3.047	2.628	2.523	17.479	17.374	19.608	19.960
43	Tc	Technetium	11.5	99	22.123	3.230	2.797	2.681	18.367	18.251	20.619	21.002
44	Ru	Ruthenium	12.37	101.7	23.229	3.421	2.973	2.844	19.279	19.150	21.656	22.072
45	Rh	Rhodium	12.41	102.905	24.365	3.619	3.156	3.013	20.216	20.073	22.723	23.173
46	Pd	Palladium	12.02	106.4	25.531	3.822	3.344	3.187	21.178	21.021	23.819	24.303
47	Ag	Silver	10.501	107.87	26.727	4.034	3.540	3.368	22.163	21.991	24.943	25.463
48	Cd	Cadmium	8.69	112.4	27.953	4.250	3.742	3.554	23.173	22.985	26.095	26.653
49	In	Indium	7.31	114.82	29.211	4.475	3.951	3.744	24.209	24.002	27.275	27.872
50	Sn	Tin	7.287	118.69	30.499	4.706	4.167	3.939	25.272	25.044	28.491	29.122
51	Sb	Antimony	6.685	121.75	31.817	4.942	4.389	4.140	26.359	26.110	29.725	30.402

(Continued)

Appendix C: Radiologic Data for Elements 1–100

TABLE C-1 RADIOLOGIC DATA FOR ELEMENTS 1–100 (Continued)

Z	SYM	ELEMENT	DENSITY (g/cm³)	AT MASS (g/mol)	K-EDGE (keV)	L-EDGES: L_I (keV)	L-EDGES: L_{II} (keV)	L-EDGES: L_{III} (keV)	Ka_1 (keV)	Ka_2 (keV)	Kb_1 (keV)	Kb_2 (keV)
52	Te	Tellurium	6.232	127.6	33.168	5.186	4.616	4.345	27.472	27.201	30.995	31.712
53	I	Iodine	4.93	126.904	34.551	5.442	4.851	4.556	28.612	28.317	32.295	33.054
54	Xe	Xenon	0.005887	131.3	35.966	5.700	5.092	4.772	29.779	29.459	33.625	34.428
55	Cs	Cesium	1.873	132.905	38.894	6.235	5.341	4.993	30.973	30.625	34.985	35.833
56	Ba	Barium	3.594	137.34	40.410	6.516	5.597	5.220	32.194	31.817	36.378	37.270
57	La	Lanthanum	6.145	138.91	41.958	6.802	5.860	5.452	33.442	33.034	37.802	38.739
58	Ce	Cerium	6.77	140.12	43.538	7.095	6.131	5.690	34.720	34.279	39.258	40.243
59	Pr	Praseodymium	6.773	140.907	45.152	7.398	6.408	5.932	36.026	35.550	40.748	41.778
60	Nd	Neodymium	7.007	144.24	46.801	7.707	6.691	6.177	37.361	36.847	42.272	43.345
61	Pm	Promethium	7.26	145	48.486	8.024	6.981	6.427	38.725	38.171	43.825	44.947
62	Sm	Samarium	7.52	150.35	50.207	8.343	7.278	6.683	40.118	39.523	45.413	46.584
63	Eu	Europium	5.243	151.96	51.965	8.679	7.584	6.944	41.542	40.902	47.036	48.256
64	Gd	Gadolinium	7.895	157.25	53.761	9.013	7.898	7.211	42.996	42.309	48.696	49.964
65	Tb	Terbium	8.229	158.924	55.593	9.365	8.221	7.484	44.481	43.744	50.382	51.709
66	Dy	Dysprosium	8.55	162.5	57.464	9.725	8.553	7.762	45.999	45.208	52.119	53.491
67	Ho	Holmium	8.795	164.93	59.374	10.097	8.894	8.046	47.547	46.699	53.878	55.308
68	Er	Erbium	9.066	167.26	61.322	10.479	9.243	8.336	49.128	48.221	55.681	57.164
69	Tm	Thulium	9.321	168.934	63.311	10.869	9.601	8.632	50.742	49.773	57.513	59.059
70	Yb	Ytterbium	6.965	173.04	65.345	11.262	9.968	8.933	52.389	51.354	59.374	60.991
71	Lu	Lutetium	9.84	174.97	67.405	11.672	10.346	9.241	54.070	52.965	61.286	62.960
72	Hf	Hafnium	13.31	178.49	69.517	12.092	10.734	9.555	55.790	54.611	63.236	64.973
73	Ta	Tantalum	16.654	180.948	71.670	12.522	11.128	9.872	57.533	56.277	65.221	67.011
74	W	Tungsten	19.25	183.85	73.869	12.968	11.535	10.199	59.318	57.982	67.244	69.100
75	Re	Rhenium	21.02	186.2	76.111	13.416	11.952	10.530	61.140	59.718	69.309	71.230
76	Os	Osmium	22.61	190.2	78.400	13.880	12.382	10.868	63.001	61.487	71.416	73.404

77	Ir	Iridium	22.56	192.2	80.729	14.353	12.824	11.215	64.896	63.287	73.560	75.620
78	Pt	Platinum	21.46	195.09	83.109	14.835	13.277	11.568	66.832	65.123	75.751	77.883
79	Au	Gold	19.282	196.967	85.532	15.344	13.739	11.925	68.804	66.990	77.985	80.182
80	Hg	Mercury	13.5336	200.5	88.008	15.863	14.215	12.290	70.819	68.894	80.261	82.532
81	Tl	Thallium	11.85	204.37	90.540	16.391	14.700	12.660	72.872	70.832	82.575	84.924
82	Pb	Lead	11.342	207.19	93.113	16.940	15.204	13.039	74.969	72.804	84.936	87.367
83	Bi	Bismuth	9.807	208.98	95.730	17.495	15.725	13.422	77.118	74.815	87.354	89.866
84	Po	Polonium-209	9.32	208.98	98.402	18.047	16.250	13.812	79.301	76.863	89.801	92.403
85	At	Astatine-210	7	209.983	101.131	18.630	16.787	14.207	81.523	78.943	92.302	94.983
86	Rn	Radon-222	0.00973	222.018	103.909	19.222	17.337	14.609	83.793	81.065	94.866	97.617
87	Fr	Francium-223	1.87	223.02	106.738	19.823	17.900	15.017	86.114	83.231	97.477	100.306
88	Ra	Radium-226	5.5	226.025	109.641	20.449	18.475	15.433	88.476	85.434	100.130	103.039
89	Ac	Actinium-227	10.07	227.028	112.599	21.088	19.063	15.854	90.884	87.675	102.846	105.837
90	Th	Thorium-232	11.72	232.038	115.606	21.757	19.688	16.283	93.358	89.952	105.611	108.690
91	Pa	Protactinium-231	15.37	231.036	118.678	22.427	20.312	16.716	95.883	92.287	108.435	111.606
92	U	Uranium-238	18.95	238.051	121.818	23.097	20.947	17.166	98.440	94.659	111.303	114.561
93	Np	Neptunium-237	20.45	237.048	125.027	23.773	21.601	17.610	101.068	97.077	114.243	117.591
94	Pu	Plutonium-239	19.84	239.052	128.220	24.460	22.266	18.057	103.761	99.552	117.261	120.703
95	Am	Americium-241	13.69	241.05	131.590	25.275	22.944	18.504	106.523	102.083	120.360	123.891
96	Cm	Curium-247	13.51	247.07	135.960	26.110	23.779	18.930	109.290	104.441	123.423	127.066
97	Bk	Berkelium-247	14.79	247.07	139.490	26.900	24.385	19.452	112.138	107.205	126.663	130.355
98	Cf	Californium-251	15.1	251.08	143.090	27.700	25.250	19.930	116.030	110.710	130.851	134.681
99	Es	Einsteinium-252	13.5	252.083	146.780	28.530	26.020	20.410	119.080	113.470	134.238	138.169
100	Fm	Fermium-257	2	257.095	150.540	29.380	26.810	20.900	122.190	116.280	137.693	141.724

Reprinted with permission from Deslattes RD, Kessler EG Jr, Indelicato P, et al. X-ray transition energies: new approach to a comprehensive evaluation. *Rev Mod Phys.* 2003;75(1):35-99. ©2003 American Physical Society. doi: 10.1103/RevModPhys.75.35.

APPENDIX D

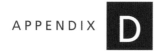

Mass Attenuation Coefficients

D-1 MASS ATTENUATION COEFFICIENTS FOR SELECTED ELEMENTS

TABLE D-1 MASS ATTENUATION COEFFICIENTS IN cm²/g (DENSITY (ρ) IN g/cm³)

ENERGY (keV)	ALUMINUM Z=13 $\rho=2.699$	CALCIUM Z=20 $\rho=1.55$	COPPER Z=29 $\rho=8.96$	MOLYBDENUM Z=42 $\rho=10.22$	RHODIUM Z=45 $\rho=12.41$	IODINE Z=53 $\rho=4.93$	TUNGSTEN Z=74 $\rho=19.3$	LEAD Z=82 $\rho=11.35$
3	7.83E+02	2.71E+02	7.47E+02	2.01E+03	4.42E+02	7.49E+02	1.92E+03	1.96E+03
4	3.58E+02	1.20E+02	3.46E+02	9.65E+02	1.17E+03	3.56E+02	9.54E+02	1.25E+03
5	1.92E+02	5.97E+02	1.89E+02	5.42E+02	6.55E+02	8.30E+02	5.51E+02	7.28E+02
6	1.15E+02	3.74E+02	1.15E+02	3.38E+02	4.11E+02	6.10E+02	3.55E+02	4.73E+02
7	7.37E+01	2.46E+02	7.48E+01	2.23E+02	2.72E+02	4.13E+02	2.36E+02	3.16E+02
8	5.04E+01	1.72E+02	5.18E+01	1.56E+02	1.90E+02	2.89E+02	1.69E+02	2.27E+02
9	3.56E+01	1.25E+02	2.76E+02	1.13E+02	1.39E+02	2.13E+02	1.24E+02	1.68E+02
10	2.60E+01	9.30E+01	2.14E+02	8.55E+01	1.05E+02	1.62E+02	9.33E+01	1.29E+02
12	1.53E+01	5.60E+01	1.35E+02	5.22E+01	6.44E+01	1.00E+02	2.10E+02	8.15E+01
14	9.73E+00	3.62E+01	8.91E+01	3.40E+01	4.21E+01	6.61E+01	1.65E+02	1.33E+02
16	6.58E+00	2.48E+01	6.20E+01	2.37E+01	2.92E+01	4.61E+01	1.17E+02	1.51E+02
18	4.65E+00	1.76E+01	4.49E+01	1.72E+01	2.10E+01	3.35E+01	8.63E+01	1.10E+02
20	3.42E+00	1.30E+01	3.36E+01	7.89E+01	1.57E+01	2.52E+01	6.56E+01	8.61E+01
25	1.83E+00	6.88E+00	1.82E+01	4.78E+01	5.29E+01	1.37E+01	3.66E+01	4.93E+01
30	1.13E+00	4.07E+00	1.09E+01	2.82E+01	3.32E+01	8.38E+00	2.28E+01	3.06E+01
35	7.69E-01	2.63E+00	7.05E+00	1.85E+01	2.21E+01	3.10E+01	1.51E+01	2.02E+01
40	5.67E-01	1.83E+00	4.85E+00	1.29E+01	1.54E+01	2.20E+01	1.06E+01	1.43E+01

45	4.46E−01	1.34E+00	3.51E+00	9.38E+00	1.12E+01	1.62E+01	7.72E+00	1.05E+01
50	3.68E−01	1.02E+00	2.62E+00	7.07E+00	8.42E+00	1.23E+01	5.84E+00	7.98E+00
55	3.15E−01	8.07E−01	2.01E+00	5.42E+00	6.52E+00	9.56E+00	4.54E+00	6.20E+00
60	2.78E−01	6.61E−01	1.60E+00	4.29E+00	5.18E+00	7.61E+00	3.62E+00	4.98E+00
65	2.52E−01	5.56E−01	1.30E+00	3.46E+00	4.20E+00	6.18E+00	2.92E+00	4.04E+00
70	2.30E−01	4.72E−01	1.06E+00	2.80E+00	3.39E+00	5.02E+00	1.09E+01	3.30E+00
75	2.14E−01	4.12E−01	9.00E−01	2.33E+00	2.84E+00	4.19E+00	9.21E+00	2.77E+00
80	2.02E−01	3.66E−01	7.63E−01	1.96E+00	2.37E+00	3.53E+00	7.80E+00	2.32E+00
85	1.92E−01	3.33E−01	6.71E−01	1.70E+00	2.05E+00	3.05E+00	6.78E+00	1.98E+00
90	1.83E−01	3.00E−01	5.80E−01	1.44E+00	1.74E+00	2.57E+00	5.78E+00	7.20E+00
95	1.77E−01	2.79E−01	5.20E−01	1.27E+00	1.53E+00	2.26E+00	5.10E+00	6.38E+00
100	1.71E−01	2.58E−01	4.60E−01	1.10E+00	1.32E+00	1.95E+00	4.42E+00	5.54E+00
110	1.61E−01	2.28E−01	3.78E−01	8.66E−01	1.04E+00	1.52E+00	3.47E+00	4.36E+00
120	1.53E−01	2.06E−01	3.23E−01	7.10E−01	8.43E−01	1.22E+00	2.83E+00	3.55E+00
130	1.47E−01	1.90E−01	2.81E−01	5.88E−01	6.95E−01	1.00E+00	2.29E+00	2.90E+00
140	1.42E−01	1.77E−01	2.47E−01	4.91E−01	5.77E−01	8.26E−01	1.89E+00	2.38E+00
150	1.38E−01	1.67E−01	2.23E−01	4.23E−01	4.94E−01	7.00E−01	1.59E+00	2.02E+00
160	1.34E−01	1.59E−01	2.03E−01	3.69E−01	4.29E−01	6.01E−01	1.36E+00	1.72E+00
170	1.31E−01	1.53E−01	1.89E−01	3.31E−01	3.82E−01	5.31E−01	1.18E+00	1.50E+00

(Continued)

Appendix D: Mass Attenuation Coefficients

TABLE D-1 **MASS ATTENUATION COEFFICIENTS IN cm²/g (DENSITY (ρ) IN g/cm³) (Continued)**

ENERGY (keV)	ALUMINUM $Z = 13$ $\rho = 2.699$	CALCIUM $Z = 20$ $\rho = 1.55$	COPPER $Z = 29$ $\rho = 8.96$	MOLYBDENUM $Z = 42$ $\rho = 10.22$	RHODIUM $Z = 45$ $\rho = 12.41$	IODINE $Z = 53$ $\rho = 4.93$	TUNGSTEN $Z = 74$ $\rho = 19.3$	LEAD $Z = 82$ $\rho = 11.35$
180	1.27E−01	1.47E−01	1.75E−01	2.93E−01	3.36E−01	4.61E−01	1.02E+00	1.29E+00
190	1.25E−01	1.42E−01	1.65E−01	2.68E−01	3.06E−01	4.14E−01	9.03E−01	1.15E+00
200	1.22E−01	1.37E−01	1.56E−01	2.43E−01	2.75E−01	3.68E−01	7.90E−01	1.00E+00
250	1.12E−01	1.22E−01	1.28E−01	1.73E−01	1.91E−01	2.40E−01	4.75E−01	6.02E−01
300	1.04E−01	1.11E−01	1.12E−01	1.38E−01	1.49E−01	1.80E−01	3.26E−01	4.07E−01
350	9.76E−02	1.04E−01	1.01E−01	1.18E−01	1.25E−01	1.43E−01	2.43E−01	2.97E−01
400	9.26E−02	9.75E−02	9.39E−02	1.04E−01	1.10E−01	1.22E−01	1.92E−01	2.33E−01
450	8.82E−02	9.26E−02	8.82E−02	9.52E−02	9.90E−02	1.07E−01	1.60E−01	1.90E−01
500	8.43E−02	8.83E−02	8.35E−02	8.83E−02	9.11E−02	9.67E−02	1.37E−01	1.61E−01
550	8.10E−02	8.45E−02	7.94E−02	8.27E−02	8.49E−02	8.89E−02	1.21E−01	1.40E−01
600	7.80E−02	8.13E−02	7.61E−02	7.82E−02	8.02E−02	8.31E−02	1.10E−01	1.26E−01
650	7.52E−02	7.83E−02	7.30E−02	7.45E−02	7.60E−02	7.79E−02	9.98E−02	1.13E−01
700	7.27E−02	7.56E−02	7.04E−02	7.13E−02	7.25E−02	7.37E−02	9.16E−02	1.02E−01
750	7.05E−02	7.34E−02	6.81E−02	6.86E−02	6.97E−02	7.05E−02	8.59E−02	9.53E−02
800	6.83E−02	7.11E−02	6.59E−02	6.61E−02	6.70E−02	6.73E−02	8.02E−02	8.82E−02

D.2 MASS ATTENUATION COEFFICIENTS FOR SELECTED COMPOUNDS

TABLE D-2 MASS ATTENUATION COEFFICIENTS IN cm²/g (DENSITY (ρ) IN g/cm³)

ENERGY (keV)	AIR $\rho = 0.001293$	WATER $\rho = 1.00$	PLEXIGLAS[a] $\rho = 1.19$	MUSCLE $\rho = 1.06$	BONE $\rho = 1.5$ TO 3.0	ADIPOSE[b] $\rho = 0.930$	50/50[b] $\rho = 0.982$	GLANDULAR[b] $\rho = 1.040$
2	5.20E+02	6.17E+02	4.04E+02	5.67E+02	5.24E+02	3.70E+02	4.60E+02	5.41E+02
3	1.63E+02	1.95E+02	1.26E+02	1.87E+02	2.42E+02	1.15E+02	1.44E+02	1.71E+02
4	7.43E+01	8.24E+01	5.23E+01	8.16E+01	1.06E+02	4.77E+01	6.04E+01	7.17E+01
5	3.84E+01	4.24E+01	2.66E+01	4.22E+01	1.34E+02	2.43E+01	3.09E+01	3.68E+01
6	2.24E+01	2.47E+01	1.54E+01	2.47E+01	8.26E+01	1.41E+01	1.79E+01	2.14E+01
7	1.40E+01	1.54E+01	9.66E+00	1.55E+01	5.36E+01	8.81E+00	1.12E+01	1.34E+01
8	9.42E+00	1.03E+01	6.46E+00	1.04E+01	3.71E+01	5.90E+00	7.50E+00	8.94E+00
9	6.62E+00	7.23E+00	4.54E+00	7.32E+00	2.68E+01	4.15E+00	5.28E+00	6.28E+00
10	4.84E+00	5.30E+00	3.34E+00	5.37E+00	1.99E+01	3.06E+00	3.87E+00	4.60E+00
12	2.87E+00	3.16E+00	2.01E+00	3.21E+00	1.19E+01	1.85E+00	2.33E+00	2.75E+00
14	1.85E+00	2.02E+00	1.31E+00	2.05E+00	7.67E+00	1.22E+00	1.51E+00	1.77E+00
16	1.29E+00	1.40E+00	9.36E-01	1.43E+00	5.26E+00	8.74E-01	1.07E+00	1.24E+00
18	9.55E-01	1.04E+00	7.12E-01	1.06E+00	3.78E+00	6.71E-01	8.03E-01	9.22E-01
20	7.43E-01	8.08E-01	5.70E-01	8.23E-01	2.82E+00	5.42E-01	6.37E-01	7.23E-01
25	4.66E-01	5.09E-01	3.86E-01	5.16E-01	1.56E+00	3.74E-01	4.22E-01	4.64E-01
30	3.46E-01	3.75E-01	3.04E-01	3.79E-01	9.80E-01	3.00E-01	3.26E-01	3.49E-01
35	2.80E-01	3.07E-01	2.60E-01	3.09E-01	6.86E-01	2.59E-01	2.75E-01	2.90E-01
40	2.44E-01	2.68E-01	2.34E-01	2.69E-01	5.20E-01	2.35E-01	2.46E-01	2.55E-01
45	2.21E-01	2.44E-01	2.19E-01	2.44E-01	4.18E-01	2.21E-01	2.28E-01	2.34E-01

(Continued)

Appendix D: Mass Attenuation Coefficients

TABLE D-2 MASS ATTENUATION COEFFICIENTS IN cm²/g (DENSITY (ρ) IN g/cm³) (Continued)

ENERGY (keV)	AIR ρ = 0.001293	WATER ρ = 1.00	PLEXIGLAS[a] ρ = 1.19	MUSCLE ρ = 1.06	BONE ρ = 1.5 TO 3.0	ADIPOSE[b] ρ = 0.930	50/50[b] ρ = 0.982	GLANDULAR[b] ρ = 1.040
50	2.05E−01	2.27E−01	2.07E−01	2.26E−01	3.53E−01	2.10E−01	2.15E−01	2.19E−01
55	1.94E−01	2.14E−01	1.98E−01	2.14E−01	3.07E−01	2.02E−01	2.05E−01	2.08E−01
60	1.86E−01	2.06E−01	1.92E−01	2.05E−01	2.75E−01	1.96E−01	1.98E−01	2.00E−01
65	1.80E−01	1.99E−01	1.87E−01	1.98E−01	2.52E−01	1.91E−01	1.92E−01	1.94E−01
70	1.74E−01	1.93E−01	1.82E−01	1.92E−01	2.34E−01	1.86E−01	1.87E−01	1.88E−01
75	1.69E−01	1.88E−01	1.78E−01	1.86E−01	2.20E−01	1.82E−01	1.83E−01	1.84E−01
80	1.65E−01	1.83E−01	1.75E−01	1.82E−01	2.08E−01	1.79E−01	1.79E−01	1.80E−01
85	1.62E−01	1.79E−01	1.72E−01	1.78E−01	2.00E−01	1.76E−01	1.76E−01	1.76E−01
90	1.59E−01	1.76E−01	1.69E−01	1.75E−01	1.92E−01	1.73E−01	1.73E−01	1.73E−01
95	1.56E−01	1.73E−01	1.66E−01	1.72E−01	1.86E−01	1.70E−01	1.70E−01	1.70E−01
100	1.54E−01	1.71E−01	1.64E−01	1.69E−01	1.80E−01	1.68E−01	1.68E−01	1.68E−01
110	1.49E−01	1.65E−01	1.59E−01	1.64E−01	1.71E−01	1.63E−01	1.63E−01	1.63E−01
120	1.45E−01	1.61E−01	1.55E−01	1.60E−01	1.64E−01	1.60E−01	1.59E−01	1.59E−01
130	1.42E−01	1.57E−01	1.52E−01	1.56E−01	1.58E−01	1.56E−01	1.55E−01	1.55E−01
140	1.38E−01	1.54E−01	1.49E−01	1.52E−01	1.53E−01	1.52E−01	1.52E−01	1.51E−01
150	1.35E−01	1.50E−01	1.46E−01	1.49E−01	1.49E−01	1.49E−01	1.49E−01	1.48E−01
160	1.33E−01	1.47E−01	1.43E−01	1.46E−01	1.45E−01	1.46E−01	1.46E−01	1.45E−01
170	1.30E−01	1.44E−01	1.40E−01	1.43E−01	1.42E−01	1.44E−01	1.43E−01	1.42E−01
180	1.27E−01	1.42E−01	1.37E−01	1.40E−01	1.38E−01	1.41E−01	1.40E−01	1.40E−01
190	1.25E−01	1.39E−01	1.35E−01	1.38E−01	1.36E−01	1.39E−01	1.38E−01	1.37E−01
200	1.23E−01	1.37E−01	1.32E−01	1.35E−01	1.33E−01	1.36E−01	1.35E−01	1.35E−01

250	1.14E-01	1.27E-01	1.23E-01	1.25E-01	1.22E-01	1.26E-01	1.25E-01	1.25E-01
300	1.07E-01	1.18E-01	1.15E-01	1.17E-01	1.14E-01	1.18E-01	1.17E-01	1.17E-01
350	1.00E-01	1.11E-01	1.08E-01	1.10E-01	1.07E-01	1.11E-01	1.11E-01	1.10E-01
400	9.53E-02	1.06E-01	1.03E-01	1.05E-01	1.02E-01	1.06E-01	1.05E-01	1.04E-01
450	9.09E-02	1.01E-01	9.82E-02	1.00E-01	9.68E-02	1.01E-01	1.00E-01	9.97E-02
500	8.70E-02	9.67E-02	9.39E-02	9.58E-02	9.26E-02	9.65E-02	9.60E-02	9.54E-02
550	8.36E-02	9.29E-02	9.03E-02	9.21E-02	8.89E-02	9.27E-02	9.22E-02	9.17E-02
600	8.05E-02	8.96E-02	8.70E-02	8.87E-02	8.56E-02	8.94E-02	8.89E-02	8.83E-02
650	7.77E-02	8.64E-02	8.39E-02	8.56E-02	8.26E-02	8.62E-02	8.57E-02	8.52E-02
700	7.51E-02	8.35E-02	8.11E-02	8.27E-02	7.98E-02	8.34E-02	8.29E-02	8.24E-02
750	7.29E-02	8.10E-02	7.87E-02	8.03E-02	7.75E-02	8.09E-02	8.04E-02	7.99E-02
800	7.06E-02	7.85E-02	7.63E-02	7.78E-02	7.51E-02	7.84E-02	7.79E-02	7.75E-02

[a] Polymethyl methacrylate, $C_5H_8O_2$.

[b] Composition data from Hammerstein GR, Miller DW, White DR, et al. Absorbed radiation dose in mammography. *Radiology* 1979;130:485–491. The 50% adipose data is presented here for reference. More recent information suggests that the typical breast is not 50%–50%, but much lower in terms of volume glandular fraction. See: Yaffe MJ, Boone JM, Packard N, Alonzo-Proulx O, Peressoti K, Al-Mayah A, Brock K. The Myth of the 50%–50% breast. *Med Phys* 2009;36:5437–5443.

Appendix D: Mass Attenuation Coefficients

D.3 MASS ENERGY ATTENUATION COEFFICIENTS FOR SELECTED DETECTOR COMPOUNDS

TABLE D-3   MASS ENERGY ATTENUATION COEFFICIENTS IN cm²/g (DENSITY (ρ) IN g/cm³)

ENERGY (keV)	Si (ELEMENTAL) $\rho = 2.33$	Se (ELEMENTAL) $\rho = 4.79$	BaFBr $\rho = 4.56$	CsI $\rho = 4.51$	Gd$_2$O$_2$S $\rho = 7.34$	YTaO$_4$ $\rho = 7.57$	CaWO$_4$ $\rho = 6.12$	AgBr $\rho = 6.47$
2	2.75E+03	3.09E+03	2.48E+03	2.11E+03	2.88E+03	2.37E+03	2.76E+03	2.24E+03
3	9.81E+02	1.11E+03	9.20E+02	7.96E+02	1.22E+03	1.49E+03	1.31E+03	8.14E+02
4	4.51E+02	5.22E+02	4.37E+02	3.80E+02	5.90E+02	7.28E+02	6.47E+02	9.89E+02
5	2.44E+02	2.88E+02	2.93E+02	5.20E+02	3.35E+02	4.14E+02	4.46E+02	5.62E+02
6	1.47E+02	1.78E+02	4.96E+02	6.44E+02	2.12E+02	2.64E+02	2.85E+02	3.52E+02
7	9.49E+01	1.16E+02	3.39E+02	4.33E+02	1.39E+02	1.74E+02	1.88E+02	2.33E+02
8	6.44E+01	8.08E+01	2.37E+02	3.04E+02	3.44E+02	1.23E+02	1.34E+02	1.63E+02
9	4.57E+01	5.81E+01	1.73E+02	2.25E+02	2.96E+02	9.01E+01	9.81E+01	1.19E+02
10	3.37E+01	4.34E+01	1.32E+02	1.71E+02	2.27E+02	1.46E+02	7.39E+01	8.99E+01
12	2.02E+01	2.64E+01	8.16E+01	1.06E+02	1.43E+02	1.38E+02	1.43E+02	5.51E+01
14	1.26E+01	1.22E+02	8.54E+01	6.97E+01	9.47E+01	9.29E+01	1.11E+02	8.36E+01
16	8.49E+00	8.66E+01	6.01E+01	4.87E+01	6.64E+01	6.70E+01	7.87E+01	5.88E+01
18	6.02E+00	6.39E+01	4.39E+01	3.54E+01	4.86E+01	6.93E+01	5.78E+01	4.31E+01
20	4.44E+00	4.80E+01	3.32E+01	2.66E+01	3.68E+01	5.26E+01	4.39E+01	3.27E+01
25	2.37E+00	2.62E+01	1.82E+01	1.45E+01	2.02E+01	2.93E+01	2.44E+01	1.77E+01
30	1.43E+00	1.60E+01	1.11E+01	8.87E+00	1.25E+01	1.82E+01	1.52E+01	2.83E+01
35	9.63E-01	1.04E+01	9.20E+00	1.82E+01	8.22E+00	1.20E+01	1.01E+01	1.91E+01
40	7.00E-01	7.17E+00	1.77E+01	2.29E+01	5.72E+00	8.40E+00	7.06E+00	1.33E+01

45	5.41E-01	5.18E+00	1.30E+01	1.69E+01	4.15E+00	6.11E+00	5.17E+00	9.68E+00
50	4.39E-01	3.88E+00	9.91E+00	1.29E+01	3.07E+00	4.61E+00	3.92E+00	7.29E+00
55	3.70E-01	2.98E+00	7.72E+00	1.00E+01	1.23E+01	3.57E+00	3.05E+00	5.64E+00
60	3.22E-01	2.35E+00	6.17E+00	7.96E+00	9.83E+00	2.84E+00	2.44E+00	4.50E+00
65	2.87E-01	1.90E+00	5.01E+00	6.46E+00	8.05E+00	2.30E+00	1.98E+00	3.62E+00
70	2.59E-01	1.54E+00	4.07E+00	5.25E+00	6.59E+00	6.42E+00	7.06E+00	2.93E+00
75	2.40E-01	1.29E+00	3.39E+00	4.37E+00	5.55E+00	5.40E+00	5.98E+00	2.44E+00
80	2.23E-01	1.09E+00	2.86E+00	3.68E+00	4.69E+00	4.57E+00	5.07E+00	2.05E+00
85	2.11E-01	9.37E-01	2.47E+00	3.18E+00	4.06E+00	3.97E+00	4.41E+00	1.77E+00
90	2.00E-01	8.12E-01	2.10E+00	2.69E+00	3.44E+00	3.40E+00	3.77E+00	1.51E+00
95	1.92E-01	7.22E-01	1.85E+00	2.37E+00	3.02E+00	3.00E+00	3.33E+00	1.33E+00
100	1.84E-01	6.31E-01	1.60E+00	2.04E+00	2.61E+00	2.61E+00	2.90E+00	1.15E+00
110	1.72E-01	5.07E-01	1.25E+00	1.59E+00	2.04E+00	2.06E+00	2.28E+00	9.05E-01
120	1.63E-01	4.23E-01	1.01E+00	1.28E+00	1.65E+00	1.68E+00	1.87E+00	7.36E-01
130	1.56E-01	3.59E-01	8.38E-01	1.05E+00	1.36E+00	1.37E+00	1.52E+00	6.13E-01
140	1.50E-01	3.08E-01	6.93E-01	8.65E-01	1.12E+00	1.13E+00	1.26E+00	5.12E-01
150	1.45E-01	2.72E-01	5.91E-01	7.33E-01	9.44E-01	9.57E-01	1.07E+00	4.40E-01
160	1.40E-01	2.43E-01	5.10E-01	6.28E-01	8.09E-01	8.21E-01	9.18E-01	3.84E-01
170	1.37E-01	2.21E-01	4.51E-01	5.54E-01	7.11E-01	7.22E-01	8.07E-01	3.43E-01
180	1.33E-01	2.02E-01	3.95E-01	4.80E-01	6.15E-01	6.26E-01	6.98E-01	3.04E-01

(Continued)

Appendix D: Mass Attenuation Coefficients

TABLE D-3 **MASS ENERGY ATTENUATION COEFFICIENTS IN cm²/g (DENSITY (ρ) IN g/cm³) (Continued)**

ENERGY (keV)	Si (ELEMENTAL) ρ = 2.33	Se (ELEMENTAL) ρ = 4.79	BaFBr ρ = 4.56	CsI ρ = 4.51	Gd₂O₂S ρ = 7.34	YTaO₄ ρ = 7.57	CaWO₄ ρ = 6.12	AgBr ρ = 6.47
250	1.16E−01	1.35E−01	2.14E−01	2.48E−01	3.06E−01	3.14E−01	3.46E−01	1.77E−01
300	1.08E−01	1.14E−01	1.63E−01	1.84E−01	2.21E−01	2.27E−01	2.48E−01	1.41E−01
350	1.01E−01	1.02E−01	1.33E−01	1.46E−01	1.72E−01	1.78E−01	1.92E−01	1.19E−01
400	9.59E−02	9.27E−02	1.15E−01	1.24E−01	1.42E−01	1.47E−01	1.58E−01	1.06E−01
450	9.14E−02	8.63E−02	1.02E−01	1.09E−01	1.23E−01	1.27E−01	1.35E−01	9.61E−02
500	8.73E−02	8.11E−02	9.30E−02	9.78E−02	1.09E−01	1.13E−01	1.19E−01	8.88E−02
550	8.38E−02	7.68E−02	8.61E−02	8.97E−02	9.91E−02	1.02E−01	1.08E−01	8.31E−02
600	8.07E−02	7.33E−02	8.09E−02	8.37E−02	9.16E−02	9.45E−02	9.93E−02	7.87E−02
650	7.78E−02	7.02E−02	7.62E−02	7.84E−02	8.51E−02	8.78E−02	9.19E−02	7.48E−02
700	7.52E−02	6.75E−02	7.23E−02	7.40E−02	7.99E−02	8.22E−02	8.58E−02	7.14E−02
750	7.29E−02	6.52E−02	6.94E−02	7.08E−02	7.60E−02	7.81E−02	8.13E−02	6.88E−02
800	7.07E−02	6.30E−02	6.64E−02	6.75E−02	7.21E−02	7.40E−02	7.69E−02	6.62E−02

ᵃSource of these coefficients is described in: Boone JM, Chavez AE. Comparison of x-ray cross sections for diagnostic and therapeutic medical physics. *Med Phys* 1996;23:1997–2005.

Effective Doses, Organ Doses, and Fetal Doses from Medical Imaging Procedures

Estimates of effective dose and organ doses for a specific diagnostic procedure extend over a range of values and are dependent on many parameters such as image quality (signal-to-noise and contrast-to-noise ratios), patient size, x-ray acquisition techniques, and the application of dose reduction technologies. Methods to reduce radiation dose include the utilization of higher quantum detection efficiency digital radiographic detectors and application of image processing algorithms to reduce noise. In CT, they include the implementation of automatic tube current modulation as a function of tube angle and patient attenuation and deployment of statistical iterative reconstruction techniques. As technology advances and improves, a trend towards lower radiation dose should occur, which for many procedures will result in lower effective doses than the values listed in these tables. The numbers of days of typical background radiation equal to the average effective dose of the examination are provided to help to place the magnitude of the exposure into perspective.

Tables E-1 and E-2 list typical adult and pediatric effective doses for various diagnostic radiology procedures. Table E-3 provides specific information for adult interventional examinations. Table E-4 provides values of effective dose for adult CT imaging, along with the numbers of annual CT procedures and CT scans as of the year 2016 (NCRP Report No. 184). Information on pediatric CT exposures is given in Tables E-5 and E-6. The values of effective dose in adult dental radiographic procedures are given in Table E-7.

Table E-8 provides information on *organ doses* based on typical techniques for adult radiography and CT procedures. Table E-9 lists *organ doses* determined from direct measurements of a 6-year-old pediatric anthropomorphic phantom for "routine" abdominal and chest CT examination techniques at seven different sites in Japan, along with the effective dose. Table E-10 lists *effective dose* estimates of various pediatric examinations including the common chest radiograph as well as CT of the head and abdomen as a function of age, from neonate to 15 years old. Table E-11 lists the conceptus dose for various CT, radiography, and fluoroscopy imaging procedures.

Appendix E: Effective Doses, Organ Doses, and Fetal Doses

TABLE E-1 ADULT EFFECTIVE DOSES FOR VARIOUS DIAGNOSTIC RADIOLOGY PROCEDURES (2016)

EXAMINATION	AVERAGE EFFECTIVE DOSE (mSv)[a]	DAYS OF EQUIVALENT BACKGROUND RADIATION[b]	NO. OF PROCEDURES
Radiography			
Urography	3.0	352	647,000
Lumbar spine	1.4	164	11,255,000
Thoracic spine	1.0	117	2,509,000
Esophagus	0.7	82	2,105,000
Abdomen	0.6	70	12,228,000
Pelvis	0.4	47	5,411,000
Hip	0.4	47	14,995,000
Cervical spine	0.36	42	4,884,000
Other head and neck	0.22	26	1,121,000
Skull	0.14	16	229,000
Chest	0.10	12	110,388,000
Shoulder	0.006	0.7	11,951,000
Knees	0.003	0.35	25,757,000
Hands and feet	<0.001	<0.12	31,194,000
Diagnostic Fluoroscopy			
Upper gastrointestinal	6.0	704	938,000
Barium enema	6.0	704	192,000
Mammography			
Mammography	0.36	42	39,252,000

[a]Based on ICRP Publication 103 radiation and tissue weighting factors.
[b]Based upon a background effective dose rate of 3.1 mSv/y.
Source: Adapted with permission from National Council on Radiation Protection and Measurements (NCRP). *Report No. 184 Medical Radiation Exposure of Patients in the United States (2019),* http://NCRPonline.org.

TABLE E-2 PEDIATRIC EFFECTIVE DOSES FOR VARIOUS DIAGNOSTIC RADIOLOGY PROCEDURES (2016)

EXAMINATION	AVERAGE EFFECTIVE DOSE (mSv)[a]	DAYS OF EQUIVALENT BACKGROUND RADIATION[b]	NO. OF PROCEDURES
Radiography			
Spine	0.60	70	1,250,000
Abdomen	0.10	12	1,250,000
Chest	0.05	6	5,000,000
Pelvis	0.05	6	1,250,000
Extremity	0.005	1	15,000,000
Diagnostic Fluoroscopy			
Contrast enema	2.0	235	156,000
Other	2.0	235	31,000
Upper gastrointestinal	1.5	176	156,000
Cystogram	0.2	23	281,000

[a]Based on ICRP Publication 103 radiation and tissue weighting factors.
[b]Based upon a background effective dose rate of 3.1 mSv/y.
Source: Adapted with permission from National Council on Radiation Protection and Measurements (NCRP). *Report No. 184 Medical Radiation Exposure of Patients in the United States (2019),* http://NCRPonline.org.

TABLE E-3 ADULT EFFECTIVE DOSES FOR VARIOUS FLUOROSCOPICALLY GUIDED INTERVENTIONAL CARDIAC PROCEDURES (2016)

EXAMINATION	AVERAGE EFFECTIVE DOSE (mSv)[a]	DAYS OF EQUIVALENT BACKGROUND RADIATION[b]	NO. OF PROCEDURES
Percutaneous intervention	23	2,699	850,000
Diagnostic arteriography	7	822	2,500,000
Electrophysiology nonpacemaker	3.2	376	350,000
Pacemaker	1	117	360,000

[a]Based on ICRP Publication 103 radiation and tissue weighting factors.
[b]Based upon a background effective dose rate of 3.1 mSv/y.
Source: Adapted with permission from National Council on Radiation Protection and Measurements (NCRP). *Report No. 184 Medical Radiation Exposure of Patients in the United States (2019),* http://NCRPonline.org.

TABLE E-4 ADULT EFFECTIVE DOSES FOR VARIOUS COMPUTED TOMOGRAPHY PROCEDURES (2016)

EXAMINATION	AVERAGE EFFECTIVE DOSE (mSv)[a]	DAYS OF EQUIVALENT BACKGROUND RADIATION[b]	NO. OF CT PROCEDURES	NO. OF CT SCANS
PET/CT	10.0	1,174	1,821,610	1,821,610
Spine	8.8	1,033	6,400,000	6,457,522
Cardiac	8.7	1,021	281,920	281,920
Abdomen and pelvis	7.7	904	20,100,000	22,137,153
CT colonography	6.6	775	200,000	200,000
Chest	6.2	728	12,700,000	13,250,657
CT angiography (non-cardiac)	5.1	599	6,600,000	13,027,708
Interventional	5.0	587	863,280	863,280
Miscellaneous	5.0	587	300,000	300,000
Lower extremity	3.2	376	1,203,716	1,223,064
SPECT/CT	3.0	352	314,206	314,206
Calcium scoring	1.7	200	57,492	57,492
Upper extremity	1.7	200	471,100	479,288
Brain	1.6	188	15,300,000	15,891,371
Head and neck	1.2	141	7,200,000	7,700,481

[a]Based on ICRP Publication 103 radiation and tissue weighting factors.
[b]Based upon a background effective dose rate of 3.1 mSv/y.
Source: Adapted with permission from National Council on Radiation Protection and Measurements (NCRP). *Report No. 184 Medical Radiation Exposure of Patients in the United States (2019),* http://NCRPonline.org.

TABLE E-5 DISTRIBUTION OF EFFECTIVE DOSE (mSv) AND PERCENTILE FROM CT BY ANATOMIC REGION AND PEDIATRIC PATIENT AGE

	HEAD			ABDOMEN/PELVIS			CHEST		
	<5 y	5–9 y	10–14 y	<5 y	5–9 y	10–14 y	<5 y	5–9 y	10–14 y
Mean	3.5	1.5	1.1	10.6	11.1	14.8	5.3	7.5	6.4
25th	1.4	0.5	0.6	3.2	3.5	6.4	2.5	2.6	3.1
50th	2.6	1.2	1.0	4.7	8.0	11.1	3.1	3.9	5.3
75th	4.8	2.0	1.6	14.4	14.8	20.0	4.8	10.5	8.6
95th	11.2	3.2	2.6	30.2	32.9	35.0	20.5	26.1	18.4
≥20 mSv (% patients)	0	0	0	13.9	15.7	25.2	5.8	8.1	3.4

Source: Adapted with permission from National Council on Radiation Protection and Measurements (NCRP). *Report No. 184 Medical Radiation Exposure of Patients in the United States (2019)*, http://NCRPonline.org.

TABLE E-6 PEDIATRIC EFFECTIVE DOSES FOR VARIOUS COMPUTED TOMOGRAPHY PROCEDURES (2016)

EXAMINATION	AVERAGE EFFECTIVE DOSE (mSv)[a]	DAYS OF EQUIVALENT BACKGROUND RADIATION[b]	EFFECTIVE DOSE RANGE (mSv)	NO. OF CT PROCEDURES
Abdominopelvis	7.0	822	2.9–10.0	1,300,000
Spine	3.5	411	2.5–5.0	520,000
Chest	3.0	352	1.3–6.0	260,000
Head	2.0	235	0.8–3.0	2,860,000
Other	2.0	235	NA	260,000

[a]Based on ICRP Publication 103 radiation and tissue weighting factors.
[b]Based upon a background effective dose rate of 3.1 mSv/y.
Source: Adapted with permission from National Council on Radiation Protection and Measurements (NCRP). *Report No. 184 Medical Radiation Exposure of Patients in the United States (2019)*, http://NCRPonline.org.

TABLE E-7 ADULT EFFECTIVE DOSES FOR VARIOUS DENTAL RADIOLOGY PROCEDURES (2016)

EXAMINATION	AVERAGE EFFECTIVE DOSE (μSv)[a]	DAYS OF EQUIVALENT BACKGROUND RADIATION[b]	NO. OF PROCEDURES
Intraoral	43	5	296,000,000
Panoramic	26	3	21,000,000
Cone beam CT	176.0	21	5,200,000
Cephalometric	5–10	0.6-1.2	<1%

[a]Based on ICRP Publication 103 radiation and tissue weighting factors.
[b]Based upon a background effective dose rate of 3.1 mSv/y.
Source: Adapted with permission from National Council on Radiation Protection and Measurements (NCRP). *Report No. 184 Medical Radiation Exposure of Patients in the United States (2019)*, http://NCRPonline.org.

TABLE E-8 TYPICAL ORGAN-SPECIFIC RADIATION DOSES RESULTING FROM VARIOUS RADIOLOGY PROCEDURES

EXAMINATION	ORGAN	ORGAN-SPECIFIC RADIATION DOSE (mGy)
PA chest radiography	Lung	0.01
Mammography	Breast	3.5
CT chest	Breast	21.4
CT coronary angiography	Breast	51.0
Abdominal radiography	Stomach	0.25
CT abdomen	Stomach	10.0
	Colon	4.0
Barium enema	Colon	15.0

Source: Reproduced from *BMJ*. Davies HE, Wathen CG, Gleeson FV. The risks of radiation exposure related to diagnostic imaging and how to minimise them. 342:d947. Copyright © 2011, with permissions from British Medical Journal Publishing Group. doi: 10.1136/bmj.d947

TABLE E-9 ORGAN DOSE AVERAGES FOR A 6-YEAR PEDIATRIC ANTHROPOMORPHIC PHANTOM USING ROUTINE TECHNIQUES AT SEVEN CT SCANNER SITES

TISSUE OR ORGAN	ORGAN DOSE (mGy) ± σ	
	Pediatric Abdomen	*Pediatric Chest*
Thyroid gland	0.3 ± 0.2	10.5 ± 6.6
Lung	4.2 ± 2.1	9.1 ± 4.2
Breast	2.3 ± 1.8	8.4 ± 4.7
Esophagus	4.2 ± 2.0	9.0 ± 4.4
Liver	8.8 ± 3.5	8.0 ± 3.7
Stomach	9.5 ± 3.9	4.7 ± 2.8
Kidneys	9.0 ± 3.5	4.3 ± 2.2
Colon	9.4 ± 3.5	0.6 ± 0.3
Ovary	9.0 ± 3.1	0.1 ± 0.1
Bladder	9.1 ± 3.3	0.1 ± 0.0
Testis	7.8 ± 3.7	0.1 ± 0.0
Bone surface	8.1 ± 2.8	8.5 ± 3.8

σ, standard deviation.
Source: Republished with permission of British Institute of Radiology from Fujii K, Aoyama T. Koyama S, et al. Comparative evaluation of organ and effective doses for paediatric patients with those for adults in chest and abdominal CT examinations. *Br J Radiol* 2007; 80[956]: 657-667.

Appendix E: Effective Doses, Organ Doses, and Fetal Doses

TABLE E-10 CTDI$_{vol}$, DLP, AND EFFECTIVE DOSE FROM PEDIATRIC CT IMAGING AS A FUNCTION OF PATIENT AGE

CT PROTOCOL	CTDI$_{vol16}$ (mGy)		DLP$_{16}$ (mGy-cm)		AVERAGE EFFECTIVE DOSE (mSv)[a]	DAYS OF EQUIVALENT BACKGROUND RADIATION[b]
	Mean	Range	Mean	Range		
Head/Brain CT						
Newborn	18.8 ± 18.2	4.2–67.2	225.0 ± 177.9	39–665	2.1	246
≤1 year	29.3 ± 17.9	8.6–71.6	439.0 ± 313.6	103–1,163	3.3	387
2–5 year	29.6 ± 15.3	13.1–56.0	401.0 ± 164.7	231–735	1.8	211
6–10 year	38.1 ± 18.0	7.01–80.6	645.0 ± 318.0	190–1,617	2.1	246
≤15 year	44.0 ± 15.0	14.9–77.3	728.0 ± 270.4	209–1,477	1.8	211
Chest CT						
Newborn	3.2 ± 2.2	1.85–5.84	37.0 ± 20.8	20–60	Not Reported	—
≤1 year	3.6 ± 2.3	0.8–7.2	720.0 ± 5.7	12–166	2.8	329
2–5 year	5.3 ± 2.2	1.8–9.4	128.0 ± 6.8	41–288	2.6	305
6–10 year	7.2 ± 3.9	3.1–15.6	205.0 ± 9.3	26–458	2.6	305
≤15 year	11.4 ± 5.9	4.0–21.8	375.0 ± 199.5	148–800	3.1	364
Abdominopelvic CT						
Newborn	5.1 ± 4.5	2.9–10.2	93.0 ± 74.8	46–205	Not Reported	—
≤1 year	5.6 ± 2.4	4.5–10.4	162.0 ± 7.5	72–324	5.0	587
2–5 year	6.7 ± 2.9	3.3–12.8	249.0 ± 137.8	88–508	5.9	692
6–10 year	10.1 ± 5.5	3.5–28.1	412.0 ± 246.5	88–972	6.3	739
≤15 year	13.1 ± 7.1	4.1–33.9	607.0 ± 371.5	172–1,714	6.0	704

[a]Values of effective dose are derived from the product of the third quartile values of DLP and the effective dose coefficients from Deak PD, Smal Y, Kalender WA. Multisection CT protocols: sex and age-specific conversion factors used to determine effective dose from dose-length product. Radiology. 2010;257:158–166.
[b]Based upon a background effective dose rate of 3.1 mSv/y.
Adapted with permission from Hwang J-Y, Do K-H, Yang D, et al. A survey of pediatric CT protocols and radiation doses in South Korean hospitals to optimize the radiation dose for pediatric CT scanning. Medicine. 2015;94(50):e2146.

TABLE E-11 ESTIMATED CONCEPTUS DOSES FROM COMMON RADIOGRAPHIC, FLUOROSCOPIC, AND CT EXAMINATIONS

ESTIMATED CONCEPTUS DOSES FROM SINGLE CT ACQUISITION

Examination	Dose Level	Typical Conceptus Dose (mGy)
Extra-Abdominal		
Head CT	Standard	0
Chest CT		
Routine	Standard	0.2
Pulmonary embolus	Standard	0.2
CT angiography of coronary arteries	Standard	0.1
Abdominal		
Abdomen, routine	Standard	4
Abdomen/pelvis, routine	Standard	25
CT angiography of aorta (chest through pelvis)	Standard	34
Abdomen/pelvis, stone protocol[a]	Reduced	10

ESTIMATED CONCEPTUS DOSES FROM RADIOGRAPHIC AND FLUOROSCOPIC EXAMINATIONS

Examination	Typical Conceptus Dose (mGy)
Cervical spine (AP, lat)	<0.001
Extremities	<0.001
Chest (PA, lat)	0.002
Thoracic spine (AP, lat)	0.003
Abdomen (AP)	
21-cm patient thickness	1
33-cm patient thickness	3
Lumbar spine (AP, lat)	1
Limited IVP[b]	6
Small-bowel study[c]	7
Double-contrast barium enema study[d]	7

[a]Anatomic coverage is the same as for routine abdominopelvic CT, but the tube current is decreased and the pitch is increased because standard image quality is not necessary for detection of high-contrast stones.
[b]Limited IVP is assumed to include four abdominopelvic images. A patient thickness of 21 cm is assumed.
[c]A small-bowel study is assumed to include a 6-min fluoroscopic examination with the acquisition of 20 digital spot images.
[d]A double-contrast barium enema study is assumed to include a 4-min fluoroscopic examination with the acquisition of 12 digital spot images.
AP, anteroposterior projection; lat, lateral projection; PA, posteroanterior projection.
Reprinted with permission from McCollough CH, Schueler BA, Atwell TD, et al. Radiation exposure and pregnancy: when should we be concerned? *Radiographics.* 2007;27:909-917. Copyright © Radiological Society of North America. doi: 10.1148/rg.274065149.

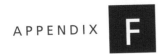

Radiopharmaceutical Characteristics and Dosimetry

TABLE F-1 METHOD OF ADMINISTRATION, LOCALIZATION, CLINICAL UTILITY, AND OTHER CHARACTERISTICS OF CURRENTLY FDA-APPROVED RADIOPHARMACEUTICALS

	RADIO-PHARMACEUTICAL	TRADE NAME (MANUFACTURER)	MEDICAL USE	METHOD OF ADMINISTRATION	DELAY BEFORE IMAGING
1	C-11 Choline	None (Various)	Diagnostic imaging	Intravenous injection	0 to 15 min
2	C-11 Urea	PYtest (Halyard Health)	Diagnostic non-imaging	Oral administration	Breath sample is taken 10 min following capsule ingestion.
3	F-18 Florbetaben	Neuraceq (Life Molecular Imaging)	Diagnostic imaging	Intravenous injection	45 to 130 min

METHOD OF LOCALIZATION/ACTION	CLINICAL INDICATIONS AND USE	PATIENT PREPARATION/ PRECAUTIONS
Radiolabeled analog of choline, a precursor molecule essential for the biosynthesis of cell membrane phospholipids. Choline is involved in synthesis of the structural components of cell membranes, as well as modulation of trans-membrane signaling.	Indicated for PET imaging of patients with suspected prostate cancer recurrence based upon elevated blood prostate-specific antigen (PSA) levels following initial therapy and non-informative bone scintigraphy, computerized tomography (CT), or magnetic resonance imaging (MRI) to help identify potential sites of prostate cancer recurrence for subsequent histologic confirmation.	Prior to administration of Choline C-11 Injection: (1) Fasting for at least 6 h is recommended to minimize the potential for dietary choline interference with radioactivity uptake in tissue. (2) Ensure that the patient is well hydrated and encourage voiding when imaging is completed.
Urea labeled with C-14 is swallowed by the patient. If gastric urease from *Helicobacter pylori* is present, urea is split to form CO_2 and NH_3 at the interface between the gastric epithelium and lumen and $^{14}CO_2$ is absorbed into the blood and exhaled in the breath.	Detection of gastric urease as an aid in the diagnosis of *H. pylori* infection in the stomach.	It is necessary for the patient to fast for 6 h before the test. The patient should also be off antibiotics and bismuth for 1 mo, and proton pump inhibitors and sucralfate for 2 wk prior to the test. Instruct the patient not to handle the capsule directly as this may interfere with the test result. The capsule should be swallowed intact. Do not chew the capsule.
Florbetaben F-18 is an F-18-labeled stilbene derivative, which binds to β-amyloid plaques in the brain. The F-18 isotope produces a positron signal that is detected by a PET scanner. 3H-florbetaben in vitro binding experiments reveal two binding sites (K_d of 16 and 135 nM) in frontal cortex homogenates from patients with AD.	Indicated for positron emission tomography (PET) imaging of the brain to estimate β amyloid neuritic plaque density in adult patients with cognitive impairment who are being evaluated for Alzheimer disease (AD) or other causes of cognitive decline.	Errors may occur in the Neuraceq estimation of brain neuritic β-amyloid plaque density during image interpretation. Image interpretation should be performed independently of the patient's clinical information. The use of clinical information in the interpretation of Neuraceq images has not been evaluated and may lead to errors. Errors may also occur in cases with severe brain atrophy that limits the ability to distinguish gray and white matter on the Neuraceq scan. Errors may also occur due to motion artifacts that result in image distortion.

(Continued)

TABLE F-1 **METHOD OF ADMINISTRATION, LOCALIZATION, CLINICAL UTILITY, AND OTHER CHARACTERISTICS OF CURRENTLY FDA-APPROVED RADIOPHARMACEUTICALS (*Continued*)**

	RADIO-PHARMACEUTICAL	TRADE NAME (MANUFACTURER)	MEDICAL USE	METHOD OF ADMINISTRATION	DELAY BEFORE IMAGING
4	F-18 Florbetapir	Amyvid (Eli Lilly)	Diagnostic imaging	Intravenous injection	30 to 50 min
5	F-18 Flortaucipir	TAUVID (Eli Lilly)	Diagnostic imaging	Intravenous injection	80 min

METHOD OF LOCALIZATION/ACTION	CLINICAL INDICATIONS AND USE	PATIENT PREPARATION/ PRECAUTIONS
Florbetapir F-18 binds to β-amyloid plaques and the F-18 isotope produces a positron signal that is detected by a PET scanner. The binding of florbetapir F-18 to β-amyloid aggregates was demonstrated in postmortem human brain sections using autoradiographic methods, thioflavin S, and traditional silver staining correlation studies as well as monoclonal antibody β-amyloid-specific correlation studies. Florbetapir binding to tau protein and a battery of neuroreceptors was not detected in in vitro studies.	Amyvid is indicated for PET imaging of the brain to estimate β-amyloid neuritic plaque density in adult patients with cognitive impairment who are being evaluated for AD and other causes of cognitive decline. A negative Amyvid scan indicates sparse to no neuritic plaques and is inconsistent with a neuropathological diagnosis of AD. A positive Amyvid scan indicates moderate to frequent amyloid neuritic plaques; neuropathological examination has shown this amount of amyloid neuritic plaque is present in patients with AD, but may also be present in patients with other types of neurologic conditions as well as older people with normal cognition.	Errors may occur in the Amyvid estimation of brain neuritic plaque density during image interpretation. Image interpretation should be performed independently of the patient's clinical information. The use of clinical information in the interpretation of Amyvid images has not been evaluated and may lead to errors. Other errors may be due to extensive brain atrophy that limits the ability to distinguish gray and white matter on the Amyvid scan as well as motion artifacts that distort the image.
Flortaucipir F-18 binds to aggregated tau protein. In the brains of patients with AD, tau aggregates combine to form NFTs, one of two components required for the neuropathological diagnosis of AD. In vivo, flortaucipir F-18 is differentially retained in neocortical areas that contain aggregated tau.	TAUVID is indicated for use with PET imaging of the brain to estimate the density and distribution of aggregated tau neurofibrillary tangles (NFTs) in adult patients with cognitive impairment who are being evaluated for AD.	TAUVID does not target β-amyloid, one of two required components of the neuropathological diagnosis of AD. TAUVID performance for detecting tau pathology was assessed in terminally ill patients, the majority of whom had AD dementia with B3 level NFT pathology. TAUVID performance for detecting tau pathology may be lower in patients in earlier stages of the pathological spectrum.

(Continued)

TABLE F-1 **METHOD OF ADMINISTRATION, LOCALIZATION, CLINICAL UTILITY, AND OTHER CHARACTERISTICS OF CURRENTLY FDA-APPROVED RADIOPHARMACEUTICALS (Continued)**

	RADIO-PHARMACEUTICAL	TRADE NAME (MANUFACTURER)	MEDICAL USE	METHOD OF ADMINISTRATION	DELAY BEFORE IMAGING
6	F-18 Fluciclovine	Axumin (Blue Earth Diagnostics)	Diagnostic imaging	Intravenous injection	3 to 5 min
7	F-18 Sodium Fluoride	None (Various)	Diagnostic imaging	Intravenous injection	1 to 2 h

METHOD OF LOCALIZATION/ACTION	CLINICAL INDICATIONS AND USE	PATIENT PREPARATION/ PRECAUTIONS
Fluciclovine F-18 is a synthetic amino acid transported across mammalian cell membranes by amino acid transporters, such as LAT-1 and ASCT2, which are up-regulated in prostate cancer cells. Fluciclovine F-18 is taken up to a greater extent in prostate cancer cells compared with surrounding normal tissues.	Axumin is a radioactive diagnostic agent indicated for PET imaging in men with suspected prostate cancer recurrence based on elevated blood PSA levels following prior treatment.	Advise the patient to avoid any significant exercise for at least 1 day prior to PET imaging. Advise patients not to eat or drink for at least 4 h (other than small amounts of water for taking medications) prior to administration of Axumin. Image interpretation errors can occur with Axumin PET imaging. A negative image does not rule out the presence of recurrent prostate cancer and a positive image does not confirm the presence of recurrent prostate cancer. The performance of Axumin seems to be affected by PSA levels. Fluciclovine F-18 uptake is not specific for prostate cancer and may occur with other types of cancer and benign prostatic hypertrophy in primary prostate cancer. Clinical correlation, which may include histopathological evaluation of the suspected recurrence site, is recommended.
Fluoride F-18 ion normally accumulates in the skeleton in an even fashion, with greater deposition in the axial skeleton (e.g., vertebrae and pelvis) than in the appendicular skeleton and greater deposition in the bones around joints than in the shafts of long bones.	Sodium Fluoride F-18 Injection is indicated for diagnostic PET imaging of bone to define areas of altered osteogenic activity.	To minimize the radiation-absorbed dose to the bladder, encourage adequate hydration. Encourage the patient to ingest at least 500 mL of fluid immediately prior and subsequent to the administration of Sodium Fluoride F-18 Injection, USP. Encourage the patient to void one half hour after administration of Sodium Fluoride F-18 Injection, USP, and as frequently thereafter as possible for the next 12 h. As with any injectable drug product, allergic reactions and anaphylaxis may occur. Emergency resuscitation equipment and personnel should be immediately available.

(Continued)

TABLE F-1 METHOD OF ADMINISTRATION, LOCALIZATION, CLINICAL UTILITY, AND OTHER CHARACTERISTICS OF CURRENTLY FDA-APPROVED RADIOPHARMACEUTICALS (Continued)

	RADIO-PHARMACEUTICAL	TRADE NAME (MANUFACTURER)	MEDICAL USE	METHOD OF ADMINISTRATION	DELAY BEFORE IMAGING
8	F-18 Fluorodeoxy-glucose (FDG)	None (various)	Diagnostic imaging	Intravenous injection	40 min
9	F-18 Fluoroestradiol	CERIANNA (Zionexa)	Diagnostic imaging	Intravenous injection	80 min

METHOD OF LOCALIZATION/ACTION	CLINICAL INDICATIONS AND USE	PATIENT PREPARATION/ PRECAUTIONS
Fluorodeoxyglucose F-18 is a glucose analog that concentrates in cells that rely upon glucose as an energy source, or in cells whose dependence on glucose increases under pathophysiological conditions. Fludeoxyglucose F-18 is transported through the cell membrane by facilitative glucose transporter proteins and is phosphorylated within the cell to [18F] FDG-6-phosphate by the enzyme hexokinase. Once phosphorylated, it cannot exit until it is dephosphorylated by glucose-6-phosphatase. Therefore, within a given tissue or pathophysiological process, the retention and clearance of Fludeoxyglucose F-18 reflect a balance involving glucose transporter, hexokinase, and glucose-6-phosphatase activities.	Fludeoxyglucose F-18 Injection is indicated for PET imaging in the following settings: (1) Oncology: For assessment of abnormal glucose metabolism to assist in the evaluation of malignancy in patients with known or suspected abnormalities found by other testing modalities, or in patients with an existing diagnosis of cancer. (2) Cardiology: For the identification of left ventricular myocardium with residual glucose metabolism and reversible loss of systolic function in patients with coronary artery disease and left ventricular dysfunction, when used together with myocardial perfusion imaging. (3) Neurology: For the identification of regions of abnormal glucose metabolism associated with foci of epileptic seizures.	To minimize the radiation absorbed dose to the bladder, encourage adequate hydration. Encourage the patient to drink water or other fluids (as tolerated) in the 4 h before their PET study. In the oncology and neurology setting, suboptimal imaging may occur in patients with inadequately regulated blood glucose levels. In these patients, consider medical therapy and laboratory testing to assure at least 2 days of normoglycemia prior to Fludeoxyglucose F-18 Injection administration.
Fluoroestradiol F-18 binds to estrogen receptors (ER).	CERIANNA is indicated for use with PET imaging for the detection of ER-positive lesions as an adjunct to biopsy in patients with recurrent or metastatic breast cancer.	Image patients with CERIANNA prior to starting systemic endocrine therapies that target ER (e.g., ER modulators and ER down-regulators). Instruct patients to drink water to ensure adequate hydration prior to administration of CERIANNA and to continue drinking and voiding frequently during the first hours following administration to reduce radiation exposure. Breast cancer may be heterogeneous within patients and across time. CERIANNA images ER and is not useful for imaging other receptors such as HER2 and PR. The uptake of fluoroestradiol F-18 is not specific for breast cancer and may occur in a variety of ER-positive tumors that arise outside of the breast, including from the uterus and ovaries. Do not use CERIANNA in lieu of biopsy when biopsy is indicated in patients with recurrent or metastatic breast cancer.

(Continued)

TABLE F-1 METHOD OF ADMINISTRATION, LOCALIZATION, CLINICAL UTILITY, AND OTHER CHARACTERISTICS OF CURRENTLY FDA-APPROVED RADIOPHARMACEUTICALS (*Continued*)

	RADIO-PHARMACEUTICAL	TRADE NAME (MANUFACTURER)	MEDICAL USE	METHOD OF ADMINISTRATION	DELAY BEFORE IMAGING
10	F-18 Flutemetamol	Vizamyl (GE Healthcare)	Diagnostic imaging	Intravenous injection	90 min
11	Ga-67 Citrate	None (Curium/Lantheus Medical Imaging)	Diagnostic imaging	Intravenous injection	Typically 24–72 h Range 6–120 h

METHOD OF LOCALIZATION/ACTION	CLINICAL INDICATIONS AND USE	PATIENT PREPARATION/ PRECAUTIONS
Flutemetamol F-18 binds to β-amyloid plaques in the brain, and the F-18 isotope produces a positron signal that is detected by a PET scanner. Selectivity of [3H]flutemetamol binding in postmortem human brain sections was demonstrated using autoradiography, silver-stained protein, and immunohistochemistry (monoclonal antibody to β-amyloid) correlation studies.	Vizamyl is indicated for PET imaging of the brain to estimate β-amyloid neuritic plaque density in adult patients with cognitive impairment who are being evaluated for AD and other causes of cognitive decline.	Hypersensitivity reactions such as flushing and dyspnea have been observed within minutes following Vizamyl administration. These reactions may occur in patients with no history of prior exposure to Vizamyl. Before administering Vizamyl, ask patients about prior reactions to drugs, especially those containing polysorbate 80. Have resuscitation equipment and trained personnel immediately available at the time of Vizamyl administration.
Gallium Citrate Ga-67, with no carrier added, has been found to concentrate in certain viable primary and metastatic tumors as well as focal sites of infection. The mechanism of concentration is unknown, but investigational studies have shown that Gallium Ga-67 accumulates in lysosomes and is bound to a soluble intracellular protein.	Gallium Citrate Ga-67 Injection may be useful to demonstrate the presence and extent of Hodgkin disease, lymphoma, and bronchogenic carcinoma. Positive Gallium Ga-67 uptake in the absence of prior symptoms warrants follow-up as an indication of a potential disease state. Gallium Citrate Ga-67 Injection may be useful as an aid in detecting some acute inflammatory lesions.	A thorough knowledge of the normal distribution of intravenously administered Gallium Citrate Ga-67 Injection is essential in order to accurately interpret pathologic states. The finding of an abnormal Gallium Ga-67 concentration usually implies the existence of underlying pathology, but further diagnostic studies should be done to distinguish benign from malignant lesions. Gallium Citrate Ga-67 Injection is intended for use as an adjunct in the diagnosis of certain neoplasms as well as focal areas of infection. Certain pathologic conditions may yield up to 40% false-negative Gallium Ga-67 studies. Therefore, a negative study cannot be definitely interpreted as ruling out the presence of disease.

(Continued)

TABLE F-1 **METHOD OF ADMINISTRATION, LOCALIZATION, CLINICAL UTILITY, AND OTHER CHARACTERISTICS OF CURRENTLY FDA-APPROVED RADIOPHARMACEUTICALS (*Continued*)**

	RADIO-PHARMACEUTICAL	TRADE NAME (MANUFACTURER)	MEDICAL USE	METHOD OF ADMINISTRATION	DELAY BEFORE IMAGING
12	Ga-68 Dotatate	NETSPOT (Advanced Accelerator Appl)	Diagnostic imaging	Intravenous injection	40 to 90 min
13	Ga-68 Dotatoc	None (University of Iowa)	Diagnostic imaging	Intravenous injection	55 to 90 min

METHOD OF LOCALIZATION/ACTION	CLINICAL INDICATIONS AND USE	PATIENT PREPARATION/ PRECAUTIONS
Ga-68 Dotatate binds to somatostatin receptors, with highest affinity for subtype 2 receptors (sstr2). It binds to cells that express somatostatin receptors including malignant cells, which overexpress sstr2 receptors.	NETSPOT, after radiolabeling with Ga-68, is a radioactive diagnostic agent indicated for use with PET for localization of somatostatin receptor–positive neuroendocrine tumors (NETs) in adult and pediatric patients.	Instruct patients to drink a sufficient amount of water to ensure adequate hydration prior to administration of Ga-68 Dotatate. Drink and void frequently during the first hours following administration to reduce radiation exposure. The uptake of Ga-68 Dotatate reflects the level of somatostatin receptor density in NETs. However, uptake can also be seen in a variety of other tumor types (*e.g.*, those derived from neural crest tissue). Increased uptake might also be seen in other pathologic conditions (*e.g.*, thyroid disease or subacute inflammation) or might occur as a normal physiologic variant (*e.g.*, uncinate process of the pancreas). The uptake may need to be confirmed by histopathology or other assessments.
Ga-68 DOTATOC binds to somatostatin receptors, with highest affinity for subtype 2 receptors (sstr2). Ga-68 DOTATOC binds to cells that express somatostatin receptors including malignant neuroendocrine cells, which overexpress sstr2 receptors.	Ga-68 DOTATOC Injection is indicated for use with PET for the localization of somatostatin receptor–positive neuroendocrine tumors (NETs) in adult and pediatric patients.	Instruct patients to drink water to ensure adequate hydration prior to administration of Ga-68 DOTATOC Injection and to continue to drink and void frequently during the first hours following administration to reduce radiation exposure. The uptake of Ga-68 DOTATOC Injection reflects the level of somatostatin receptor density in NETs; however, uptake can also be seen in a variety of other tumors that also express somatostatin receptors. Increased uptake might also be seen in other non-cancerous pathologic conditions that express somatostatin receptors including thyroid disease or in subacute inflammation, or might occur as a normal physiologic variant (*e.g.*, uncinate process of the pancreas).

(Continued)

TABLE F-1 METHOD OF ADMINISTRATION, LOCALIZATION, CLINICAL UTILITY, AND OTHER CHARACTERISTICS OF CURRENTLY FDA-APPROVED RADIOPHARMACEUTICALS (Continued)

	RADIO-PHARMACEUTICAL	TRADE NAME (MANUFACTURER)	MEDICAL USE	METHOD OF ADMINISTRATION	DELAY BEFORE IMAGING
14	In-111 Chloride	None (Curium)	Diagnostic imaging		
15	In-111 Oxyquinoline (Labeled Leukocytes)	None (BWXT/GE Healthcare)	Diagnostic imaging	Intravenous injection	24 h
16	In-111 Pentetate (DTPA)	None (GE Healthcare)	Diagnostic imaging	Intrathecal administration	1 to 3 h

METHOD OF LOCALIZATION/ACTION	CLINICAL INDICATIONS AND USE	PATIENT PREPARATION/ PRECAUTIONS
	Indium In-111 Chloride is a diagnostic radiopharmaceutical intended for radiolabeling OncoScint (satumomab pendetide) or ProstaScint (capromab pendetide) used for in vivo diagnostic imaging procedures and for radiolabeling Zevalin (ibritumomab tiuxetan) in preparations used for radioimmunotherapy procedures. It is supplied as a sterile, pyrogen-free solution of Indium (^{111}In) Chloride in 0.04 M HCl. Each milliliter is supplied at a radioactive concentration of 370 MBq, 10 mCi of Indium In-111 Chloride at time of calibration.	
Indium forms a saturated (1:3) complex with oxyquinoline. The complex is neutral and lipid-soluble, which enables it to penetrate the cell membrane. Within the cell, indium becomes firmly attached to cytoplasmic components; the liberated oxyquinoline is released by the cell. It is thought likely that the mechanism of labeling cells with indium In-111 oxyquinoline involves an exchange reaction between the oxyquinoline carrier and subcellular components, which chelate indium more strongly than oxyquinoline.	Indicated for radiolabeling autologous leukocytes that may be used as an adjunct in the detection of inflammatory processes to which leukocytes migrate, such as those associated with abscesses or other infection.	The content of the vial of indium In-111 oxyquinoline solution is intended only for use in the preparation of indium In-111 oxyquinoline labeled autologous leukocytes, and is not to be administered directly. Autologous leukocyte labeling is not recommended in leukopenic patients because of the small number of available leukocytes.
After intrathecal administration, the radiopharmaceutical is absorbed from the subarachnoid space as described below and the remainder flows superiorly to the basal cisterns within 2 to 4 h and subsequently will be apparent in the Sylvian cisterns, in the inter-hemispheric cisterns, and over the cerebral convexities. In normal individuals, the radiopharmaceutical will have ascended to the parasagittal region within 24 h with simultaneous partial or complete clearance of activity from the basal cisterns and Sylvian regions.	For use in radionuclide cisternography. This test is used to diagnose a cerebrospinal fluid (CSF) leak. It can be ordered with pledgets (for CSF leaks of the head) or without (for spinal leaks or normal-pressure hydrocephalus).	Since the drug is excreted by the kidneys, caution should be exercised in patients with severely impaired renal function. Aseptic meningitis and pyrogenic reactions have been rarely (<0.4%) observed following cisternography with Pentetate Indium Disodium In-111.

(Continued)

TABLE F-1 **METHOD OF ADMINISTRATION, LOCALIZATION, CLINICAL UTILITY, AND OTHER CHARACTERISTICS OF CURRENTLY FDA-APPROVED RADIOPHARMACEUTICALS (Continued)**

	RADIO-PHARMACEUTICAL	TRADE NAME (MANUFACTURER)	MEDICAL USE	METHOD OF ADMINISTRATION	DELAY BEFORE IMAGING
17	In-111 Pentetreotide	Octreoscan (GE Healthcare)	Diagnostic imaging	Intravenous injection	24 h
18	I-123 Iobenguane	MIBG/AdreView (GE Healthcare)	Diagnostic imaging	Intravenous injection	18 to 30 h

METHOD OF LOCALIZATION/ACTION	CLINICAL INDICATIONS AND USE	PATIENT PREPARATION/ PRECAUTIONS
Pentetreotide is a DTPA conjugate of octreotide, which is a long-acting analog of the human hormone, somatostatin. Indium In-111 pentetreotide binds to somatostatin receptors on cell surfaces throughout the body. Within an hour of injection, most of the dose of indium In-111 pentetreotide distributes from plasma to extravascular body tissues and concentrates in tumors containing a high density of somatostatin receptors. After background clearance, visualization of somatostatin receptor–rich tissue is achieved. In addition to somatostatin receptor–rich tumors, the normal pituitary gland, thyroid gland, liver, spleen, and urinary bladder also are visualized in most patients, as is the bowel, to a lesser extent. Excretion is almost exclusively via the kidneys.	An agent for the scintigraphic localization of primary and metastatic neuroendocrine tumors bearing somatostatin receptors	The sensitivity of scintigraphy with indium In-111 pentetreotide may be reduced in patients concurrently receiving therapeutic doses of octreotide acetate. Consideration should be given to temporarily suspending octreotide acetate therapy before the administration of indium In-111 pentetreotide and to monitoring the patient for any signs of withdrawal.
Iobenguane is similar in structure to the antihypertensive drug guanethidine and to the neurotransmitter norepinephrine (NE). Iobenguane is, therefore, largely subject to the same uptake and accumulation pathways as NE. Iobenguane is taken up by the NE transporter in adrenergic nerve terminals and stored in the presynaptic storage vesicles. Iobenguane accumulates in adrenergically innervated tissues such as the adrenal medulla, salivary glands, heart, liver, spleen, and lungs as well as tumors derived from the neural crest. By labeling iobenguane with the isotope iodine 123, it is possible to obtain scintigraphic images of the organs and tissues in which the radiopharmaceutical accumulates.	AdreView is a diagnostic radiopharmaceutical agent for γ-scintigraphy. It is indicated for use in the detection of primary or metastatic pheochromocytoma or neuroblastoma as an adjunct to other diagnostic tests.	Before administration of AdreView, administer Potassium Iodide Oral Solution or Lugol's Solution (equivalent to 100 mg iodide for adults, body-weight adjusted for children) or potassium perchlorate (400 mg for adults, body-weight adjusted for children) to block uptake of iodine 123 by the patient's thyroid. Administer the blocking agent at least 1 h before the dose of AdreView. To minimize radiation dose to the bladder, prior to and following AdreView administration, encourage hydration to permit frequent voiding. Encourage the patient to void frequently for the first 48 h following AdreView administration.

(Continued)

TABLE F-1 **METHOD OF ADMINISTRATION, LOCALIZATION, CLINICAL UTILITY, AND OTHER CHARACTERISTICS OF CURRENTLY FDA-APPROVED RADIOPHARMACEUTICALS (*Continued*)**

	RADIO-PHARMACEUTICAL	TRADE NAME (MANUFACTURER)	MEDICAL USE	METHOD OF ADMINISTRATION	DELAY BEFORE IMAGING
19	I-123 Ioflupane	DaTscan (GE Healthcare)	Diagnostic imaging	Intravenous injection	3 to 6 h
20	I-123 Sodium Iodine Capsules	None (Cardinal Health/Curium)	Diagnostic imaging	Oral administration	6 h

METHOD OF LOCALIZATION/ACTION	CLINICAL INDICATIONS AND USE	PATIENT PREPARATION/ PRECAUTIONS
In vitro, ioflupane binds reversibly to the human recombinant dopamine transporter (DaT). Autoradiography of postmortem human brain slices exposed to radiolabeled ioflupane shows concentration of the radiolabel in striatum (caudate nucleus and putamen). The specificity of the binding of ioflupane I-125 to dopamine transporter was demonstrated by competition studies with the DaT inhibitor GBR 12909 (a dopamine reuptake inhibitor), the serotonin reuptake inhibitor citalopram, and the norepinephrine reuptake inhibitor desipramine in postmortem human brain slices exposed to radiolabeled ioflupane. Citalopram reduced binding in the neocortex and thalamus with only minor effects in the striatum. This indicated that the binding in the cortex and thalamus is mainly to the serotonin reuptake sites.	DaTscan is a radiopharmaceutical indicated for striatal dopamine transporter visualization using single photon emission computed tomography (SPECT) brain imaging to assist in the evaluation of adult patients with suspected parkinsonian syndromes (PS). In these patients, DaTscan may be used to help differentiate essential tremor from tremor due to PS (idiopathic Parkinson disease, multiple system atrophy. and progressive supranuclear palsy). DaTscan is an adjunct to other diagnostic evaluations.	Before administration of DaTscan, administer Potassium Iodide Oral Solution or Lugol's Solution (equivalent to 100 mg iodide) or potassium perchlorate (400 mg) to block uptake of iodine 123 by the patient's thyroid. Administer the blocking agent at least 1 h before the dose of DaTscan. Hypersensitivity reactions have been reported following DaTscan administration. The reactions have generally consisted of skin erythema and pruritus and have resolved either spontaneously or following the administration of corticosteroids and anti-histamines. Prior to administration, question the patient for a history of prior reactions to DaTscan.
Sodium iodide I-123 is readily absorbed from the upper gastrointestinal tract. Following absorption, the iodide is distributed primarily within the extracellular fluid of the body. It is trapped and organically bound by the thyroid and concentrated by the stomach, choroid plexus, and salivary glands. It is excreted by the kidneys. The fraction of the administered dose that is accumulated in the thyroid gland may be a measure of thyroid function in the absence of unusually high or low iodine intake or administration of certain drugs that influence iodine accumulation by the thyroid gland.	Administration of sodium iodide I-123 is indicated as a diagnostic procedure to be used in evaluating thyroid function and/or morphology.	To date there are no known contraindications to the use of sodium iodide I-123 capsules. Females of childbearing age and pediatric patients should not be studied unless the benefits anticipated from the performance of the test outweigh the possible risk of exposure to the amount of ionizing radiation associated with the test.

(Continued)

TABLE F-1 **METHOD OF ADMINISTRATION, LOCALIZATION, CLINICAL UTILITY, AND OTHER CHARACTERISTICS OF CURRENTLY FDA-APPROVED RADIOPHARMACEUTICALS (*Continued*)**

RADIO-PHARMACEUTICAL	TRADE NAME (MANUFACTURER)	MEDICAL USE	METHOD OF ADMINISTRATION	DELAY BEFORE IMAGING
21 I-125 Human Serum Albumin (HSA)	Jeanatope (IsoTex Diagnostics)	Diagnostic non-imaging	Intravenous injection	Blood sample drawn after 5 and 15 min postinjection.
22 I-125 Iothalamate	Glofil-125 (IsoTex Diagnostics)	Diagnostic non-imaging	(1) Continuous intravenous infusion or (2) single intravenous injection (Cohen Method)	30 to 60 min are allowed for equilibration of plasma activity concentration.

METHOD OF LOCALIZATION/ACTION	CLINICAL INDICATIONS AND USE	PATIENT PREPARATION/ PRECAUTIONS
Following intravenous injection, radioiodinated serum albumin is uniformly distributed throughout the intravascular pool within 10 min; extravascular distribution takes place more slowly. Labeled albumin also can be detected in the lymph and in certain body tissues within 10 min after injection, but maximum distribution of radioactivity throughout the extravascular space does not occur until 2 to 4 days after administration.	Jeanatope I-125 is indicated for use in the determination of total blood and plasma volume.	(1) Inject the dose into a large vein in patient's arm. Measure the residual radioactivity in the syringe and needle. (2) Destroy syringe after injecting. Do not attempt to resterilize. (3) At 5 to 15 min after injecting the dose, withdraw blood samples from the patient's other arm with a sterile heparinized syringe. (4) Take a known aliquot from each blood sample and determine radioconcentration in net cpm/mL. (5) Plot the 5- and 15-min sample counts (net cpm/mL) on semilog graph paper using the average count value of each sample and determine the radioconcentration at injection time (zero time) by drawing a straight line through the 15- and 5-min points to zero time. The x ordinate of the graph is the sample withdrawal time and the logarithmic y ordinate is radioconcentration in net cpm/mL. (6) Calculate patient's blood volume (in mL) using the following formula: (Net cpm/mL reference solution/Net cpm/mL patient' s blood sample) $\times$ DF = blood volume (in mL).
The renal clearance of sodium iothalamate closely approximates that of inulin. The compound is cleared by glomerular filtration without tubular secretion or reabsorption. Following infusion administration of I-125 iothalamate, the effective half-life is about 0.07 days.	GLOFIL-125 (Sodium Iothalamate I-125 Injection) is indicated for evaluation of glomerular filtration in the diagnosis or monitoring of patients with renal disease.	There are no reported adverse reactions. (1) Adequate diuresis (a urine flow exceeding 3 mL/min) is established, preferably by an oral water load of 1,500 mL 2 h prior to the beginning of the clearance study. (2) It is not necessary to withhold breakfast or admit the patient the night before.

(Continued)

TABLE F-1 METHOD OF ADMINISTRATION, LOCALIZATION, CLINICAL UTILITY, AND OTHER CHARACTERISTICS OF CURRENTLY FDA-APPROVED RADIOPHARMACEUTICALS (*Continued*)

	RADIO-PHARMACEUTICAL	TRADE NAME (MANUFACTURER)	MEDICAL USE	METHOD OF ADMINISTRATION	DELAY BEFORE IMAGING
23	I-131 Human Serum Albumin	Megatope (IsoTex Diagnostics)	Diagnostic non-imaging	Intravenous injection	Blood sample drawn after 5 and 15 min postinjection.
24	I-131 Iobenguane	AZEDRA (Progenics Pharmaceuticals)	Therapy	Intravenous injection	NA
25	I-131 Sodium Iodide	HICON (DRAXIMAGE) None (International Isotopes)	Therapy	Oral administration	NA

METHOD OF LOCALIZATION/ACTION	CLINICAL INDICATIONS AND USE	PATIENT PREPARATION/ PRECAUTIONS
Following intravenous injection, radioiodinated albumin human is uniformly distributed throughout the intravascular pool within 10 min; extravascular distribution takes place more slowly. Iodinated I-131 albumin can also be detected in the lymph and in certain body tissues within 10 min after injection but maximum distribution of radioactivity throughout the extravascular space does not occur until 2 to 4 days after administration.	Megatope (Iodinated I-131 Albumin Injection) is indicated for use in determinations of total blood and plasma volumes, cardiac output, and cardiac and pulmonary blood volumes and circulation times, and in protein turnover studies, heart and great vessel delineation, localization of the placenta, and localization of cerebral neospasms.	A few instances of hyperpyrexia and aseptic (chemical) meningeal irritation have been reported with the use of iodinated I-131 in cisternography. Iodinated I-131 Albumin injection is not approved for use in cisternography.
AZEDRA is an I-131 labeled iobenguane. Iobenguane is similar in structure to the neurotransmitter norepinephrine (NE) and is subject to the same uptake and accumulation pathways as NE. Iobenguane is taken up by the NE transporter in adrenergic nerve terminals and accumulates in adrenergically innervated tissues, such as the heart, lungs, adrenal medulla, salivary glands, liver, and spleen as well as tumors of neural crest origin. Pheochromocytoma and paraganglioma (PPGL) are tumors of neural crest origin that express high levels of the NE transporter on their cell surfaces. Following intravenous administration, AZEDRA is taken up and accumulates within pheochromocytoma and paraganglioma cells, and radiation resulting from radioactive decay of I-131 causes cell death and tumor necrosis.	AZEDRA is indicated for the treatment of adult and pediatric patients 12 y and older with iobenguane scan positive, unresectable, locally advanced or metastatic pheochromocytoma or paraganglioma who require systemic anticancer therapy.	Administer inorganic iodine starting at least 24 h before and continuing for 10 days after each AZEDRA dose. Instruct patients to increase fluid intake to at least 2 L a day starting at least 1 day before and continuing for 1 wk after each AZEDRA dose to minimize irradiation to the bladder. Adverse reactions can include myelosuppression, secondary myelodysplastic syndrome, leukemia, other malignancies, hypothyroidism, elevations in blood pressure, renal toxicity, and pneumonitis.
Sodium iodide is readily absorbed from the gastrointestinal tract. Following absorption, the iodide is distributed primarily within the extracellular fluid of the body. It is concentrated and organified by the thyroid, and trapped but not organified by the stomach and salivary glands. It is also promptly excreted by the kidneys.	Sodium iodide I-131 Therapeutic may be indicated in the treatment of hyperthyroidism and selected cases of carcinoma of the thyroid. Palliative effects may be seen in patients with papillary and/or follicular carcinoma of the thyroid. Stimulation of radioiodide uptake may be achieved by the administration of thyrotropin.	Vomiting and diarrhea represent contraindications to the use of radioiodide.

(Continued)

TABLE F-1 METHOD OF ADMINISTRATION, LOCALIZATION, CLINICAL UTILITY, AND OTHER CHARACTERISTICS OF CURRENTLY FDA-APPROVED RADIOPHARMACEUTICALS (Continued)

	RADIO-PHARMACEUTICAL	TRADE NAME (MANUFACTURER)	MEDICAL USE	METHOD OF ADMINISTRATION	DELAY BEFORE IMAGING
26	Lu-177 Dotatate	LUTATHERA (Advanced Accelerator Applications)	Therapy	Intravenous injection	NA
27	Molybdenum Mo-99 Generator	Ultra-TechneKow V4 (Curium) TechneLite (Lantheus Medical Imaging) RadioGenix (NorthStar Medical Radioisotopes)			
28	N-13 Ammonia	None (Various)	Diagnostic imaging	Intravenous injection	3 min
29	Ra-223 Dichloride	Xofigo (Bayer HealthCare Pharmaceuticals)	Therapy	Intravenous injection	NA

METHOD OF LOCALIZATION/ACTION	CLINICAL INDICATIONS AND USE	PATIENT PREPARATION/PRECAUTIONS
Lutetium Lu-177 Dotatate binds to somatostatin receptors with highest affinity for subtype-2 receptors (ssrt2). Upon binding to somatostatin receptor–expressing cells, including malignant somatostatin receptor-positive tumors, the compound is internalized. The β emission from Lu-177 induces cellular damage by formation of free radicals in somatostatin receptor–positive cells and in neighboring cells.	LUTATHERA is indicated for the treatment of somatostatin receptor–positive gastroenteropancreatic neuroendocrine tumors (GEP-NETs), including foregut, midgut, and hindgut neuroendocrine tumors in adults. Administration: 7.4 GBq (200 mCi) every 8 wk for a total of four administrations.	The following serious adverse reactions are described elsewhere in the labeling: myelosuppression, secondary myelodysplastic syndrome and leukemia, renal toxicity, hepatotoxicity, and neuroendocrine hormonal crisis. Before initiating LUTATHERA: Discontinue long-acting somatostatin analogs (e.g., long-acting octreotide) for at least 4 wk prior to initiating LUTATHERA. Administer short-acting octreotide as needed; discontinue at least 24 h prior to initiating LUTATHERA
See Chapter 16		
Ammonia N-13 Injection is a radiolabeled analog of ammonia that is distributed to all organs of the body after intravenous administration. It is extracted from the blood in the coronary capillaries into the myocardial cells where it is metabolized to glutamine N-13 and retained in the cells. The presence of ammonia N-13 and glutamine N-13 in the myocardium allows for PET imaging of the myocardium.	Ammonia N-13 Injection is indicated for diagnostic PET imaging of the myocardium under rest or pharmacologic stress conditions to evaluate myocardial perfusion in patients with suspected or existing coronary artery disease.	To increase renal clearance of radioactivity and to minimize radiation dose to the bladder, ensure that the patient is well hydrated before the procedure and encourage voiding as soon as a study is completed and as often as possible thereafter for at least 1 h.
The active moiety of Xofigo is the alpha particle–emitting isotope radium-223 (as radium Ra-223 dichloride), which mimics calcium and forms complexes with the bone mineral hydroxyapatite at areas of increased bone turnover, such as bone metastases. The high linear energy transfer of alpha emitters (80 keV/μm) leads to a high frequency of double-strand DNA breaks in adjacent cells, resulting in an anti-tumor effect on bone metastases. The alpha particle range from radium-223 dichloride is < 100 μm (< 10 cell diameters), which limits damage to the surrounding normal tissue.	Xofigo is indicated for the treatment of patients with castration-resistant prostate cancer, symptomatic bone metastases, and no known visceral metastatic disease.	**Bone Marrow Suppression**: Measure blood counts prior to treatment initiation and before every dose of Xofigo. Discontinue Xofigo if hematologic values do not recover within 6 to 8 wk after treatment. Monitor patients with compromised bone marrow reserve closely. Discontinue Xofigo in patients who experience life-threatening complications despite supportive care measures.

(Continued)

TABLE F-1 **METHOD OF ADMINISTRATION, LOCALIZATION, CLINICAL UTILITY, AND OTHER CHARACTERISTICS OF CURRENTLY FDA-APPROVED RADIOPHARMACEUTICALS (*Continued*)**

RADIO-PHARMACEUTICAL	TRADE NAME (MANUFACTURER)	MEDICAL USE	METHOD OF ADMINISTRATION	DELAY BEFORE IMAGING
30 Rb-82 Chloride	Cardiogen-82 (Bracco Diagnostics) Ruby-Fill (DRAXIMAGE)	Diagnostic imaging	Intravenous injection	2 to 7 min
31 Sm-153 Lexidronam	Quadramet (Lantheus Medical Imaging)	Therapy	Intravenous injection	NA

METHOD OF LOCALIZATION/ACTION	CLINICAL INDICATIONS AND USE	PATIENT PREPARATION/ PRECAUTIONS
Following intravenous administration, rubidium Rb-82 rapidly clears the blood and is extracted by myocardial tissue in a manner analogous to potassium. In human studies, myocardial activity was noted within the first minute after injection. When areas of myocardial infarction are detected with rubidium chloride Rb-82 injection, they are visualized within 2 to 7 min after injection as photon-deficient or "cold areas" on the myocardial scan. Uptake is also observed in kidney, liver, spleen, and lung.	Rubidium chloride Rb-82 injection is a myocardial perfusion agent that is useful in distinguishing normal from abnormal myocardium in patients with suspected myocardial infarction.	Caution should be used during infusion as patients with congestive heart failure may experience a transitory increase in circulatory volume load. These patients should be observed for several hours following the Rb-82 procedure to detect delayed hemodynamic disturbances.
Quadramet (Samarium Sm-153 EDTMP) has an affinity for bone and concentrates in areas of bone turnover in association with hydroxyapatite. In clinical studies employing planar imaging techniques, more Quadramet accumulates in osteoblastic lesions than in normal bone lesion-to-normal bone ratio of approximately 5. The mechanism of action in relieving the pain of bone metastases is not known.	Quadramet is a therapeutic agent consisting of radioactive Sm-153 and a tetraphosphonate chelator EDTMP. Quadramet is indicated for relief of pain in patients with confirmed osteoblastic metastatic bone lesions that enhance on radionuclide bone scans.	Quadramet is contraindicated in patient who have known hypersensitivity to EDTMP or similar phosphonate compounds. Quadramet causes bone marrow suppression. Before administration, consideration should be given to the patient's current clinical and hematologic status and bone marrow response history to treatment with myelotoxic agents.

(*Continued*)

TABLE F-1 **METHOD OF ADMINISTRATION, LOCALIZATION, CLINICAL UTILITY, AND OTHER CHARACTERISTICS OF CURRENTLY FDA-APPROVED RADIOPHARMACEUTICALS (*Continued*)**

RADIO-PHARMACEUTICAL	TRADE NAME (MANUFACTURER)	MEDICAL USE	METHOD OF ADMINISTRATION	DELAY BEFORE IMAGING
32 Sr-89 Chloride	Metastron (Q BioMed)	Therapy	Intravenous injection	NA
33 Tc-99m Bicisate (ECD)	Neurolite (Lantheus Medical Imaging)	Diagnostic imaging	Intravenous injection	30 to 60 min

METHOD OF LOCALIZATION/ACTION	CLINICAL INDICATIONS AND USE	PATIENT PREPARATION/ PRECAUTIONS
Following intravenous injection, soluble strontium compounds behave like their calcium analogs, clearing rapidly from the blood and selectively localizing in bone mineral. Uptake of strontium by bone occurs preferentially in sites of active osteogenesis; thus primary bone tumors and areas of metastatic involvement (blastic lesions) can accumulate significantly greater concentrations of strontium than surrounding normal bone. Strontium-89 Chloride is retained in metastatic bone lesions much longer than in normal bone, where turnover is about 14 days. In patients with extensive skeletal metastases, well over half of the injected dose is retained in the bones.	Strontium Chloride Sr-89 Injection is indicated for the relief of bone pain in patients with painful skeletal metastases.	Use of Strontium-89 Chloride Injection in patients with evidence of seriously compromised bone marrow from previous therapy or disease infiltration is not recommended unless the potential benefit of the treatment outweighs its risks. Bone marrow toxicity is to be expected following the administration of Strontium-89, particularly white blood cells and platelets. The extent of toxicity is variable. It is recommended that the patient's peripheral blood cell counts be monitored at least once every other week. Typically, platelets will be depressed by about 30% compared to pre-administration levels. White blood cells are usually depressed to a varying extent compared to pre-administration levels. Thereafter, recovery occurs slowly, typically reaching pre-administration levels 6 mo after treatment unless the patient's disease or additional therapy intervenes.
Technetium Tc-99m Bicisate is metabolized by endogenous enzymes to the mono- and di-acids of Technetium Tc-99m Bicisate that can be detected in blood and urine. No studies have been performed to compare the concentration of Technetium Tc-99m Bicisate or its metabolites in normal, ischemic, and infarcted cells.	Neurolite single photon emission computerized tomography (SPECT) is indicated as an adjunct to conventional CT or MRI imaging in the localization of stroke in patients in whom stroke has already been diagnosed. Neurolite is not indicated for assessment of functional viability of brain tissue. Also, Neurolite is not indicated for distinguishing between stroke and other brain lesions.	Patients should be encouraged to drink fluids and to void frequently during the 2–6 h immediately after injection to minimize radiation dose to the bladder and other target organs. Contents of the vials are intended only for use in the preparation of Technetium Tc-99m Bicisate and are not to be administered directly to the patient without first undergoing the preparation procedure.

(Continued)

TABLE F-1 METHOD OF ADMINISTRATION, LOCALIZATION, CLINICAL UTILITY, AND OTHER CHARACTERISTICS OF CURRENTLY FDA-APPROVED RADIOPHARMACEUTICALS (*Continued*)

	RADIO-PHARMACEUTICAL	TRADE NAME (MANUFACTURER)	MEDICAL USE	METHOD OF ADMINISTRATION	DELAY BEFORE IMAGING
34	Tc-99m Exametazime (HMPAO)	None (DRAXIMAGE) Ceretec (GE Healthcare)	Diagnostic imaging	Intravenous injection	2 to 4 h
35	Tc-99m Macroaggregated Albumin (MAA)	Pulmotech (Curium) None (DRAXIMAGE)	Diagnostic imaging	Intravenous injection	Immediately following injection

METHOD OF LOCALIZATION/ACTION	CLINICAL INDICATIONS AND USE	PATIENT PREPARATION/ PRECAUTIONS
When technetium Tc-99m pertechnetate is added to exametazime in the presence of stannous reductant, a lipophilic technetium Tc-99m complex is formed. This lipophilic complex is the active moiety. It converts at approximately 12%/h to less lipophilic species. When the secondary complex is separated from the lipophilic species, it is unable to cross the blood-brain barrier. The useful life of the reconstituted agent is limited to 30 min. The in vitro addition of methylene blue to the Tc-99m-exametazime will stabilize the complex for 4–6 h. Methylene blue may be added to Tc-99m for cerebral imaging. Methylene blue should not be used in the preparation of Tc-99m-exametazime labeled leukocytes.	Technetium Tc-99m exametazime scintigraphy (with or without methylene blue stabilization) may be useful as an adjunct in the detection of altered regional cerebral perfusion in stroke. Tc-99m exametazime without methylene blue stabilization is indicated for leukocyte labeled scintigraphy as an adjunct in the localization of intraabdominal infection and inflammatory bowel disease.	As with any injected product, acute hypersensitivity or allergic reactions are possible. Limited reports have been received of hypersensitivity reactions following administration of Tc-99m labeled leukocytes prepared using Tc-99m exametazime. However, the materials used in leukocyte cell separation may cause hypersensitivity reactions. It is essential that cells are washed free of sedimentation agents before they are reinjected into the patient.
Immediately following intravenous injection, more than 80% of the albumin aggregated is trapped in the pulmonary alveolar capillary bed. The imaging procedure can thus be started as soon as the injection is complete. Assuming that a sufficient number of radioactive particles has been used, the distribution of radioactive aggregated particles in the normally perfused lung is uniform throughout the vascular bed, and will produce a uniform image. Areas of reduced perfusion will be revealed by a corresponding decreased accumulation of the radioactive particles, and are imaged as areas of reduced photon density.	Technetium Tc-99m Albumin Aggregated Injection is a lung imaging agent that may be used as an adjunct in the evaluation of pulmonary perfusion in adults and pediatric patients. Technetium Tc-99m Albumin Aggregated Injection may be used in adults as an imaging agent to aid in the evaluation of peritoneovenous (LeVeen) shunt patency.	Technetium Tc-99m Albumin Aggregated Injection should not be administered to patients with severe pulmonary hypertension. The use of Technetium Tc-99m Albumin Aggregated Injection is contraindicated in persons with a history of hypersensitivity reactions to products containing human serum albumin.

(Continued)

TABLE F-1 **METHOD OF ADMINISTRATION, LOCALIZATION, CLINICAL UTILITY, AND OTHER CHARACTERISTICS OF CURRENTLY FDA-APPROVED RADIOPHARMACEUTICALS (*Continued*)**

	RADIO-PHARMACEUTICAL	TRADE NAME (MANUFACTURER)	MEDICAL USE	METHOD OF ADMINISTRATION	DELAY BEFORE IMAGING
36	Tc-99m Mebrofenin	Choletec (Bracco Diagnostics) None (Pharmalucence)	Diagnostic imaging	Intravenous injection	5 to 10 min
37	Tc-99m Medronate (MDP)	MDP-25 (DRAXIMAGE) MDP Multidose (GE Healthcare) None (Pharmalucence)	Diagnostic imaging	Intravenous injection	1 to 4 h

METHOD OF LOCALIZATION/ACTION	CLINICAL INDICATIONS AND USE	PATIENT PREPARATION/ PRECAUTIONS
Mebrofenin is an iminodiacetic acid (HIDA) derivative with no known pharmacologic action at the recommended doses. Following intravenous administration in normal subjects, Technetium Tc-99m Mebrofenin was rapidly cleared from the circulation. The mean percent injected dose remaining in the blood at 10 min was 17%. The injected activity was cleared through the hepatobiliary system with visualization of the liver by 5 min and maximum liver uptake occurring at 11 min postinjection. Hepatic duct and gallbladder visualization occurred by 10 to 15 min and intestinal activity was visualized by 30 to 60 min in subjects with normal hepatobiliary function.	Technetium Tc-99m Mebrofenin is indicated as a hepatobiliary imaging agent.	The patient should be in a fasting state; 4 h is preferable. False positives (non-visualization) may result if the gallbladder has been emptied by ingestion of food. An interval of at least 24 h should be allowed before repeat examination. Patients with hepatocellular disease may show non-visualization or delayed visualization of the gallbladder. Delayed intestinal transit may also be noted in such patients. Juvenile hepatitis may be associated with gallbladder non-visualization and the failure to visualize activity in the intestine.
Following intravenous administration of Technetium Tc-99m Medronate, skeletal uptake occurs as a function of blood flow to bone and bone efficiency in extracting the complex. Bone mineral crystals are generally considered to be hydroxyapatite, and the complex appears to have an affinity for the hydroxyapatite crystals in the bone. The rapid blood clearance provides bone to soft-tissue ratios that favor early imaging. The skeletal uptake is bilaterally symmetrical and is greater in the axial skeleton than in the long bones. Areas of abnormal osteogenesis show altered uptake making it possible to visualize a variety of osseous lesions.	Technetium Tc-99m Medronate may be used as a bone imaging agent to delineate areas of altered osteogenesis.	This class of compounds is known to complex cations such as calcium. Particular caution should be used with patients who have, or who may be predisposed to, hypocalcemia (*i.e.*, alkalosis).

(Continued)

TABLE F-1 METHOD OF ADMINISTRATION, LOCALIZATION, CLINICAL UTILITY, AND OTHER CHARACTERISTICS OF CURRENTLY FDA-APPROVED RADIOPHARMACEUTICALS (*Continued*)

	RADIO-PHARMACEUTICAL	TRADE NAME (MANUFACTURER)	MEDICAL USE	METHOD OF ADMINISTRATION	DELAY BEFORE IMAGING
38	Tc-99m Mertiatide	TechneScan MAG3 (Curium) None (Pharmalucence)	Diagnostic imaging	Intravenous injection	None
39	Tc-99m Oxidronate	TechneScan HDP (Curium)	Diagnostic imaging	Intravenous injection	1 to 4 h

METHOD OF LOCALIZATION/ACTION	CLINICAL INDICATIONS AND USE	PATIENT PREPARATION/ PRECAUTIONS
Following intravenous injection of technetium Tc-99m mertiatide, the appearance, concentration, and excretion of the tracer in the kidney can be monitored to assess renal function. Although technetium Tc-99m mertiatide is highly plasma protein bound following intravenous injection, the protein binding is reversible and the tracer is rapidly excreted by the kidneys via active tubular secretion and glomerular filtration. Following intravenous injection of technetium Tc-99m mertiatide in normal volunteers, 89% of the tracer was plasma protein bound. In healthy subjects with normal renal function (mean serum creatinine 1.2 mg/dL) technetium Tc-99m mertiatide was rapidly cleared from the blood.	Technetium Tc-99m mertiatide is a renal imaging agent for use in the diagnosis of congenital and acquired abnormalities, renal failure, urinary tract obstruction, and calculi in adults and pediatric patients. It is a diagnostic aid in providing renal function, split function, renal angiograms, and renogram curves for whole kidney and renal cortex.	There are no known contraindications. The following adverse reactions have been reported: nausea, vomiting, wheezing, dyspnea, itching, rash, tachycardia, hypertension, shaking chills, fever, and seizure.
During the 24 h following injection, Tc-99m oxidronate is rapidly cleared from blood and other non-osseous tissues and accumulates in the skeleton and urine in humans. Blood levels are about 10% of the injected dose at 1-h postinjection and continue to fall to about 6%, 4%, and 3% at 2, 3, and 4 h, respectively. When measured at 24-h following administration, skeletal retention is approximately 50% of injected dose. Tc-99m oxidronate exhibits its greatest affinity for areas of altered osteogenesis and actively metabolizing bone.	TechneScan HDP Tc-99m is a diagnostic skeletal imaging agent used to demonstrate areas of altered osteogenesis in adult and pediatric patients.	Some hypersensitivity reactions, as well as nausea and vomiting, have been infrequently associated with Tc-99 oxidronate.

(Continued)

TABLE F-1 METHOD OF ADMINISTRATION, LOCALIZATION, CLINICAL UTILITY, AND OTHER CHARACTERISTICS OF CURRENTLY FDA-APPROVED RADIOPHARMACEUTICALS (Continued)

	RADIO-PHARMACEUTICAL	TRADE NAME (MANUFACTURER)	MEDICAL USE	METHOD OF ADMINISTRATION	DELAY BEFORE IMAGING
40	Tc-99m Pentetate (DTPA)	None (DRAXIMAGE)	Diagnostic imaging	Intravenous injection or inhalation	None
41	Tc-99m Pyrophosphate	TechneScan PYP (Curium) None (Pharmalucence)	Diagnostic imaging	Intravenous injection	1 to 6 h
42	Tc-99m Red Blood Cells	UltraTag (Curium)	Diagnostic imaging	Intravenous injection	None

METHOD OF LOCALIZATION/ACTION	CLINICAL INDICATIONS AND USE	PATIENT PREPARATION/ PRECAUTIONS
Intravenous Administration: Following intravenous administration for brain and renal imaging, Technetium Tc-99m pentetate is distributed in the vascular compartment. It is cleared by the kidneys, which results in the ability to image the kidney. **Aerosolized Inhalation Administration:** Following inhalation of the aerosol, Technetium Tc-99m pentetate deposits on the epithelium of ventilated alveoli.	**Brain Imaging:** Brain imaging in adults by intravenous administration **Renal Scintigraphy:** Renal visualization, assessment of renal perfusion, and estimation of glomerular filtration rate in adult and pediatric patients by intravenous administration **Lung Ventilation Imaging:** Lung ventilation imaging and evaluation of pulmonary embolism when paired with perfusion imaging in adult and pediatric patients when administered by nebulizer for inhalation	Hypersensitivity reactions, including anaphylaxis, have been reported during postapproval diagnostic use of Technetium Tc-99m pentetate injection. Monitor all patients for hypersensitivity reactions and have access to cardiopulmonary resuscitation equipment and personnel.
When injected intravenously, TechneScan PYP Tc-99m has a specific affinity for areas of altered osteogenesis. It is also concentrated in the injured myocardium, primarily in areas of irreversibly damaged myocardial cells.	TechneScan PYP Tc-99m is a skeletal imaging agent used to demonstrate areas of altered osteogenesis, and a cardiac imaging agent used as an adjunct in the diagnosis of acute myocardial infarction.	Reports indicate impairment of brain images using sodium pertechnetate Tc-99m, which have been preceded by a bone image. The impairment may result in false positives or false negatives. It is recommended, where feasible, that brain imaging precede bone imaging procedures.
In vitro Tc-99m red blood cell labeling is accomplished by adding 1–3 mL of autologous whole blood, anticoagulated with heparin or anticoagulant citrate dextrose solution (ACD) to the reaction vial. A portion of the stannous ion in the reaction vial diffuses across the red blood cell membrane and accumulates intracellularly.	Tc-99m-labeled red blood cells are used for blood pool imaging, including cardiac first pass and gated equilibrium imaging and for detection of sites of gastrointestinal bleeding.	No known contraindications

(Continued)

TABLE F-1 METHOD OF ADMINISTRATION, LOCALIZATION, CLINICAL UTILITY, AND OTHER CHARACTERISTICS OF CURRENTLY FDA-APPROVED RADIOPHARMACEUTICALS (*Continued*)

	RADIO-PHARMACEUTICAL	TRADE NAME (MANUFACTURER)	MEDICAL USE	METHOD OF ADMINISTRATION	DELAY BEFORE IMAGING
43	Tc-99m Sestamibi	None (Cardinal Health) None (DRAXIMAGE) Cardiolite (Lantheus Medical Imaging) None (Pharmalucence)	Diagnostic imaging	Intravenous injection	30 to 60 min
44	Tc-99m Sodium Pertechnetate	None (Curium) None (Lantheus Medical Imaging) None (NorthStar Medical Radioisotopes)	Diagnostic imaging	Intravenous injection or oral administration	None (angio or venography). Other applications 30 min to 1 h.

METHOD OF LOCALIZATION/ACTION	CLINICAL INDICATIONS AND USE	PATIENT PREPARATION/ PRECAUTIONS
Technetium Tc-99m Sestamibi is a cationic Tc-99m complex that has been found to accumulate in viable myocardial tissue in a manner analogous to that of thallous chloride Tl-201. Scintigraphic images obtained in humans after the intravenous administration of the drug have been comparable to those obtained with thallous chloride Tl-201 in normal and abnormal myocardial tissue. The mechanism of Tc-99m Sestamibi localization in various types of breast tissue (*e.g.*, benign, inflammatory, malignant, fibrous) has not been established.	**Myocardial Imaging:** Technetium Tc-99m Sestamibi Injection is a myocardial perfusion agent that is indicated for detecting coronary artery disease by localizing myocardial ischemia (reversible defects) and infarction (non-reversible defects), in evaluating myocardial function and developing information for use in patient management decisions. **Breast Imaging:** Technetium Tc-99m Sestamibi is indicated for planar imaging as a second line diagnostic drug after mammography to assist in the evaluation of breast lesions in patients with an abnormal mammogram or a palpable breast mass.	In studying patients in whom cardiac disease is known or suspected, care should be taken to assure continuous monitoring and treatment in accordance with safe, accepted clinical procedure. Infrequently, death has occurred 4 to 24 h after Tc-99m Sestamibi use and is usually associated with exercise stress testing
The pertechnetate ion distributes in the body similarly to the iodide ion, but is not organified when trapped in the thyroid gland. Pertechnetate tends to accumulate in intracranial lesions with excessive neovascularity or an altered blood-brain barrier. It also concentrates in the thyroid gland, salivary glands, gastric mucosa, and choroid plexus. However, in contrast to the iodide ion, the pertechnetate ion is released unchanged from the thyroid gland. After intravascular administration, the pertechnetate ion remains in the circulatory system for sufficient time to permit blood pool measurement, organ perfusion, and major vessel studies. It gradually equilibrates with the extravascular space. A small fraction is promptly excreted via the kidneys.	Sodium pertechnetate Tc-99m injection is used in adults as an agent for brain imaging including cerebral radionuclide angiography; thyroid imaging; salivary gland imaging; placenta localization; blood pool imaging including radionuclide angiography; urinary bladder imaging (direct isotopic cystography) for detection of vesicoureteral reflux; and nasolacrimal draining system imaging (dacryoscintigraphy).	There are no known contraindications. Allergic reactions including anaphylaxis have been reported infrequently following the administration of sodium pertechnetate Tc-99m.

(Continued)

TABLE F-1 METHOD OF ADMINISTRATION, LOCALIZATION, CLINICAL UTILITY, AND OTHER CHARACTERISTICS OF CURRENTLY FDA-APPROVED RADIOPHARMACEUTICALS (*Continued*)

	RADIO-PHARMACEUTICAL	TRADE NAME (MANUFACTURER)	MEDICAL USE	METHOD OF ADMINISTRATION	DELAY BEFORE IMAGING
45	Tc-99m Succimer (DMSA)	None (GE Healthcare)	Diagnostic imaging	Intravenous injection	1 to 2 h
46	Tc-99m Sulfur Colloid	None (Pharmalucence)	Diagnostic imaging	Oral administration	20 min

METHOD OF LOCALIZATION/ACTION	CLINICAL INDICATIONS AND USE	PATIENT PREPARATION/ PRECAUTIONS
After intravenous administration, technetium Tc-99m succimer (DMSA) injection is distributed in the plasma, apparently bound to plasma proteins. There is negligible activity in the red blood cells. The activity is cleared from the plasma with a half-time of about 60 min and concentrates in the renal cortex. Approximately 16% of the activity is excreted in the urine within 2 h. At 6 h, about 20% of the dose is concentrated in each kidney.	Tc-99m DMSA is to be used as an aid in the scintigraphic evaluation of renal parenchymal disorders.	There are no known contraindications. Rare instances of syncope, fever, nausea, and maculopapular skin rash have been reported.
Following intravenous administration, Technetium Tc-99m Sulfur Colloid Injection is rapidly cleared by the reticuloendothelial system from the blood with a nominal clearance half-life of approximately 2 1/2 min. Uptake of the radioactive colloid by organs of the reticuloendothelial system is dependent upon both their relative blood flow rates and the functional capacity of the phagocytic cells. In the average patient, 80% to 90% of the injected collodial particles are phagocytized by the Kupffer cells of the liver, 5% to 10% by the spleen, and the balance by the bone marrow.	Technetium Tc-99m Sulfur Colloid Injection is used in adults and children as an agent for imaging areas of functioning reticuloendothelial cells in the liver, spleen, and bone marrow. It is used orally in adults and children for esophageal transit studies, for gastroesophageal reflux scintigraphy, and for the detection of pulmonary aspiration of gastric contents. Technetium Tc-99m Sulfur Colloid may be used in adults as an imaging agent to aid in the evaluation of peritoneo-venous (LeVeen) shunt patency.	The following adverse reactions have been reported associated with the use of Technetium Tc-99m Sulfur Colloid Injection: cardiopulmonary arrest, seizures, anaphylactic shock, hypotension, dyspnea, abdominal pain, fever, chills, bronchospasm, nausea, vomiting, perspiration, and redness.

(Continued)

TABLE F-1 METHOD OF ADMINISTRATION, LOCALIZATION, CLINICAL UTILITY, AND OTHER CHARACTERISTICS OF CURRENTLY FDA-APPROVED RADIOPHARMACEUTICALS (Continued)

	RADIO-PHARMACEUTICAL	TRADE NAME (MANUFACTURER)	MEDICAL USE	METHOD OF ADMINISTRATION	DELAY BEFORE IMAGING
47	Tc-99m Tetrofosmin	Myoview (GE Healthcare)	Diagnostic imaging	Intravenous injection	15 min (stress) and 30 min (rest)
48	Tc-99m Tilmanocept	Lymphoseek (Cardinal Health)	Diagnostic imaging	Subcutaneous, intradermal, subareolar, or peritumoral injection	Administer Lymphoseek at least 15 min prior to initiating intraoperative lymphatic mapping and sentinel node biopsy; complete these procedures within 15 h

METHOD OF LOCALIZATION/ACTION	CLINICAL INDICATIONS AND USE	PATIENT PREPARATION/ PRECAUTIONS
When technetium Tc-99m pertechnetate is added to tetrofosmin in the presence of stannous reductant, a lipophilic, cationic technetium Tc-99m complex is formed, Tc-99m tetrofosmin. This complex is the active ingredient in the reconstituted drug product, on whose biodistribution and pharmacokinetic properties the indications for use depend. Studies in normal volunteers have demonstrated rapid myocardial uptake of Tc-99m tetrofosmin, and rapid blood, liver, and lung clearances. Uptake in the myocardium reaches a maximum of about 1.2% of the injected dose (i.d.) at 5 min and approximately 1% of the i.d. at 2 h, respectively. Background activities in the blood, liver, and lung were < 5% of the administered activity in whole blood at 10 min postinjection, < 4.5% i.d., after 60 min, and < 2% i.d. after 30 min. Approximately 66% of the injected activity is excreted within 48 h postinjection, with approximately 40% excreted in the urine and 26% in the feces.	MYOVIEW is indicated for scintigraphic imaging of the myocardium following separate administrations under exercise and/or resting conditions. It is useful in the delineation of regions of reversible myocardial ischemia in the presence or absence of infarcted myocardium. MYOVIEW is also indicated for scintigraphic imaging of the myocardium to identify changes in perfusion induced by pharmacologic stress in patients with known or suspected coronary artery disease. MYOVIEW is also indicated for the assessment of left ventricular function (left ventricular ejection fraction and wall motion) in patients being evaluated for heart disease.	In studying patients with known or suspected coronary artery disease, care should be taken to ensure continuous cardiac monitoring and the availability of emergency cardiac treatment. Pharmacologic induction of cardiovascular stress may be associated with serious adverse events such as myocardial infarction, arrhythmia, hypotension, bronchoconstriction, and cerebrovascular events. Caution should be used when pharmacologic stress is selected as an alternative to exercise; it should be used when indicated and in accordance with the pharmacologic stress agent's labeling.
Lymphoseek (technetium Tc-99m tilmanocept) is a radioactive diagnostic agent. It accumulates in lymphatic tissue and selectively binds to mannose binding receptors (CD206) located on the surface of macrophages and dendritic cells. Technetium Tc-99m tilmanocept is a macromolecule consisting of multiple units of diethylenetriaminepentaacetic acid (DTPA) and mannose, each covalently attached to a 10 kDa dextran backbone. The mannose acts as a ligand for the receptor, and the DTPA serves as a chelating agent for labeling with technetium Tc-99m.	Lymphoseek is a radioactive diagnostic agent indicated with or without scintigraphic imaging for: (1) Lymphatic mapping using a handheld γ counter to locate lymph nodes draining a primary tumor site in patients with solid tumors for which this procedure is a component of intraoperative management, and (2) Guiding sentinel lymph node biopsy using a handheld γ counter in patients with clinically node negative squamous cell carcinoma of the oral cavity, breast cancer, or melanoma.	Lymphoseek may pose a risk of hypersensitivity reactions due to its chemical similarity to dextran. Serious hypersensitivity reactions have been associated with dextran and modified forms of dextran (such as iron dextran drugs).

(Continued)

TABLE F-1 METHOD OF ADMINISTRATION, LOCALIZATION, CLINICAL UTILITY, AND OTHER CHARACTERISTICS OF CURRENTLY FDA-APPROVED RADIOPHARMACEUTICALS (*Continued*)

	RADIO-PHARMACEUTICAL	TRADE NAME (MANUFACTURER)	MEDICAL USE	METHOD OF ADMINISTRATION	DELAY BEFORE IMAGING
49	Tl-201 Chloride	None (Curium) None (GE Healthcare) None (Lantheus Medical Imaging)	Diagnostic imaging	Intravenous injection	Injected at maximum stress. Image 10–15 min later. Redistribution image at 4 h after stress image.
50	Xe-133 Gas	None (Curium) None (Lantheus Medical Imaging)	Diagnostic imaging	Inhalation	None

METHOD OF LOCALIZATION/ACTION	CLINICAL INDICATIONS AND USE	PATIENT PREPARATION/ PRECAUTIONS
Thallium images have been found to visualize areas of infarction as "cold" or non-labeled regions, which are confirmed by electrocardiographic and enzyme changes. When the "cold" or non-labeled regions constitute a substantial portion of the left ventricle, the prognosis for survival is unfavorable. Regions of transient myocardial ischemia corresponding to areas perfused by coronary arteries with partial stenoses have been visualized when Thallous Chloride Tl-201 Injection was administered in conjunction with an exercise stress test. Body habitus may interfere with visualization of the inferior wall.	Thallous Chloride Tl-201 Injection may be useful in myocardial perfusion imaging using either planar or SPECT (single photon computed tomography) techniques for the diagnosis and localization of myocardial infarction. It may also have prognostic value regarding survival, when used in the clinically stable patient following the onset of symptoms of an acute myocardial infarction, to assess the site and size of the perfusion defect. Thallous Chloride Tl-201 Injection may also be useful in conjunction with exercise stress testing as an adjunct in the diagnosis of ischemic heart disease (atherosclerotic coronary artery disease). It is usually not possible to differentiate recent from old myocardial infarction, or to differentiate between recent myocardial infarction and ischemia.	In studying patients in whom myocardial infarction or ischemia is known or suspected, care should be taken to assure continuous clinical monitoring and treatment in accordance with safe, accepted procedure. Exercise stress testing should be performed only under the supervision of a qualified physician and in a laboratory equipped with appropriate resuscitation and support apparatus.
Xenon Xe-133 is a readily diffusible gas that is neither utilized nor produced by the body. It passes through cell membranes and freely exchanges between blood and tissue. It tends to concentrate more in body fat than in blood, plasma, water, or protein solutions. In the concentrations used for diagnostic purposes it is physiologically inactive. Inhaled Xenon Xe-133 Gas will enter the alveolar wall and enter the pulmonary venous circulation via the capillaries. Most of the Xenon Xe-133 that enters the circulation from a single breath is returned to the lungs and exhaled after a single pass through the peripheral circulation.	Inhalation of Xenon Xe-133 Gas is used for the evaluation of pulmonary function and for imaging the lungs. It may also be applied to assessment of cerebral flow.	No reported adverse reactions

(Continued)

TABLE F-1 **METHOD OF ADMINISTRATION, LOCALIZATION, CLINICAL UTILITY, AND OTHER CHARACTERISTICS OF CURRENTLY FDA-APPROVED RADIOPHARMACEUTICALS (*Continued*)**

	RADIO-PHARMACEUTICAL	TRADE NAME (MANUFACTURER)	MEDICAL USE	METHOD OF ADMINISTRATION	DELAY BEFORE IMAGING
51	Y-90 Chloride	None (Eckert & Ziegler Nuclitec)			
52	Y-90 Ibritumomab Tiuxetan	Zevalin (Acrotech Biopharma)	Therapy	Intravenous injection preceded by infusions of rituximab (see dosing schedule).	Pretherapy imaging with In-111 Zevalin to determine patient biokinetics and to compute therapeutic dose

METHOD OF LOCALIZATION/ACTION	CLINICAL INDICATIONS AND USE	PATIENT PREPARATION/ PRECAUTIONS
	Yttrium-90 Chloride Sterile Solution is a component intended for use in the preparation of radiolabeled monoclonal antibodies.	Not to be administered directly to patients
Ibritumomab tiuxetan binds specifically to the CD20 antigen. The CD20 antigen is expressed on pre-B and mature B lymphocytes and on >90% of B-cell non-Hodgkin lymphomas (NHL). The CD20 antigen is not shed from the cell surface and does not internalize upon antibody binding.	Zevalin is indicated for the treatment of relapsed or refractory, low-grade or follicular B-cell non-Hodgkin lymphoma (NHL). Zevalin is also indicated for the treatment of untreated follicular NHL in patients who achieve a partial or complete response to first-line chemotherapy.	Patient complications can include (1) serious infusion reactions, (2) prolonged and sever cytopenias, (3) severe cutaneous and mucocutaneous reactions, and (4) leukemia and myelodysplastic syndrome.

Appendix F: Radiopharmaceutical Characteristics and Dosimetry

TABLE F-2 SUMMARY OF TYPICALLY ADMINISTERED ADULT DOSE; ORGAN RECEIVING THE HIGHEST RADATION DOSE AND ITS DOSE; GONADAL DOSE; EFFECTIVE DOSE, AND EFFECTIVE DOSE PER ADMINISTERED ACTIVITY FOR FDA-APPROVED RADIOPHARMACEUTICALS

RADIOPHARMACEUTICAL	TYPICAL ADULT ADMINISTERED ACTIVITY		ORGAN RECEIVING HIGHEST DOSE	ORGAN DOSE		GONADAL DOSE			EFFECTIVE DOSE		EFFECTIVE DOSE COEFFICIENT		SOURCE
	MBq	mCi		mGy	rad	mGy		rad	mSv	rem	mSv/MBq	rem/mCi	
C-11 Choline	555 (370–740)	15 (10–20)	Pancreas	16	1.6	0.75 / 1.1	ts / ov	0.075 / 0.11	2.4	0.24	0.0044	0.016	PI
C-11 Urea (PYtest)	0.037	0.001	BE	1.22E−03	1.22E−04	8.88E−04 / 8.88E−04	ts / ov	8.88E−05 / 8.88E−05	1.15E−03	1.15E−04	0.031	0.115	ICRP P128
F-18 Florbetaben (Neuraceq)	300	8.1	UB wall	21	2.1	2.7 / 4.8	ts / ov	0.27 / 0.48	5.7	0.57	0.019	0.070	PI
F-18 Florbetapir (Amyvid)	370	10	GB wall	53	5.3	2.6 / 6.7	ts / ov	0.26 / 0.67	7.0	0.70	0.019	0.070	PI
F-18 Flortaucipir (TAUVID)	370	10	Upper large Intestine wall	36	3.6	2.6 / 7.8	ts / ov	0.26 / 0.78	8.9	0.89	0.024	0.089	PI
F-18 Fluciclovine (Axumin)	370	10	Pancreas	38	3.8	6.3 / 4.8	ts / ov	0.63 / 0.48	8.1	0.81	0.022	0.081	PI
F-18 Sodium Fluoride	375 (300–450)	10 (8–12)	UB wall	56	5.6	2.3 / 3.1	ts / ov	0.23 / 0.31	6.4	0.64	0.017	0.063	ICRP P128
F-18 Fluorodeoxyglucose (FDG)	280 (185–370)	7.6 (5–10)	UB wall	36	3.6	3.1 / 3.9	ts / ov	0.31 / 0.39	5.3	0.53	0.019	0.070	ICRP P128
F-18 Fluoroestradiol (CERIANNA)	222 (111–222)	6 (3–6)	Liver	28	2.8	2.7 / 4.0	ts / ov	0.27 / 0.40	4.9	0.49	0.022	0.081	PI
F-18 Flutemetamol (Vizamyl)	185	5	GB wall	53	5.3	1.5 / 4.6	ts / ov	0.15 / 0.46	5.9	0.59	0.032	0.118	PI
Ga-67 Citrate	130 (74–185)	3.5 (2–5)	BE	82	8.2	7.3 / 11	ts / ov	0.73 / 1.1	13	1.3	0.100	0.370	ICRP P128

Radiopharmaceutical	MBq	mCi	Critical Organ				ts / ov						Source
Ga-68 Dotatate (NETSPOT)	150 (2 MBq/kg)	4.1 (0.05 mCi/kg)	Spleen	16	1.6	1.5 / 2.4	ts / ov	0.15 / 0.24	3.2	0.32	0.021	0.078	PI
Ga-68 Dotatoc	148	4	UB wall	18	1.8	2.1 / 2.1	ts / ov	0.21 / 0.21	3.1	0.31	0.021	0.078	PI
In-111 Chloride (Used only for radiolabeling—see Appendix F-1)													
In-111 Oxyquinoline (Labeled Leukocytes)	13 (7.4–18.5)	0.35 (0.2–0.5)	Spleen	200	20	0.14 / 2.0	ts / ov	0.014 / 0.20	3.7	0.37	0.170	0.629	PI
In-111 Pentetate (DTPA)	18.5	0.5	UB wall	4.6	0.46	0.22 / 0.33	ts / ov	0.022 / 0.033	0.46	0.046	0.025	0.093	ICRP P53
In-111 Pentetreotide (Octreoscan)	222 (SPECT)	6 (SPECT)	Kidneys	91	9.1	3.8 / 6.0	ts / ov	0.38 / 0.6	12	1.2	0.054	0.200	ICRP P128
I-123 Iobenguane (MIBG)	370	10	Liver	25	2.5	2.1 / 3.0	ts / ov	0.21 / 0.30	4.8	0.48	0.013	0.048	ICRP P80
I-123 Ioflupane (DaTscan)	148 (111–185)	4 (3–5)	UB wall	7.9	0.79	1.3 / 2.5	ts / ov	0.13 / 0.25	3.2	0.32	0.021	0.079	PI
I-123 Sodium Iodine Capsules	9.3 (3.7–14.8)	0.25 (0.1–0.4)	Thyroid	37	3.7	0.037 / 0.065	ts / ov	0.0037 / 0.0065	2.0	0.20	0.220	0.814	ICRP P128 (medium uptake)
I-125 Human Serum Albumin (HSA)				Organ dosimetry not provided in PI Whole-body dose estimated at 0.25 mSv									
I-125 Iothalamate	0.74 (0.37–1.11)	0.02 (0.01–0.03)	UB wall	0.6	0.06	0.021 / 0.0085	ts / ov	0.0021 / 0.00085	0.011	0.0011	0.015	0.056	PI
I-131 HSA (Megatope)	1.85	0.05	Thyroid (blocked)	13	1.3	1 / 4.5	ts / ov	0.10 / 0.45	0.5	0.05	0.270	1.00	PI
I-131 Iobenguane (AZEDRA)	18,500 (Therapy)	500	Salivary glands	2.8E+04	2.8E+03	1,129 / 2,331	ts / ov	113 / 233	Not Applicable				PI

(Continued)

TABLE F-2 SUMMARY OF TYPICALLY ADMINISTERED ADULT DOSE; ORGAN RECEIVING THE HIGHEST RADIATION DOSE AND ITS DOSE; GONADAL DOSE; EFFECTIVE DOSE, AND EFFECTIVE DOSE PER ADMINISTERED ACTIVITY FOR FDA-APPROVED RADIOPHARMACEUTICALS *Continued*

RADIOPHARMACEUTICAL	TYPICAL ADULT ADMINISTERED ACTIVITY MBq	mCi	ORGAN RECEIVING HIGHEST DOSE	ORGAN DOSE mGy	rad	GONADAL DOSE mGy		rad	EFFECTIVE DOSE mSv	rem	EFFECTIVE DOSE COEFFICIENT mSv/MBq	rem/mCi	SOURCE
I-131 Sodium Iodide	3,700 (Therapy)	100	Thyroid (not blocked)	1.6E+06	1.6E+05	ts 85 ov 133		8.5 13.3	Not Applicable				ICRP P128 (medium uptake)
Lu-177 Dotatate (LUTATHERA)	4 × 7,400 (Therapy)	4 × 200	Spleen	2.5E+04	2.5E+03	ts 800 ov 900		80 90	Not Applicable				PI
Molybdenum Mo-99 Generator				See Chapter 16									
N-13 Ammonia	555 (370–740)	15 (10–20)	UB wall	4.5	0.45	ts 1.0 ov 0.94		0.10 0.094	1.50	0.15	0.003	0.010	ICRP P53
Ra-223 Dichloride (Xofigo)	3.5	0.095	BE	4,032	403	ts 0.28 ov 1.72		0.028 0.172	Not Applicable				PI
Rb-82 Chloride	2,220	60	Kidneys	21	2.1	ts 0.58 ov 1.1		0.058 0.11	2.4	0.24	0.0011	0.0041	ICRP P128
Sm-153 Lexidronam (Quadramet)	2,590	70	BE	1.73E+04	1.73E+03	ts 14 ov 22		1.4 2.2	Not Applicable				PI
Sr-89 Chloride (Metastron)	148	4	BE	2,516	252	ts 115 ov 115		11.5 11.5	Not Applicable				ICRP P53
Tc-99m Bicisate (ECD)	740 (370–1,110)	20 (10–30)	UB wall	37	3.7	ts 2.0 ov 5.8		0.20 0.58	5.7	0.57	0.0077	0.0285	ICRP P128
Tc-99m Exametazime (HMPAO)	590 (260–925)	16 (7–25)	Kidneys	20	2.0	ts 1.4 ov 3.9		0.14 0.39	5.5	0.55	0.0093	0.0344	ICRP P128
Tc-99m MAA	93 (37–148)	2.5 (1–4)	Lung	6.1	0.61	ts 0.10 ov 0.17		0.01 0.017	1.02	0.102	0.011	0.041	ICRP P128

Radiopharmaceutical	Administered Activity (MBq / mCi)	Critical Organ										Reference
Tc-99m Mebrofenin (Choletec)	130 (74–185) / 3.5 (2–5)	GB wall	14	1.4	ts	0.13	0.013	2.1	0.21	0.016	0.059	ICRP P128
					ov	2.3	0.23					
Tc-99m Medronate (MDP)	555 (370–740) / 15 (10–20)	UB wall (Normal uptake/excretion)	26	2.6	ts	1.3	0.13	2.7	0.27	0.0049	0.0181	ICRP P128
					ov	2.0	0.20					
Tc-99m Mertiatide (MAG3)	280 (185–370) / 7.6 (5–10)	UB wall (Normal renal function)	31	3.1	ts	1.0	0.10	2.0	0.20	0.007	0.026	ICRP P128
					ov	1.5	0.15					
Tc-99m Oxidronate (HDP)	555 (370–740) / 15 (10–20)	UB wall (Normal uptake/excretion)	26	2.6	ts	1.3	0.13	2.7	0.27	0.0049	0.0181	ICRP P128
					ov	2.0	0.20					
Tc-99m Pentetate (DTPA)	555 (370–740) / 15 (10–20)	UB wall (Normal renal function)	34	3.4	ts	1.6	0.16	2.7	0.27	0.0049	0.0181	ICRP P128
					ov	2.3	0.23					
Tc-99m Pyrophosphate (TechneScan)	370 (185–555) / 10 (5–15)	UB wall (Normal uptake/excretion)	17	1.7	ts	0.9	0.09	1.8	0.18	0.0049	0.0181	ICRP P128
					ov	1.3	0.13					
Tc-99m Red Blood Cells (UltraTag)	555 (370–740) / 15 (10–20)	Heart wall	13	1.3	ts	1.3	0.13	3.9	0.39	0.007	0.026	ICRP P128
					ov	2.1	0.21					
Tc-99m Sestamibi	740 (370–1,110) / 20 (10–30)	GB wall (Resting subject)	29	2.9	ts	2.8	0.28	6.7	0.67	0.009	0.033	ICRP P128
					ov	6.7	0.67					
Tc-99m Sodium Pertechnetate	740 (18.5–1,110) / 20 (0.5–30)	Upper large intestine wall (IV admin/no blocking agent)	41	4.1	ts	2.1	0.21	9.6	0.96	0.013	0.048	ICRP P128
					ov	7.3	0.73					
Tc-99m Succimer (DMSA)	148 (72–222) / 4 (2–6)	Kidneys	27	2.7	ts	0.27	0.027	1.3	0.13	0.0088	0.0326	ICRP P128
					ov	0.52	0.052					

(Continued)

TABLE F-2 SUMMARY OF TYPICALLY ADMINISTERED ADULT DOSE; ORGAN RECEIVING THE HIGHEST RADIATION DOSE AND ITS DOSE; GONADAL DOSE; EFFECTIVE DOSE, AND EFFECTIVE DOSE PER ADMINISTERED ACTIVITY FOR FDA-APPROVED RADIOPHARMACEUTICALS (Continued)

RADIOPHARMACEUTICAL	TYPICAL ADULT ADMINISTERED ACTIVITY		ORGAN RECEIVING HIGHEST DOSE	ORGAN DOSE		GONADAL DOSE				EFFECTIVE DOSE		EFFECTIVE DOSE COEFFICIENT		SOURCE
	MBq	mCi		mGy	rad	mGy		rad		mSv	rem	mSv/MBq	rem/mCi	
Tc-99m Sulfur Colloid	240 (37–444)	6.5 (1–12)	Spleen (Normal liver function)	18	1.8	0.13 0.53	ts ov	0.013 0.053		2.2	0.22	0.0091	0.034	ICRP P128
Tc-99m Tetrofosmin (Myoview)	740 (185–1,221)	20 (5–33)	GB wall (Resting subject)	27	2.7	2.3 6.5	ts ov	0.23 0.65		5.9	0.59	0.008	0.030	ICRP P128
Tc-99m Tilmanocept (Lymphoseek)	18.5	0.5	Breast (injection site) (Breast cancer)	1.7	0.17	0.05 0.19	ts ov	0.005 0.019		0.33	0.033	0.018	0.067	PI
Tl-201 Chloride	56 (37–74)	1.5 (1–2)	Kidneys	27	2.7	10 6.7	ts ov	1.0 0.67		7.8	0.78	0.140	0.518	ICRP P128
Xe-133 Gas	740 (370–1,110)	20 (10–30)	Lungs (Single inhalation)	0.61	0.061	0.070 0.074	ts ov	0.007 0.007		0.13	0.013	0.00018	0.00067	ICRP P128
Y-90 Chloride (Used only for radiolabeling)														
Y-90 Ibritumomab Tiuxetan	1,184	32	Spleen	11,130	1,113	1,776 474	ts ov	178 47		Not Applicable				Package Insert

Note: PI = Package Insert

TABLE F-3A EFFECTIVE DOSE PER UNIT ACTIVITY ADMINISTERED TO PEDIATRIC PATIENTS (1, 5, 10, AND 15 YEARS) FOR FDA-APPROVED RADIOPHARMACEUTICALS

	RADIOPHARMACEUTICAL	EFFECTIVE DOSE COEFFICIENT									
		15-Year-Old		10-Year-Old		5-Year-Old		1-Year-Old		SOURCE
		mSv/MBq	rem/mCi	mSv/MBq	rem/mCi	mSv/MBq	rem/mCi	mSv/MBq	rem/mCi	
8	F-18 Fluorodeoxyglucose (FDG)	0.024	0.089	0.037	0.137	0.056	0.207	0.095	0.352	ICRP P128
11	Ga-67 Citrate	0.130	0.481	0.200	0.740	0.330	1.221	0.640	2.368	ICRP P128
16	In-111 Pentetate (DTPA)	0.031	0.115	0.045	0.167	0.067	0.248	0.120	0.444	ICRP P53
17	In-111 Pentetreotide (Octreoscan)	0.071	0.263	0.100	0.370	0.160	0.592	0.280	1.036	ICRP P128
18	I-123 Iobenguane (MIBG)	0.017	0.063	0.026	0.096	0.037	0.137	0.068	0.252	ICRP P80
20	I-123 Sodium Iodine Capsules	0.350	1.295	0.520	1.924	1.100	4.070	2.100	7.770	ICRP P128
25	I-131 Sodium Iodide	35	130	53	196	110	407	180	666	ICRP P128
33	Tc-99m Bicisate (ECD)	0.010	0.037	0.015	0.056	0.022	0.081	0.040	0.148	ICRP P128
34	Tc-99m Exametazime (HMPAO)	0.011	0.041	0.017	0.063	0.027	0.100	0.049	0.181	ICRP P128
35	Tc-99m MAA	0.016	0.059	0.023	0.085	0.034	0.126	0.063	0.233	ICRP P128
36	Tc-99m Mebrofenin (Choletec)	0.020	0.074	0.027	0.100	0.043	0.159	0.100	0.370	ICRP P128
37	Tc-99m Medronate (MDP)	0.0057	0.021	0.0086	0.032	0.012	0.044	0.018	0.067	ICRP P128
38	Tc-99m Mertiatide (MAG3)	0.009	0.033	0.012	0.044	0.012	0.044	0.022	0.081	ICRP P128
40	Tc-99m Pentetate (DTPA)	0.0063	0.023	0.0094	0.035	0.012	0.044	0.016	0.059	ICRP P128
42	Tc-99m Red Blood Cells (UltraTag)	0.009	0.033	0.014	0.052	0.021	0.078	0.039	0.144	ICRP P128
43	Tc-99m Sestamibi	0.012	0.044	0.018	0.067	0.028	0.104	0.053	0.196	ICRP P128
44	Tc-99m Sodium Pertechnetate	0.017	0.0629	0.026	0.0962	0.042	0.1554	0.079	0.2923	ICRP P128
45	Tc-99m Succimer (DMSA)	0.011	0.041	0.015	0.056	0.021	0.078	0.037	0.137	ICRP P128
46	Tc-99m Sulfur Colloid	0.012	0.0444	0.018	0.0666	0.027	0.0999	0.049	0.1813	ICRP P128
49	Tl-201 Chloride	0.200	0.740	0.560	2.072	0.790	2.923	1.300	4.810	ICRP P128
50	Xe-133 Gas	0.00026	0.00096	0.00040	0.00148	0.00065	0.00241	0.00130	0.00481	ICRP P128

TABLE F-3B NORTH AMERICAN CONSENSUS GUIDELINES FOR PEDIATRIC ADMINISTERED RADIOPHARMACEUTICAL ACTIVITIES—2016 UPDATE

RADIOPHARMACEUTICAL	IMAGING TASK	NOTES	ADMINISTERED ACTIVITY (AA)		MINIMUM AA		MAXIMUM AA	
			(MBq/kg)	*(mCi/kg)*	*(MBq)*	*(mCi)*	*(MBq)*	*(mCi)*
I-123 MIBG	Cancer detection	A	5.2	0.14	37	1.0	370	10.0
Tc-99m MDP	Bone imaging	A	9.3		37	1.0		
F-18 FDG	Body imaging	A, B	3.7–5.2	0.10–0.14	26	0.7		
	Brain imaging	A, B	3.7	0.10	14	0.37		
Tc-99m DMSA	Kidney function	A	1.85	0.05	18.5	0.5	100	2.7
Tc-99m MAG3	Without flow study	A, C	3.7	0.10	37	1.0	148	4.0
	With flow study	A	5.55	0.15				
Tc-99m IDA	Hepatobiliary Imaging	A, D	1.85	0.05	18.5	0.5		
Tc-99 MAA	Ventilation study	A	2.59	0.07				
	No ventilation study	A	1.11	0.03	14.8	0.4		
Tc-99m Pertechnetate	Meckel diverticulum imaging	A	1.85	0.05	9.25	0.25		
F-18 Sodium Fluoride	Bone imaging	A	2.22	0.06	14	0.38		
Tc-99m Pertechnetate	Cystography	E	No weight-based dose		37	1.0	37	1.0
Tc-99m Sulfur Colloid	Oral liquid gastric emptying	F	No weight-based dose		9.25	0.25	37	1.0
Tc-99m Sulfur Colloid	Solid gastric empyting	F	No weight-based dose		9.25	0.25	18.5	0.5
Tc-99m HMPAO (Ceretec)	Brain perfusion		11.1	0.3	185	5	740	20
Tc-99m ECD (Neurolite)	Brain perfusion		11.1	0.3	185	5	740	20
Tc-99m Sestamibi (Cardiolite)	Myocardial perfusion (single/first of two)		5.55	0.15	74	2	370	10
Tc-99m Tetrofosmin (Myoview)	Myocardial perfusion (single/first of two)		5.55	0.15	74	2	370	10
Tc-99m Sestamibi (Cardiolite)	Myocardial perfusion (second of two)		16.7	0.45	222	6	1,110	30

Tc-99m Tetrofosmin (Myoview)	Myocardial perfusion (second of two)	16.7	0.45	222	6	1,110	30
I-123 NaI	Thyroid imaging	0.28	0.0075	1	0.027	11	0.3
Tc-99m Pertechnetate	Thyroid imaging	1.1	0.03	7	0.19	93	2.5
Tc-99m RBC	Blood pool imaging	11.8	0.32	74	2	740	20
Tc-99m WBC	Infection imaging	7.4	0.2	74	2	555	15
Ga-68 DOTATOC G	Neuroendocrine tumor imaging	2.7	0.074	14	0.38	185	5
Ga-68 DOTATATE G	Neuroendocrine tumor imaging	2.7	0.074	14	0.38	185	5

Notes: This information is intended as a guideline only. Local practice may vary depending on patient population, choice of collimator, and specific requirements of clinical protocols. Administered activity may be adjusted when appropriate by order of the nuclear medicine practitioner. For patients who weigh 0.70 kg, it is recommended that the maximum administered activity not exceed the product of the patient's weight (kg) and the recommended weight-based administered activity. Some practitioners may choose to set a fixed maximum administered activity equal to 70 times the recommended weight-based administered activity, expressed as MBq/kg or mCi/kg (e.g., <10 mCi [370 MBq] for 18F-FDG body imaging). The administered activities assume use of a low-energy high-resolution collimator for ^{99m}Tc radiopharmaceuticals and a medium-energy collimator for ^{123}I-MIBG. Individual practitioners may use lower administered activities if their equipment or software permits them to do so. Higher administered activities may be required in selected patients. No recommended administered activity is given for intravenous 67Ga-citrate; intravenous ^{67}Ga-citrate should be used very infrequently and only in low doses.

[A] The EANM Dosage Card 2014 version 2 administered activity may also be used.

[B] The low end of the dose range should be considered for smaller patients. Administered activity may take into account patient mass and time available on the PET scanner. The EANM Dosage Card 2014 version 2 administered activity may also be used.

[C] Administered activities assume that image data are reframed at 1 min/image. Administered activity may be reduced if image data are reframed at a longer time per image.

[D] A higher administered activity of 1 mCi may be considered for neonatal jaundice.

[E] ^{99m}Tc-sulfur colloid, ^{99m}Tc-pertechnetate, ^{99m}Tc-DTPA, or possibly other ^{99m}Tc radiopharmaceuticals may be used. There is a wide variety of acceptable administration and imaging techniques for ^{99m}Tc cystography, many of which will work well with lower administered activities. An example of appropriate lower administered activities is found in the 2014 revision of the EANM Paediatric Dose Card 2.

[F] The administered activity may be based on patient weight or on the age of the child.

[G] The administered activity is based on the EANM Dosage Card 2014 version 2 dosage for a 60-kg patient, using the minimum and maximum doses from the EANM Dosage Card. There was little experience with this radiopharmaceutical in children in North America at the time of preparation of this dosage table.

Appendix F: Radiopharmaceutical Characteristics and Dosimetry

TABLE F-4A SUMMARY OF ABSORBED DOSE ESTIMATES TO THE EMBRYO/FETUS PER UNIT ACTIVITY ADMINISTERED TO THE MOTHER FOR SOME COMMONLY USED RADIOPHARMACEUTICALS

RADIOPHARMACEUTICAL	DOSE AT DIFFERENT STAGES OF GESTATION							
	Early		3 months		6 months		9 months	
	mGy/MBq	rad/mCi	mGy/MBq	rad/mCi	mGy/MBq	rad/mCi	mGy/MBq	rad/mCi
Co-57 Vitamin B$_{12}$ also known as Schilling test	1.0	3.7	0.68	2.516	0.84	3.108	0.88	3.256
F-18 Sodium fluoride	0.022	0.081	0.017	0.063	0.008	0.028	0.007	0.025
F-18 Fluoro-deoxyglucose	0.022	0.081	0.022	0.081	0.017	0.063	0.017	0.063
Ga-67 Citrate	0.093	0.344	0.2	0.74	0.18	0.666	0.13	0.481
I-123 Sodium iodide	0.02	0.074	0.014	0.052	0.011	0.041	0.01	0.036
I-125 Albumin	0.25	0.925	0.078	0.289	0.038	0.141	0.026	0.096
I-131 Sodium iodide	0.072	0.266	0.068	0.252	0.23	0.851	0.27	0.999
In-111 Pentetreotide also known as Octreoscan	0.082	0.303	0.06	0.222	0.035	0.13	0.031	0.115
In-111 White blood cells	0.13	0.481	0.096	0.355	0.096	0.355	0.094	0.348
Tc-99m Disofenin also known as HIDA (iminodiacetic acid)	0.017	0.0629	0.0150	0.056	0.012	0.044	0.007	0.025
Tc-99m DMSA (dimercaptosuccinic acid) also known as succimer	0.005	0.019	0.005	0.017	0.004	0.015	0.003	0.013
Tc-99m Exametazime also known as Ceretec and HMPAO	0.009	0.032	0.007	0.025	0.005	0.018	0.004	0.013
Tc-99m Macroaggregated albumin (MAA)	0.003	0.01	0.004	0.015	0.005	0.019	0.004	0.015
Tc-99m Medronate also known as Tc-99m Methylene diphos-phonate (MDP)	0.006	0.023	0.005	0.02	0.003	0.01	0.002	0.009
Tc-99m Mertiatide also known as MAG3	0.018	0.067	0.014	0.052	0.006	0.02	0.005	0.019
Tc-99m Bicisate also known as ECD and Neurolite	0.011	0.041	0.008	0.03	0.004	0.014	0.004	0.013

Tc-99m Pentetate also known as Tc-99m DTPA	0.012	0.044	0.009	0.032	0.004	0.015	0.005	0.017
Tc-99m Pyrophosphate	0.006	0.022	0.007	0.024	0.004	0.013	0.003	0.011
Tc-99m Red Blood Cells	0.006	0.024	0.004	0.016	0.003	0.012	0.003	0.01
Tc-99 Sestamibi also known as Cardiolite (rest)	0.015	0.056	0.012	0.044	0.008	0.031	0.005	0.02
Tc-99 Sestamibi also known as Cardiolite (stress)	0.012	0.044	0.01	0.035	0.007	0.026	0.004	0.016
Tc-99m Sodium Pertechnetate	0.011	0.041	0.022	0.081	0.014	0.052	0.009	0.034
Tc-99m Sulfur Colloid	0.002	0.007	0.002	0.008	0.003	0.012	0.004	0.014
Tc-99 Tetrofosmin also known as Myoview	0.01	0.036	0.007	0.026	0.005	0.02	0.004	0.013
Tc-99m WBC	0.004	0.014	0.003	0.01	0.003	0.011	0.003	0.01
Tl-201 Thallous Chloride (rest)	0.097	0.359	0.058	0.215	0.047	0.174	0.027	0.1
Xe-133 Xenon gas (rebreathing for 5 min)	0.00041	0.00152	0.00005	0.00018	0.00004	0.00013	0.00003	0.0001

Reprinted with permission from Stabin M.G., Blackwell R., Brant R.L., Donnelly E., Kinf V.A., Lovins K., Stovall M. *Fetal Radiation Dose Calculations. ANSI N13.54 2008.* Washington, DC: American National Standards Institute, 2008.

TABLE F-4B EFFECTIVE DOSE TO THE NEWBORN AND INFANT PER UNIT ACTIVITY ADMINISTERED FROM THE MOTHER'S BREAST MILK[a]

RADIOPHARMACEUTICAL	NEWBORN mSv/MBq (rem/mCi)	1-YEAR-OLD mSv/MBq (rem/mCi)
[67]Ga-citrate	1.2 (4.4)	0.490 (1.81)
^{99m}Tc-DTPA	0.030 (0.111)	0.014 (0.052)
^{99m}Tc-MAA	0.17 (0.63)	0.068 (0.252)
[99m]Tc-pertechnetate	0.14 (0.52)	0.062 (0.229)
[131]I-NaI[b]	5,400 (20,000)	3,900 (14,400)
[51]Cr-EDTA	0.028 (0.104)	0.012 (0.044)
^{99m}Tc-DISIDA	0.22 (0.81)	0.095 (0.35)
[99m]Tc-glucoheptonate	0.080 (0.30)	0.036 (0.13)
^{99m}Tc-HAM	0.20 (0.74)	0.083 (0.31)
^{99m}Tc-MIBI	0.14 (0.52)	0.065 (0.24)
^{99m}Tc-MDP	0.063 (0.23)	0.026 (0.096)
^{99m}Tc-PYP	0.066 (0.24)	0.028 (0.10)
^{99m}Tc-RBC in vivo labeling	0.070 (0.26)	0.031 (0.12)
^{99m}Tc-RBC in vitro labeling	0.071 (0.26)	0.031 (0.12)
[99m]Tc-sulfur colloid	0.092 (0.34)	0.042 (0.16)
[111]In-white blood cells	5.5 (20)	2.2 (8.1)
[123]I-NaI	2.7 (10)	1.9 (7.0)
^{123}I-OIH	0.051 (0.19)	0.022 (0.081)
^{123}I-MIBG	2.7 (10)	1.9 (7.0)
^{125}I-OIH	0.20 (0.74)	0.082 (0.30)
^{131}I-OIH	0.23 (0.85)	0.093 (0.34)
^{99m}Tc-DTPA aerosol	0.052 (0.19)	0.022 (0.081)
^{99m}Tc-MAG3	0.027 (0.10)	0.012 (0.044)
[99m]Tc-white blood cells	0.20 (0.74)	0.074 (0.27)
[201]Tl-chloride	3.6 (13)	2.1 (7.8)

[a]Effective Dose to infant per unit activity administered intravenously to infant. (*i.e.*, assumes 100% of the activity ingested by the infant is instantaneously absorbed). Calculation based on ICRP 60 methodology. See below for narrative and sample calculation of effective dose to the infant based on serial measurements of activity in the breast milk.

[b]Dose to infant's thyroid per unit activity administered intravenously (or orally) to infant.

DTPA, diethylenetriamine pentaacetic acid; MAA, macroaggregated albumin; EDTA, ethylenediaminetetraacetic acid; DISIDA, disofenin (iminodiacetic acid derivative); HAM, human albumin microspheres; MIBI, methoxyisobutyl isonitrile; MDP, methylene diphosphonate; PYP, pyrophosphate; RBC, red blood cells; WBC, white blood cells; OIH, orthoiodohippurate; MIGB, metaiodobenzylguanidine; MAG3, mercaptoacetyltriglycine.

This research was original published in JNM. Stabin MG, Breitz HB. Breast milk of radiopharmaceuticals: mechanisms, findings, and radiation dosimetry. *J Nucl Med.* 2000;41(5):863-873. Table 2. © SNMMI.

TABLE F-4C BREAST DOSE FROM RADIOPHARMACEUTICALS EXCRETED IN BREAST MILK

RADIOPHARMACEUTICAL	ADMINISTERED ACTIVITY IN MBq (mCi)	BREAST DOSE (Gy)	
		Best Case[a]	*Worst Case*[a]
^{67}Ga-citrate	185 (5.0)	2.18E−04	1.10E−02
^{99m}Tc-DTPA	740 (20)	6.09E−06	1.20E−04
^{99m}Tc-MAA	148 (4)	1.55E−05	1.21E−03
^{99m}Tc-pertechnetate	1,110 (30)	1.86E−05	2.52E−03
^{131}I-NaI	5,550 (150)	–	1.96E+00
^{51}Cr-EDTA	1.85 (0.05)	4.21E−09	2.52E−08
^{99m}Tc-DISIDA	300 (8)	1.94E−05	5.98E−05
^{99m}Tc-glucoheptonate	740 (20)	3.58E−05	7.40E−05
^{99m}Tc-HAM	300 (8)	8.48E−06	2.33E−04
^{99m}Tc-MIBI	1,110 (30)	5.54E−06	5.09E−05
^{99m}Tc-MDP	740 (20)	2.69E−05	3.76E−05
^{99m}Tc-PYP	740 (20)	4.16E−05	2.26E−04
^{99m}Tc-RBC in vivo	740 (20)	2.46E−06	1.14E−03
^{99m}Tc-RBC in vitro	740 (20)	9.25E−06	1.61E−05
^{99m}Tc-sulfur colloid	444 (12)	3.17E−05	4.64E−04
^{111}In-WBCs	18.5 (0.5)	5.03E−06	2.52E−05
^{123}I-NaI	14.8 (0.4)		4.74E−04
^{123}I-OIH	74 (2)	7.50E−05	5.84E−04
^{123}I-MIBG	370 (10)		2.71E−04
^{125}I-OIH	0.37 (0.01)		8.46E−07
^{131}I-OIH	11.1 (0.3)	4.97E−05	3.22E−04
^{99m}Tc-DTPA aerosol	37 (1)	1.22E−07	2.49E−06
^{99m}Tc-MAG3	185 (5)	3.04E−06	6.01E−05
^{99m}Tc-WBCs	370 (10)	1.11E−04	1.51E−02
^{201}Tl-chloride	111 (3)	2.35E−05	4.14E−05

[a]Best and worst case as observed from the literature.
DTPA, diethylenetriamine pentaacetic acid; MAA, macroaggregated albumin; EDTA, ethylenediaminetetraacetic acid; DISIDA, disofenin (iminodiacetic acid derivative); HAM, human albumin microspheres; MIBI, methoxyisobutyl isonitrile; MDP, methylene diphosphonate; PYP, pyrophosphate; RBC, red blood cells; WBC, white blood cells; OIH, orthoiodohippurate; MIGB, metaiodobenzylguanidine; MAG3, mercaptoacetyltriglycine. E, exponential (e.g., 2.18E−04 = 2.18 × 10⁻⁴).
This research was original published in JNM. Stabin MG, Breitz HB. Breast milk of radiopharmaceuticals: mechanisms, findings, and radiation dosimetry. *J Nucl Med.* 2000;41(5):863-873. Table 4. © SNMMI.

NARRATIVE AND EXAMPLE[1]

Recommended duration of interruption of breast-feeding following radiopharmaceutical administration to a patient who is nursing an infant or child was provided in Chapter 21, Table 21-9. The interruption schedules for the nursing infant were derived using a dose criterion of 1 mSv effective dose to the infant. However, Stabin

[1]*Source:* Stabin MG, Breitz HB. Breast milk excretion of radiopharmaceuticals: mechanisms, findings and radiation dosimetry. *J Nucl Med.* 2000;41(5):863-873.

and Breitz recommend taking breast milk samples from subjects when possible to determine, on an individual basis, the best recommendation for the duration of interruption. According to their recommendations in the article cited above, breast milk samples should be obtained: "(1) at about 3 h after administration (this is when the peak concentrations have most often been observed); (2) then, as many more samples as the patient is willing and able to give, over 2 to 3 effective half-times of the radiopharmaceutical in the body. If there is uncertainty about the biologic half-time, the radionuclide physical half-life may be used to estimate this overall time period. A minimum of two more samples (after the first sample at 3 h) should be obtained to calculate a good estimate of the retention half-time in the milk. Once the peak concentration and rate of decrease of the activity are determined, some approximate calculations can be performed by any physician or physicist to estimate the amount of activity that the infant will ingest starting at different points in time. One can set up a calculation in a simple spreadsheet that sums, for whatever sampling schedule the mother suggests that the infant is likely to follow, the amounts of activity likely to be ingested, using the observed concentrations and rate of elimination." Then, the dose conversion factors in Appendix F-4B can be used to calculate the infant dose.

This technique is illustrated in the following example from the Stabin and Breitz article: assume that for an administration of Tc-99m pertechnetate the breast-milk concentration reported at 3 h after administration to the mother is 2×10^{-2} MBq/mL. Three more samples, taken over the next 8 h, show a clearance biologic half-time of 20 h. The effective half-time is

$$(6 \text{ h} \times 20 \text{ h})/(6 \text{ h} + 20 \text{ h}) = 4.6 \text{ h}.$$

The mother wants to feed the baby (a newborn) approximately every 4 h. The volume ingested per feeding is assumed to be in feedings of 142 mL every 4 h (i.e., ~850 mL/d). Thus for the following times, starting at 12 h after administration (we are already at 11 h after administration), the baby's intakes for the next seven feedings would be

T (h)	A_t (MBq)
12	0.735
16	0.403
20	0.221
24	0.121
28	0.067
32	0.036
36	0.02
40	0.011
	Total activity = 1.62 MBq

Each value of A_t is given by the expression:

$$A_t = (142 \text{ mL} \times 0.02 \text{ MBq/mL}) \times e^{-0.693} \times (T-3)/(4.6).$$

A_t (MBq) is the activity ingested by the infant at the feeding at time T (h). We are assuming that the peak concentration (0.02 MBq/mL) occurred at 3 h and then decreased with the effective half-time (4.6 h) thereafter. We took the calculations out to 40 h, when the concentration seemed to have diminished to the point that further contributions would be negligible. The sum of the activity values listed previously is 1.62 MBq. In Appendix F-4B, we find a dose value for Tc-99m pertechnetate of

0.14 mSv/MBq for a newborn. The cumulative dose, assuming that feeding started at 12 h, would be 1.62 MBq × 0. 14 mSv/MBq = 0.23 mSv.

This dose is within the 1 mSv guideline used here, and one would conclude that breast-feeding could resume safely at 12 h after administration. If the dose had turned out to be too high, the calculation could be repeated easily, simply excluding some of the values in the table shown above from the sum, starting at 16 h, then at 20 h, and so on, until an acceptable dose value was obtained. The time at which this value was obtained would represent the time at which breast-feeding could be resumed.

Convolution and Fourier Transforms

Both convolution and Fourier transform operations are crucial for understanding the mathematical underpinning of imaging. In this appendix we review the basic definitions of these operators and their application to filtered backprojection, the modulation transfer function, aliasing, and noise power. Sampling effects are also described, but it should be noted that many details of numerical implementation for these concepts are beyond the scope of this appendix.

G.1 CONVOLUTION

Convolution is the mathematical property that describes blurring processes in medical imaging, among other physical phenomenon. It is the basis of physical optics and much of imaging physics, and it is also the basis of many image processing procedures. For a function $f(x)$ and a convolution kernel $h(x)$, convolution is an integral resulting in the function $g(x)$:

$$g(x) = \int_{-\infty}^{\infty} f(x')h(x - x')\,dx', \qquad \text{[G-1a]}$$

where x' is a *dummy* variable used for integration. The shorthand symbol for convolution is described in Equation G-1b:

$$g(x) = f(x) \otimes h(x), \qquad \text{[G-1b]}$$

where $\otimes$ is the mathematical symbol for convolution. The convolution process can be extended to two dimensions via a double integral:

$$g(x,y) = \int_{y'=-\infty}^{\infty} \int_{x'=-\infty}^{\infty} f(x',y')h(x - x', y - y')\,dx'dy'. \qquad \text{[G-1c]}$$

Figure G-1 shows a one-dimensional convolution, and it is straightforward to extend convolution to a three-dimensional function as well. With the advent of near-isotropic three-dimensional image data sets, three-dimensional convolution techniques are used with increasing utility for many imaging applications.

Figure G-1 illustrates the effect of a 0.4-mm rectangular (RECT) convolution kernel, $h(x)$, on an input signal $f(x)$ with some considerable noise. The output function $g(x)$ is much *smoother* than the input signal, but the edges are not as sharp. The RECT kernel is illustrated in the inset. A RECT kernel used in convolution is also known as a boxcar average. If the kernel is normalized to integrate to 1, as in this case ($0.4 \times 2.5 = 1$), the total amplitude of the convolved function will be equal to that of the input function. Convolution kernels that have all positive values (as in Fig. G-1) will always result in some degree of smoothing of the input function. Other kernels with all positive elements (such as a triangle function or a bell-shaped function) will also result in smoothing to some degree.

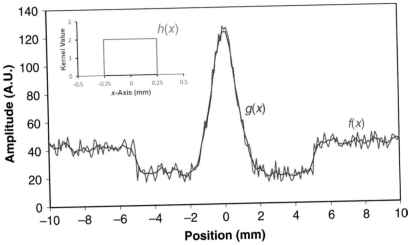

■ **FIGURE G-1** This figure illustrates the impact of convolution with a noise-suppressing kernel. The original signal $f(x)$ was convolved with the five element RECT kernel $h(x)$ shown in the inset, resulting in the smoothed function $g(x)$.

Convolution can be used to enhance edges as well, and Figure G-2 illustrates this with a kernel that has negative side lobes (see inset). In this case, the noise in the input function $f(x)$ is made worse by the convolution procedure resulting in the output function $g(x)$. Although the noise in the signal is amplified, the edges are enhanced as well. Edge enhancement (also known as high pass filtering) is a key part of filtered backprojection reconstruction in tomographic imaging applications where there is a trade-off between balancing the sharpness of the image and controlling acquisition noise.

The convolution operation can perform a number of interesting mathematical procedures on an input signal. Figure G-3 shows a convolution procedure with an antisymmetric kernel. In this case, the output function, $g(x)$, is similar to a derivative of the input function $f(x)$. Notice that in this example the integral

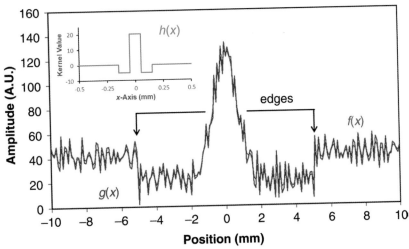

■ **FIGURE G-2** The role of an edge-enhancing kernel, $h(x)$, is illustrated. The original signal $f(x)$ was convolved with $h(x)$, resulting in the noisier function $g(x)$. While $g(x)$ is noisier than the original function, the two edges (arrows) have also been enhanced.

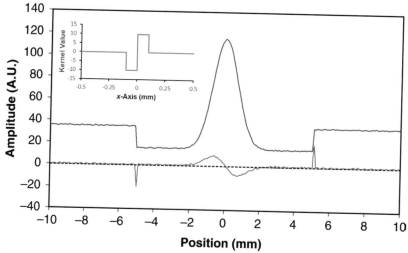

■ **FIGURE G-3** This figure illustrates the original signal (blue) with only a small amount of noise, and the kernel (inset) was used to compute the derivative signal (magenta). The numerical derivative was computed using convolution.

of the kernel is zero, and the average value of the output function $g(x)$ also becomes zero.

The convolution operation has a number of shifting and scaling properties. Figure G-4 illustrates a convolution kernel with an impulse function at 0.5 mm that points in the negative direction with a magnitude of -0.5. Convolution with this kernel produces an output function, $g(x)$, that is shifted laterally relative to the input function. And because the impulse function has a negative direction, the entire output function has its polarity flipped relative to the input function, $f(x)$. Finally, because the amplitude of the kernel has a magnitude of 0.5, the output function is scaled to be 50% of the amplitude of the input function (albeit in the negative direction due to the negative direction of the kernel).

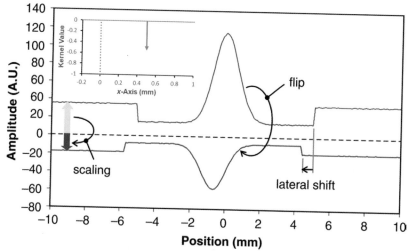

■ **FIGURE G-4** This figure illustrates three different effects of convolution—(1) because the total amplitude of the kernel was negative, the convolved function is flipped downward relative to the input signal (*i.e.*, it has become negative); (2) because the amplitude of the kernel was 0.5, the convolved function has half of the (negative) amplitude as the original; and (3) because the *d-function* used (see kernel—inset) was shifted from zero, the convolved function is shifted laterally compared to the original function.

G.2 THE FOURIER TRANSFORM

In the analysis of time-based signals, the Fourier transform converts from the time domain (x-axis labeled in seconds) to the temporal frequency domain (x-axis labeled in s^{-1}). While time-series analysis has applications in radiological imaging in Doppler ultrasound and magnetic resonance imaging, here we focus on input signals that are in the spatial domain (x-axis labeled typically in mm), which is pertinent to most anatomical medical images. The Fourier transform of a spatial domain signal converts it to the *spatial frequency* domain (x-axis labeled in mm^{-1}).

The one-dimensional Fourier transform of a spatial domain signal input function, $f(x)$, is given by

$$F(v) = \int_{-\infty}^{\infty} f(x)e^{-2\pi ivx}\,dx, \qquad [\text{G-2a}]$$

where $F(v)$ is the Fourier transform of $f(x)$ and is in the units of amplitude versus spatial frequency v (mm^{-1}), and where i is the imaginary unit, equal to $\sqrt{-1}$. As with convolution, the Fourier transform can be performed in two dimensions as described by

$$F(v, \upsilon) = \int_{y=-\infty}^{\infty}\int_{x=-\infty}^{\infty} f(x,y)e^{-2\pi i(vx+\upsilon y)}\,dx\,dy. \qquad [\text{G-2b}]$$

Three-dimensional Fourier transforms can also be performed.

For simplicity, only one-dimensional Fourier transforms are described below. The shorthand notation for the Fourier transform in Equation G-2a is given by

$$F(v) = FT\big[f(x)\big]. \qquad [\text{G-3a}]$$

Of course, other functions such as $h(x)$ can be transformed as well:

$$H(v) = FT\big[h(x)\big]. \qquad [\text{G-3b}]$$

An important result of linear systems theory is that multiplication of the two frequency domain functions $F(v)$ and $H(v)$ is the equivalent of convolution in the spatial domain. In terms of Equation G-1b, we can say that

$$G(v) = F(v) \times H(v). \qquad [\text{G-4}]$$

The product, $G(v)$, then needs to be converted back to the spatial domain, which is accomplished using the inverse Fourier transform (shorthand FT^{-1}[]):

$$g(x) = \int_{-\infty}^{\infty} G(v)e^{2\pi ixv}\,dv. \qquad [\text{G-5}]$$

Notice that the use of the Fourier transform and its inverse in Equations G-3a, G-3b, G-4, and G-5 provides the same result as the convolution function described in Equation G-1a. Explicitly:

$$g(x) = f(x) \otimes h(x) = FT^{-1}\big\{FT\big[f(x)\big] \times FT\big[h(x)\big]\big\}. \qquad [\text{G-6}]$$

For most applications, these equations are implemented numerically using Fast Fourier transform algorithms,[1] and this has led to the widespread use of the Fourier transform in image processing, image reconstruction, and other image analysis operations.

---

[1] The Fast Fourier Transform is the principal tool used for computer implementation of the Fourier Transform, as it achieves computational efficiency over a general Discrete Fourier Transform.

G.3 THE FOURIER TRANSFORM IN FILTERED BACKPROJECTION

The purpose of this section is to tie the discussion of convolution and Fourier transforms into previous discussions on filtered backprojection in tomographic reconstruction (Chapters 10 and 19). The backprojection procedure results in a characteristic $1/r$ blurring phenomenon, and the filtering component in filtered-backprojection reconstruction is a mathematical operation of the sort described in Equation G-6 that corrects for this blurring. In the case of filtered backprojection, $h(x)$ is a convolution kernel that corrects for the $1/r$ blurring—and hence it can be called a "deconvolution" kernel. Deconvolution simply refers to convolution when it is used to correct for a specific effect (such as blurring). In the image reconstruction literature, it is common to talk about the filtering function $h(x)$ in the frequency domain, that is, FT($h(x)$) or $H(v)$. As was seen in Chapter 10, $h(x)$ is an edge-enhancing kernel, more complicated (with long tails) but similar conceptually to that shown here in Figure G-2. In the frequency domain, $H(v)$ is a ramp filter that always has an additional high-frequency roll-off term as well in clinical CT imaging to control for noise. Thus, $H(v) = R(v) A(v)$, where $R(v)$ is the RAMP filter (thus $R(v) = \alpha v$, where α is a scalar) and $A(v)$ is an apodization filter that approaches zero as v approaches the maximum desired frequency. Typically this is the Nyquist frequency, determined by the sampling size of the discrete image elements.

G.4 THE FOURIER TRANSFORM AND THE MODULATION TRANSFER FUNCTION

The rigorous assessment of spatial resolution as discussed in Chapter 4 involves the measurement of the modulation transfer function (MTF) of an imaging system. There are several approaches to this, but the most widely used method is to measure the line spread function (LSF), and from it, the MTF is computed as a function of spatial frequency: MTF(v). In this section, more details about this process are provided. The line spread function, LSF(x), is measured or synthesized as discussed in Chapter 4. Recall that the LSF represents the average intensity of illumination in a line going across (*i.e.*, perpendicular to) a slit illumination. Here we show the analytic description of MTF calculation. But in most practical situations, computer programs are used that perform the mathematics in a discrete manner. The first step of MTF assessment is to normalize the area of LSF(x) to unity, which involves setting a positive scaling constant, s, so that:

$$s = \int_{-\infty}^{\infty} \text{LSF}(x)\, dx. \tag{G-7}$$

The Fourier transform of the line spread function is then computed, resulting in the optical transfer function, OTF(v).

$$\text{OTF}(v) = \frac{1}{s} \int_{-\infty}^{\infty} \text{LSF}(x) e^{-2\pi\, ifx}\, dx. \tag{G-8}$$

The line spread function is a real function, whereas the OTF(v) can be a complex function; that is, it has real and imaginary components. As a reminder, a complex number c has a real component, a, and an imaginary component, b, where $c = a + bi$, and as mentioned earlier, $i = \sqrt{-1}$. The MTF(v) is computed as:

$$\text{MTF}(v) = \sqrt{\Re\{\text{OTF}(v)\}^2 + \Im\{\text{OTF}(v)\}^2}, \tag{G-9}$$

where $\Re\{OTF(v)\}$ is the real component of the OTF and $\Im\{OTF(v)\}$ is the imaginary component. With this transformation, the MTF(v) represents the modulus of the OTF and as such is a real function. Another way to write Equation G-9 is

$$MTF(v) = \|OTF(v)\|. \qquad [G\text{-}10]$$

Because of the properties of the Fourier transform, since LSF(x) is normalized to 1, the MTF(v) value at $v = 0$ is also unity, that is, MTF(0) = 1.

G.4.1 Fourier Transform Pairs

There are a number of well-known functions for which the Fourier transform is also relatively well known. These are often referred to as Fourier Transform pairs. We review a few of the most common pairs below.

Impulse

We have seen in Figure G-4 how an impulse function can be used in a convolution to shift, flip, and scale a function. Technically, the impulse (often called a Dirac Delta Function) is not actually a function itself; it is the limit of a sequence of functions that get more and more narrow, while also getting taller and taller in such a way that they always integrate to 1. For example, consider the smoothing kernel in Figure G-1, and imagine that the width of the kernel was 1/N, while the height was equal to N (The kernel in G-1 occurs when $N = 2$). As N gets larger, the width of the function gets smaller while simultaneously the height gets taller, and the area under it will always be 1 (= $N \times 1/N$). The limit as N goes to infinity is an impulse.

The critical property of impulse functions is something called the "sifting property," which means that they pick out specific values of a function in an integral. Mathematically, let us define the impulse at a point, x_0, as $\delta(x - x_0)$, and integrate this against a function $f(x)$. We find that

$$\int \delta(x - x_0) f(x) dx = f(x_0). \qquad [G\text{-}11]$$

The sifting property of the impulse function refers to the idea that the impulse "sifts" through all the values of the function, $f(x)$, and picks out the value at $x = x_0$. Note that in Figure G-4, the convolution kernel is $h(x) = -(1/2)\delta(x - 1/2)$.

The sifting property of the impulse makes it an easy Fourier transform to calculate,

$$F(v) = \int_{-\infty}^{\infty} \delta(x - x_0) \exp(-2\pi i x v) dx = \exp(-2\pi i x_0 v). \qquad [G\text{-}12]$$

Note that when $x_0 = 0$, the Fourier transform is just the constant function, $F(v) = 1$.

Gaussian

The Fourier transform of a gaussian function is also a gaussian, but generally with a different amplitude and width. Because the line spread function in many settings is well approximated by a gaussian function, that example will be used here to illustrate the utility of Fourier transform pairs. A set of three hypothetical line spread functions is shown in Figure G-5. These LSF(x) plots correspond loosely to those for three imaging modalities—analog screen film radiography (curve A), computed tomography (curve B), and single photon emission computed tomography (SPECT, curve C). The full width at half maximum of these curves is approximately 0.14, 0.6, and 6 mm, respectively. The MTFs of these three LSF(x) curves are shown in Figure G-6. It can be seen that the widest LSF(x) (curve C) in Figure G-5 has the worst MTF in Figure G-6 (i.e., it has the most rapid decay to zero). Note that the limiting resolution for the three MTFs shown in Figure G-6 (at the 5% dashed line) corresponds approximately to 0.2, 1.4, and 6.6 mm^{-1}.

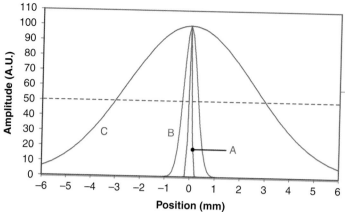

■ **FIGURE G-5** A number of gaussian line-spread functions are illustrated (A, B, and C). This figure shows the gaussian functions in the spatial domain, with the wider functions blurring the resulting signal more.

Let the spatial domain function LSF(x) be given by

$$LSF(x) = e^{-(\pi x^2)/a^2},$$ [G-13a]

where a is a constant that affects the width of the line spread function. The integral of the LSF, as in Equation G-7, yields a value of a, and so the scaling constant needed to normalize the LSF is $s = a$. After scaling, the analytical Fourier transform of Equation G-13a is given by

$$OTF(v) = FT\left[\frac{1}{s}LSF(x)\right] = e^{-\pi v^2 a^2}.$$ [G-13b]

Note that the value of a in Equation G-13b is the same as that in Equation G-13a for the Fourier transform pair. In this case, the OTF is real-valued (there is no i in Equation G-13b) and positive, and so MTF = OTF. The LSF/MTF curves shown in Figures G-5 and G-6 (respectively) were produced with values of a corresponding to 0.15, 0.68, and 6.0 (for curves A, B, and C as labeled in these figures).

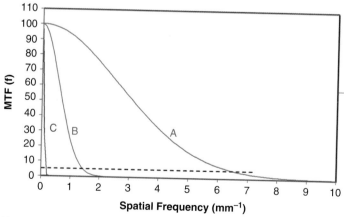

■ **FIGURE G-6** These gaussian functions are the Fourier transforms of the gaussian functions seen in Figure G-5. Notice that the widest gaussian in Figure G-5 results in the narrowest function on this plot. While the relationship between the gaussian functions shown in Figure G-5 and their FT counterparts in this figure is general and illustrates Fourier transform pairs, if the functions in Figure G-5 are considered to be line spread functions, then the functions illustrated here in Figure G-6 are the corresponding MTFs. Note that the widest LSF results in the greatest degree of frequency attenuation in the MTF.

The LSF/MTFs shown in Figures G-5 and G-6 were meant to illustrate the use of the Fourier transform in image science, but they also illustrate gaussian Fourier transform pairs. It should be noted that gaussian FT pairs are not limited to LSFs and MTFs, but rather this is a general relationship. In addition, there are many LSFs and MTFs that do not fit a gaussian function.

RECT

The rectangle function, or $\text{RECT}\left(\dfrac{x}{a}\right)$, is an important function in image science for a variety of reasons. In the absence of other sources of blur, the $\text{RECT}\left(\dfrac{x}{a}\right)$ function describes how a detector element (dexel) of width a integrates a signal incident upon it. It was also seen to be the smoothing kernel in Figure G-1. $\text{RECT}\left(\dfrac{x}{a}\right)$ is defined for a specific width by

$$\text{RECT}\left(\frac{x}{a}\right) = \begin{cases} 1 & |x| < \dfrac{a}{2} \\ 0 & \text{elsewhere} \end{cases}. \qquad \text{[G-14]}$$

With this definition, the limits of integration of the Fourier transform can be modified resulting in the following analytical derivation:

$$F(v) = \int_{-\infty}^{\infty} \text{RECT}\left(\frac{x}{a}\right) e^{-2\pi i v x}\, dx = \int_{-a/2}^{a/2} e^{-2\pi i v x}\, dx = \frac{\sin(\pi a v)}{\pi v}. \qquad \text{[G-15]}$$

The SINC function is defined as

$$\text{SINC}(x) = \frac{\sin(\pi x)}{\pi x}. \qquad \text{[G-16]}$$

And thus Equation G-16 can be written as

$$F(v) = a\,\text{SINC}(av). \qquad \text{[G-17]}$$

The above derivation illustrates that $\text{RECT}\left(\dfrac{x}{a}\right)$ and $a\,\text{SINC}(av)$ are Fourier transform pairs.

The SINC function oscillates like a sine wave, but also decays to zero as $1/x$. Figure G-7 shows the MTFs for three hypothetical LSFs that have RECT function profiles with different apertures ($a = 0.4, 0.2,$ and 0.1 mm). Note that because of the absolute value in the definition of the MTF, the *SINC* function "bounces" at zero values. As the aperture gets smaller and the RECT function gets narrower, the spatial resolution (MTF) improves (*i.e.*, extends further into the frequency domain). Indirect detector systems that use an x-ray phosphor have other significant sources of resolution loss (optical blur), but for direct x-ray detectors, the RECT function can provide a reasonable characterization of the detector's response to the incident x-ray beam and thus the SINC function approximates the MTF of indirect detector systems. For a direct x-ray detector, the aperture (a) may also be considered the sampling width as well (in the absence of any dead space between detectors). In this case, the Nyquist frequency (see below) is given by $F_{\text{Nyq}} = 1/(2a)$, it can be seen that the theoretical SINC-function MTF extends well beyond the Nyquist frequency. This shows that aliasing, as described in the next section, remains an issue in direct detector systems.

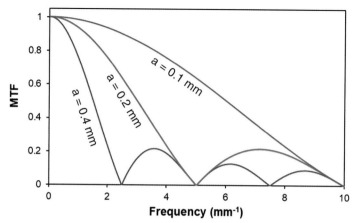

■ **FIGURE G-7** These are three MTFs that result from various RECT functions being the LSF. Note that the MTF plots the absolute value of the LSF Fourier transform, and so the oscillating SINC functions appear to "bounce" in the MFT plots.

G.4.2 Digital Sampling and Aliasing

The continuously defined functions used above are helpful for describing imaging principles at a conceptual level. The discrete analogs of the Fourier Transform, convolutions, MTF, etc. require an investment of effort to learn the appropriate notation and methods related to sampling. In this section these topics will be selectively and briefly presented to illustrate two fundamental and important concepts from sampling theory as they apply to imaging. These are the concept of the Nyquist frequency, and aliasing. These concepts are critical for understanding when an imaging system suffers from undersampling.

Sampling converts a continuously defined function, such as $g(x)$ in Equation G-1, into a list of numbers that represent the value of the function at a set of sample points. When the sample points are separated by a fixed sampling length, Δ, the function is considered *regularly* sampled, also referred to as *uniformly* sampled. In this case we can define the sampled values as $g_n = g(n\Delta)$. This process is shown graphically in Figure G-8A. However, sampling introduces ambiguity into our understanding of the underlying function. In Figure G-8B another function that is equally consistent with the sampled values is shown. Understanding this ambiguity is key for evaluating the adequacy of sampling in imaging systems.

The difference between the two functions in Figure G-8B is seen to oscillate relatively rapidly with respect to the sampling width. The ambiguity introduced by sampling concerns the inability to resolve components of a function that are highly oscillatory (*i.e.*, contain high spatial frequencies). This is not an issue if we can safely assume that the underlying function does not contain any of these high frequencies. The Nyquist frequency, $F_{Nyq} = 1/2\Delta$, for a regular sampling scheme gives the highest frequency that can be unambiguously identified for a given sampling width. Frequencies that are greater than the Nyquist frequency will be aliased when the function is sampled.

Imaging systems with a decaying MTF pass a bounded range of frequencies that may be fully characterized after sampling, assuming the sample width is well matched to the MTF. As an example, consider the MTFs shown in Figure G-6, and a sample width of 0.25 mm. The resulting Nyquist frequency is 2.0 mm^{-1}. For the gaussian LSF that is 6 mm wide (labeled C), the MTF is seen to fall off well before 2.0 mm^{-1}.

A. The Sampling Process

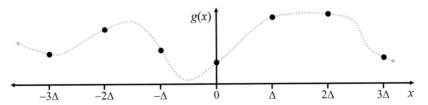

B. Sampling Ambiguity

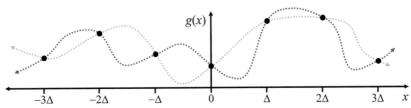

■ **FIGURE G-8 A** illustrates the sampling of a function with a center-to-center spacing of Δ. **B** shows two functions that are both consistent with the sampled values, illustrating the potential for ambiguity in a sampled system.

In this case, a sample width of 0.25 mm is oversampling the signal. Oversampling is not a problem itself, although it may indicate that the bandwidth of the detector is being potentially wasted on frequencies that do not contain any signal. For the 0.6-mm LSF (labeled B), the MTF has essentially fallen off right at 2 mm^{-1}, and the signal may be considered critically sampled. This is generally considered ideal and is often the goal of an analysis of sampling, although it is important to have a clear notion of what "fallen off" means in this context. Finally, the narrow 0.14-mm LSF (labeled A) extends well past 2 mm^{-1}. In this case the signal will be undersampled by a sample width of 0.25 mm.

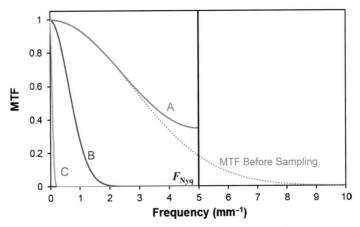

■ **FIGURE G-9** The effects of sampling on MTF plots are shown for the LSFs of Figure G-5, and at a sampling width of 0.25. The widest LSF has fallen off to zero well before the Nyquist frequency of 2 mm^{-1}, indicating oversampling. The mid-width LSF falls off right at the Nyquist frequency, indicating critical sampling. And the narrowest LSF has not decayed by the Nyquist frequency, indicating undersampling and showing evidence of aliasing as a departure from the unsampled MTF.

Recognizing an oversampled or undersampled system often comes down to diagnosing the issue from a sampled MTF. Figure G-9 shows sampled MTFs for the three LSFs shown in Figure G-6. The MTFs are sampled at a width of 0.1 mm, resulting in a Nyquist frequency of 5 mm^{-1}. Both of the wider LSFs decay to zero well in advance of Nyquist, suggesting oversampling. However, the narrowest LSF starts to decay, but then levels out and flattens near the Nyquist frequency, where it terminates. This is the signature of undersampling and aliasing in a sampled MTF. The deviation from the continuous MTF is due to aliasing, and represents higher frequencies in the LSF that get "folded" into the sampled MTF.

SUGGESTED READING AND REFERENCES

Barrett HH, Swindell W. *Radiological Imaging: The Theory of Image Formation, Detection, and Processing.* Vol. 1. New York, NY: Academic Press; 1981.

Dainty JC, Shaw R. *Image Science.* London: Academic Press; 1974.

Ji WG, Zhao W, Rowlands JA. Digital x-ray imaging using amorphous selenium: reduction of aliasing. *Med Phys.* 1998;25(11):2148-2162.

Radiation Dose: Perspectives and Comparisons

This appendix was prepared as a resource to provide ready access to radiation protection quantities as well as an overview of the variety of types and extent of radiation sources and exposures encountered in medical and public settings. The aim is to assist in placing radiation exposure into perspective and to guide the reader towards some of the contemporary risk communication tools that are available.

Table H-1 provides the ICRP tissues and tissue weighting factors (w_T) that were used in the calculation of effective dose equivalent (H_E) in ICRP report 26 (ICRP 1977) and effective dose (E) in ICRP report 60 (ICRP 1990) and ICRP report 103 (ICRP 2007).

Figure H-1 shows the relationships between the emission of radiation and the various quantities described in previous chapters to express radiation exposure; kerma; absorbed dose; equivalent dose (from which the dose to tissues and organs can be used along with other risk-modifying variables such as age at the time of exposure and gender to estimate cancer incidence and mortality risk to an individual); and effective dose to the body, which can be used to estimate the stochastic health risk for a group that has the same general age and gender distribution as the general population.

Figure H-2 provides an example of estimated effective doses and weighted organ equivalent doses from some standard cardiac radionuclide and CT diagnostic studies using ICRP report 103 (2007) and ICRP report 60 tissue weighting factors.

Figure H-3 provides a comparison of estimated effective doses (mSv) for standard myocardial perfusion imaging protocols, determined with the use of ICRP and manufacturers' package insert dose coefficients.

Tables H-2 to H-7 and Figures H-4 and H-5 are presented to help put radiation exposure into perspective by providing examples of other sources of radiation, the doses from those sources as well as comparison of typical effective doses from common imaging examinations, as well as other public health risks and their relative magnitude. Several of these also introduce proposed qualitative terminology that could be used to convey the general level of risk from imaging procedures.

Table H-2 provides information on doses from several sources of public and occupational radiation exposure from data obtained in the United States. Table H-3 presents information on the average and range of effective doses from several naturally occurring sources worldwide. Table H-4 provides some examples of the amount of natural radioactivity encountered in daily life and the identity and typical quantities of naturally occurring radioactive material in the human body. Figure H-4 illustrates the variation in the annual effective dose from cosmic radiation in North America. Figure H-5 compares the average annual effective dose from natural background radiation sources in the United States to that of a number of European countries.

Tables H-5 and H-6 present an example of terminology that can be used to provide a qualitative perspective as a means of communicating different levels of hypothetical increase in the risk of cancer mortality and incidence (respectively) following radiation exposure. Table H-7 applies the terminology in Table H-6 associated with

TABLE H-1 ICRP TISSUE WEIGHTING FACTORS w_T (ICRP 1977; ICRP 1990; ICRP 2007)

ICRP REPORT	ICRP 26	ICRP 60	ICRP 103	ICRP 26	ICRP 60	ICRP 103
YEAR	1977	1990	2007	Tissues Included in Remainder Tissues		
Quantity	EDE	ED	ED	—	—	Adipose tissue
Tissue	Tissue Weighting Factors, w_T			—	Adrenals	Adrenals
Gonads	0.25	0.2	0.08	—	Brain	STWF
Breast	0.15	0.05	0.12	—	—	Connective tissue
Red bone marrow	0.12	0.12	0.12	—	—	Extrathoracic airways
Lung	0.12	0.12	0.12	—	—	Gallbladder
Thyroid	0.03	0.05	0.04	—	Brain	IMT
Bone surfaces	0.03	0.01	0.01	—	—	Heart wall
Colon	—	0.12	0.12	—	Kidney	Kidney
Stomach	—	0.12	0.12	—	—	Lymphatic nodes
Bladder	—	0.05	0.04	—	Muscle	Muscle
Esophagus	—	0.05	0.04	Liver	STWF	STWF
Liver	—	0.05	0.04	LLI	STWF	STWF
Brain	—	—	0.01	—	—	Pancreas
Salivary Glands	—	—	0.01	—	—	Prostate
Skin	—	0.01	0.01	SG	—	IMT
Remainder tissues[a]	0.3	0.05	0.12	SI	SI	SI wall
Total	**1.0**	**1.0**	**1.0**	Stomach	STWF	STWF
				—	Spleen	Spleen
				—		Thymus
				ULI	ULI	STWF

[a]Tissues selected to represent the remainder in ICRP reports 26, 60, and 103 are shown on the right side of the table.
EDE, effective dose equivalent (H_E); ED, effective dose (E); STWF, see tissue weighting factor table; LLI, lower large intestine; SG, salivary glands; SI, small intestine; ULI, upper large intestine.
ICRP 26: ICRP Publication 26. *Recommendations of the International Commission on Radiological Protection.* Oxford, England: Pergamon Press; 1977.
ICRP 60: ICRP Publication 60. International Commission on Radiological Protection. *1990 Recommendations of the International Commission on Radiological Protection. Ann ICRP.* 1991;21(1-3).
ICRP 103: ICRP Publication 103. The 2007 Recommendations of the International Commission on Radiological Protection. *Ann ICRP.* 2007;37:1-332.

the estimated increase in age- and sex-averaged additional cancer incidence risk for a variety of imaging procedures. Table H-8 presents a proposed qualitative terminology that could be used to convey the general level of risk at four different ages for some common pediatric examinations. Table H-9 presents the estimated loss of life expectancy from several health risks including an estimate for the risk from background radiation. It is important to be aware of the assumptions incorporated into the values presented and limitations inherent in making risk comparisons (see table footnotes).

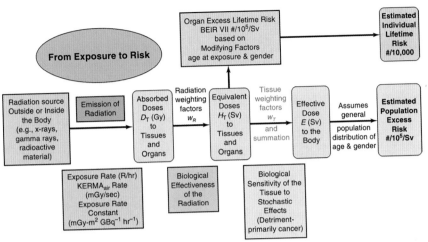

■ **FIGURE H-1** Relationships between the emission of radiation and the various physical and radiological protection dose quantities described in Chapter 3 and discussed throughout the text. (Data from ICRP. The 2007 Recommendations of the International Commission on Radiological Protection, ICRP Publication 103. *Ann ICRP.* 2007;37:1-332.)

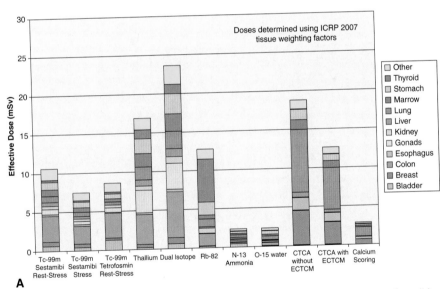

A

■ **FIGURE H-2** Estimated effective doses and weighted organ equivalent doses from cardiac radionuclide and CT studies. **A.** Doses determined using ICRP Publication 103 (2007) tissue weighting factors.

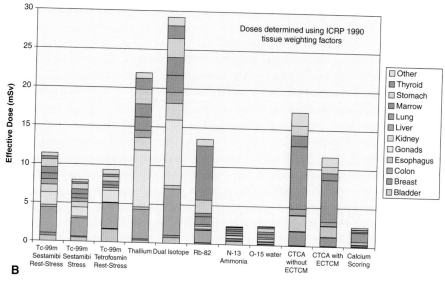

■ FIGURE H-2 (*Continued*) **B.** Doses determined using ICRP Publication 60 (1990) tissue weighting factors. CTCA indicates 64-slice computed tomography coronary angiogram; CaSc, calcium scoring; and ECTCM, ECG-controlled tube current modulation. Calculations were performed with ImpactDose (VAMP GmbH, Erlangen, Germany); for Siemens Sensation 64 scanner with retrospective gating, the voltage was 120 kV, pitch 0.2, and scan length 15 cm. For CTCA, slice thickness was 0.6 mm and tube current-time product was 165 mAs; ECTCM was simulated by reducing tube current by a third, to 110 mAs. For CaSc, collimation was 20 × 1.2 mm, and tube current-time product was 27 mAs. Doses shown are arithmetic means of doses to standard-ized male and female phantoms. (Reprinted with permission from Einstein AJ, Moser KW, Thompson RC, et al. Radiation dose to patients from cardiac diagnostic imaging. *Circulation* 2007;116:1290–1305. doi: 10.1161/CIRCULATIONAHA.107.688101.)

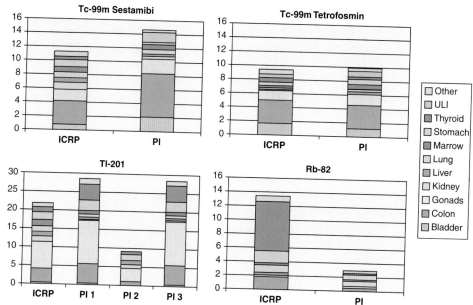

■ FIGURE H-3 Comparison of estimated effective doses (mSv) for standard myocardial perfusion imaging protocols, determined with the use of ICRP and manufacturers' package insert dose coefficients. Weighted equivalent doses were determined with the use of ICRP Publication 60 tissue weighting factors. ULI indicates upper large intestine. Some notable differences exist between effective doses estimated with the use of ICRP dose coefficients and those estimated with the use of dose coefficients provided in package inserts (PI), as illustrated above. Most PIs were initially issued at the time of approval of a radiopharmaceutical, and dosimetry information included in subsequent revisions has not been updated to reflect new biokinetic data or changes in the ICRP dosimetry system. Note that in some cases there can also be substantial discordance in dose es-timates between different manufactures' PIs (*e.g.*, Tl-201). In general, the most recent ICRP data should be used for dosimetry estimates. PI should only be used as the source of dose information for new radiopharma-ceuticals for which ICRP dosimetry data have not yet been published. (Reprinted with permission from Einstein AJ, Moser KW, Thompson RC, et al. Radiation dose to patients from cardiac diagnostic imaging. *Circulation* 2007;116:1290 -1305. doi: 10.1161/CIRCULATIONAHA.107.688101.)

TABLE H-2 DOSES FROM SEVERAL SOURCES OF PUBLIC AND OCCUPATIONAL RADIATION EXPOSURE

RADIATION EXPOSURE	TYPICAL EFFECTIVE DOSE (mSv)
US annual average *per capita* dose from natural background radiation	3.1
US annual average *per capita* dose from medical radiation exposure	3
Total US annual average *per capita* dose from all sources	6.2
Commercial aviation aircrew average annual dose from cosmic radiation	3
Radiation workers annual average occupational dose	2–5
Whole-body x-ray airport scanner (1 scan)	0.00003–0.0001
Flying on an airplane at 35,000 ft (per hour)	0.0024

Data taken from NCRP Report 160 and NCRP Commentary 16 with permission of the National Council on Radiation Protection and Measurements, http://NCRPonline.org.

TABLE H-3 ANNUAL AVERAGE RADIATION DOSES AND RANGES PER PERSON WORLDWIDE

SOURCE OR MODE	ANNUAL AVERAGE DOSES WORLDWIDE AND THEIR TYPICAL RANGES (mSv[a])
Natural Sources of Exposure	
Inhalation (radon gas)	1.26 (0.2–10)[b]
Ingestion (food and drinking water)	0.29 (0.2–1)
External terrestrial	0.48 (0.3–1)[c]
Cosmic radiation	0.39 (0.3–I)[d]
Total natural	**2.4 (1–13)[e]**

[a]mSv: millisievert, a unit of measurement of effective dose.
[b]The dose is much higher in some dwellings.
[c]The dose is higher in some locations.
[d]The dose increases with altitude.
[e]Large population groups receive 10–20 mSv.
Adapted from *Communicating Radiation Risks in Paediatric Imaging: Information to Support Healthcare Discussions about Benefit and Risk*, © World Health Organization 2016. Available at: https://www.who.int/ionizing_radiation/pub_meet/radiation-risks-paediatric-imaging/en/. Accessed June 9, 2020.

TABLE H-4 **EXAMPLES OF LEVELS OF NATURAL RADIOACTIVITY IN THE DAILY LIFE ARE PROVIDED BELOW**

	NATURAL RADIOACTIVITY IN FOOD			TYPICAL AMOUNT OF NATURAL RADIOACTIVITY IN THE BODY[a]
FOOD	^{40}K (POTASSIUM)	^{226}Ra (RADIUM)	NUCLIDE	
Banana	130 Bq/kg	0.037 Bq/kg	Uranium	1.1 Bq
Brazil Nuts	207 Bq/kg	37–260 Bq/kg	Thorium	0.11 Bq
Carrot	130 Bq/kg	0.02–0.1 Bq/kg	Potassium	4.4 kBq
White Potato	130 Bq/kg	0.037–0.09 Bq/kg	Radium	1.1 Bq
Beer	15 Bq/kg	NA	Carbon	3.7 kBq
Red Meat	110 Bq/kg	0.02 Bq/kg	Tritium	23 Bq
Raw	170 Bq/kg	0.07–0.2 Bq/kg	Polonium	37 Bq

[a]The typical amount of disintegrations per second (DPS) in the human body from naturally occurring radioactivity is approximately 7,400 DPS.
Adapted from *Communicating Radiation Risks in Paediatric Imaging: Information to Support Healthcare Discussions about Benefit and Risk*, © World Health Organization 2016. Available at: https://www.who.int/ionizing_radiation/pub_meet/radiation-risks-paediatric-imaging/en/. Accessed June 9, 2020.

TABLE H-5 **EXAMPLES OF A QUALITATIVE APPROACH TO COMMUNICATE DIFFERENT LEVELS OF RISK OF CANCER INCIDENCE COMPARED WITH THE LIFETIME BASELINE RISK OF CANCER INCIDENCE**

RISK QUALIFICATION	APPROXIMATE LEVEL OF ADDITIONAL RISK OF CANCER INCIDENCE	PROBABILITY OF DEVELOPING CANCER IN THE GENERAL POPULATION (% LBR)[a]	PROBABILITY OF DEVELOPING CANCER IN THE GENERAL POPULATION IF ADDING THIS EXTRA LEVEL OF RISK (% LBR + % LAR)
Negligible	<1 in 500,000	42	42.00
Minimal	Between 1 in 500,000 and 1 in 50,000	42	42.00
Very low	Between 1 in 50,000 and 1 in 5,000	42	42.02
Low	Between 1 in 5,000 and 1 in 500	42	42.25
Moderate	Between 1 in 500 and 1 in 250	42	42.50

[a]The 42% presented in this column is a sex-averaged rounded value of LBR for cancer incidence due to leukemia and solid cancer based on BEIR VII Table 12-4. BEIR. *Health Risks from Exposure to Low Levels of Ionizing Radiation: BEIR VII Phase 2.* Washington, DC: National Academy of Sciences; 2006.
LBR, lifetime baseline risk; LAR, lifetime attributable risk.
Reprinted from *Communicating Radiation Risks in Paediatric Imaging: Information to Support Healthcare Discussions about Benefit and Risk*, © World Health Organization 2016. Available at: https://www.who.int/ionizing_radiation/pub_meet/radiation-risks-paediatric-imaging/en/. Accessed June 9, 2020.

TABLE H-6 AGE- AND SEX-AVERAGED ADDITIONAL CANCER INCIDENCE RISK ASSOCIATED WITH RADIOLOGICAL PROCEDURES IN CHILDREN COMPARED WITH BASELINE CANCER RISK

RISK QUALIFICATION	PROBABILITY OF CANCER INCIDENCE IN THE GENERAL POPULATION (% LBR)[a]	PROBABILITY OF CANCER INCIDENCE IN THE GENERAL POPULATION IF ADDING THIS EXTRA LEVEL OF RISK (% LBR + % LAR)	PROPOSED RISK QUALIFICATION
Catheterization interventional	42	42.36	Moderate
Catheterization diagnostic	42	42.25	Low[b]
CT angiography head	42	42.16	Low
CT chest	42	42.15	Low
CT abdomen	42	42.12	Low
CT angiography abdomen	42	42.12	Low
CT pelvis	42	42.10	Low
CT head	42	42.06	Low
Barium swallow esophagus	42	42.05	Low
Barium enema colon	42	42.04	Low
Perfusion lung scan	42	42.04	Low
Fluoroscopy tube placement	42	42.04	Low
Chest PA and lateral	42	42.00	Negligible

[a]The 42% presented in this column is a sex-averaged rounded value of LBR for cancer incidence due to leukemia and solid cancer based on BEIR VII Table 12-4. BEIR. Health Risks from Exposure to Low Levels of Ionizing Radiation: BEIR VII Phase 2. Washington, DC: National Academy of Sciences; 2006.
[b]Level of risk between low and moderate needs to consider the patient age in the risk-benefit discussion.
LBR, lifetime baseline risk; LAR, lifetime attributable risk.
Reprinted from *Communicating Radiation Risks in Paediatric Imaging: Information to Support Healthcare Discussions about Benefit and Risk*, © World Health Organization 2016. Available at: https://www.who.int/ionizing_radiation/pub_meet/radiation-risks-paediatric-imaging/en/. Accessed June 9, 2020.

The annual outdoor effective dose (µSv) from cosmic radiation for Canada and the U.S.

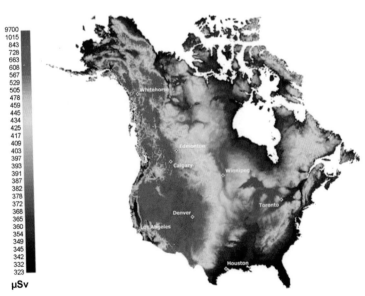

■ FIGURE H-4 Color plot of the annual outdoor effective dose from cosmic radiation (in microsievert) in North America. (From Grasty RL, Lamarre JR. The annual effective dose from natural sources of ionizing radiation in Canada. *Radiat Protect Dosim* 2004;108(3):215–226, by permission of Oxford University Press. doi: 10.1093/rpd/nch022)

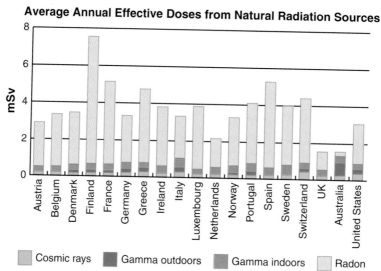

Average Annual Effective Doses from Natural Radiation Sources

Legend: Cosmic rays | Gamma outdoors | Gamma indoors | Radon

■ **FIGURE H-5** Examples of variation in natural background and the sources of the variation. (Adapted from Green BMR, Hughes JS, Lomas PR, et al. Natural radiation atlas of Europe. *Radiat Protect Dosim.* 1992;45: 491-493, by permission of Oxford University Press. doi: 10.1093/rpd/45.1-4.491.)

TABLE H-7 PROPOSED QUALITATIVE PRESENTATION OF RISK AT THREE DIFFERENT AGES FOR SOME COMMON PEDIATRIC EXAMINATIONS BASED ON DATA PRESENTED IN THIS SECTION

EXAMINATION	AGE 1 YEAR	AGE 5 YEARS	AGE 10 YEARS
Dental intra-oral	NA	Negligible	Negligible
Chest x-ray	Negligible	Negligible	Negligible
Head CT	Low	Low	Low
Chest CT	Low	Low	Low
Abdominal CT	Moderate	Low	Low
FDG PET CT	Moderate	Moderate	Moderate

NA, not applicable; FDG, fludeoxyglucose; PET, positron emission tomography.
Reprinted from *Communicating Radiation Risks in Paediatric Imaging: Information to Support Healthcare Discussions about Benefit and Risk*, © World Health Organization 2016. Available at: https://www.who.int/ionizing_radiation/pub_meet/radiation-risks-paediatric-imaging/en/. Accessed June 9, 2020.

TABLE H-8 TYPICAL EFFECTIVE DOSES FROM ADULT AND PEDIATRIC CT IMAGING AS A FUNCTION OF PATIENT AGE FOR DIAGNOSTIC IMAGING EXAMINATIONS AND THEIR EQUIVALENCE IN TERMS OF NUMBER OF CHEST X-RAYS AND DURATION OF EXPOSURE TO NATURAL BACKGROUND RADIATION

CT EXAM PROTOCOL[a,b]	AVERAGE EFFECTIVE DOSE (mSv)	DAYS OF EQUIVALENT BACKGROUND RADIATION[c]	EQUIVALENT NUMBER OF ADULT CHEST X-RAY EXAMS[d]
Head/brain CT (adult)	**1.6**	188	32
Newborn	2.1	246	42
≤1 year	3.3	387	66
2–5 years	1.8	211	36
6–10 years	2.1	246	42
≤15 years	1.8	211	36
Chest CT (adult)	**6.6**	775	132
Newborn	Not Reported	—	—
≤1 year	2.8	329	56
2–5 years	2.6	305	52
6–10 years	2.6	305	52
≤15 years	3.1	364	62
Abdominopelvic CT (adult)	**7.7**	904	154
Newborn	Not Reported	—	—
≤1 year	5.0	587	100
2–5 years	5.9	692	118
6–10 years	6.3	739	126
≤15 years	6.0	704	120
DENTAL EXAMINATIONS[e]			
Intra-oral radiography (adult)	**0.081**	10	2
Intra-oral radiography	0.051	6	1
Panoramic (adult)	**0.350**	41	7
Panoramic	0.210	25	4
Craniofacial cone-beam CT (adult)[f]	**0.176**	21	4
Craniofacial cone-beam CT (5-year-old)[f]	0.103	12	2
FLUOROSCOPY			
Fluoroscopic cystogram (adult)[b]	**0.2**	23	4
Fluoroscopic cystogram (5-year-old)[g]	0.5	59	10
NUCLEAR MEDICINE EXAMINATIONS			
FDG PET CT (adult)[h]	**10.0**	1,174	200
FDG PET CT (5-year-old)[i]	20.0	2,347	400
Tc-99m DMSA (adult)[h]	**1.3**	153	26
Tc-99m DMSA (5-year-old)[i]	0.77	90	15.4

(Continued)

TABLE H-8 TYPICAL EFFECTIVE DOSES FROM ADULT AND PEDIATRIC CT IMAGING AS A FUNCTION OF PATIENT AGE FOR DIAGNOSTIC IMAGING EXAMINATIONS AND THEIR EQUIVALENCE IN TERMS OF NUMBER OF CHEST X-RAYS AND DURATION OF EXPOSURE TO NATURAL BACKGROUND RADIATION (*Continued*)

CT EXAM PROTOCOL[a,b]	AVERAGE EFFECTIVE DOSE (mSv)	DAYS OF EQUIVALENT BACKGROUND RADIATION[c]	EQUIVALENT NUMBER OF ADULT CHEST X-RAY EXAMS[d]
NUCLEAR MEDICINE EXAMINATIONS			
Tc-99m MDP (adult)[h]	**1.8**	**211**	**36**
Tc-99m bone scan (5-year-old)[i]	2.2	258	44

[a]Values of CT pediatric effective dose are derived from the product of the third quartile values of DLP and the effective dose coefficients from Deak PD, Smal Y, Kalender WA. Multisection CT protocols: sex and age-specific conversion factors used to determine effective dose from dose-length product. *Radiology.* 2010;257:158-166.
[b]Adult effective doses are from Mettler et al.: Patient exposure from radiologic and nuclear medicine procedures in the United States: procedure volume and effective dose for the period 2006–2016. *Radiology.* 2020;295(2):418-427.
[c]Based upon a background effective dose rate of 3.1 mSv/y.
[d]The equivalent number of adult chest x-ray exams at 0.05 mSv per exam is provided as a crude comparison of the amount of radiation used in each of the exams. It should not be taken as a risk comparison for a number of reasons. In addition to the fact that the metric used in effective dose which (as explained in Chapter 3) does not provide an adequate assessment of individual risk from diagnostic imaging examinations, children are, in general, at higher risk per unit dose for stochastic risks (*e.g.*, cancer) from radiation exposure than adults.
[e]Ludlow JB, Timothy R, Walker C, et al. Effective dose of dental CBCT—a meta analysis of published data and additional data for nine CBCT units. *Dentomaxillofac Radiol.* 2015;44(1):20140197.
[f]Shin HS, et al. Effective doses from panoramic radiography and CBCT (cone beam CT) using dose area product (DAP) in dentistry. *Dentomaxillofac Radiol.* 2014;43(5):20130439. doi: 10.1259/dmfr.20130439.
[g]Ward VL, Strauss K, Barnewolt CE, et al. Pediatric radiation exposure and effective dose reduction during voiding cystourethrography. *Radiology.* 2008;249(3):1002-1009
[h]Adult effective dose from Appendix F, Table F-2.
[i]Chawla SC, Federman N, Zhang D, et al. Estimated cumulative radiation dose from PET/CT in children with malignancies: a 5-year retrospective review. *Pediatr Radiol.* 2010;40(5):681-686.
[j]Five-year-old effective dose based on administered activity as recommended in MBq/kg for a 20-kg child (see Appendix F, Table F3-B).

TABLE H-9 ESTIMATED LOSS OF LIFE EXPECTANCY FROM HEALTH RISKS

HEALTH RISK[a]	ESTIMATES OF AVERAGE DAYS (YEARS) OF LIFE EXPECTANCY LOST
Smoking 20 cigarettes/d	2,250 (6.2 y)
All accidents combined	366 (1 y)
Auto accidents	207
Alcohol consumption	125
Home accidents	74
Drowning	24
Natural background radiation	30
Medical diagnostic x-rays	30

[a]With the exception of smoking, all risks are expressed as the loss of life expectancy averaged over the U.S. population.
Data from Cohen BL. Catalog of risks extended and updated. *Health Phys.* 1991;61(3):317-335. It is important to note that there are a lot of assumptions that are incorporated into the numerical values presented in this table. The original text should be consulted for the details and caution should be exercised when comparing a risk from one source or activity to another (see Covello VT. Risk comparisons and risk communication: issues and problems in comparing health and environmental risks. In: Kasperson RE, Stallen PJM, eds. *Communicating Risks to the Public: International Perspectives.* London, UK: Kluwer Academic; 1991:79-124; Covello VT, Sandman PM, Slovic P. *Risk Communication, Risk Statistics, and Risk Comparisons: A Manual for Plant Managers.* Washington, DC: Chemical Manufacturers Association; 1988; Covello VT, Sandman PM, Slovic P. Appendix B risk comparison tables and figures. http:// www.psandman.com/articles/cma-appb.htm#. Accessed June 17, 2020.)

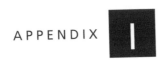 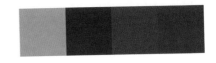
Radionuclide Therapy Home Care Guidelines

 GENERAL SAFETY GUIDE FOR OUTPATIENTS RECEIVING RADIOIODINE THERAPY: LESS THAN 10 mCi

The radioactive iodine that you have been treated with is for your benefit. You need to take some precautions so that others do not receive unnecessary radiation exposure.

A. Please follow the instructions below.

1. Breast-feeding your infant must be discontinued.
2. Drink plenty of liquids.
3. Women of childbearing potential must have a negative pregnancy test before therapy. Results ⎯⎯⎯⎯⎯⎯⎯⎯⎯.

B. Please follow the steps below during the first 2 days after your treatment.

1. Most of the remaining radioiodine in your body will come out through the urine. A small portion of radioactivity will be found in your saliva and sweat. To decrease the spread of radioactivity:
   a. Use paper drinking cups, plates, and plastic utensils. Put these items in the trash when you are done with them.
   b. Use towels and washcloths that only you will touch.
   c. You should sleep in a separate bed.
   d. At the end of 2 days wash your laundry separately. This need only be done once.
   e. Avoid touching and hugging babies and pregnant women.
2. Most of the radioactivity is in the urine during these first 2 days. If urine should be spilled or splashed, wash and rinse the affected area three times, using paper towels or tissue. Be sure to carefully wash your hands after using the bathroom.
3. Breast-Feeding: Breast-feeding must be discontinued. Your physician will advise you when you may resume.

C. During the rest of the week.

Your body will still contain some radioactivity. Avoid sitting close to others for hours at a time. This will reduce their radiation exposure. Do not be concerned about being close to people for a few minutes. Avoid holding babies or young children for a long time each day.

If you have problems or questions about the above, please call: ⎯⎯⎯⎯⎯⎯⎯⎯⎯, M.D.

Nuclear Medicine Division—Ph. No. ⎯⎯⎯⎯⎯⎯⎯⎯⎯

I.2 GENERAL SAFETY GUIDE FOR OUTPATIENTS RECEIVING RADIOIODINE THERAPY: MORE THAN 10 mCi

The radioactive iodine that you have been treated with is for your benefit. You need to take some precautions so that others do not receive unnecessary radiation exposure.

A. **Please follow the instructions below.**
  Young people are more sensitive to radiation. To minimize possible effects from radiation, do not hold children or spend time near pregnant women during the next week.

  1. Go directly home. Do not stay at a hotel.
  2. Sit as far from anyone as practical during your ride home from the hospital. Let us know if your trip is longer than 3 hours.
  3. Breast-feeding your infant must be discontinued.
  4. Drink plenty of liquids.
  5. Women of childbearing potential must have a negative pregnancy test before therapy. Results _____.

B. **Please follow the steps below during the first 4 days after your treatment.**
  1. Most of the radioiodine in your body will come out in the urine and stool. A small portion of radioactivity will be found in your saliva and sweat. To decrease the spread of radioactivity:
    a. If possible, use a separate bathroom.
    b. Flush the toilet two times after each use.
    c. Men should sit down when urinating.
    d. If urine is spilled/splashed, wash and rinse the spill area three times, using paper towels or tissue.
    e. Menstruating women should consider the use of tampons that can be flushed down the toilet.
    f. Be sure to carefully wash your hands after using the bathroom.
    g. Do not share utensils or food with others. (For example, do not drink from the same glass or share a sandwich.)
    h. Use dedicated towels and washcloths that only you will touch.
    i. Run water in the sink while brushing your teeth or shaving and rinse the sink well after use.
    j. Nausea following therapy is very rare. However, if you feel sick to your stomach, try to vomit into the toilet. If necessary, wash and rinse any spill areas three times, using paper towel/tissue.
    k. At the end of 4 days wash your laundry, including the pillowcases, separately from others. This need only be done once.
  2. To decrease the radiation exposure to others:
    a. You should sleep in a separate bed. Cover the pillow with two pillowcases.
    b. Remain in your home for the first 4 days.
    c. Young people are more sensitive to radiation so do not hold children or spend time near pregnant women.
    d. Family members should stay six feet or more from you. After the first 2 days, they may be closer for brief periods such as a few minutes.
    e. Avoid sexual relations.

C. **Please follow the steps below until the end of the first week after your treatment.**

Your body will still contain some radioactivity. To minimize radiation exposure to other people, you should:

1. Avoid sitting close (within a foot) to others for hours at a time.

2. Minimize the use of public transportation (bus, airplane, etc.) and going to public gatherings such as movies, plays, etc. Do not be concerned about being close to people for short times (less than an hour).

3. To minimize possible effects from radiation, avoid holding babies or children.

D. **Please follow the steps below for the next 6 to 12 months.**

1. Avoid becoming pregnant for the next 12 months or fathering a child for the next 6 months.

2. If you are hospitalized or require emergency medical treatment within the next 2 weeks, please inform the doctor or nurse that you have been treated with _____ mCi of radioactive iodine on _____. Please contact the Nuclear Medicine Department at _____ as soon as possible. After hours, call the hospital operator at _____ and ask for the Nuclear Medicine on-call physician.

_____, M.D.   _____, M.D.

                                          Nuclear   Medicine   Physician

Nuclear Medicine Physician Signature   Printed Name

Date: _____

I understand the above instructions that have been discussed with me and I agree to follow them.

_____   _____

           Patient's Signature   Date

Index

Note: Page numbers followed by *f* indicate figures; page numbers followed by *t* indicate tables.

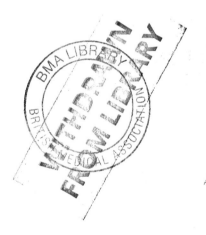